Body Contouring

Juarez Moraes Avelar • Ricardo Cavalcanti Ribeiro
Editors

Body Contouring

Current Concepts and Best Practices

Springer

Editors
Juarez Moraes Avelar
Brazilian Scientific Institute of Plastic and Reconstructive Surgery
São Paulo, Brazil

Ricardo Cavalcanti Ribeiro
Plastic and Reconstructive Surgery
Federal University of the State of Rio de Janeiro
Rio de Janeiro, Brazil

ISBN 978-3-031-42801-2 ISBN 978-3-031-42802-9 (eBook)
https://doi.org/10.1007/978-3-031-42802-9

This Springer imprint is published by the registered company Springer Nature Switzerland AG
The registered company address is: Gewerbestrasse 11, 6330 Cham, Switzerland

Foreword

This wonderful book opens a new era in the field of body contouring surgery edited by two renowned Brazilian plastic surgeons, Dr. Juarez Avelar and Dr. Ricardo Ribeiro. Both have an unquestionable experience in presenting scientific productions around the world, they have produced many papers of an outstanding value and published in peer review journals a remarkable contribution. We can distinguish four important papers published by Dr. Juarez: the "Mercedes" umbilicoplasty without external scar that appears in the first issue of the APS Journal. A second one about the histoanatomical research done in the subcutaneous abdominal flap that earned the first price from the APS Journal in 1988. A third one in 1999 about abdominoplasty combining with assisted liposuction without undermining the abdomen wall that contributed to so many surgeons from our country to start with similar procedures. And a fourth one about ear reconstruction that is a "landmark" from him. He has edited 23 scientific books and many other chapters with emphasizes in body countering and facial surgeries. Besides these extensive scientific production, he served as National President of our Brazilian Society of Plastic Surgery for two times (1986/87 and 1990/91).

Dr. Ricardo Ribeiro from Rio is the second Editor with a great experience on research publishing many papers focusing on breast and body contouring surgeries. He has on his career edited 9 books and 42 scientific chapters. He is Head of the Division of Plastic and Reconstructive Surgery of Federal University of Rio de Janeiro State (UNIRIO)and member of many plastic surgery societies around the world.

Dr. Juarez and Dr. Ricardo have done a wonderful job to edit this book, around 500 pages like a compendium, distributed in 61 chapters. They have invited 82 renowned plastic surgeons from Brazil and abroad to bring the most important advances of our specialty. Enriched with very nice pictures the subjects come together with an extensive bibliographic reference to be prospected. This is a book that certainly will enrich our knowledge and directly reach the young plastic surgeons and residents who are seeking for new ideas and horizons on their career. It is something that certainly deserves to be in our libraries.

Division of Plastic Surgery
PUCRS University
Porto Alegre, Brazil

Carlos Oscar Uebel

Foreword

It is with great pleasure that I write the foreword of "body contouring," one more book edited by Juarez Avelar. He is not only a skilled plastic surgeon but also a prolific writer whose energetic mind does not stop creating new scientific projects. I have been fortunate to be part of Juarez's creations since 1982, when I helped him organize and edit the annals of our first symposium for the Brazilian Society of Plastic Surgery, and he has not stopped creating and innovating.

In this book, Juarez Avelar and Ricardo C. Ribeiro summarize everything the modern plastic surgeon should know to be up to date with the newest techniques in body contouring.

Starting with the surgical fundamentals for body contour surgery, a review of the anatomy, and eight chapters about several abdominoplasty techniques. We cannot forget that it was Avelar who, in 1999, established a new way of performing lipoabdominoplasty, preserving perforators and lymphatics, a technique copied and modified by many authors.

The modern vertical mammoplasty technique created in 1957 by George Arié was soon modified by Ivo Pitanguy, transforming it into an inverted T, and became known as the Arié-Pitanguy breast technique. Over the last six decades, many modifications appeared and the nine chapters dedicated to breast surgery create a full panorama on how to reduce and lift the female breast and gynecomastia.

Avelar was among the first Brazilians to start performing liposuction in the early 1980s in São Paulo. Not only that, he was responsible for bringing Yves Gérard Illouz and Pierre Fournier to perform surgical demonstrations in the congresses I helped him organize in São Paulo in 1983 and 1984. Avelar and Illouz published the first Brazilian book on liposuction in 1986.

For this book, the editors have commissioned seven chapters from prominent surgeons on liposuction and liposculpture and six on fat grafting, covering all aspects of these landmark techniques with special attention to safety and correction of irregularities.

Massive weight loss patients represent today another branch of plastic surgery, the post-bariatric surgery techniques, for body lift, thigh lift, gluteoplasty, torsoplasty, flank and armplasty. The surgeons invited to contribute chapters are highly experienced professionals who teach us the steps on how to perform these difficult procedures with careful planning. We know there are many books on body contouring. The experienced surgeon, however, will find here all the necessary steps towards obtaining a good result. Both editors and all authors of the chapters are outstanding Brazilian plastic surgeons teaching refinements and updating techniques concerning the subject of this book.

I wish you good reading and even better results.

Luiz Toledo
MMC Aesthetics
Plastic and Reconstructive Surgery Department
Dubai, UAE

Tribute to Prof. Ivo Pitanguy and Prof. Yves G. Illouz

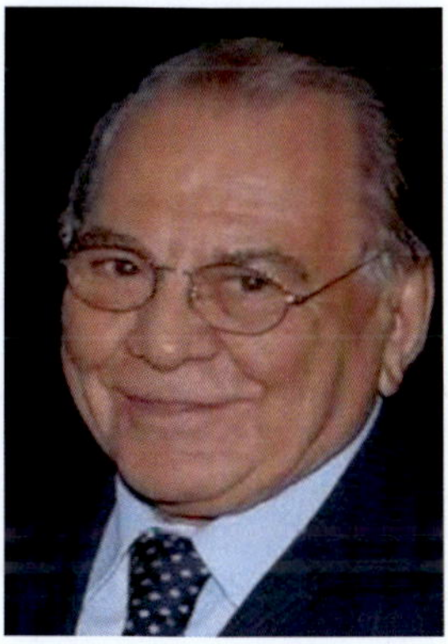

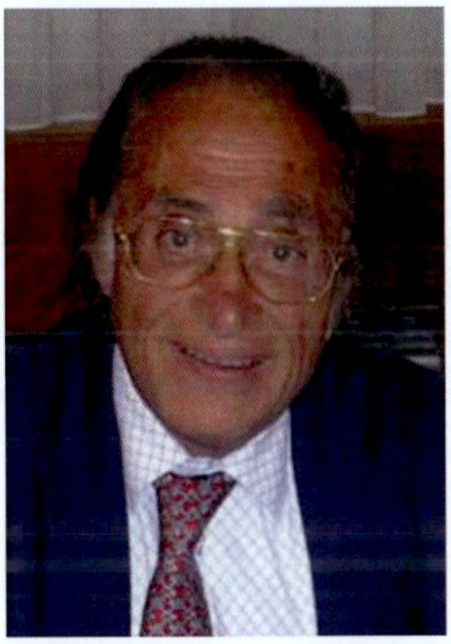

We dedicate this book to the memories of Profs. Pitanguy and Illouz for their constant incentive for scientific development of plastic surgery through their talents and creativities transmitted in their numerous publications. Besides, to teach their knowledge both were always happy to stimulate scientific contributions conscious of the progress and the future of our specialty. Although they are not among us anymore, since both passed away in 2016, we felt their presence during preparation of this book. Definitely, if they were here both would be writing once more their remarkable chapters concerning their superb scientific contributions to plastic surgery. We are so sad since they are not in our world, but we are very happy to dedicate this book to their memories with our gratitude for their permanent devotion to stimulate plastic surgery to all specialists all around the world.

Homage to Prof. Ivo Pitanguy

It is our privilege to pay homage to Prof. Ivo Pitanguy for his remarkable contribution to body contouring surgery since his publication in 1964 concerning surgical treatment of trochanteric lipodystrophy. He used to perform combined surgeries resulting in outstanding improvement remodeling the silhouette and created the expression—body contouring. In fact, to perform breast reduction combined with abdominoplasty since 60 years, before liposuction technique, means reshaping the body contour.

Prof. Pitanguy during all his professional activities devoted so much effort performing associated procedures, even writing useful scientific articles as well as giving lectures all around the world teaching to all plastic surgeons his personal contributions.

Although he is not among us in our world, but wherever he is, he is still stimulating everyone to dedicate improving plastic surgery.

While we were preparing the manuscripts for this book, we felt the presence of Prof. Pitanguy in our spirit to follow our hard work to offer scientific knowledge to plastic surgeons from Brazil and from all other countries. He is not physically close to us, but wherever he is, we are constantly asking him to bless us to follow his way, sharing our knowledge.

With the essence of our heart, we homage to Prof. Ivo Pitanguy simultaneously with our gratitude for his superb work developed during all his life giving up the chance to learn his personal techniques as well as the Noble attitude to transmit knowledge to the readers.

Sincerely,
Juarez Moraes Avelar, MD
Ricardo Cavalcanti Ribeiro, MD

Homage to Prof. Yves G. Illouz

Publishing this book is the representation of the fulfillment of our desire to transmit knowledge to plastic surgeons wishing to improve their body contouring skills and techniques. Regarding this subject, it is an honor for us to pay homage to Prof. Yves G. Illouz for his memorable contribution to plastic surgery developing and publishing liposuction technique. We had the great privilege to learn from him one of the most revolutionary procedures introduced to plastic surgery during the last decades of twentieth century. Prof. Illouz was a brilliant French plastic surgeon, but he used to come several times to Brazil teaching his remarkable method that he became almost a Brazilian.

Since 1980 when Prof. Illouz came for the first time to teach his fantastic technique during the Brazilian Congress held in Fortaleza, state of Ceará, we have developed a special ambience to learn it. He was always happy to attend our invitations to come to our country to participate at our events to share his knowledge with our colleagues.

Liposuction developed and worldwide popularized by Prof. Illouz changed the concepts of plastic surgery. Instead of leaving long scars to remove the volume of localized adiposities, his method leaves inconspicuous ones. Reshaping the silhouette of the body by fat suction, liposuction, represents an immense contribution to our filed, therefore with pleasure and warm feelings we pay homage to Prof. Illouz in this book—Body Contouring.

Sincerely,
Juarez Moraes Avelar, MD
Ricardo Cavalcanti Ribeiro, MD

Preface

Since I was realizing the dream of my life of graduating in Medicine in December 1968, I took an unusual decision to work in Amazon Forest as a volunteer physician to help poor people, even Indians inside of the jungle. I used to attend many patients expecting to solve all kinds of health problems. Some of them used to see me just to touch my hands or my arms to certify that I was a human being similar to them, since they had never seen a doctor. Recognizing such a strange situation gave me one more special reason to be there. So far, among different patients, when I saw someone presenting overweight with fatty abdomen, arms, legs, and buttocks that shocked me deeply, since it was impossible to help them there. I could not operate them since I was not technically prepared to perform any procedure to remodel their body. Although I was not able to do it, their strange physical appearance remained in my mind and in my soul.

After I concluded my volunteer job in the interior of the jungle, I returned to Rio de Janeiro to start my Plastic Surgery Post Graduation Course with Professor Pitanguy's Infirmary at Santa Casa da Misericódia (General Hospital) as well as in his world renowned Clinic. Ever since I was his resident, quite often I used to see some patients presenting similar deformities that I had seen in the interior of the Amazon Forest. It was fascinating to observe Professor Pitanguy performing his technique to repair those complex body deformities achieving very smooth and harmonious surgical results. Meantime, I used to hear from him the term body contouring surgery and facial contouring surgery as well. It was clear in my mind that those expressions were related to combined procedures improving body and facial contour respectively. In fact, I did not perform any operations on those patients I saw in Amazon, but that unusual body image remained in my mind, even now when I am preparing the manuscripts having Prof. Ricardo Cavalcanti Ribeiro as my partner for this book.

These body contouring concepts impressed me very much during the period of my training as well as when Professor Pitanguy was invited to perform a surgical demonstration at the Hadassah Hospital in Jerusalem (Israel) during the Second Congress of ISAPS held in June 1973. While I was there, he asked me to participate in a surgical demonstration of his technique of trochanteric lipodystrophy with outstanding surgical results.

So far, when I started my professional activities in São Paulo City I became motivated to organize the Brazilian Symposium of Abdominoplasty in 1982 and on the next year the Brazilian Symposium on Facial Contouring in which Prof. Pitanguy gave a lecture and wrote two remarkable chapters about both subjects. In fact, associated operations were performed frequently during the period of my training at his clinic under excellent team organization in the operating room as well as with outstanding surgical results improving very much body and facial contouring.

When one looks fifty years back in the history of plastic surgery concerning body contouring, it is evident that good surgical results were possible to achieve in breast surgery. However, concerning abdominoplasty there were several challenges specially about complications during and after surgery.

So far, in 1980 Illouz developed and published liposuction which is one of the most revolutionary techniques during the last decades of twentieth century with deep changes on concepts in plastic surgery. The complex deformities on trochanteric lipodystrophy became possible remodeling body contouring through liposuction approach leaving only some punctiform scars. Even other regions of the human body such as abdomen and torso received so much improvement employing liposuction. However, the combination of Illouz's method with traditional abdominoplasty presented a very high rate of complications which bother very much patients and surgeons.

I was worried about these problems, therefore, I dedicated so much effort performing anatomical research trying to improve surgical results as well as minimizing complications. After a long time, in 1999 I found that it would be possible to perform abdominoplasty combined with liposuction as long as the abdominal panniculus is not undermined with preservation of perforator vessels. Therefore, I achieved my anatomical research and published "new concepts on abdominoplasty" as well as further applications as lipoabdominoplasty.

To publish this book is an accomplishment of my professional activities started during my period of specialization with Professor Pitanguy with intense effort all the way through my practice.

To organize this publication, Professor Ricardo Cavalcanti and I, besides writing our chapters, we invited outstanding Brazilian plastic surgeons to participate in the Table of Contents with useful chapters about multiple aspects concerning body contouring in order to present to readers the most updated contribution. I take this opportunity to thank all of our colleagues for the important participation in this book expressing the most advanced techniques as well as concepts about the subject.

São Paulo, Brazil Juarez Moraes Avelar

Preface

Body contour is one of the most fascinating chapters in plastic surgery due to variation of procedures. To perform such kind of operations, surgeons must have skills for dealing with different body regions.

During the last decades, many new procedures have been incorporated to achieve better results. One example was liposuction which appeared changing dramatically the outcomes and increasing the possibilities. Less invasive approaches, substitute conventional surgeries, where results were only obtained by skin and fat removal. Many surgeons refused to incorporate the technique in the very first moment, however, with the learning curve, they gained confidence on the surgery, and it became an indispensable tool in body surgery armamentarium.

With time, studies were conducted improving safety and effectiveness in liposuction. Physiological knowledge and understanding the body response to fat removal turned this surgery asequible in the vast majority of body contour procedures around the world.

Furthermore, new technologies are being developed constantly reducing complications rates and time consumption.

Body surgery is one of the most performed operations among Brazilian plastic surgeons. Personally, during my participation in international events for the last three decades, I have perceived that it is always a Brazilian surgeon sharing expertise and new ideas for improving body contouring techniques and long term results.

Avelar and I have accepted the challenges of editing a book, which involves time consumption, knowledge of each part of content, as well critical analyses to turn the subject a continuously source of learning for the readers.

Thinking in terms of currents concepts as the main topic for a book, along with inviting a constellation of experienced collaborators, whom have a tied agenda, was a difficult task, however, after our first request, all of them agreed enthusiastically to share their experience.

Thus, we tried to gather up to date contents covering all the body regions and we believe in a constant development on this field.

We must express our gratitude to all of those colleagues for their contribution in the diffusion of Brazilian plastic surgery.

Rio de Janeiro, Brazil Ricardo Cavalcanti Ribeiro

Acknowledgment

Although my parents Anisio and Maria Ana are not anymore in this world, I am deeply thanking them for the constant enthusiasm during all of our lives. Due to their warm and comforting presence I have had the courage to follow my way, my gratitude to both.

To my lovely son Thiago and my wife Gloria, who have been a constant source of inspiration for this publication and permanent witnesses to my scientific activities.

I am deeply thankful to Prof. Pitanguy, although he is not beside me during preparation of this book, but wherever he is, I feel his presence providing inspiration and organization to prepare this publication.

To Dr. Edgar Bollanho, for his outstanding work on technical illustrations in this book, and other projects along of my career.

Juarez Moraes Avelar

First, I want to express my gratitude to my parents for believing in me and giving me the opportunity to be a doctor of medicine.

As surgical specialists, continous training is of utmost importance, which requires patience, resiliency, and mentorship. Fortunately, I had the privilege to learn with many masters, such as Virmar Ribeiro Soares, Ewaldo Bolivar, John Bostwick, Ruy Vieira, Ives Gerard Illouz, Al Ali, among others. My learning curve in body contouring was done by understanding principles and key points during international meetings, surgical demonstrations, and fellowship periods.

From my residents, I have been learning to absorb fresh and new ideas of the young minds. Always, I try to understand their ways of thinking, encouraging them to pursue and develop their ideas. For me this coexistence is great mental exercise and a way to learn more.

I want to thank my wife Luciana for her patience and understanding of my absences due to several calls and meetings during this job.

Finally, I want to express my gratitude to Dr. Luis Fernandez de Córdova Rio de La Loza for his invaluable assistance and support during the book's elaboration.

Ricardo Cavalcanti Ribeiro

Contents

Part I
Introduction: Surgical Fundaments for Body Contouring Surgery

Chapter 1
Surgical Principles for Body-Contouring Approaches

Juarez Moraes Avelar

Abstract Ever since I was a resident at Prof. Pitanguy's clinic, I used to often hear Pitanguy say the terms *body-contouring surgery* and *facial-contouring surgery*. Those expressions were related to combined procedures improving body and facial contours, respectively. These new concepts impressed me so much that at the beginning of my career, I became motivated to organize the Brazilian Symposium of Abdominoplasty and the Brazilian Symposium on Facial Contouring, at which Prof. Pitanguy delivered a lecture and wrote a remarkable chapter about it. In fact, the associated operations were frequently performed during the period of my training under excellent team organization in the operating room and with outstanding surgical results, greatly improving body and facial contouring.

Such operations were performed daily at his clinic according to Pitanguy's technique, on thighs, buttocks, and the trochanteric lipodystrophy regions. His memorable approach opened up a new era for body surgery in that it became possible to remove redundant skin and localized adiposities, which used to be removed through vertical incisions on the lateral and inner aspect of the thigh.

During my residency, people, both female and male, had constant demands for their physical appearance, as they still do today. In addition to food administration, diet, and physical activities, surgery is used to eliminate the signs of obesity and actual obesity to achieve desirable physical appearances. During the last decade, obesity has been replaced by people looking to reshape their bodies after weight loss, which is an important field with a large number of patients.

Thanks to the liposuction technique introduced by Illouz, it became possible to remove excess localized adiposity without redundant skin, leaving only inconspicuous scars. The accumulation of adipose tissue on abdominal walls presenting with excess cutaneous tissue was not treated. So far, a combination of liposuction with conventional abdominoplasty has been able to improve body contouring by remov-

J. M. Avelar (✉)
Brazilian Scientific Institute of Plastic and Reconstructive Surgery, São Paulo, Brazil

J. M. Avelar, R. Cavalcanti Ribeiro (eds.), *Body Contouring*,
https://doi.org/10.1007/978-3-031-42802-9_1

ing the accumulation of fat through the new approach. However, such a combined procedure has come with a very high incidence of complications, such as seroma formation, hematoma, slough from the panniculus, and others. Those undesirable situations occurred because the wide undermining of the abdominal panniculus used to be performed to remove the excess cutaneous covering. Those complications seriously concern me and other plastic surgeons. After a very short period of time, I decided not to perform such a combined procedure of liposuction and resecting the redundant panniculus. Later, I dedicated to conduct research on my previous anatomic dissections and introduced new concepts for abdominoplasty without panniculus undermining while preserving the perforator vessels, which work as multiples pedicles, providing adequate blood supply to the remaining abdominal panniculus. A similar procedure may be employed for remodeling other regions to improve body contouring on areas such as the flanks, torsos, medial thighs, arms, and axilla.

Keywords Liposuction · Trochanteric region · Body conoturing · Conventional resection · Remodeling the body

Introduction

New techniques for body-contouring surgery were introduced by Pitanguy (1964, 1977) for remodeling the abdominal wall, medial thigh, buttocks, and trochanteric regions (Fig. 1.1). Such surgical techniques impressed me during my period of training at Prof. Pitanguy's clinic (where I worked from 1970 to 1972). Currently, combined operations are still performed very often at his clinic under excellent team organization in the operating room, achieving outstanding surgical results in greatly improving body and facial contouring.

I used to often hear Pitanguy say the terms *body-contouring surgery* and *facial-contouring surgery*, which were related to the combined procedures for improving body and facial contouring. In addition to hearing those expressions, I also participated in some scientific articles on these techniques. I had such expressions in mind that even at the beginning of my career, such as when I had some female patients presenting severe buttock deformities caused by infection after injection. They presented very deep depressions, which were repaired by using mammary silastic prostheses, achieving good surgical results (Fig. 1.2) (Avelar 1974a, b, c). Notably, we didn't have gluteal prostheses at the time, because they wouldn't be developed until several years later. A paper on this subject was presented as my thesis for me to become a full member of the Brazilian Society of Plastic Surgery.

Concerning the expression *body contouring*, I organized the Brazilian Symposium on Abdominoplasty and the Brazilian Symposium of Facial Contouring, at which Prof. Pitanguy delivered two brilliant lectures and about which he wrote two useful chapters (Pitanguy 1982, 1983). Moreover, he wrote a useful chapter concerning body contouring in our book *Liposuction*, featuring the fundaments and surgical principles concerning his new technique (Pitanguy 1986). Localized adipose tissue as an accumulation of fat on abdominal walls and on the lateral, posterior, and

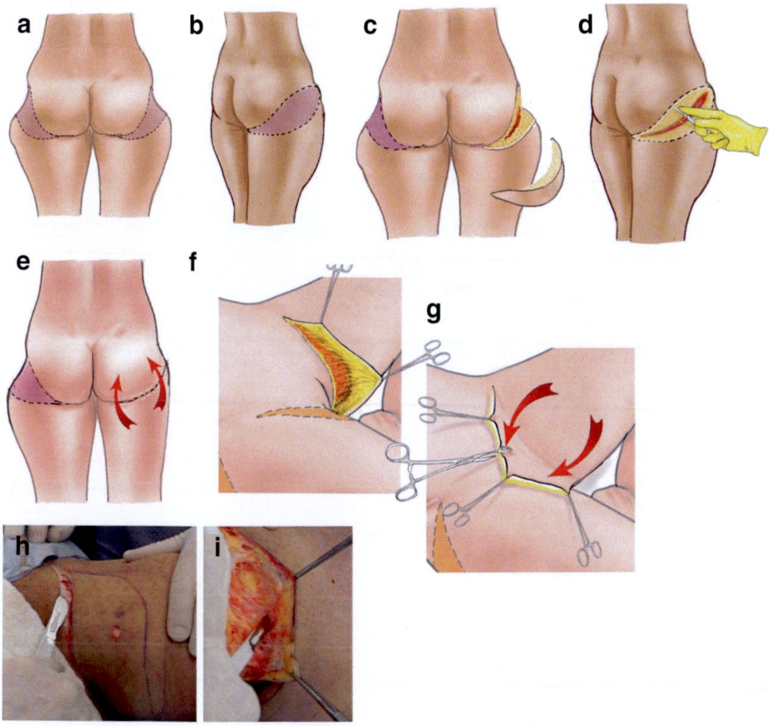

Fig. 1.1 Sequential drawings to illustrate Pitanguy's technique for surgical treatment of trochanteric lipodystrophy. (**a**) Posterior view with typical deformities, and demarcations; (**b**) posterolateral view showing the incision extending anteriorly; (**c**) a wedge of panniculus is resected on right side; (**d**) reduced area of cutaneous undermining on each border is done; (**e**) after suture on right side showing advancement of lower flap indicated by arrows. When the medial thigh presents deformities associated with lipodystrophy the posterior cutaneous incision extends into the inguinal crease. (**f**) Diagram shows tunnelization of the cutaneous flaps of the incision on anterior aspect of the thigh; (**g**) after reduced area of cutaneous undermining the cutaneous flap is pulled and advanced upwards for resection the excess medially and anteriorly indicted by arrows. (**h, i**) Perioperative photos showing cutaneous incisions on inguinal crura using knife. The final scar lies on inguinal sulcus

medial aspects of the thighs and buttocks may damage the contouring of these regions, producing unaesthetic and inelegant appearances. Such abnormalities were described by Pitanguy (1964, 1977) as trochanteric lipodystrophy, or the "riding breeches" deformity. It could be repaired through his new techniques because those deformities used to be removed through vertical incisions on the lateral and inner aspect of the thigh (Farina et al. 1960).

In addition to the accumulation of adiposity, very often a depression is present on the posterior and lateral aspect of the buttocks (Fig. 1.1). A similar accumulation of fat is quite frequently apparent on the inner side of the thighs, which may be accompanied by the flaccidity of the skin and subcutaneous tissue. Owing to this accumulation of localized adiposities, the buttocks may droop, caused by musculocutaneous flaccidity; secondary to aging, this droop may bring an even-more-unaesthetic appearance to the region. The original technique described by Pitanguy (1964,

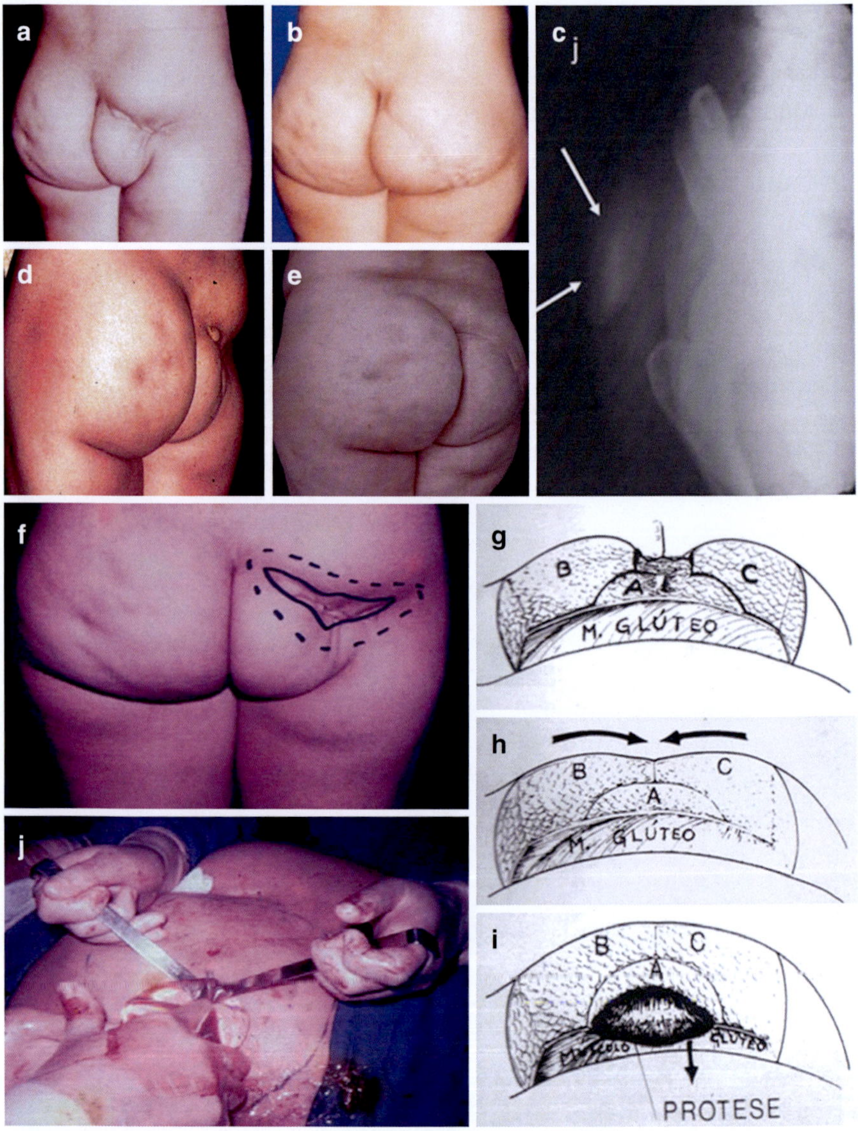

Fig. 1.2 A 19-year-old female patient with severe deformities on right buttock caused by infection after injection in infancy which was repaired in two surgical stages with mammary silastic prosthesis in 1972. Photos (**a, d**) before operation; (**b, e**) 1 year after surgery; (**c**) an X-ray 1 year after operation where one can see the prosthesis indicated by arrows; (**f**) before the first stage the fibrotic scar tissues are demarcated with continuous black line to be resect and doted lines indicate the area of the panniculus to be undermined; (**g**) scheme in profile view showing the scar tissue area of resection during first stage; (**h**) scheme after first stage the flaps B and C after undermining were sutured over the flap A underneath; scheme (**i**) it is showing the prosthesis placed below the flap A; (**j**) photo perioperative when prosthesis was introduced through a lateral cutaneous incision

1977) treated the localized adiposity along the lateral side of the thighs and corrected the depression in the buttocks. Although extensive scars remained on the trochanteric and buttocks regions after surgery, it was possible to reshape the abnormalities, which was an important development for body-contouring surgery (Pitanguy 1964, 1977) (Fig. 1.1).

A few years later, Illouz (1980, 1983a, b, 1984) introduced and popularized the liposuction method, which was one of the most revolutionary procedures in plastic surgery in the twentieth century. Therefore, removing accumulations of fat, especially on the abdominal walls and buttocks, became a much simpler procedure that resulted in only very small scars (Fig. 1.3). However, quite often, there were evident redundancies of skin after liposuction on abdominal walls, which were real problems and constant challenges. Such excesses of cutaneous covering, which bothered me and my patients, were solved through skin resection (Avelar 1985a, b, 1986), which became a new approach. Although such combined approaches did not bring any new sorts of complications, they came with very high incidences of seroma formation and other adverse situations. Because of such complications and after a very short period of time, I made the definitive decision to not perform those combined procedures anymore (Avelar 1988).

Aiming to solve those problems motived me to develop new techniques for abdominoplasty that may be used to remodel several other regions of the human body, as I described in my publications on my new technique for abdominoplasty (Avelar 1999a, b, c, d, e, 2000a, b) (Figs. 1.4 and 1.5). Even for

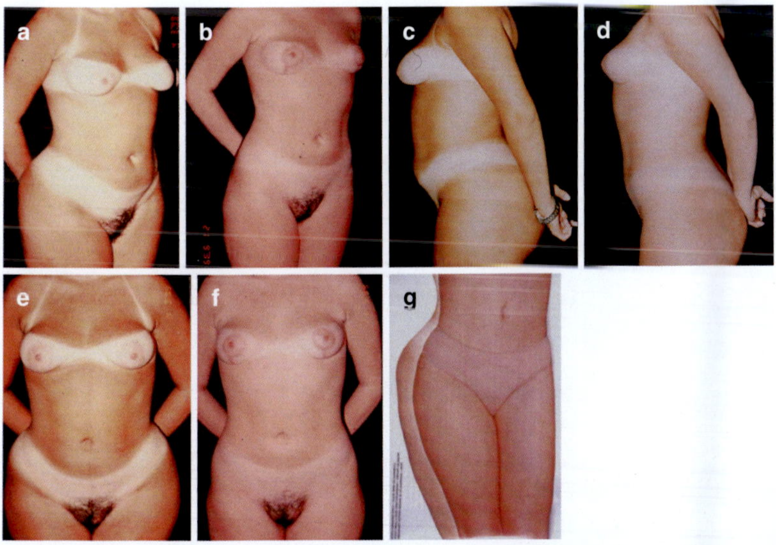

Fig. 1.3 Liposuction procedure improving body contouring in a 24-year-old patient after two pregnancies presenting complex accumulation of localized adiposities on abdomen, buttocks, flanks, and trochanteric regions. Photos (**a, c, e**) before surgery presenting severe alterations on body contour. Photos (**b, d, f**) after liposuction on abdomen, buttocks, and trochanteric regions combined with mastopexy. On photo (**g**) it is a superposition of the silhouette after surgery comparing with her body contouring before liposuction

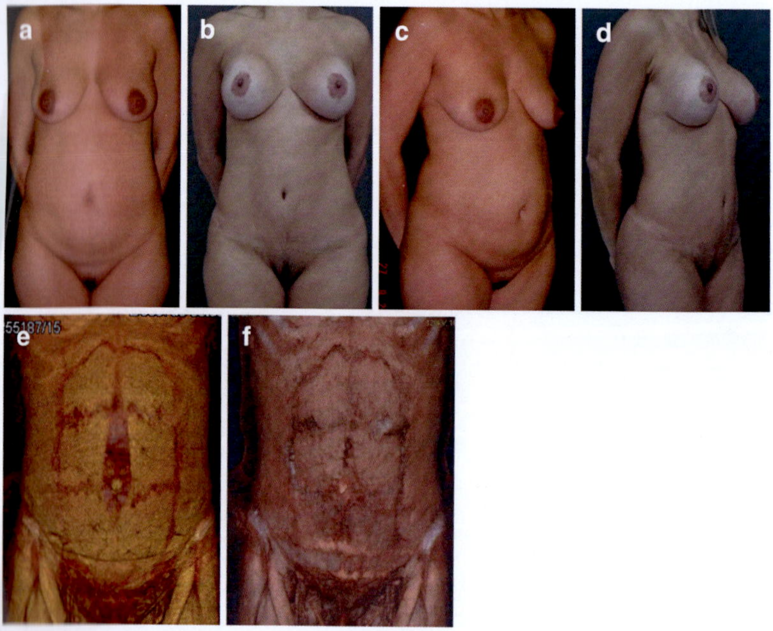

Fig. 1.4 A 39-year-old patient underwent lipoabdominoplasty with plication of the musculoaponeurotic wall combined with augmentation mastoplasty and mastopexy. Photos (**a, c**) before surgery; (**b, d**) post-operatory view showing improvement of body contouring; (**e**) tomography of the muscular abdominal wall showing diástases of the muscles; (**f**) same patient after operation

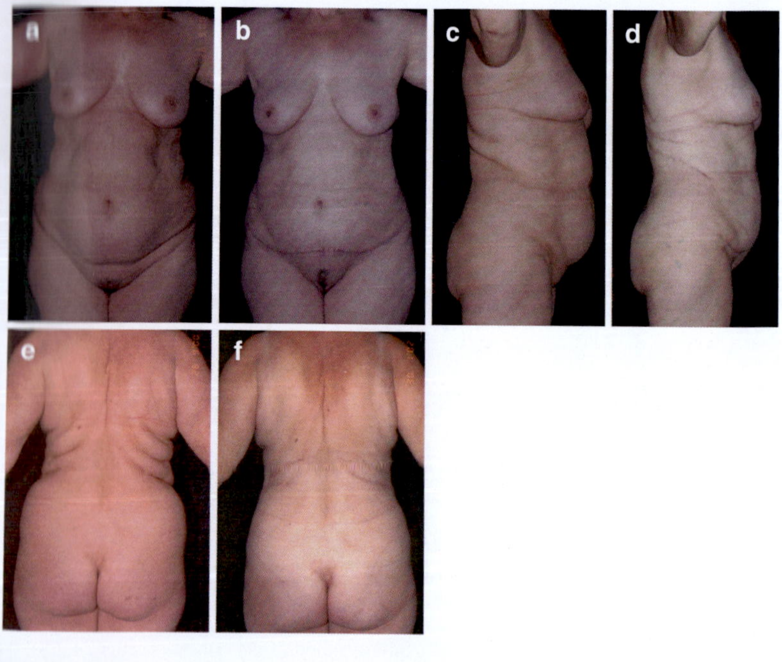

Fig. 1.5 A 54-year-old patient underwent upper and lower lipoabdominoplasty combined with torso lipoplasty. Photos (**a, c, e**) before surgery; (**b, d, f**) after operation

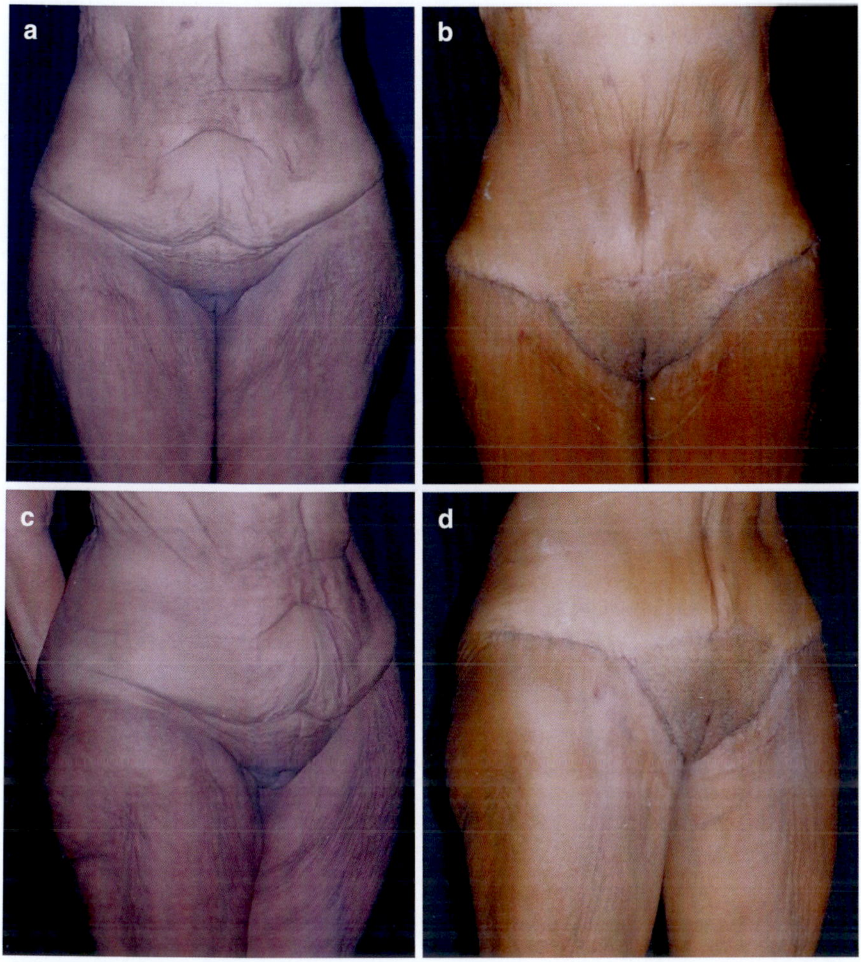

Fig. 1.6 A 65-year-old female patient underwent lipoabdominoplasty and 6 months later medial thigh lifting was performed to achieve harmonious body contouring. Same patient in oblique view showing improvement of the abdomen and thigh

patients who have undergone severe weight loss, this technique could be used to simultaneously treat several regions, achieving harmonious body contouring (Fig. 1.6).

Technique

Each patient must undergo a full-body analysis in a standing position and in front of mirrors for them to be properly evaluated for adequate surgical treatment to improve their body contouring (Fig. 1.7). As several regions may be in disharmony with the other segments of the body, there is no gold-standard procedure to employ. For these

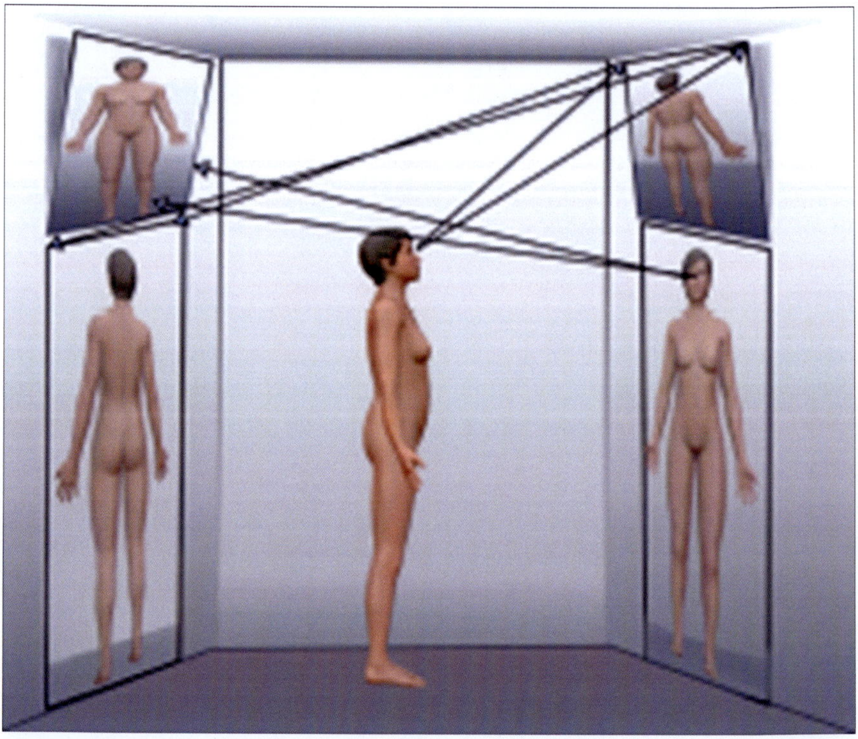

Fig. 1.7 Examining room in my clinic there are two vertical mirrors, one in front of the other and two other ones placed 45° above them. In this drawing one can see that a patient in stand position in front of one vertical mirror she or he can observe in front view. When the patient looks at the superior mirror placed 45° she or he can see the posterior side as well as the whole body contouring

reasons, each patient must be treated according to their unique physical imperfections when improving body contouring.

Abdominoplasty

Abdominoplasty is one of the most frequently used procedures to improve body contouring, and it is performed either alone or in combination with other techniques (Figs. 1.5 and 1.6). A combination of liposuction with abdominoplasty and without panniculus undermining has been introduced, achieving smooth surgical results and minimizing complications (Avelar 1999a, b, c, 2000a, b). In this modality of lipoabdominoplasty, the umbilicus is transposed and a new umbilical area is created. The selection of patients before surgery is a fundamental step for the surgeon to evaluate the possibility of removing all skin in suprapubic region, and the cutaneous area above the umbilicus may be pulled downward to be sutured to the inferior border of the surgical incision (Figs. 1.4 and 1.6). Finally, abdominoplasty may be performed according to the techniques designed by Callia (1965), Pitanguy (1967), Sinder (1975), or others, bringing considerable refinements to aesthetic body contouring.

Reduction or Augmentation Via Mastoplasty

Large breasts or small breasts may cause unsatisfaction for female patients, motivating them to undergo aesthetic procedures to reshape their body's silhouette (Fig. 1.8). Each surgeon may follow their own techniques which are more used to performing in order to remodel of the body. Reduction mastoplasty, which is also used to improve the shape of the breasts, can provide harmony to all segments of the body (Fig. 1.9).

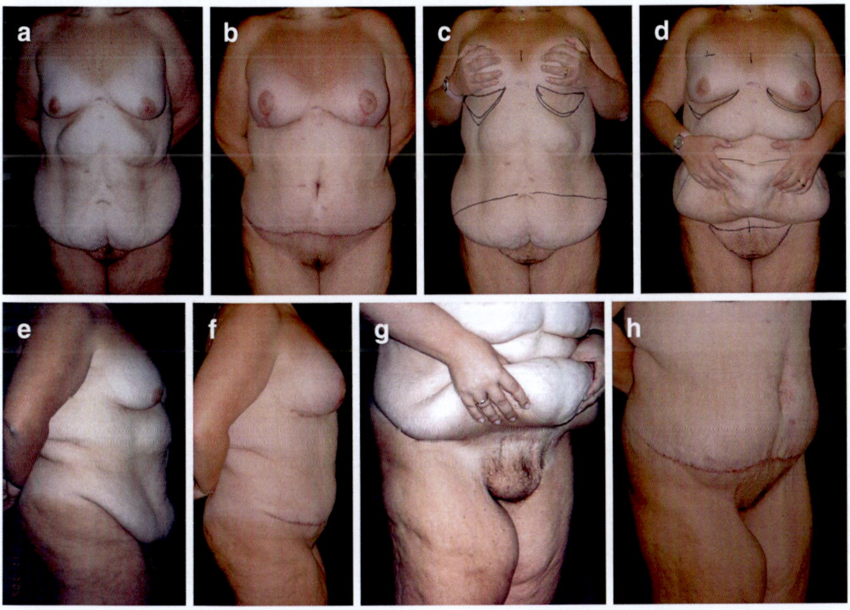

Fig. 1.8 A 42-year-old patient after bariatric surgery presenting improvement of body contouring through mastopexy with prosthesis inclusion associated with upper and full-lipoabdominoplasty. Photos (**a, c, e, g**) before operation; (**b, d, f, h**) postoperative photos after associated procedures. Photos (**c, d**) one can see surgical planning of upper and full-lipoabdominoplasty

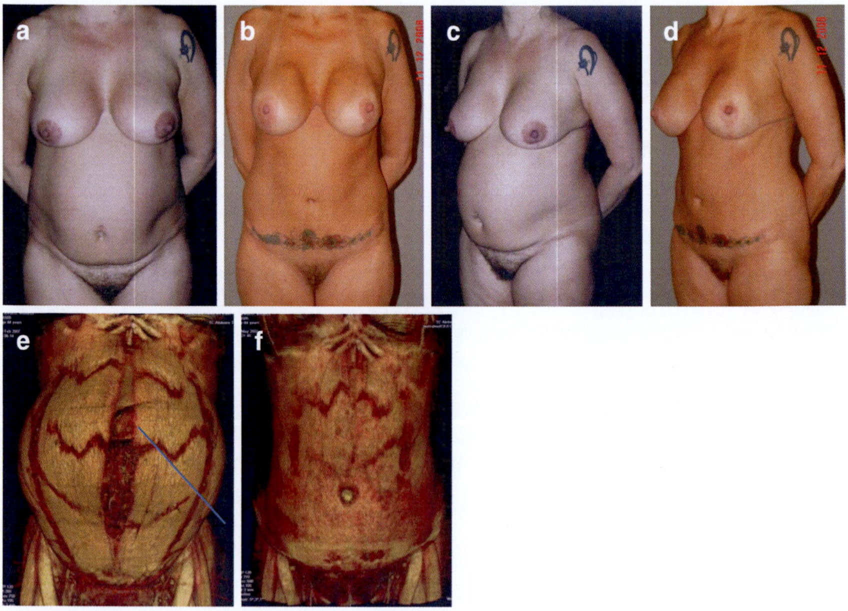

Fig. 1.9 Mastopexy combined with lipoabdominoplasty and medial and lateral plication of the musculoaponeurotic structures. Photos (**a, c**) before surgery; (**b, d**) after combined procedures improving body contouring; (**e**) TC of the abdominal structures before plication shows diástases on medline and lateral as well; (**f**) TC after reinforcement of the abdominal wall

The Accumulation of Localized Adiposities

Abdominal walls may present the accumulation of localized adipose tissue, as may the lateral and posterior aspects of the thighs and buttocks, producing unaesthetic and inelegant appearances. Such imperfections were described as trochanteric lipodystrophies or the "riding breeches" deformities (Pitanguy 1964, 1977). Quite often, the bulging area of adiposity develops a depression in the posterior lateral aspects of the buttocks (Fig. 1.1). A similar deformity is frequently apparent on the inner side of the thighs, usually accompanied by the flaccidity of the skin and subcutaneous tissue. The drooping of the buttocks secondary to musculocutaneous flaccidity from aging is another type of deformity that has shown significant improvement after a combination of remodeling via skin resection and tunnelization without panniculus undermining (Avelar 1999a, b, c, d, e, f) (Figs. 1.10 and 1.11).

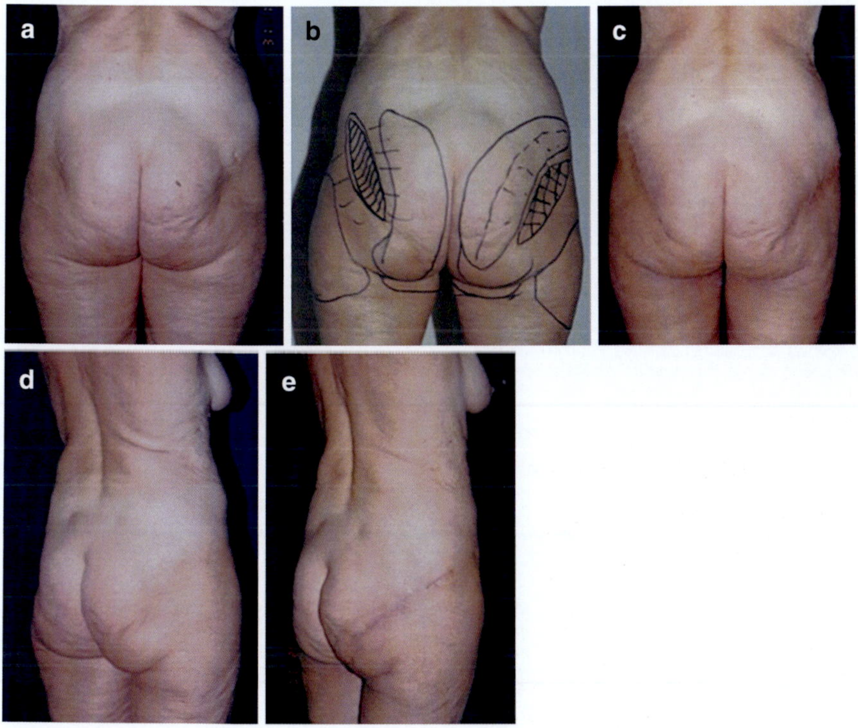

Fig. 1.10 Correction of unaesthetic deformities caused by previous surgery on buttocks. I employed liposuction combined with my surgical principles without panniculus undermining. Photos (**a**) preoperative of a 69-year-old female patient presenting bilateral unaesthetic depression with scars secondary to previous surgery; (**b**) surgical demarcations following Pitanguy's technique with two segments of skin resection bilaterally and the area for liposuction; (**c**) final result of aesthetic reparation; (**d**) posterolateral view showing depression caused by previous operation; (**e**) final result on posterolateral on right side

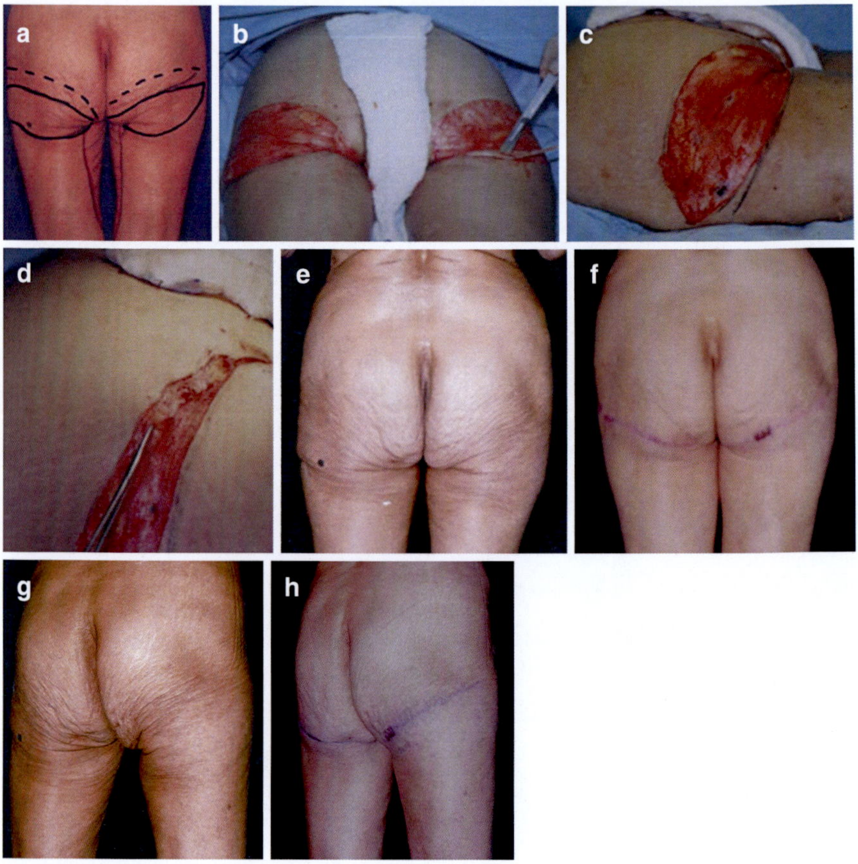

Fig. 1.11 Correction of flaccidity of buttocks and trochanteric regions employing new procedure without panniculus undermining following Pitanguy's technique. Photos (**a**) posterior view showing surgical demarcation on gluteal folds and inner aspect of the thigh; (**b**) after tunnelization with cannula the excess of skin was resected; (**c**) wide raw area after cutaneous resection; (**d**) the raw area was sutured by inverted stitches folded over itself; (**e**) preoperataive on posterior view; (**f**) postoperative; (**g**) oblique posterolateral view before surgery; (**h**) same patient 6 months after surgery. Six months later she underwent silastic prosthesis inclusion on inner side of the thigh performed by Dr. Montellano

Liposuction

The liposuction operation introduced and popularized by Illouz (1980, 1983a, b, 1986a, b), which opened up a new era of body-contouring surgery, is doubtless an important step in improving and remodeling the body's contours. On one hand, some deformities from the severe accumulation of adiposities in certain regions may yield important surgical results when isolated liposuction is performed (Figs. 1.3 and 1.12). On the other, other deformities require procedures to achieve harmonious aesthetic results (Figs. 1.10, 1.11, and 1.13).

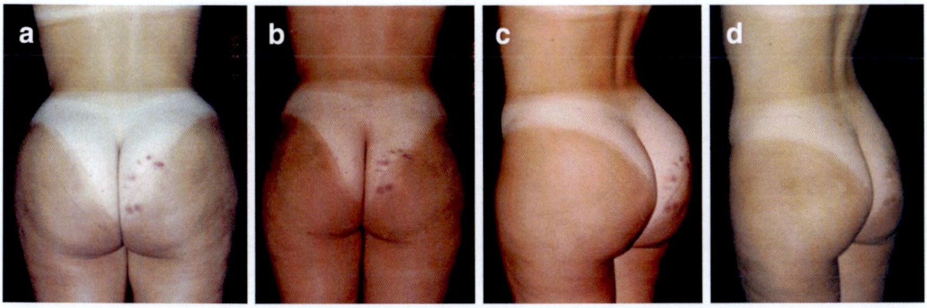

Fig. 1.12 Isolated liposuction of the flanks and buttocks without skin resection in a 19-year-old girl presented excessive accumulation of fat with unaesthetic appearance. Photos (**a, c**) before operation; (**b, d**) after liposuction on the buttocks

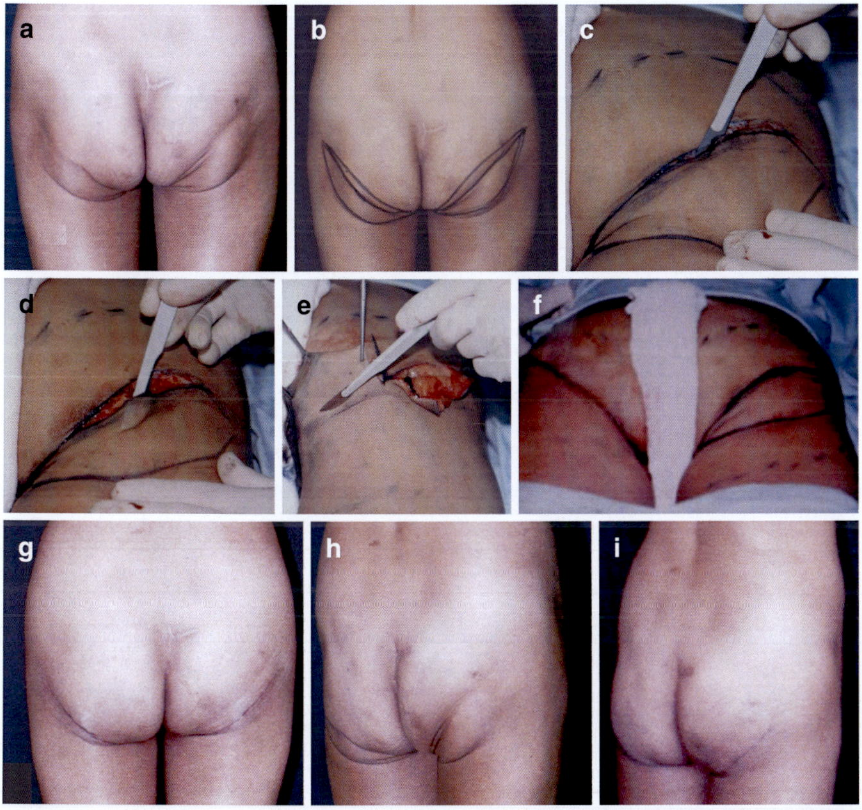

Fig. 1.13 Unaesthetic deformities of buttocks caused by unsuccessful silastic prosthesis inclusion. Photos (**a**) posterior view showing severe scars with ungraceful appearance of the buttock; (**b**) demarcation of the procedure according to Pitanguy's technique; (**c**) cutaneous incisions following demarcations; (**d**) cutaneous undermining with knife; (**e**) traction upwards of the inferior segment and resection of the excess of skin followed by internal suture to approximate the borders; (**f**) final suture on left side of the patient one can see the improvement comparing with the right one; (**g**) same patient 1 year after surgery on posterior view; (**h**) posterior oblique view on right side with unaesthetic aspect of the buttocks and ungraceful scars caused by extrusion of silastic prosthesis; (**i**) final result with reshaping of the buttocks

Buttock Remodeling

The remodeling of an accumulation of localized adiposities on gluteal regions has shown good improvement on body contouring under liposuction, with inconspicuous scarring and harmonious surgical results (Figs. 1.3 and 1.12). Several kinds of deformities of the buttocks require surgical corrections for reparation with resections of the cutaneous covering (Figs. 1.10 and 1.11). Some patients have undergone unsuccessful operations, such as silastic implants in the gluteal region with unaesthetic results (Fig. 1.13). For correcting such reparation, Pitanguy's technique (Pitanguy 1964, 1977) is an excellent support in order to demarcate the skin resection, to orient the skin undermining, and to resect, even when remodeling the buttocks (Fig. 1.13). Mammary silastic implants have been employed for the reconstruction of severe deformities to the buttocks Fig. 1.2) (Avelar 1974a, b, 1977), improving body contouring. Later, a new prosthesis was developed specifically to improve the aesthetics of gluteal implants.

Torsoplasty

The posterior aspect of the torso has a peculiar anatomy in the subcutaneous panniculus that requires the appropriate technique to improve body contouring (Fig. 1.14). Some localized adiposity along the posterior regions of the torso may be remodeled via isolated liposuction when there is no redundant skin (Fig. 1.15). The accumulation of localized fat has so far required skin resection associated with the liposuction procedure when performed under new approaches without panniculus undermining (Avelar 1999a, b, 2000a, b) (Figs. 1.5 and 1.16). Many kinds of body asymmetry may be remediated by employing isolated liposuction or a combination of it with skin resection to achieve good harmonious contouring to the torso and abdomen (Fig. 1.17).

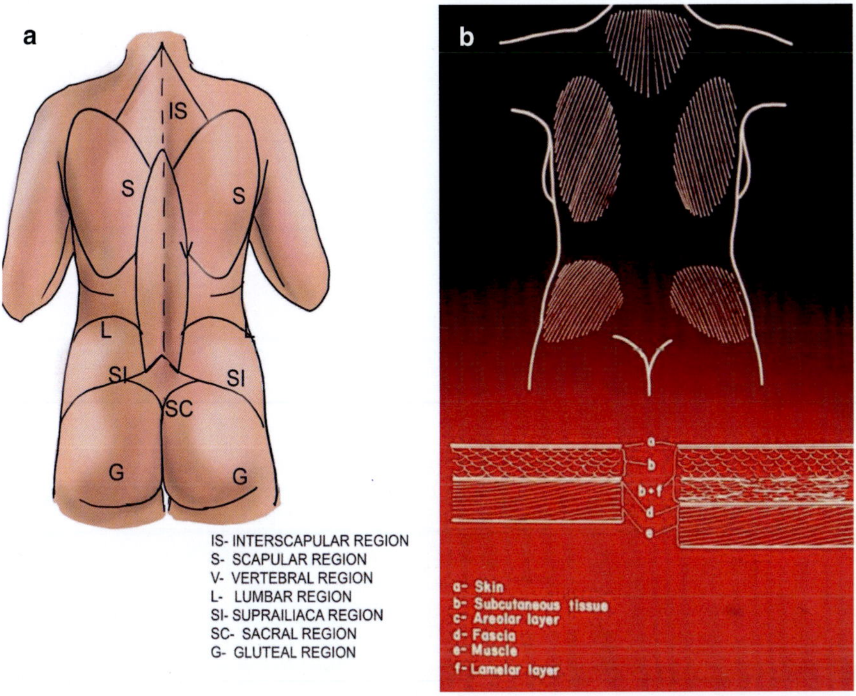

Fig. 1.14 Regions of the posterior regions of the torso. Diagram (**a**) one can observe the three odd (interscapular, vertebral, and sacral) and three even (scapular, lumbar, and suprailiac); (**c**) shows the most frequent regions presenting localized adiposities on posterior side of the torso, inside of the fascia superficialis

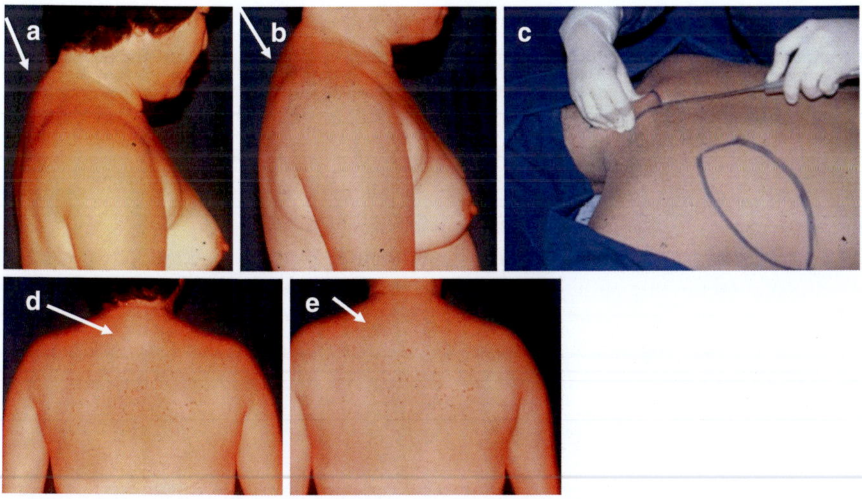

Fig. 1.15 Accumulation of localized adiposities on interscapular region and its treatment; (**a, d**) preoperatory photos indicating the adiposities by arrows; (**b, e**) postoperative photos showing correction of deformities; (**c**) photo during operation with the patient on ventral position on operating table the cannula works through a cutaneous incision on lower border of the interscapular region with adiposities

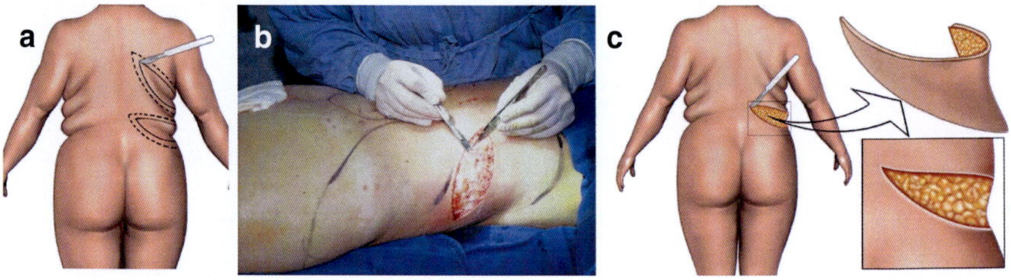

Fig. 1.16 Torso lipoplasty performed as combined procedure of skin resection plus liposuction without panniculus undermining. Diagram (**a**) shows surgical planning on right side: demarcation of skin resection and lipoplasty; (**b**) preoperatory photo shows full-thickness skin resection as well as demarcations for liposuction; (**c**) diagram demonstrates full-thickness skin resection indicated by arrow

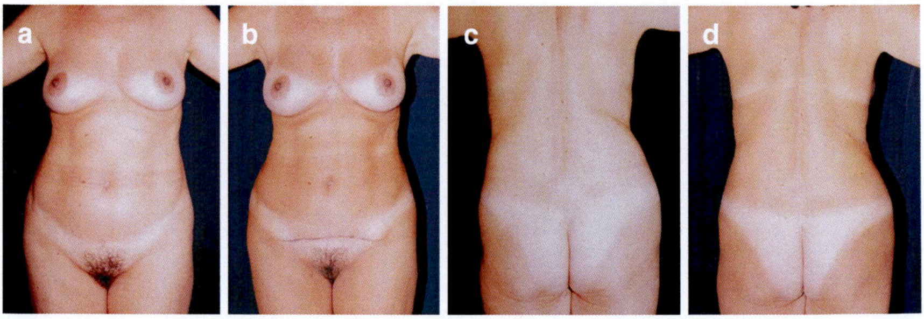

Fig. 1.17 Liposuction procedure repairing asymmetric body contouring. Photos (**a, c**) a 42-year-old female patient presenting complex asymmetry of the body in front view as well as on posterior one. Photos (**b, d**) after liposuction combined with lower abdominoplasty and liposuction on posterior regions of the torso

Aesthetic Surgery on Thighs and Buttocks

The appearance of aging may occur all over of the human body. Any region may present skin flaccidity, striae, redundancy, or the accumulation of local adiposities. Before Illouz introduced the liposuction technique in the 1980s (Illouz 1980, 1983a, b, 1984), such deformities could be treated with Pitanguy's technique (Figs. 1.10 and 1.11) (Pitanguy 1964, 1977). Later, both procedures, liposuction alone and liposuction combined with panniculus resection, may be employed, without panniculus undermining, by following the surgical method that I previously described (Fig. 1.18) (Avelar 1999a, b). Ever since this liposuction technique was introduced, several deformities have been adequately treated to achieve harmonious body contouring (Figs. 1.3, 1.12, 1.15, 1.17, and 1.18).

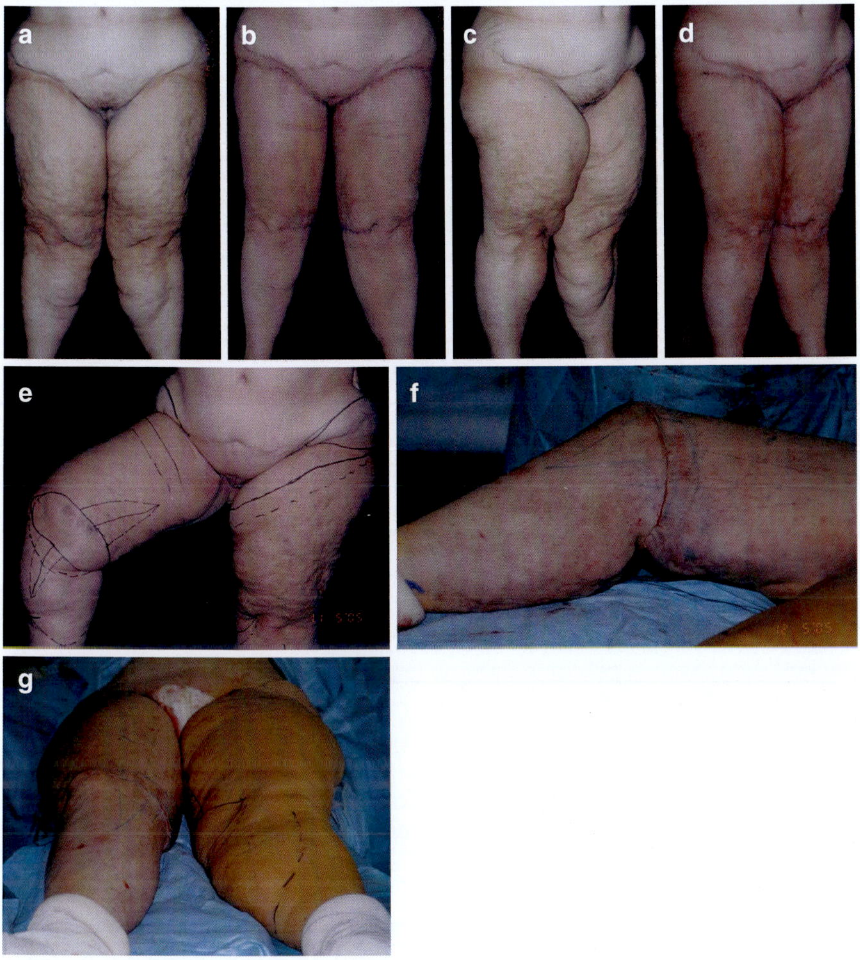

Fig. 1.18 Female patient with lipodystrophy of the lower extremities presenting improvement of body contouring through Pitanguy's demarcations associated with medial thigh lifting without panniculus undermining (Avelar 1999b). Photos (**a, c**) unaesthetic appearance; (**b, d**) surgical result with scars on inguinal sulcus

Abdominoplasty Combined with Aesthetic Surgery on Thighs and Buttocks

When adiposities accumulate on the abdominal walls of the external and inner sides of the thighs, the treatment is performed as a combination of surgeries on all the affected regions. My preference is to perform my procedures without panniculus undermining (Figs. 1.6, 1.8, and 1.18) (Avelar 1999a, b, c, 2000a, b)

Discussion

The combined procedure for reshaping body contouring was introduced by Pitanguy (1977, 1982, 1986). Ever since I was a resident at Prof. Pitanguy's clinic, I used to often hear him say the terms *body-contouring surgery* and *facial-contouring surgery*. Those expressions were related to combined procedures meant to improve body contouring and facial contouring, respectively. At the beginning of my career, I was so impressed with those concepts that I became motivated to organize the Brazilian Symposium of Abdominoplasty and Facial Contouring, and Prof. Pitanguy delivered lectures at each of those events and wrote two memorable chapters about those fields (Pitanguy 1982, 1983). In fact, associated operations were performed frequently during the period of my training at Pitanguy's clinic, under outstanding surgical team organization in the operating room and yielding excellent surgical results showing great improvements to body and facial contouring. Given all the knowledge that I gained from Pitanguy; our warm professional relationship; and my deep and sincere gratitude, at an event that I organized in São Paulo, I paid him homage (Fig. 1.19). After the liposuction technique had been introduced by Illouz (1980, 1983a, b, 1984, 1986a, b), body-contouring surgeries received important support to achieve better surgical results. Again, given the opportunity I had had to learn the liposuction technique and our later partnership in several professional activities, even together publishing a book (*Liposuction*), I offered Prof. Illouz my deep recognition and ardent thanks (Fig. 1.20).

Nevertheless, the techniques of associated operations were regularly performed at Pitanguy's clinic—on thighs, buttocks, and the trochanteric regions—according to Pitanguy's technique (Pitanguy 1964, 1977). His memorable approaches opened up a new era for body surgery because the removal of redundant skin and localized adiposities became possible, which used to be removed through vertical incisions on the lateral and inner aspect of the thigh (Farina et al. 1960).

Nowadays, people are exposed to two antithetical propagandas: a wide and intense variety of food with lessons on how to prepare delicious dishes that

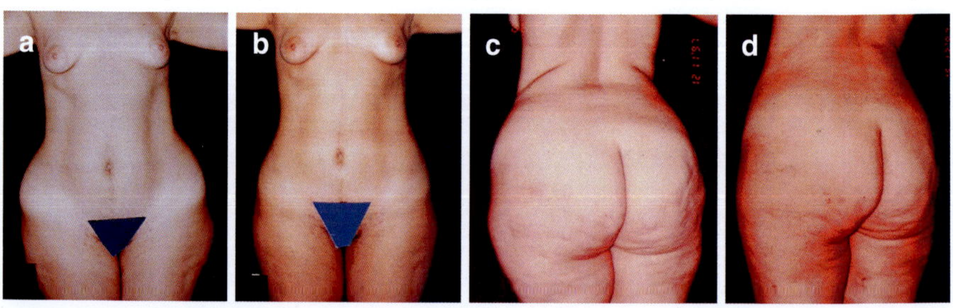

Fig. 1.19 My homage to Prof. Pitanguy during a Symposium in São Paulo (Brazil) August 2002. Photo (**a**) during the ceremony specially dedicated to give Prof. Pitanguy a surgical instrument (a knife) made in gold; (**b**) photo of the instrument with a plac in gold with my sentence: "To Prof. Pitanguy, my gratitude to teach me how to work with this surgical instrument. São Paulo, August 2002"

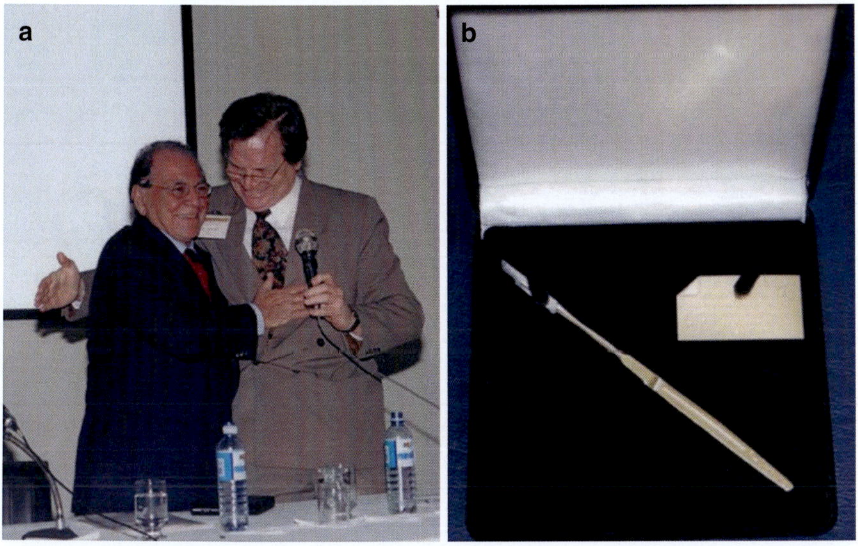

Fig. 1.20 During the First Congress of the Prof. Illouz Association (PIA), held in Brasilia (Brazil) in 2008, our homage to Prof. Illouz. Photos (**a**) I gave him a plac made in gold as my gratitude; (**b**) photo of the plac with the map of Brazil with a canula from Fortaleza (where he made his first lecture) pointing to São Paulo (where we organized several events to teach liposuction); (**c**) a certificate from the Board of Prof. Illouz Association to him. Few years later during an ISAPS event in Paris I was invited for a reception at Illouz' office, he was so happy to show and he said to everybody my gifts with a map of Brazil that I offered as a symbol of my gratitude

stimulate people to eat more and more on one hand and on the other constant information about diet and physical exercises to eliminate the signs of obesity and real obesity, both for appearance and for improving health conditions. Consequently, there is a constant demand from people, female and male, for a desirable physical appearance.

Over the past few decades, bariatric surgeries have been performed more and more to treat obesity, and plastic surgeons perform reparations for people after weight loss (Figs. 1.6, 1.8, and 1.11). In such way, all regions of the body require intense effort from plastic surgeons aiming to remodel the body's contours (Figs. 1.3, 1.4, 1.5, and 1.12). Ever since the liposuction technique introduced by Illouz (1980, 1983a, b, 1984, 1986a, b) made possible the removal of excess localized adiposities, leaving inconspicuous scars, it has been an important procedure for removing accumulations of adipose tissue from abdominal walls and other regions. So far, redundancy of cutaneous tissue has not been treated, but a combination of liposuction with conventional abdominoplasty has improved body contouring (Avelar 1985a, b, 1986).

However, such a combined procedure comes with very high incidences of complications, such as seroma formation, hematoma, slough from the panniculus, and others. Aiming to avoid these sorts of complications motivated me to search for new techniques for abdominoplasty. Therefore, after a long period of research, I concluded that the abdominal panniculus may be undermined as long as the perforator vessels are preserved; these vessels work as multiple pedicles to the remaining panniculus, providing adequate blood supply (Avelar 1999a, b, c, 2000a, b) (Figs. 1.4, 1.5, 1.6, 1.8, 1.9, and 1.13).

My anatomical studies gave me adequate support to perform combined procedures (liposuction with panniculus resection) with minimal complications. Similar procedures may be employed for remodeling other regions, such as flanks, torsos, medial thighs, arms, and axilla (Figs. 1.5, 1.6, 1.8, 1.9, 1.10, 1.11, 1.16, 1.17, and 1.18) (Avelar 1999a, b, c)

At the beginning of my career, I employed mammary silastic implants for the reconstruction of severe acquired deformities on the buttocks from complex infections caused by injections into the gluteal regions (Fig. 1.2) (Avelar 1974a, b, 1977) Although these prostheses were not made specifically for gluteal regions, they still improved body contouring. Later, a new prosthesis was developed specifically to improve the aesthetics of gluteal implants.

Conclusions

Body-contouring surgeries have undergone an evolution over the past few decades. Direct approaches to removing localized adiposities on the lateral and inner side of the thighs (Farina et al. 1960) have been replaced by horizontal and anatomic incisions on the gluteal sulcus (Pitanguy 1964, 1977) to remodel the trochanteric regions. A few years later, Illouz (1980, 1983a, b, 1984, 1986a, b) introduced the revolutionary method of liposuction, yielding outstanding surgical results with minimal complications (Figs. 1.3, 1.12, 1.15, 1.17, 1.18, and 1.21). Nevertheless, liposuction leaves redundant skin that requires treatment, which opened up another modality for body contouring and introduced new techniques for abdominoplasty (Avelar 1985a, b, 1986). So far, the very high rates of seroma formation and other sorts of complications after combined procedures of liposuction with the resection of the excess cutaneous covering motivated me to research new approaches (Avelar 1999a, b, c, 2000a, b) (Figs. 1.4, 1.5, 1.6, 1.8, and 1.9).

After a long period of research and anatomical study, I found the key to avoiding those frequent complications during and after operations, where the abdominal panniculus is undermined but the perforator vessels are preserved during surgery, providing normal vascularization to the remnant panniculus and thus avoiding seroma formation and other sorts of complications. The new techniques originated as lipoabdominoplasty (Figs. 1.4, 1.5, 1.6, 1.8, and 1.9), and the same surgical principles may be employed for remodeling other regions, such as thighs and buttocks (Figs. 1.10, 1.11, 1.13, and 1.18), arms, axilla, and torsos, achieving smooth shapes and thus improving body contouring.

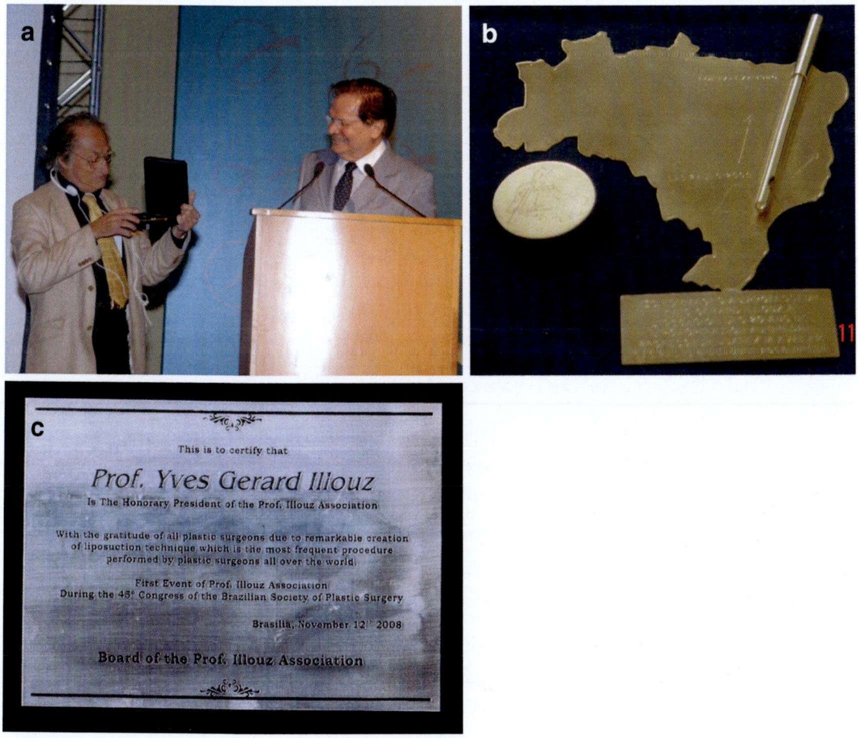

Fig. 1.21 Isolated liposuction of the flanks, supra iliac, trochanteric, and gluteal regions leaving inconspícuos scars, without skin resection in a 22-year-old patient presented accumulation of fat with unaesthetic appearance. Photos (**a, c**) before operation; (**b, d**) after liposuction on the buttocks, supra iliac, flanks, and trochanteric regions

References

Avelar JM (1974a) Reparation of Buttocks deformities using mammary prosthesis. (Reparação de deformidades de nádega com emprego de próteses mamárias). Presented at Brazilian Congress of Plastic Surgery (BSPC) (as thesis to be full member of the BSPC), Belo Horizonte (Brazil), May

Avelar JM (1974b) Reparation of severe Buttocks deformity employing mammary prosthesis. (Reparación de severa deformidad de náldegas con emplego de próteses mamárias). Presented at V Congress of the Mexican Association of Plastic Surgery (Associación Mexicana de Cirugia Plástica. Acapulco (México), October.

Avelar JM (1977) Buttocks reconstruction. (Reconstrução de nádega) Braz. Journ of Medicine (Jornal Bras. de Medicina). Fevereiro, 43–55

Avelar JM (1985a) Combined liposuction with traditional surgery in abdomen Lipodystrophy. XXIV Instructional Course of Aesth Plast Surg of ISAPS, Madrid.

Avelar JM (1985b) Fat-suction versus abdominoplasty. Aesthetic Plast Surg 9:265–276

Avelar JM (1985c) Fat-Suction of the Submental and Submandibular Regions. Aesth Plast Surg 9:257–263

Avelar JM (1986) Liposuction of Abdominal Wall (Lipoaspiração da Parede Abdominal). In Liposuction (Lipoaspiração). Ed. by Avelar JM. & Illouz YG. Sao Paulo (Brasil). Editora Hipócrates 27:158–176.
Avelar JM (1988) Abdominoplasty – Reflections and Bio-psychological Perspectives (Abdominoplastia – reflexões e perspectivas biopsicológicas). Rev Soc Bras Cir Plast 3(2):152–154.
Avelar JM (1999a) New concepts for abdominoplasty. (Novos conceitos para abdominoplastia). Paper presented at the 36th congress of the Brazilian Society of Plastic Surgery, Rio de Janeiro, November.
Avelar JM (1999b) A new technique for abdominoplasty – closed vascular system of subdermal flap folded over itself combined to liposuction (Uma nova técnica para Abdominoplastia – Sistema vascular fechado de retalho subdérmico dobrado sobre si mesmo combinado com lipoaspiração). Rev Bras Cir 88/89(1/6):3–20.
Avelar JM (1999c) Abdominoplastia: nuevos conceptos para una nueva técnica (Abdominoplasty: new concepts for a new technique). XXVI Annual international symposium of aesthetic plastic surgery, Chairman: Prof. Jose Guerrerosantos, Puerto Vallarta, pp 10–13.
Avelar JM (1999d) Aesthetic Plastic in the Inner Side of the Thigh – New Concepts and Technique without Cutaneous or Subcutaneous Undermining. (Cirurgia Plástica de Face Interna de Coxas – novos conceitos e técnica7 minutos sem descolamento cutâneo e subcutâneo). Rev Bras Cir 88/89(1/6):57–67.
Avelar JM (1999e) Aesthetic plastic in the inner side of the thigh – new concepts and technique without cutaneous or subcutaneous undermining. (Cirurgia Plástica de Face Interna de Coxas – novos conceitos e tecnica sem descolamento cutâneo e subcutâneo). Rev Bras Cir 88/89(1/6):57–67.
Avelar JM (1999f) Flankplasty and torsoplasty – a new surgical approach. (Flancoplastia e Torsoplastia - Nova Abordagem Cirúrgica). Rev Bras Cir 88/89(1/6):21–35.
Avelar JM (2000a) Abdominoplasty: a new technique without panniculus undermining and without panniculus resection. 57th Instructional Course of ISAPS, Chairman: Lloyd Carlsen, in Montreal, Canada.
Avelar JM (2000b) Abdominoplasty: a new technique without undermining and fat layer removal (Abdominoplastia: uma nova técnica sem descolamento e remoção da camada de gordura). Arq Catarinense de Med 29:147–149
Callia WEP (1965) Contribuição ao estudo de correção cirúrgica do abdomen pêndulo e globus (contribution to the study of surgical correction of the pendulum abdomen and globus). original art. Doctoral Thesis Fac Med USP, São Paulo.
Farina R, Baroudi R, Coleman B. & Castro O (1960) Riding trousersilke type of pelvicrual lipodistrophy (trochanteric lipomatosis). Brit. J. Plast. Surg. XIII(2): July.
Illouz Y (1980) Une nouvelle technique pour les lipodystrophies localisées. Rev Chir Esthet 4:19.
Illouz YG (1983a) Instructional Course on Liposuction Technique First Course of Liposuction. Organized by Dr. Juarez M. Avelar, Sponsored by Brazilian Society of Plastic Surgery (São Paulo Section) Heled at São Paulo Hospital, Service of Prof. Andrews at Escola Paulista de Medicina. October São Paulo (Brazil).
Illouz YG (1983b) Body contouring by lipolysis: 5 years experience with over 3,000 cases. Plast Reconstr Surg 72(5):591–597.
Illouz YG (1984) My technique of Liposuction – 4 years evolution. Second Course of Liposuction. (Minha Técnica de Lipoaspiração – 4 Anos de Evolução. 2° Curso de Lipoaspiração) - Heled at "9 de Julho Hospital". Organized by Juarez M. Avelar, Sponsored By Brazilian Society of Plastic Surgery. September, São Paulo (Brazil).
Illouz YG (1986a) Basic Principles of liposuction technique (Princípios básicos da técnica de lipoaspiração). Liposuction (Lipoaspiração). Ed. by AvelarJM. & Illouz YG. Sao Paulo (Brasil). Editora Hipócrates 3:22–225.

Illouz YG (1986b). Study of the Adipocite in Lipodistrophy (Estudo do Adipócito nas Lipodistrogias). In Liposuction (Lipoaspiração). Ed. by AvelarJM. & Illouz YG. Sao Paulo (Brasil). Editora Hipócrates 4:19–23.

Pitanguy I (1964) Trochanteric lipodystrophy. Plast Reconstr Surg 34:280.

Pitanguy I (1977) Dermolipectomy of the abdominal wall, thighs, buttocks and upper extremity – In: Reconstructive Plastic Surgery. Ed. By Converse JM. pg. 3.800-3.823 – Ed. W.B. Saunders Company (Philadelphia and London).

Pitanguy I (1982) Phylosophic and Psychological Perspectives of the Abdomen. (Perspectivas Filosóficas e Psicológicos do Abdomen). In Annals of Brazilian Symposio of Abdominoplasty (Anais do Simpósio Brasileiro de Abdominoplastia), Ed. by Juarez M. Avelar, Sponsored by Brazilian Society of Plastic Surgery-Regional São Paulo, (Patrocinado pela Sociedade Brasileira de Cirurgia Plástica – Regional São Paulo). 1:15–24. Editora Cidade, Rio de Janeiro – Brazil.

Pitanguy I (1983) Philosophical and Psychological Aspects of the Facial Contouring Surgery (Aspectos Filosóficos e Psicológicos da Cirurgia do Contorno Facial). In Annals of the Brazilian Symposium of Facial Contouring (Anais do Simpósio Brasileiro Do Contorno Facial), Ed. By Juarez M. Avelar, Sponsored by Brazilian Society of Plastic Surgery-Regional São Paulo (Patrocinado pela Sociedade Brasileira de Cirurgia Plástica- Regional São Paulo), 1:2–9. Editora Cidade, Rio de Janeiro Brasil.

Pitanguy I (1986) Philosophical and Psychosocials Perspectives of the Body Contouring. (Perspectivas Filosóficas e Psicossociais do Contorno Corporal). In Liposuction (Lipoaspiração), Ed. By Avelar and Illouz, - 1:3–7 - Editora Hipócrates - São Paulo (Brasil).

Pitanguy I (1967) Abdominal lipectomy: an approach to it through an analysis of 300 consecutive cases. Plast Reconstr Surg 40(4):38

Sinder R (1975) Plastic Surgery of the abdomen - Técnica pessoal de abdominoplastia, com prévio deslocamento de retalho supraumbilical (antes da ressecção infraumbilical) e uso de retalho dermoadiposo, – VI International Congress of Plastic and Reconstructive Surgery, Paris (France) August

Chapter 2
Anatomy of the Subcutaneous Layers in the Human Body

Juarez Moraes Avelar

Abstract Ever since I learned the liposuction technique, the subcutaneous compartment of the human has obviously needed to be studied so that the new method for reshaping the face and body can be performed. I dedicated much effort to studying it, performing anatomic dissections on cadavers and even performing liposuction on them to determine the subcutaneous layers. Created and popularized by Illouz, liposuction remains one of the most recent, important methods introduced in plastic surgery to improve body contouring. As soon as I learned such a revolutionary procedure directly from its creator in early 1982, two concerns immediately came to my mind: (1) the unknown anatomy of the subcutaneous layer and (2) the behavior of the tissue after the liposuction procedure. More specifically, my concerns on the anatomical descriptions of the subcutaneous panniculus centered on a lack of sufficient information in textbooks and other publications on the relevant anatomy. I did not feel comfortable performing liposuction procedures without having sufficient knowledge about the anatomy underneath the cutaneous covering of the abdomen wall and other regions concerning body contouring.

At that time, I found information on anatomical dissections performed on cadavers of various ages, sexes, levels of adipose tissue, heights, and ethnicities. I found enough important anatomical information in publications to clarify the specific and detailed findings to plastic surgeons. The distribution of the adipose tissue in the subcutaneous layer was described. After I started performing anatomic dissections on cadavers that had undergone liposuction, I found peculiar characteristics in each region of the human body; a careful evaluation of the adipose tissue revealed specific distributions, which were well described. I mentioned in my earlier publications that there are two layers: the areolar layer and the lamellar layer, which are separated by fascia superficialis all over the subcutaneous panniculus. Later, another author described fascia superficialis in thigh lifting. The behavior of the subcutane-

J. M. Avelar (✉)
Brazilian Scientific Institute of Plastic and Reconstructive Surgery, São Paulo, Brazil

J. M. Avelar, R. Cavalcanti Ribeiro (eds.), *Body Contouring*,
https://doi.org/10.1007/978-3-031-42802-9_2

ous tissue after an operation frequently produces a thick and hard fibrosis, which shows that liposuction should be performed on the lamellar layers. This type of fibrotic tissue in the subcutaneous areola layer often brings about irregularities and inelegant waves on the skin surface.

Keywords Fat tissue · Distribution of adiposities · Subcutaneous layers · Areolar layer · Lamellar layer · Fascia superficialis · Behavior of subcutaneous tissue

Introduction

As soon as I learned the liposuction technique for face and body contouring, I figured out that the subcutaneous layer was an unknown compartment of the human body (Avelar 1983, 1986c). Also, I noticed that there was cutaneous redundance after liposuction on the abdomen. Those circumstances motivated me to dedicate my time to researching the anatomy of the subcutaneous compartments all over the human body (Avelar 1986a, 1987, 1989). The excess skin left after liposuction gave me the inspiration to resect it, which opened up the new field for abdominoplasty (Avelar 1985a, b, 1986b).

The liposuction technique became popular among plastic surgeons all around the world thanks to the intense efforts of Illouz's publications, lectures, and surgical demonstrations (Illouz 1980, 1983a, b, c, 1984). Ever since I started to perform the liposuction technique, my curiosity has been directed toward learning about the anatomy where the cannulas work underneath the skin in order to remove excess fat tissue. Testut's textbooks (Testut and Jacob 1975, 1984), Gray (1974), Spaltroltz (1970), and Sobotta (1977) contained little information on the subcutaneous panniculus. Only two layers were mentioned: the **areolar** layer, which is more superficial and external and which is situated just below the skin, and the **lamellar** layer, which is just beneath the areolar layer.

I immediately started to study the subcutaneous segment in order to obtain anatomic information that had not been well described at the time. I found a specific distribution and peculiar characteristics in each particular region of the human body that I studied, and I have described all of them (Avelar 1986a, 1987, 1989) (see Fig. 2.1).

My anatomical dissections and my liposuctions on the abdominal regions, torsos, and upper and lower extremities of several corpses aimed to learn more about this field so that I could better perform liposuction. In my first publication on this subject (Avelar 1986a), I described the measurements of the subcutaneous layers in several regions of the human body associated with the liposuction technique. I compared fat people and thin people to determine the thickness of the subcutaneous tissue (Avelar 1987). I found (Fig. 2.2) wide variation in the thickness of the lamellar and areolar layers in all regions of the body concerning the thickness of the subcutaneous adipose tissue (Fig. 2.3). The thickness of the layers in children also presents peculiar variations because the lamellar and areolar layers are not well

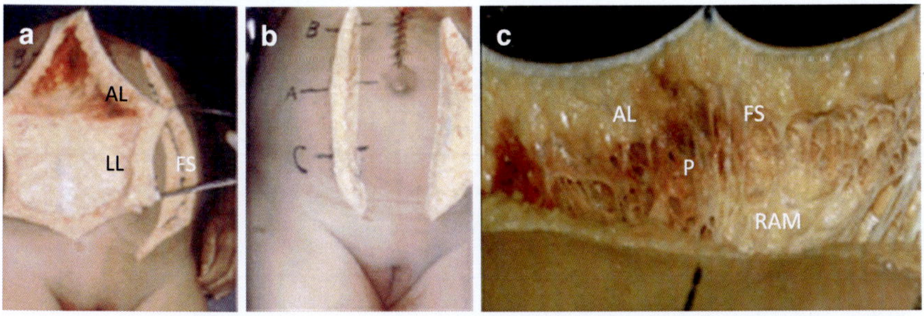

Fig. 2.1 Anatomical study on dissection on cadaver showing the perforator vessels preserved after liposuction on abdominal wall. Photo (**a**) liposuction was done in lamellar layer (LL) on right side showing remaining areolar layer (AL) and on left side of the cadaver fascia superficialis is marked with black ink; (**b**) the remaining panniculus lies on muscles with demarcation of A, B, C for anatomical study; (**c**) the panniculus after liposuction is pulled upwards where one can see the preserved areolar layer (AL) and perforator vessels between rectus abdominalis muscle (RAM) and fascia superficialis (FS)

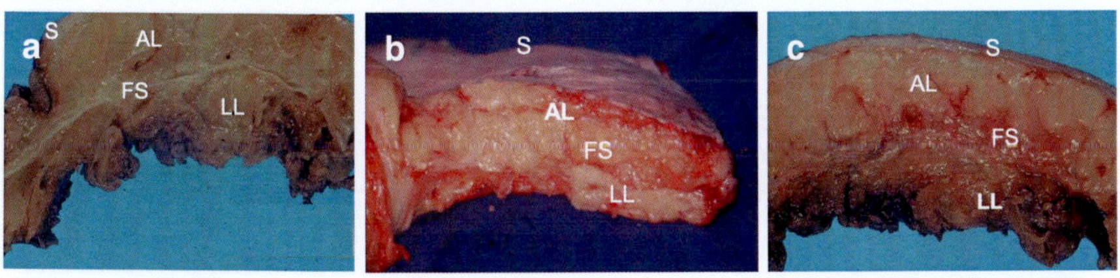

Photo a – abdominal panniculus of a thin cadaver

Photo b – abdominal panniculus of a thin patient

Photo c – abdominal panniculus of a patient with localized adiposity afer liposuction on lamelar layer

Fig. 2.2 Comparison of the anatomical segments of the abdominal panniculus between a thin cadáver, a thin patient, and a patient after liposuction showing relationship of its layers: *S* skin, *AL* areolar layer, *FS* fascia superficialis, *LL* lamellar layer. Photo (**a**) a section of a thin cadaver showing very thin lamellar layer; (**b**) a section of a thin patient; (**c**) a section of fat patient after liposuction on lamellar layer. It is important to emphasize that lamellar layer is very thin one and fascia superficialis in all abdominal panniculus is well identified

identified. For this reason, performing liposuction in infancy is not advisable (Avelar 1986b).

Ever since I completed anatomic studies, I found that between those two adipose layers is a connective structure with vessels, namely the fascia superficialis (Fig. 2.4). In fact, it separates the two adipose layers where arterial, venous, and lymphatic vessels and the nerves are. According to the anatomic information I found, the liposuction technique can be combined with panniculus undermining as long as the perforator vessels do not incur damage (Avelar 1999a). Some years later, another author described the fascia superficialis in thigh lifting (Lockwood 1995). In my previous publications, I have described that the behavior of the subcutaneous tissue after an operation develops a thick and hard fibrosis, which shows that liposuction should be performed on the lamellar layers. I also described that the areolar

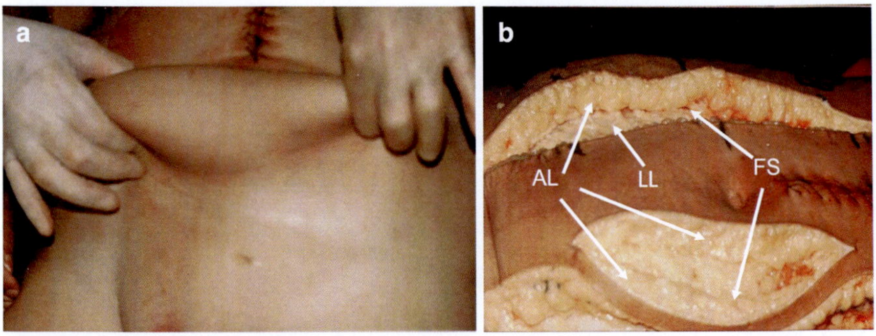

Fig. 2.3 Anatomical study in cadaver to show by Illouz's "pinch test" the modifications of the thickness of the panniculus in the abdominal wall after liposuction procedure. (**a**) Frontal view of the abdomen after liposuction performed on left side of the cadaver. With my hands pinching the panniculus one can see the difference of thickness with the right side without liposuction procedure. (**b**) In the same cadaver an incision was done on left side and another on right. On left side the areolar layer (AL) is preserved, since liposuction was properly performed on lamellar layer. The fascia superficialis (FS) with perforator vessels was preserved on the lamellar layer (LL) lie smoothly on the muscular abdominal wall. On right side the areolar layer (AL), fascia superficialis (FS), and lamellar layer (LL) are identified

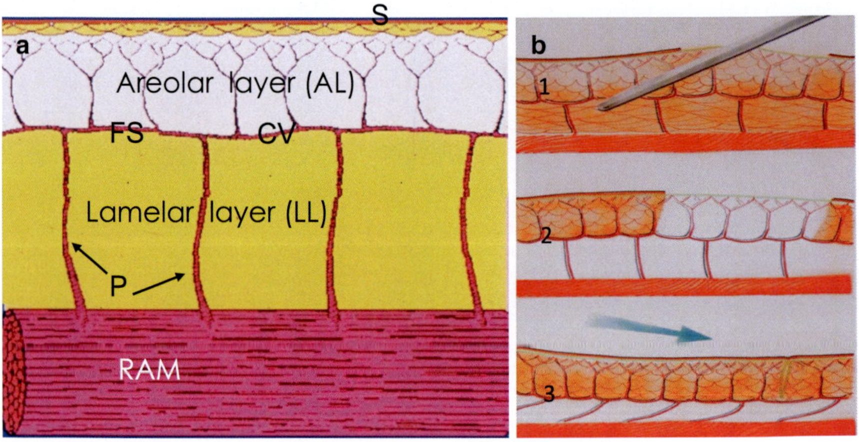

Fig. 2.4 Drawings showing the anatomical structures of the abdominal panniculus and proper level of liposuction. (**a**) Diagram of the panniculus from top to bottom: skin (S), areolar layer (AL), fascia superficialis (FS) with communicating vessels (CV) which work as a "peripheric heart," lamellar layer (LL) with perforator vessels (P) that must be preserved during liposuction and rectus abdominalis muscle (RAM); (**b**) the proper level to perform liposuction: (*1*) (on top) the cannula is introduced through the skin incision with its tip in the lamellar layer (LL), below fascia superficialis, (*2*) the perforator vessels are preserved without fat in lamellar layer and in areolar (AL) where skin resection is done, (*3*) on bottom the areolar layer is pulled downwards with inclination of the perforator vessels which work as multiple pedicle to blood supply to remain panniculus

layer is formed by large, round, and turgid cells that are piled together where small vessels pass to irrigate the subdermal layer and the deep aspect of the skin (Fig. 2.2). On the opposite side, the lamellar layer contains much smaller, empty, and horizontally elongated fat cells (Avelar 1986a).

I described that the thick vessel coming from the aponeurosis and muscular plane perpendicularly crosses the lamellar layer and perforates in the direction of the fascia superficialis. The connective tissue that forms the fascia superficialis behaves in a distinct manner in each region of the human body (Fig. 2.4).

Finally, I confirmed that the subcutaneous panniculus is formed by two specific layers: the areolar layer and the lamellar layer, each of which has a different thickness depending on the region of the human body that it is in. Obviously, the tissue's behavior varies depending on the degree of nutrition and the excess of adiposity in the organism. After studying the same region in fat people and thin people, I notice a great difference that is relevant to liposuction (Fig. 2.2).

Another important role of the subcutaneous cellular tissue is to protect the body's surface, creating a smooth contour. This structure has a peculiar behavior in different areas, where it can produce more protection in regions of attrition, such as in the plantar, palmar, and digital areas.

Anterior Abdominal Wall

Ever since my first liposuction procedure, the abdominal wall has motivated me to study the anatomy of the subcutaneous compartment. In fact, the anterior abdominal panniculus shows immense variation in anatomic constitutions, which were described for performing liposuction to remodel the body's contours (Avelar 1986a, 1987, 1989). The abdominal panniculus contains a complex variety of anatomical changes, which is crucial information to have before performing liposuction (Avelar 1986a, 1987, 1989).

The anterior abdominal wall can be divided into the following regions: three odd, namely epigastric, umbilical, and hypogastric, and three even, namely hypochondriac, lumbar, and inguinal (Fig. 2.5). The main anatomical structures include the fascia superficialis and the perforator vessels. The odd regions present more alterations than the even ones do and even more so in fat people than in thin people (Fig. 2.6a, b).

The fascia superficialis in those regions contains several layers separated by adipose tissue in patients with localized adiposity (Figs. 2.7 and 2.8). The measurement of and the variation of thickness in the areolar and lamellar layers have been described in different types of persons to determine indications for liposuction.

The thicker zone of the abdomen corresponds to the projection of the rectus abdominalis muscle, from which the large perforating vessels come and in which they are situated (Figs. 2.5 and 2.6). The thickness of the lamellar layer progressively decreases in the lateral regions of the abdomen (Figs. 2.7 and 2.8). When the

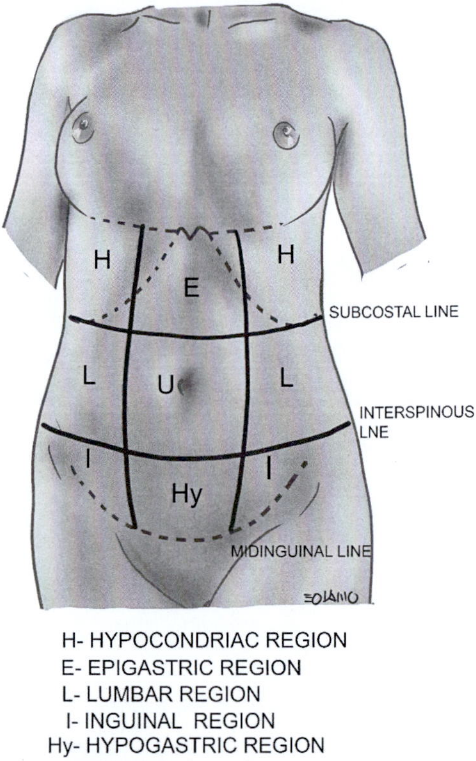

Fig. 2.5 The anterior abdominal is divided into nine regions: three odd (epigastric, umbilical, and hypogastric; six even: hypochondriac, lumbar, and inguinal)

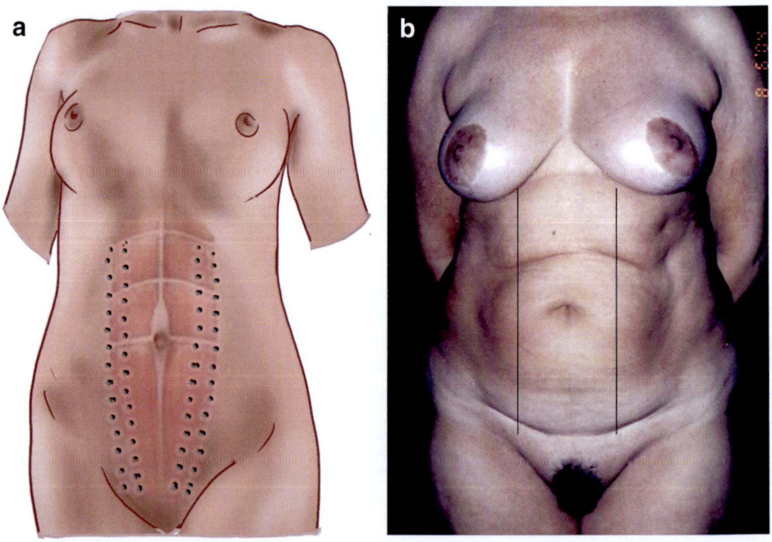

Fig. 2.6 Location of the perforator vessels on abdominal wall coming from rectus abdominalis muscle (RAM). (**a**) Diagram showing the perforator vessels coming from the rectus abdominalis; (**b**) photo of a patient with projection of the perforator vessels where the areolar layer is thick which is adequate to perform insulin injections using short needle

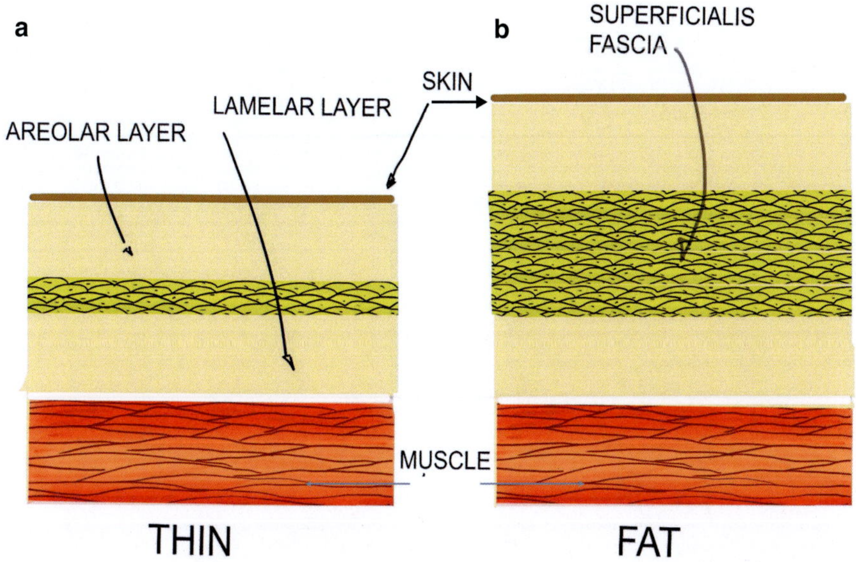

Fig. 2.7 Schemas showing a comparison between the layers of the abdominal panniculus of a thin person and another with localized adiposity. (**a**) A thin person presents a compact fascia superficialis separating the areolar layer and lamellar one; (**b**) on a person with localized adiposity presents a thick fascia superficialis due to localized adiposity which divides into several layers

lamellar layer is thick, the panniculus firmly adheres to the muscular level underneath, which can also be observed through the Illouz's "pinch test" (Illouz 1983a) (Fig. 2.3). However, in regions with a thin lamellar layer, the panniculus easily slides over the abdominal musculature (Fig. 2.7). On the other hand, the lateral regions on the right and the left (Fig. 2.5) do not present significant anatomical variations; rather, the areolar and lamellar layers show regular thickness, even in fat people. Once again, the fascia superficialis shows firm structures separating both layers. It shows several layers that make a network with vessels passing between them (Figs. 2.4, 2.7, and 2.8). And it is very rare in some people with localized adiposity (Avelar 1986a, 1987, 1989).

When liposuction is correctly performed, the areolar layer maintains the same thickness because the operation must be performed on the lamellar layer. The final result for patients is a lamellar layer devoid of adipose tissue. The cicatricial tissue is developed in the lamellar layer, making a very hard fibrotic tissue. The behavior of the subcutaneous tissue is shown by the thick layer of cicatricial tissue (Fig. 2.2c). Also, the perforating vessels are not damaged by the cannula during liposuction (Figs. 2.4 and 2.9). The areolar layer must be totally preserved. If it is damaged it may develop similar fibrotic tissue after liposuction resulting some ungraceful irregularities below the skin producing waves on the surface of the skin covering.

Such fibrotic tissue makes a strong and thick layer, which makes a secondary liposuction on the same region difficult and dangerous to perform. It is possible to do but should be done carefully because the hard thickness of the cicatricial tissue

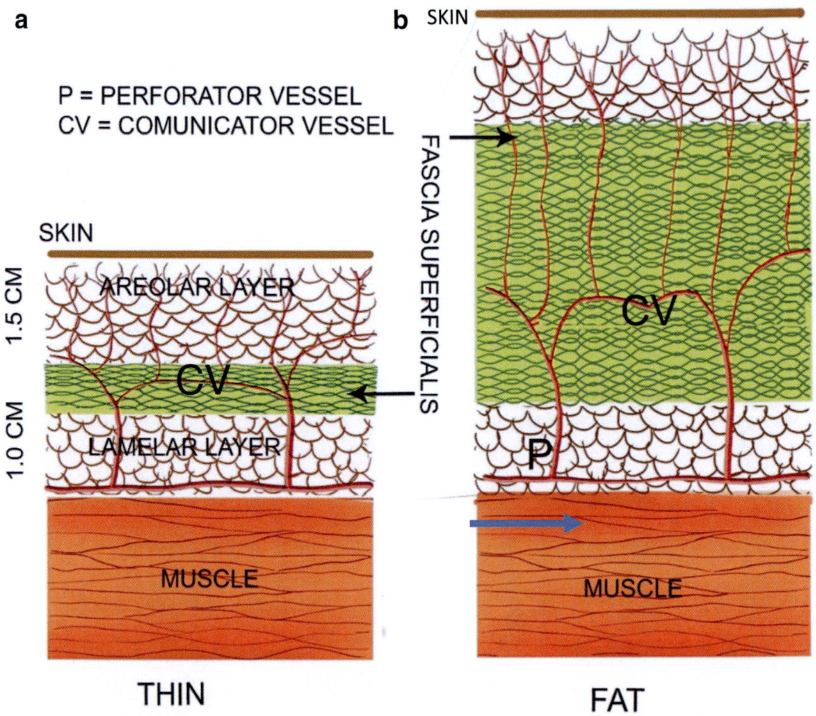

Fig. 2.8 Diagrams showing a comparison of the vascularization of the abdominal panniculus between a thin person and another with localized adiposity. (**a**) A thin person presents a compact fascia superficialis separating the areolar layer and lamellar one; (**b**) on a person with localized adiposity presents a thick fascia superficialis due to localized adiposity which divides into several layers: *P* perforator vessels coming from muscle; *CV* communicating vessels which work similar to a "peripheric heart" to supply smooth vascularization to areolar and subdermal layers as well as to dermis as well

does not allow the cannula to cross through it (Fig. 2.2c) and because the second stage may damage the areolar layer, producing irregularities on the skin surface.

Therefore, liposuction should be performed on the deep layer (lamellar), maintaining the regular and harmonious thickness of the areolar layer and thus preserving the perforator vessels (Figs. 2.9, 2.10, and 2.11). The final result shows the relief of the abdominal musculature through the cutaneous panniculus, which indicates a natural and elegant body contouring.

Besides anatomic knowledge, knowing the difference between fat tissues is crucial to performing liposuction, even when some kind of injection is carried out inside each layer. Because of the sophisticated vascularization of the panniculus, insulin injection with short, thin needles as a treatment for diabetes must be performed inside the areolar layer; otherwise, the constitution of the fat tissue may absorb the medical product. Even when using very thin needle, if the injection is performed inside the lamellar layer of any other region of the body with a minimal areolar layer, the abortion of insulin is not absorbed. Such a phenomenon is due to

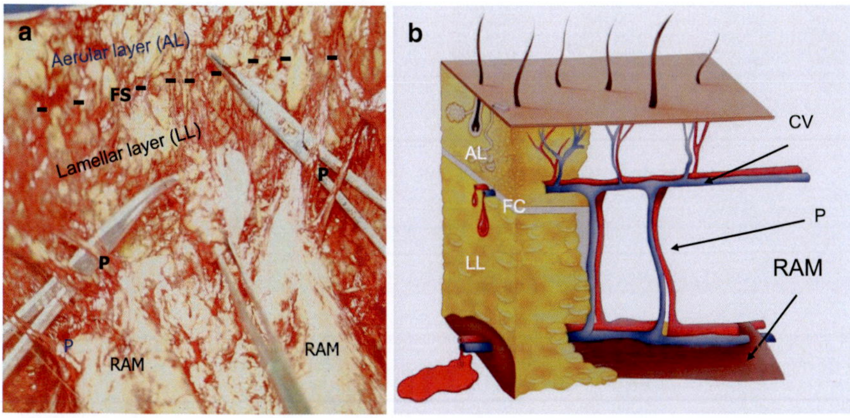

Fig. 2.9 Surgical principles on anatomic structures of the abdominal panniculus. Photo (**a**) the panniculus of a patient who underwent liposuction 6 months before to perform conventional abdominoplasty showing preservation of the perforator vessels (P) indicated by forceps, fascia superficialis (FS) between areolar layer (AL) and lamellar layer (LL), rectus abdominalis (RAM); (**b**) scheme of the panniculus: fascia superficialis (FS) and the communicated vessels (CV) which work similar to a "peripheric heart" creating an arch between the perforator vessels (P) from where small vessels go perpendicularly through the areolar layer (AL) to vascularize the cutaneous and subdermal layers. The lamellar layer (LL) is placed between the rectus abdominalis muscle (RAM) and fascia superficialis (F) where is the correct level to perform liposuction technique

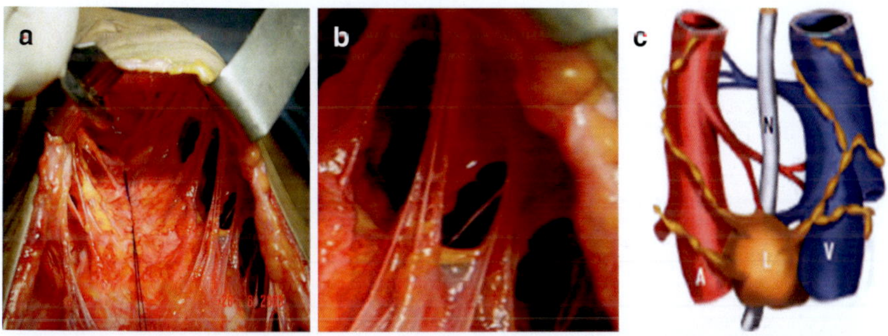

Fig. 2.10 Constitution of an anatomic unit of a neuro-vascular pedicle of a perforator vessel. Photos (**a**) internal perioperative view from the abdominal panniculus after liposuction procedure performed on lamellar layer showing the preserved perforator vessels coming from rectus abdominalis bilaterally; (**b**) photo in close up that one can see the perforator vessels; (**c**) schema showing the neuro-vascular structures of the pedicle formed by: *A* artery, *V* vein, *N* nerves, *L* lymphatics

the type of adipose tissue in the areolar layer, which has round and turgid fat cells, as described previously (Avelar 1986a, b, c, 1989) (Figs. 2.2b, 2.3b, and 2.4a). Such an observation is crucial because the areolar layer of the abdominal wall is the preferable region for injecting insulin, and it must be carried out inside this layer (Figs. 2.4a, 2.6b, and 2.12).

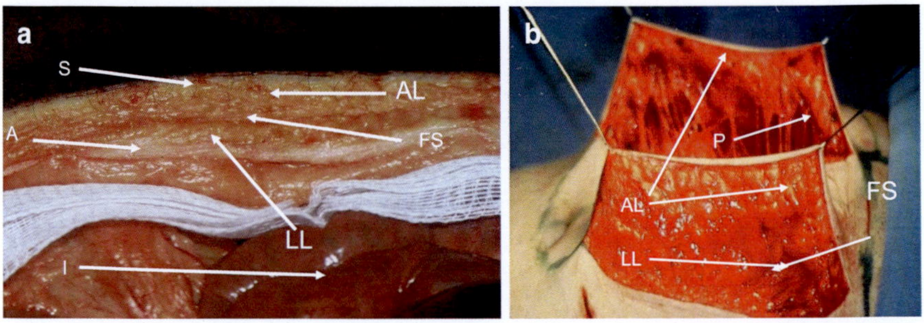

Fig. 2.11 Anatomical study in cadavers to show relationship of the subcutaneous panniculus layers in the abdominal wall. Photo (**a**) the whole panniculus was sectioned where one can see all layers and internal viscera in the abdominal cavity of a cadaver without localized adiposity: skin (S), areolar layer (AL), fascia superficialis (FS), lamellar layer (LL) muscular-aponeurosis of the abdomen (A), internal viscera (I); (**b**) photo of a fresh cadaver after liposuction performed on left side of the abdomen and the whole thickness of the panniculus on right side without liposuction. On left side of the abdomen the perforator vessels (P) and areolar layer were preserved. On right side one can see the areolar layer (AL), fascia superficialis (FS) as well as the lamellar layer (LL) with perforator vessels included. The panniculus of both side is pulled by two hooks

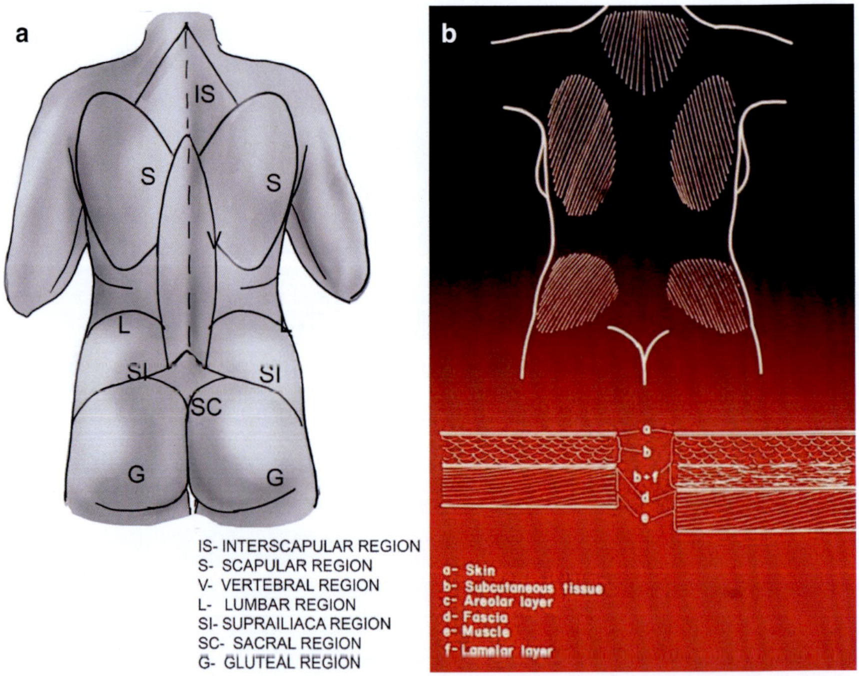

Fig. 2.12 Diagram demonstrating the correct injection of insulin in areolar layer (between skin and fascia superficialis)

Because I am diabetic, two unusual situations have happened to me from the injection of insulin. Once, I rapidly developed severe hypoglycemia symptoms immediately after I injected insulin into the subcutaneous level of my abdomen. I concluded that the tip of the needle damaged some small vessels during injection and that the insulin was absorbed in an erratic way. Because I was at home, I ingested several units of sugar to treat the symptoms. My physician agreed with me about the possibility of accidental damage to the vessels, but such an abnormal occurrence is extremely rare. Another complex situation happened despite three regular daily injections of insulin: my glycemia level progressively became too elevated. Although I injected higher and higher doses of insulin, the level of glycemia was out of control. I concluded that the injections were inserted into a lamellar layer, where small vessels are in a lower proportion of adipose tissue, so the insulin was not regularly absorbed. Afterward, I was assured that the injections were inserted into my abdominal panniculus, inside the areolar layer, and after four days, the glycemia level normalized. Therefore, the anatomy of the panniculus is also important because such injections must be carried out within the areolar layer in order for the absorption to occur normally.

Posterior Regions of the Trunk

The posterior regions of the torso are as follows: three odd, namely interscapular (IS), vertebral (V), and sacral (SC), and three even, namely scapular (S), lumbar (L), and suprailiac (SI) (Fig. 2.13a). Also, the regions that most frequently present localized adiposities can be identified to prove that adiposity occurs inside the fascia superficialis (Fig. 2.13b).

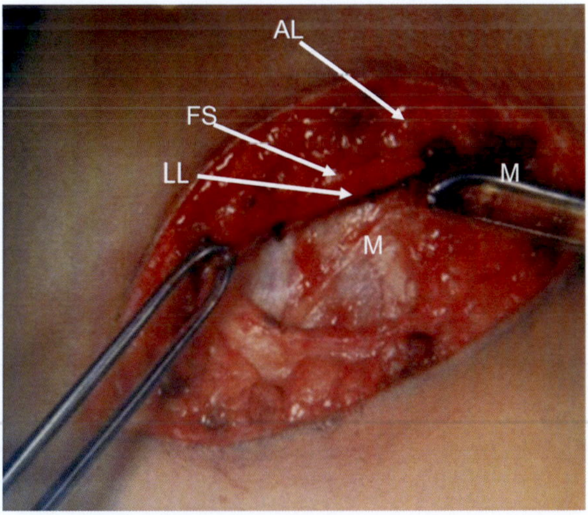

Fig. 2.13 Regions of the torso. Diagram (**a**) one can see the three odd regions: interscapular (IS), vertebral (V), and sacral (SC) and three even regions: scapular (S), lumbar (L) and suprailiac regions (SI); (**b**) shows the most frequent regions presenting localized adiposities, inside the fascia superficialis

All the regions of the posterior aspect of the trunk feature the ideal anatomical constitution to perform liposuction on localized adiposities. Usually, the areolar layer is very thick and the fascia superficialis is quite close to the muscular aponeurotic level, but not in those regions with localized adiposities in the lamellar layer, whose distribution is quite similar to that in abdominal walls (Figs. 2.4a, 2.6b, and 2.13b).

There are some relationships between the anterior regions of the abdominal wall and some between the posterior ones (Avelar 1989). Therefore, plastic surgeons must examine the torso every time a patient complains about any problem in the abdominal wall. The abdomen must be also evaluated when the problem is in the torso (Figs. 2.5, 2.6, and 2.13).

All the regions of the posterior aspect of the trunk present a similar constitution in both cutaneous and subcutaneous tissue. Thin people show a thick and firm areolar layer, and the lamellar layer is also thin. Patients presenting localized adiposity show a noticeable growth in the lamellar layer, which is responsible for the alterations in unaesthetic shapes requiring liposuction for their remodeling (Figs. 2.6b and 2.13b).

In all regions of the torso, the panniculus is very thick, but it is not uniform, because each one presents peculiarities on which liposuction can be performed. The final results may present outstanding surgical contouring, providing a smooth appearance when the selection of patients and adequate indications are performed preoperatively. Some regions present external alterations—for example, the lamellar layer has shown increased thickness in cases of localized adiposity (Fig. 2.13b).

On one hand, some areas of the torso, such as the lumbar region, seldom show the accumulation of adiposity because the lamellar layer does not present anatomical characteristics for those abnormalities. On the other, the suprailiac regions may present the accumulation of localized adiposities, which are good indications for requiring remodeling via liposuction (Fig. 2.13b). The scapular regions of the torso may present accumulations of adipose tissues in the lamellar layer, which may help reshape the body's contouring (Fig. 2.13a, b). The areolar layer shows peculiar regularity without any alterations in thickness.

The interscapular region is another area that may present localized adiposities on lamellar layer which may achieve smooth surgical result ever since deep liposuction is performed (Fig. 2.13a, b). The regions on the anterior aspect of the chest present panniculus constitutions similar to those of the posterior ones: The lamellar layer is very thin, and the fascia superficialis is quite close to the muscular level, presenting the thick areolar layer (Fig. 2.14).

During examination, the surgeon should identify that when the lamellar layer shows localized adiposity, the subcutaneous panniculus does not slide over the muscular plane.

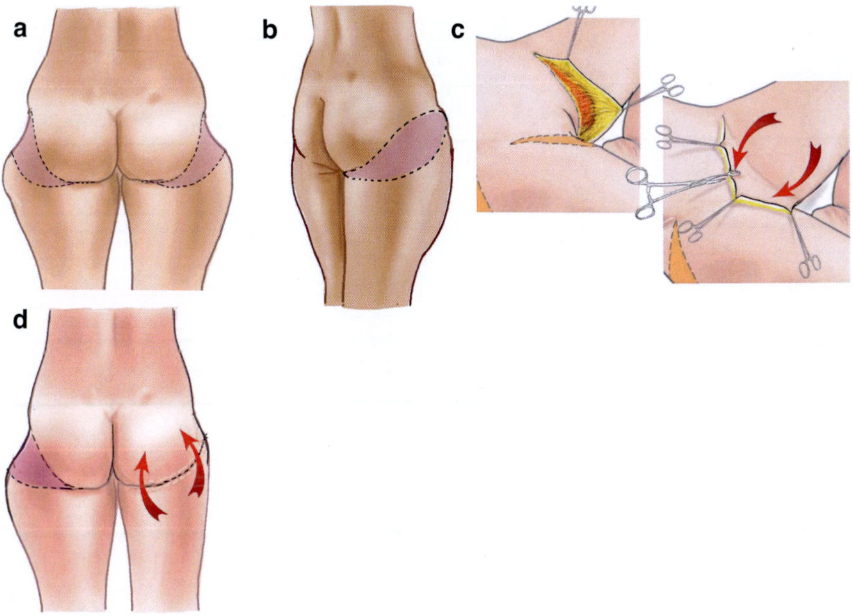

Fig. 2.14 Photo during surgery showing the subcutaneous panniculus of the chest wall. Areolar layer (AL) is the full thickness of the panniculus, since the lamellar layer (LL) is very thin associated with fascia superficialis (FS) which slides easily on the muscles (M) underneath. One can see the fascia superficialis (F) is held with a forceps

The Trochanteric and Gluteal Regions

Trochanteric lipodystrophy and gluteal lipodystrophy used to be treated through panniculus resection via the vertical approach (Farina et al. 1960). Later, Pitanguy introduced new techniques via incisions after remodeling the gluteal sulcus in both the trochanteric region and the gluteal region (Pitanguy 1964, 1977). By using this technique, the gluteal and trochanteric regions can be reshaped, but the final result leaves a long scar on the subgluteal fold and the inguinal sulcus (Fig. 2.15). Later, a new era of liposuction was introduced by Illouz (1980, 1983a, b, 1984), leaving only inconspicuous scars while improving body contouring (Fig. 2.16).

Deformities in the trochanteric and gluteal regions are usually localized to the subcutaneous cellular compartment with inelegant shapes in the lower segment of the body. Usually, people without localized adiposity show a good proportion and a good relationship between the areolar and lamellar layers. So far, heavier patients without localized adiposity in this region show a proportional augmentation in both layers, keeping well-balanced shapes in the body contours. However, localized adiposity may be caused by the excessive augmentation of the lamellar layer, which

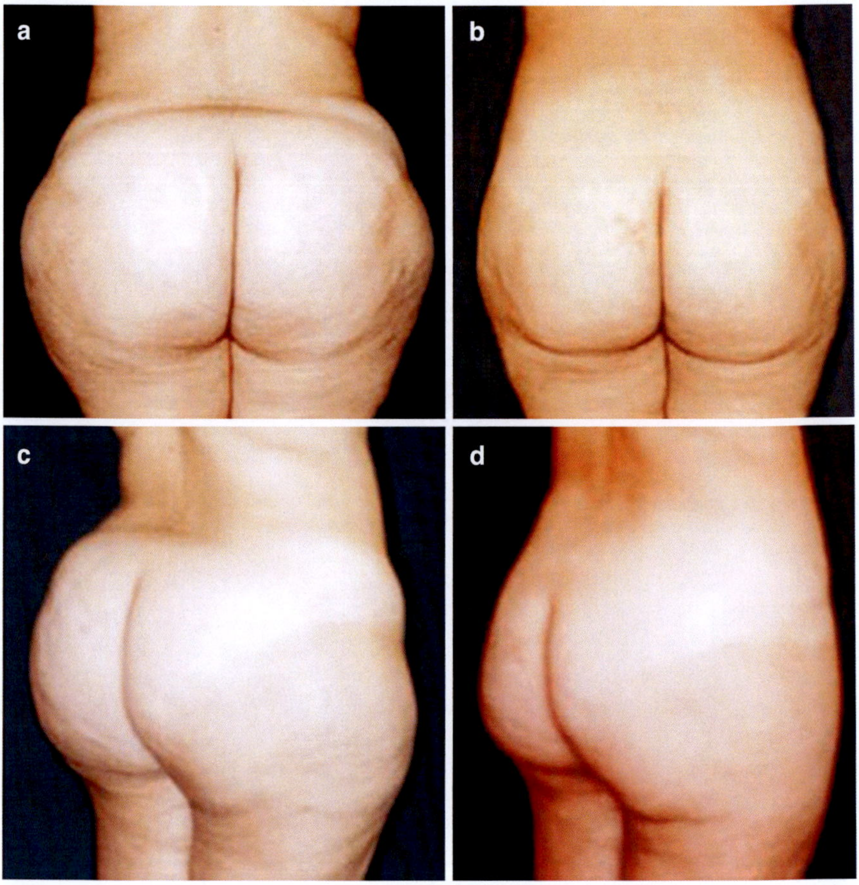

Fig. 2.15 Diagrams showing trochanteric lipodystrophy combined with dysmorphy of the gluteal regions remodelling by Pitanguy's technique. (**a**) Posterior view with asymmetric deformities with surgical demarcations of the technique; (**b**) oblique view showing the incision extending anteriorly; (**c**) demarcation goes to the upper internal thigh for correction of typical deformities; (**d**) after suture on right side showing advancement of lower flap indicated by arrows

can be much thicker than that in people without localized adiposity, while the areolar layer presents few alterations in its thickness. Ever since the introduction of liposuction, it has been performed in such a way as to achieve harmonious surgical results (Fig. 2.16). Nowadays, a combination of it with fat grafting is an excellent approach to reshaping the trochanteric gluteal regions when carried out according to specific deformities and with adequate surgical planning.

A clinical examination should be carefully carried out to evaluate each region that shows an abnormal accumulation of adipose tissue. All the data from physical examinations are useful for elaborating surgical planning before performing any operations. Each surgeon must follow their own orientation to prepare their surgical planning, which is essential before performing any operations.

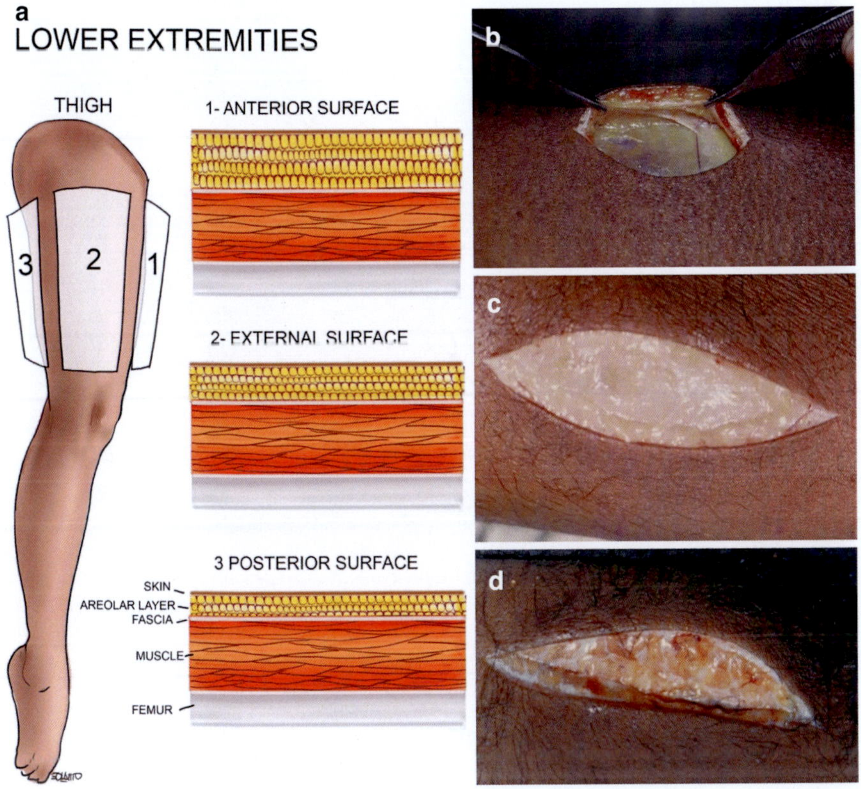

Fig. 2.16 Unaesthetic deformities of the buttocks and trochanteric regions due to accumulation of adiposities treated by liposuction procedure. Photos (**a, c**) preoperative showing ungraceful appearance due to extensive trochanteric lipodystrophy; (**b, d**) post-operative view after isolated liposuction remodelling gluteal trochanteric lipodystrophy

Lower Extremities

In Testut's classic *Treatise on Human Anatomy* (1975, 1984), the thigh has been divided into two surfaces: anterior and posterior. Now that I have performed anatomical research, I consider dividing it into four surfaces—namely anterior, posterior, external, and internal—more convenient because each of them presents peculiar histological characteristics (Fig. 2.17a). The anterior surface of the thigh is an extensive and regular region because the panniculus has a thick areolar layer and thin lamellar one. The fascia superficialis is underneath the areolar layer and immediately above the aponeurosis. The panniculus slides over the muscular level because the cutaneous and subcutaneous layers are regular and quite near the muscles. Therefore, this region does not often undergo liposuction, because if the areolar layer were damaged, it might develop severe irregularities on the cutaneous surface

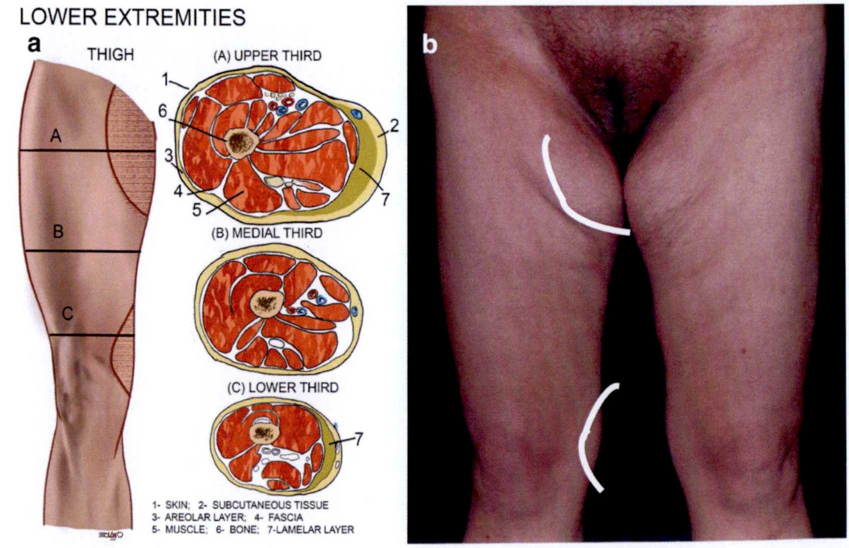

Fig. 2.17 Anatomic constitution and variation of thickness of the panniculus in the three surfaces of the thigh. (**a**) Scheme shows the situation on three surfaces: (*1*) anterior, (*2*) external, (*3*) posterior. (**b–d**) Photos show cutaneous incisions on the thigh where one can see the panniculus of a cadaver with variation of the thickness on the anterior, external, and posterior surfaces. (**b**) The forceps hold the fascia superficialis and one can see that the lamellar layer is very thin and close to muscles underneath. (**c**) The external surface of the thigh where areolar layer, fascia superficialis, and lamellar layer make a compact structure. (**d**) The posterior surface of the thigh where areolar layer is quite thick, the fascia superficialis and lamellar layer make a compact structure

(Fig. 2.17b). The external surface of the thigh has some similarity to the anterior one, but the areolar layer is thinner and the lamellar layer does not exist or is too thin to observe. The fascia superficialis is between the areolar and the aponeurosis. For this reason, the panniculus slides on the muscular level (Fig. 2.17c). Also, the posterior surface has the same anatomical and histological distribution as the anterior surface (Fig. 2.17d). Therefore, liposuction is not a good technique to be performed on those regions.

On another hand, the internal surface of the thigh can be divided into three segments: superior, middle, and inferior. The upper third has very thin skin and a soft and thin areolar layer. The lamellar layer is present even in thin patients. One can estimate the lamellar layer because it contains adiposities (Fig. 2.18). Therefore, this region quite often undergoes liposuction. Also, excess skin from the upper internal thigh is removed according to the technique proposed by Pitanguy (1964, 1977) (Fig. 2.15a, c). Some years later, other procedures were described that confer smooth contouring to internal thigh (Avelar 1996, 1999b).

When the lower third of the thigh presents localized adiposity, that is an adequate indication for liposuction (Fig. 2.18). So far, it has not been adequate to

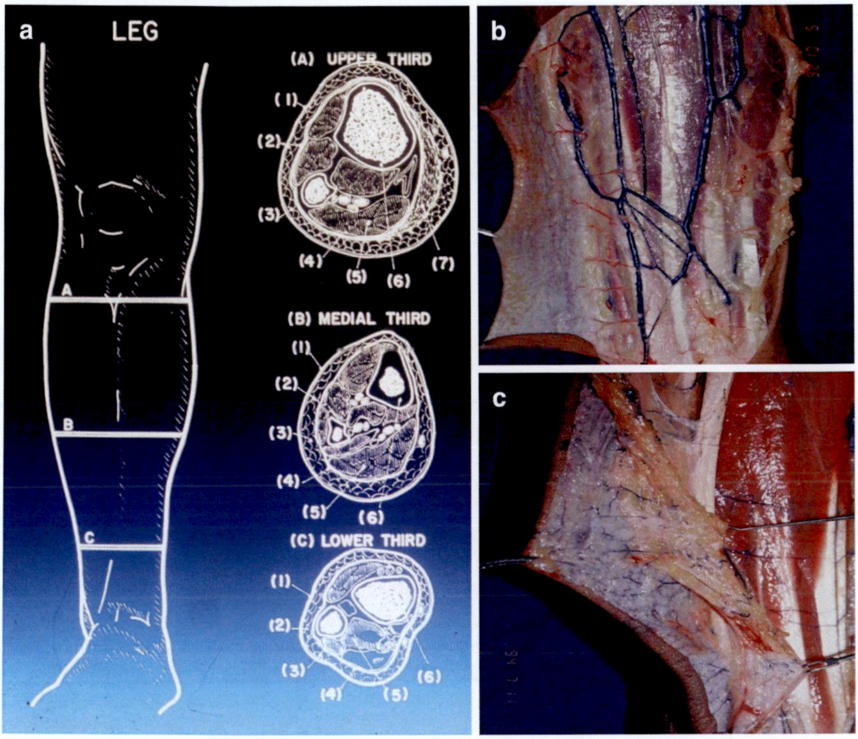

Fig. 2.18 Diagram and photo of the localized adiposities on lower extremity. (**a**) Scheme showing internal surface of the thigh. The upper and lower third present thick lamellar layer as is demonstrated in sections A and C, since section B shows the middle third which presents insignificant thickness of lamellar layer; (**b**) photo of a female patient presenting localized adiposities indicated by white lines on upper and lower third of internal thigh

perform this procedure on the medial third of the internal thigh in absence of the accumulation of adipose tissue, because in this scenario, the lamellar layer is very thin.

Legs

The legs are the segments of the lower extremities that normally do not present localized adiposity in that the areolar and lamellar layers are normally quite thin (Fig. 2.19a). Consequently, it is quite unusual to perform liposuction on these segments. The anatomy presents fascia superficialis with a rich network of arterial, venous, and lymphatic vascularization (Fig. 2.19b, c).

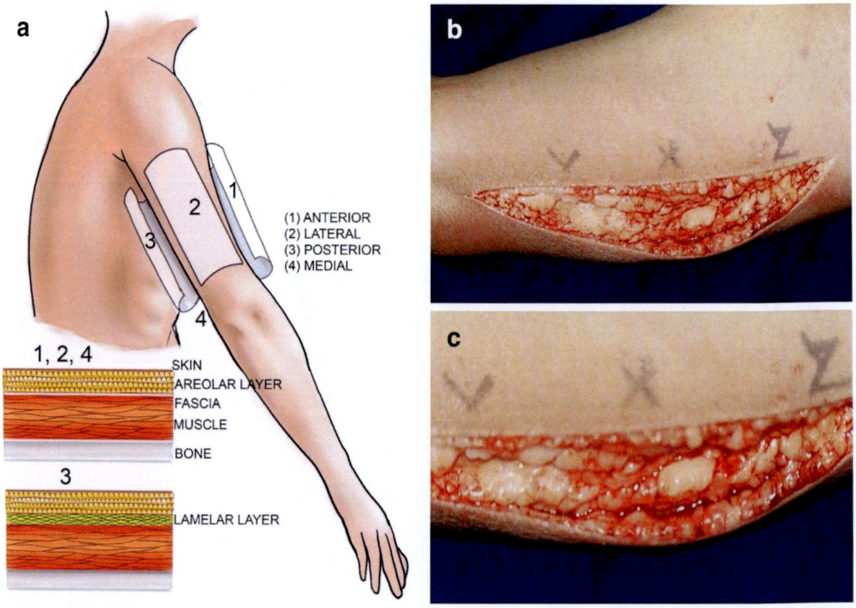

Fig. 2.19 Diagram and anatomic dissections on cadaver's photos of the right leg. In the diagram (**a**) shows the cutaneous and subcutaneous layers in three levels: upper, medial, and lower; (**b**) the skin of the leg was incised and undermined just above the fascia superficialis which lies on the muscles; (**c**) the fascia superficialis is rotated laterally to show the muscles underneath

Upper Extremities

Arms

The posterior surface of the upper arm is the only one that is a candidate for liposuction because it contains a thick lamellar layer. Testut's book (1982) divides the arm into anterior and posterior sections. After performing anatomical dissections, I suggested dividing it into four surfaces—anterior, external, internal, and posterior (Fig. 2.20a)—because each one has specific anatomical characteristics in its panniculus. The posterior surface of the arm should be considered because it may contain thick lamellar and areolar layers in patients with localized adiposities (Fig. 2.20b, c). So far, both layers are quite thin in people without localized adiposities. Nevertheless, patients with such abnormalities may present enough accumulation of fat for liposuction, even for a resection of the panniculus, especially after severe weight loss.

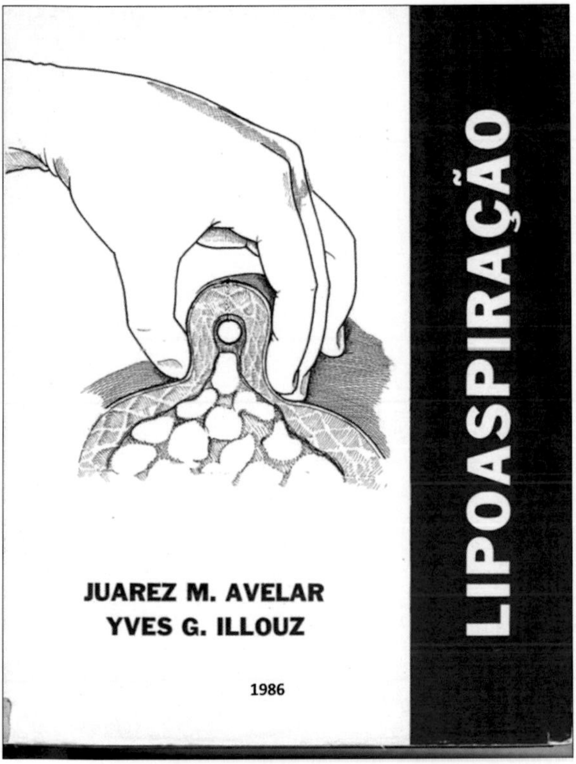

Fig. 2.20 Anatomical study showing the constitution and variation of thickness of the panniculus in the four surfaces of the arm. (**a**) Scheme shows the situation on the four surfaces: (*1*) anterior, (*2*) external and four internal present thin thickness of lamellar layer with very thin fascia superficialis, (*3*) the posterior surface present very thick thickness of the lamellar where usually may present accumulation of fat; photos (**b, c**) of a fresh cadaver showing cutaneous incision on the posterior surface (*3*) of the arm where one can see the panniculus with accumulated fat on lamellar layer. It is marked with black ink on the skin (V, X, and Z) three levels of circumferences of the arm as references study. It demonstrates that usually the posterior surface of the arm is the most common surface to present a localized adiposity

Discussion

According to the anatomic dissections that I performed on cadavers, the subcutaneous tissue in patients with localized adiposity clearly varies depending on the region (Figs. 2.5, 2.6, and 2.13). The lamellar layer increases in thickness thanks to the accumulated adipose tissue. The areolar layer does not change in thickness as much as the lamellar one does (Figs. 2.2, 2.7, and 2.8). With Illouz's "pinch test" (Illouz 1983a, b, c, 1986), the thickness of the panniculus and that of a thick lamellar layer can be estimated (Fig. 2.3). When the panniculus slides over the aponeurotic layer, there are no localized adiposities and the perforator vessels are very thin. When this layer is thick, the panniculus does not slide, because of the numerous perforating vessels (Fig. 2.8).

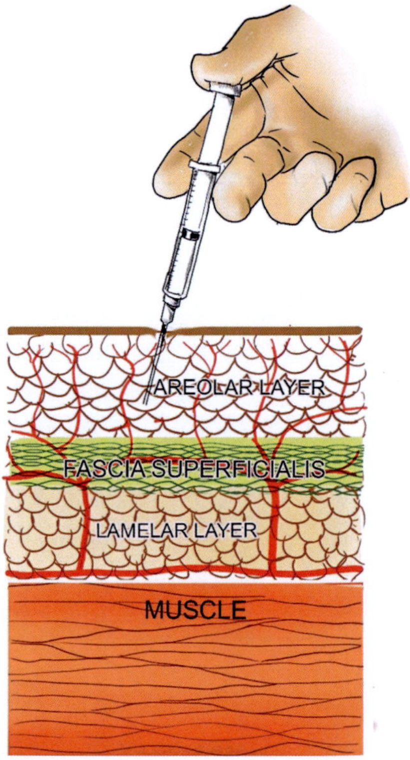

Fig. 2.21 Cover of our book (LIPOSUCTION) published in São Paulo (Brazil) with didactic information about the position of surgeon's left hand with the cannula between his fingers without damaging the areolar layer

Classic anatomy does not describe in detail the subcutaneous tissue over the entire human body. Because the canula of liposuction technique works on subcutaneous tissue, as soon as I started to perform the new method in 1983, I felt it necessity to study such compartments in human body. Thus, I performed a considerable number of anatomic dissections and liposuctions on cadavers to study the thickness and distribution of the adipose tissue in every region while performing the new technique (Figs. 2.1, 2.2, 2.3, and 2.11). The tissue's characteristics vary widely from one region to another. Even each region may vary from person to person, depending on the degree of nutrition.

After I performed this anatomical research, I was able to gain specific knowledge on superficial body contouring, which gave me enough information to create the cover of our book, published in association with Prof. Illouz in 1986 (*Liposuction*, edited by Avelar and Illouz) (Fig. 2.21). On the cover, my left hand is holding the abdominal panniculus with a cannula between my fingers to demonstrate the level that the main surgical instrument should be at during a liposuction procedure.

In my previous publications (Avelar 1986a, 1987, 1989), I reached some conclusions, which I repeat here:

1. The areolar layer is more resistant, and it is responsible for the terminal vascularization of the skin (Fig. 2.4a).
2. Daily injections of insulin must be carried out in the areolar layer because fat cells are round, large, and full of fatty liquid inside and because it is well vascularized (Figs. 2.3b and 2.11).

3. The lamellar layer contains a large number of connective tissue layers that form "bridges" through which larger vessels pass, giving softness to the tissues (Figs. 2.4a, 2.8, and 2.10).
4. The regular thickness of the areolar layer must be preserved (Figs. 2.1, 2.2, and 2.3) because traumatism during the liposuction of the local tissue causes cutaneous depressions.
5. The lamellar layer is the region that can be aspirated. The larger vessels do not suffer the local effects caused by the traumatism of the cannula (Figs. 2.4a and 2.9a).
6. In the regions featuring thin skin, the cannula can be used superficially if regularity is maintained (Fig. 2.13).

In the regions featuring thick and firm skin, liposuction has to go deeper, leaving more thickness in the dermal-fat flap (Fig. 2.18).

Conclusions

The distribution and characteristics of fat tissue in the subcutaneous layer have been described after intensive research via dissection and liposuction on cadavers. Each region of the surface of human body has a specific anatomic composition that is vital in body-contouring surgery (Figs. 2.5, 2.6, and 2.13). There are differences between the areolar and lamellar layers, and each layer has specific anatomic characteristics (Figs. 2.7 and 2.8). The areolar one is formed by large, round, and turgid cells that are piled together where small vessels pass to irrigate the subdermal layer and the deep aspect of the skin (Figs. 2.4a, 2.8, and 2.9a). To identify localized adiposities, careful examinations, careful patient selections, and region-specific evaluations for treatment options are recommended before surgery. The behavior of the subcutaneous tissue after surgery shows that it develops a thick and hard fibrosis, indicating that liposuction should be performed on the lamellar layer when the accumulation of adipose tissue occurs (Fig. 2.2). This sort of fibrotic tissue on the areolar layer will cause irregularities and unsightly waves on the skin's surface.

References

Avelar JM (1983) Submentonean and Submandibular Adiposity – Liposuction X Lipectomy (Adiposidade Submentoniana e Submandibular – Lipoaspiração X Lipectomia). In: Annals of the Brazilian Symposium on Facial Contouring, organized by Dr. Juarez Avelar, Sponsored by Brazilian Society of Plastic Surgery (Section of São Paulo), September pag. 69–72

Avelar JM (1985a) - Fat-suction versus abdominoplasty. Aesth Plast Surg 9:265–276, 1985.

Avelar JM (1985b) - Combined liposuction with traditional surgery in abdomen lipodystrophy. XXIV Instructional Course of Aesthetic Plastic Surgery of the ISAPS. Madrid, September 19.

Avelar JM (1986a) - Surgical Anatomy and Distribution of Adipose Tissue on Human Body (Anatomia cirúrgica e distribuição do tecido celular no organismo humano). In: Liposuction (Lipoaspiração), ed. by Avelar and Illouz, Ed. Hipócrates, São Paulo (Brazil) 9:45–57.

Avelar JM (1986b) Liposuction of Abdominal Wall (Lipoaspiração da Parede Abdominal). In Liposuction (Lipoaspiração). Ed. by Avelar JM. & Illouz YG. Sao Paulo (Brasil). Editora Hipócrates 27:158–176.
Avelar JM (1986c) Liposuction of the Submental and Submandibular Regions (Lipoaspiração das Regiões Submentoniana e Submandibular). In Liposuction (Lipoaspiração). Ed. by AvelarJM. & Illouz YG. Sao Paulo (Brasil). Editora Hipócrates 24:139–147.
Avelar JM (1987) - Study of the anatomy of the subcutaneous adipose tissue applied for fat-suction technique. In: Maneksha RJ (ed): Trans IX Int Congr Plast Reconstr Surg. New Delhi, India, March 1–6, pp 377–379.
Avelar JM (1989) Regional distribution and behavior of the subcutaneous tissue concerning selection and indication for liposuction. Aesth Plast Surg 13:155–165.
Avelar JM (1996) Creation of a Natural and Definitive Inguino-Crural Crease During Lifting of the Upper Medial Thigh (Criação de Natural e Definitivo Sulco Inguino-Crural no Lifting da Face interna da Coxa). Rev Bras Cirug 86(5):213–228
Avelar JM (1999a) A new technique for abdominoplasty – closed vascular system of subdermal flap folded over itself combined to Liposuction. (Uma nova técnica de abdominoplastia – sistema vascular fechado de retalho subdérmico dobrado sobre si mesmo combinado com lipoaspiração). Rev Bras Cir 88/89(1/6):3–20.
Avelar JM (1999b) Aesthetic plastic in the inner side of the thigh – new concepts and technique without cutaneous or subcutaneous undermining. (Cirurgia Plástica de Face Interna de Coxas – novos conceitos e tecnica sem descolamento cutâneo e subcutâneo). Rev Bras Cir 88/89(1/6):57–67.
Farina R., Baroudi R., Coleman B., & Castro O. (1960) Riding trousersilke type of pelvicrual lipodistrophy (trochanteric lipomatosis). Brit. J. Plast. Surg. XIII(2): July.
Gray H (1974) - Anatomy, descriptive and surgical. Philadelphia: Running Press.
Illouz YG (1980) Une nouvelle technique pour les lipodystrophies localisées. Rev Cir Esth Franc 6(9)
Illouz YG (1983a) Liposuction - My technique and applications. First Course of Liposuction. Organized by Dr. Juarez M. Avelar, heled at São Paulo Hospital, Service of Prof. Andrews at Escola Paulista de Medicina. Sponsored By Brazilian Society of Plastic Surgery (São Paulo Section) October São Paulo (Brazil).
Illouz YG (1983b) - My technique of suction lipectomy. Meeting of the American Society of Aesthetic and Plastic Surgeons and Instructional Course, April
Illouz YG (1983c) Body contouring by lipolysis: 5 years' experience with over 3,000 cases. Plast Reconstr Surg 72(5):591–597
Illouz YG (1984) – My technique of Liposuction – 4 Years Evolution. Second Course of Liposuction. Heled at 9 de Julho Hospital. Organized by Juarez M. Avelar, Sponsored By Brazilian Society of Plastic Surgery. September, São Paulo (Brazil).
Illouz YG (1986) - Basic principles of liposuction technique (Princípios básicos da técnica de lipoaspiração). In Lipoaspiração (Liposuction), ed. by Avelar and Illouz, Ed. Hipócrates, São Paulo (Brazil) 3:13–18
Lockwood T (1995) High lateral-tension abdominoplasty with superfi cial fascial system suspension. Plast Reconstr Surg 96:603–615.
Pitanguy I (1964) - Trochanteric lipodystrophy. Plast Re-const Surg 34:280, 1964
Pitanguy I (1977) – Dermolipectomy of the Abdominal Wall, Thighs, Buttocks, and Upper Extremity. In Plastic and Reconstructive Surgery, Ed. by Converse JM, Ed. W. B.Saunders Company – Philadelphia and London, 92:3800-3823.
Sobotta, Figge (1977) Atlas of human anatomy. Baltimore: Urban & Schwarzenber.
Spalteholz W (1970) - Atlas de anatomia humana, (Atlas of Human Anatomy) 5th ed. Espanha: Editora Labor.
Testut L, Jacob O (1975) - Tratado de Anatomia Topográfica. (Compedia of Topografic Anatomy) Barcelona, – Madrid, Bogota, Buenos Airees, Rio de Janeiro.: Salvat Editores, 1975
Testut L, Jacob O (1984) - Tratado de Anatomia Topográfica. Salvat Editores. Barcelona, Madrid, Bogota, Buenos Airees, Rio de Janeiro. 1984.

Chapter 3
Importance and Behavior of Fascia Superficialis for Body-Couturing Surgery

Juarez Moraes Avelar

Abstracts The human body contains the fascia superficialis, which is between the skin and muscular or bony level in almost all the body's regions, with peculiar characteristics in each one. The anatomy and behavior of the fascia superficialis are so important that it may be considered as a "second skin" because it is present in mostly regions, providing adequate vascularization to the dermis and to the subdermal layer. Anatomically, the fascia superficialis is a very thin structure containing connective tissue in several layers, with vessels between them. This anatomical structure is between the skin and the muscular plane at one of two levels: (1) In some regions, it is in the middle of the subcutaneous structures, and (2) in other regions, it is near the muscle or bone level.

1. The fascia superficialis is in the middle of the subcutaneous panniculus structures. The main anatomical characteristic is that it may present localized adiposities only in some regions: the abdominal walls, the upper and lower third of the medial thigh, the posterior side of the arms, the gluteal regions, the suprailiac regions, and all regions of the posterior aspects of the torso. When the panniculus is incised during an operation, in those regions, it is necessary to suture the fascia superficialis to reinstate the subcutaneous layers. If it is not correctly sutured, the anatomical structure will be damaged, which may develop unaesthetic surgical scarring with retraction and contraction.
2. The fascia superficialis close to the muscle or bone level. It may occur in most of the regions of the upper and lower extremities and underneath the scalp. The fascia superficialis on the scalp has a peculiar anatomical composition in that the vessels (arteries, veins, and lymphatics) connect a wide network similar to those between the areolar and lamellar layers on the abdominal wall. In cranial regions, the fascia superficialis is an important anatomical structure that I created tempo-

J. M. Avelar (✉)
Brazilian Scientific Institute of Plastic and Reconstructive Surgery, São Paulo, Brazil

J. M. Avelar, R. Cavalcanti Ribeiro (eds.), *Body Contouring*,
https://doi.org/10.1007/978-3-031-42802-9_3

roparietal fascial flaps for, to improve ear reconstruction they are excellent and useful surgical resource options for craniofacial surgery.

Keywords Fascia · Fascia superficialis · Antomical structure

Introduction

In almost all regions of the human body, there is a fascia superficialis, and each one exhibits a peculiar distribution. The fascia superficialis is formed through connective tissue in multiple layers through which run the arterial, venous, and lymphatic vessels. Owing to its constant presence, it may be considered as a second skin because it is present in almost all regions, providing adequate vascularization to the dermis and the subdermal layer. In the traditional textbooks on anatomy, such as those by Testut and Jacob (1975, 1984), Gray (1974), Spalteholz (1970), and Sobotta (1977), there is little information on the subcutaneous panniculus and few words concerning the fascia superficialis. Anatomically, the fascia superficialis is a very thin connective tissue structure in several layers with vessels between them. This anatomical structure is between the skin and the muscular or bone planes at one of two levels: (1) In some regions, the fascia superficialis is in the middle of the subcutaneous structures, and (2) in other regions, it is near the muscle or bone level.

1. There are some regions where the fascia superficialis is situated between the areolar and lamellar layers, which are in the middle of the subcutaneous panniculus structures. Its main anatomical characteristic is that it may be in localized adiposities in regions of the abdominal wall, the upper and lower third of the medial thigh, the posterior side of the arms, the gluteal regions, the suprailiac regions, and some regions of the posterior aspects of the torso. My anatomic research (Avelar 1986a, b, 1987, 1989a, b, 1996, 2000) features a comparison between the panniculus of a person without localized adiposities and that of other person presenting with localized adiposities (Fig. 3.1). In fact, in those regions, the fascia superficialis is located between the areolar and lamellar layers, where it may be present with localized adiposities. Fat cells in the lamellar layer are elongated when there is no fat inside. However, when there are localized adiposities, those fat cells (inside of lamellar layer) become rounded, presenting considerable increase to the thickness of the panniculus, dividing the fascia superficialis into several layers of connective tissue (Fig. 3.2). Liposuction may be performed only in those areas presenting with localized adiposities between layers of the fascia superficialis.
2. The fascia superficialis is close to the muscle or bone level. It may appear in most regions of the upper and lower extremities and underneath the scalp (Fig. 3.3b–g). In those regions, during surgery, it is necessary to suture the fascia superficialis to avoid bleeding afterward—even when a fascial flap is raised to cover another anatomical segment, as happens during ear reconstruction. The vessels inside the fascia superficialis create a wide network between the tempo-

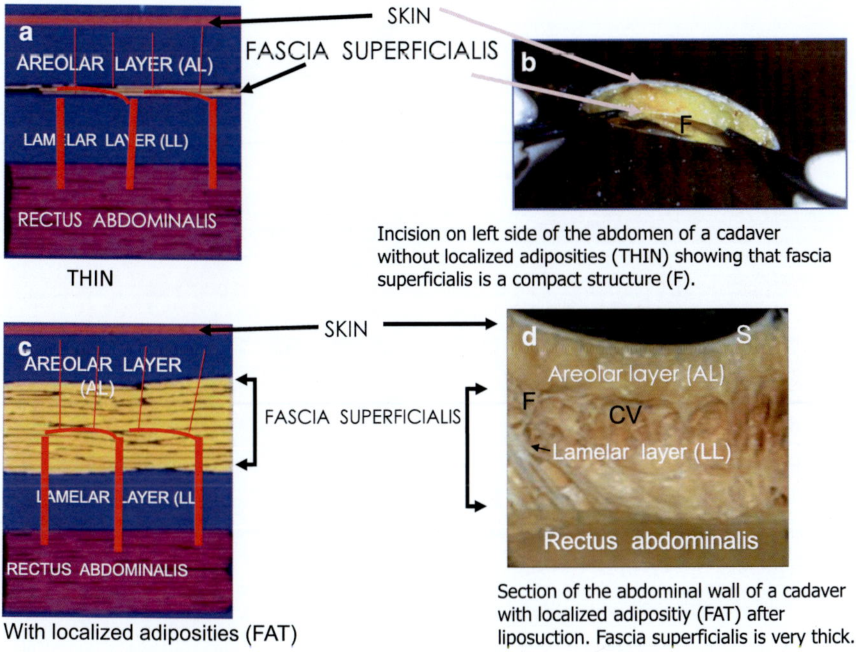

Fig. 3.1 Diagrams: (**a, c**) research in cadaver: (**b, d**) this is a comparison between THIN person (without localized adiposities) (**a, b**) and FAT person (with localized adiposities) (**c, d**)

ral superficial artery and the posterior auricular artery, which work like communicating vessels (CVs), similar to a "peripheric heart" that provides the well-balanced blood pressure of terminal vascularization to the subdermal layer and to the cutaneous covering of the scalp (Fig. 3.3g–j).

Because of the localization of the vessels, dissecting the cutaneous covering of the scalp to create fascial flaps on the temporoparietal regions is quite difficult. Just below the subdermal level and above the fascia superficialis are very small vessels coming from the communicating vessels inside the fascia. It is advisable to not carry out local infiltration, because doing so may damage the vascular network. I recommend performing a careful dissection with a knife to preserve the vascular network inside the fascia superficialis. Do not use an electric cauterization, because it will damage the communicating vessels underneath, causing bleeding after the operation. The dissection must be carried out precisely between the fascia superficialis and the subdermal layer to preserve the full thickness of the cutaneous covering (Fig. 3.3e, g).

Hair follicles are essential anatomical references because they cannot be damaged during undermining, as one can observe on scalp flaps. In the temporoparietal region, the presence of the fascia superficialis is an important anatomical detail for which I created useful temporoparietal flaps to improve ear reconstruction (Fig. 3.3) (Avelar 1977a, b, 1978). Also, the temporoparietal fascia flaps are excellent surgical options for craniofacial surgery, as described in my publications (Avelar 1983, 1992; Avelar and Psillakis 1981).

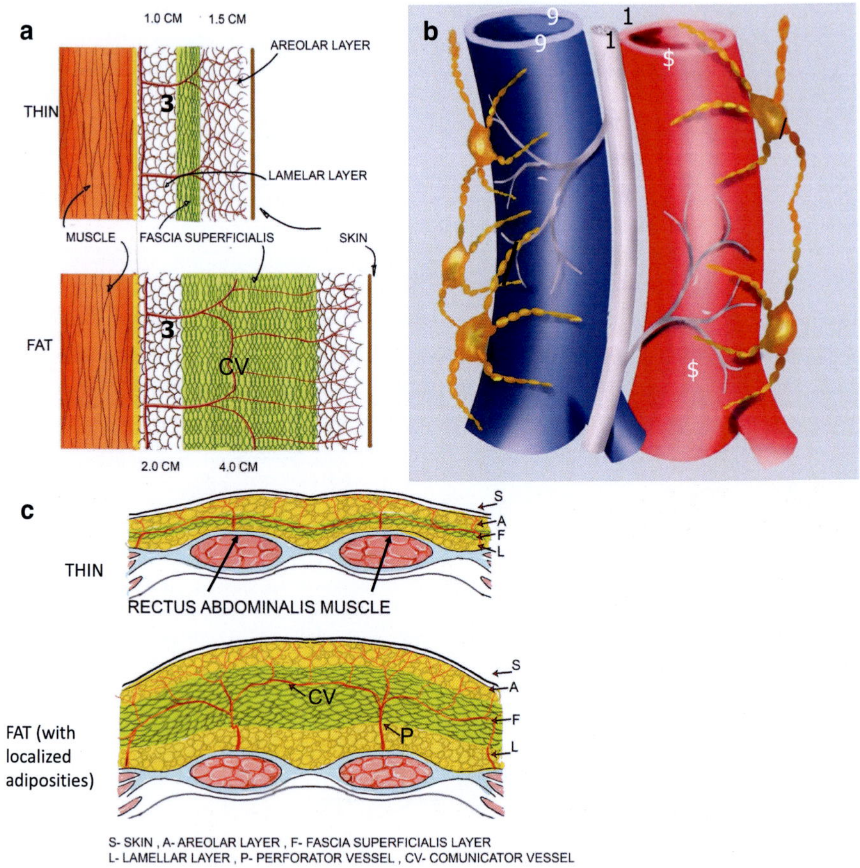

Fig. 3.2 Diagram (**a**) demonstrates a comparison of the subcutaneous panniculus between a thin person (above) and a person with localized adiposity (below). The fascia superficialis and lamellar layer in person with localized adiposity (below) increases the thickness much more than the areolar layer. Perforator vessels (P) coming from the muscle cross the lamellar layer until to reach fascia superficialis creating communicator vessels (CV) which work as a "periferic heart" to provide smooth vascularization to subdermis layer and dermis as well; diagram (**b**) anatomic unit of a perforator vessel, presenting: *V* vein, *A* artery, *L* lymphatic, *N* nerve

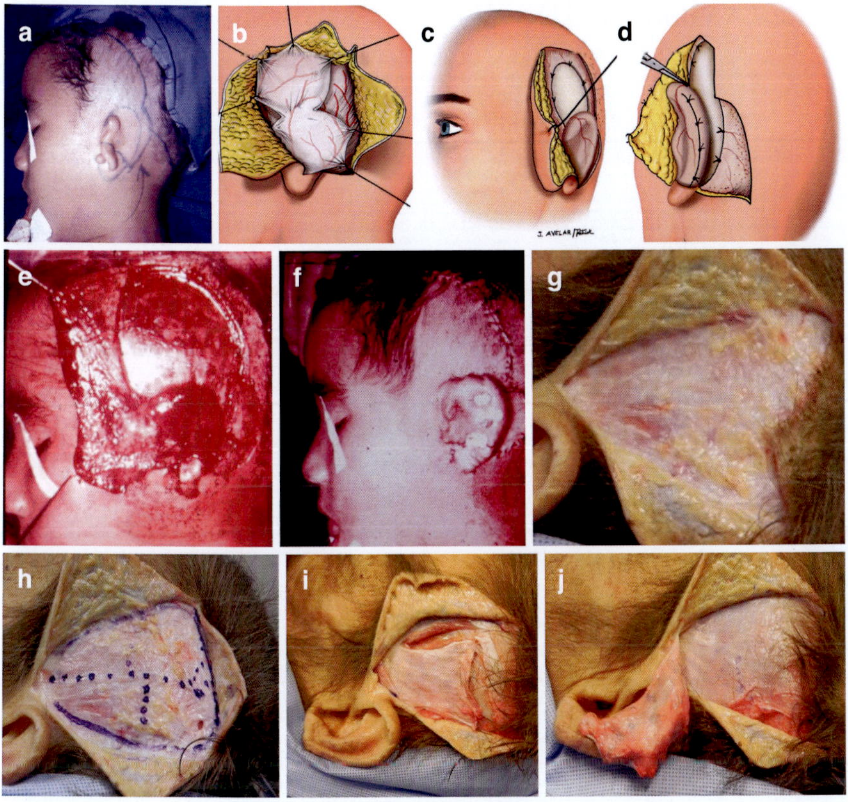

Fig. 3.3 Drawings on transverse sections showing a comparison of the subcutaneous panniculus of a thin person (above) and a person with localized adiposity (below). The fascia superficialis and lamellar layer in person with localized adiposity increases the thickness much more than the areolar layer. The perforator vessels coming from rectus abdominalis muscle crossing perpendicularly the lamellar layer reaching fascia superficialis where create the communicating vessels (CV) which provide smooth vascularization to subdermal layer and dermis as well. Due to my anatomical research in cadaver I created two fascial flaps for ear reconstruction which became possible to perform in one single stage: one supplied by temporal superficial artery and other one by posterior auricular artery. Sequential photos and illustrations during surgery: (**a**) patient with microtia on left side; (**b–d**) diagrams showing rotation of the two fascial flaps covering the new cartilagem auricular framework; (**e**) perioperative photo shows the fascial flap already rotated covering the new auricular framework; (**f**) final surgical reconstruction of the ear with skin graft on posterior side. Sequential photos of dissection on cadaver to demonstrate creation of the temporal fascia flap on left side to be used on ear reconstruction and cranio-facial surgeries as well. Photo (**g**) incision on scalp was done followed by cutaneous undermining just below the hair follicles without any damage to them. The scalp flap is raised from its place in order to create the temporal fascial flap supplied by temporal superficial artery; (**h**) the temporal fascia flap is demarcated with blue ink; (**i**) the fascia superficialis flap is already raised; (**j**) the temporal fascia flap having temporal superficial artery in its pedicle is already rotated and covering the left auricle demonstrating its use during ear reconstruction

Surgical Anatomy and Distribution of Fascia Superficialis

The fascia superficialis is an anatomical structure formed through connective tissue layers, one on top of another, with vessels between them. The arteries come from underneath the muscular plane in those regions and may have localized adiposities in specific regions.

Anatomically, the fascia superficialis is a very thin connective tissue structure formed of several layers with vessels between them. Its sophisticated distribution is a peculiar and important anatomical structure that appears between the skin and the muscular or bone planes at one of two levels: (1) In some regions, the fascia superficialis is in the middle of the subcutaneous structures, and (2) in other regions, it is near the muscle or bone level.

1. The fascia superficialis is in the middle of the subcutaneous structures. All the regions of the anterior aspect of the abdominal wall (Fig. 3.4a) feature a peculiar distribution in several layers, where fat cells increase the thickness because of the accumulation of fat inside them, as I have demonstrated in my anatomical research with perforator vessels on the projection of the rectus abdominalis (Figs. 3.1, 3.2, and 3.5) (Avelar 1986a, b, 1987, 1989a). On the posterior aspect of the torso (Fig. 3.4b), among the 11 regions are eight that may present with localized adiposities: two odd, namely interscapular and sacral, and three even, namely scapular, suprailiac, and gluteal (Fig. 3.4c).

   During an operation, when the skin and subcutaneous panniculus are incised and the fascia superficialis has not been correctly sutured, it may develop scar

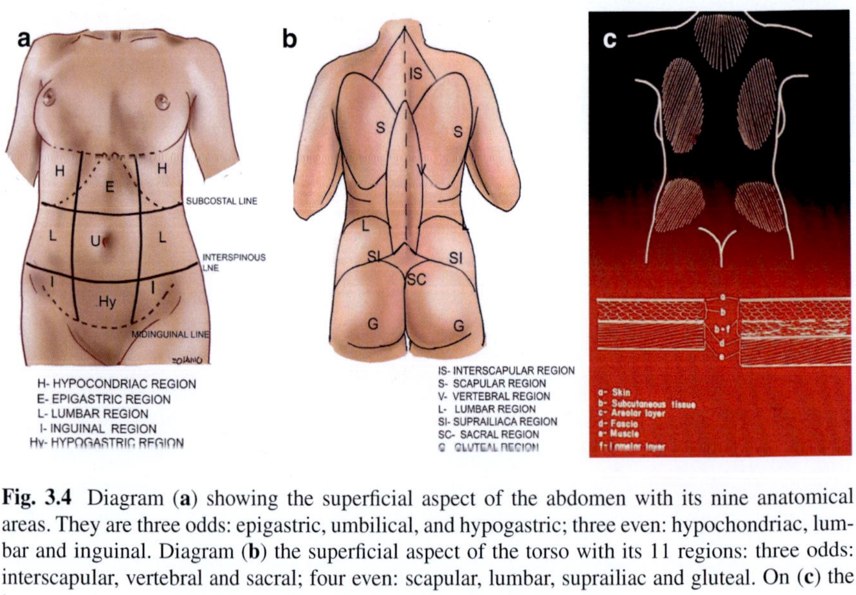

Fig. 3.4 Diagram (**a**) showing the superficial aspect of the abdomen with its nine anatomical areas. They are three odds: epigastric, umbilical, and hypogastric; three even: hypochondriac, lumbar and inguinal. Diagram (**b**) the superficial aspect of the torso with its 11 regions: three odds: interscapular, vertebral and sacral; four even: scapular, lumbar, suprailiac and gluteal. On (**c**) the interscapular, scapular and suprailiac may present localized adiposities

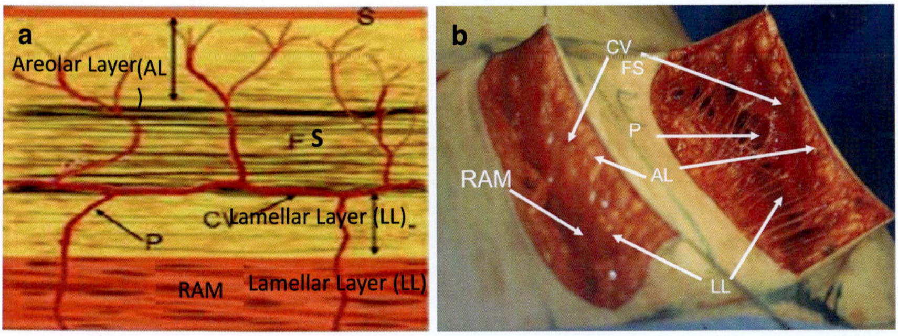

Fig. 3.5 Drawing and anatomical study in fresh cadaver to show relationship of the layers of the subcutaneous panniculus in the abdominal wall. (**a**) Scheme of the panniculus: skin (S), Areolar Layer (AL), Fascia Superficialis (FS) Communicated Vessels (CV), Perforator Vessels (P) crossing perpendicularly Lamellar Layer (LL). The communicated vessels (CV) create an arch between the perforator vessels (P) from where small vessels go perpendicularly through the areolar layer (AL) to vascularize the areolar and subdermal layers. The lamellar layer (LL) is placed between the rectus abdominalis muscle (RAM) and fascia superficialis (F) where is the correct level to perform liposuction technique; (**b**) photo of the cadaver's panniculus after liposuction performed on left side of the abdomen—CV, FS, AL, P and LL. The right side of the abdomen was incised but liposuction was not performed, where one can see the full-thickness of the panniculus with all anatomic elements

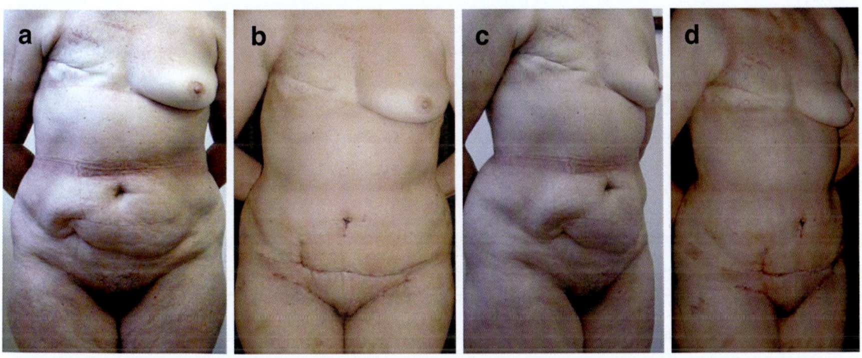

Fig. 3.6 A 59-year-old patient with unaesthetic surgical scars on abdomen caused by previous operations when fascia superficialis was not properly sutured and the areolar layer lost the anatomical structure causing depression, retraction and contraction scars. Photos (**a, c**) one can see unaesthetic scars on abdominal wall with deep and retracted surgical scars; (**b, d**) after surgery performed with adequate reparation of the fascia superficialis

retraction and contraction with inelegant results (Figs. 3.6, 3.7, 3.8, and 3.9). In such circumstances, the areolar layer loses the important anatomic support naturally provided by the fascia superficialis, causing a deep collapse, an unaesthetic surgical scar with irregularities, depression, retraction, and even contraction. If the fascia superficialis has not been properly sutured, the final scar may present inelegant irregularities caused by the absence of its reparation, which is itself

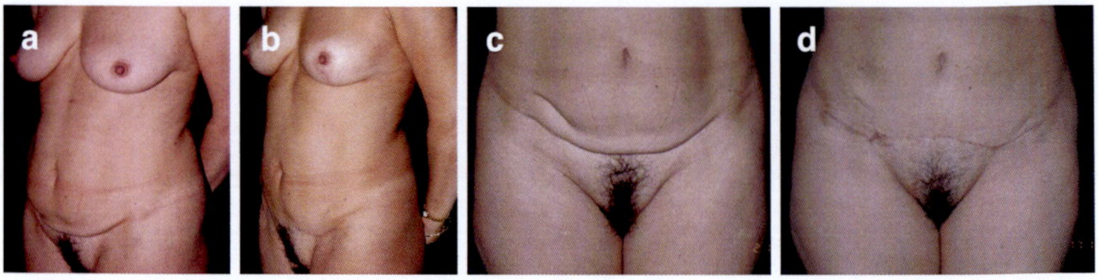

Fig. 3.7 A 46-year-old patient with ungraceful and deep surgical scars on abdomen caused by previous operations. It is evident that the fascia superficialis was not properly sutured during original surgery. Photos (**a, c**) the scars are so deep, retracted and unaesthetic on abdominal wall; (**b, d**) after lower lipoabdominoplasty performed with adequate reparation of the fascia superficialis

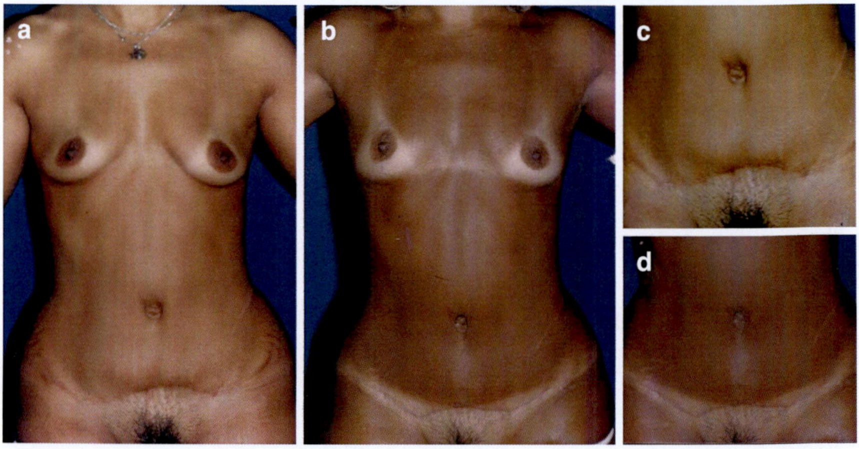

Fig. 3.8 A 41-year-old patient presenting deep and unaesthetic surgical scars on supra pubic region due to previous abdominoplasty performed elsewhere and the fascia superficialis was not sutured correctly during operation. Even the umbilical region was too wide and ungraceful. Photos (**a, c**) unaesthetic scars secondary to previous abdominoplasty performed in other service presenting deep scar and ungraceful umbilicus; (**b, d**) after correction of the scars with adequate suture of the fascia superficialis and reparation of the umbilical scar following my technique

due to a disturbance in the vascularization of the areolar layer and the subdermal layer (Fig. 3.10e–g).

During surgery, each anatomical structure must be sutured with the same one on the other border of the wound, particularly for the abdominal wall and all the regions of the anterior aspects of the chest to reinstate all layers of the panniculus. When the anatomical architecture of the panniculus has been correctly sutured, it avoids an unaesthetic depression or retractile scars because the fascia superficialis is the basis of the areolar layer, which prevents abnormalities from forming after healing has completed (Fig. 3.11a–c, e–g).

During a medial tight lift procedure, the fascia superficialis is an important structure and must be sutured to achieve the adequate suspension of the

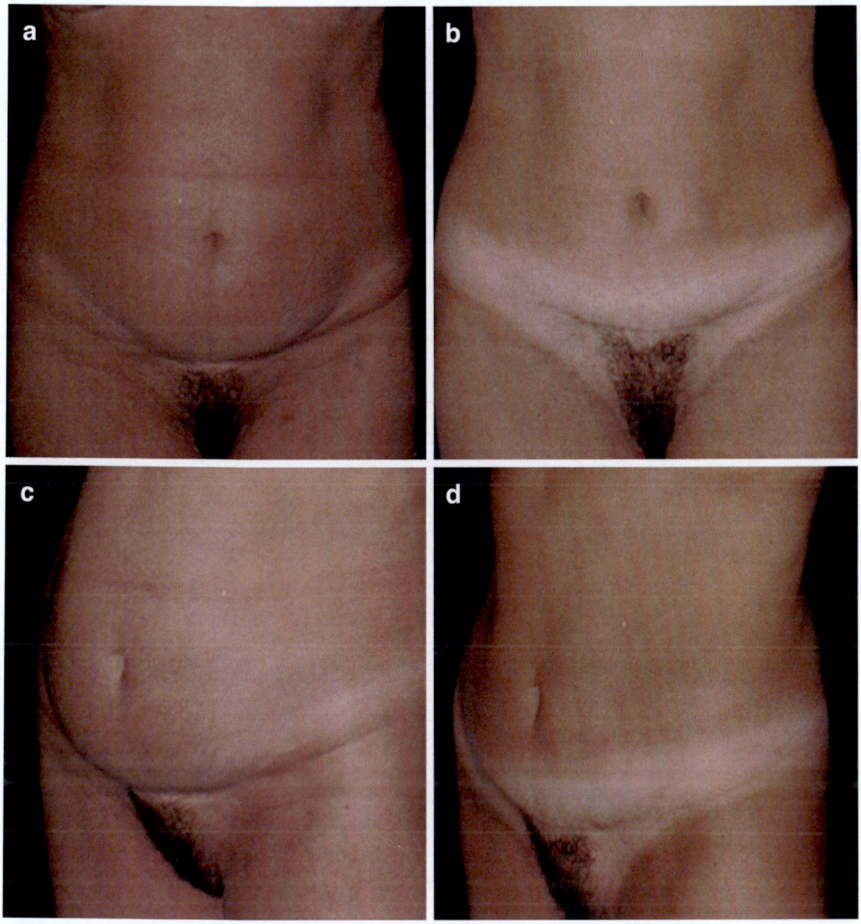

Fig. 3.9 A 36-year-old patient with deep surgical scar on supra pubic region caused by previous intra cavity operation performed by gynecologist. The fascia superficialis was not properly sutured during surgery. Photos (**a, c**) the scar is deep with retraction and ungraceful appearance; (**b, d**) after lower lipoabdominoplasty performed with adequate suture of the fascia superficialis

panniculus (Figs. 3.12 and 3.13). Such a suture works as a strong suspension to maintain the panniculus in the proper position, as I previous described (Avelar 1997, 1999a, b). Regarding medial thigh suspension, a similar report was published by other authors (Lockwood 1995).

2. The fascia superficialis is close to the muscle or bone level. It may appear in most regions of the upper and lower extremities (Fig. 3.14) and underneath the scalp (Fig. 3.3). In those regions, during surgery, it is also necessary to suture the fascia superficialis. In the temporoparietal region, the presence of the fascia superficialis is an important anatomical structure for which I created useful temporoparietal flaps to improve ear reconstruction (Figs. 3.3 and 3.15) (Avelar 1977a, b, 1978). Also, the temporoparietal fascia flaps are excellent surgical

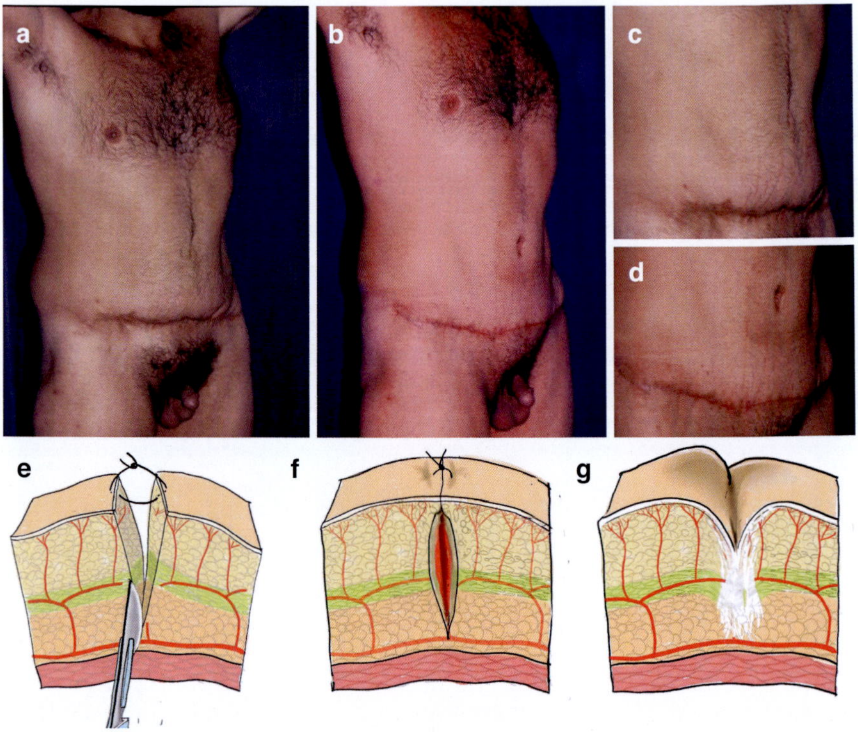

Fig. 3.10 A 49-year-old male patient with unaesthetic surgical scars on abdomen caused by previous operations performed elsewhere when the fascia superficialis was not properly sutured. Photos (**a, c**) one can see deep and unaesthetic scars on abdominal wall presenting deep and retracted surgical scars; (**b, d**) after surgery performed with adequate reparation of the fascia superficialis. (**e**) Scheme showing incision of the panniculus with inadequate suture of the subcutaneous layers; (**f**) as far as only skin was sutured, both sides of the fascia superficialis are not correctly repaired indicate by arrow; (**g**) final aspect of the wrong suture of the wound, since fascia superficialis was not sutured it does not reinstate the normal anatomy of the panniculus and areolar layer collapsed downwards causing fibrosis, local depression with retraction and contraction of the scar, because

options for craniofacial surgery (Avelar 1992; Avelar and Padovez 1982; Avelar and Psillakis 1981). Each flap contains a single pedicle supplied by the temporo-superficial artery, and the other one contains the posterior auricular artery. In my first publications, because of vital vascularization, performing reconstruction on the auricle in only one stage became possible (Figs. 3.3 and 3.15) (Avelar 1977a, b, 1978).

Nevertheless, I later found an anatomical opportunity to perform primary ear reconstruction without employing the temporoparietal fascial flaps. My preference since that time is to preserve the temporoparietal region and all the structures inside the fascia superficialis for other situations, such as the treatment of eventual complications that may occur after the first or second stage of ear reconstruction (Avelar 1979; Avelar and Psillakis 1980) So far, it has been very

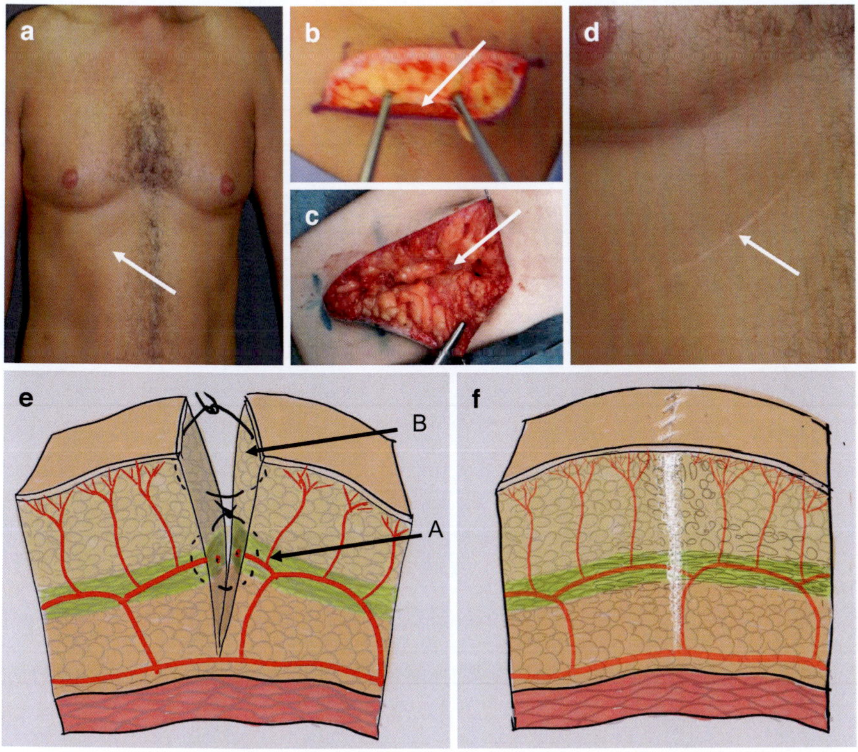

Fig. 3.11 A surgical scar on chest wall of a male patient 5 years after removal of rib cartilage on right side in which the fascia superficialis and all layers of panniculus were properly sutured during surgery. Photo (**a**) the arrow indicates the final scar; (**b**) perioperative photo shows incision on the panniculus of the chest with arrow indicates the fascia superficialis held by two forceps; (**c**) after correct suture of the fascia superficialis (indicates by arrow) providing important anatomical support for areolar layer; (**d**) photo in close up of the same patient showing on photo (**a**) the scar with excellant healing due to adequate suture of the fascia superficialis providing normal anatomical structure of the panniculus. (**e**) Scheme demonstrating the correct sutures of the panniculus on regions presenting fascia superficialis between thick areolar and lamellar layers.One can see the suture A is done repairing the fascia superficialis, and the suture B is done repairing the dermis; (**f**) demonstrates that the fascia superficialis is well repaired creating an adequate support for areolar layer, since the final scar on the skin is smooth without retraction or contraction to the cutaneous surface

useful for secondary ear reconstruction and complex deformities caused by the traumatic amputation of the auricle, for which the temporoparietal flaps may be primarily employed during first stage of reconstruction (Avelar 1997).

In some regions, the fascia superficialis is quite close to the cutaneous covering, with very few layers, and its behavior here is similar to that in other regions. An excellent example is in the mastoid region: Here, the fascia superficialis is just above the periosteum and is quite close to the skin. Such knowledge is important when ear reconstruction (on congenital or traumatic amputations) is

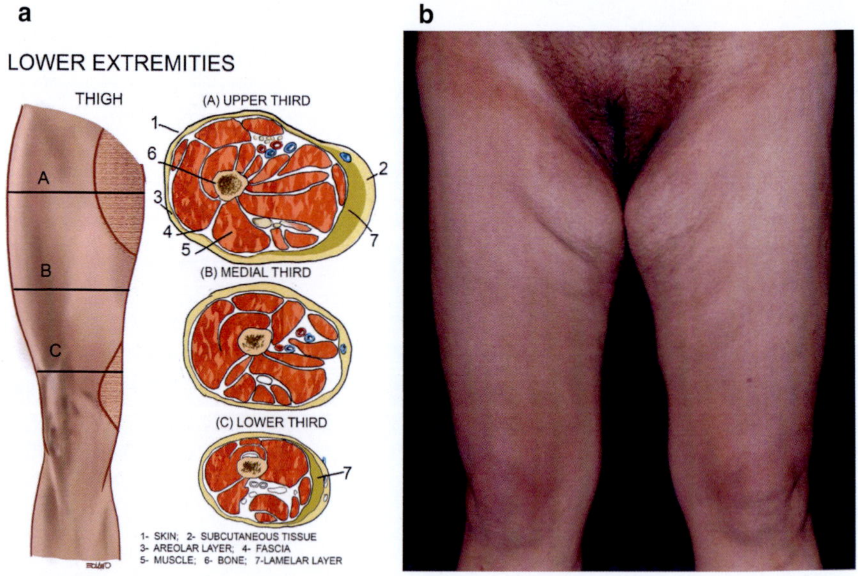

Fig. 3.12 Diagram and photo of the thigh. (**a**) Internal surface of the thigh. The upper and lower third present thick lamellar layer as is shown in sections A and C. Section B shows the middle third which does not have a lamellar; (**b**) photo of a female patient presenting localized adiposity on upper third of internal thigh

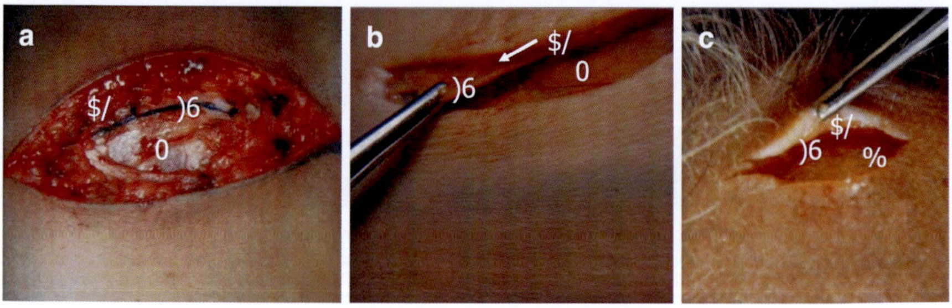

Fig. 3.13 Comparison between location of the fascia superficialis in panniculus of chest, anterior side of the thigh and scalp. Photo (**a**) transoperatory of the right side of the chest for removal of cartilage. One can see: areolar layer (AL), fascia superficialis (FS) is marked with blue ink, muscle (M) underneath; (**b**) photo of the anterior side of the thigh showing the fascia superficialis (FS) is held by a forceps, the areolar layer (AL) is very thin and attached to the dermis, muscle (M) on depth; (**c**) incision on scalp showing the fascia superficialis (FS) and areolar layer (AL) are very close to each other and just above the bone (B) of the cranium

performed because it is necessary to undermine the skin in order to create a subcutaneous tunnel to embed the new auricular framework in (Avelar 1979; Avelar and Psillakis 1980, 1981). Such a detachment must be carried out just underneath the subdermal layer and above the fascia superficialis, and surgeons must

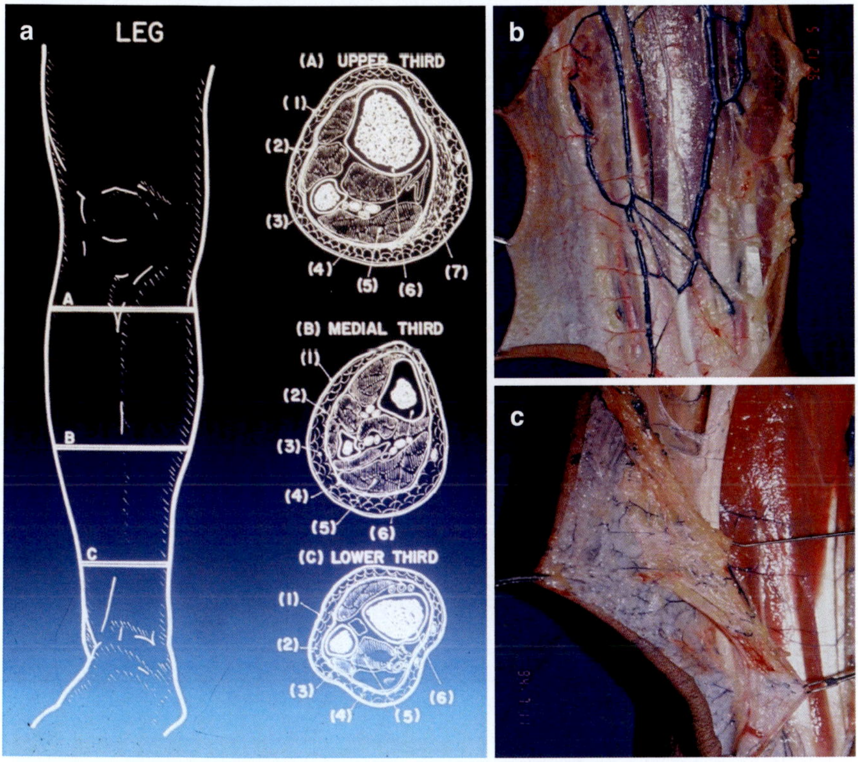

Fig. 3.14 Diagram and anatomic dissections on cadaver's photos of the right leg. In the diagram (**a**) shows the cutaneous and subcutaneous layers in three levels: upper, medial and lower; (**b**) the skin of the leg was incised and undermined just above the fascia superficialis which lies on the muscles; (**c**) the fascia superficialis is rotated laterally to show the muscles underneath

avoid damaging the vessels inside so that enough blood supply is provided to the cutaneous covering (Fig. 3.3e, g). When such a procedure is carried out on the correct level, there is no bleeding during or after the operation. For this reason, it is not necessary to use any kind of postoperative drainage after ear reconstruction. To find an adequate level, inject saline solution with a thin needle just underneath the skin in a parallel position. Cutaneous incision and undermining must both be performed while the surface of the skin shows elevation from the injection of the saline solution.

In all regions of the face, the fascia superficialis is also quite close to the skin. When cutaneous undermining is performed during a face lift, select the level that is just below the fascia superficialis to preserve adequate vascularization to the subdermal layer and to the skin. This structure is above the superficial musculo-aponeurotic system (SMAS), according to Mitz and Perronie (1976).

Usually, in the upper and lower extremities, the fascia superficialis is quite close to the muscular level, except on the posterior surface of the arm and on the

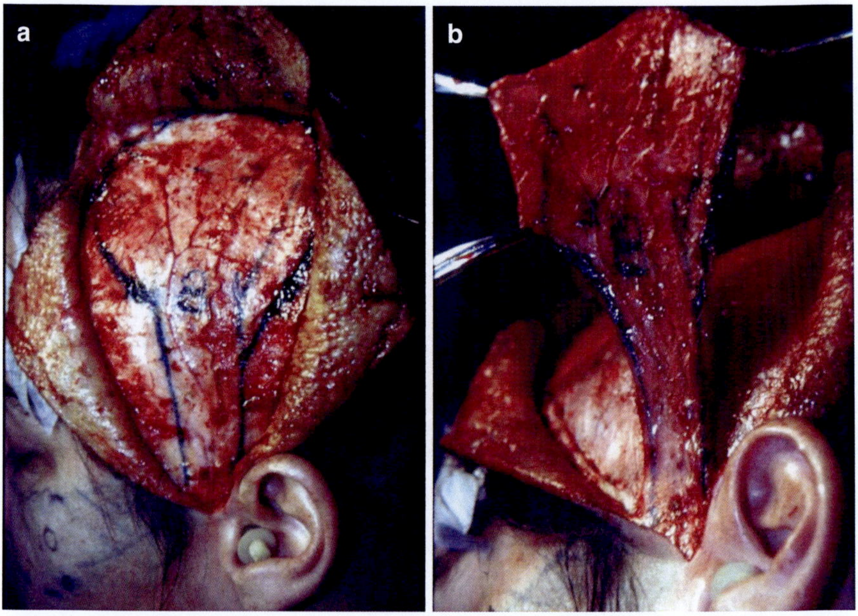

Fig. 3.15 Creation of the fascial flaps on temporal and parietal regions during anatomical dissections on fresh cadaver. Photo (**a**) the flap is marked with ink, having its pedicle supplied by temporal superficial artery; (**b**) the long flap is raised from scalp showing its pedicle

upper and lower thirds of the internal surface of the thigh (Fig. 3.12). Once again, in these areas, the fascia superficialis is divided into several layers thanks to the presence of localized adiposities.

In all the regions of the lower and upper extremities, the fascia superficialis features a peculiar distribution that is very close to the musculoaponeurotic level, where arterial and venous vascularization is present (Fig. 3.13).

Discussion

Ever since I started my professional activities in 1973, I've noticed that several fields in plastic surgery still require further technical development to achieve better aesthetic results and to reduce the incidence of complications. Among those fields were two that came with challenges requiring new techniques to incorporate updated technical knowledge:

1. Ear reconstruction
2. Abdominoplasty

In both fields, I concluded that such technical development requires gaining more anatomic information to achieve scientific progress.

1. For the reconstruction of the auricle, significant technical improvements have been published by outstanding authors such as Gillies (1937), Converse (1958a, b, 1963), Tanzer (1959), Psillakis et al. (1990), Tanzer (1978) and Pitanguy (1967), Pitanguy et al. (1972), with good aesthetic results. Nevertheless, each reconstruction was a challenge because it requires performing several surgical stages to achieve the final result and because it comes with a very high incidence of complications.

   Therefore, at that time, I dedicated much time to studying the anatomy of a normal auricle and its neighboring areas. In addition to reading textbooks, I improved my knowledge by performing anatomic dissections on cadavers, and I found out important information on the neighboring regions of the auricle, especially those concerning arterial and venous vascularization (Figs. 3.3 and 3.15). In the beginning, I identified that the temporal superficial artery and the posterior auricular artery could be transferred to the ear in order to improve blood supply, by providing better vascularization to the reconstructed organ. During my anatomical dissections, I concluded that I could perform such a vascular transposition without causing any local damage because those vessels were between the fascia superficialis.

   Thanks to such anatomical information, I designed two flaps: one supplied by the temporal superficial artery and the other supplied by the posterior auricular artery (Avelar 1977a, b). Each contained a very small vascular pedicle and the wide surface of the fascia superficialis with a rich vascular network between the connective layers. Because of the wide surface of the anatomical structure, I named this flap the "racquet-shaped flap" (Figs. 3.3 and 3.15). It was such a crucial anatomical finding to my research that it became possible to perform ear reconstruction in one surgical stage (Avelar 1977a, b). Therefore, at the beginning of my career, I demonstrated that it was possible to reduce ear reconstruction surgery from six or eight surgical stages to one surgical stage (Fig. 3.3). In addition to reducing it to one surgical stage, this technique minimizes complications and improves aesthetic refinements to the reconstructed auricles (Avelar 1978, 1979, 1986a, b). Since those publications, I have performed ear reconstruction following the same surgical principles, with necessary variations according to each deformity (congenital or acquired).
2. Abdominoplasty is an aesthetic surgery of the abdominal wall. There were several problems that required new ideas and new concepts to add to the basic techniques to minimize the high incidence of complications during and after operations. At the beginning of my practice, those problems motivated me to establish the Brazilian Symposium of Abdominoplasty in 1982 with the participation of all outstanding Brazilian plastic surgeons and some renowned specialists from other countries. Besides the event, we also published the annals of the event, with participation from all the attending surgeons and featuring their updated knowledge on the subject (Avelar and Padovez 1982). In the scientific program concerning the techniques for abdominoplasty, the speakers presented a high level of information. However, many questions regarding complications during and after operation did not convince given that many problems remained after all the discussions (Guerrerosantos 1982; Mélega 1982; D'Assumpção 1982).

At that moment, once again, I was sure that abdominoplasty presented multiple challenges to plastic surgeons all over of the world. In my reflections and brainstorming, I identified three main problems with the operation: (1) the creation of a new umbilical region; (2) complications during and after the operation; and (3) remaining adiposities after surgery. First, I had already presented a new method that makes triangular incisions around it to avoid leaving a circular scar after surgery and thus resulting in smooth surgical results (Avelar 1976a, b, 1978, 1979, 1983). Second, complications during and after abdominoplasty were even more difficult to solve. I concluded that abdominoplasty was a field that still required technical improvements to minimize complications. Third, the remaining adiposities after abdominoplasty were reduced thanks to development of liposuction by Illouz (1980, 1983a, b, 1984, 1986).

In 1983, I went to Paris to learn the liposuction technique by observing Illouz's performing his technique. When I performed my operations, the cannulas worked inside an unknown anatomical compartment of the human body. At that time, I decided to study the anatomy of the subcutaneous layers in order to gain more-precise anatomical knowledge. I performed anatomic research on cadavers to find new information, when possible, so that I could identify the lamellar layer, which was close to the muscles, and the areolar layer, which was superficially separated by the fascia superficialis.

This structure had rich vascularization coming from the perforator vessels, which I call the communicating vessels (CVs), as a "peripheric heart"," because the blood pressure decreases to irrigate the areolar layer and the subdermal layer (Figs. 3.1a, c, 3.2, and 3.5). I performed dissections on several cadavers of various ages, sexes, levels of adipose tissue, heights, and ethnicities and used liposuction to look for new information and explore the behavior of the subcutaneous compartment after liposuction (Avelar 1986a, b, 1987, 1989a, b).

The fascia superficialis is an anatomical structure between the areolar and lamellar layers with peculiar characteristics in abdominal wall and with differences between each region and between thin people and people with localized adiposities. A similar anatomy was found in upper and lower thirds of the medial thighs (Fig. 3.12) and in some regions of the torso. On the abdominal wall and in the posterior regions of the torso, the fascia superficialis is well identified on computerized tomography (CT) when the image is well analyzed on same level while observing the bone structures as anatomic references (Fig. 3.16).

The fascia superficialis must be well sutured during surgeries on the abdominal wall to repair the architecture of the panniculus (Fig. 3.10e–g). If it is not adequately sutured, the areolar layer will not reinstate the anatomical structure, thus leaving behind unaesthetic and inelegant surgical scars (Figs. 3.6, 3.7, 3.8, 3.9, and 3.10a, c).

The fascia superficialis in the scalp regions contains a rich vascular network supplied mostly by the temporal superficial artery, the posterior auricular artery, and the occipital artery. They run between the connective tissue layers of the fascia superficialis, providing vascularization to the areolar and subdermal lay-

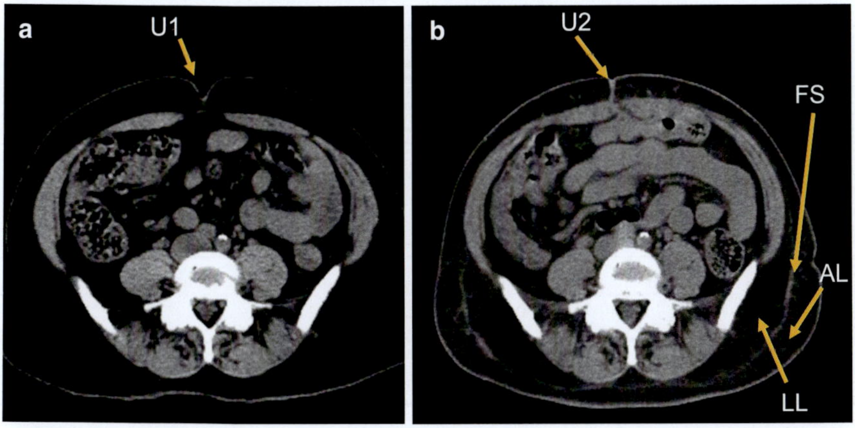

Fig. 3.16 Computerized Tomography (CT) of a patient, before and one year after full lipoabdominoplasty combined with reinforcement of the abdominal muscular aponeurotic wall. One can see that both images are on the same level as showing the references of the bone structures. The fascia superficialis is well identified on supra iliac region. Photo (**a**) image of CT before operation showing diastasis of the muscles on umbilicus indicated by arrow (U1); (**b**) CT of the same patient 1 year after full lipoabdominoplasty combined with reinforcement of the muscular wall repairing umbilical region (U2), and thick layer of fascia superficialis (FS) which is placed between areolar layer (AL) and lamellar layer (LL)

ers and the dermis, similar to how the CVs operate. The fascia superficialis in the temporoparietal region (galea) is useful for ear reconstruction (Avelar 1977a, b, 1978) and the reparation of cranial defects (Avelar 1983). Those flaps must be designed with a knife without local infiltration to avoid damaging the vascular network.

The subdermal fat layer must remain attached to the dermis to preserve vascularization to scalp. I have had the opportunity to attend some patients presenting with defects on the cranium that the neurosurgeon intended to remove by using cranial fascial (galea) as a graft to replace the defect. Members on a neurosurgeon's staff accepted my surgical plan for repairing the cranial defect without performing a graft of the cranial fascial structure. Instead of following their surgical plan, I suggested rotating the full thickness of the scalp with the cranial fascia flap, where rotation is carried out from the back to the anterior in order to cover the cranial defect (Fig. 3.17). The full thickness of the scalp flap is supplied with blood by the posterior auricular artery and the occipital artery, providing adequate vascularization to the wide area of the scalp flap. If neurosurgeons had resected the temporoparietal fascia and grafted on the cranial defect in order to cover the brain tissue, the scalp flap could certainly not have been rotated. If the temporoparietal fascia is removed from the scalp, it will damage the blood supply of the scalp and it will therefore no longer be available for use as a wide flap. After all, the fascia superficialis on the cranium's surface is in charge of the vascularization of the scalp through a wide arterial and venous network of communicating vessels.

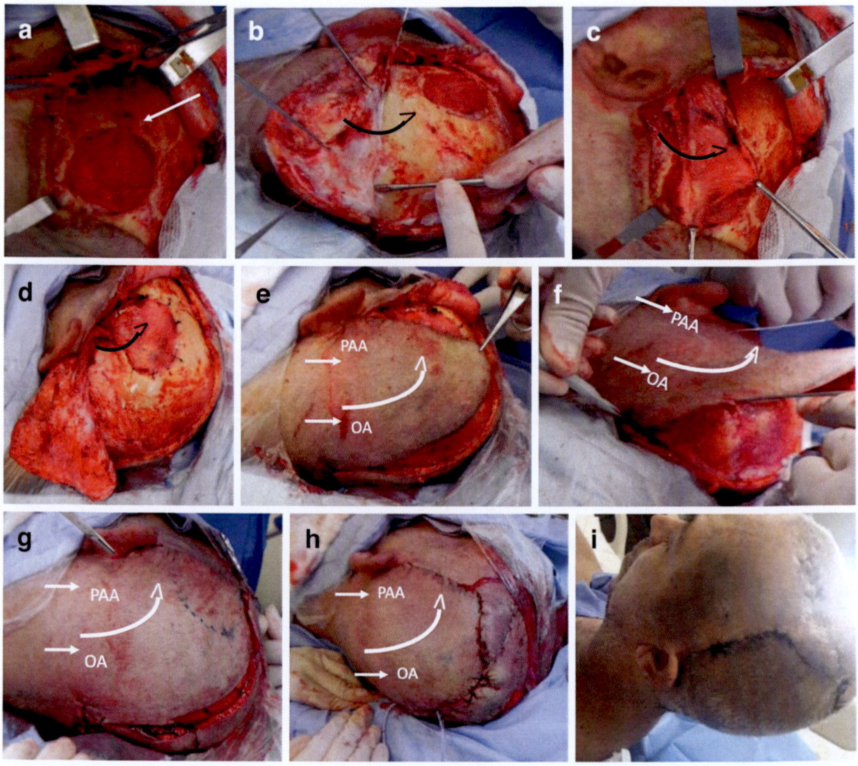

Fig. 3.17 Perioperative photos showing rotation of the temporal muscle flap for reparation of 10 cm defect on temporal bone with exposition of brain. Photo (**a**) a defect missing 10 cm diameter on temporal bone with exposition of the brain indicated by arrow; (**b, c**) arrows indicate the rotation arch of the temporal muscle flap; (**d**) the flap is already sutured covering exposition of the brain through bone defect. Members of neurosurgeon's staff intended to remove the tempo-parietal fascia for grafting to cover the cranium defect, but proposed to rotate a composite scalp flap to repair the defect. Photo (**e**) the scalp is already raised with its pedicle supplied by posterior auricular artery (PAA) and occipital artery (AO) with arrow indicates the rotation arch; (**f**) a 3 cm incision is done to provide rotation of the flap; (**g**) the flap is rotated from back forward; (**h**) the scalp flap is already sutured covering the bone defect; (**i**) the same patient one month after surgery

Conclusions

The fascia superficialis is a sophisticated anatomical structure that is present in almost all the regions of the human body between the skin and the muscular or bone levels (Figs. 3.1, 3.2, and 3.3). Because of its importance and peculiar behavior after surgery, it can be considered as second skin." During operations on the abdominal wall, the posterior aspect of the torso, and the posterior side of the arm—regions where the fascia superficialis is between the areolar and lamellar layers—the fascia superficialis should be sutured to reinstate the full thickness of the panniculus (Fig. 3.11). If it is not adequately sutured during surgery, it may leave unaesthetic and retractile scars because it could damage the areolar layer and even cause vascular alterations in the subdermal level (Figs. 3.6, 3.7, 3.8, 3.9, and 3.10).

The fascia superficialis, which is just above the muscles and on bone structures, also must be sutured from border to border to reinstate it, although the areolar and lamellar layers are too thin (Figs. 3.3, 3.14, and 3.15). These anatomical characteristics appear on the upper and lower extremities—except on the upper and lower thirds of the media thigh (Fig. 3.13) and except on the posterior side of the arm, where the fascia superficialis is between thick layers of the areolar and lamellar layers, which is described in more detail in Chap. 2.

References

Avelar JM (1976a) Umbilicoplasty – a technique without external scar. (Umbilicoplastia – uma técnica sem cicatriz externa). 13° Congr Bras Cir Plast, 1° Congr Bras Cir Estética 13th Braz. Congr. of Plastic Surgery and First Braz. Congr. of Aesthetic Surgery, Porto Alegre, pp 81–82

Avelar JM (1976b) Umbilicoplasty. A technique without external scar. Cahiers de Chirurgie Esthétique. Journees internationals de Chirurgie Esthetique. Vendredi 21 mai, pp 5–25.

Avelar JM (1977a) Total reconstruction of the auricular pavilion in one stage (Reconstrução total do pavilhão auricular num único tempo cirúrgico). Rev Bras Cir 67:139

Avelar JM (1977b) One stage – total reconstruction of the ear. In: Presented at the Second Congress of the Asian Pacific Section of the International Conference for Plastic and Reconstructive Surgery. August, Tokyo (Japan).

Avelar JM (1978) Total reconstruction of the ear in one single stage – technical variation with cutaneous flap with inferior pedicle. Folha Med 76:457–467 (Brazil).

Avelar JM (1979) Microtia: simplified technique for total reconstruction of the auricle in one single stage. In: Transactions of the Seventh International Congress of Plastic and Reconstructive Surgery. Ed. By Fonseca Ely J, Ed. Cartgraf, Rio de Janeiro, p 353 (Brasil).

Avelar JM, Psillakis JM (1980) Surgical Techniques for Reconstruction of Auricular Pavillon (Técnicas Cirúrgicas de Reconstrução do Pavilhão Auricular). Rev Bras Otorrinolaringol 46(3):262–281.

Avelar JM, Psillakis JM (1981) Microtia: total Reconstructio of the Auricle in One Single Operation. Br J Plast Surg 34:224

Avelar JM and Padovez JC (1982) – Mamoplasty combined with Abdominoplasty – Analises of 40 consecutive cases. (Mamaplastia e Abdominoplastia Combinadas – Análise de 40 Casos Consecutivos) In: Annals of Brazilian Symposio of Abdominoplasty. (Anais do Simpósio Brasileiro de Abdominoplastia), ed. by Juarez M. Avelar, Sponsored by Brazilian Society of Plastic Surgery-Regional São Paulo, (Patrocinado pela Sociedade Brasileira de Cirurgia Plástica – Regional São Paulo). 1:141–148. Editora Cidade, Rio de Janeiro – Brazil.

Avelar JM (1983) A new fascial flap for use in craniofacial surgery. Ann Acad Med Singapore 2:382–387

Avelar JM (1986a) Surgical anatomy and distribution of the cellular tissue on human organism. (Anatomia cirúrgica e distribuição do tecido celular no organismo humano) In: Liposuction (Lipoaspiração). Ed. By Avelar JM and Illouz IG. Editora Hipócrates, São Paulo, pp 45–57.

Avelar JM (1986b) – Importance of Ear Reconstruction for the Aesthetic Balance of the Facial Contour. Aesth Plast Surg 10:147–156

Avelar JM (1987) - Study of the Anatomy of the Subcutaneous Adipose Tissue Applied for Fat-suction Technique. In: Maneksha RJ (ed): Trans IX Int Congr Plast Reconstr Surg. New Delhi, India, March 1-6, pp 377–379.

Avelar JM (1989a) Regional Distribution and Behavior of the Subcutaneous Tissue Concerning Selection and Indication for Liposuction. Aesthetic Plast Surg 13:155–165

Avelar JM (1989b) Cranean Fascial (galea) Flap – Anatomy, Planning and Surgical Aplication (Retalho da Fascia Craniana (gálea). Anatomia, Planejamento e Aplicação Cirúrgica. In: Cirurgia Plástica na Infância, ed. By Juarez M. Avelar. Ed. Hipócrates, São Paulo, pp 314–326

Avelar JM (1992) The use of fascial flap in ear reconstruction. In: Transactions of the X Congress of the Inter Conf for Plastic and Reconst Surgery. Ed. By Hinderer UT, Ed. Excepta Medica, Madrid, p 265–268

Avelar JM (1996) Creation of a Natural and Definitive Inguino-crural Crease during Lifting of the Upper Medial Thigh (Criação de natural e definitivo sulco ínguino-crural no "lifting" da face interna da coxa). Rev. Bras. Cirurg 86(5):213–228.

Avelar JM (1997) Secondary Reconstruction of the Ear. In Creation of the Auricle. Ed. by Juarez M. Avelar. Ed. Hipócrates, São Paulo (Brasil) 14:267–291.

Avelar JM (1999a) Aesthetic plastic in the Inner Side of the Thigh – New concepts and Technique without Cutaneous or Subcutaneous Undermining. (Cirurgia Plástica de Face Interna de Coxas – Novos Conceitos e Técnica sem Descolamento Cutâneo e Subcutâneo). Rev Bras Cir 88/89(1/6):57–67.

Avelar JM (1999b) Flankplasty and torsoplasty – a new surgical approach. (Flancoplastia e Torsoplastia - Nova Abordagem Cirúrgica). Rev Bras Cir 88/89(1/6):21–35.

Avelar JM (2000) Cirurgia Plástica: Obrigação de meio e não obrigação de fim ou de resultado. Ed. Hipócrates, São Paulo, pp 237–265

Converse JM (1958a) Reconstruction of the auricle: part I. Plast Reconstr Surg 22:150

Converse JM (1958b) Reconstruction of the auricle: part II. Plast Reconstr Surg 22:230

Converse JM (1963) Construction of the auricle in congenital microtia. Plast Reconstr Surg 32:425

D'Assumpção EA (1982) Three Common Complictions in Abdominoplasty: Infeccion, Deiscence and Seroma Formation. (Três Complicações Comuns em Abdominoplastias: Infecção, Deiscência e Seroma). In: Annals of the Brazilian Symposio of Abdominoplasty (Simpósio Brasileiro de Abdominoplastia), organized and ed. by Juarez M. Avelar, Sponsored by Brazilian Society of Plastic Surgery-Regional São Paulo, (Patrocinado pela Sociedade Brasileira de Cirurgia Plástica – Regional São Paulo), pág. 77–82. Editora Cidade, Rio de Janeiro – Brazil.

Gillies HD (1937) Reconstruction of the external ear with special references to the use of maternal ear cartilage as the supporting structure. Rev Chir Structive 7:169

Gray H (1974) - Anatomy, descriptive and surgical. Philadelphia: Running Press.

Guerrerosantos J (1982) Necrosis of Abdominal Wall Post-Abdominoplasty – Etiology, Profilaxis and Treatment (Necrose de Parede Pós-Abdominoplastia – Etiologia, Profilaxia e Tratamento). Presented at the Brazilian Symposio of Abdominoplasty (Simpósio Brasileiro de Abdominoplastia), organized and ed. by Juarez M. Avelar, Sponsored by Brazilian Society of Plastic Surgery-Regional São Paulo, (Patrocinado pela Sociedade Brasileira de Cirurgia Plástica – Regional São Paulo). Section "E" Round Table. Editora Cidade, Rio de Janeiro – Brazil.

Illouz YG (1980) Une nouvelle technique pour les lipodystrophies localisées. Rev Cir Esth Franc 6(Illouz YG (eds) Lipospiração. Ed. Hipocrates, São Paulo, pp 45–57

Illouz YG (1983a) – Liposuction - My technique and applications. First Course of Liposuction. Organized by Dr. Juarez M. Avelar. Heled at São Paulo Hospital, Service of Prof. Andrews at Escola Paulista de Medicina., Sponsored by Brazilian Society of Plastic Surgery (São Paulo Section) October São Paulo (Brazil).

Illouz YG (1983b) Body contouring by lipolysis: 5 years' experience with over 3,000 cases. Plast Reconstr Surg 72(5):591–597.

Illouz YG (1984) – My Technique of Liposuction – 4 years evolution. Second Course of Liposuction. (Minha Técnica de Lipoaspiração 4 Anos de Evolução. 2° Curso de Lipoaspiração) - Heled at "9 de Julho Hospital." Organized by Juarez M. Avelar, Sponsored by the Brazilian Society of Plastic Surgery. September, São Paulo (Brazil)

Lockwood T (1995) High lateral-tension abdominoplasty with superficial fascial system suspension. Plast Reconstr Surg 96:603

Mélega JM (1982) Thromboembolism as a complication of abdominoplasty: etiology, prevention and treatment. (Tromboembolismo Como complicação de abdominoplastia: etiologia, prevenção e tratamento) In: Annals of the Brazilian Symposium of Abdominoplasty. Ed. by Juarez M Avelar. Sponsored by Brazilian Society of Plastic Surgery (Regional São Paulo) pp 73–76.
Mitz V, Perronie M (1976) The superficial musculoaponeurotic system; (SMAS) in the parotid and check area. Plast Reconstr Surg; 58(1):80–8.
Pitanguy I (1967) Dysplasia auricularis. In: Savenero- Roselli G, Boggio-Robutti G (eds) Transactions of the fourth International Congress of Plastic and Reconstructive Surgeons. Excerpta Medica International Congress, Rome, p 660
Pitanguy I, Cansanção A, Avelar JM (1972) Reconstrução do lobo: contribuição técnica através do uso do retalho pré-auricular. Rev Bras Cir 62(l/2):51–55. Bol Cir Plast 5
Psillakis JM, Avelar JM, Perssonelli J (1990) Galeal flaps. In: Vasconez SB, Hall-Findlay E (eds) Encyclopedia oí Flaps. Little, Brown and Co., Boston, pp 389–392
Sobotta, Figge (1977) - Atlas of human anatomy. Baltimore: Urban & Schwarzenber.
Spalteholz W (1970) - Atlas de anatomia humana, (Atlas of Human Anatomy) 5th ed. Espanha: Editora Labor
Tanzer RC (1959) Total reconstruction of the external ear. Plast Reconstr Surg 23:1
Tanzer RC (1978) Microtia: along term follow-up of forty-four reconstructed auricles. Plast Reconstr Surg 61:161
Testut L, Jacob O (1975) - Tratado de Anatomia Topográfica. (Compedia of Topografic Anatomy) Barcelona, – Madrid, Bogota, Buenos Airees, Rio de Janeiro.: Salvat Editores, 1975
Testut L, Jacob O (1984) - Tratado de Anatomia Topográfica. Salvat Editores. Barcelona – Madrid, Bogota, Buenos Airees, Rio de Janeiro. 1984.

Part II
Abdominoplasty on Body Contouring

Chapter 4
Sinder's Technique: A Useful and Safe Approach for Abdominoplasty

Juarez Moraes Avelar

Abstract The first abdominoplasty was credited to Kelly when he performed a panniculus resection of the lower segment of the abdominal wall. According to Sinder, in 1890 Demars and Marx described a resection of skin and the subcutaneous abdominal wall. During the twentieth century, several authors developed substantial developments in different types of panniculus resections. A remarkable operation was introduced by Vernon, who performed the reimplantation of the umbilicus on the cutaneous abdominal wall. A memorable abdominoplasty was described by Callia as a cutaneous incision on the suprapubic region followed by panniculus undermining. Later, Pitanguy performed wider panniculus undermining by using reinforcement from the musculoaponeurotic wall to reinstate the body contouring.

Sinder introduced new concepts to abdominoplasty by bringing more security to the operation, starting with the detachment of the abdominal panniculus through a supraumbilical incision. Afterward, the cutaneous flap of the upper abdominal wall is pulled downward so that an appropriate location for the skin incision in the suprapubic region can be determined. Therefore, the resection of the abdominal panniculus is carried out once the surgeon has properly evaluated its extension into the infraumbilical area. The plication of the musculoaponeurotic wall is performed after the abdominal panniculus undermining has been completed according to surgical planning. Sinder's method also to introduced a new, safe technique for abdominoplasty.

Keywords Abdominoplasty · New technique · Upper undermining · Safe approach · First superior incision

J. M. Avelar (✉)
Brazilian Scientific Institute of Plastic and Reconstructive Surgery, São Paulo, Brazil

J. M. Avelar, R. Cavalcanti Ribeiro (eds.), *Body Contouring*,
https://doi.org/10.1007/978-3-031-42802-9_4

Introduction

For patients with cutaneous flaccidity, unaesthetic skin surgical scars, or a voluminous abdomen, the operation will leave a horizontal scar localized to the suprapubic region (Pitanguy 1967). But when there is poor elasticity and less flaccidity in the supraumbilical region, there may be some difficulty in bringing the supraumbilical flap to the suprapubic edge of the incision. If the suture is made under strong tension, it poses a risk of causing dehiscence in the central part of the wound and other complications.

To avoid this risk, Sinder (1975a, b) introduced new concepts to abdominoplasty through adequate surgical planning (Fig. 4.1). He started his operation by first performing the detachment of the supraumbilical area, creating a cutaneous flap (Fig. 4.2). Afterward, the upper abdominal flap is pulled on in a downward direction, and the surgeon may then properly evaluate the correct location for an incision in the suprapubic region (Fig. 4.3). Once the surgeon has completed their evaluation, the infraumbilical panniculus can then be correctly demarcated for a final cutaneous incision in the suprapubic region (Fig. 4.4a). The skin of the umbilicus is isolated on all sides by making triangular incisions (Avelar 1976a, b, 1979, 1983,

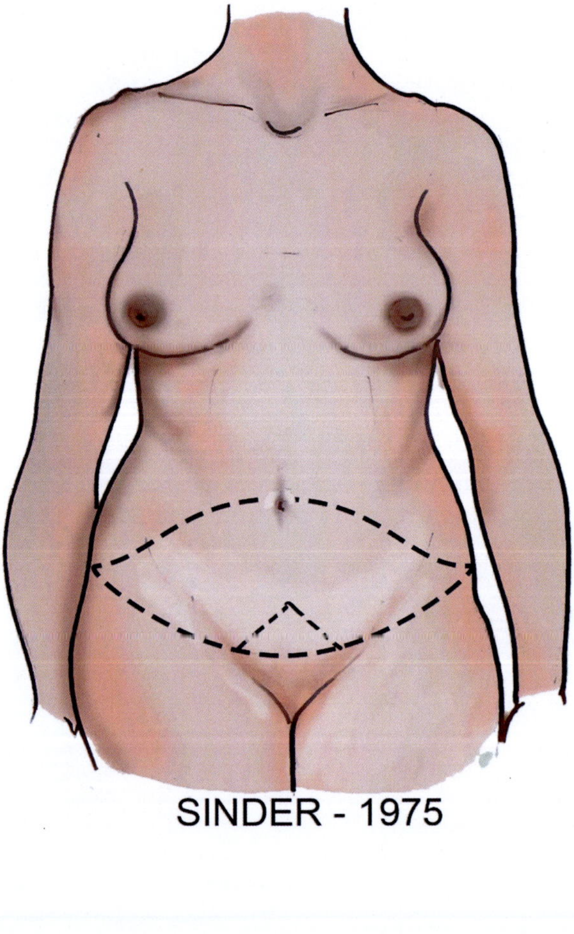

Fig. 4.1 Surgical demarcations before operation of Sinder's technique. A triangular area with base on the lower line is drawn inside of the area of skin resection to provide adequate surgical support to the abdominal flap

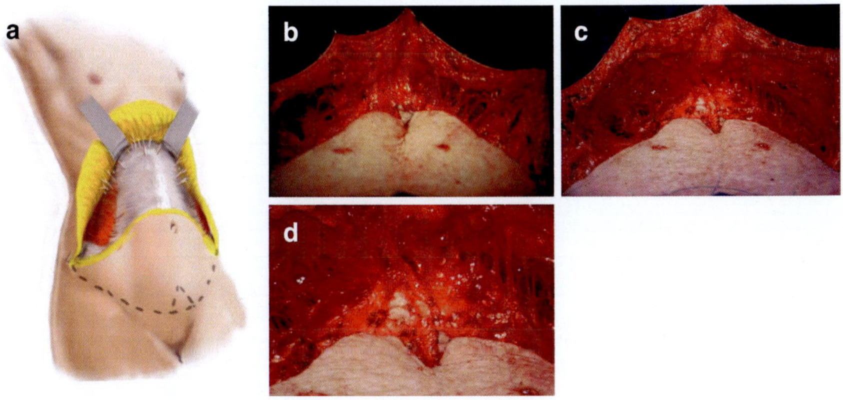

Fig. 4.2 The first incision is done on superior line of the surgical demarcations following panniculus undermining up to the rib margin. (**a**) Scheme of the technique on right oblique view showing the superior flap is already undermined until costal margin; perioperative photo (**b**) one can see the superior incision was done passing through the umbilical region and the upper abdominal panniculus starts undermining, with three triangular incisions around the umbilicus were done following Avelar's technique; (**c**) the superior abdominal flap is already undermined with the umbilicus incised; (**d**) close up shows the triangular surface of the umbilicus according to the technique

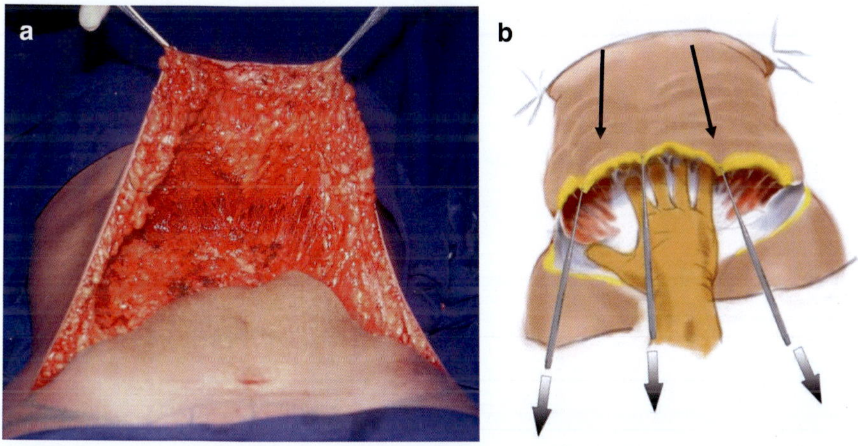

Fig. 4.3 The superior flap is already undermined until to reach the costal margin. (**a**) Perioperative photo demonstrates that the superior panniculus flap is pulled upwards showing the rib margin; (**b**) scheme shows the superior panniculus flap is undermined and pulled downwards indicating by arrows and the surgeon's hand is placed on the raw area in order to pull it properly

1999a, b) in order to keep it in its natural position on the musculoaponeurotic wall for its later reimplantation into the abdominal wall. Making an adequate evaluation of the panniculus resection is the main surgical principle introduced by Sinder, R. (1975a, b, c), which represents an important approach in that it avoids exerting excessive tension on the abdominal flap after the final suture (Figs. 4.2a, 4.3b, and 4.4a).

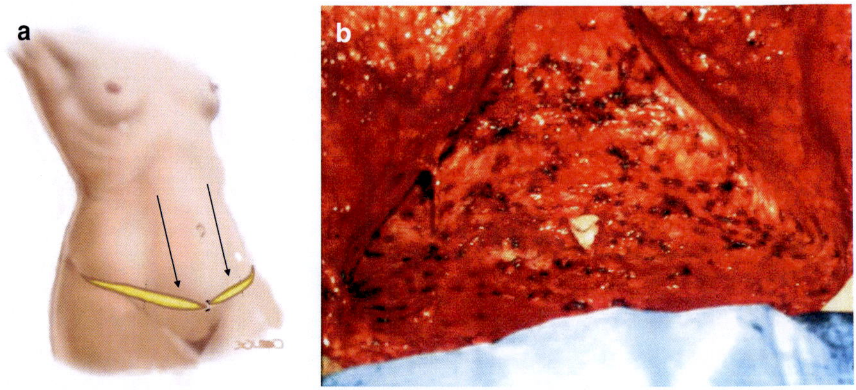

Fig. 4.4 Traction of the superior abdominal panniculus flap and resection of the infra umbilical cutaneous area. (**a**) Diagram showing traction downwards of the superior flap to determine the adequate cutaneous incision on supra pubic region. The arrows indicate the direction of traction with a temporary stich on midline; (**b**) perioperative photo where one can see the raw area of the abdominal area after ressecção of the infra umbilical panniculus when reinforcement of muscular aponeurotic wall was done

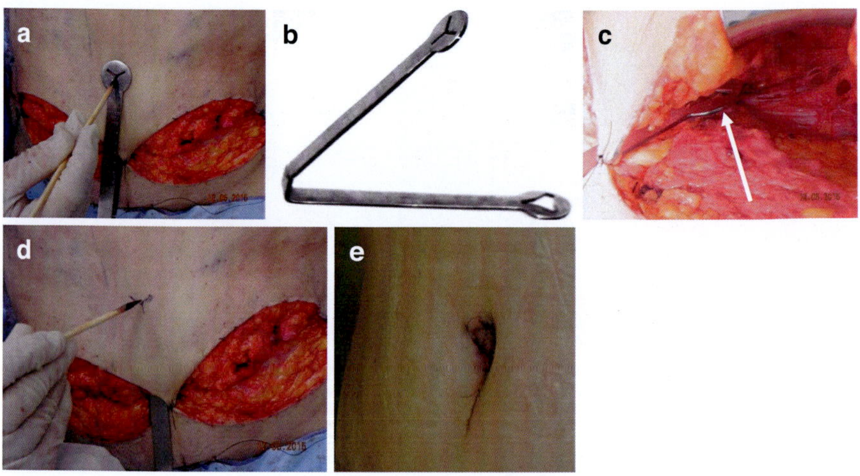

Fig. 4.5 Perioperative photos demonstrating creation and demarcation of the new umbilical region during abdominoplasty. Photo (**a**) one can see a temporary stitch is done on midline and the superior segment of my surgical instrument is placed on the abdominal flap to demarcate the new umbilical area; (**b**) photo of my instrument with two segments articulated between them; (**c**) the arrow indicates the lower segment of the instrument placed on the umbilicus to project the new location of the umbilical area on the abdominal panniculus flap; (**d**) the new umbilical region is determined with three triangular flaps; (**e**) close up of the new umbilical region one week after surgery

After properly resecting the infraumbilical panniculus, the plication of the musculoaponeurotic structures is conducted to reshape the body contouring. The umbilicus is then reimplanted into the abdominal flap by employing my surgical instrument (Fig. 4.5) (Avelar 1983).

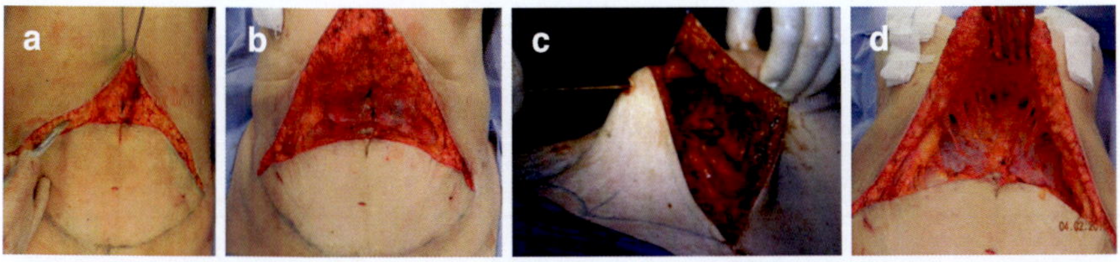

Fig. 4.6 Photos showing liposuction procedure on the supra umbilical panniculus during lipoabdominoplasty through Sinder's technique. Photo (**a**) Sinder's incision was done passing through umbilicus and the supra umbilical flap is puling upwards; (**b**) the upper flap is then pulled upwards; (**c**) left profile view showing the upper abdominal panniculus is held by surgeon's left hand and the cannula passes between his fingers with forth and backwards movements below fascia superficialis; (**d**) wide view from bottom showing the superior abdominal panniculus is lifted where one can see preservation of all perforator vessels

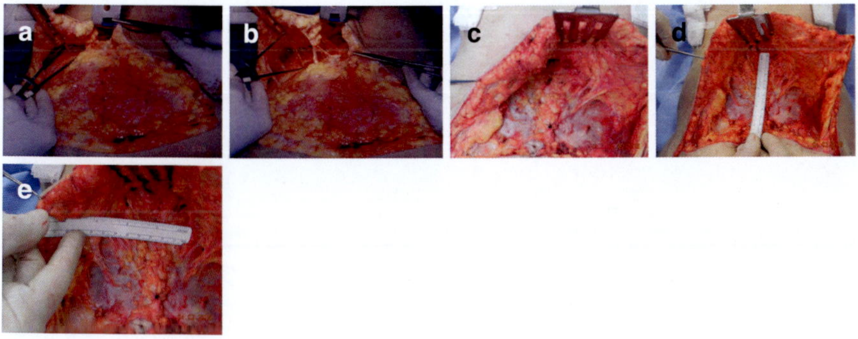

Fig. 4.7 Photos perioperative showing preservation and elongation of the perforator vessels during lipoabdominoplasty performed through Sinder's technique associated with Avelar's method without panniculus undermining. Photo (**a**) a compass shows length of the perforator vessels; (**b**) under traction of the abdominal flap they elongate without any damage; (**c**) wide view of the upper abdominal area; (**d**) with a ruler and measurement of the vertical distance from umbilical to xyphoid process is about 20 cm; (**e**) the lateral distance is about 14 cm without any damage to the perforator vessels as it is the main surgical principle of Avelar's method

However, I also used to employ Sinder's technique, without panniculus undermining (Avelar 1999, 2000a, b), but in combination with liposuction (Fig. 4.6), which is also a safe surgical option. In such an associated procedure, the surgical demarcation is similar to that already described above, but the operation is performed without panniculus undermining, following previous descriptions (Avelar 1999, 2000a, b). The surgery starts by making cutaneous incisions into the umbilicus, followed by liposuction on the superior abdominal panniculus flap while preserving the perforator vessels, which is the essential surgical principle of my method (Figs. 4.6 and 4.7). Resecting the infraumbilical panniculus is performed without undermining, as described in my original publications (Fig. 4.8). The plication of the musculoaponeurotic wall is carried out while preserving the perforator vessels, which provides adequate vascularization to the remaining abdominal panniculus (Fig. 4.9). The method to create this new umbilical region follows the descriptions above (Fig. 4.10) (Avelar 1999, 2000a, b).

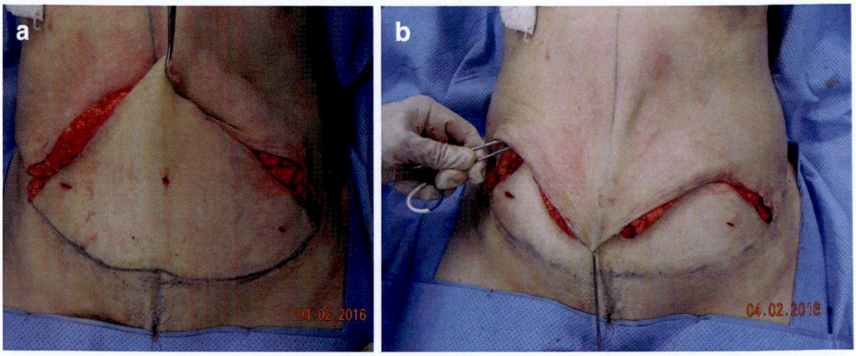

Fig. 4.8 Perioperative photos demonstrating another procedure to demarcate the adequate level of the incision on supra pubic region for resection of the abdominal panniculus. Photo (**a**) using a forceps to hold the superior border of the panniculus to be resected; (**b**) with one hand the surgeon pushs it upwards as high as possible and with another hand the supra umbilical panniculus flap is pulling downwards to determine the safe position of the lower incision

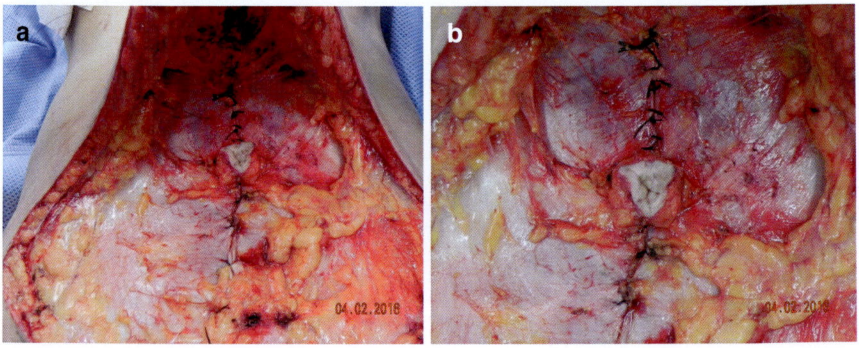

Fig. 4.9 Photos perioperatives demonstrating reinforcement of the muscular aponeurotic abdominal wall during lipoabdominoplasty through Sinder's technique. Photo (**a**) wide view of the raw area of the abdominal surface with plication is performed without any bleeding all over with preservation of the perforator vessels; (**b**) close up of the umbilicus with its cutaneous surface triangular shape (Avelar technique)

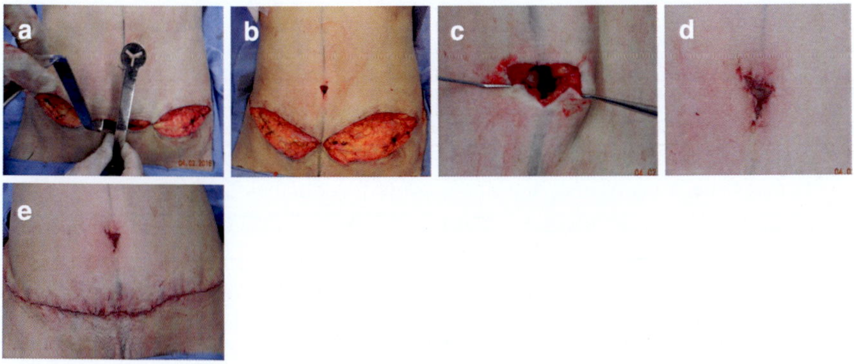

Fig. 4.10 Photos perioperatives demonstrating demarcating the new location of the umbilicus on abdominal flap after reinforcement of the muscular aponeurotic abdominal wall during lipoabdominoplasty through Sinder's technique. Photo (**a**) a temporary stitch is done approximating the inferior border of the superior flap to the border of the supra pubic region with Avelar's instrument introduced below the flap; (**b**) through the superior segment of the instrument the umbilical region is already incised creating three cutaneous small triangular flaps; (**c**) close up of the umbilical region that it is possible to see the umbilicus underneath; (**d**) the umbilicus is already sutured to triangular flaps coming from abdominal flap; (**e**) final suture of the wound

Technique

Surgical planning is an essential step to take before any operation, even more when abdominoplasty is to be performed because several circumstances must be previously evaluated. Measuring the anatomic references points of the abdomen is required to gain sufficient indications before an operation and to conclude the final examination. All these preparations must be carried out during consultation, giving all the information to the patient about their operation.

Surgical Demarcation

Predemarcation is a useful procedure when the patient is already in the hospital and awake as long as it occurs before they have been given medication. When the patient is in the operating room under general or epidural anesthesia, the definitive marks are made. The lower line lies on the suprapubic region with lateral prolongation up to the iliac spine (Fig. 4.1). Another curve line is made by passing by umbilicus with lateral prolongation until it has reached the end of the previous one. The umbilicus can also be demarcated by following Avelar's technique (Avelar 1976a, b, 1979, 1983), which should be used to create a natural umbilical region while avoiding leaving a circular scar around it.

The Operation

Once the patient is under anesthesia the definitive demarcations are done following the previous ones. Local infiltration is done with lidocaine plus epinephrine following the lines of demarcations to avoid bleeding during surgery. The operation starts by cutaneous incisions on the superior line until to reaches the muscular aponeurotic plan followed by panniculus undermining up to rib costal cartilage (Fig. 2) as the original Sinder`s descriptions (1979).

This surgical stage may also be performed without panniculus undermining (Fig. 4.6). The umbilicus is isolated by making triangular incisions around it by following to my technique (Avelar 1976a, b, 1979, 1983). Once the upper abdominal flap has been detached, the surgical table must be bent so that the patient's torso is elevated enough to carry out the next steps of the operation (Fig. 4.2). A similar procedure is part of a surgery performed without panniculus undermining (Figs. 4.7 and 4.8).

The surgeon pulls the upper undermined abdominal flap downward until it has reached the suprapubic region (Figs. 4.3 and 4.4). Afterward, the inferior incision of the abdominoplasty is demarcated. Next, the infraumbilical panniculus is resected and careful hemostasis is carried out. Following the operation, the musculoaponeurotic wall is reinforced from the xyphoid process to the pubic region.

A temporary stitch is used suture from the upper abdominal flap to the lower edge on the suprapubic region (Figs. 4.3b and 4.4a). Afterward, using my surgical instrument, the new location of the umbilicus is reached, at which point triangular incisions are made, creating three small flaps to be sutured to the other three coming from the umbilicus (Fig. 4.5) (Avelar 1976a, b, 1979). Moreover, when lipoabdominoplasty is performed by using Sinder's technique, the perforator vessels are not damaged, which is the essential surgical principle of my method (Figs. 4.7, 4.8, and 4.9) (Avelar 1999, 2000a, b) after the plication of the musculoaponeurotic wall has been completed.

Next, the new umbilical region is demarcated by using Avelar's surgical instrument, creating three small triangular flaps on the abdominal flap (Fig. 4.10), and the wound is next sutured as a part of a routine procedure.

Creating a Triangular Dermal-Adipose Flap

In thin people, the belly clearly has a peculiar superficial anatomy, with depressions or folds corresponding to the weakness of the rectus abdominalis muscle and musculoaponeurotic structures. Importantly, the supraumbilical area, called the linea albae (at the midline), contains very thin adipose layers. Here, the thickness of the subcutaneous layer of fat (adipose tissue) is not uniform, and it is thinner at the level of the umbilicus. To treat such a lack of adipose tissue, some surgeons (myself including) used to suture both sides of the borders to improve the tissue's thickness.

However, following Sinder's technique, a triangular dermal-adipose flap is adequately prepared in the suprapubic region to embed it underneath the abdominal panniculus flap, which will expand its thickness. Quite often, the protuberance or salience at the level of the muscle masses, the suprapubic adipose tissue, or the mons pubis do not meet enough of the anatomic conditions to improve the thickness of the abdominal flap.

Instead of these resources, Sinder (1975a, b) prefers to prepare a suprapubic triangular dermal-adipose flap with an inferior pedicle at the beginning of the operation, and after the musculoaponeurotic plane has been sufficiently reinforced, he imbeds it underneath the medial part of the large lowering flap, initially corresponding to the supraumbilical region called the linea albae. Finally, the border of the upper abdominal flap is sutured to the inferior edge of the suprapubic incision. The triangular dermal-adipose flap is introduced underneath the panniculus of the abdominal flap to yield a smooth result (Figs. 4.5 and 4.10). The aesthetic results are similar if the abdominoplasty is performed by using Sinder's technique with a wide undermining of the abdominal flap or if it is carried out without panniculus undermining. The advantages of each method are similar (Figs. 4.11, 4.12, and 4.13).

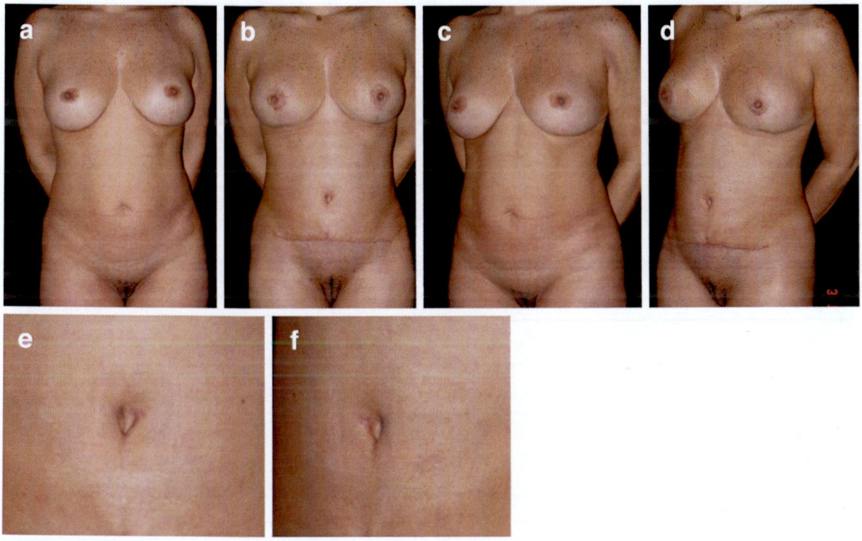

Fig. 4.11 A 49-year-old patient underwent abdominoplasty through Sinder's technique, combined with secondary mastopexy. Photos (**a, c**) pre-operative; (**b, d**) after operations. The triangular dermo adipose flap according to Sinder's technique was created on supra pubic region to provide adequate support to the abdominal flap; (**e**) close up in frontal view of the umbilical region created through Avelar's technique; (**f**) the same umbilical region in left oblique view shows the surgical result with natural appearence

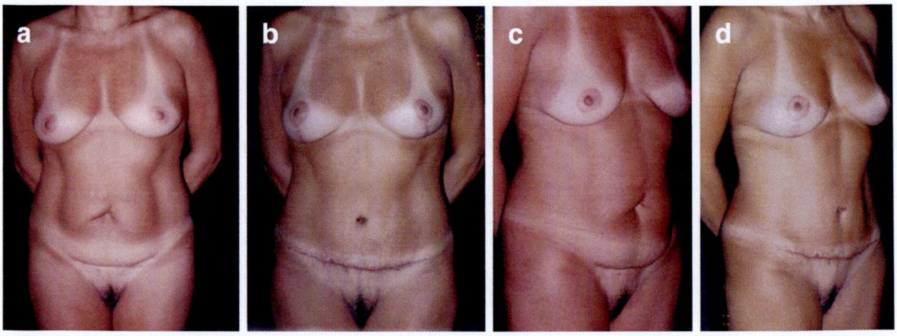

Fig. 4.12 A 51-year-old patient with unaesthetic and deep surgical scars on supra pubic region underwent abdominoplasty according to Sinder's technique, combined with mastopexy without prosthesis implant. Photos (**a, c**) pre-operative; (**b, d**) 6 months after operations. The new location of the umbilicus was determined following Avelar's technique. A triangular dermo adipose flap was created following Sinder's technique and imbedded underneath of the panniculus of the abdominal flap

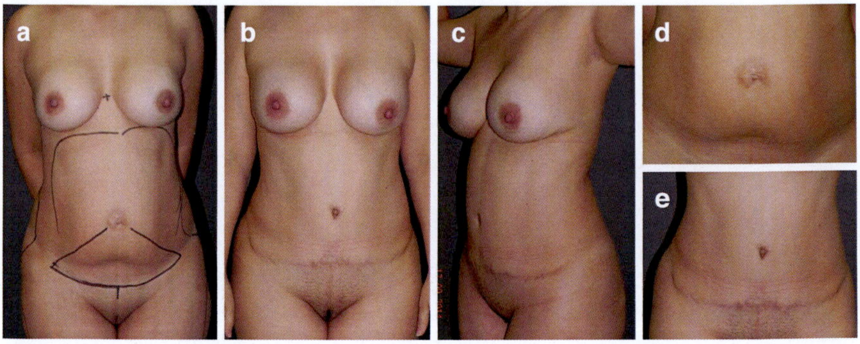

Fig. 4.13 A 48-year-old patient with deep and unaesthetic surgical scars on supra pubic region and on the umbilicus as well, underwent abdominoplasty by Sinder's technique, Photos (**a, d**) pre-operative showing unaesthetic scars on supra pubic region and on umbilicus as well, (**b, c, e**) post-operative photos. A triangular dermo adipose flap was created according to Sinder's technique and imbedded it underneath the panniculus of the abdominal flap. The new umbilical region was created following Avelar's technique achieving natural and harmonious aesthetic appearance

Discussion

At the beginning of my career, I used to employ Pitanguy's technique (Figs. 4.14 and 4.15) as a continuation of the useful knowledge that I absorbed from the author (Pitanguy 1967, 1974; Pitanguy et al. 1974). However, as soon as I learned Sinder's technique, I started using it. Especially in patients with a flaccid or voluminous abdomen, it is helpful for planning and operating by leaving a horizontal scar on the suprapubic region. When I introduced lipoabdominoplasty (Avelar 1999, 2000a, b), I could perform a similar procedure with wide abdominal panniculus undermining

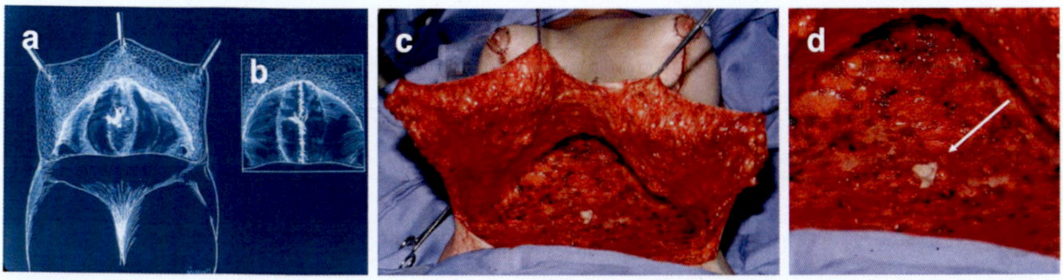

Fig. 4.14 Wide panniculus undermined during abdominoplasty performed by Pitanguy's technique. Diagram (**a**) shows wide undermining of the abdominal panniculus with severe diastasis of the rectus abdominalis; (**b**) after reinforcement of the musculo-aponeutic wall; (**c**) perioperative photo where one can see the abdominal flap already undermined is pulled upwards showing the triangular surface of the umbilicus according to my personal technique; (**d**) the arrow indicating the triangular surface of the umbilicus according to the technique

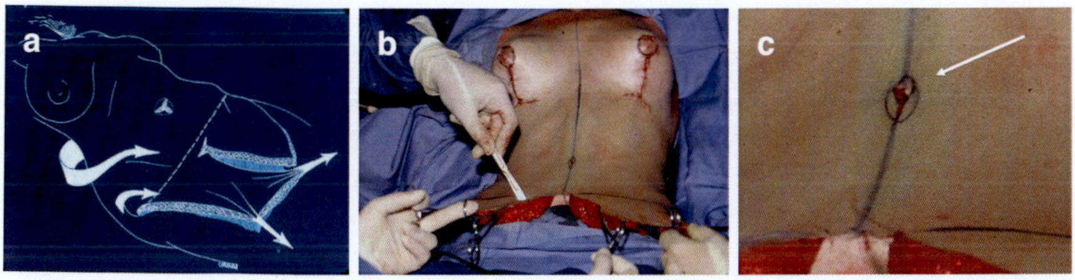

Fig. 4.15 Traction of the panniculus during abdominoplasty performed by Pitanguy's technique. Diagram (**a**) the arrows indicate traction and rotation of the abdominal panniculus from back forward, showing the triangular incision on the umbilical area; (**b**) perioperative photo where one can see the flap pulled from up downwards with resection of the excess of the abdominal panniculus being resected with knife; (**c**) photo in detail showing the three triangular small flaps of the umbilicus according to Avelar's technique

(Figs. 4.2, 4.3, 4.4, and 4.5) or without panniculus undermining (Figs. 4.6, 4.7, 4.8, 4.9, and 4.10). However, when there is poor elasticity and less flaccidity in the supraumbilical region, some difficulty may be encountered when bringing the upper abdominal flap to the suprapubic edge of the incision. If the suture is made under strong tension, it risks causing dehiscence in the central part of the wound and other complications. To avoid this risk, Sinder (1975a, b) introduced new concepts to abdominoplasty without any difficulty or excess tension in the suture of the operatory wound. If this is not the case, the inferior incision of the skin to be resected should be dislocated more upward in order to avoid excess tension in the suture (Figs. 4.11, 4.12, and 4.13).

When the flaccidity and/or excess of the skin is located in the infraumbilical portion or when there is little elasticity in the supraumbilical skin, Sinder's technique (1975a, b) is a useful approach. Sinder (1979) prefers to perform a simple suprapubic horizontal crescent-shaped resection with cranial concavity and without transposing the navel, as suggested by Jolly (1911) and Thorek (1942). In fact, the transposition of the umbilicus was introduced by Vernon (1957), which opened up a new era for abdominoplasty. If the navel is abnormally high, the umbilical pedicle is cut to its depth or to the aponeurotic fixation, and without any skin incision around it, a new navel fixation is lowered into position, according to normal anatomy (Callia 1965). This technique is described in detail in Chap. 12.

Conclusion

Sinder's technique is a very useful and safe approach for performing abdominoplasty. The operation starts by making an incision into the superior border of the area to be resected and according to the surgical plan (Figs. 4.1, 4.2, and 4.3). The superior panniculus is then undermined on the supra-aponeurotic level until it has reached the border of the rim's costal cartilage. Meticulous hemostasia must be caried out (Fig. 4.4b). At this time in the operation, bend the surgical table such that the extension of the resection of the lower panniculus can be properly evaluated. After correct demarcation, the panniculus of the infraumbilical region is removed, and the new umbilical region is marked by using my surgical instrument (Fig. 4.5) (Avelar 1976a, b, 1983). A similar procedure may be performed for a type of lipoabdominoplasty where the abdominal panniculus is not undermined, which is the basic surgical principle of this method (Figs. 4.6, 4.7, 4.8, 4.9, and 4.10). If the patient already has some abdominal scars caused by previous surgeries, then, depending their location and size, use Sinder's technique to determine the adequate placement of the final surgical scar (Figs. 4.11 and 4.12).

At the beginning of an operation that uses Sinder's technique, a suprapubic triangular dermal-adipose flap with an inferior pedicle should be prepared to embed it underneath the medial part of the abdominal panniculus flap. The behavior of the dermal-adipose flap replaces the thickness of the supraumbilical zone, or the linea albae.

References

Avelar JM (1976a) Umbilicoplasty – a technique without external scar (Umbilicoplastia uma técnica sem cicatriz externa). 13rd Bras Cong of Plast Surg and First Brazilian Cong of Aesthetic Surgery. (13° Congresso Brasileiro de Cirurgia Plástica e 1° Congr Bras Cir Estética), Porto Alegre – RS (Brazil) 81–82

Avelar JM (1976b) Umbilicoplasty - A technique without external scar. Cahiers de chirurgie Esthétique. Journees internationals de Chirurgie Esthetique. Vendredi 21 mai.

Avelar JM (1979) Umbilical scar – its importance and technique for creating during abdominoplasty (Cicatriz umbilical – da sua importância e da técnica de confecção nas abdominoplastias). Rev Bras Cir 1(2):41–52.

Avelar JM (1983) Abdominoplasty: technical refinements and analysis of 130 cases in 8 years' follow-up. Aesth Plast Surg 7:205–212.

Avelar JM (1999) Uma nova técnica de abdominoplastia – sistema vascular fechado de retalho subdérmico dobrado sobre si mesmo combinado com lipoaspiração (A new technique for abdominoplasty – closed vascular system of subdermal flap folded over itself combined to liposuction). Rev Bras Cir 88/89(1/6):3–20.

Avelar JM (1999a) Abdominoplasty: new concepts for a new technique. (Abdominoplastia: Nuevos conceptos para una nueva técnica). XXVI Annual International Symposium of Aesthetic Plastic Surgery, Chairman: Prof. Jose Guerrerosantos, Puerto Vallarta, Mexico.
Avelar JM (1999b) New concepts for abdominoplasty. (Novos conceitos para abdominoplastia). Paper presented at the 36th Congress of the Brazilian Society of Plastic Surgery, Rio de Janeiro, Brazil.
Avelar JM (2000a) Abdominoplasty without undermining (Abdominoplastia sem descolamento). São Paulo: XX Jorn. Paulista Cir Plast.
Avelar JM (2000b) Abdominoplasty: a new technique without undermining and fat layer removal (Abdominoplastia: uma nova técnica sem descolamento e remoção da camada de gordura). Arq Catarinense de Med 29:147–149.
Callia WE (1965) Contribuição ao estudo de correção cirúrgica do abdomen pêndulo e globus (contribution to the study of surgical correction of the pendulum abdomen and globus). original art. Doctoral Thesis Fac Med USP, São Paulo.
Jolly R (1911) Die operation des Fettbauches. Berl Klin Wochenschr 29:1317.
Pitanguy I (1967) Abdominal lipectomy: an approach to it through an analysis of 300 consecutive cases. Plast Reconstr Surg 40:384–391
Pitanguy I (1974) Yabar AA, Pires CEB, Motta SR Aspectos atuais em lipectomia abdominal. Rev Bras Cir 64(5/6):147–167.
Pitanguy I et al. (1974) Aspectos atuais em lipectomia abdominal. Rev Bras Cir 64(4/5): 49–164
Sinder R (1975a) Plastic surgery of the abdomen – personal technique with prior undermining of the supraumbilical flap – before infraumbilical resection and the use of the dermoadipose flap. (Cirurgia Plastica do Abdomen – Tecnica Pessoal com prévio descolamento do retalho supraumbilical – antes da Ressecção Infraumbilical e uso de retalho dermoadiposo) VI Int Congr of Plast and Reconstructive Surg, Paris, 25 Aug.
Sinder R (1975b) Plastic Surgery of the Abdomen. Personal technique. In: Abstracts of the 6th International Congress of plastic and reconstructive surgery. Masson, Paris, pp 584–591.
Sinder R (1975c) Use of a decorticated dermo-adipose fl ap in abdominoplasty. Abstracts of the sixth international congress of plastic and reconstructive surgery, Paris, 24–29
Sinder R (1979) Abdominal plastic surgery. (Cirurgia plástica abdominal) Ed. by Sinder, Niteroi. Rio de Janeiro, Brasil.
Thorek M (1942) Plastic surgery of the breast and abdominal wall. Ed. Charles C. Thomas, Springfield.
Vernon S (1957) Umbilical transplantation upward and abdominal contouring in lipectomy. Am J Surg 94:490–492.

Chapter 5
The Beginning, Development, and Current Status of Lipoabdominoplasty: New Concepts for Abdominoplasty

Juarez Moraes Avelar

Abstract Ever since I started my professional activates in 1973, I noticed that there were several fields in plastic surgery that needed technical improvements to solve multiple problems. In my opinion, abdominoplasty was one of those areas that required new surgical fundaments and other techniques to achieve better results and minimize complications.

At that time, I identified three essential topics that needed new surgical approaches for abdominoplasty: (1) the creation of a new umbilical region; (2) adiposities remaining in the silhouette of the body; and (3) the high incidence of local and systemic complications. I concluded that those three topics required new anatomic studies and new techniques to achieve better surgical, more-aesthetic results.

1. The creation of the new umbilical region was needed for the transposition of the umbilicus and for other techniques that leave circular scars around the incisions, which may lead to retraction and contraction scars. To avoid circular scars, I developed a new method of making triangular incisions.
2. Remaining local adiposities were improved through the liposuction technique introduced by Illouz which reshaped the body's contouring. However, redundant skin after liposuction on the abdomen bothers patients and surgeons. My first operations inspired me to consider two problems: (1) the unknown anatomy of the subcutaneous compartment and (2) the redundant skin of the abdominal wall after liposuction.

   To study the anatomy of the abdominal wall, I performed dissections combined with liposuction on cadavers, which enabled me to describe the areolar and lamellar layers and the fascia superficialis between them. Concerning redundant skin after liposuction, I performed this combined procedure to remove it, and in this way, a new procedure was introduced.

J. M. Avelar (✉)
Brazilian Scientific Institute of Plastic and Reconstructive Surgery, São Paulo, Brazil

J. M. Avelar, R. Cavalcanti Ribeiro (eds.), *Body Contouring*,
https://doi.org/10.1007/978-3-031-42802-9_5

3. Complications after and during abdominoplasty, especially in combination with liposuction, remained great challenges. After my anatomical study, I concluded that I could combine those two procedures as long as the perforator vessels did not sustain damage during surgery. Therefore, I described and introduced a new technique, namely lipoabdominoplasty, which reduced complications and achieved smooth body contouring.

Keywords Abdominoplasty · Liposuction · Lipoabdominoplasty · Combined approach · Without undermining

Introduction

When I looked back on 50 years of performing plastic surgery, I noticed that several fields still required technical changes to improve aesthetics of surgical results. At that time, I identified that abdominoplasty was one of the areas that had several complications that hampered achieving better surgical results. Among surgeries, abdominoplasty was one of the most complex and presented challenges to all plastic surgeons around the world.

The first abdominoplasty was performed by Kelly (1899), which was the beginning of a long and rich history of such surgeries over the past century, followed by many other authors' improving the aesthetic outcomes of surgeries on the abdominal wall. Horizontal incisions were described by Malbec (1948), Callia (1965), Pontes (1965, 1982), Pitanguy (1967, 1977, 1982), Avelar (1976a, b, 1983a, b, 1985a, b, 1999a, b, 2000a, b), Guerrerosantos (1982a, b), Guerrerosantos et al. (1980), Planas (1982), Sinder (1975, 1982), Hinderer (1982), and Cavalcanti and Cavalcanti (1982), among others. Vertical incisions were described by Babcock (1916). The circular approach was proposed by Gonzales-Ulloa (1959, 1982), Vilain and Dubousset (1964), and Vilain (1982). Submammary incisions were described by Thorek (1939), Rebello et al. (1972), and Rebello (1982). More recently, I intro duced (Avelar 1999a, b, 2000a, b) a crescent-shaped skin resection on bilateral submammary folds combined with liposuction to improve the aesthetics of upper abdominoplasty.

According to my analysis and reflections, there have been three main complications for every plastic surgeon: new ideas to add to basic techniques, new concepts for abdominoplasty, and more anatomical knowledge. In my opinion, surgical performance should minimize complications during and after surgery and improve the aesthetics of surgical results. In my practice, meeting these demands has been complex ever since I started my professional activities in 1973. These complications needed specific approaches to give plastic surgeons more enthusiasm for performing abdominoplasty. The anterior abdominal wall is a specific anatomical structure that protects the internal organs and gives an aesthetic image to the human body.

When performing any surgery on this area, remodeling the body's contouring was a constant challenge.

Since the beginning of my practice, I have identified three essential topics that needed new surgical approaches for abdominoplasty: (1) the creation of a new umbilical region; (2) the remaining adiposities leaving behind an inelegant silhouette of the body; (3) the high incidence of local and systemic complications. I concluded that those three topics required new anatomic studies and new techniques to achieve better surgical aesthetic results and minimize patients' suffering.

1. In all cases of full abdominoplasty, a new umbilical area must be created because the umbilicus is transposed to that new location (Vernon 1957). Ever since I started my professional activities, I have devoted considerable effort to trying to avoid leaving behind a final circular scar around the new umbilicus, which was the final result of every technique. Therefore, I developed a new method making triangular incisions around the umbilicus, similar to atypical Z-plasty (Avelar 1976a, b, 1978, 1979, 1983a, b). Following my procedure, the final scar is not a circular one, the aim of which is to avoid retraction and contraction, which themselves may leave an inelegant appearance. Therefore, in my hands and publications, one of the three main complications in abdominoplasty had been solved. My method was well understood and employed by other surgeons for the reconstruction of a new umbilicus (Lessa 1982), even as a routine approach during abdominoplasty (Daher 1982).
2. Remaining adiposities leave behind an inelegant silhouette of the body, but this has been improved through the liposuction technique introduced by Illouz (1980, 1983a, b, 1984, 1986a, b), yielding better aesthetic results on body contouring. After I went to Paris in early 1983 with the specific purpose of observing Illouz's operations to learn his new technique, I noted two problems: first, the unknown anatomy of the subcutaneous compartment where the cannulas worked during the liposuction procedure, and second, the redundant skin of the abdominal wall after liposuction.
3. The high incidence of local and systemic complications during and after abdominoplasty were still great challenges to solve, as reported by Guerrerosantos (1982a, b), Guerrerosantos et al. (1980), D'Assumpção (1982), Mélega (1982), and Martins (1982).

When I observed Illouz's operations and performed my first liposuction operations on the abdominal wall, I concluded that the cannula worked in an unknown compartment of the subcutaneous panniculus. Since the beginning, I decided to research the anatomy of this region by performing several anatomical dissections and liposuctions on cadavers to study the subcutaneous layers and the behavior of these tissues after liposuction (Avelar 1986a, b, c, 1987, 1989).

On the other hand, to treat the excess skin on the abdominal wall after liposuction, I decided to simultaneously resect it. In this way, a new approach was developed for abdominoplasty that became well understood by and earned the acceptance of plastic surgeons (Avelar 1985a, b, 1986b). A new field was thus introduced: aesthetic surgery on the abdominal wall as a complementary procedure to solve the excess of panniculus after liposuction. However, liposuction on the submentonian and submandibular regions in patients without cutaneous flaccidity, even in association with rhytidoplasty, did not present redundant skin after liposuction, or those complications arose after abdominoplasty (Avelar 1983b, 1985c).

The combined procedure of liposuction with resecting excess skin during abdominoplasty didn't bring new kinds of complications, but the high incidence of seroma, the slough and necrosis of the panniculus, local infection, and hyperpigmentation of the skin remained. In light of these frequent complications, after a short period of time, I made the radical decision to no longer perform such combined procedures (Avelar 1988). Over a period of 10 years, I no longer combined both procedures during abdominoplasty, but rather, I returned to my previous anatomical research on the abdominal wall (Avelar 1986a, b, c, 1987, 1989), looking for a way to solve the problems stemming from this combination of liposuction with resecting the redundant skin of the abdominal wall. In my previous anatomical study, I described and recommended that liposuction should be performed primarily on lamellar layer (the deeper one) in order to preserve the perforator vessels during surgery (Figs. 5.5d and 5.6d, e, f). This technical principle has been recommended ever since I described the anatomy of the abdominal wall. After 10 years of reviewing my previous anatomic study and reflecting on the aforementioned complications, I finally concluded that I could combine those two procedures simultaneously (liposuction and the resection of redundant skin of the abdomen wall) as long as the perforator vessels (arteries, veins, and lymphatics) did not sustain damage during surgery, thus avoiding dead space (Avelar 1999a, b, c, 2000a, b, 2001a, b).

All these surgical principles are part of an evolution in abdominoplasty where the perforator vessels work as multiple pedicles that provide adequate arterial blood supply to the remaining abdominal panniculus, preserve venous circulation and lymphatic circulation, and avoid seroma formation. Thanks to the perforator vessels and because there is no dead space around the abdomen, no internal suture from the panniculus to the aponeurosis is needed.

Therefore, I described and introduced new concepts to minimize complications during and after surgery and to improve the aesthetics of the surgical results. Such a combined procedure is called lipoabdominoplasty, for which I established new surgical principles after a long time as the result of my anatomical research into solutions for some of the perioperative and postoperative complications. So, my dream at the beginning of my career in 1973 became a reality. When liposuction was introduced by Illouz (1980, 1983a, b, 1984, 1986a, b), I proposed a combination of his new technique with traditional abdominoplasty to solve several complications during and after surgery (Avelar 1985a, b, 1986b).

Technique

Surgical Planning: Classification

According to clinical evaluations and patient selections, the surgical planning for lipoabdominoplasty with reduced panniculus undermining may be classified in four types of operations: lower lipoabdominoplasty, upper lipoabdominoplasty, upper and lower lipoabdominoplasty, and full lipoabdominoplasty (which is described in Chap. X). Also, Erfon created a classification system that is an excellent guideline for reaching an adequate orientation before surgery (Erfon 2000). The subject of this chapter is restricted to full lipoabdominoplasty, through which all skin above the suprapubic region and below the umbilicus must be resected. In fact, the whole abdomen wall is treated, but the perforator vessels are not cut, because in my original descriptions (Avelar 1999a, b, c, 2000a, b), the remaining panniculus is not to be undermined. That is the main difference between my technique and the conventional abdominoplasty, where wide undermining is performed and all the perforator vessels are cut.

Surgeons *must* carry out a preoperative evaluation before planning any operation (Fig. 5.1) to take an adequate measurement of the anatomical points at the location of the umbilicus, and the patient may follow the surgeon's evaluation. The surgeon must hold the panniculus below the umbilicus and be sure that they can resect it and that the skin of the periumbilical area can reach the suprapubic incision. It means that the upper abdomen may be pulled downward to cover the entire area of the abdominal wall. Also, the surgeon should examine the patient in a standing position in this evaluation. I have mirrors strategically positioned in my examination room so that patients can see all the anatomical abnormalities in their bodies' contours (Fig. 5.2) (Avelar 1986a, b, c).

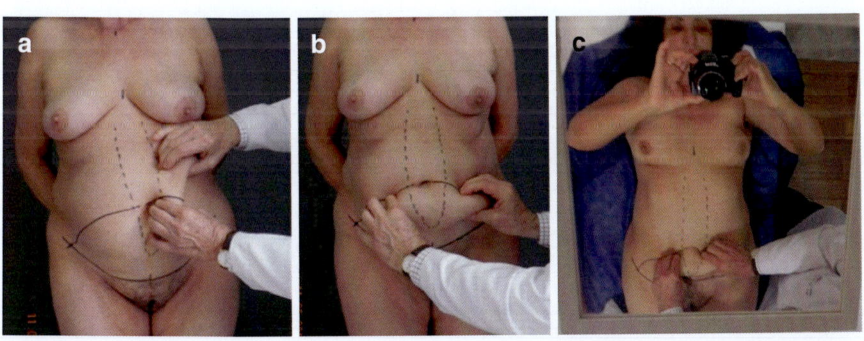

Fig. 5.1 Pre-operatory examination and demarcation for full lipoabdominoplasty. Photo (**a**) patient in standing position the abdominal panniculus is held in order to evaluate its thickness on upper abdominal wall; (**b**) muscular diastasis is demarcated on each side of the rectus abdominalis and the infraumbilical area is pulled downwards to evaluate the possibility of its resection during operation; (**c**) the patient with a camera takes photo through a mirror placed on ceiling of the examining room, following preoperatory examination and demarcation as well

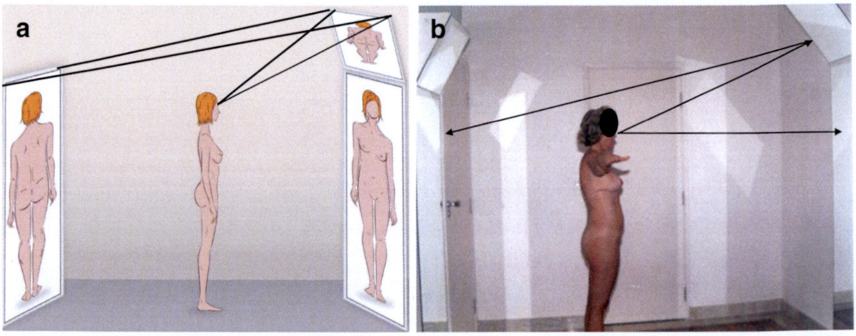

Fig. 5.2 A set of mirrors in the examining room at my clinic in order the patient can see herself or himself in frontal, posterior, and lateral view simultaneously. Photo (**a**) a diagram to demonstrate my examining; (**b**) photo of a patient in front of one vertical mirror and she can see herself in all sides

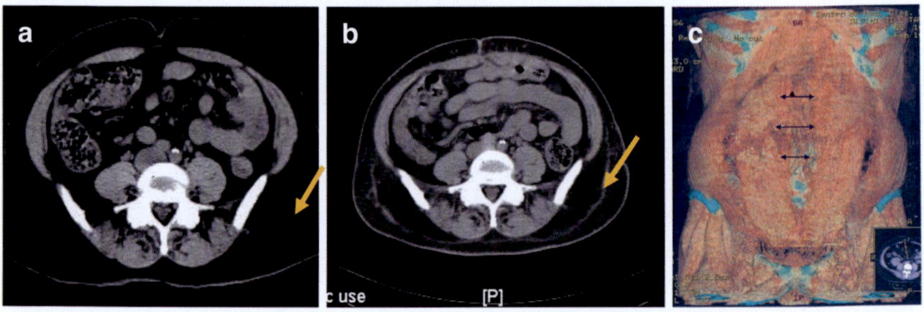

Fig. 5.3 Computerized tomography is a useful rotinaire exam before lipoabdominoplasty for confirmation the surgical evaluation of patient presenting diastasis of the rectus abdominalis muscle on the umbilical region. Photo (**a**) before surgery showing diastasis of the rectus. The arrow indicates the fascia superficialis all around the abdominal wall; (**b**) same patient after operation with reinforcement of the muscular aponeurotic wall. The arrow shows the fascia superficialis is very close to muscular aponeurotic wall, however in supra iliac regions it is well preserved in the middle of the panniculus; (**c**) front view of TC showing diastasis of the rectus abdominis

The Operation

After completing the above steps, the surgeon might have enough information to choose the appropriate technique for lipoabdominoplasty. Each patient must present normal blood tests and must have undergone a fundamental clinical evaluation performed by physician that includes an electrocardiogram (ECG) and other specific exams, such as computerized tomography (CT), when they are necessary to evaluate the diastasis of the rectus abdominalis (Fig. 5.3). A complete series of photos of the regions to be treated must have already been taken.

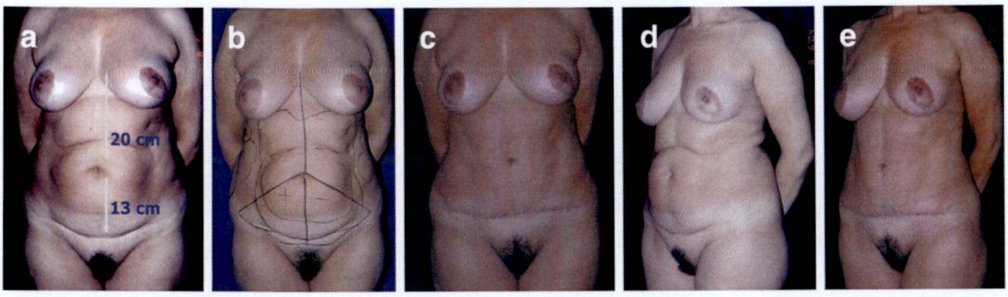

Fig. 5.4 A 65-year-old patient underwent full lipoabdominoplasty following the technique described. Photos (**a, b**) mesurement and technical demarcations prior surgery; (**c**) after full lipoabdominoplasty; (**d**) same patient in left oblique view; (**e**) after full lipoabdominoplasty with creation of the new umbilical region

Preliminary Demarcations

All my operations are performed at the hospital under epidural or general anesthesia, where patients stay for at least 24 h. I prefer to demarcate the patient's body the day before the operation. Because I have a useful set of mirrors, my patient can see and follow my demarcations (Fig. 5.4). Patient should see their deformities once more, and surgeons must explain the relevant surgical details to them. The patient must stay in a standing position in front of the mirrors in order to follow my drawing on their body (Avelar 1986c). After a careful analysis, all the deformities are drawn. Two areas must be well demarcated: (1) the area for full-thickness skin resection where liposuction will be performed on the panniculus and the location of the final scars and (2) the areas for deep liposuction (below the fascia superficialis) on the upper abdomen wall, the lateral sides, and the posterior regions (Fig. 5.4). Premedication is a matter of a routine and is prescribed by an anesthesiologist after a clinical evaluation has been completed before surgery.

Full Lipoabdominoplasty

Full lipoabdominoplasty is the most frequently performed procedure in abdominoplasty; it is combined with liposuction and skin resection on the entire suprapubic region to repair abnormalities in the abdominal wall. In this modality of lipoabdominoplasty, the umbilicus is transposed and a new umbilical area is created. Once again, the selection of patients before surgery is a fundamental step for the surgeon to evaluate whether to remove all the skin of the suprapubic region, and the cutaneous area above the umbilicus may be pulled downward to be sutured to the inferior border of the surgical incision.

Surgical Demarcations During Surgery

Two areas must be well demarcated to reach an adequate orientation during surgery:

1. The area for skin resection corresponding to the whole segment on the suprapubic region that is below the umbilicus needs demarcation. My preferred technique for drawing is similar to Callia's technique (Callia 1965). Therefore, the final scar will be as small as possible where the lateral segment is placed on the inguinal folds on each side and a convex line is placed on the pubic area (Fig. 5.4).
2. The area for liposuction on the abdominal wall above the umbilicus and on the lateral and posterior aspects of the torso also need demarcation. Therefore, all deformities (localized adiposities and skin excess) must be drawn on the day before surgery.

Liposuction Procedure

The patient on the operating table stays in the supine position, and after anesthesia, the abdomen and lateral aspects of the torso are prepared. Before starting the liposuction procedure, local infiltration with a special solution is carried out according to surgical planning. My preference of solution is a serum of 1000 mL, plus 2 mg of epinephrine—or 2 mg per 1000 mL. Usually, at this volume, the abdomen and lateral sides of the torso can be infiltrated as well. The infiltration is performed at two levels on two areas:

1. In all the regions where liposuction is performed, the infiltration is deep (in the lamellar layer, below the fascia superficialis)
2. In the area for skin resection, the infiltration is carried out in the suprapubic region underneath the skin and the full thickness of the panniculus (in the areolar and lamellar layers) (Fig. 5.5).

After infiltration, the surgeon should wait at least 15 min before starting the liposuction procedure, which is performed at two levels in those two previously demarcated areas:

1. Full-thickness liposuction is conducted on all the areas in the suprapubic region and below the umbilicus (Fig. 5.5). Afterward, the perforator vessels and connective tissues are preserved, and that area becomes deep because of the absence of adipose tissue (Fig. 5.6).
2. Deep liposuction (below the fascia superficial) is performed on all the regions where the abdominal panniculus remains with its normal cutaneous covering. Therefore, all the adipose tissue in the lamellar layer is aspirated (Fig. 5.7). I already described that liposuction must first be performed on half of the abdominal wall until the ideal thickness has been reached. The other side undergoes liposuction only after the first procedure has concluded. Thus, the surgeon may

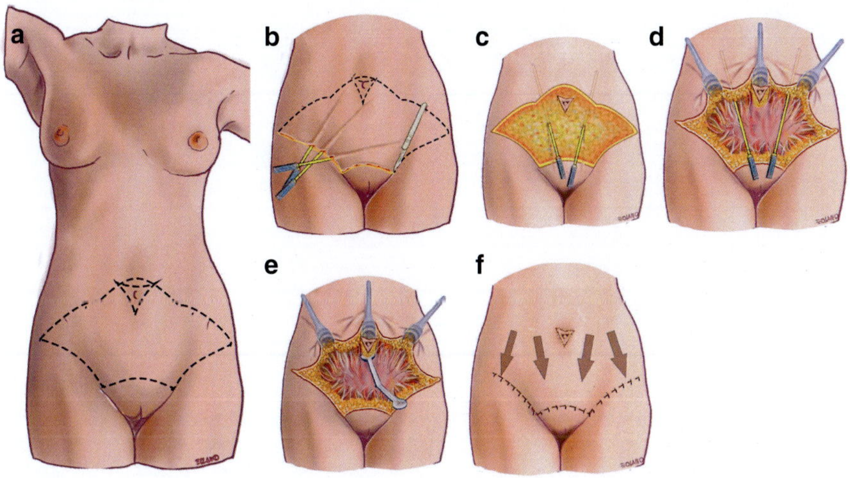

Fig. 5.5 Sequential drawing showing the technique of full lipoabdominoplasty. (**a**) Preoperatory demarcation of the area of skin resection, even my triangular incisions around the umbilicus; (**b**) liposuction is performed on full-thickness of the panniculus on supra pubic region; (**c, d**) skin resection was done following by deep liposuction (below fascia superficialis) on supra umbilical region; (**e**) my surgical instrument is placed on the umbilicus in order to demarcate its new location on the remaining abdominal flap; (**f**) the superior abdominal panniculus flap is pulled downwards indicated by arrows and the new umbilical region is already created

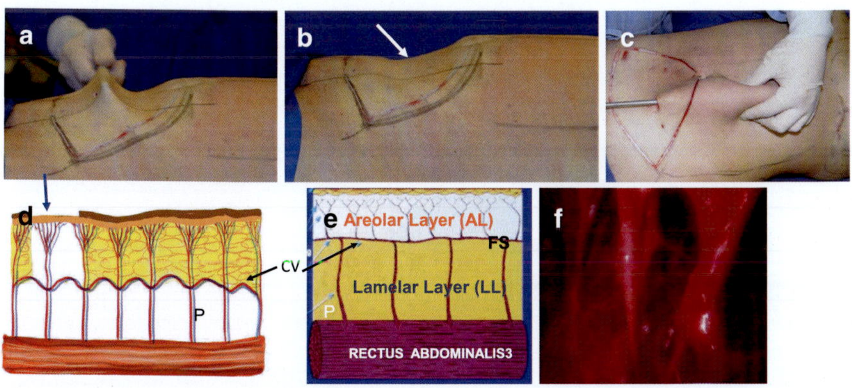

Fig. 5.6 Sequential photos (**a–c**) and diagrams (**d, e**) showing liposuction on full lipoabdominoplasty. Photo (**a**) profile view showing that the suprapubic region until the umbilicus is done in full thickness of the lamellar (LL) and areolar one (AL); (**b**) on the same patient one can see a depression in all infra umbilical region, indicated by arrow, caused by absence of the panniculus all over the region; (**c**) one can see deep liposuction (below fascia superficialis) (FS) on segment without cutaneous resection; (**d, e**) diagrams show that liposuction was done in all thickness of the panniculus on infra umbilical region (indicated by arrow) one can see the perforator vessels (P) coming from rectus abdominalis muscle (RAM), are preserved; (**f**) photo from inside of the panniculus during surgery showing perforator vessels are preserved

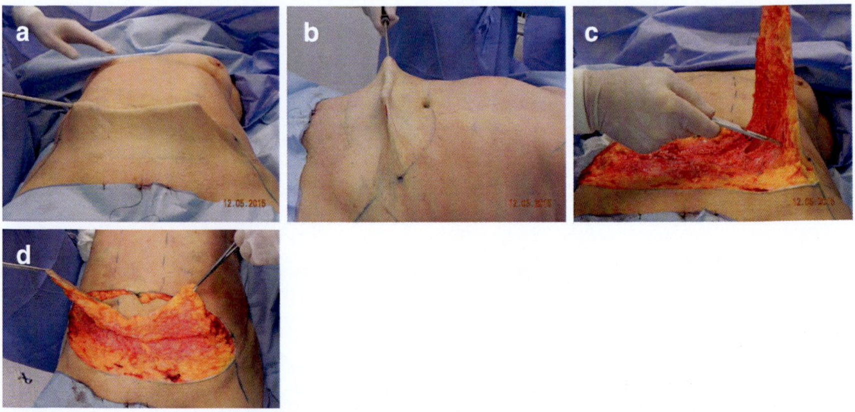

Fig. 5.7 Perioperative photos demonstrating full lipoabdominoplasty. Liposuction is done on full thickness of the panniculus of the supra pubic region. Photo (**a**) from bottom one can see the cannula below the skin; (**b**) on lateral view after liposuction showing that the skin is free of adipose tissue; (**d**) resection of the skin after liposuction; (**c**) the skin is being resected; (**d**) one can see the raw area without panniculus

evaluate and compare the thickness of both sides (Avelar 1985b, 1986b, 1999a, b, c).

After deep liposuction, the abdominal subcutaneous panniculus easily slides over the musculoaponeurotic wall, keeping all the perforator vessels as multiple pedicles (Figs. 5.6 and 5.7). This situation is similar to that on a child's panniculus because they don't have adiposity in the lamellar layer on any of the regions of the abdominal panniculus (Avelar 1986a, b, c, 1989). The areolar layer must be preserved to achieve the regular thickness of the remaining panniculus, yielding a harmonious result and a good balance in the body contouring (Fig. 5.6). However, in some cases, a surgeon may perform superficial liposuction on the upper panniculus flap to reduce its thickness.

Full-Thickness Skin Resection

After performing liposuction, the first step is to incise the umbilicus according to my procedure (Avelar 1976a, b, 1978, 1979), in which a star-shaped incision is made inside the umbilical region. In order to facilitate the umbilical incisions and to avoid the accidental perforation of the deep structures of the abdominal cavity, I created a double half-circular instrument (Fig. 5.8). It is introduced into one part on each side of the umbilicus, which joins around the umbilical pedicle and is pulled upward (Avelar 1983a). Cutaneous incisions are carried out on the umbilical cavity with a number 11 knife, followed by the anatomical dissection of the umbilical pedicle. Afterward, a cutaneous resection is performed with this knife on the entire

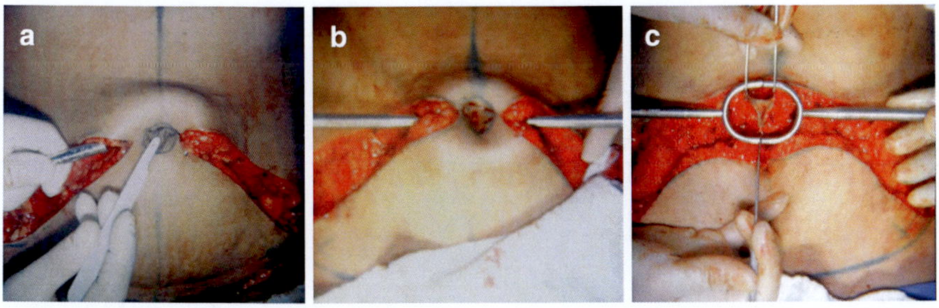

Fig. 5.8 Photos during surgery demonstrating that creation of the new umbilical region starts with triangular incisions around the umbilicus. Photo (**a**) using my surgical instrument with two half circles which are articulated around the umbilicus and cutaneous incisions are done with bladder. 11; (**b**) all incisions are already done; (**c**) the umbilicus is in the center of my double half circle instrument

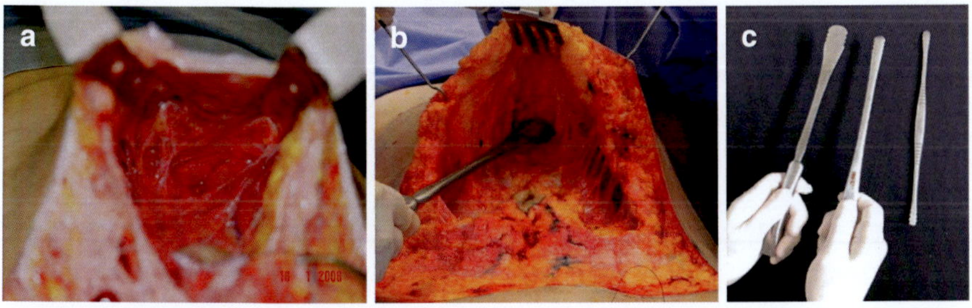

Fig. 5.9 Tunnelization of the midline on superior abdomen for reinforcement of the muscular abdominal wall during full lipoabdominoplasty. Photo (**a**) after liposuction of full thickness of the panniculus on infraumbilical region one can see preservation of the perforator vessels and the umbilicus was isolated with triangular incisions; (**b**) using special surgical instruments to create a subcutaneous tunnel on midline without undermining; (**c**) my surgical instruments developed to avoid panniculus undermining

area around the suprapubic region by retracing the demarcations (Fig. 5.7c, d). The subdermal structures and the perforator vessels underneath are preserved during this liposuction procedure. After full-thickness skin resection has been performed, the vessels of the previous panniculus are left undamaged, showing no bleeding during or after the skin resection (Fig. 5.6d, e, f).

Finally, a fundamental aspect of my method is that after liposuction on the full thickness of the panniculus has been carried out, the only anatomical structures that remain are the connective tissues, all the perforator vessels (arterial, venous, and lymphatic), and the nerves (Figs. 5.5d and 5.6f).

Afterward, the surgeon's assistant pulls the remaining panniculus upward with strong hooks to show the perforator vessels and connective tissues coming from the muscular level to the panniculus, which is now possible because the lamellar layer was previously aspirated (Fig. 5.9). I created special dissectors to be introduced from the midline above the umbilicus to the xyphoid process (where there

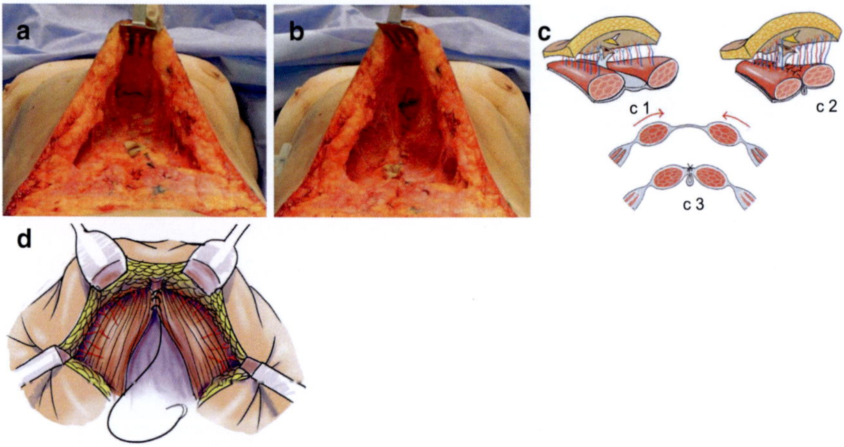

Fig. 5.10 Plication of the muscular abdominal wall during full lipoabdominoplasty. Photo (**a**) internal image after tunnelization on midline on upper abdomen one can see preservation of the perforator vessels on each side; (**b**) after plication the rectus abdominalis the perforator vessels are preserved; (**c**) sequential diagrams showing plication: (*c1*) before plication; (*c2*) after reinforcement; (*c3*) details of plication on midline; (**d**) scheme demonstrating plication of the rectus abdominalis on upper abdomen

are no perforator vessels), according to my previous descriptions (Fig. 5.9c) (Avelar 1986a, b, c, 1987, 1989). Therefore, only the connective tissues are dissected when the instruments are introduced into the fourth and backward movements, without any lateral ones (Fig. 5.9b). The perforator vessels can be seen on each side of the tunnel that was created by the dissectors on the superior segments of the muscles of the rectus abdominalis. In fact, they indicate the location of the muscles for reinforcement sutures (Fig. 5.10). When conventional abdominoplasty is performed, a wide undermined area is formed that cut all perforator vessels.

Reinforcing the Rectus Abdominalis and Aponeurotic Wall

According to my previous publications (Avelar 1983a, 1987), the treatment represented by reinforcing the musculoaponeurotic abdominal wall isn't a routine procedure in conventional abdominoplasty. It is a useful surgical step when the patient presents with moderate or severe muscular flaccidity, diastasis in the rectus abdominalis, or herniation in the abdominal wall, as mentioned by Pontes (1965) and emphasized and popularized by Pitanguy (1967, 1977, 1982)

Although the abdominal panniculus isn't undermined during full lipoabdominoplasty, the plication of the abdominal aponeurotic structures can be performed on the midline and laterally to reinforce the muscular wall and to treat the diastasis of the rectus abdominalis (Figs. 5.10 and 5.11) (Avelar 2000a, b). This surgical step

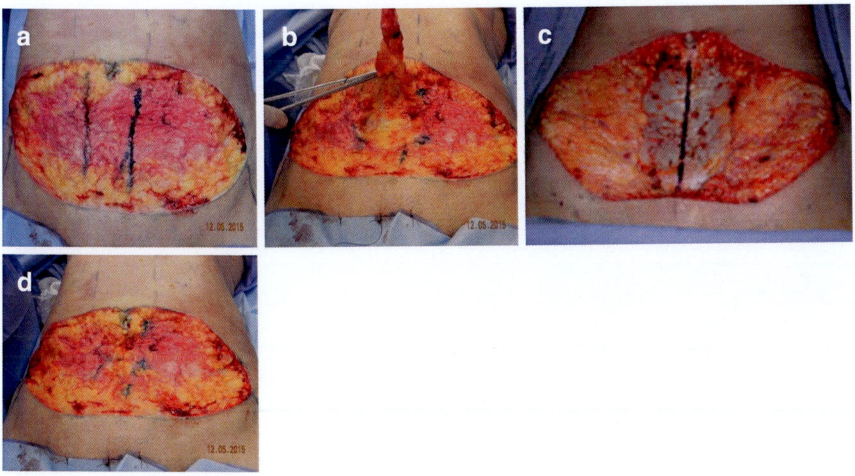

Fig. 5.11 Perioperative photos showing plication of the infra umbilical segment following Erfon's approach. Photo (**a**) demarcation two vertical line with blue ink; (**b**) resection of the fascia superficialis on midline; (**c**) after resection the midline is demarcated with blue ink; (**d**) the infra umbilical segment after plication on midline

wasn't described in my original publication (Avelar 1999a, b, c), because my first 22 patients did not show any indications for this. However, Leão presented plication on the midline of the abdominal wall via the tunnel approach without panniculus undermining (Leão 2000a, b). Afterward, I found a good indication for plication in some of my patients who underwent lipoabdominoplasty without panniculus undermining because they presented the diastasis of the rectus abdominalis, from the xyphoid process to the suprapubic region. Although I can identify the diastasis and an umbilical hernia, I always ask patients to undergo a CT scan in order to demonstrate the abnormality to them, which is useful for patients to gain support from their private health insurance (Fig. 5.3). I ask to measure the distance between the rectus abdominalis from the xyphoid process to the pubis bone and to evaluate the presence of herniation on the umbilicus and on the area of diastasis. Also, I measure, via a CT scan, the thickness of the abdominal panniculus and the muscles.

Therefore, when there is such an indication, reinforcement via the plication of the musculoaponeurotic abdominal wall is simultaneously performed with my new lipoabdominoplasty procedure. Because there is a wide distance between the rectus abdominalis from the diastasis, there is also a wide distance from the perforator vessels on one side to those on the other (Figs. 5.3 and 5.10). I don't perform any undermining on the midline, because by using my special dissector, I can identify the inner border of the muscles on each side. The shorter width of the diastasis of the rectus abdominalis, the less chance that the perforator vessels will be damaged. Therefore, the plication is 5 to 6 cm and is performed from the xyphoid process to the umbilical region by using isolated stitches. The pedicle of the umbilicus isn't routinely shortened, except in patients who have undergone massive weight lost and who have very long segments of pedicle.

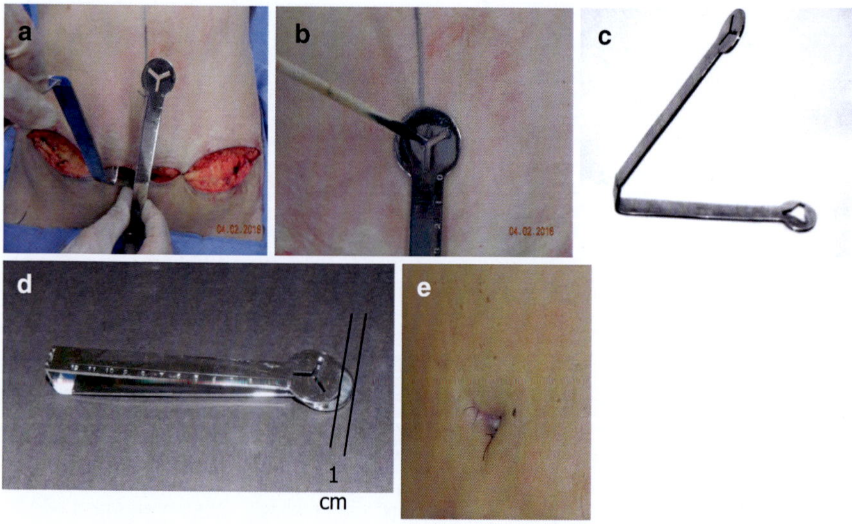

Fig. 5.12 Perioperative photos for demarcation of the new umbilical region on abdominal flap after its downward traction. Photos (**a, b**) the lower segment of my surgical instrument is placed on umbilicus; (**b**) the other segment lies on the abdominal flap and the new umbilicus is drawn; (**c**) lateral view of my surgical instrument with two segments; (**d**) oblique view with one segment on the other, the superior one is 1 cm shorter than the inferior one; (**e**) a new umbilicus 1 week after surgery with natural depression on the umbilical region

The creation of the new umbilical region during full lipoabdominoplasty is described in Chap. X (Figs. 5.8 and 5.12).

Traction for the Remaining Panniculus and the Demarcation of the New Umbilical Area

After reinforcing the musculoaponeurotic wall, the operating table needs to be bent. The upper abdominal flap is pulled downward over the infraumbilical area until it has reached the lower incision (Fig. 5.12). A temporary stitch is applied on the midline, and another one is applied on each side of the previous one. Afterward, the table needs to be returned to the straight position so that the abdominal flap is in its normal position, at which point the future umbilical area can be demarcated. I created a new surgical instrument to establish a new umbilical area (Avelar 1983a). My instrument has two segments like a pair of forceps. One segment is introduced through the inferior border of the abdominal flap and placed on the umbilicus close to the muscles on the midline. The other segment of the instrument lies on the abdominal flap so that the natural projection of the umbilicus can be determined. The upper segment is made 1 cm shorter than the inferior one so that the new umbilical area can be marked 1 cm lower than the projection of the umbilicus on the middle of the abdominal flap (Figs. 5.5e and 5.12d).

After the demarcation of the new umbilical area, a 2 cm diameter circle is drawn, which is divided into three equal skin flaps (Fig. 5.12b) (Avelar 1976a, b, 1978, 1983a, b). One of them is superior and the other two are inferior on the left and the right, and they are alternately stitched with the other three of the umbilicus.

After suturing the triangular flaps, a dry gauze is placed inside the umbilicus, which is kept for 1 week—that is, until the patient returns to the office for their first instance of postoperative care. Afterward, a new gauze is placed inside the umbilicus, which is changed every 10 to 15 days during the first 2 months after surgery. The final aspect of the new umbilicus is a natural depression with the triangular skin flaps on the side of the cavity.

The final step of the operation is the suture of the wound is performed with absorbent material and with isolated stitches in three or four layers. According to the above description, the raw area preserves the connective tissues, the fascia superficialis, and all the perforator vessels. It is important to suture the fascia superficialis from the border of the upper panniculus flap to the lower border of the fascia superficialis, where liposuction is not performed.

Afterward, the subdermal layers are also sutured with separate stitches, and finally a running intradermal suture is applied by using absorbent material. On top of it, adhesive tapes are used to cover the surgical wound.

Bandaging

I don't use any kind of drainage after lipoabdominoplasty, because no preoperative damage is caused to the perforator vessels and because there is no bleeding during or after the operation. A thick layer of cotton is placed on the patient's abdomen, and a comfortable garment is dressed as a final bandaging. The patient may leave the hospital the next day provided that they keep the bandaging for 1 week, at which time they return to the office for their first instance of postoperative care. The final result after full lipoabdominoplasty takes about 6 months to 1 year (Figs. 5.13, 5.14, and 5.15).

Discussion

Kelly (1899) has been credited with performing the first operation whose treatment reinstated the aesthetics of the abdomen wall. Since then, so much attention has been paid to finding a procedure that can achieve better results. The transposition of the umbilicus proposed by Vernon (1957) was an important step for abdominoplasty. Afterward, the wide undermining of the abdominal panniculus was introduced by Callia (1965), and Pitanguy (1967) and improved the approach by reinforcing the muscular abdominal wall (Figs. 5.3, 5.10, 5.11, and 5.13). However, the very high rates of complications have been severe impediments to performing abdominoplasty because the perforator vessels are cut to achieve wide undermining. Local and systemic complications have been reported by Grazer and Goldwyn

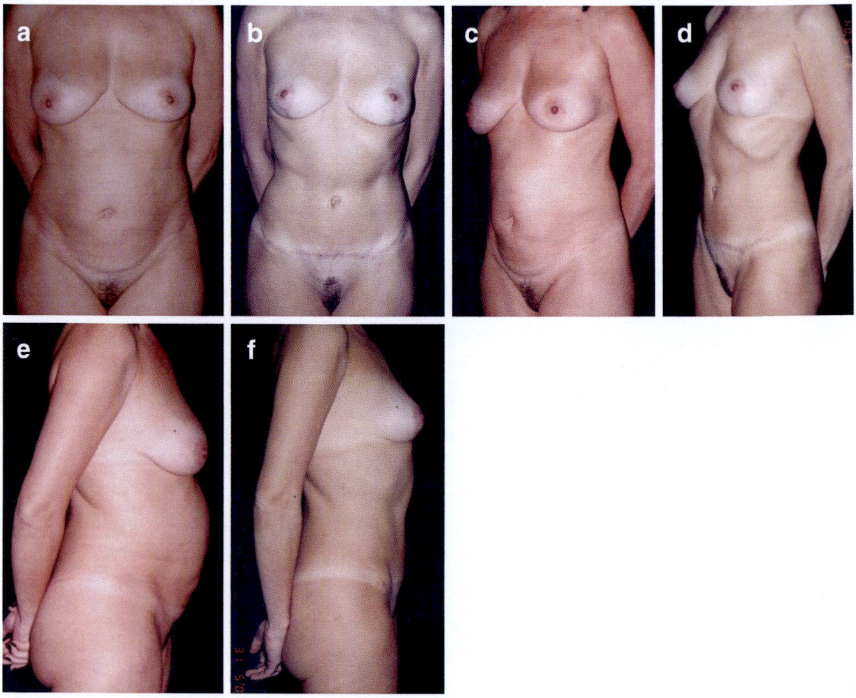

Fig. 5.13 A 59-year-old patient underwent full lipoabdominoplasty according to the described technique. Photos (**a, c, e**) before operation; photos (**b, d, f**) after full lipoabdominoplasty with creation of the new umbilical region

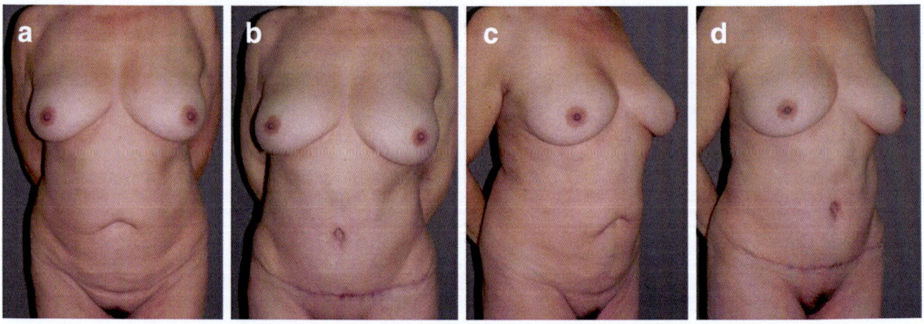

Fig. 5.14 A 63-year-old patient underwent full lipoabdominoplasty according to the technique described. Photos (**a, c**) frontal and oblique view before operation; (**b, d**) after full lipoabdominoplasty with creation of the new umbilical region

(1977), Lodovici (1982), Guerrerosantos (1982a, b), Guerrerosantos et al. (1980), Mélega (1982), and D'Assumpção (1982), among other authors.

Since the beginning of my career, I have identified several challenges to abdominoplasty: (1) the creation of a new umbilical region, (2) complications during and after the operation, and (3) adiposities remaining after surgery.

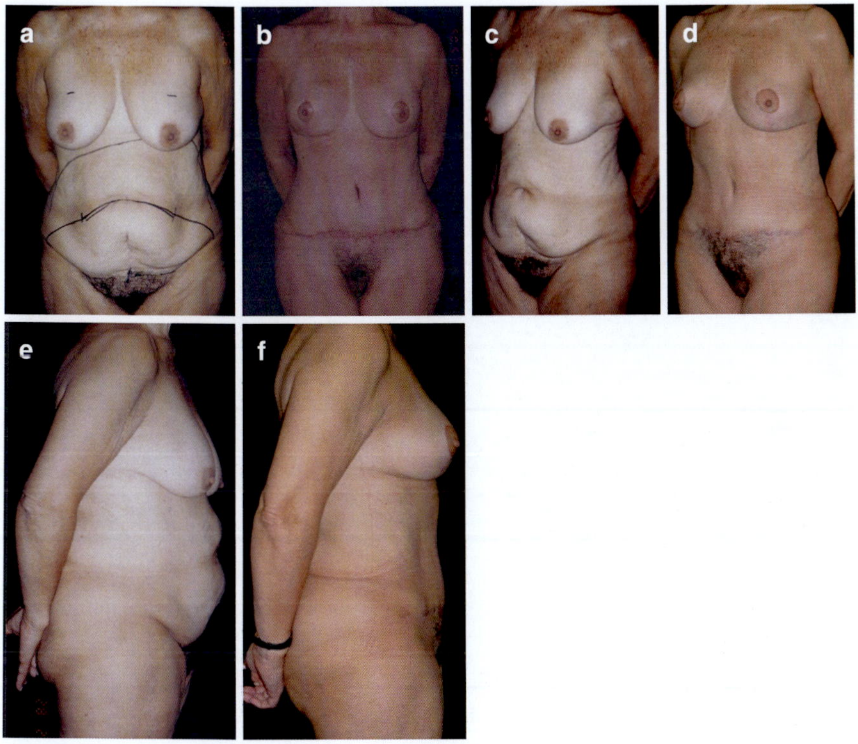

Fig. 5.15 A 66-year-old patient underwent full lipoabdominoplasty according to the described technique. Photos (**a, c, e**) before surgery; photos (**b, d, f**) after full lipoabdominoplasty with creation of the new umbilical region

First, I presented a new technique that makes triangular cutaneous incisions around the umbilicus (Avelar 1976a, b, 1978 1979, 1983a, b) to avoid leaving a circular scar after surgery; such scars have been reported by Grazer and Goldwyn (1977), Lodovici (1982), and others.

Second, complications during and after abdominoplasty were even more difficult to solve, which motivated me to organize the Brazilian Symposium of Abdominoplasty featuring renowned foreign and Brazilian plastic surgeons to serve as a remarkable panel for discussion (Fig. 5.16). My purpose at that time was to try to find a solution, but those severe complications were challenges for all plastic surgeons, according to a discussion among 19 panelists. At that time, I concluded once more that abdominoplasty was a field that still required technical improvements to minimize complications. It was quite often performed as a combination of procedures (Avelar and Padovez 1982) and as an approach for breast augmentation (Hinderer 1982).

Third, the remaining adiposities after abdominoplasty were improved via the development of liposuction by Illouz (1980, 1983a, b, 1984, 1986a, b). In early 1983, I went to Paris to learn the liposuction technique by observing Illouz perform his

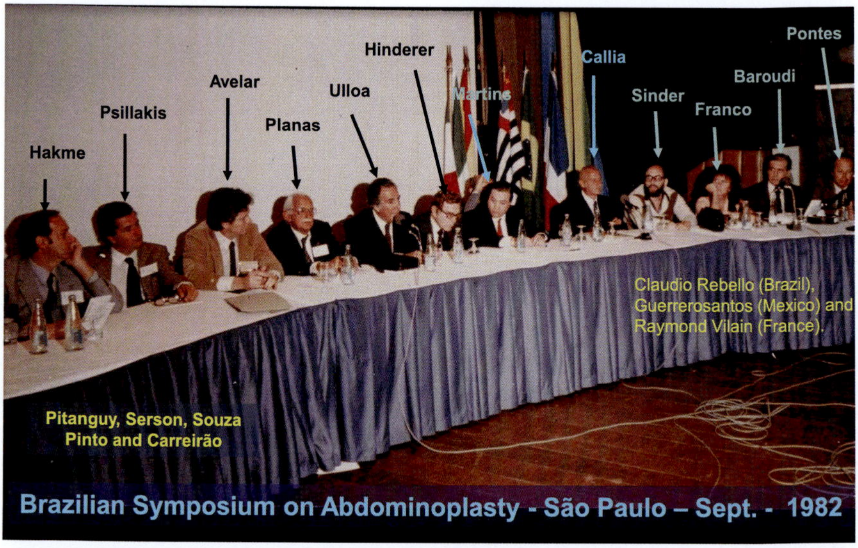

Fig. 5.16 Photo of a panel during the symposium with several authors of articles about abdominoplasty. The Panel had also: Souza Pinto (President), Pitanguy and Serson Neto (Moderators), Carreirão (Secretary). The panelists: from left to right: Hakme, Jorge Psillakis, Juarez Avelar (Brazil), Jaime Planas (Spain), Mario Gonzalles Ulloa (Mexico), Ulrich Hinderer (Spain), Luiz C. Martins, Willian Callia, Ramil Sinder, Talita Franco, Ricardo Baroudi and Ronaldo Pontes (Brazil). Besides the pannelists in the photo, there were also: Claudio Rebello (Brazil), Guerrerosantos (Mexico), and Raymond Vilain (France)

revolutionary approach. When I started to perform my first operations, I recognized that the cannulas worked inside an unknown anatomical compartment of the human body. I immediately started to study the anatomy of the subcutaneous layers to gain more anatomical knowledge. I devoted considerable time to anatomic research on cadavers to find new information, after which I could identify the lamellar layer, which is close to the muscles, and the areolar layer, which is more superficial.

Those layers are separated by the fascia superficialis, which features such rich vascularization that I called the vessels communicating vessels (CVs). They serve as a "peripheric heart" because the very high blood pressure inside the perforator vessels is what decreases the communicating vessels' ability to irrigate the areolar and subdermal layers (Fig. 5.6d, e, f). The perforator vessels are quite thick because they come from the epigastric artery running inside the rectus abdominalis muscles that perpendicularly cross the lamellar layer (Fig. 5.6d, e, f). I performed dissections on several cadavers of various ages, sexes, levels of adipose tissue, heights, and ethnicities. I also performed liposuction on them while looking for new anatomic information and documenting the behavior of the subcutaneous compartment after liposuction (Avelar 1986a, b, c, 1987, 1989).

According to my publications, the fascia superficialis is a sophisticated anatomical structure between the areolar and lamellar layers with peculiar characteristics in the abdominal wall. Each region's layers is different from the others, and more differences appear between thin people and people with localized adiposities.

A similar anatomy was found in the upper and lower thirds of the medial thighs and in some regions of the torso. On the abdominal wall and the posterior regions of the torso, the fascia superficialis is well identified on CT when the image is well analyzed on the same level while using the bone structures as anatomic references (Fig. 5.3). Later, Lockwood (1995) described the importance of the fascia superficialis in media thigh lifting. Also, an outstanding anatomic study was performed by Levy, the details of which appear in Chap. X, concerning the differences in thickness and the histological alterations of the subcutaneous tissue after severe weight loss. He also described the difference between weight loss from diet and that from bariatric surgery.

The aesthetic treatment of the abdominal wall introduced by Illouz (1980, 1983a, b, 1984, 1986a, b) employing the liposuction procedure has been improved, but there was another problem, namely the excess skin of the abdominal wall after surgery. As soon as I started to perform liposuction on the abdominal wall, I recognized that the excess skin would need to be resected (Avelar 1985a, b, 1986a, b, c). Thus, a new aesthetic procedure was introduced for abdominoplasty: an approach combining liposuction with the resection of cutaneous redundance. Therefore, the surgical results on body contouring were greatly improved. Such a combined procedure has highly increased the incidence of complications (e.g., seroma, the slough and necrosis of the panniculus, and infection). However, those sorts of complications didn't occur on the face and neck when associated procedures of liposuction with rhytidoplasty were performed (Avelar 1983a, 1985c). So, in 1988, I made an extreme decision not to perform combined procedures of liposuction with the resection of the excess skin during abdominoplasty (Avelar 1988).

Although I didn't perform any more combinations of these techniques, I started to think about and to study my previous anatomical descriptions on the panniculus of the abdominal wall (Avelar 1986a, b, c, 1987, 1989). Finally, I concluded that I could perform liposuction with the resection of the redundant skin as long as the perforator vessels were not cut because they preserve normal blood supply to the remaining abdominal panniculus, thus avoiding dead space underneath (Fig. 5.6d, e, f). Another technical improvement was described by Matarasso (Matarasso 2000) after he heard my presentation at the ISAPS course in Montreal (Avelar 2000a), namely lipoabdominoplasty as a new technique in abdominoplasty (Avelar 1999a, b, c, 2000a, b). My descriptions in publications and during presentations were clear enough and the surgical principles well understood enough that they were accepted by several other surgeons (Ribeiro 2016); as a result, nowadays, lipoabdominoplasty has become a common operation (Erfon 2000; Leão 2000a, b; Saldanha 2002).

Conclusions

Since 1999, abdominoplasty has undergone significant technical improvements in that it can now be performed in combination with a liposuction procedure that preserves the perforator vessels; this is the main surgical principle of lipoabdominoplasty (Fig. 5.6d, e, f) (Avelar 1999a, b, 2000a, b). As long as the perforator vessels are not damaged during the operation, the blood supply to the remaining abdominal panniculus is maintained, whose multiple pedicles avoid dead space (Figs. 5.9 and 5.10). This is my surgical contribution, and it comes with a minor rate of complications because the operation can be carried out without panniculus undermining and without resection.

Those surgical principles are essential in order for the lipoabdominoplasty procedure to improve body contouring (Avelar 1999a, b, c, 2000a, b) and for it to include several other regions, as long as my original descriptions on aesthetic surgeries on the axillary regions are followed (Avelar 1999d, e), even for flankplasty and torsoplasty (Avelar 1999f) and for medial tight lifting (Avelar 1999g). Also, I employ similar surgical principles to perform face lifts, ear reconstruction, reverse lower blepharoplasty, and surgeries on other segments of the human body. Such a combined approach is so important in plastic surgery because it doesn't cut the arterial, venous, and lymphatic structures, thus yielding smooth and aesthetic results.

Finally, I was able to solve the problems that I identified 50 years ago in the field of abdominoplasty and surgeries on other regions to improve body contouring. Therefore, I described a new method to create the umbilical region during abdominoplasty (Avelar 1976a, b, 1979, 1983a, b). Also, I introduced new concepts to solve the problems of the unaesthetic aspect of the abdominal wall from the accumulation of local adiposities after liposuction combined with cutaneous resection (Avelar 1985a, b, 1986b). My recent contribution to abdominoplasty came in the last year of the twentieth century, which was a new procedure for lipoabdominoplasty (Avelar 1999a, b, c, d, e, f, g, 2000a, b). Following this technique, there are minimal local and systemic complications thanks to its maintaining normal blood supply to the remaining abdominal panniculus coming from the perforator vessels, which are preserved in this technique (Figs. 5.6, 5.9, and 5.10).

References

Avelar JM (1976a) Umbilicoplasty – a technique without external scar (Umbilicoplastia uma técnica sem cicatriz externa). 13rd Bras Cong of Plast Surg and First Brazilian Cong of Aesthetic Surgery. (13° Congresso Brasileiro de Cirurgia Plástica e 1° Congr Bras Cir Estética), Porto Alegre – RS (Brazil) 81–82

Avelar JM (1976b) Umbilicoplasty – A istema without external scar. Cahiers de chirurgie Esthétique. Journees internationals de Chirurgie Esthetique. Vendredi 21 – Paris (France) mai.

Avelar J (1978) Abdominoplasty – systematization of a technique without external umbilicalscar. Aesthet Plast Surg 2:141

Avelar JM (1979) Umbilical scar – its importance and technique for creating during abdominoplasty (Cicatriz umbilical – da sua importância e da técnica de confecção nas istemalasties). Rev Bras Cir 1(2):41–52.

Avelar JM and Padovez JC (1982) – Mamoplasty combined with Abdominoplasty – Analises of 40 consecutive cases. (Mamaplastia e Abdominoplastia Combinadas – Análise de 40 Casos Consecutivos) In: Annals of Brazilian Symposio of Abdominoplasty. (Anais do Simpósio Brasileiro de Abdominoplastia), ed. by Juarez M. Avelar, Sponsored by Brazilian Society of Plastic Surgery-Regional São Paulo, (Patrocinado pela Sociedade Brasileira de Cirurgia Plástica – Regional São Paulo). 1:141–148. Editora Cidade, Rio de Janeiro – Brazil.

Avelar JM (1983a) Abdominoplasty: technical refinements and analysis of 130 cases in 8 years follow-up. Aesthetic Plast Surg 7:205–212.
Avelar JM (1983b) Submentonean and Submandibular Adiposity – Liposuction X Lipectomy (Adiposidade Submentoniana e Submandibular – Lipoaspiração X Lipectomia). Brazilian Symposium on Facial Contouring, organized and edited by Dr. Juarez Avelar. Sponsored by Brazilian Society of Plastic Surgery (Section of São Paulo), September pag. 69–72
Avelar JM (1985a) Combined liposuction with traditional surgery in abdomen Lipodystrophy. XXIV Instructional Course of Aesth Plast Surg of ISAPS, Madrid (Spain) May.
Avelar JM (1985b) Fat-suction versus abdominoplasty. Aesthetic Plast Surg 9:265–276.
Avelar JM (1985c) – Fat-Suction of the Submental and Submandibular Regions. Aesth Plast Surg 9:257–263
Avelar JM (1986a) Surgical anatomy and distribution of the cellular tissue on human organism. (Anatomia cirúrgica e distribuição do tecido istema no istema humano). In: Liposuction (Lipoaspiração). Ed; by Avelar JM and Illouz IG. Editora Hipócrates, São Paulo, pp 45–57.
Avelar JM (1986b) – Liposuction of the Abdominal Wall. (Lipoaspiração da Parede Abdominal). In: Liposuction (Lipoaspiração), ed. by Avelar and Illouz, Ed. Hipócrates, São Paulo (Brazil) 27:157–176.
Avelar JM (1986c) – Photografic standardization as Method for Cientific Documentation (Padronização fotográfica como Método de Documentação Científica). In: Liposuction (Lipoaspiração), ed. by Avelar and Illouz, Ed. Hipócrates, São Paulo (Brazil) 13:80–86.
Avelar JM (1987) Study of the subcutaneous adipose tissue applied for fat-suction technique. In: Manesksha RJ (ed) Trans. IX Int. Congr. Plast. Reconstr. Surg, New Delhi, 1–6 Mar, pp 377–379.
Avelar JM (1988) Abdominoplasty – Reflections and bio-psychological perspectives (Abdominoplastia – reflexões e perspectiva biopsicológicas). Revista Soc Bras Cir Plast 3(2)
Avelar JM (1989) Regional distribution and behaviour of the subcutaneous tissue concerning selection and indication for liposuction. Aesthetic Plast Surg 13:155–156.
Avelar JM (1999a) New concepts for abdominoplasty. (Novos conceitos para abdominoplastia). Paper presented at the 36th congress of the Brazilian Society of Plastic Surgery, Rio de Janeiro, November.
Avelar JM (1999b) A new technique for abdominoplasty – closed vascular system of subdermal flap folded over itself combined to Liposuction. (Uma nova técnica de abdominoplastia – istema vascular fechado de retalho subdérmico dobrado sobre si mesmo combinado com lipoaspiração). Rev Bras Cir 88/89(1/6):3–20.
Avelar JM (1999c) Abdominoplasty: new concepts for a new technique (Abdominoplastia: Nuevos conceptos para una nueva técnica). XXVI annual international symposium of aesthetic plastic surgery, Chairman: Prof. Jose Guerrerosantos – Puerto Vallarta, pp 10–13.
Avelar JM (1999d) Aesthetic Plastic Surgery of the Axilla (Cirurgia Plástica e Estética de Axila) Rev Bras Cir 88/89(1/6):41–54
Avelar JM (1999e) Aesthetic Plastic Surgery of the Axilla. Presented at the XV Congress of the International Society of Aesthetic Plastic Surgery (ISAPS, Tokyo (Japan) April 2.000
Avelar JM (1999f) Flankplasty and torsoplasty – a new surgical approach. (Flancoplastia e Torsoplastia – Nova Abordagem Cirúrgica). Rev Bras Cir 88/89(1/6):21–35
Avelar JM (1999g) Plastic Surgery in Internal Medial Thigh (Cirurgia Plástica de Face Interna de Coxas) Rev Bras Cir 88/89(1/6):57–67
Avelar JM (2000a) Abdominoplasty: a new technique without panniculus undermining and without panniculus resection. 57th Instructional Course of ISAPS, Chairman: Lloyd Carlsen, in Montreal, Canada.
Avelar JM (2000b) Abdominoplasty: a new technique without undermining and fat layer removal (Abdominoplastia: uma nova técnica sem descolamento e remoção da camada de gordura). Arq Catarinense de Med 29:147–149
Avelar JM (2001a) The new abdominoplasty and derived technique. ISAPS and ASERF Annual Meeting. The Aesthetic Meeting, New York.

Avelar JM (2001b) Abdominoplasty without lipectomy. Mini Course of ISAPS with Aesthetic Plastic Surgery Congress of Spain, Valladolid.

Callia WE (1965) Contributions for the surgical correction of the pendulous and globose abdomen: original technique. Doctor's thesis, Medicine Medical School, São Paulo University, Sao Paulo.

Cavalcanti MA and Cavalcanti M (1982) Abdominoplasty on Corrections of Severe Cases (Abdominopastias nas Correções de Casos Graves). In: Annals of the Brazilian Symposio of Abdominoplasty (Simpósio Brasileiro de Abdominoplastia), organized and ed. by Juarez M. Avelar, Sponsored by Brazilian Society of Plastic Surgery-Regional São Paulo, (Patrocinado pela Sociedade Brasileira de Cirurgia Plástica – Regional São Paulo), pág. 185–192. Editora Cidade, Rio de Janeiro – Brazil.

Daher JC (1982) Onphaloplasty in Abdominoplasty (Onfaloplastias nas Abdominoplastias). In: Annals of the Brazilian Symposio of Abdominoplasty (Simpósio Brasileiro de Abdominoplastia), organized and ed. by Juarez M. Avelar, Sponsored by Brazilian Society of Plastic Surgery-Regional São Paulo, (Patrocinado pela Sociedade Brasileira de Cirurgia Plástica – Regional São Paulo), pág. 68–70. Editora Cidade, Rio de Janeiro – Brazil.

D'Assumpção EA (1982) Three Common Complictions in Abdominoplasty: Infeccion, Deiscence and Seroma Formation. (Três Complicações Comuns em Abdominoplastias: Infecção, Deiscência e Seroma). In: Annals of the Brazilian Symposio of Abdominoplasty (Simpósio Brasileiro de Abdominoplastia), organized and ed. by Juarez M. Avelar, Sponsored by Brazilian Society of Plastic Surgery-Regional São Paulo, (Patrocinado pela Sociedade Brasileira de Cirurgia Plástica – Regional São Paulo), pg. 77–82. Editora Cidade, Rio de Janeiro – Brazil.

Erfon JA (2000) Resection of the lower abdominal fascia to improve plication of infraumbilical aponeurosis during lipoabdominoplasty without panniculus undermining (Ressecção da fascia abdominal inferior para plicatura infra umbilical em lipoabdominoplastia sem descolamento do panículo). Second Courese of Abdominoplasty at the Heart Hospital (2° Curso de Abdominoplastia), Hospital do Coração –, São Paulo (Brazil)

Gonzales-Ulloa, M (1959) Circular Lipectomy wirh Transposition of the umbilicus and aponeurotic Technique. Cirug Y Ciruj 27:394–409

Gonzales-Ulloa M (1982) Circular Abdominoplasty (Abdominoplastia Circular) Presented at the Brazilian Symposio of Abdominoplasty (Simpósio Brasileiro de Abdominoplastia), organized and ed. by Juarez M. Avelar, Sponsored by Brazilian Society of Plastic Surgery-Regional São Paulo, (Patrocinado pela Sociedade Brasileira de Cirurgia Plástica – Regional São Paulo). Section "I" Round Table. Editora Cidade, Rio de Janeiro – Brazil.

Grazer FM, Goldwyn RM (1977) Abdominoplasty assessed by the survey, with emphasis on complications. Plast Reconstr Surg 59(4):513–517

Guerrerosantos J, Spaillat L, Morales F, Dickeheet S (1980) Some problems and solutions in abdominoplasty. Aesthetic Plast Surg 4:227

Guerrerosantos J (1982a) Necrosis of Abdominal Wall Post-Abdominoplasty – Etiology, Profilaxis and Treatment (Necrose de Parede Pós-Abdominoplastia – Etiologia, Profilaxia e Tratamento). Presented at the Brazilian Symposio of Abdominoplasty (Simpósio Brasileiro de Abdominoplastia), organized and ed. by Juarez M. Avelar, Sponsored by Brazilian Society of Plastic Surgery-Regional São Paulo, (Patrocinado pela Sociedade Brasileira de Cirurgia Plástica – Regional São Paulo). Section "E" Round Table. Editora Cidade, Rio de Janeiro – Brazil.

Guerrerosantos J (1982b) Tecnichal Refinments in Abdominoplasty (Refinamentos Técnicos nas Abdominoplastia). Presented at the Brazilian Symposio of Abdominoplasty (Simpósio Brasileiro de Abdominoplastia), organized and ed. by Juarez M. Avelar, Sponsored by Brazilian Society of Plastic Surgery-Regional São Paulo, (Patrocinado pela Sociedade Brasileira de Cirurgia Plástica – Regional São Paulo). Section "B" Round Table. Editora Cidade, Rio de Janeiro – Brazil.

Hinderer UT (1982) Treatment of the Mammary Hypoplasia Combined with Abdominal Lypodistrofia (Tratamento de la Hipoplasia Mamaria Combindo con Lipodistrofia Abdominal). In: Annals of the Brazilian Symposio of Abdominoplasty (Simpósio Brasileiro de Abdominoplastia), organized and ed. by Juarez M. Avelar, Sponsored by Brazilian Society

of Plastic Surgery-Regional São Paulo, (Patrocinado pela Sociedade Brasileira de Cirurgia Plástica – Regional São Paulo), pág. 55–57. Editora Cidade, Rio de Janeiro – Brazil.
Illouz YG (1980) Une nouvelle technique pour çles lipodystrophies localisées. Rev Chir Esth Franc 6:19
Illouz YG (1983a) – Liposuction – My technique and applications. First Course of Liposuction. Organized by Dr. Juarez M. Avelar. Heled at São Paulo Hospital, Service of Prof. Andrews at Escola Paulista de Medicina., Sponsored by Brazilian Society of Plastic Surgery (São Paulo Section) October São Paulo (Brazil).
Illouz YG (1984) – Refinements in Liposuction to improve body contour. Theory and Practical Course with surgical demonstrations at "Nove de Julho Hospital". Organized by Dr. Juarez M. Avelar. Sponsored by Brazilian society of Plastic Surgery with collaboration of Regional São Paulo. São Paulo (Brazil), May.
Illouz YG (1986a) Basic Principles of liposuction technique (Princípios básicos da técnica de lipoaspiração). Liposuction (Lipoaspiração). Ed. by AvelarJM. & Illouz YG. São Paulo (Brasil). Editora Hipócrates 3:22–225.
Illouz YG (1986b). Study of the Adipocite in Lipodistrophy (Estudo do Adipócito nas Lipodistrogias). In Liposuction (Lipoaspiração). Ed. by AvelarJM. & Illouz YG. São Paulo (Brasil). Editora Hipócrates 4:19–23.
Kelly HA (1899) Report of gynecological cases. John Hopkins Med J 10:197
Leão CF (2000a) Plication of the musculoaponeurotic wall through a tunnel on the superior abdominal on the midline during lipoabdominoplasty without panniculus undermining (Plicatura da parede músculo-aponeurótica por um tunel no abdômen superior na linha média em lipoabdominoplastia sem descolamento). Presented at the 2nd Course of Abdominoplasty at Heart Hospital (Hospital do Coração), São Paulo, October. (2° Curso de abdominoplastia, no Hospital do Coração, outubro – São Paulo, organizado por Dr. Juarez M. Avelar) no Hospital do Coração, São Paulo, October
Leão CF (2000b) Plicatura da parede músculo-aponeurótica por um tunel criado abaixo do panículo abdominal na linha média em lipoabdominoplastia sem descolamento. 37° Congresso Brasileiro de Cirurgia Plástica, novembro – Porto Alegre. (Reinforcement of the musculoaponeurotic wall through a tunnel created below the abdominal panniculus during lipoabdominoplasty). 37th Brazilian Congress of Plastic Surgery, Porto Alegre, November
Lockwood T (1995) High lateral-tension abdominoplasty with superfi cial fascial system suspension. Plast Reconstr Surg 96:603–615
Lodovici O (1982) Hypertrofic or Keloidean Umbilicl Scar in Abdominoplasty (Cicatriz Umbilical Hipertrófica ou Queloidiana na Abdominoplastia) In: Annals of the Brazilian Symposio of Abdominoplasty (Simpósio Brasileiro de Abdominoplastia), organized and ed. by Juarez M. Avelar, Sponsored by Brazilian Society of Plastic Surgery-Regional São Paulo, (Patrocinado pela Sociedade Brasileira de Cirurgia Plástica – Regional São Paulo), pág. 83–85. Editora Cidade, Rio de Janeiro – Brazil.
Malbec EF (1948) Lipectomia abdominal. La Prensa Méd Arg 35(26)
Martins LC (1982) Respiratory Problems on Pre and Post-Operatory of the Abdominoplasty (Problemas Respiratorios no Pré e Pós-Operatório das Abdominoplastias) In: Annals of the Brazilian Symposio of Abdominoplasty (Simpósio Brasileiro de Abdominoplastia), organized and ed. by Juarez M. Avelar, Sponsored by Brazilian Society of Plastic Surgery-Regional São Paulo, (Patrocinado pela Sociedade Brasileira de Cirurgia Plástica – Regional São Paulo), pág. 86–89. Editora Cidade, Rio de Janeiro – Brazil.
Matarasso A (2000) Liposuction as an adjunct to full abdominoplasty revised. Plast Reconstr Surg 106:1197–1206
Mélega JM (1982) Thromboembolism as a complication of abdominoplasty: etiology, prevention and treatment. (Tromboembolismo Como complicação de abdominoplastia: etiologia, prevenção e tratamento) In: Annals of the Brazilian Symposium of Abdominoplasty. Ed. by Juarez M Avelar. Sponsored by Brazilian Society of Plastic Surgery (Regional São Paulo) pp 73–76.
Pitanguy I (1967) Abdominal lipectomy: an approach to it through an analysis of 300 consecutive cases. Plast Reconstr Surg 40(4):384–391

Pitanguy I (1977) Dermolipectomy of the abdominal wall, thighs, buttocks, and upper extremity. In: Converse JM (ed) Reconstructive plastic surgery, 2nd edn. Saundrs, Philadelphia, pp 3800–3823

Pitanguy I (1982) Phylosophic and Psychological Perspectives of the Abdomen. (Perspectivas Filosóficas e Psicológicos do Abdomen). In Annals of Brazilian Symposio of Abdominoplasty. (Anais do Simpósio Brasileiro de Abdominoplastia), Ed. by Juarez M. Avelar, Sponsored by Brazilian Society of Plastic Surgery-Regional São Paulo, (Patrocinado pela Sociedade Brasileira de Cirurgia Plástica – Regional São Paulo). 1:15–24. Editora Cidade, Rio de Janeiro – Brazil.

Planas J (1982) Abdominoplasty through upper incision (Abdominoplastia por Incisão Superior). Presented at the Brazilian Symposio of Abdominoplasty (Simpósio Brasileiro de Abdominoplastia), organized and ed. by Juarez M. Avelar, Sponsored by Brazilian Society of Plastic Surgery-Regional São Paulo, (Patrocinado pela Sociedade Brasileira de Cirurgia Plástica – Regional São Paulo). Section "C" Round Table. Editora Cidade, Rio de Janeiro – Brazil.

Pontes R (1965) Abdominal plastic. importance of its association with the correction of incisional hernias (Plástica abdominal: importância da sua associação com a correção de hérnia incisional). Rev Bras Cir 52:8.

Pontes R (1982) Abdominal Plastic – Unsatisfactory Results (Plástica Abdominal – Resultados Insatisfatórios). In: Annals of Brazilian Symposio of Abdominoplasty. (Anais do Simpósio Brasileiro de Abdominoplastia), Ed. by Juarez M. Avelar, Sponsored by Brazilian Society of Plastic Surgery-Regional São Paulo, (Patrocinado pela Sociedade Brasileira de Cirurgia Plástica – Regional São Paulo). 2:47–51. Editora Cidade, Rio de Janeiro – Brazil.

Rebello C, Lion P, Franco T (1972) Abdominopalsty through submammary incision. International Congress of ISAPS. Rio de Janeiro. Ed. Publicaciones Comntroladas, 58, Madrid

Rebello C (1982) – Abdominoplasty through submammary approach (Abdominoplastia por incisão submamária In: Annals of Brazilian Symposio of Abdominoplasty. (Anais do Simpósio Brasileiro de Abdominoplastia), Ed. by Juarez M. Avelar, Sponsored by Brazilian Society of Plastic Surgery-Regional São Paulo, (Patrocinado pela Sociedade Brasileira de Cirurgia Plástica – Regional São Paulo). 52–53. Editora Cidade, Rio de Janeiro – Brazil.

Ribeiro R (2016) Modified Lipoabdominoplasty: Updating Concepts. Plat Recont Surg 138(1):38e-47e DOI:https://doi.org/10.1097/PRS.0000000000002321.

Sinder R (1975) Plastic Surgery of the abdomen - Técnica pessoal de abdominoplastia, com prévio deslocamento de retalho supraumbilical (antes da ressecção infraumbilical) e uso de retalho dermoadiposo, – VI International Congress of Plastic and Reconstructive Surgery, Paris (France) August

Sinder R (1982) – Technical Variations of Abdominoplasty -– Generalities About Plastic Surgery of Abdomen (Variações Técnicas das Abdominoplastias Generalidades Sobre Cirurgia Plástica do Abdome. In Annals of Brazilian Symposio of Abdominoplasty. (Anais do Simpósio Brasileiro de Abdominoplastia), Ed. by Juarez M. Avelar, Sponsored by Brazilian Society of Plastic Surgery-Regional São Paulo, (Patrocinado pela Sociedade Brasileira de Cirurgia Plástica – Regional São Paulo). 2:31–40. Editora Cidade, Rio de Janeiro – Brazil.

Saldanha O R (2002) Lipoabdominoplasty. In: Abdominoplasty Without Panniculus Undermining and Resection, ed. by Avelar J M, Ed Hipócrates Pg 315–322 – São Paulo

Thorek M (1939) Modern operative technique. J.P. Lippincott-Phil, London

Vernon S (1957) Umbilical transplantation upward and abdominal contouring in lipectomy. Am J Surg 94:490–492

Vilain R, Dubousset J. (1964) Technique et indications de la lipectomie circulaire. 150 observations. Ann Chir 18:289–300.

Vilain R (1982) Circular Abdominoplasty (Abdominoplastia Circular). In Annals of Brazilian Symposio of Abdominoplasty (Anais do Simpósio Brasileiro de Abdominoplastia), Ed. by Juarez M. Avelar, Sponsored by Brazilian Society of Plastic Surgery-Regional São Paulo, (Patrocinado pela Sociedade Brasileira de Cirurgia Plástica – Regional São Paulo). 6:152–153. Editora Cidade, Rio de Janeiro – Brazil.

Chapter 6
Personal Experience with Abdominoplasty Without Undermining and Its Modifications

Ricardo Cavalcanti Ribeiro, Wilson Novaes, and Luis Fernandez de Cordova

Abstract Abdominoplasty is a very common aesthetic surgery performed worldwide. Data from the American Society of Plastic Surgeons have shown that it ranks as one of the most cosmetic surgical procedures performed in the United States. With the appearance of liposuction in the 1980s, classical abdominoplasty was modified using both techniques to improve body contour. At the end of the 1990s and the beginning of 2000, Avelar (New concepts for abdominoplasty, 1999a, Rev Bras Cir 88/89(1/6):3–20, 1999b, Abdominoplasty: new concepts for a new technique, 1999c) published several articles reporting a new approach called "abdominoplasty without undermine" that was proven to be safe, with good results. We have been using this technique since 2003 with excellent outcomes; however, some details were added because of significant shortcomings, including the lack of treatment of the pubic area and flanks, presence of a high-position scar, and, in some cases, a bulging inferior abdomen. Thus, after a long period of performing this technique, some improvements were made to the original surgical technique that included deep liposuction in the lower abdomen, pubic liposuction, liposuction of

R. C. Ribeiro (✉)
Plastic and Reconstructive Surgery, Federal University of the State of Rio de Janeiro, Rio de Janeiro, Brazil
e-mail: rribeiro@centroin.net.br

W. Novaes
Plastic and Reconstructive Surgery, Carlos Chagas Institute, Rio de Janeiro, Brazil

Brazilian Society of Plastic Surgery, Rio de Janeiro, Brazil

L. F. de Cordova
Plastic and Reconstructive Surgery, Carlos Chagas Institute, Rio de Janeiro, Brazil

Division of Plastic and Reconstructive Surgery, Casa de Portugal Rio de Janeiro, Rio de Janeiro, Brazil

Division of Plastic and Reconstructive Surgery, Global Plastic Surgery, México City, Mexico

J. M. Avelar, R. Cavalcanti Ribeiro (eds.), *Body Contouring*,
https://doi.org/10.1007/978-3-031-42802-9_6

the flanks or dorsum with power-assisted liposuction (PAL), Scarpa's fascia removal in the inferior abdomen, lipoplasty and Mons lipolifting, and pubic fixation. We present a retrospective study since that time on patients who underwent surgery with these related improvements. For global harmonization of the body contour, abdominoplasty using Avelar's principles was routinely associated with lipoplasty of the flanks or dorsum and outer thigh and fat graft in the gluteal-trochanteric regions. Taking into consideration these key points, a multi-pedicle flap was created, vessels were preserved, and less dead space was created, reducing the number of most common complications. Using these advances allowed us to overcome difficulties and optimize the outcomes.

Keywords Abdominoplasty · Liposuction · Body contour · Flanks · Abdomen

Introduction

Demars and Marx reported the first dermolipectomy in France in 1890; they reported it as an isolated procedure (Gemperli et al. 1992). Later, in 1899, Kelly, a gynecologic surgeon at Johns Hopkins University (Baltimore, MD, USA), published the first attempt to correct excess abdominal skin and fat, making a horizontal wedge resection that included the umbilicus (Kelly 1899). Although abdominoplasty is a very common procedure, few modifications have been observed over the last 50 years. Most publications related to the subject have referred to the scar position, as well as the changing of its size and direction (Ribeiro 2010).

In 1965, the modern era of abdominoplasty began with the contribution of Callia (1965), who described the scar at the pubic area and lateral extension of the down crural arcades. Later, in 1967, Pitanguy indicated treatment of the abdominal rectus muscle without the approach to the aponeurosis. He published 300 cases of consecutive abdominoplasty, referring to techniques, results, and complications (Pitanguy 1967). In 1975, he published a large study, which included 539 abdominoplasty cases (Pitanguy 1975).

In the mid-1980s, with the incorporation of liposuction, a significant improvement of body contouring was observed in abdominoplasty. Hakme (1985) and Wilkinson and Swartz (1986), associated liposuction with abdominal plastic surgery involving a small skin resection. Avelar, in 1985, described a technique of liposuction associated with abdominoplasty for patients who have a prominent abdomen and muscular laxity (Avelar 1985). Bozola and Psilakis (1988) and Matarasso (1991), created a clinical abdomen classification, suggesting a specific treatment for each type. Later, in 1999 (Avelar 1999c), Avelar described abdominoplasty without undermining and removal of fat through liposuction, with skin and fat resection below, in the belly button (Avelar 2000; Graf et al. 2006). In 2000, Matarasso described liposuction in combination with abdominoplasty to preserve the blood supply of the abdominal flap (Matarasso 1991, 2000).

Preservation of Scarpa's fascia has been suggested in order to lower complications associated with conventional abdominoplasty; thus, Saldanha et al. have proposed a new name for the procedure—lipoabdominoplasty (Saldanha et al. 2001)—according to the same principles previously proposed by Avelar (1999a).

With time and learning curve, some changes could be introduced to refine the technique. We have been performing this technique since 2003 with good results; however, over the years, some details and problems have been found. Therefore, in 2010, important approaches and improvements were introduced to optimize the postsurgical results, including the following: deep liposuction in the lower abdomen; power-assisted liposuction (PAL) of the pubic region, flanks, or dorsum; Scarpa's fascia removal in the inferior abdomen; lipoplasty; Mons lipolifting; and pubic fixation, where we observed a better harmony of body contouring.

Selection of Patients

In our experience, you can expect positive outcomes with women with an age ranging between 24 and 69 years, and American Society of Anesthesiologists (ASA) Physical Status I (ASA I), with an indication of classical abdominoplasty or lipoabdominoplasty. All the patients were treated using the lipoabdominoplasty technique and the abovementioned improvements, and fat removal by liposuction ranges from 1.5 l to 2.5 l, and surgical time ranges from 2 to 3 h.

Exclusion criteria were as follows: post-bariatric patients, ASA III patients, BMI above 30, combined general or gynecological surgeries and patients with skin laxity and stretch marks above the umbilicus.

Surgical Technique

Prior to the surgery with the patient standing, the adipose tissue disposition estimated to be liposuctioned included the hypochondrium, pubic area, and flanks. A skin fuse to be removed was calculated with the patient sitting down, and then a low abdominal curved line was designed 6 to 8 cm from the labia major vertex. If the patient had previous scars, the size was maintained as best as possible and was increased to the necessary amount.

Saline solution and epinephrine (1:500,000) were infiltrated in all areas previously marked for lipoaspiration and undermined to help reduce bleeding.

Power-assisted liposuction (PAL) was performed increasing cannulas' size from 3.5 to 4.0 mm and, less frequently, 5 mm. The liposuction began in the prone decubitus position, allowing access to the dorsal region and flanks.

The patients were rotated to the supine position, and PAL was performed, reaching the medial and deep layer in the superior abdomen, including the ribcage. Deep fat excess was removed through liposuction. Liposuction was intensified at the transition of the rectus and oblique abdominis muscles to achieve better body contour.

Pubic incision and undermining of the lower abdomen with Scarpa's fascia removal were performed until umbilical region. From the supraumbilical region to the xiphoid appendix, narrow undermining was performed, just leaving a tunnel. Thus, a selective area of the diastasis region along the medial margins of the rectus muscles is undermined preserving the perforator vessels. The umbilicus was completely isolated removing the entire fat surrounding its stalk.

From the xiphoid appendix to the suprapubic area, the rectus muscle diastasis was corrected in two lines of aponeurotic plications. The umbilicus was fixated at the midline.

In the Fowler position, the superior flap was transported down to the inferior flap, evaluated, and then closed with sutures, trying to generate the least possible tension between the two flaps. During that surgical time, excessive skin at the lower region was removed if required.

Prior to the closure, the pubic flap was immobilized and fixed with 3-0 nylon sutures separated to prevent its ascent. When the patient had a significant amount of fatty tissue on the pubis, liposuction was performed in this area, avoiding uneven surface between the region and lower abdomen.

An aspiration drainage was placed before closure of the abdominal wall and remained there until the collection was less than 30 mL for the day. The superior and inferior flaps were closed using subcutaneous and intradermic stitches, made with 3-0 and 4-0 sutures. In the supine position, the umbilicus was exteriorized and trimmed and placed back into the skin. The umbilical scar was closed, leaving a 3- to 4-cm scar at the hypogastrium region. Omphaloplasty was performed with different sketches according to the body contouring of the patient.

Sterile Micropore tape was placed over the scar, and the patient was dressed in a compression garment that covered the areas that were treated for 30 uninterrupted days. The patient remained hospitalized for 1 day. Early ambulation within 24 h was encouraged for mobilization of third-space fluid shifts to expedite recovery and prevent deep vein thrombosis. Antibiotics, analgesics, and anti-inflammatory medications were used for 7 days after surgery.

Clinical Data and Results

In the last 19 years, we have performed this technique in more than 800 patients, all with indications for classical abdominoplasty or lipoabdominoplasty. The women ranged in age between 24 and 69 years (Figs. 6.1 and 6.2).

The complication rates were as follows 1.00% (eight patients, skin necrosis), 1.11% (nine patients, seroma), and 0.12% (one patient, hematoma) (Table 6.1). The results improved due to correct positioning of the suprapubic scar and previously mentioned reasons. However, scar revision and "dog ear" correction were required in two (0.25%) patients. Late complications such as hypertrophic scars occurred in six (0.75%) patients. Another important result was absence of sensibility loss in the lower abdomen in all patients of the study.

Additional rare complications included fat embolism, thromboembolism, fluid imbalance, perforation of the viscera, and death, which were not present in our patients.

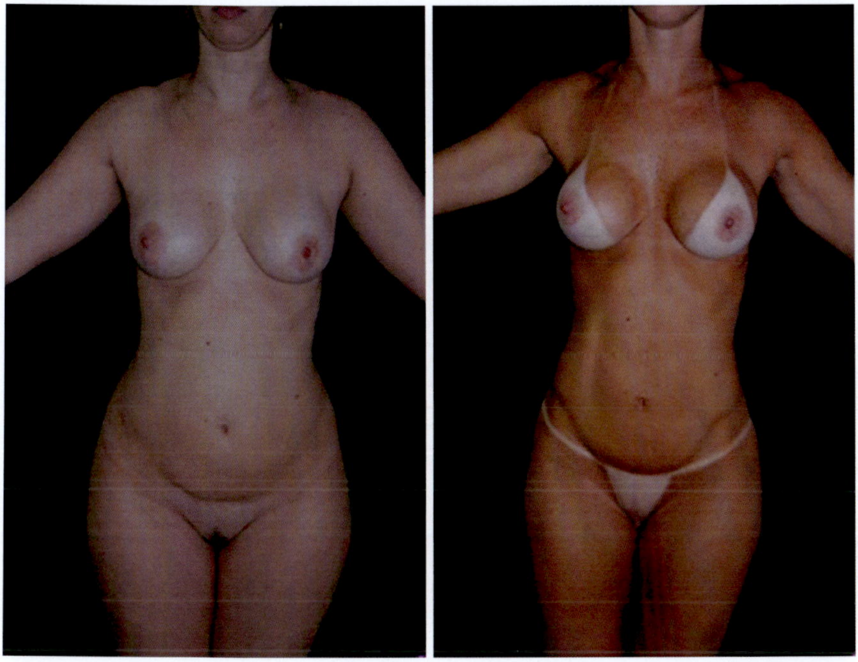

Fig. 6.1 Before and after pictures, 3 months post-op, woman in the fifth decade of life

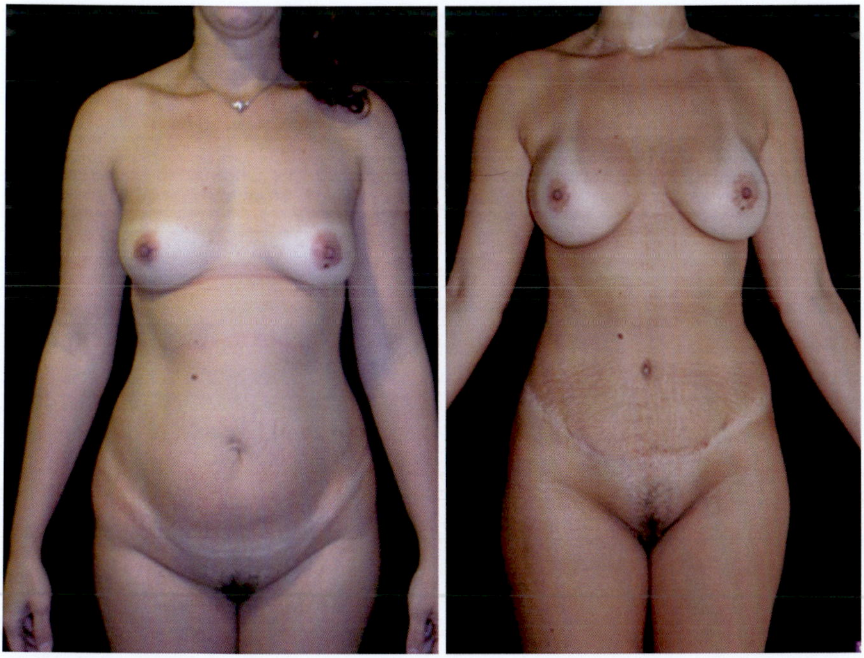

Fig. 6.2 Before and after pictures, 3 months post-op, woman in the fourth decade of life

Table 6.1 Complications

Complications	No. of patients	%
Seroma	9	1.11
Skin necrosis	8	1.00
Hypertrophic scar	6	0.75
Scar revision (dog ear)	2	0.25
Hematoma	1	0.12
Infection	0	0
Thromboembolism	0	0
Suprapubic epidermolysis	0	0
Loss of sensibility	0	0

Discussion

Several body contouring techniques, including liposuction, combined with abdominoplasty have been developed in the last decades, making contributions and progress in lipoabdominoplasty. Since 2003, we have been using lipoabdominoplasty and have found that the procedure results in a broadened vascularized flap and decreases the incidence of complications, such as hematoma, epitheliosis, and necrosis.

The principles and foundations of lipoabdominoplasty are based on preservation of the anatomy of the vascular, lymphatic, and nervous systems of the abdominal wall, involving the two layers of the adipose tissue and muscular groups (Ribeiro 2010; Graf et al. 2006; Saldanha et al. 2001). We observe the global improvement of the technique with less seroma formation, more appropriate body contouring, and a decrease in the incidence of devascularization in the central area of the abdomen, associated with necrosis of the skin and dehiscence.

We used PAL (power-assisted liposuction) using the tumescent technique, which has been shown to be effective and safe for small- to large-volume liposuction cases for body contouring purposes, to be superior in the ease and speed of fat extraction, and to demonstrate shorter procedure times with less surgeon fatigue and a lower incidence of touch-up secondary procedures than traditional liposuction. The same results were observed in studies performed by Fodor in the 1990s (Fodor and Vogt 1999).

Through superficial and deep lipoplasty, we dissected the two layers of the abdominal fat and reached the abdominal flap with fewer traumas than with dissection using a Bovie, which splits up the perforator vessels emerging from the rectoabdominal muscles. Currently, this principle is used in all of our cases. Even in those cases in which the adipose tissue was thin (4% of cases), we preferred to perform divulsion with lipoplasty suction cannulas without a vacuum for the flap (Novaes and Cavalcanti 2006), a maneuver we called lipo undermining.

Selective undermining performed only in the diastasis region of the rectoabdominal muscle allowed plication, and this divulsion did not reach the perforator arteries, which were located 2 cm from the rectoabdominal muscle external edge. Dissection using lipoplasty and selective undermining for plication replaced the large-scale dissections of conventional abdominoplasty and lipectomy (Saldanha

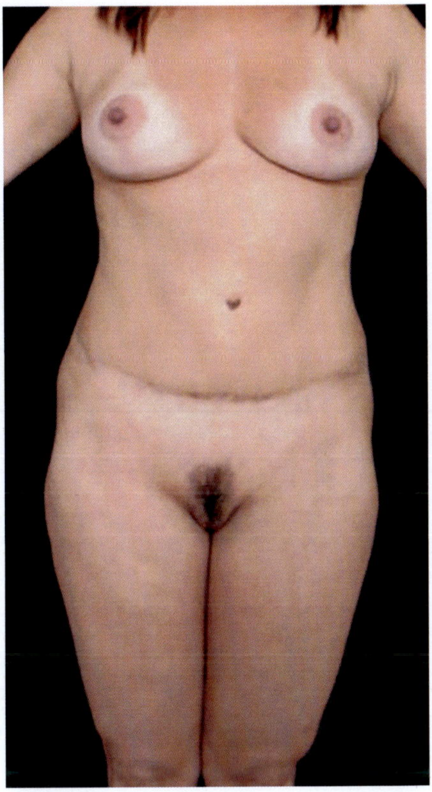

Fig. 6.3 Postoperative of conventional abdominoplasty, leaving a high scar with an unsatisfactory aesthetic result

2003; Lockwood 1995). We maintained the same principles reported by Avelar (1999a, b, c) because we believed that less dissection allows the preservation of vascularity.

Lipoabdominoplasty is a safe and very effective technique, and its results led to the reduction of complications, including seroma, hematoma, and skin necrosis, caused by large skin detachments.

A multi-pedicle flap is created, vessels are preserved, and less dead space is observed, reducing the number of complications commonly observed during abdominoplasty. However, isolated selective undermining may restrain flap movement to the pubic area, resulting in higher scar positioning (Fig. 6.3). To avoid this, we made a modification to the original technique, creating lipoplasty, Mons lipolifting, and pubic fixation.

We routinely associated lipoabdominoplasty with lipoplasty of the flanks or dorsum and outer thigh and lipografting in the gluteal-trochanteric regions, allowing global enhancement of the body contour. Additionally, 2000 units of hyaluronidase were included to help improve the absorption of adipose tissue collected during liposuction. In patients who had undergone great weight loss, lipoabdominoplasty enables thinning of the skin flap, prevents wide undermining, improves the final result, and reduces the complication rate. We can also apply this technique in cases

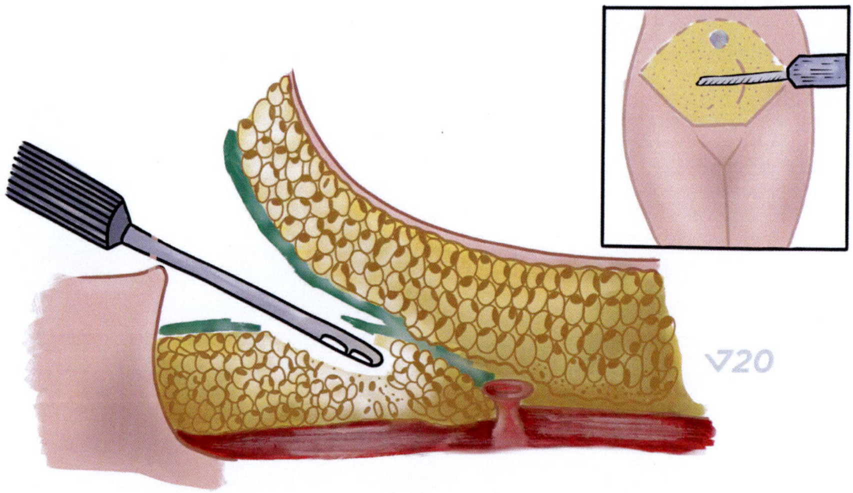

Fig. 6.4 Modified lipoabdominoplasty with removal of the Scarpa's fascia below the navel

of secondary abdominoplasty, when it is necessary to remove the fatty tissue and remaining excessive skin.

Saldanha's technique advocated that it is necessary to perform deep liposuction above the belly button and perform superficial liposuction below it (Saldanha et al. 2001). The liposuction difference in the upper and lower abdomen in terms of depth in the fatty tissue may present an inconvenience in many patients regarding uneven surfaces. We believe this technique impedes the creation of a uniform junction plane, particularly in the lower abdomen. To correct this alteration, we conducted a superficial and deep lipoaspiration in the upper region of the abdomen, deep lipoaspiration in the lower abdomen, and pubic lipoaspiration.

Saldanha et al. also reported complete Scarpa's fascia preservation in the lower abdomen because they believed that preserving the perforating and lymph vessels reduces the complications, such as seroma, hematoma, epitheliosis, and necrosis of the skin, caused by large detachments (Saldanha et al. 2001). However, this preservation can result in the union of the fascia with the superior abdomen, creating a type of "sandwich fascia capsulation" and leading to prolonged edema and bulging. To correct these complications, we modified the surgical technique and performed deep liposuction in the lower abdomen and pubic liposuction. In addition, we proposed that Scarpa's fascia removal in the lower abdomen helps to accommodate the upper abdomen tissue and avoids creating "sandwich fascia capsulation" (Fig. 6.4).

The preservation of structures in the lower abdominal deep fat is important for superior flap accommodation, and it is another relevant foundation of the technique because, anatomically and histologically, the lymphatic vessels are more numerous in this region. We believe that maintenance of the lymphatic system using this method is the main factor in the decrease in the incidence of seroma in the patient subgroup treated according to these principles, as evidenced by some studies (Kelly 1899; Ribeiro 2010; Graf et al. 2006; Marcello et al. 2010).

Conclusion

According to our experience, we have observed important key points that allowed us to overcome difficulties, as well as evolve and progress this technique. By introducing the treatment of flanks with liposuction, an improvement in the quality of the result and a more appropriate body contour have been shown. Using the same principle, patients with Mons pubis lipodystrophy and flaccidity must be treated because it is important for the aesthetic result of this region.

Another fundamental principle in the modification of the technique is the removal of Scarpa's fascia in the inferior flap, thus avoiding the formation of the "fascia sandwich capsulation."

To reduce the number of complications related to the procedure, resection of adipose tissue is recommended through the lipoplasty cannula and selective undermining, allowing the preservation of vascular, lymphatic, and nervous tissue associated with the abdomen. Similarly, the reduction in surgical trauma is the main factor in the decrease in the seroma, hematoma, and necrosis rates.

Finally, the learning curve was fast because the described procedures use techniques and methods that are already familiar to most plastic surgeons.

References

Avelar JM (1999a) New concepts for abdominoplasty. (Novos conceitos para abdominoplastia). Paper presented at the 36th congress of the Brazilian Society of Plastic Surgery, Rio de Janeiro, November.

Avelar JM (1999b) A new technique for abdominoplasty – closed vascular system of subdermal flap folded over itself combined to liposuction. (Uma nova técnica de abdominoplastia – sistema vascular fechado de retalho subdérmico dobrado sobre si mesmo combinado com lipoaspiração). Rev Bras Cir 88/89(1/6):3–20.

Avelar JM (1999c) Abdominoplasty: new concepts for a new technique (Abdominoplastia: Nuevos conceptos para una nueva técnica). XXVI annual international symposium of aesthetic plastic surgery, Chairman: Prof. Jose Guerrerosantos - Puerto Vallarta, pp 10–13.

Gemperli R, Neves RI, Tuma P, et al. Abdominoplasty combined with other intraabdominal procedures. Ann Plast Surg, 1992, 29(1):18–22.

Kelly, H. A.: Johns Hopkins Med. J. 10:197, 1899.

Ribeiro, RC. Evolution of Abdominoplasty. Baker And Gordon Symposium. 2010. EUA.

Callia W. Contribuição para o estudo da correção cirúrgica do abdome pêndulo e globoso—Técnica original [dissertation]. Faculty of the Medical University of São Paulo, 1965.

Pitanguy I. Abdominal lipectomy: an approach to it through an analysis of 300 consecutive cases. Plast Reconst Surg, 1967, 40(4):384–391.

Pitanguy I Abdominal lipectomy. Clin Plast Surg, 1975, 2(3):401–410.

Hakme F (1985) Technical details in the liposuction associated with abdominoplasty. Rev Bras Cir 75:331.

Willkinson TS, Swartz BE: Individual modification of body contour surgery: the "limited" abdominoplasty. Plast Reconstr Surg 77:779, 1986.

Avelar JM: Fat suction versus abdominoplasty. Aesth Plast Surg 9:265–276, 1985.

Bozola AR, Psilakis JN: Abdominoplasty: New concept and classification for treatment. Plast Reconst Surg 82:983–993, 1988

Matarasso A (1991) Abdominoplasty: a system of classification and treatment for combined abdominoplasty and suction-assisted lipectomy. Aesthetic Plast Surg 15:111

Matarasso A: Liposuction as an adjunct to full abdominoplasty revisited. Plast Reconstr Surg 106:1197–1206, 2000

Avelar JM: Abdominoplasty: A new technique without undermining and fat layer removal. Arq Catarinense Med 29:147–149, 2000

Graf R, Araujo L, Rippel R, et al. Lipoabdominoplasty: Liposuction with Reduced Undermining and Traditional Abdominal Skin Flap Resection. Aesth. Plast. Surg. 2006. 30:1–8.

Saldanha OR, de Souza Pinto EB, Mattos WN Jr, et al. Lipoabdominoplasty without undermining. Aesthetic Surg J. 2001; 21: 518–526.

Fodor PB, Vogt PA. Power-assisted lipoplasty (PAL): A clinical pilot study comparing PAL to traditional lipoplasty (TL). Aesth Plast Surg 1999; 23:379–385.

Novaes M. Wilson, Cavalcanti R. Ricardo. Classification for Indications of Lipoabdominoplasty and its Variations; Aesthetic Surgery Journal. 2006: 417–431.

Saldanha OR. Lipoabdominoplasty with selective and safe undermining. Aesthetic plast Surg. 2003;27:322–327.

Lockwood T. High lateral-tension abdominoplasty with superficial fascial system suspension. Plast Reconstr Surg 1995;96:603–608.

Di Martino Marcello, Nahas, F; Barbosa Marcus et al. Seroma in Lipoabdominoplasty and Abdominoplasty: A Comparative Study Using Ultrasound. Plastic & Reconstructive Surgery. 2010;126:1742–1751.

Chapter 7
Surgical Principles and Classification of Lipoabdominoplasty

Juarez Moraes Avelar and Ricardo Cavalcanti Ribeiro

Abstract Kelly is credited with the first publication on abdominoplasty and panniculus resection performed on the elliptical horizontal skin, a publication where he coined the term *abdominal lipectomy*. Following his surgical principles, several other authors have described other approaches. Moreover, remarkable improvements came with liposuction, introducing revolutionary concepts that improved body-contouring procedures.

However, by employing liposuction, the accumulation of fat could be removed, but the redundant skin required conventional resection, which did not cause new sorts of complications. Such combined approaches have increased the rate of some complications, such as seroma formation, the slough and necrosis of the panniculus, and local infections, among others. Because of those uncomfortable situations, after a short period of time, I made a radical decision to not perform both procedures anymore. Nevertheless, I obsessively looked for a solution to those complex problems. In trying to solve such complications, I envisioned finding a new approach to perform the combined procedures. Thinking about a safe technique, I returned to my previous anatomical study of the abdominal panniculus and concluded that I could combine liposuction with conventional abdominoplasty as long as the perforator vessels didn't sustain damage. After 10 years of intensive study and research, I discovered new concepts in abdominoplasty that I presented and published, and with them, I could combine both procedures: liposuction with abdominoplasty. After such persistent research, I found new approaches for the treatment of the abdominal wall that reduced complications. Thus, the aesthetic results for the abdominal wall were improved in lower, upper, and lower and upper abdomino-

J. M. Avelar
Brazilian Scientific Institute of Plastic and Reconstructive Surgery, São Paulo, Brazil

R. C. Ribeiro (✉)
Plastic and Reconstructive Surgery, Federal University of the State of Rio de Janeiro, Rio de Janeiro, Brazil
e-mail: rribeiro@centroin.net.br

J. M. Avelar, R. Cavalcanti Ribeiro (eds.), *Body Contouring*,
https://doi.org/10.1007/978-3-031-42802-9_7

plasty and in full abdominoplasty. In all modalities of this operation, the surgical principle of preserving the perforator vessels was the key to the procedure.

Keywords Abdominoplasty · Lipoabdominoplasty · Surgical principles · Classification · Lower abdominoplasty · Upper abdominoplasty

Introduction

Abdominoplasty was quite a new procedure in plastic surgery at the end of the nineteenth century, when some publications reported on the aesthetic treatment of the abdominal wall while still searching for a harmonious balance for the body. The credit was given to Kelly (1899), but Demars and Marx published a procedure earlier, in 1890 (Sinder 1979).

In his first publication, Kelly (1899) performed elliptical horizontal skin resection on the adipose tissue of the abdominal wall, including the umbilical area, and in this publication, he coined the term *abdominal lipectomy*. His original publication popularized the operation, and his name is a symbol of abdominoplasty. That marks the beginning of a long history of abdominoplasty, which has since been followed by many other scientific publications all over the world. Abdominoplasty has undergone a remarkable evolution of improving the surgical results for body contouring.

Following Kelly's resection, several other authors have since published in the medical literature different modalities of panniculus resection for the reparation of the abdominal wall and the abnormalities of the torso, as described by Sinder (1979). The various types of incisions can be classified into five modalities: horizontal incisions, vertical incisions, circular incisions, submammary incisions, and half-moon skin resections on the bilateral submammary folds.

1. Horizontal incisions are the most frequently performed in abdominoplasty, first because the majority of patients present with some sort of scars from previous operations on the lower segment of the abdominal wall in the suprapubic area and second because the first description of abdominoplasty, by Kelly, was a type of horizontal incision for the reparation of unaesthetic scars to rebuild the abdominal wall. Several authors, such as Jolly (1911), Malbec (1948), Callia (1965), Pontes (1965, 1982), Pitanguy (1967a, b, 1982), Planas (1982), Serson Neto (1970, 1982), Sinder (1975, 1982), Guerrerosantos (1982a, b), and Avelar (1976a, b, 1983a, b, 1985a, b, 1999a, b, 2000a, b), have since described their approaches to the aesthetic surgery of the abdomen wall, among other procedures introduced by other surgeons.
2. Vertical incisions have been credited to Babcock (1916), but they leave long scars on the midline of the abdomen. With this approach, the abdomen can be reshaped, particularly for patients who've undergone severe weight loss.
3. Circular incisions were introduced by Gonzales-Ulloa (1959), the first author to describe such an approach, which he called belt lipectomy (1967, 1982), and few years later, Vilain (1964, 1982, 1986) called it lipectomie circulaire. Such a procedure is performed quite often for remodeling the entire body on patients

who have undergone severe weight loss, achieving well-balanced body contouring.

4. Submammary incisions are part of an unusual approach described by Thorek (1942a, b) to remove the excess panniculus on the superior segment of the abdomen. The author did not precisely draw the skin resection on the submammary fold, but the objective of the operation was to remove the panniculus on the upper abdomen below the breasts. Three decades later, Rebello et al. (1972) and Rebello (1982) described the submammary incisions in selected patients presenting with abnormalities on the panniculus of the upper abdomen. In their descriptions, a wide undermining on the supra-aponeurotic level is performed, followed by superior traction for resection.
5. Half-moon skin resections on the bilateral submammary folds constitute the final modality. When I introduced a combination of abdominoplasty with liposuction, I had several patients presenting with unaesthetic bilateral abnormalities on the submammary folds. Since my previous scientific publications (Avelar 1999a, b, 2000a, b, 2001a, b, 2002) on abdominoplasty associated with liposuction, a new approach has been designed and new concepts described. So far, my incisions have not joined the midline of the sternal region but rather isolated ones on each side of the submammary folds (Fig. 7.1).

   A half-moon skin is resected on each side of the hypochondriac region in order to treat the upper abdominal wall by making upper incisions without panniculus undermining (Figs. 7.2, 7.3, and 7.4).

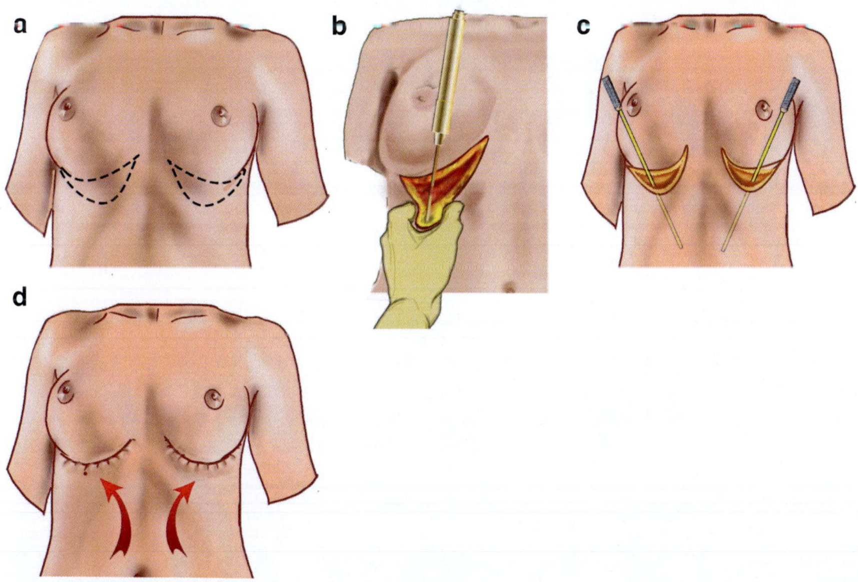

Fig. 7.1 Squamatization of upper lipoabdominoplasty technique. Drawing (**a**) surgical demarcations of the operation delimitating two areas of full-thickness of liposuction below the submammary sulcus; (**b**) liposuction procedure is firstly done on area for skin resection; (**c**) afterwards it is done on lamellar layer, on superior panniculus below the fascia superficialis; (**d**) finally the wounds are sutured by layers leaving two scars on submammary sulcus

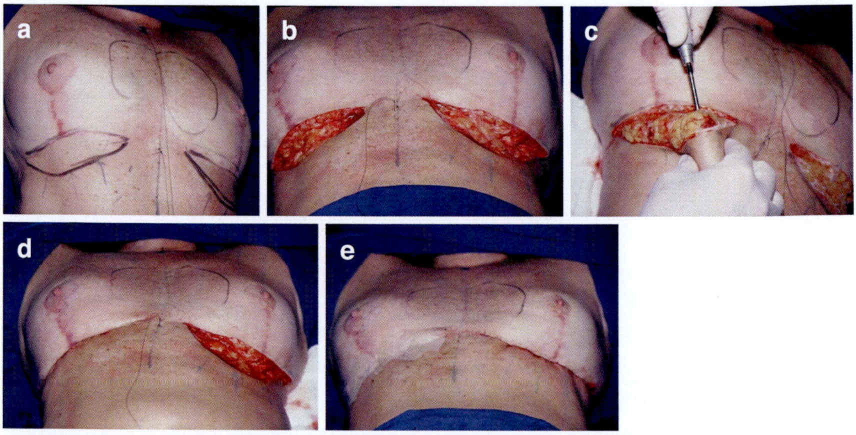

Fig. 7.2 Perioperative photos demonstrating the technique of upper lipoabdominoplasty. Photo (**a**) surgical demarcations of a half-moon area on submammary regions; (**b**) after full-thickness of the panniculus on the half-moon "island"; (**c**) deep liposuction (below the fascia superficialis) is done on remaining panniculus from up downwards; (**d**) the border of the wound is already sutured on right side; (**e**) suture was performed on both sides

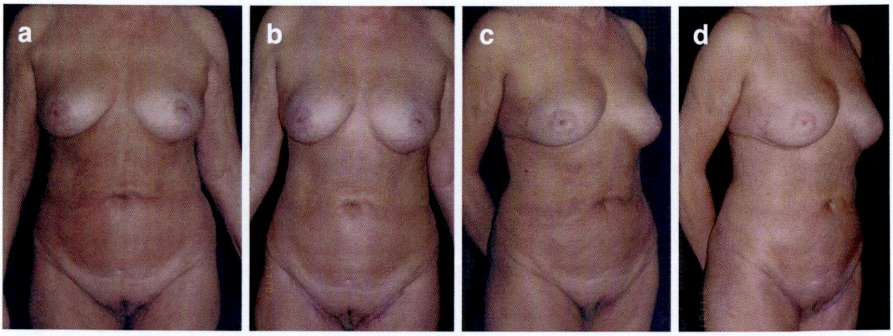

Fig. 7.3 Correction of superior region of the abdominal wall through upper lipoabdominoplasty. (**a, c**) Before operation showing localized adiposities on superior abdominal wall; (**b, d**) after upper lipoabdominoplasty

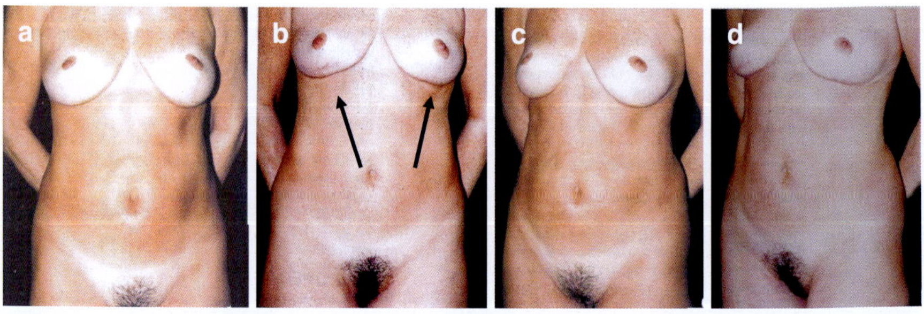

Fig. 7.4 A 39-year-old patient underwent lipoplasty of the abdominal wall performed elsewhere presenting irregularities caused by previous liposuction performed elsewhere. Photos (**a, c**) before surgery; (**b, d**) after operation of upper lipoabdominoplasty

New Concepts for Abdominoplasty Associated with Liposuction Without Panniculus Undermining

Until 1999, all the types of abdominoplasty were performed through the wide undermining of the abdominal panniculus in order to resect its excess. Such a concept was employed no matter which incisions were made in all techniques. In this way, in the traditional procedures, all the perforator vessels coming from the muscular level are cut to reach the wide area of the abdomen.

The liposuction technique, created and popularized by Illouz (1980, 1983a, b, 1984, 1986a, b), is one of the most revolutionary surgical techniques for the aesthetic treatment of the abdominal wall after abdominal lipectomy, which was first described by Kelly in 1899. The use of liposuction bought substantial improvements to the aesthetic treatment of the abdominal wall, with excellent and suitable results and very low rates of complications during and after surgery. The liposuction method is very useful for removing localized adiposity because the correction of excess skin on the abdominal wall used to be resected through panniculus undermining; I have previously described such a combined procedure (Avelar 1985a, b, 1986a, b, c). So far, the associated approaches have not presented new sorts of complications, but they have greatly increased the rate of seroma formation, the slough and necrosis of the panniculus, local infections, and other uncomfortable complications. Given such very high incidences of local complications after abdominoplasty, I decided after a short period of time to not perform it anymore (Avelar 1988). However, isolated liposuction on the submentonian and submandibular regions combined with rhytidoplasty did not present any new kinds of complications, although they have been encountered on the abdomen (Avelar 1983b, 1985c). Although I did not perform such associated procedures of liposuction with traditional abdominoplasty during that time, I devoted considerable study and thought to devising a technical solution that would avoid those uncomfortable complications. I worked obsessively for several years on my previous anatomical research (1986a, b, c, 1987, 1989), looking for an appropriate way to remove the excess skin associated with liposuction.

At the end of nineteenth century, Kelly (1899) published the first abdominoplasty method, and at the end of twentieth century, I (Avelar 1999a, b, c) published a combination of abdominoplasty with liposuction that preserves the perforator vessels to avoid all those complications (Fig. 7.5). Those are the roots of lipoabdominoplasty that developed from intensive and deep study and research (Avelar 1999a, b, c, 2000a, b).

Over the course of 10 years of studying the anatomy of the abdominal panniculus (from 1988 to 1998), I developed and published a new method, which is a new surgical procedure that removes the excess skin of the redundant panniculus with minimal rates of complications. Therefore, the surgical principles of conventional abdominoplasty through lipectomy are not performed in my method, because in mine, the perforator vessels are preserved to provide adequate vascularization to the remaining abdominal panniculus (Fig. 7.5) (Avelar 1999a, b, c, 2000a, b, 2001a, b, 2002).

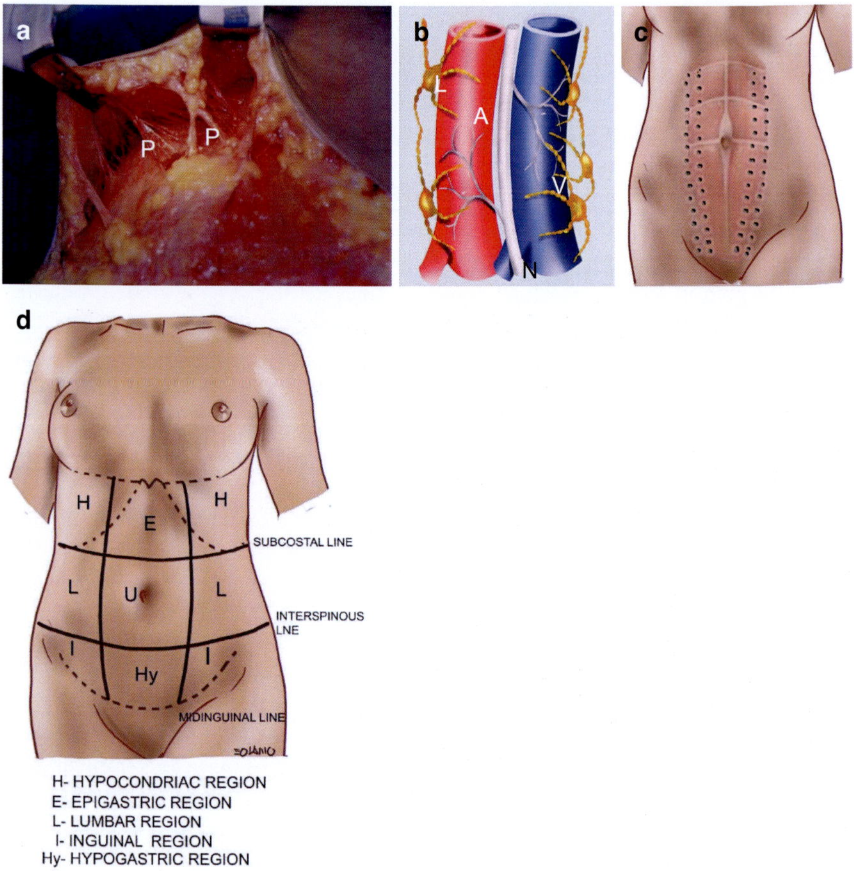

Fig. 7.5 The main surgical principles of abdominoplasty without panniculus undermining are preservation of the perforator vessels which work as multiplex pedicles for the remaining panniculus providing adequate blood supply (arterial, venous, and lymphatics). Photo (**a**) perioperative showing several perforator vessels preserved during abdominoplasty; (**b**) diagram showing the composition of the anatomic unit of a perforator vessel: *A* artery, *V* vein, *L* lymphatic, *N* nerve; (**c**) diagram showing location of the perforator vessels coming from rectus abdominalis muscle; (**d**) the abdominal wall is divided into nine regions: three odds (epigastric, umbilical, hypogastric) and three even hipochondriac, lumbar, and inguinal

Surgical Principles

Until my publications, the surgical principles of my method had not been described in the medical literature. For this reason, I present to the reader the following new concepts as surgical principles that improve abdominoplasty. My technique is recommended for patients presenting with excess skin, localized adiposities, a redundant panniculus, muscular flaccidity, and diastasis in the rectus abdominalis (Fig. 7.6). Knowing the anatomy of the abdominal panniculus, particularly of the vascularization described in my previous publications (Avelar 1986a, b, c, 1989), is

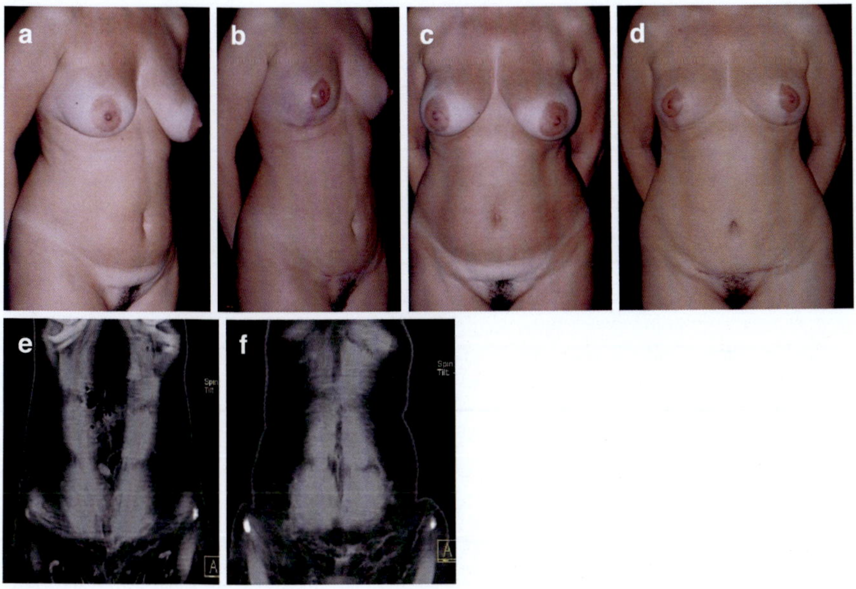

Fig. 7.6 Lower lipoabdominoplasty in a 32-year-old patient combined with plication of the muscular abdominal wall. Photos (**a, c, e**) before surgery; (**b, d, f**) post-operative photos showing reinforcement of the rectus abdominalis and its aponeurosis

fundamental to performing this procedure. Key elements of the technique are described below:

1. The operation is performed as a closed vascular system, which represents a new technique that is based on new concepts for improving body contouring (Avelar 1999a, b, c, 2000a, b). Because in this method the vascular network is not damaged, the perforator vessels supply the abdominal panniculus as multiple pedicles (Figs. 7.5 and 7.7).
2. The cutaneous excess is treated via the full-thickness skin resection of the suprapubic (Figs. 7.1, 7.2, and 7.8), infraumbilical, and/or submammary regions.
3. Deep liposuction is performed before skin resection on all the abdominal regions that present with localized adiposities. Very often, other regions of the posterior and lateral aspects of the torso must be simultaneously treated to achieve a good aesthetic balance in body contouring.
4. In the area of skin resection (suprapubic, submammary, or infraumbilical), liposuction is performed before the full-thickness skin resection (Figs. 7.1, 7.2, 7.8, 7.9, and 7.10).
5. The connective tissue and all vessels of the resected skin area are also preserved. This prevents the destruction of the perforator vessels and prevents small vessels from coursing perpendicularly to the communicating vessel network in the fascia superficial (Figs. 7.5 and 7.7b) provided by the subdermal vascularization.

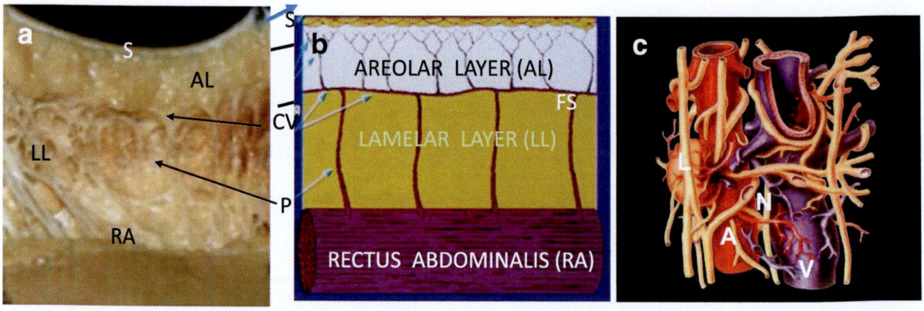

Fig. 7.7 Anatomic study of the abdominal panniculus demonstrating the basic principles of lipoabdominoplasty. Photo (**a**) abdominal panniculus of a cadaver after liposuction one can see: skin (S), with preservation of the areolar layer (AL), lamellar layer (LL), communicating vessels (CV), perforator vessels (P), rectus abdominalis (RA); (**b**) diagram showing all anatomical structures; (**c**) diagram of the anatomic unit of a perforator vessel: *A* artery, *V* vein, *L* lymphatics, *N* nerve

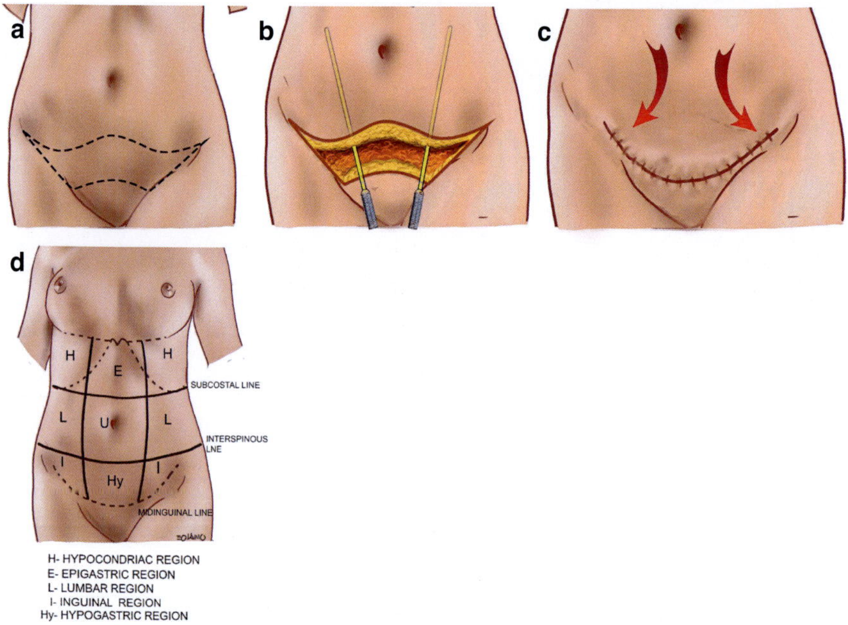

Fig. 7.8 Schemas demonstrating lower lipoabdominoplasty technique. Drawing (**a**) surgical demarcations of the operation delimitating the area of full-thickness of liposuction; (**b**) liposuction procedure is firstly done on area for skin resection, afterwards on lamellar layer, below the fascia superficialis on the remaining panniculus; (**c**) finally the wound is sutured by layers leaving a scar on supra pubic region; (**d**) diagram showing all regions of the abdominal wall

6. All the perforator vessels work as multiple pedicles to supply normal vascularization (through the arterial, venous, and lymphatic vessels) to the remaining abdominal panniculus (Figs. 7.5, 7.7, and 7.9).

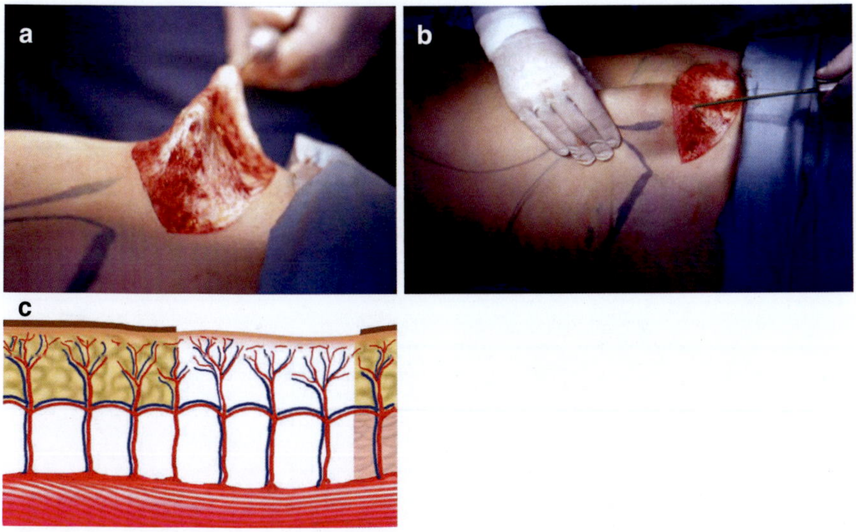

Fig. 7.9 Liposuction procedure of the abdominal panniculus is performed on two layers. Perioperative photos demonstrating: (**a**) full-thickness where skin resection is done; (**b**) deep liposuction, below fascia superficialis, all over the remaining panniculus; (**c**) diagram shows liposuction on full thickness of the panniculus where skin resection is done and deep liposuction under the remaining panniculus

7. The lymphatic vessels, which surround the arteries and veins, are preserved because the perforator vessels are not cut. Therefore, the lymph coming from the abdominal panniculus maintains its normal circulation after surgery, avoiding seroma formation (Figs. 7.5, 7.7, and 7.9).
8. Cauterization during surgery is not necessary, because this method doesn't damage the blood vessels.
9. Unlike the classical abdominoplasty—in which postoperative drainage is an important procedure that may need to be applied many times for 3, 5, or 7 days and sometimes for longer than 3 weeks—this new surgical technique does not require drainage, because it doesn't cause bleeding during or after surgery and doesn't allow seroma formation (Figs. 7.5, 7.7, and 7.9).
10. Blood transfusion is unnecessary because there is no bleeding during or after surgery.

Nevertheless, in some patients presenting with localized adiposities associated with the flaccidity of the muscular wall of the abdomen, liposuction is performed in combination with abdominoplasty to treat all the problems of the regions (Fig. 7.6). Concerning liposuction for the treatment of the abdominal wall, several authors have introduced their contributions to this field. In fact, Illouz's (1980) technique opened up a new era in body-contouring surgery, particularly on the abdominal wall. I also contributed by presenting and publishing my approach as a combination of conventional abdominoplasty with liposuction (Avelar 1985a, b, 1986a, b). Even

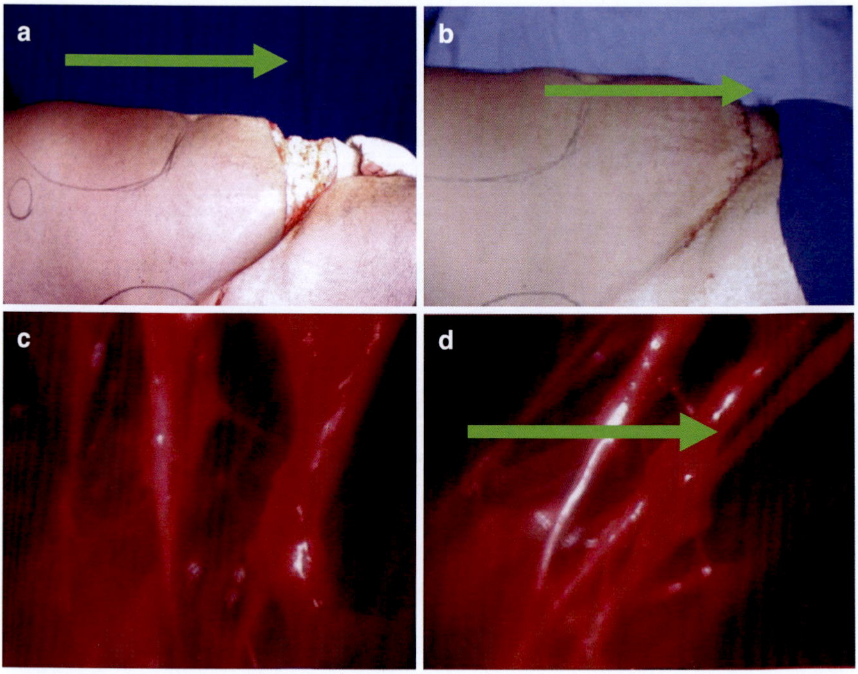

Fig. 7.10 Perioperatives photos demonstrating deep liposuction (below fascia superficialis) with preservation of perforator vessels. (**a**) Liposuction was done on suprapubic area with arrow indicating downward direction of the traction; (**b**) after traction and suture; (**c**) internal photo showing the perforator vessels after liposuction on perpendicular position; (**d**) after traction the perforator vessels are inclined due to traction of the panniculus, working as multiple pedicles to the remaining panniculus

before incorporating liposuction, I introduced my method for the creation of a natural umbilicus during abdominoplasty (Avelar 1976a, b, 1979, 1983a, b). Furthermore, I carried out careful anatomical research on corpses, which brought significant information on the alterations and behavior of the subcutaneous tissue after liposuction (Figs. 7.5 and 7.7).

Classification of Lipoabdominoplasty

The abdominal wall can be anatomically divided into nine regions: three odd, and single namely epigastric, umbilical, and hypogastric, and three even, right and left, namely hypochondriac, flank, and inguinal (Fig. 7.5d) (Avelar 1989). Aesthetic surgery can be classified into only two segments: superior and inferior (above and below the umbilical area, respectively). A careful analysis of my patients who have undergone abdominoplasty without panniculus undermining and resection shows that abdominoplasty can be classified into four types:

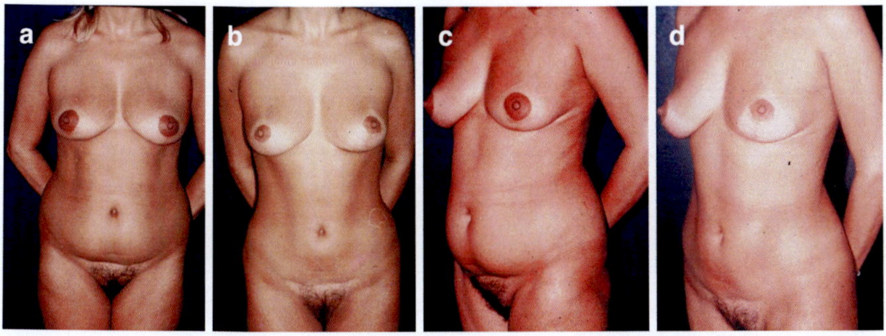

Fig. 7.11 A 48-year-old patient underwent lower lipoabdominoplasty. Photos (**a, c**) before surgery showing localized adiposities on upper and lower abdominal wall with previous surgical scars on supra pubic region; (**b, d**) after lower lipoabdominoplasty

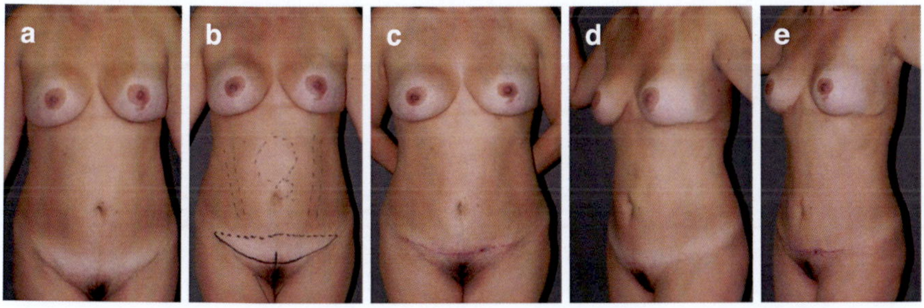

Fig. 7.12 A 39-year-old patient underwent lower lipoabdominoplasty presenting previous scars on suprapubic region and irregularities caused by previous liposuction performed elsewhere. Photos (**a, d**) before surgery; (**b**) surgical demarcations of the areas of remaining adiposities as well as the area for skin resection; photos (**c, e**) after operation of lower lipoabdominoplasty

1. Lower abdominoplasty (Figs. 7.6, 7.7, 7.8, 7.9, 7.10, 7.11, 7.12, and 7.13)
2. Upper abdominoplasty (Figs. 7.1, 7.2, 7.3, and 7.4)
3. Lower and upper abdominoplasty (combined procedure) (Figs. 7.14, 7.15, 7.16, and 7.17)
4. Full abdominoplasty (Figs. 7.18, 7.19, and 7.20)

Lower abdominoplasty must be employed for the correction of unaesthetic deformities on the inferior segment of the abdomen (Figs. 7.6, 7.7, 7.8, 7.9, 7.10, 7.11, 7.12, and 7.13). According to surgical demarcation, the area in the suprapubic region is adequately demarcated (Fig. 7.8a, b, c) and the operation may be performed under general or epidural anesthesia combined with local infiltration. Two levels of local infiltration must be carried out: a deep infiltration on the supramuscular parts of all regions for liposuction and superficial infiltration on the area for skin resection. The solution of infiltration is determined by the routine of each surgeon. The first step of the operation is to perform two types of liposuction: one on the full thickness of the panniculus in the suprapubic region where skin resection

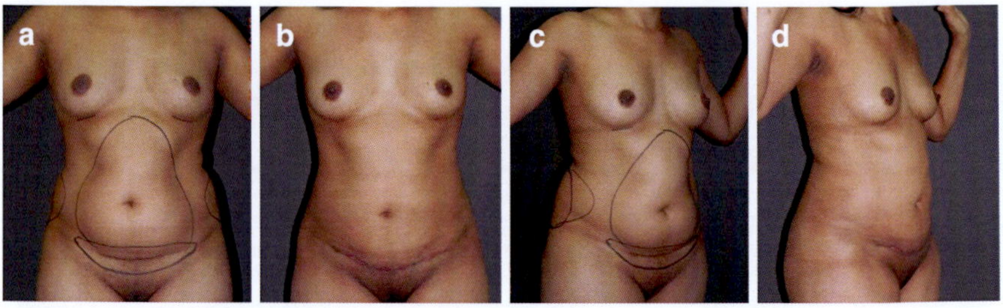

Fig. 7.13 Lower lipoabdominoplasty in a 36-year-old patient without transposition of the umbilicus. Photos (**a, c**) before surgery; (**b, d**) 6 months after lower lipoabdominoplasty

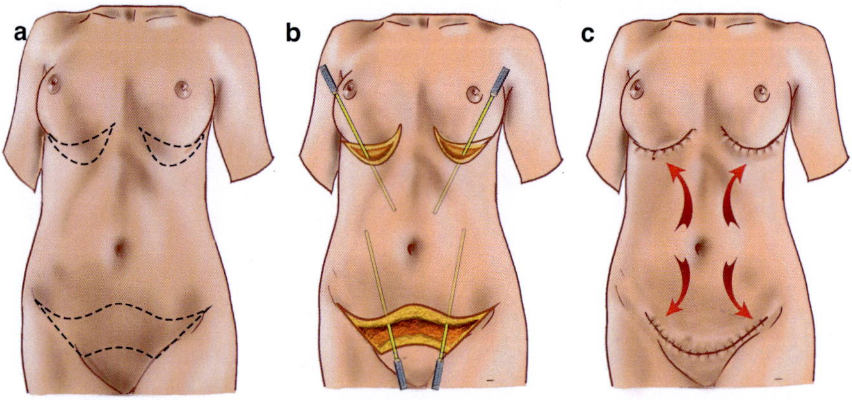

Fig. 7.14 Diagrams demonstrating upper and lower lipoabdominoplasty. (**a**) Surgical demarcations: on upper abdominal wall a half-moon area is drawing below submammary sulcus; (**b**) full-thickness liposuction of the panniculus is done on areas where skin resection is performed and deep liposuction (below the fascia superficialis) is done on remaining panniculus; (**c**) suture on submammary sulcus and supra pubic region

will be performed (Figs. 7.8a and 7.9a) and one at a deep level over all the areas presenting with localized adiposities (Figs. 7.8b and 7.9b, c).

After liposuction has been completed, the connective tissues and all the perforator vessels remain attached to the musculoaponeurotic plane, which creates a depression on the suprapubic area (Fig. 7.10a). Following the liposuction procedure on the full thickness of the panniculus, a deep liposuction is conducted on the lamellar layer (below the fascia superficialis) on all the regions of the abdominal wall presenting with localized adiposities for which skin resection will not be performed (Fig. 7.9b, c), as described in my previous publications (Avelar 1999a, b). As long as the areolar layer is well preserved, the final aspect of the abdomen wall will show a harmonious surface. The remaining panniculus easily slides over the musculoaponeurotic plane because the lamellar layer does not present with any adiposities and because all the perforator vessels are preserved, which work as multiple pedicles that supply blood to the remaining abdominal panniculus (Figs. 7.9c and 7.10c, d).

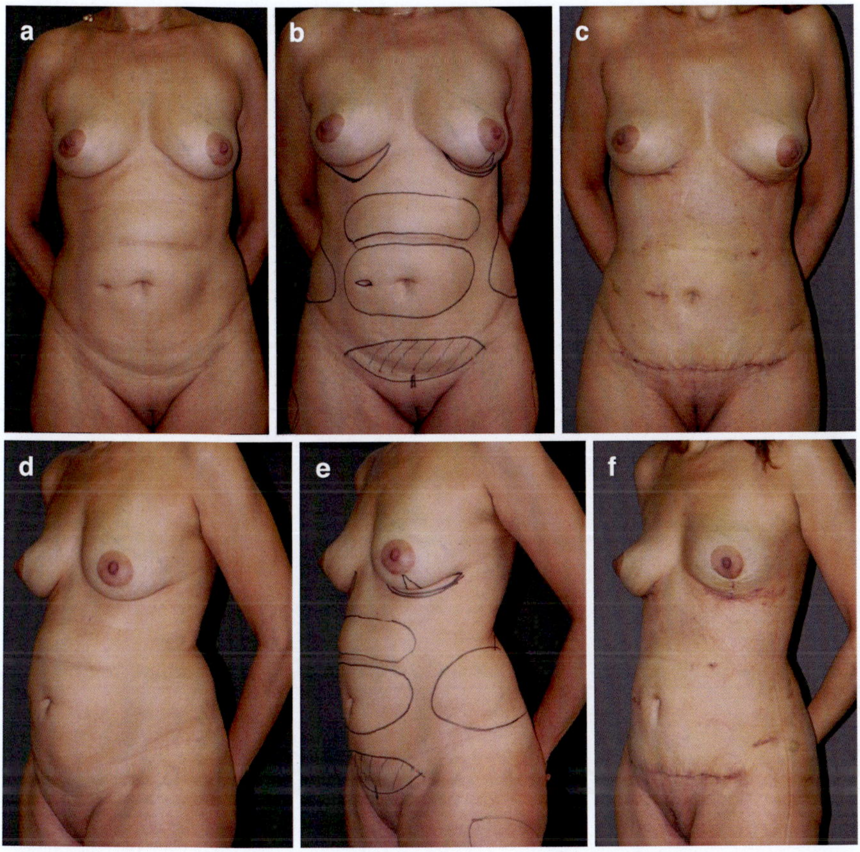

Fig. 7.15 A 49-year-old female patient before and after combined upper and lower lipoabdominoplasty. Photos (**a, d**) before operation; (**b, e**) demarcations of the areas for skin resection on half-moon shaped below the breasts and on supra pubic areas, also localized adiposities on umbilical, supra umbilical and supra iliac. She presented a transversal scar on upper abdominal region which is adverse condition for full lipoabdominalplsty. Photos (**c, f**) post-operatory view six months after operation regions

The plication of the musculoaponeurotic wall may be performed according to surgical planning when the patient presents with diastasis in the rectus abdominalis or when it shows up on computerized tomography (CT scan), which is a routine preoperative exam.

The next step of the operation is to pull the remaining panniculus downward (Fig. 7.10b), to be sutured to the inferior border of the raw area. The wound must be sutured on three levels: on the fascia superficialis, on the subdermal layer, and on the dermis (Fig. 7.10b). If necessary, a running suture is performed in the dermis, and adhesive tapes are applied on the surgical scars without any traction. Surgeons should use a garment covering over the whole area of the abdominal wall, which is maintained for the 1 week before the patient returns for the removal of their dressing

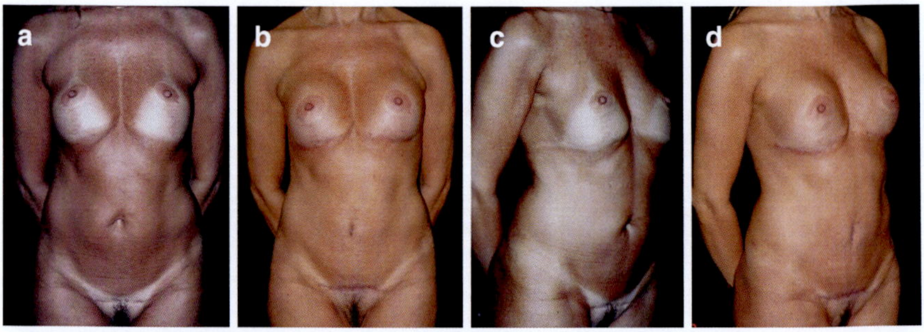

Fig. 7.16 A 51-year-old female patient underwent upper and lower lipoabdominoplasty. Photos (**a, c, e**) before operation showing unaesthetic shape of the breasts and adiposities on superior and inferior abdomen; (**b, d, f**) after operation. One can see the projection of the breasts as well as the aesthetic improvement on the superior and inferior regions of the abdomen. The final scars are located on submammary sulcus and on supra pubic region

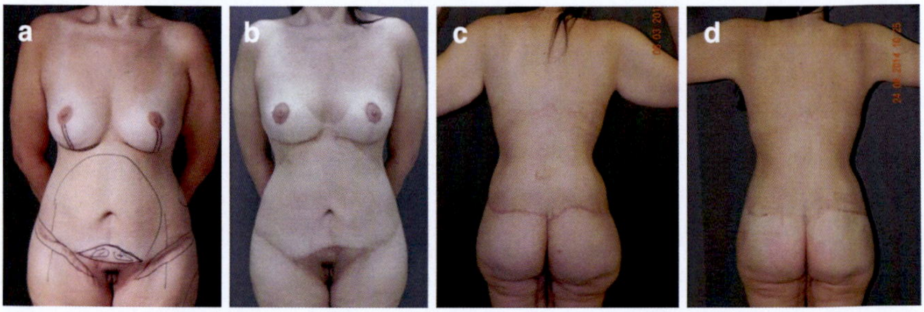

Fig. 7.17 A patient underwent upper and lower lipoabdominoplasty for reparation of previous surgeries on abdomen and breasts. Photos (**a, c**) before operation showing unaesthetic shape of the breasts and adiposities on superior and inferior abdomen, on arms, on posterior aspects of the torso as well; (**b, d**) after operation. One can see improvement of the breasts, on the superior and inferior regions of the abdomen, as well as on arms and posterior regions of the torso

and the application of new adhesive tapes, which are changed once every 2 weeks for the next 2 months. The final result may be evaluated 6 months to 1 year later (Figs. 7.11, 7.12, and 7.13).

Upper abdominoplasty should be performed when a patient presents with deformities localized specifically on the upper segment, above the umbilical region (Figs. 7.1, 7.2, 7.3, and 7.4). Upper lipoabdominoplasty is a less-common modality for aesthetic surgery on the abdomen wall. As always, this procedure requires adequate surgical planning and careful, correct demarcation before the operation (Figs. 7.1a and 7.2a). Two areas for skin resection are marked on the superior abdomen, where two crescent shapes are drawn bilaterally below the submammary fold. In addition, other areas for liposuction are marked all over the abdominal wall to indicate where to remove localized adiposities.

This surgery must be performed in a hospital or a clinic with all the necessary equipment for an operation. It may be carried out under general anesthesia or

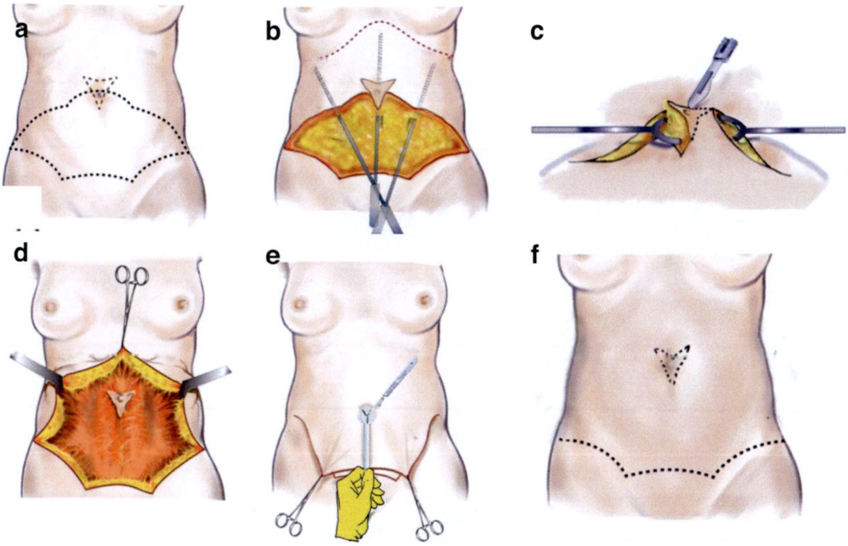

Fig. 7.18 Technical systematization of full lipoabdominoplasty. (**a**) Preoperatory demarcation of the area for skin resection and the triangular incisions on the umbilicus; (**b**) liposuction on full-thickness of the panniculus; (**c**) cutaneous incisions around the umbilicus; (**d**) skin resection was done following by deep liposuction on supra umbilical region; (**e**) a special instrument is placed to demarcate the new umbilicus on the abdominal flap; (**f**) the upper abdominal flap is pulled downwards and the suture was done

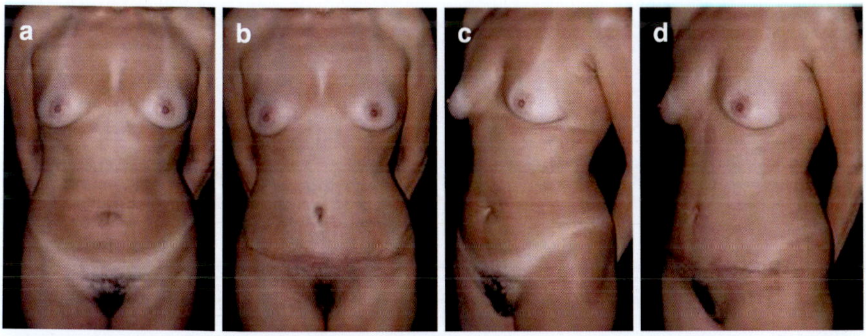

Fig. 7.19 A 54-year-old patient presenting localized adiposities and panniculus flaccidity on all regions of the abdominal wall underwent full lipoabdominoplasty. Fotos (**a, c**) before surgery; (**b, d**) after full lipoabdominoplasty

epidural associated with local infiltration. Following surgical demarcation, two levels of local infiltration must be carried out: a deep one on the supramuscular parts of all the regions for liposuction and a superficial one on the full thickness of the panniculus where liposuction will be performed. The solution of infiltration is determined by the routine of each surgeon.

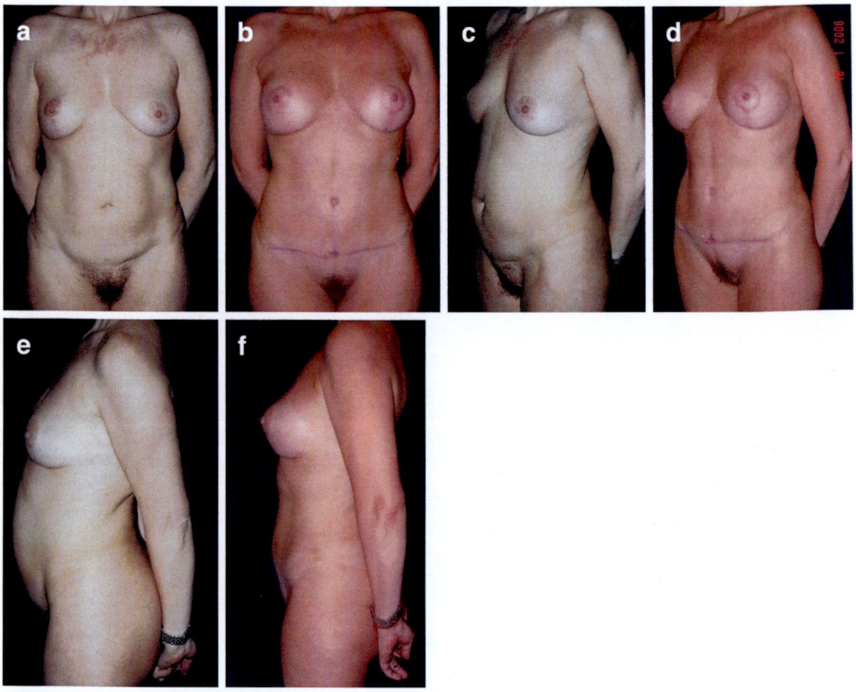

Fig. 7.20 A 51-year-old patient underwent full lipoabdominoplasty without panniculus undermining combined with mastopexy with mammary implant. Photos (**a, c, e**) before surgery operation; photos (**b, d, f**) after full lipoabdominoplasty with creation of the new umbilical region

The operation starts with two types of liposuction: a bilateral one on the full thickness of the panniculus on the submammary areas that have crescent-shaped demarcation where skin resection will be performed and a deep level one below the fascia superficialis and over all the areas presenting with localized adiposities (Figs. 7.1b, c, and 7.2c). Only connective tissue and some perforator vessels remain attached to the musculoaponeurotic level. Usually, a depression may be noticed just below the submammary folds after full-thickness liposuction (Fig. 7.2b). Through the same area below the breasts, deep liposuction is carried out on the lamellar layer (below the fascia superficialis) over all the regions presenting with localized adiposities on the abdominal wall. The cannula must be introduced below the fascia superficialis, from the top downward (Figs. 7.1b, c, and 7.2c) (Avelar 1999a, b).

After liposuction, full-thickness skin resection is performed bilaterally on the crescent-shaped areas. Usually, this operation doesn't cause any bleeding, because no vessels are damaged. The remaining panniculus slides over the musculoaponeurotic level because no fat appears below the fascia superficialis, and all the perforator vessels are preserved, which work as multiple pedicles to the abdominal panniculus. In selected cases, the plication of the musculoaponeurotic wall is performed when indications are present. Finally, the wound is sutured according to anatomical plans, where the fascia superficialis is the most important for reinstating the full thickness of the panniculus (Fig. 7.2d). Afterward, the subdermal level and the dermis are sutured. The final scar lies naturally on the submammary areas, which are postoperatively inconspicuous (Figs. 7.3 and 7.4).

Upper and lower abdominoplasty is a type of combined procedure that is indicated when both segments (the superior and the inferior) of the abdomen need to be simultaneously repaired and is performed on patients presenting with a very high navel, which makes the transposition of the umbilicus impossible (Figs. 7.14, 7.15, 7.16, and 7.17). This procedure requires adequate surgical demarcation before surgery, and it should be carried out after meticulous measurement (Figs. 7.14, 7.15, 7.16, and 7.17). The areas for skin resection are inferiorly marked on the suprapubic region and on the superior abdomen; here, two crescent-shaped areas are drawn bilaterally below the submammary fold. Also, the areas for liposuction are marked on the abdominal wall.

The operation may be performed while the patient is under general anesthesia or is administered an epidural combined with local infiltration. Two levels of local infiltration must be carried out: a deep infiltration on the supramuscular areas in all regions for liposuction and a superficial infiltration on areas for skin resection. The solution is determined by each surgeon.

The first step of the operation is to perform two types of liposuction: one on the full thickness of the panniculus where skin resection will be performed and one at deep level over all the areas presenting with localized adiposities (Figs. 7.14 and 7.15). Afterward, the connective tissue and all the perforator vessels remain attached to the musculoaponeurotic plane without any fat, which creates a depression on the suprapubic area and below the submammary fold.

Afterward, deep liposuction is carried out on the lamellar layer (below the fascia superficialis) on all the regions of the abdominal wall presenting with localized adiposities where skin resection will not be performed (Figs. 7.15, 7.16, and 7.17), according to my previous publications (Avelar 1999a, b, 2000a, b). Also, preserving the areolar layer yields a smooth and harmonious surface to the areas where skin resection is not performed.

Following the operation, skin resection is carried out on the local depressions corresponding to the areas of liposuction performed on the full thickness of the panniculus. The remaining panniculus easily slides over the musculoaponeurotic wall because there is no fat below the fascia superficialis, and all the perforator vessels are preserved, which work as multiple pedicles to the abdominal panniculus. The plication of the musculoaponeurotic wall may be performed, and it is a useful procedure during abdominoplasty if it's part of the surgical plan or when indications show up on a computerized tomography (CT) scan (Fig. 7.6). By following these technical steps, the final scar will be smooth on the submammary sulcus and the suprapubic region (Figs. 7.15, 7.16, and 7.17).

Full abdominoplasty is performed when there is an indication to perform conventional abdominoplasty because there are abnormalities on the superior and inferior segments of the abdomen, and the transposition of the umbilicus must also be performed. It is the most complex type of abdominoplasty without panniculus undermining and resection, in that it requires resecting the entire skin of the infraumbilical area. The complete description of this procedure appears in the following chapters (Figs. 7.18, 7.19, and 7.20).

Discussion

Before performing any procedure for body contouring, the appropriate technique for the specific patient must be chosen. In fact, the decision to opt for upper and lower abdominoplasty is a matter of selection according to the correct criteria:

1. When a patient presents with only isolated accumulations of fat on the anterior aspect of the abdominal wall without skin flaccidity or any other abnormality, isolated liposuction is the appropriate procedure.
2. In the case of accumulated fat on the anterior side of the abdominal wall plus skin flaccidity with a redundant panniculus localized only on the lower segment of the abdomen that presents with a high navel implantation and without the enlargement of the musculoaponeurotic abdominal wall, the adequate technique is lower abdominoplasty combined with liposuction without reinforcing the abdominal muscular structures (Fig. 7.11).When the patient presents with flaccidity in the muscular wall, plication may be combined with lower lipoabdominoplasty (Figs. 7.6 and 7.12).
3. If a patient presents with accumulated fat on the upper abdominal wall plus skin flaccidity with redundant panniculus and without flaccidity in the musculoaponeurotic abdominal wall, the appropriate technique is upper abdominoplasty (Figs. 7.1, 7.2, 7.3, and 7.4).
4. When a patient presents with accumulated fat on the lower and upper abdominal wall plus skin flaccidity with a redundant panniculus and with flaccidity in the musculoaponeurotic abdominal wall, the appropriate technique is lower and upper abdominoplasty combined with reinforcing the muscular wall (Figs. 7.15 and 7.16).
5. In cases where the patient presents with indications for full conventional abdominoplasty, the appropriate technique is full lipoabdominoplasty.

In early 1983, when I watched Illouz perform liposuction and I started performing my first operations, I noticed that the cannula worked in an unknown anatomical subcutaneous compartment of the abdominal wall. For this reason, I dedicated considerable research to the anatomy of the panniculus, even performing liposuction on cadavers, which yielded substantial knowledge about the area (Avelar 1986a, b, c, 1989). After performing some operations on the abdominal wall, I noticed that some patients had unwanted redundant skin. To solve that problem, a new approach involving the resection of the excess skin combined with liposuction was developed (Avelar 1985a, b, 1986a, b, c).

Some complications, particularly seroma formation and other circumstances, dissatisfied me and my patients. Although I used to have a very high incidence of seroma formation after abdominoplasty, I never had any severe consequences during its treatment, which was performed via syringe aspiration once a week.

After a few years, I decided not to no longer perform both procedures simultaneously (Avelar 1988). I also decided to look for a solution to those uncomfortable complications. I suspect that these problems could be solved by studying the anatomy of the panniculus. Therefore, I dedicated considerable time to reviewing my previous anatomical dissections on cadavers and also my perioperative photos of my patients, hoping to find a way to determine the cause of those complications. After some years, I concluded that I could perform liposuction with abdominoplasty because the perforator vessels would not be cut in this way, unlike what occurs when wide undermining is performed all over the abdominal wall. My conclusion was based on technical recommendations that liposuction must be performed on the lamellar layer when the perforator vessels are regularly preserved (Figs. 7.7, 7.9, and 7.10) (Avelar 1999a, b, 2000a, b). In my publications, I recommended performing abdominoplasty in association with liposuction without panniculus undermining, which is the lipoabdominoplasty that would later performed and published by other authors (Erfon 2002; Leão 2000).

As my patients presented with wide variations in their respective accumulations of adiposities, I used to perform the combined operation to remove specific areas of localized adiposities, which allowed me to classify four types of abdominoplasty: lower, upper, lower and upper, and full.

Conclusion

The nomenclature of this classification is very useful in that the operation may be indicated and performed to repair the anatomical alterations on one segment, on the other segment, or on both. The correct choice of technique is essential because the selection determines the level of aesthetic improvement to all regions of the abdomen as a whole. For this reason, each patient must undergo a physical examination to evaluate all their deformities as part of their surgical planning before undergoing abdominoplasty.

References

Avelar JM (1976a) Umbilicoplasty – a technique without external scar. (Umbilicoplastia – uma técnica sem cicatriz externa). 13th Braz. Congr. of Plastic Surgery and First Braz. Congr. of Aesthetic Surgery (13° Congr Bras Cir Plast, 1° Congr Bras Cir Estética). Porto Alegre, pp 81–82.

Avelar JM (1976b) Umbilicoplasty. A technique without external scar. Cahiers de chirurgie Esthétique. Journees internationals de Chirurgie Esthetique. Vendredi 21 mai, Paris (France) pp 5–25.

Avelar JM (1979) Cicatriz umbilical – da sua importância e da técnica de confecção nas abdominoplastias (Umbilical scar – its importance and technique for creating during abdominoplasty). Rev Bras Cir 1(2):41–52.
Avelar JM (1983a) (Abdominoplasty: Technical Refinements and Analysis of 130 cases in 8 Years Follow-up). Aesth Plast Surg 7: 205–212
Avelar JM (1983b) Submentonean and Submandibular Adiposity – Liposuction X Lipectomy (Adiposidade Submentoniana e Submandibular – Lipoaspiração X Lipectomia). In: Annals of the Brazilian Symposium on Facial Contouring. Organized and ed. by Dr. Juarez Avelar. Sponsored by Brazilian Society of Plastic Surgery (Section of São Paulo), September pag. 69–72
Avelar JM (1985a) Combined liposuction with traditional surgery in abdomen Lipodystrophy. XXIV Instructional Course of Aesth Plast Surg of ISAPS, Madrid (Spain) May.
Avelar JM (1985b) Fat-suction versus abdominoplasty. Aesthetic Plast Surg 9:265–276.
Avelar JM (1985c) – Fat-Suction of the Submental and Submandibular Regions. Aesth Plast Surg 9:257–263
Avelar JM (1986a) - Surgical Anatomy and Distribution of Adipose Tissue on Human Body (Anatomia cirúrgica e distribuição do tecido celular no organismo humano). In: Liposuction (Lipoaspiração), ed. by Avelar and Illouz, Ed. Hipócrates, São Paulo (Brazil) 9:45–57.
Avelar J (1986b) – Liposuction of the Abdominal Wall. (Lipoaspiração da Parede Abdominal). In: Liposuction (Lipoaspiração), ed. by Avelar and Illouz, Ed. Hipócrates, São Paulo (Brazil) 27:157–176.
Avelar J (1986c) – Liposuction of the Torso (Lipoaspiração do Dorso). In: Liposuction Lipoaspiração, ed. by Avelar and Illouz, Ed. Hipócrates, São Paulo (Brazil) 28:177–186.
Avelar JM (1987) - Study of the anatomy of the subcutaneous adipose tissue applied for fat-suction technique. In: Maneksha RJ (ed): Trans IX Int Congr Plast Reconstr Surg. New Delhi, India, March 1–6, pp 377–379.
Avelar JM (1988) Abdominoplasty – Reflections and Bio-Psychological Perspectives (Abdominoplastia – reflexões e perspectivas biopsicológicas). Rev Soc Bras Cir Plast 3(2):152–154.
Avelar JM (1989) Regional distribution and behavior of the subcutaneous tissue concerning selection and indication for liposuction. Aesth Plast Surg 13:155–165.
Avelar JM (1999a) Abdominoplastia: nuevos conceptos para una nueva técnica (Abdominoplasty: new concepts for a new technique). XXVI Annual international symposium of aesthetic plastic surgery, Chairman: Prof. Jose Guerrerosantos, Puerto Vallarta, pp 10–13
Avelar JM (1999b) New Concepts for Abdominoplasty (Novos conceitos para abdominoplastia). Paper presented at the 36th Congress of the Brazilian Society of Plastic Surgery. Rio de Janeiro.
Avelar JM (1999c) A new technique for abdominoplasty – closed vascular system of subdermal flap folded over itself combined to Liposuction. (Uma nova técnica de abdominoplastia – sistema vascular fechado de retalho subdérmico dobrado sobre si mesmo combinado com lipoaspiração). Rev Bras Cir 88/89(1/6):3–20.
Avelar JM (2000a) Abdominoplasty: a new technique without undermining and fat layer removal (Abdominoplastia: uma nova técnica sem descolamento e remoção da camada de gordura). Arq Catarinense de Med 29:147–149
Avelar JM (2000b) Abdominoplasty Without Undermining (Abdominoplastia sem descolamento).: XX Jorn. Paulista Cir Plast. São Paulo (Brazil) - May
Avelar JM (2001a) Abdominoplasty without lipectomy. Mini Course of ISAPS with Aesthetic Plastic Surgery Congress of Spain, Valladolid (Spain). September.
Avelar JM (2001b) The new abdominoplasty and derived technique. ISAPS and ASERF Annual Meeting. The Aesthetic Meeting, New York
Avelar JM (2002) Upper and lower abdominoplasty without panniculus undermining and resection. In: Avelar JM (ed) Abdominoplasty without panniculus undermining and resection. Editora Hipocrates, São Paulo, pp 183–198
Babcock WW (1916) On diseases of women and children. Am J Obstet 74:596. 1916 – Babcock – xiphoid-pubic fusiform cutaneous adipose excision, including the navel (Fig. 26.1) [19].

Callia WEP (1965) Contribuição ao estudo de correção cirúrgica do abdomen pêndulo e globus (contribution to the study of surgical correction of the pendulum abdomen and globus). original art. Doctoral Thesis Fac Med USP, São Paulo.
Erfon J. Abdominoplasty through a closed vascular system associated to liposuction: Avelar's technique. In: Avelar JM, ed. Abdominoplasty. São Paulo. Hipócrates, 2002. p.299–307.
Gonzales-Ulloa, M (1959) Circular Lipectomy wirh Transposition of the umbilicus and aponeurotic Technique. Cirug Y Ciruj 27:394–409
Gonzales-Ulloa M (1967) Belt Lipectomy. Brit. J. Plast. Surg. 13:179–186
Gonzales-Ulloa M (1982) Circular Abdominoplasty (Abdominoplastia Circular) Presented at the Brazilian Symposio of Abdominoplasty (Simpósio Brasileiro de Abdominoplastia), Ed. by Juarez M. Avelar, Sponsored by Brazilian Society of Plastic Surgery-Regional São Paulo, (Patrocinado pela Sociedade Brasileira de Cirurgia Plástica – Regional São Paulo). Section "I" Round Table. Editora Cidade, Rio de Janeiro – Brazil.
Guerrerosantos J (1982a) Necrosis of Abdominal Wall Post-Abdominoplasty – Etiology, Profilaxis and Treatment (Necrose de Parede Pós-Abdominoplastia – Etiologia, Profilaxia e Tratamento). Presented at the Brazilian Symposio of Abdominoplasty (Simpósio Brasileiro de Abdominoplastia), Ed. by Juarez M. Avelar, Sponsored by Brazilian Society of Plastic Surgery-Regional São Paulo, (Patrocinado pela Sociedade Brasileira de Cirurgia Plástica – Regional São Paulo). Section "E" Round Table. Editora Cidade, Rio de Janeiro – Brazil.
Guerrerosantos J (1982b) Tecnichal Refinments in Abdominoplasty (Refinamentos Técnicos nas Abdominoplastia). Presented at the Brazilian Symposio of Abdominoplasty (Simpósio Brasileiro de Abdominoplastia), ed. by Juarez M. Avelar, Sponsored by Brazilian Society of Plastic Surgery-Regional São Paulo, (Patrocinado pela Sociedade Brasileira de Cirurgia Plástica – Regional São Paulo). Section "B" Round Table. Editora Cidade, Rio de Janeiro – Brazil.
Illouz YG (1980) Une nouvelle technique pour les lipodystrophies localisées. Rev Cir Esth Franc 6(9)
Jolly (1911) – transversal infraumbilical cutaneous adipose excision, resembling a "slice of melon" or proximal concavity crescent [87]. Jolly R Die operation des Fettbauches. Berl Klin Wochenschr 29:1317.
Kelly HA (1899) Report of gynecological cases. John Hopkins Med J 10:197
Leão CF (2000) Plicatura da parede músculo-aponeurótica por um tunel criado abaixo do panículo abdominal na linha média em lipoabdominoplastia sem descolamento. 37 Congresso Brasileiro de Cirurgia Plástica, novembro - Porto Alegre. (Reinforcement of the musculoaponeurotic wall through a tunnel created below the abdominal panniculus during lipoabdominoplasty). 37th Brazilian Congress of Plastic Surgery, Porto Alegre.
Malbec EF (1948) Lipectomia abdominal. La Prensa Méd Arg vol. XXXV - (26) 1948. In: Historia, Ciencia y Arte En Cirugia Estetica. Ed. by Juarez M. Avelar and Ernesto F. Malbec. Ed. Hipócrates. Pag. 605–608, 1990.
Pitanguy I (1967a) Abdominal lipectomy: an approach to it through an analysis of 300 consecutives cases. Plast Reconstr Surg 40(4):384–391
Pitanguy I (1967b) Abdominoplastias. O Hospital, Rio de Janeiro 71(6):1541–1556 105.
Pitanguy I (1982) – Phylosophic and Psychological Perspectives of the Abdomen. (Perspectivas Filosóficas e Psicológicos do Abdomen). In Annals of Brazilian Symposio of Abdominoplasty. (Anais do Simpósio Brasileiro de Abdominoplastia), Ed. by Juarez M. Avelar, Sponsored by Brazilian Society of Plastic Surgery-Regional São Paulo, (Patrocinado pela Sociedade Brasileira de Cirurgia Plástica – Regional São Paulo). 1:15–24. Editora Cidade, Rio de Janeiro – Brazil.
Planas J (1982) Abdominoplasty through upper incision (Abdominoplastia por Incisão Superior). Presented at the Brazilian Symposio of Abdominoplasty (Simpósio Brasileiro de Abdominoplastia), ed. by Juarez M. Avelar, Sponsored by Brazilian Society of Plastic Surgery-Regional São Paulo, (Patrocinado pela Sociedade Brasileira de Cirurgia Plástica – Regional São Paulo). Section "C" Round Table. Editora Cidade, Rio de Janeiro – Brazil.
Pontes R (1965) Plástica abdominal: importância da sua associação com a correção de hérnia incisional (abdominal plastic: importance of its association with the correction of incisional hernias). Rev Bras Cir 52:8.

Rebello C, Lion P, Franco T (1972) Abdominopalsty through submammary incision. International Congress of ISAPS. Rio de Janeiro. Ed.Publicaciones Comntroladas, 58, Madrid
Rebello C (1982) – Abdominoplasty through submammary approach (Abdominoplastia por incisão submamária) In: Annals of Brazilian Symposio of Abdominoplasty. (Anais do Simpósio Brasileiro de Abdominoplastia), ed. by Juarez M. Avelar, Sponsored by Brazilian Society of Plastic Surgery-Regional São Paulo, (Patrocinado pela Sociedade Brasileira de Cirurgia Plástica – Regional São Paulo). 52-53. Editora Cidade, Rio de Janeiro – Brazil.
Serson Neto D (1970) Abdominal Dermolipectomies – Geometric Approaches (Dermolipectomias abdominais - Abordagem geométrica) Rev. CBC 10:17–20, março-abril.
Serson Neto D (1982) Abdominoplasty – Geometric Approach (Abdominoplastia - Técnica Geométrica). In Annals of Brazilian Symposio of Abdominoplasty. (Anais do Simpósio Brasileiro de Abdominoplastia), ed. by Juarez M. Avelar, Sponsored by Brazilian Society of Plastic Surgery-Regional São Paulo, (Patrocinado pela Sociedade Brasileira de Cirurgia Plástica – Regional São Paulo). 2:25–30. Editora Cidade, Rio de Janeiro, Brazil.
Sinder R (1975) Plastic Surgery of the abdomen - Técnica pessoal de abdominoplastia, com prévio deslocamento de retalho supraumbilical (antes da resseccão infraumbilical) e uso de retalho dermoadiposo, – VI International Congress of Plastic and Reconstructive Surgery, Paris (France) August
Sinder R (1979) Abdominal plastic surgery. (Cirurgia plástica abdominal), ed. by Sinder, Niteroi. Rio de Janeiro, Brasil.
Sinder R (1982) – Technical Variations of Abdominoplasty –– Generalities About Plastic Surgery of Abdomen (Variações Técnicas das Abdominoplastias Generalidades Sobre Cirurgia Plástica do Abdome. In Annals of Brazilian Symposio of Abdominoplasty. (Anais do Simpósio Brasileiro de Abdominoplastia), ed. by Juarez M. Avelar, Sponsored by Brazilian Society of Plastic Surgery-Regional São Paulo, (Patrocinado pela Sociedade Brasileira de Cirurgia Plástica – Regional São Paulo). 2:31–40. Editora Cidade, Rio de Janeiro – Brazil.
Thorek M (1942a) Plastic surgery of the breast and abdominal wall. Charles C. Thomas. Ed, Springfi eld, III, 120
Thorek M (1942b) Modern surgical technique, one volume war edition. J. B. Lippincott Company, Philadelphia, pp. 1264–1266
Vilain R (1964) A propos de la chirurgie réparatrice de la paroi abdominale. Bul Mens Soc Chir Paris 54:290–294Vilain R, Dubousset J. Technique et indications de la lipectomie circulaire. 150 observations. Ann Chir 18:289–300.
Vilain R (1982) Circular Abdominoplasty (Abdominoplastia Circular). In Annals of Brazilian Symposio of Abdominoplasty (Anais do Simpósio Brasileiro de Abdominoplastia), ed. by Juarez M. Avelar, Sponsored by Brazilian Society of Plastic Surgery-Regional São Paulo, (Patrocinado pela Sociedade Brasileira de Cirurgia Plástica – Regional São Paulo). 6:152–153. Editora Cidade, Rio de Janeiro – Brazil.
Vilain S (1986) Alternatives to the classic abdominoplasty. Ann Plast Surg 17(3):247.

Chapter 8
Lipoabdominoplasty: Classification

João Erfon, Claudio Mauricio M. Rodrigues, and Aleksandra Markovic

Abstract Background: Since 2001, the author has been using a simple and didactic classification, for patients who are candidates for liposuction and lipoabdominoplasty surgery, based on skin flaccidity, lipodystrophy, and diastasis of the rectus abdominis muscles and the extent of scars necessary for surgical correction, grouping patients into four groups, with the respective indication of the type of surgery for each group.

Methods: A retrospective study was performed evaluating patients who underwent abdominoplasty with liposuction and minimal undermining or only liposuction from July 2001 to January 2021. A total of 2076 procedures were carried out with 1066 using liposuction only and 1010 lipoabdominoplasty technique. Eight hundred one patients were submitted to full lipoabdominoplasty, 112 were submitted to mini-lipoabdominoplasty, and 97 underwent mid-lipoabdominoplasty. The mean age of patients was 36.4 years. The mean weight of skin resection was 465.48 g, and the mean volume of liposuction was 2578 mL in the cases of lipoabdominoplasty and 2886 mL in the patients who were performed liposuction only.

Conclusions: The author concludes that lipoabdominoplasty was a great change to the abdominoplasty technique in the last 60 years. Joining two great techniques (liposuction and abdominoplasty) with minimal undermining, preserving the main vascularization of the superior abdominal flap and the secondary vascularization of the lower abdomen lateral areas and skin resection in the central area up to the muscle fascia, permitting safe plication, improving the aesthetic results, and turning lipoabdominoplasty safer than the traditional abdominoplasty. The mid-lipoabdominoplasty is a new idea that when well indicated allows for safe surgery and more skin resection than in mini-lipoabdominoplasty.

Level of Evidence IV: This journal requires that authors assign a level of evidence to each article. For a full description of these Evidence-Based Medicine ratings, please refer to the Table of Contents or the online Instructions to Authors www.springer.com/00266.

J. Erfon (✉) · C. M. M. Rodrigues · A. Markovic
ArtClinic, Fortaleza, Ceará, Brazil

J. M. Avelar, R. Cavalcanti Ribeiro (eds.), *Body Contouring*,
https://doi.org/10.1007/978-3-031-42802-9_8

Keywords Lipoabdominoplasty classification · Mid-lipoabdominoplasty · Minimal undermining · Superficial fascia · Safe plication · Secondary vascularization

Introduction

Since 2001, the senior author has been using the abdominoplasty with liposuction without undermining as described by Avelar (1999) to the cases of mini-abdominoplasty introducing resection of the superficial fascia and subcutaneous tissue on the central third of the lower abdomen (Erfon 2001). He later used the same idea to perform full abdominoplasty as recommended by Saldanha that also introduced the term lipoabdominoplasty (Saldanha et al. 2001). The author suggests, from the beginning, a simple and didactic classification, for patients who are candidates for this surgery, based on skin flaccidity, lipodystrophy, and diastasis of the rectus abdominis muscles and the extent of scars necessary for surgical correction, grouping patients into four groups, with the respective indication of the type of surgery for each group: Group 1, liposuction; Group 2, mini-lipoabdominoplasty; Group 3, mid-lipoabdominoplasty; and Group 4, full lipoabdominoplasty (Table 8.1). *The author* also suggests the possibility of safe plication and reducing the amount of superficial fascia and subcutaneous tissue to be preserved in the lower abdomen and the term mid-lipoabdominoplasty. *He* also developed his own markings, dividing the lower abdomen into three areas: in the two lateral areas, the

Table 8.1 The author classified the patients to perform liposuction alone or lipoabdominoplasty into four groups: (a) G1, liposuction; (b) G2, mini-lipoabdominoplasty; (c) G3, mid-lipoabdominoplasty; and (d) G4, full lipoabdominoplasty

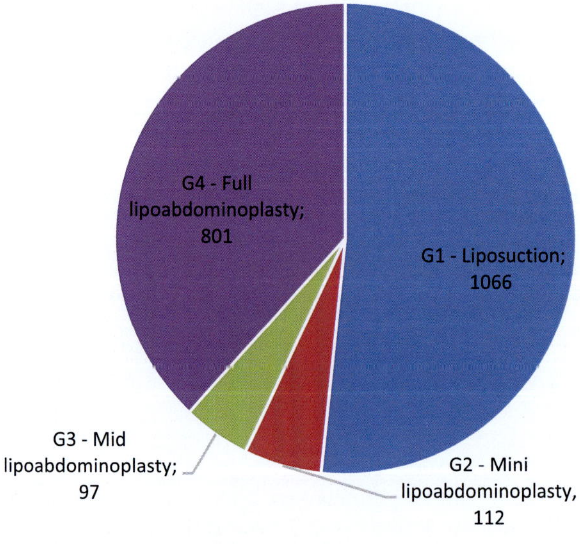

superficial fascia will be preserved, and in the central region, the skin resection goes up to the muscle fascia permitting a safe muscle plication without damage of the main and secondary vascularization of the abdominal flap. After the plication, there is no dead space and drains are not used. Another contribution was the partial transverse pubectomy that was introduced by the senior author. When comparing the aesthetic results using the lipoabdominoplasty with the traditional abdominoplasty technique, the aesthetic results are better, and the number of complications is reduced.

Mcthods

A retrospective study was performed in 2076 cases, where 2028 female patients and 48 males underwent lipoabdominoplasty, by the senior author from July 2001 to January 2021. Patients *were* classified into four groups: Group 1 (G1) patients with abdominal and/or flank lipodystrophy, without cutaneous flaccidity and without diastasis of the rectus abdominis muscles (Fig. 8.1a–c); Group 2 (G2) patients with abdominal and/or flank lipodystrophy, with small supra-pubic skin flaccidity, the navel positioned so that it is impossible to lower the upper abdominal skin flap to the pubis, with or without diastasis of the rectus abdominis muscles (Fig. 8.2a–c); Group 3 (G3) patients with lipodystrophy of the abdomen and/or flanks and skin sagging greater than in the previous group, including supra-pubic region or not, but with sagging on the sides of the lower abdomen, as well as supra-umbilical, as well as navel in an elevated position in the abdomen unable to lower the upper abdominal skin flap to the pubis, with or without diastasis of the rectus abdominis muscles (Fig. 8.3a–c); and Group 4 (G4) patients with lipodystrophy of the abdomen and flanks with great abdominal skin flaccidity, diastasis of the rectus abdominis

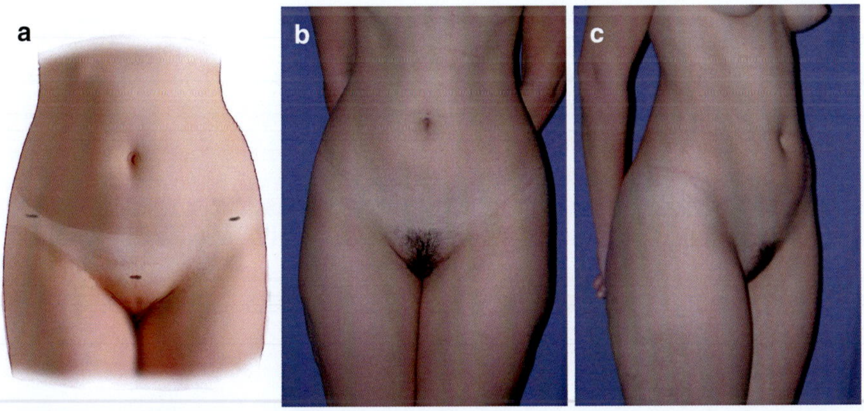

Fig. 8.1 G1. (**a**) Liposuction planning. (**b**) Kind of deformity with indication for liposuction. (**c**) Type of deformity with indication for liposuction (oblique view)

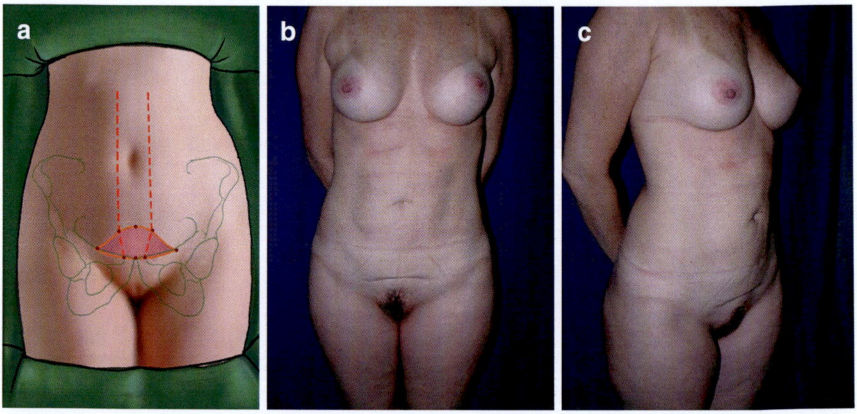

Fig. 8.2 G2. (**a**) Planning for mini-lipoabdominoplasty. (**b**) Type of deformity with indication for mini-lipoabdominoplasty. (**c**) Type of deformity with indication for mini-lipoabdominoplasty (oblique view)

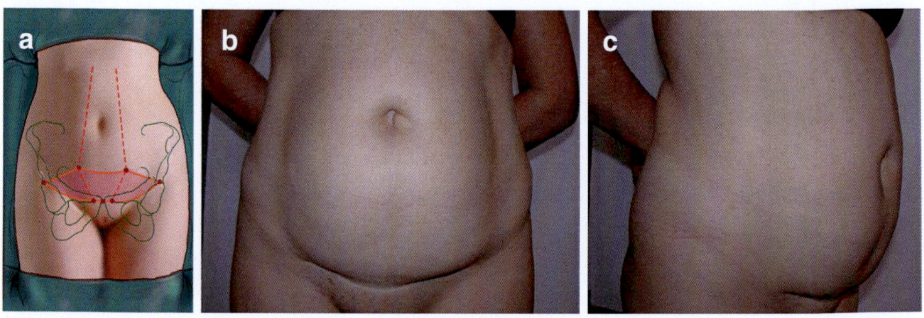

Fig. 8.3 G3. (a) Planning for mid-lipoabdominoplasty.. (**b**) Type of deformity with indication for mini-lipoabdominoplasty. (**c**) Type of deformity with indication for mid-lipoabdominoplasty (oblique view)

muscles, and navel in position that allows traction of the upper abdominal skin flap to the pubis, preserving an adequate extension of it (around 6 cm), and without vertical supra-pubic scar (Fig. 8.4a–c) (Saldanha et al. 2001; Erfon 2002, 2009, 2011; Erfon and Mauricio 2016). The surgery indicated for each group was as follows: G1, liposuction in 1066 patients; G2, mini-lipoabdominoplasty in 112 cases; G3, mid-lipoabdominoplasty in 97 patients; and G4, full lipoabdominoplasty in 801 cases.

Regarding this, the inclusion criteria were patients with indication to abdominoplasty surgery and liposuction from 19 to 70 years of age, BMI less than 30, lipodystrophy in the abdomen and flanks, skin flaccidity or not, and abdominal muscle diastasis in most of the cases. Smokers were advised to stop for at least 1 week prior and 1 week postoperatively. All patients underwent preoperative necessary routine exams, including ultrasound of the abdominal wall.

This study was carried out in accordance with the 1964 Helsinki Declaration for research in human subjects and subsequent amendments. All patients provided written informed consent for surgery and the use of photographs.

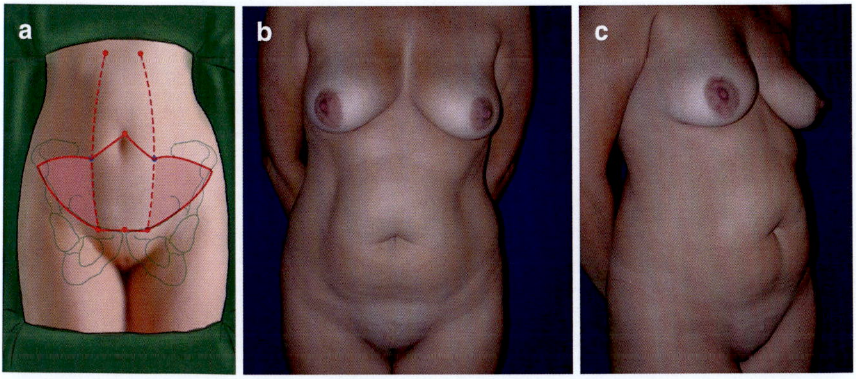

Fig. 8.4 G4. (**a**) Planning of full lipoabdominoplasty. (**b**) Type of deformity with indication for full lipoabdominoplasty. (**c**) Type of deformity with indication for full lipoabdominoplasty

Technique

Group 1: Liposuction – with the patient standing up in the hospital room, preoperative photos and areas where liposuction will be performed are marked in the flanks and abdomen. With the patient under dorsal position and general anesthesia on the operating table, marking continues. The subcutaneous space is infiltrated with a saline solution (adrenaline saline 1:1000 mL) in the whole abdomen and flanks (areas where liposuction is to be performed) up to 1.5 or 2.0 L. The surgery begins with small incisions in the pubis and iliac regions (1 cm in length), and deep liposuctions are performed in the whole abdomen and *flanks* (Fig. 8.1a). The incisions are sutured with mono-nylon 4-0.

Group 2: Mini-lipoabdominoplasty – markings are drawn only inside the pubic region. In the center of the pubis and 6 to 7 cm from the vaginal cleft, the central point is marked, and from this point laterally, two segments of lines are drawn up to the lateral borders of this region on each side. One semicircle is *marked* uniting the lateral extreme points of the pubic line, with convexity upward, according to the amount of skin to be resected in each case. Two oblique lines are drawn from semicircle downward to 2 cm laterally to the central point of the pubis dividing the marked area into three segments (Fig. 8.4a) and without navel incisions (Fig. 8.2a). The subcutaneous space is infiltrated with a saline solution (adrenaline saline 1:1000 mL) in the whole abdomen and flanks (areas where liposuction is to be performed) up to 1.5 or 2.0 L. The surgery begins with small incisions in the pubis and iliac regions (1 cm in length), and deep and superficial liposuctions are performed in the whole abdomen and flanks. After liposuction, a total skin resection is carried out in these lower lateral abdominal regions preserving the whole superficial fascia as well as the vascularization and lymphatic system (Fig. 8.5). Now the skin resection in the central area of the lower abdomen up to the muscle fascia is carried out. A narrow tunnel from the upper border of the superior skin incision up to the xiphoid appendix is dissected preserving the abdominal myocutaneous perforating vessels. The navel is freed from the muscle wall. Plication is carried out using a double zero

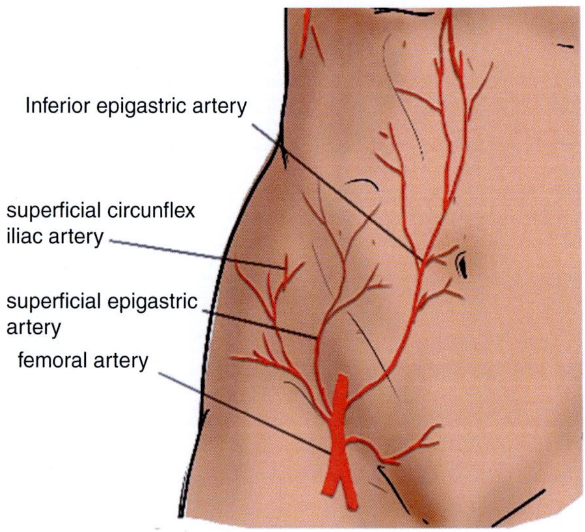

Fig. 8.5 Secondary vascularization for lipoabdominoplasty technique (superficial epigastric artery and superficial iliac circumflex artery)

mono-nylon in "X" separated stitches from the xiphoid appendix to the pubis. The umbilicus is fixed using two stitches in its upper and lower extremity. The superficial fascia is sutured in the middle line of the lower abdomen using 3-0 colorless mono-nylon. Now the table is set to 45°. The superior abdominal flap is pulled down to be sutured in the pubic region using five stitches with zero mono-nylon and continued with subcutaneous points using 3-0 colorless mono-nylon. At this time, a complementary liposuction is performed when necessary.

Group 3: Mid-lipoabdominoplasty – markings seem to be the same as used in mini-lipoabdominoplasty, but the superior central line is drawn with inverted convexity downward, improving the umbilicus-pubic distance and the lateral markings going beyond the pubis according to the amount of skin to be resected in each patient, permitting more skin resection than in mini-lipoabdominoplasty, without umbilicus incisions (Fig. 8.3a). Surgery is carried out as described in mini-lipoabdominoplasty.

Group 4: Full lipoabdominoplasty – with the patient standing up in the hospital room, preoperative photos and areas where liposuction will be performed are marked in the flanks and abdomen. With the patient under dorsal position and general anesthesia on the operating table, marking continues: the table is set to horizontal position. In the center of the pubis and 6 to 7 cm from the vaginal cleft, the central point is marked, and from this point laterally, two segments of lines are drawn up to the lateral borders of this region on each side, and they are extended laterally into the lower abdominal sulcus according to the amount of skin to be resected. The umbilical marks are *drawn* in a diamond shape, and from the top of it, two segments of lines the same size as the pubic lines are marked laterally in oblique position according to the skin flaccidity. From the lateral points of these two segments, two markings are drawn on each side: one to conclude demarcation uniting with the markings in the lower abdominal groove and another downward in oblique direction to the center of the pubis, approximately 1 or 2 cm laterally to this central point, ending up with three marked areas in the lower abdomen (Fig. 8.4a).

The subcutaneous space is infiltrated with a saline solution (adrenaline saline 1:1000 mL) in the whole abdomen and flanks (areas where liposuction is to be performed) up to 1.5 or 2.0 L. The surgery begins with small incisions in the pubis and iliac regions (1 cm in length), and deep liposuctions are performed in the whole abdomen. Deep and superficial liposuction continues in the flanks and in the lower lateral abdominal areas previously marked. After liposuction, a total skin resection is carried out in these lower lateral abdominal regions preserving the whole superficial fascia as well as the vascularization and lymphatic system. Now the skin resection in the central area of the lower abdomen and a transverse strip of the pubis reducing its length is performed up to the muscle fascia. A tunnel from the upper border of the superior skin incision up to the xiphoid appendix is dissected preserving the abdominal myocutaneous perforating vessels. The umbilicus is separated from the abdominal wall. The width of the tunnel varies according to the diastasis of the rectus abdominis muscle up to 2 cm laterally over its medial borders. Plication is carried out using a double zero mono-nylon in "X" separated stitches from the xiphoid appendix to the pubis. The umbilicus is fixed using two stitches in its upper and lower extremity, leaving 1 cm freed from the abdominal wall. The superficial fascia is sutured in the middle line of the lower abdomen using 3-0 colorless mono-nylon. Now the table is set to 45°. The superior abdominal flap is pulled down to be sutured starting with five stitches in the pubic region using zero mono-nylon. A "V" incision is performed on the navel new position, and it is sutured on its new position at this time using internal stitches with 4-0 colorless mono-nylon or Monocryl. Suture is concluded using subcutaneous separated stitches with 3-0 colorless mono-nylon or Monocryl in the whole inferior abdominal incision. At this time, a complementary liposuction is carried out where necessary. Drains are not used. Dresser with dry gauze and elastic belt is used for 2 months.

Results

From July 2001 to January 2021, a retrospective study was carried out. A total of 2076 lipoabdominoplasty or only liposuction cases were performed by the senior author using this described technique, in which 1066 were of liposuction only (Fig. 8.6), 112 of mini-lipoabdominoplasty (Fig. 8.7), 97 of mid-lipoabdominoplasty (Fig. 8.8), and 801 of full lipoabdominoplasty (Fig. 8.9). Patients' ages ranged from

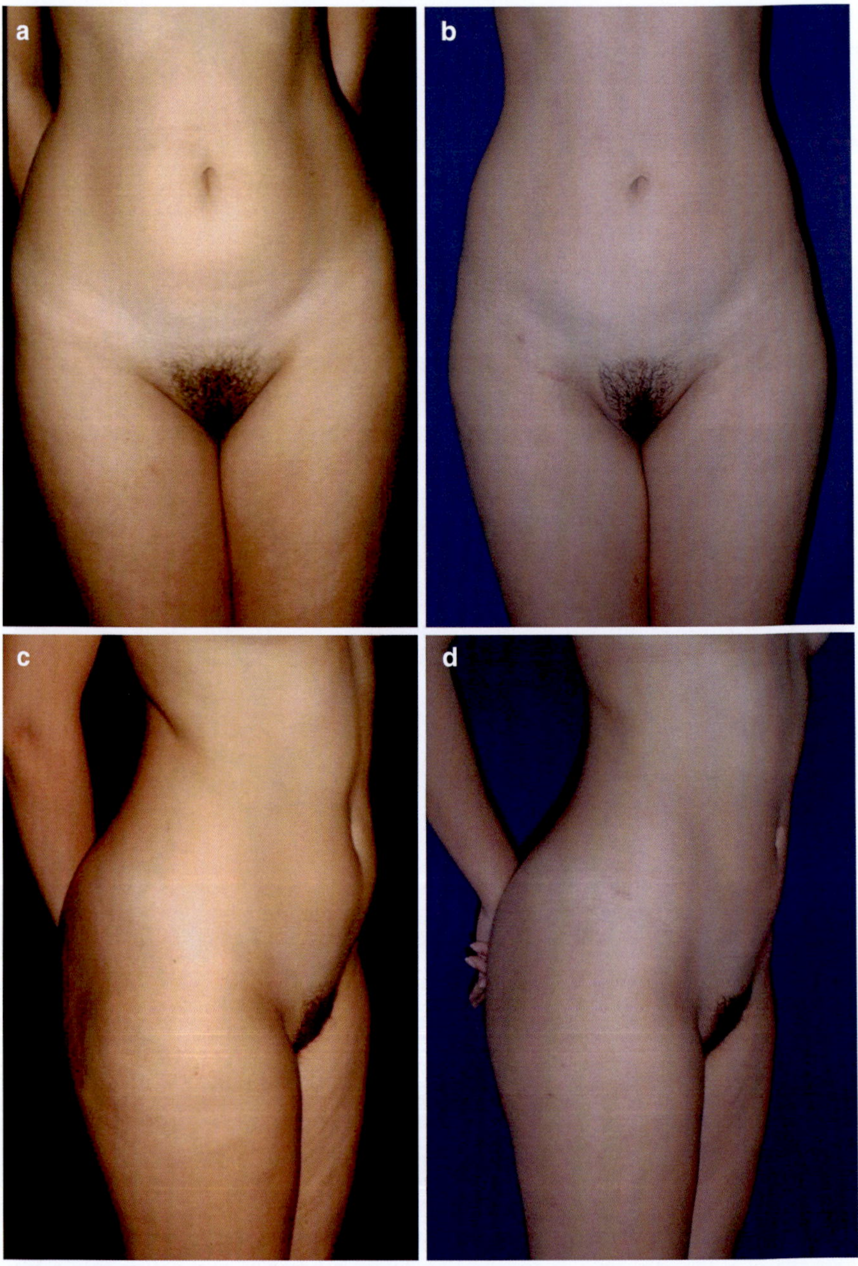

Fig. 8.6 (a) Patient with lipodystrophy (pre-op for liposuction). (**b**) 6 months post-op. (**c**) Pre-op for liposuction. (**d**) 6 months post-op

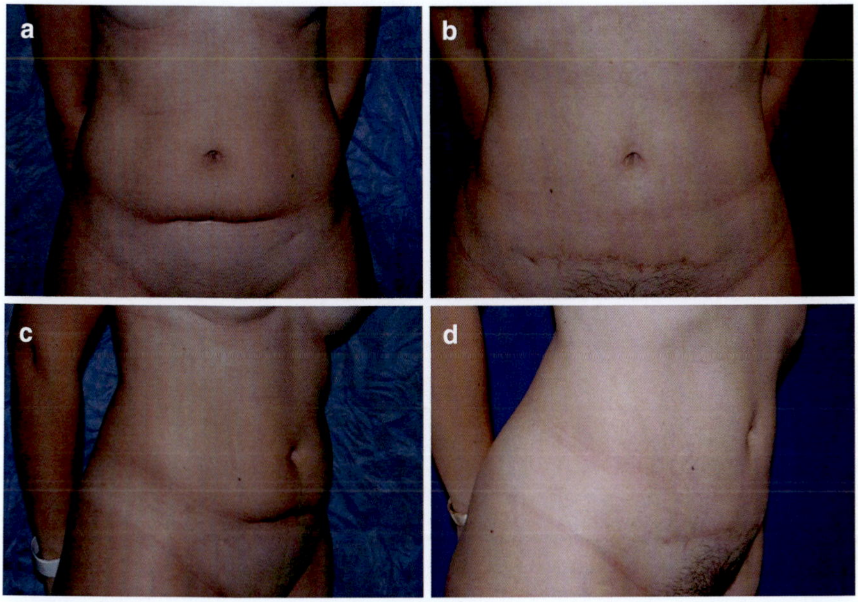

Fig. 8.7 Patient submitted to mini-lipoabdominoplasty: (**a, c**) pre-op view. (**b, d**) 6 months post-op

19 to 70 years (the average age was 36.4 years). The weight of skin resection varies from 105 to 850 g (the mean weight of skin resection was 465.48 g): full lipoabdominoplasty 704.40 g, mid-lipoabdominoplasty 498.10 g, and mini-lipoabdominoplasty 156.55 g, respectively. The liposuction volume ranged from 550 to 3850 mL (the mean volume was 2765.43 mL): full lipoabdominoplasty 3255 mL, mid-lipoabdominoplasty 3065 mL, and mini-lipoabdominoplasty 1845 mL. The time of surgery varies from 1:30 to 3:00 h (mean of 2:00 h). Drains are not used (Fig. 8.3g). The time of follow-up was 6 months or more when post-op photography was taken (Figs. 8.4, 8.5, 8.6, and 8.7).

Since 2001 when he began this technique, the senior author has observed better results and less complications using lipoabdominoplasty when compared with the traditional abdominoplasty technique that he used to perform before, from January 1980 to June 2001.

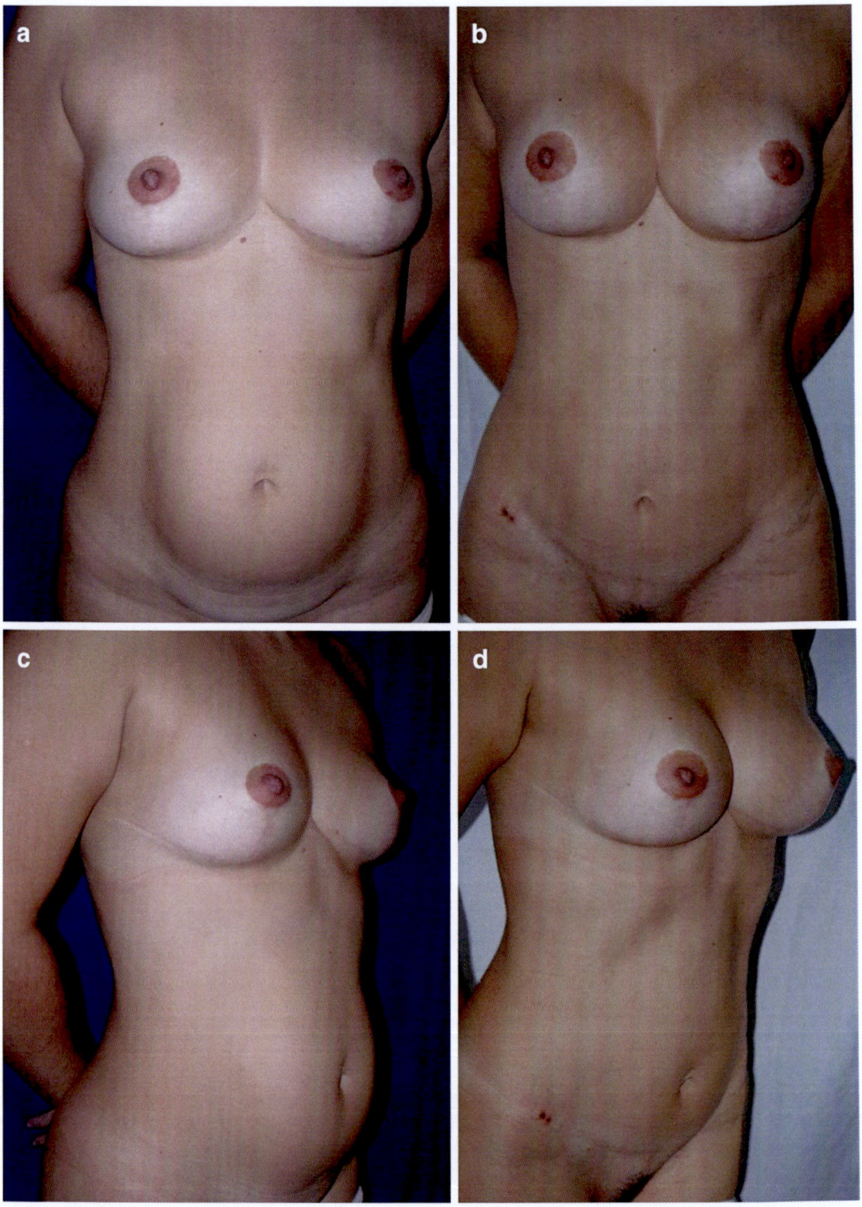

Fig. 8.8 Patient submitted to mid-lipoabdominoplasty: (**a, c**) pre-op view. (**b, d**) Results 1 year later

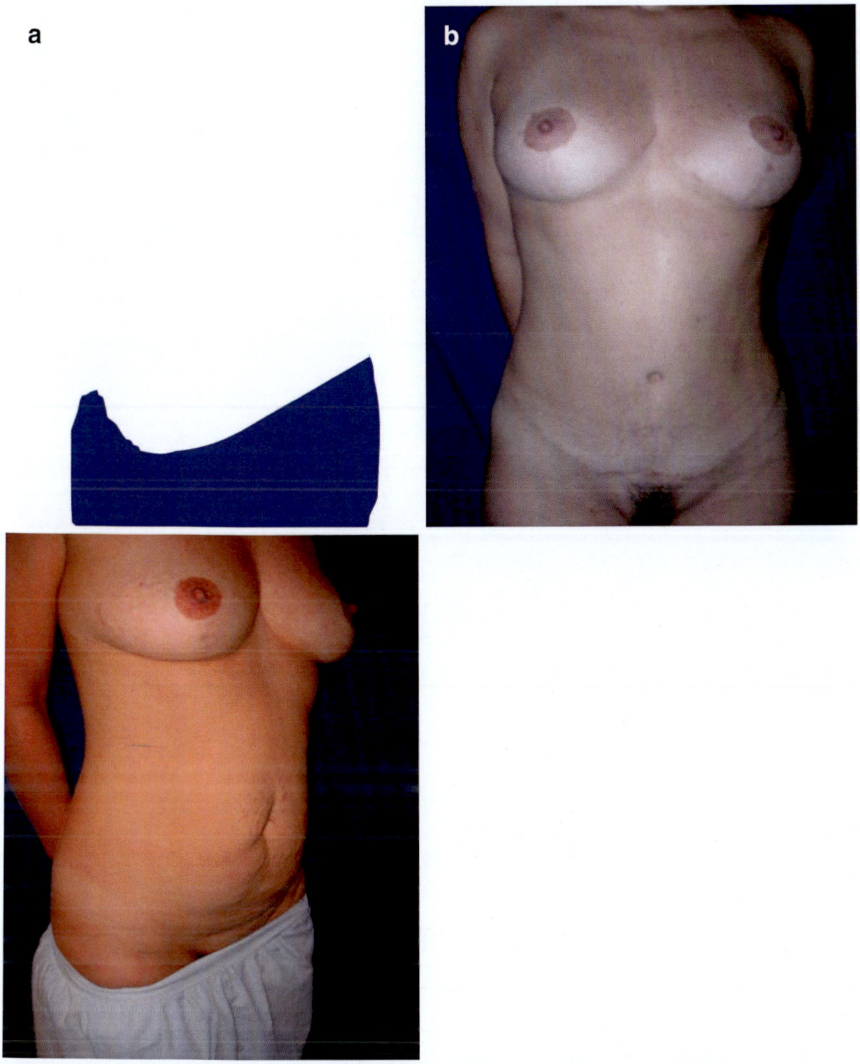

Fig. 8.9 Patient submitted to full lipoabdominoplasty: (**a, c**) pre-op view. (**b, d**) 6 months post-op

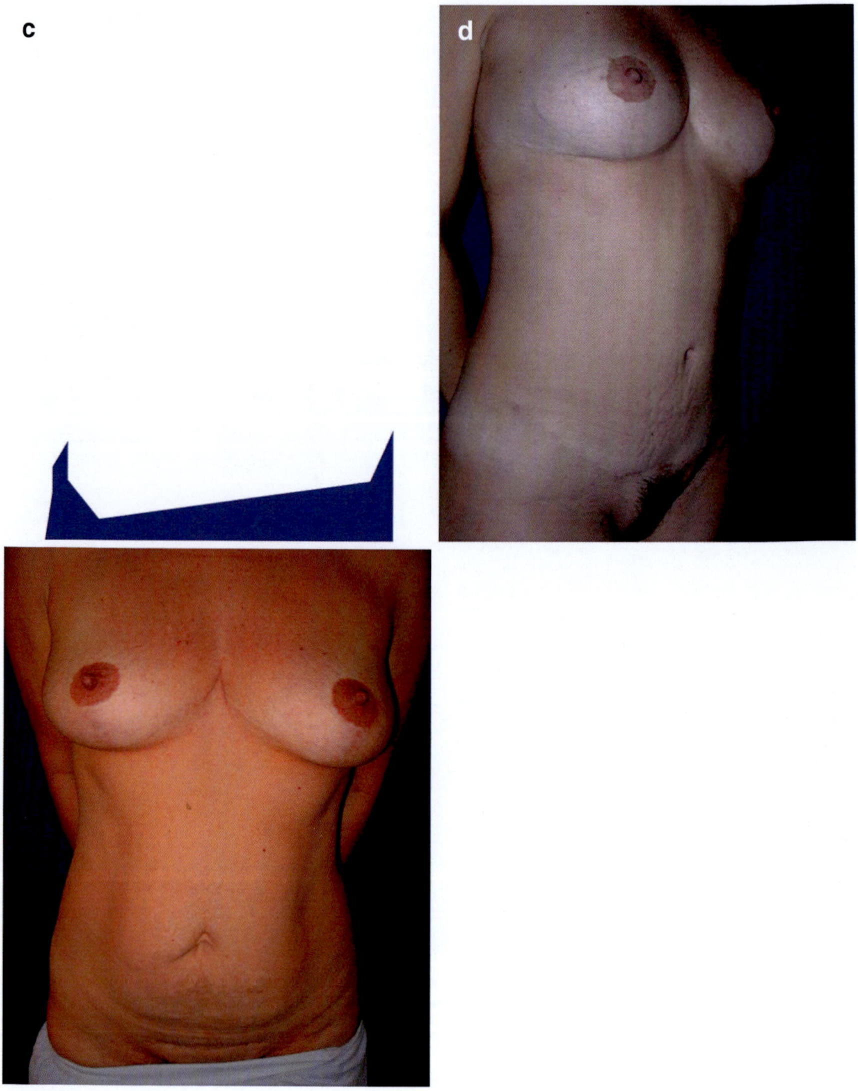

Fig. 8.9 (continued)

Complications

Since 2001, the senior author has been using the lipoabdominoplasty technique and observed one important reduction in the number of complications when compared with the traditional abdominal technique. He used to have more than 60% of seroma using the traditional technique, which reduces to 0.40% using lipoabdominoplasty technique. Considering the 1010 cases of lipoabdominoplasty (Groups 2, 3, and 4), localized hematomas occurred in 0.30% of the cases, all of which were treated with syringe aspiration only in the office: two cases in patients submitted to full lipoabdominoplasty (0.20%) and one case in mid-lipoabdominoplasty (0.10%); skin necrosis occurred in the same patient submitted to mid-lipoabdominoplasty that had hematoma, in 2 cm at the distal end of the lower abdominal flap that needed reoperation with sedation and local anesthesia, with good results; one case (0.10%) of skin allergy to chlorhexidine occurred on the fifth day of post-op that needed hospitalization and intensive treatment with satisfactory results but with spots on the skin in the whole area where the antisepsis was done that were still being treated and slowly evolving; hypertrophic scar occurred in 22 (2.21%) cases where most of them were treated with triamcinolone and 7 (0.70%) of these needed surgical revision and beta therapy (radiation therapy) and trans-operative application of intra-scar triamcinolone; and secondary surgeries were performed in 52 (5.22%) of the cases for complementary liposuction, and in 3 (0.30%) of these patients, more skin resection was carried out too.

For Group 1: 1066 patients undergoing liposuction alone, the main complication was the 92 (8.63%) cases that required re-operation to improve aesthetic results.

Discussion

Since 2001, the senior author has been using the abdominoplasty with liposuction without undermining as described by Avelar (1999) to the cases of mini-abdominoplasty introducing resection of the superficial fascia and subcutaneous tissue on the central third of the lower abdomen (Erfon 2001). He later used the same idea to perform full abdominoplasty as recommended by Saldanha that also introduced the term lipoabdominoplasty (Saldanha et al. 2001). *The author* suggests, from the beginning, a simple and didactic classification for patients who are candidates for this surgery, based on skin flaccidity, lipodystrophy, and diastasis of the rectus abdominis muscles and the extent of scars necessary for surgical correction, grouping the patients into four groups, with the respective indication of the type of surgery for each group: Group 1, liposuction; Group 2, mini-lipoabdominoplasty; Group 3, mid-lipoabdominoplasty; and Group 4, full lipoabdominoplasty. The author started dividing the lower abdomen into three areas: the two lateral regions where the total skin was resected and the superficial fascia and important anatomical structures were preserved and the central area that is resected from the skin up to the muscle fascia including a transverse strip of the pubis reducing its length (Erfon 2002, 2009, 2011). The tunnel for plication is carried out from the umbilicus up to 1 or 2 cm over the xiphoid appendix and the width of this tunnel up to 2 cm lateral to the medial borders of the rectus abdominis muscles, preserving the abdominal myocutaneous perforating vessels, permitting a good vascularization of the abdominal flap and a safe plication (Erfon and Mauricio 2016). At the same time, the term mid-lipoabdominoplasty was introduced to special cases that it's impossible to pull down the superior abdominal flap as is usual in full lipoabdominoplasty and needs more skin resection than in mini-lipoabdominoplasty, avoiding supra-pubic or very high scars (Erfon 2001, 2002).

In the cases of mid-lipoabdominoplasty, the senior author recommends an adequate umbilicus-pubic distance of 6 cm or more to improve the aesthetic results using the superior curved incision with convexity downward (Fig. 8.3a). Also the incisions are extended beyond the pubis on the lower abdominal sulcus according to the amount of skin to be resected in each case, without umbilical incisions (Fig. 8.3a). The superior markings are curved in direction to the flank regions to permit more skin resection (Fig. 8.3a). The superficial fascia and the most important anatomical structures will be preserved in the two lateral regions, and in the central area, the skin will be resected up to the rectus fascia muscle, permitting safe plication and reducing the amount of tissue to be preserved in the lower abdomen, improving the aesthetic results (Fig. 8.8). In most of the cases, one transversal strip of the pubis is resected to maintain its length to about 6 to 7 cm (transversal pubectomy), avoiding higher scars. The navel is dissected from the abdominal wall as performed in mini-lipoabdominoplasty. Plication on the superior abdominal muscle fascia is performed with reduced undermining preserving the abdominal myocutaneous perforating vessels and continues up to the pubis approaching the two preserved superficial fascia segments (Erfon and Mauricio 2016). After the muscle plication, both lateral segments of the preserved superficial fascia (Scarpa's fascia) are sutured together with 3-0 colorless mono-nylon in the lower abdomen. After this suture, there is no dead space and there is no necessity of drains. Liposuction in the flank areas can be performed as the same surgery using a special position described by the senior author, avoiding prone position. After the final sutures, a complementary liposuction is carried out to improve the aesthetic results.

Avelar (1999) described the use of liposuction associated with mini-abdominoplasty on the whole abdominal wall and flanks, with skin resection on the pubis and on the sub-mammary groove, preserving the abdominal muscle cutaneous perforating vessels in the upper abdomen and the superficial fascia in the whole lower abdomen without panicle undermining. Joining two great techniques in one new idea publishing new concepts to the classical abdominoplasty, starting a new era in the abdominoplasty approach (Avelar 1999).

Saldanha (2001) introduced the lipoabdominoplasty technique associating superficial and deep liposuction in the whole abdomen with skin resection from the pubis to the umbilicus (full lipoabdominoplasty) preserving the abdominal muscle-cutaneous perforating vessels and the lymphatic system, concluding that this approach reduces the complications and improves the aesthetic results compared to the traditional abdominoplasty technique (Saldanha et al. 2001).

The preservation of the whole superficial fascia and the important anatomical structures in the lower abdomen as recommended by Avelar (1999, 2002) and late by Saldanha (Saldanha et al. 2001) is important to avoid seromas and also is a secondary vascularization as described by Erfon (2001, 2002, 2009, 2011; Erfon and Mauricio 2016) and Almeida (Almeida et al. 2016). The connection of this vessels with their deep homonyms is an important accessory vascularization especially in the cases of mid- and mini-lipoabdominoplasty (Erfon and Mauricio 2016) late confirmed by Barcelos (Barcelos et al. 2017). It is also important the resection of the central area of the lower abdomen up to muscle fascia permitting a safe plication (without a risk of penetrating the abdominal cavity) and reducing the amount of tissue to be accommodated, improving the aesthetic results as published by Erfon (2001; Erfon and Mauricio 2016).

Illouz (1980) described the possibility of treatment of lipodystrophies in the body contour using the technique named liposuction, changing concepts about aesthetic plastic surgery in the whole body regions (Illouz 1980). Illouz (1992) also published a technique of abdominoplasty without undermining and liposuction in the upper abdomen with skin resection in the lower area to be used on obese patients (Illouz 1992).

Stuckey (1979) used for the first time the term "midabdomen abdominoplasty" to describe a surgery with skin resection using a transverse incision involving the umbilical region. "The skin was undermined above, below, and on both sides" and "the excessive skin was excised transversely as an ellipse" with local anesthesia to avoid a traditional abdominoplasty (Stuckey 1979). The senior author has been using the term mid-lipoabdominoplasty to describe a new approach since 2001 (Erfon 2001). The indications are the special cases where it's impossible to pull down the superior abdominal flap and needs more skin resection than in mini-lipoabdominoplasty.

The markings described by the senior author dividing the lower abdomen into three segments, permitting the preservation of the superficial fascia and the whole important anatomical structures on both lateral segments and the resection of the central segment up to the muscle fascia, below the umbilicus, permitting a safe plication was named by Avelar (2016a) a set contribution to the lipoabdominoplasty technique.

Uebel (1994) recommended a smaller detachment of the tunnel for plication, reducing the complications such as seromas and preserving nerves and vascularization from the flanks (Uebel 1994). The same author (2009) published that the incisions start in the supra-umbilical area and go to the xiphoid appendix through a narrow tunnel for plication and also recommends to place the patient in the Fowler position to pull down the superior abdominal flap and test the appropriate skin resection before the inferior incisions are carried out (Uebel 2009).

Pontes (2004) recommended the geometrical inferior skin flap block resection (Pontes 2004). The senior author has been performing the skin resection in the lateral areas of the lower abdomen after liposuction preserving the superficial fascia.

Hakme (1983) published his contribution to abdominoplasty technique using a peri- and supra-umbilical lipectomy from the navel to the xiphoid appendix producing a resultant depression in this central region and natural aspect. He also recommends a diamond shape to the umbilicus (Hakme 1983).

Ishida (2011) analyzed the strength of different abdominal fascia in different sutures used in abdominoplasty and concluded that the vertical suture is more resistant than the horizontal due to the distribution and arrangement of muscle fibers (Ishida et al. 2011). Since the beginning, the senior author has recommended the "X" separated stitches using mono-nylon 0 (zero) from 1 cm above the xiphoid process to the pubis (Erfon 2011; Erfon and Mauricio 2016). Also the plication of the superficial fascia in the lower abdomen is carried out using 3-0 colorless mono-nylon with the following advantages: there is no dead space or necessity of drain and the seromas and the length of the final scars are reduced (Avelar 1999; Saldanha et al. 2001; Erfon and Mauricio 2016).

Baroudi (Baroudi and Ferreira 1998) introduced internal stitches fixing the abdominal flap to the abdominal wall reducing the dead space and also the seroma, an important contribution to the abdominoplasty technique (Baroudi and Ferreira 1998). When the superficial fascia is preserved in the lower abdomen associated with small undermining of the tunnel for plication, these kinds of stitches are not necessary.

Koller (Koller and Hintringer 2012) concluded with anatomical study that the superficial fascia preservation prevents seromas (Koller and Hintringer 2012), as recommended by the senior author and others (Erfon 2002; Avelar 2002; Barcelos et al. 2017).

Caprini (2005) recommends a low molecular weight heparin, 40 mg/day for 10 days, to reduce thrombotic events (Caprini 2005). The senior author uses this protocol to all his patients and phlebopressor on the legs during their hospitalization and early de-ambulation (Erfon and Mauricio 2016).

Faria-Correa (1992) published the possibility of a video-endoscopic approach to perform muscle plication, reducing the scars in cases of mini-abdominoplasty (Faria-Corrêa 1992). This was also suggested late by Avelar (1999).

Nahas (2001) published an objective classification based on subcutaneous and skin deformities (Nahas 2001), allowing scar above the pubis line, in its type II. The senior author inverted the incision convexity in his Group 3 to avoid high scars.

Faria-Correa (2016) also introduced the possibility of plication of the rectus abdominis muscle using robotic approach, permitting a minimally invasive surgery associated with minimal incisions at remote sites (Faria Correa 2016).

Bozolla (Bozolla and Psillakis 1988) published important new classification of abdominoplasty deformities in five types and indication of surgery for each type (Bozolla and Psillakis 1988). The senior author classified his patients into four groups with his respective surgical indications.

Avelar (2016a, b) drew attention to the anatomical principles of his technique giving special attention to the description of the vascularization of the skin and musculoaponeurotic wall and his classification of abdominoplasty in order to improve a safest abdominoplasty (Avelar 2016b).

Yacoub (2016) published the extended reverse abdominoplasty in which a complete abdominoplasty is performed with a transversal sub-mammary incision and extended dissection of the skin flap up to the pubis region using in special cases the flap to breast reconstruction (Yacoub 2016). This approach was performed by senior author in rare cases.

Hunstad (Hunstad and Jones 2011) recommends the circumferential body liposuction associated with abdominoplasty with tumescent infiltration (Hunstad and Jones 2011).

Graf (2006) using Doppler published important evidence that abdominoplasty with small undermining and preserving the abdominal myocutaneous perforating vessels reduces complications such as necroses and seromas (Graf et al. 2006).

Barcelos (2017) published a study showing 86.7% reduction in the rate of seroma when comparing lipoabdominoplasty with classical abdominoplasty (Barcelos et al. 2017). The senior author also described the importance of the superficial fascia preservation and the reduction on the rate of complication such as skin necrosis and seroma and secondary liposuction in the lipoabdominoplasty compared with traditional abdominoplasty technique (Erfon 2002, 2009, 2011; Erfon and Mauricio 2016).

Conclusion

The senior author concludes that lipoabdominoplasty was a great evolution to the abdominoplasty technique in the last 60 years. Joining two great techniques, liposuction and abdominoplasty, with minimal undermining, preserving the main vascularization to the superior abdominal flap and the secondary vascularization to the lower abdomen lateral areas and skin resection in the central area up to the muscle fascia, permitting safe plication and reducing the amount of tissue to be preserved in the lower abdomen, improving the aesthetic results, and turning the lipoabdominoplasty technique safer than the traditional abdominoplasty. He suggests, from the beginning, a simple and didactic classification, for patients who are candidates for this surgery, based on skin flaccidity, lipodystrophy, and diastasis of the rectus abdominis muscles and the extent of scars necessary for surgical correction, grouping patients into four groups, with the respective indication of the type of surgery for each group: Group 1, liposuction; Group 2, mini-lipoabdominoplasty; Group 3, mid-lipoabdominoplasty; and Group 4, full lipoabdominoplasty. He also introduced the term mid-lipoabdominoplasty to the special cases where more skin resection is necessary than in mini-lipoabdominoplasty without umbilicus incisions and it's impossible to pull down the superior abdominal flap (full lipoabdominoplasty), configuring a simple and didactic classification for the lipoabdominoplasty technique based on lipodystrophy, the length of the scars, the amount of skin to be resected, and the diastasis of the rectus abdominis muscle.

Compliance with Ethical Standards

Conflict of Interest The authors have no conflict of interest, commercial associations, or financial interests to disclose.

Ethics Statement This study was performed in accordance with the 1964 Helsinki Declaration for research in human subjects and its later amendments or comparable ethical standards. All procedures performed in studies involving human participants were in accordance with ethical standards of the institutional research committee. All patients provided written informed consent for surgery and use of photographs.

References

Avelar JM (1999) – Uma nova técnica de abdominoplastia: sistema vascular fechado de retalho subdérmico dobrado sobre si, combinado com lipoaspiração. Rev Bras Cir 6:3–20

Erfon J (2001) – Abdominoplastia por sistema vascular fechado associado à lipoaspiração. Apresentado na XVI Jornada Norte-Nordeste de Cirurgia. Plástica. Costa do Sauípe-Bahia, Brasil 13 a 15 Set

Saldanha OR, Pinto EB, Matos WN Jr, Lucon RL, Magalhães F, Bello EM (2001) – Lipoabdominoplasty without undermining. Aesthet Surg J 21(6):518–526

Erfon J (2002) – Abdominoplasty through a closed vascular system associated to liposuction: Avelar's technique. In: Avelar JM, ed. Abdominoplasty. Hipócrates. São Paulo, Brasil 299–307
Erfon J (2009) – Abdominoplasty with Liposuction and Minimal Undermining. 11th Espras Congress. Book of Abstracts. Rhodes, Greece. 20–27 September 291–294
Erfon J (2011) Abdominoplasty with Liposuction and Minimal Undermining. Rev Bras Cir Plást 26(1): 116–120
Erfon J, Mauricio C (2016) Plication of the Abdominal Wall in Lipoabdominoplasty. In Avelar JM (ed.), New Concepts on Abdominoplasty and Further Applications. Springer, Switzerland 303–315
Avelar JM (2002) Anatomy of the abdominal panniculus. In: Avelar JM, ed, Abdominoplasty without panniculus undermining and resection, Hippócrates, São Paulo 59–86
Almeida CLA, Vieira LFDF, Leite LAS, Oliveira JAV, Ataide RF, Oliveira EJB, Brandt CT(2016) Importância da preservação da artéria ilíaca circunflexa superficial do abdome na prevenção das necroses da parede abdominal em pacientes submetidas a miniabdominoplastias: estudo anatômico cirúrgico descritivo prospectivo Rev Bras Cir Plast 31(2):178–185
Barcelos FVT, Avelar LET, Bordoni LS, Barcelos RVT(2017) Anatomical analysis of abdominoplasty Rev Bras Cir Plast 32(2):272–281
Illouz YG (1980) – Une nouvelle technique pour les lipodystrophies localiseés. Rev Chir Esth France 6(9): Ap
Illouz YG (1992) A new safe and aesthetic approach to suction abdominoplasty Aesthetic Plastic Surgery 16:237–245
Stuckey JG (1979) – Midabdomen Abdominoplasty Plastic Reconstructive Surgery. March: 333–335.
Avelar JM (2016a) New Concepts in Abdominoplasty: Origin and Evolution. In: Avelar JM (ed.), New Concepts on Abdominoplasty and Further Applications. Springer, Switzerland 3–17
Uebel CO (1994) – Cirurgia do abdome associada à lipoescultura. In: Tourniex AAB Ed. Atualização em Cirurgia Plástica Estética. São Paulo, Brasil: Robe Editorial. PP.483–489.
Uebel CO (2009) Lipoabdominoplasty: Revisiting the Superior Pull-Down Abdominal Flap and New Approaches Aesthetic Plastic Surgery 33:366–376
Pontes R(2004) Variantes das abdominoplastias em bloco. In: Pontes R (ed) Abdominoplastia: ressecção em bloco e sua aplicação em lifting de coxa e torsoplastia. Revinter, Rio de Janeiro, pp 25–54
Hakme F (1983) Abdominoplasty: Peri- and Supra-umbilical Lipectomy Aesthetic Plastic Surgery 7:213–220
Ishida LH, Gemperli R, Longo MV, Alves HR, da Silva PH, Ishida LC, Ferreira MC (2011 Aug) – Analysis of the strength of the abdominal fascia in different sutures used in abdominoplasties. Aesthetic Plastic Surgery. 35(4):435–438
Baroudi R, Ferreira CA (1998) - Seroma: how to avoid it and how to treat it. Aesthet Surg J. 18(6):439–441
Koller M, Hintringer T (2012) – Scarpa fascia or rectus fascia in abdominoplasty flap elevation: A prospective clinical trial. Aesthetic Plastic Surgery 36:241–243
Caprini, JA(2005) Thrombosis risk assessment as a guide to quality patient care Dis Mon 51(2-3):70–78
Faria-Corrêa MA (1992) Videoendoscopic Abdominoplasty (Subcutaneoscopy). Rev Bras Cir Plást. 7:32–34
Nahas FX (2001) A Pragmatic Way to Treat Abdominal Deformities Based on Skin and Subcutaneous Excess Aesthetic Plastic Surg 25:365–371
Faria Correa MA (2016) Robotic Procedure for Plication of the Muscle Aponeurotic Abdominal Wall. In Avelar JM (ed.), New Concepts on Abdominoplasty and Further Applications. Springer, Switzerland 161–177
Bozolla A, Psillakis J (1988) Abdominoplasty: a new concept and a classification for treatment Plastic Reconstructive Surgery 82(6):983–993

Avelar JM (2016b) Surgical Principles and Classification of Abdominoplasty or Lipoabdominoplasty. In Avelar JM (ed.), New Concepts on Abdominoplasty and Further Applications. Springer, Switzerland 31–45

Yacoub CD (2016) Extended Reverse Abdominoplasty: A Technical Alternative for Breast Reconstruction. In Avelar JM (ed.), New Concepts on Abdominoplasty and Further Applications. Springer, Switzerland 555–570

Hunstad JP, Jones SR (2011) Abdominoplasty with thorough concurrent circumferential abdominal tumescent liposuction Aesthetic Surgery J 31(5):572–590

Graf R, Araujo LR, Rippel R, Neto LG, Pace DT, Cruz GA (2006) – Lipoabdominoplasty: liposuction with reduced undermining and traditional abdominal skin flap resection. Aesthetic Plastic Surgery. 30(1):1–8

Chapter 9
Classification for Indications of Lipoabdominoplasty

Wilson Novaes Matos Jr, Ricardo Cavalcanti Ribeiro, and Luis Fernandez de Córdova

Abstract Lipoabdominoplasty, the combination of lipoplasty with classical abdominoplasty, since published by Avelar at the end of the 1990s, presented opportunities for the treatment of body contour enhancing the aesthetics of flanks and abdomen. According to the indications for the most appropriate technique in each case, we identified and classified the patients into nine different groups, which ranged from those presenting with mild fat with good-quality skin to massive weight loss patients with a high degree of flaccidity. The techniques described by the authors included lipoplasty and abdominoplasty alone, and four variations of lipoabdominoplasty.

The classification of lipoabdominoplasty indications offers a better understanding for treatment of the abdominal region. Lipoplasty, selective undermining, and maintenance of Scarpa's fascia help reduce surgical trauma that is the main risk factor of hematoma and necrosis. This classifications is easy to learn since the described procedures are already familiar to most plastic surgeons.

Keywords Abdominoplasty · Liposuction · Lipoabdominoplasty · Body contour · Reverse abdominoplasty

W. N. Matos Jr
Plastic and Reconstructive Surgery, Plastic Day Hospital, Sao paulo, Brazil

R. C. Ribeiro (✉) · L. F. de Córdova
Plastic and Reconstructive Surgery, Federal University of the State of Rio de Janeiro, Rio de Janeiro, Brazil
e-mail: rribeiro@centroin.net.br

J. M. Avelar, R. Cavalcanti Ribeiro (eds.), *Body Contouring*,
https://doi.org/10.1007/978-3-031-42802-9_9

Introduction

Abdominal plastic surgery has evolved greatly from its original description (Callia, 1965) to the introduction of lipoplasty (Illouz, 1980; the combination of lipoplasty and a small skin resection (Hakme, 1985); and the association od lipoplasty and full abdominoplasty (Matarasso, 1991). Since 2000, when it was proposed the overall treatment of the abdominal subcutaneous fat pad with deep lipoplasty, without undermining and without fat pad resection (Avelar 2000), using video endoscopic diastasis suturing (Corrêa, 1995), we have used this technique to treat the abdominal region. Finally in 2001 Saldanha proposed associating lipoplasty and classical abdominoplasty naming has technique *lipoabdominoplasty*. The varied indications were the basis for changes in surgical strategy and technique, depending on the need for treatment of the abdominal structures. The classification of lipoabdominoplasty indications enabled us to standardize and systemize the associated lipoplasty and classical abdominoplasty techniques. It is based on five sequential surgical phases or steps:

1. Dissection and sculpturing of the subcutaneous deep layer and superficial layer through lipoplasty
2. Selective undermining and plication of the anterior rectus sheath
3. Preservation of the perforator vessels
4. Preservation of Scarpa's fascia and deep fat
5. Skin resection and umbilical transposition

Based on this analysis, we propose a new clinical-therapeutic abdomen classification to indicate the best technique for each case (Table 9.1, Fig. 9.1).

Table 9.1 Classification of lipoabdominoplasty and variations

Procedure	Subgroup	Skin	Muscles
Lipoplasty		No flaccidity	No diastasis
Lipominiabdominoplasty	I: Lipoplasty, suprapubic resection with or without lower plication	Light/mild infra-umbilical flaccidity	With/without lower diastasis
	II: Lipoplasty, suprapubic resection and total or infra-umbilical plication, downward traction of the umbilicus	Light/mild infra- and supraumbilical flaccidity	Partial or total diastasis
	III: Lipoplasty, suprapubic resection, plication, transposition of the umbilicus	Mild infra- and supraumbilical flaccidity, high umbilicus	Partial or total diastasis
Lipoabdominoplasty	Lipoplasty, total plication, supraumbilical resection	Excessive skin over the entire abdomen	Total diastasis
Classical abdominoplasty	Dermolipectomy, herniorrhaphy, plication	Excessive skin over the entire abdomen	Diastasis, ventral hernia

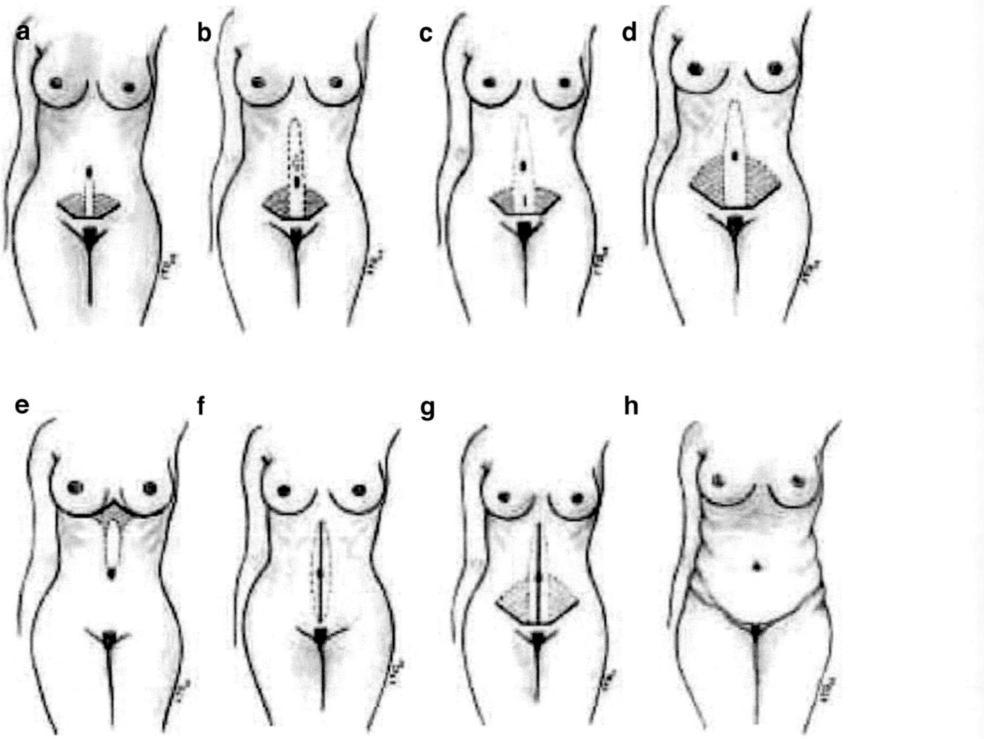

Fig. 9.1 Lipoabdominoplasty classification. (**a**) Lipominiabdominoplasty, type I. (**b**) Lipominiabdominoplasty, type II. (**c**) Lipominiabdominoplasty, type III. (**d**) Lipoabdominoplasty. (**e**) Reverse lipoabdominoplasty. (**f**) Vertical lipoabdominoplasty. (**g**) Anchor lipoabdominoplasty. (**h**) Postbariatric lipoabdominoplasty

Preoperative Evaluation

Note that skin features, such as elasticity, laxity, wrinkles, surface irregularities, and presence of scars, must be taken. The umbilical scar must be positioned taking into consideration the navel's position, its distance in relation to the pubis and xiphoid appendix, and scarring in the hypogastrium. The same parameters indicate the amount of skin to be removed. Through pinch test, the thickness, amount, and disposal of the fatty tissue are evaluated to estimate the volume of fat to be aspirated. Diagnosis of rectoabdominal diastasis for plication as well as its location, infra-umbilical or supraumbilical, to better determine the best technique to be used must be performed. Body contouring lipodystrophies in other areas are evaluated.

Surgical Technique

Saline solution and epinephrine at a concentration of 1:1,000,000 are infiltrated. The abdomen is aspirated by the "scanner" technique, with the cannula holes turned laterally, using short circular movements into the superficial and deep layers rather than conventional undermining.

Infra-umbilical skin resection, plication of the rectoabdominal muscles, and mobilization of the umbilicus are performed, depending on the circumstances of each case. Scarpa's fascia is always preserved, except during classical abdominoplasty, to keep the superficial fatty layer flat, preserving lymphatic drainage and suprapubic sensibility. Aspirative drainage is used postoperatively, with the closed suction drain placed into the selected undermining region, and is to be removed by the third to fifth postoperative day in all cases in which lipoplasty is performed.

Lipoplasty

It is indicated exclusively for those patients who present with a light or mild fat panniculus and good-quality skin.

Lipoabdominoplasty I

This technique could be considered for patients who present with none to mild skin flaccidity in the infra-umbilical region, with or without inferior diastasis. After lipoplasty of the abdomen and surrounding areas, an elliptical fuse of the skin located in the suprapubic area (Uebel, 1987), as well as the entire superficial fatty layer, is removed for the flap to be advanced over the preserved Scarpa's fascia (Fig. 9.2a). When inferior abdominal diastasis was present, Scarpa's fascia was removed at the medial line to perform the rectoabdominal muscle plication in the inferior region and suture the superficial fascia borders (Fig. 9.2b).

Lipoabdominoplasty II

This procedure is indicated for patients with mild skin flaccidity at the upper and lower abdomen in whom partial or total diastasis and high positioning of the umbilical scar are present. Following lipominiabdominoplasty as described above, the umbilicus is "floated" by cutting it free from the underlying fascial attachments. Selective upper undermining at the region of diastasis for the plication is performed, and the umbilicus is repositioned 2 to 5 cm lower and fixed to the aponeurosis of the

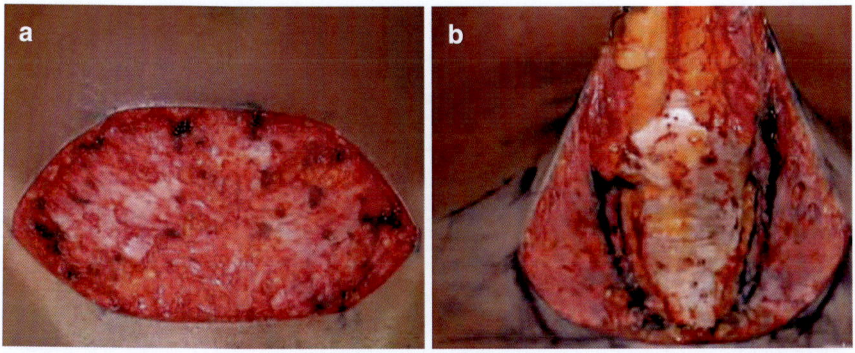

Fig. 9.2 Lipominiabdominoplasty type I. (**a**) After deep and superficial lipoplasty of the abdominal region, Scarpa's fascia is visible, preserved with the deep fat tissue. (**b**) An elliptical incision is made in Scarpa's fascia for performance of the rectoabdominal muscle plication in the inferior abdominal region

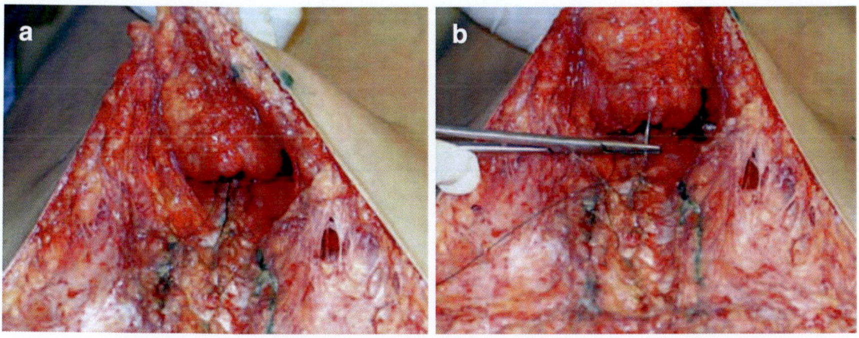

Fig. 9.3 Lipominiabdominoplasty type II. (**a**) After deep and superficial lipoplasty of abdominal region, Scarpa's fascia is visible, preserved with the deep fat tissue in the hypogastrium. (**b**) Umbilical suture in the midline before rectoabdominal plicature in patients with superior abdominal skin flaccidity

rectus abdominal muscle (Delerm, 1982) (Fig. 9.3). Excessive skin at the lower region is removed by means of a suprapubic elliptical fuse.

This technique can only be used in patients whose umbilicus position is originally high in relation to the pubis. Its goal was to treat the mild upper abdominal skin flaccidity that might occur after lipoplasty.

Lipominiabdominoplasty III

It is indicated for patients with severe skin flaccidity at the supra- and infra-umbilical region lacking sufficient excess skin to enable flap traction to the pubic region due to a high umbilicus position. After lipoplasty, selective undermining at the midline,

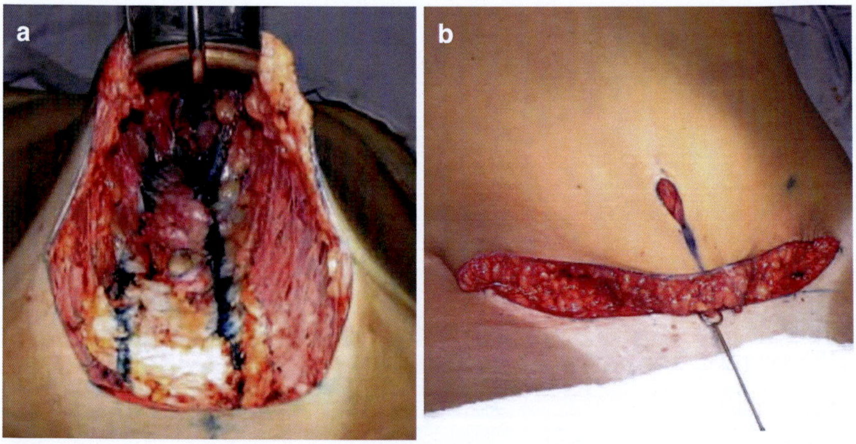

Fig. 9.4 Lipominiabdominoplasty type III. (**a**) After deep and superficial lipoplasty of the entire abdomen, selective undermining was performed in the area of diastasis for plicature. Scarpa's fascia is visible, preserved with the perforating vessels in the inferior abdomen. (**b**) An enlarged skin incision was made in the infra-umbilical region (hypogastrium), resulting in a vertical scar. Then extended elliptical resection of the suprapubic skin was performed with transposition of the umbilicus and omphaloplasty. The umbilical orifice was closed, leaving a 3- to 4-cm scar at the hypogastrium region

and partial or total plication, an extended elliptical resection of suprapubic skin is performed, followed by transposition of the umbilicus and omphaloplasty. The umbilical orifice is closed, leaving a 3- to 4-cm scar at the hypogastrium region (Fig. 9.4).

Lipoabdominoplasty

Lipoabdominoplasty is indicated for patients with skin flaccidity over the entire abdomen and mild to severe lipodystrophy with or without abdominal muscle diastasis (Marques, 1996). Following aspiration of the deep and superficial abdomen and flank layer, the umbilicus is isolated, and the infra-umbilical skin is resected as in a traditional abdominoplasty, preserving Scarpa's fascia; the venous, arterial, and lymphatic vessels; and the innervation. Selective undermining at the medial diastasis area is performed close to the internal rectus abdominis muscle borders, preserving the abdominal perforating vessels. The partial resection of Scarpa's fascia at the mid-infra-umbilical line exposed the aponeurosis for conventional plication of the entire muscle diastasis. The navel is transposed to achieve the "star-shaped" omphaloplasty. Closing of the abdomen is performed in three planes: the superficial fat, deep dermis, and superficial skin (Fig. 9.5). In cases of difficult traction, it is possible to complete the procedure with a small inverted "T" scar at the lower region (Baroudi 1995; Cardoso, 1987).

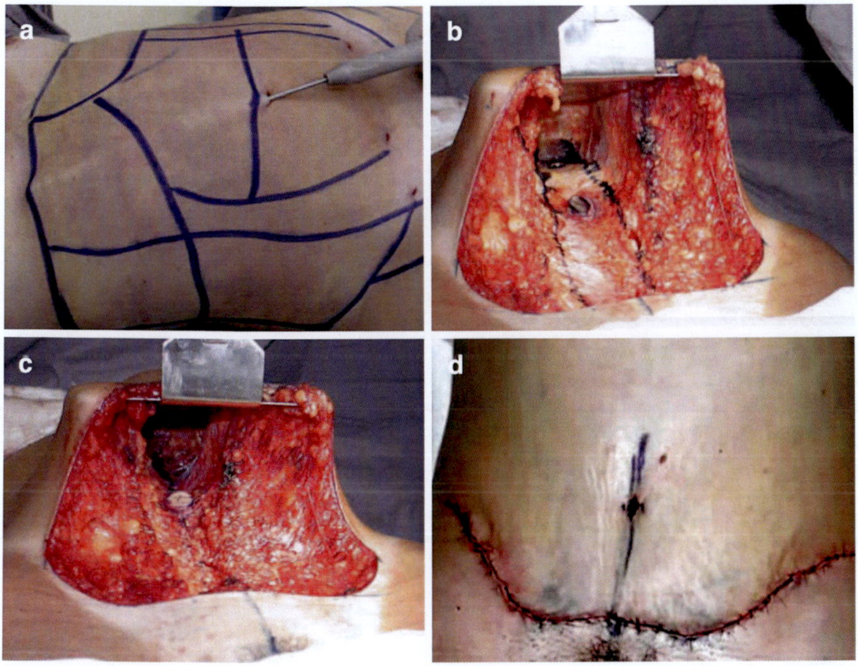

Fig. 9.5 Lipoabdominoplasty. (**a**) Deep and superficial lipoplasty. (**b**) Lipoplasty of the superficial layer in the inferior abdomen with Scarpa's fascia and the fat deep tissue preserved. Selective undermining was performed with a bistoury only in the diastasis region of the rectoabdominal muscle for plication in the superior abdomen and elliptical incision of Scarpa's fascia in the inferior abdomen for the plicature. (**c**) Rectoabdominal plicature and Scarpa's fascia suture. Deep fat tissue over the inferior abdomen. (**d**) Final result before elliptical skin resection and omphaloplasty

Lipoabdominoplasty in the Atypical Abdomen

In patients with atypical abdominal variations related to the presence of pre-existing scars in the abdomen or to massive weight loss, we adapted the techniques in the previously described categories to the individual needs of each case.

Reverse Lipoabdominoplasty and Anchor or Vertical Abdominoplasty

In patients in whom a high degree of flaccidity of the inframammary fold is present, the excessive skin is removed through the inframammary reverse approach, and, if necessary, selective undermining with diastasis plication should be performed (Rebelo, 1972). It is possible to associate the suprapubic resection without transposing the umbilicus in cases of lower region flaccidity, as described by Avelar, Hakme,

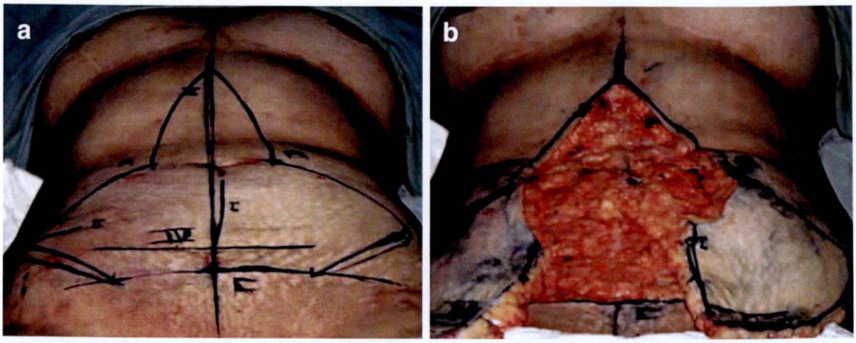

Fig. 9.6 Anchor lipoabdominoplasty. (**a**) Marking of the skin resection before lipoplasty. (**b**) Skin resection after lipoplasty without flap undermining

and Shestack. The same strategy is used with skin resection in a vertical or anchor lipoabdominoplasty (Carreirão, 1983), depending on the position and location of the scars, and preserving the irrigation through the undermining by lipoplasty (Fig. 9.6).

Postbariatric Lipoabdominoplasty

In treating patients who had undergone massive weight loss, in whom great skin excess and adipose tissue are present, lipoabdominoplasty is performed, using lipoplasty to undermine and thin out the flap, removing the skin according to the need of each case. A fuse of Scarpa's fascia and deep fatty layers may be removed from the midline. The borders are to be sutured, even in those cases when there is no need to expose the aponeurosis for the plication. Physical examination and abdominal ultrasound may diagnose hernias and scar adherences in the abdominal wall, which would contraindicate lipoplasty.

Abdominoplasty

Lipoplasty was contraindicated in the presence of abdominal wall hernias. In such cases, the traditional flap undermining, herniorrhaphy, abdominal muscle plication, and conventional dermolipectomy are the technique of choice.

Discussion

A thorough preoperative evaluation of the abdominal region is essential for the diagnosis, classification, and selection of the technique most appropriate to each case. The principles and foundations of this classification system are based on preservation of the anatomy of the vascular, lymphatic, and nervous systems of the abdominal wall, involving the two layers of the adipose tissue and the muscular groups. Through superficial and deep lipoplasty, the basic lipoabdominoplasty techniques, we can dissect the two layers of the abdominal fat and reach the abdominal flap with less trauma compared with dissection using a Bovie, which splits up the perforator vessels emerging from the rectoabdominal muscles. Currently, this principle is used in 99.06% of our cases (Table 9.2). Even in those cases in which the adipose tissue is thin, we prefer to perform divulsion with lipoplasty suction cannulas without vacuum for flap undermining.

Selective undermining performed with a bistoury only in the diastasis region of the rectoabdominal muscle for plication does not reach the perforator arteries, which are located 2 cm from the rectoabdominal muscle edge. Dissection by means of lipoplasty and selective undermining for plication replace the large-scale dissections of conventional abdominoplasty and lipectomy. Since we began using these techniques, we have found that they result in a broadened vascularized flap and decrease the incidence of complications, such as hematoma, epitheliosis, and necrosis.

The preservation of Scarpa's fascia and of the lower abdominal deep fat is important for the superior flap accommodation, and it is another important foundation of the technique, because anatomically and histologically speaking, the lymphatic vases are more numerous in this region. We believe that maintenance of the lymphatic system through this method is the main factor in the decrease in the incidence of seroma in the patient subgroup treated according to these principles. In those lipoabdominoplasty cases in which Scarpa's fascia of the suprapubic region was removed completely, exposing the aponeurosis, we encountered seroma and observed a difference in elevation of the lower abdomen in relation to the pubis. Another important result was the lack of any sensibility loss in the lower abdomen in any of the cases. We routinely associate lipoabdominoplasty and its variations with lipoplasty of the flanks and outer thigh and lipografting in the gluteal-trochanteric regions, which allows for global harmonization of the body contour. In patients who have undergone great weight loss, lipoabdominoplasty enables thinning of the skin flap, prevents wide undermining, improves the final result, and reduces the complication rate. We can also apply this technique in cases of secondary abdominoplasty, when it is necessary to remove the fatty tissue and remaining excessive skin.

Table 9.2 Incidence of the indications

Surgical technique	% of indications
Lipoabdominoplasty	79.65
Lipoabdominoplasty in atypical abdomen	9.95
Lipominiabdominoplasty I	4.73
Lipominiabdominoplasty III	2.84
Lipominiabdominoplasty II	1.89
Classical abdominoplasty–herniorrhaphy	0.94

Conclusions

The preoperative evaluation and the correct indication of lipominiabdominoplasty, lipoabdominoplasty, and variations offer good options for abdominal region treatment, resulting in a more youthful appearance to the abdomen with less scarring and a lower incidence of major complications than traditional abdominal aesthetic surgery. We observed good results and high patient satisfaction with respect to abdominal profile appearance (Figs. 9.7, 9.8, 9.9, 9.10, 9.11, 9.12, and 9.13). Resection of adipose tissue through the lipoplasty cannula, selective undermining, and maintenance of Scarpa's fascia and deep fat permit a better preservation of the vascular,

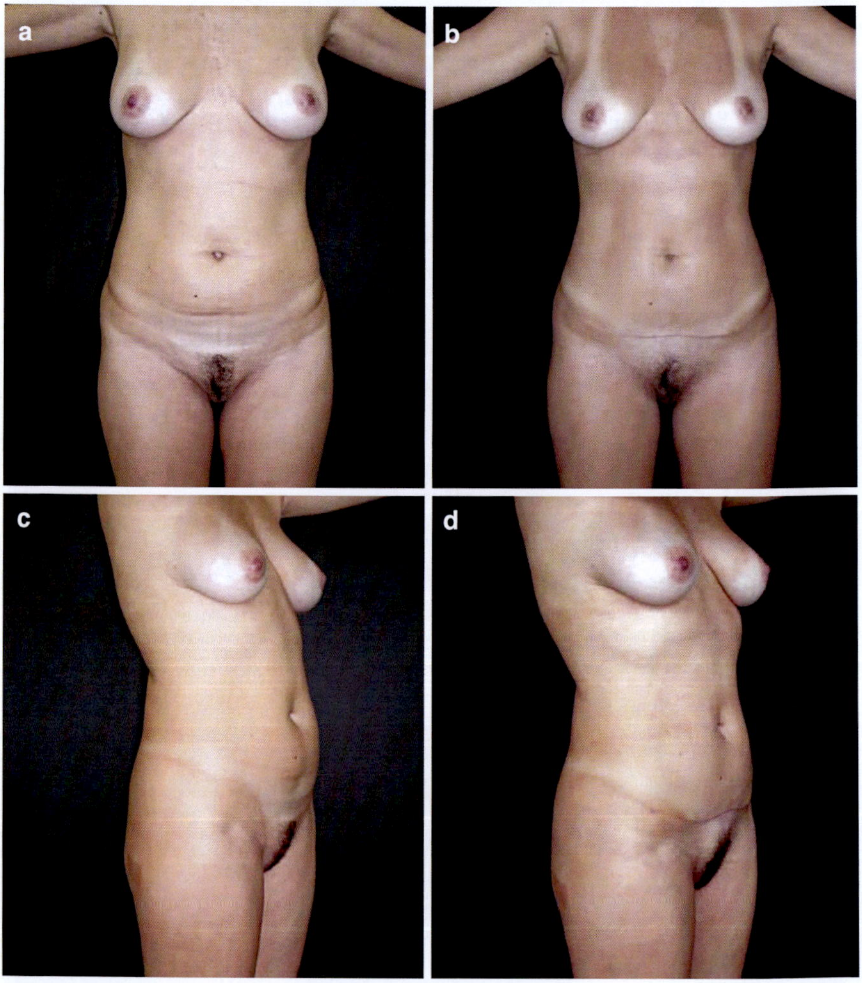

Fig. 9.7 (**a, c**) Preoperative views of a 36-year-old woman with one previous pregnancy, mild abdominal lipodystrophy, and a flaccid inferior abdominal region. (**b, d**) Postoperative views 8 months after lipominiabdominoplasty type I and lipoplasty of the flanks and legs

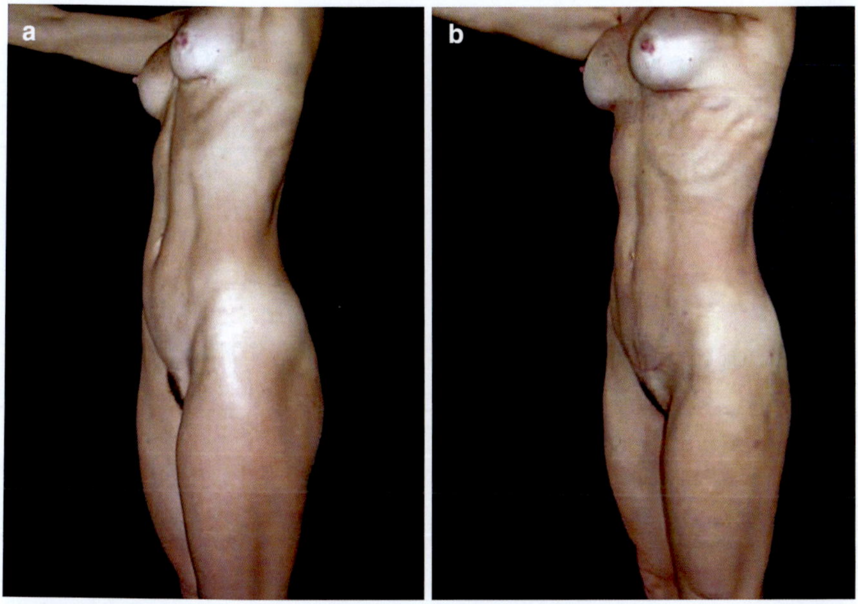

Fig. 9.8 (**a**) Preoperative view of a 48-year-old woman with two previous pregnancies, previous breast augmentation, and inferior diastasis of the rectoabdominal muscles. (**b**) Postoperative view 13 months after lipominiabdominoplasty type I with plicature. Her breast implants were also replaced with round, high-profile silicone gel implants placed under the muscle

lymphatic, and nervous systems associated with the abdomen. The resulting decrease in surgical trauma is the main factor in the decrease of hematoma and necrosis rates.

The learning curve is fast because the described procedures utilize techniques and methods already familiar to most plastic surgeons.

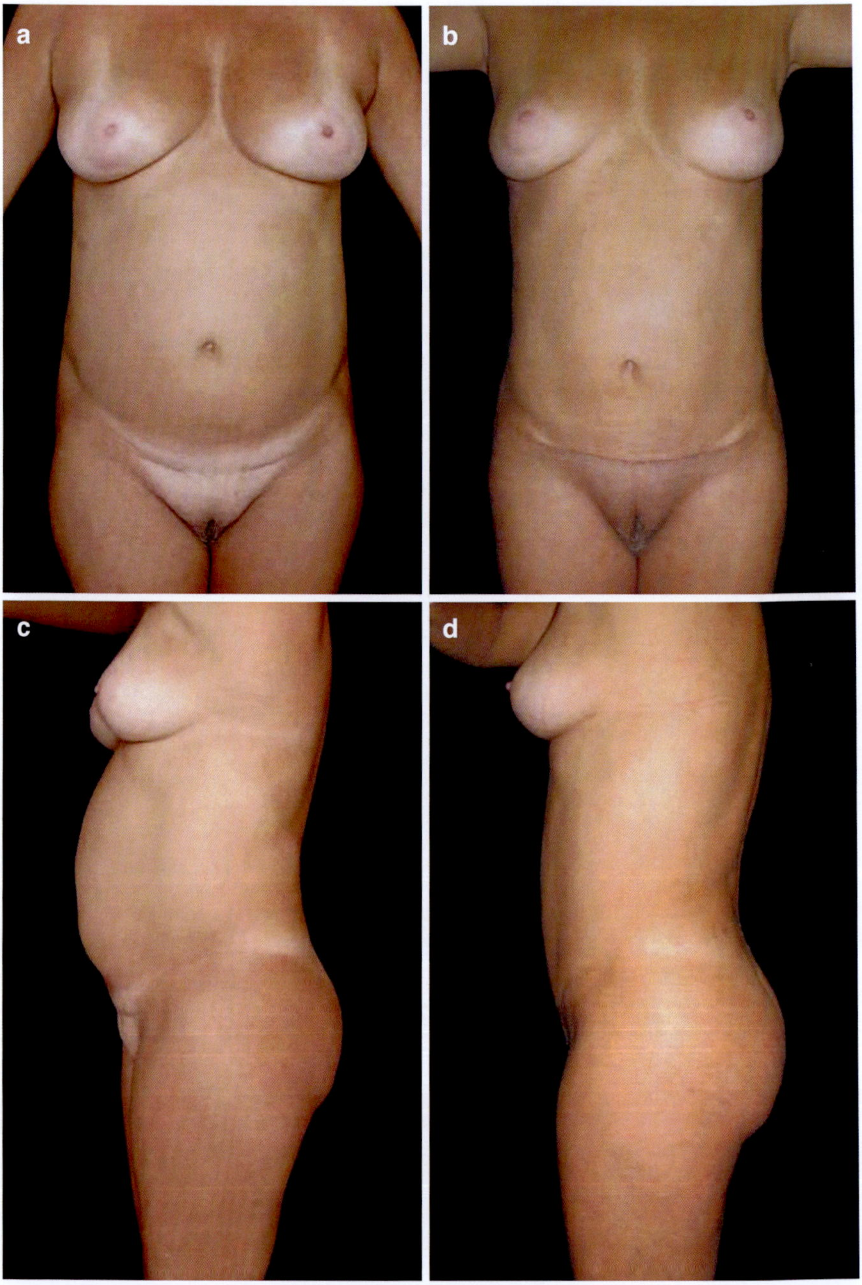

Fig. 9.9 (**a, c**) Preoperative views of a 45-year-old woman with one previous pregnancy, an inferior scar, abdominal lipodystrophy, excessive skin, and diastasis of the rectoabdominal muscles. (**b, d**) Postoperative views 1 year after lipominiabdominoplasty type II and lipoplasty of the waist

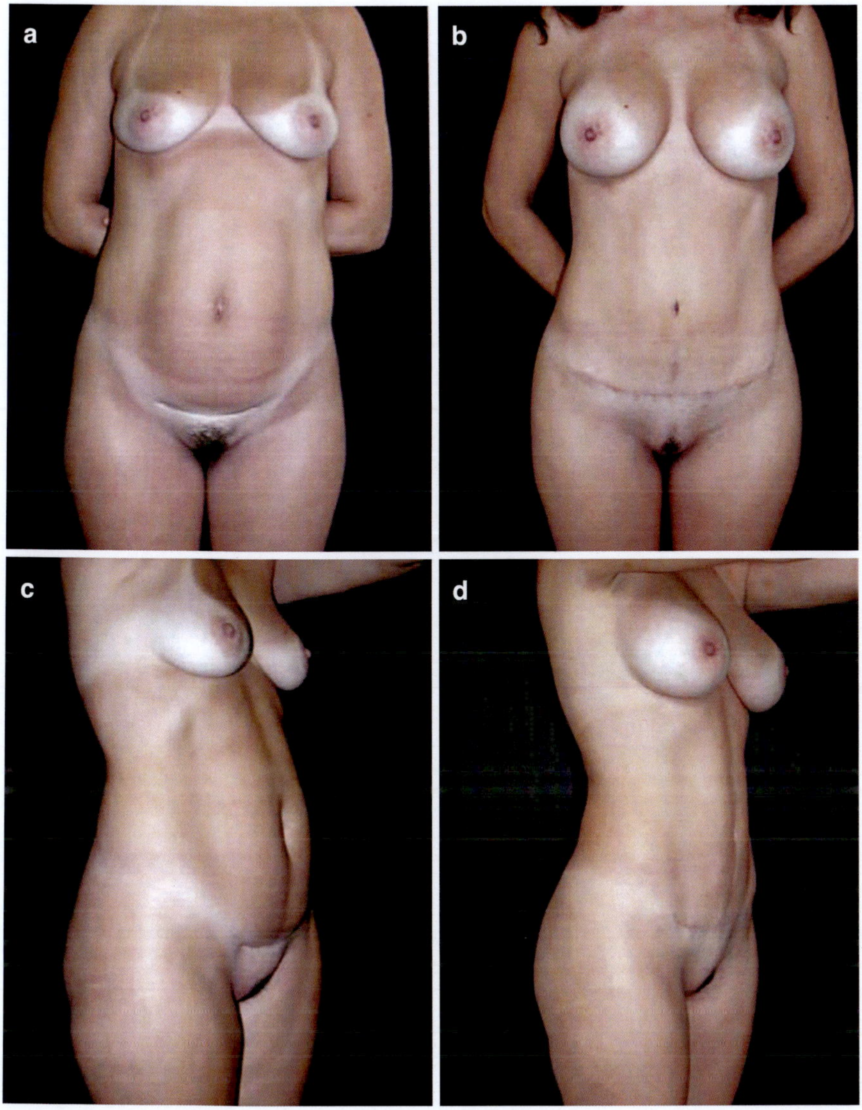

Fig. 9.10 (**a, c**) Preoperative views of a 42-year-old woman with two previous pregnancies, an inferior scar, abdominal lipodystrophy, excessive skin, and diastasis of the rectoabdominal muscles. (**b, d**) Postoperative views 1 year after lipominiabdominoplasty type III, breast augmentation, and lipoplasty of the waist

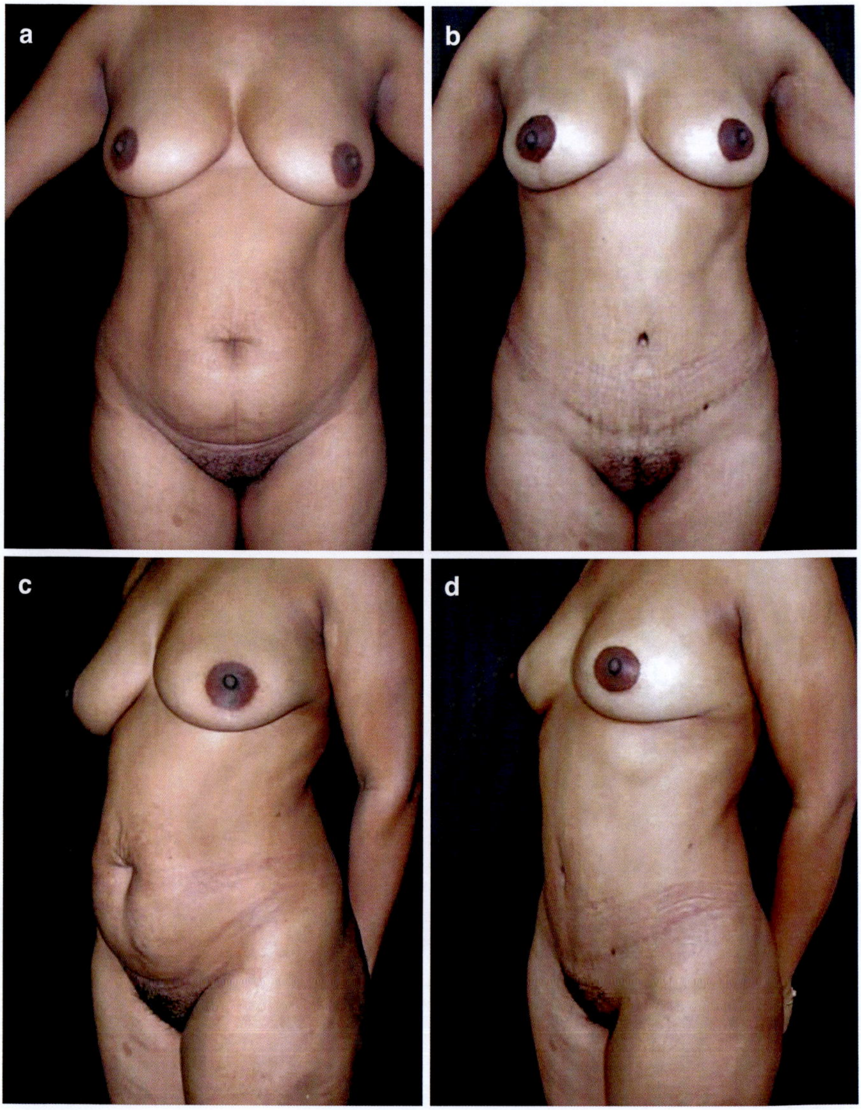

Fig. 9.11 (**a, c**) Preoperative views of a 45-year-old woman with three previous pregnancies, an inferior abdominal scar, excessive skin, and diastasis of the rectoabdominal muscles. (**b, d**) Postoperative views 1 year after lipoabdominoplasty and associated mastopexy

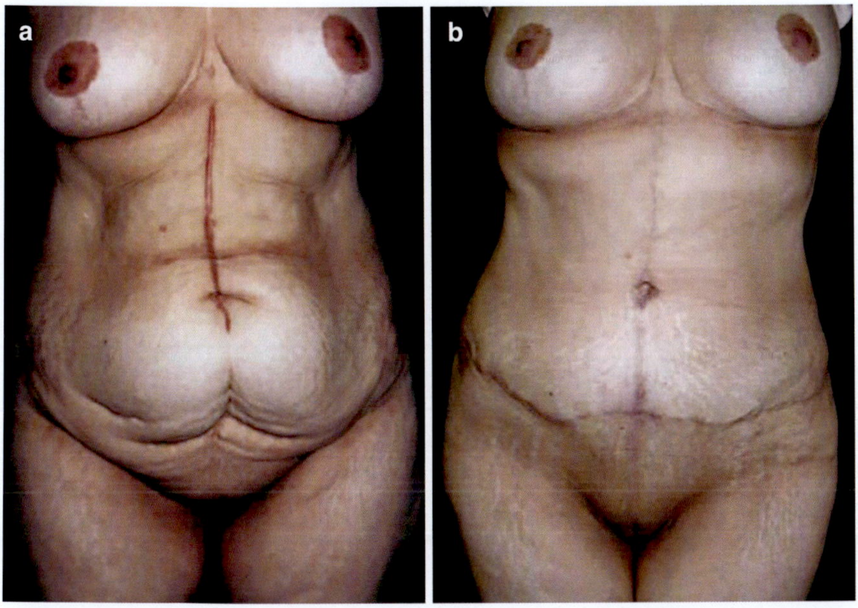

Fig. 9.12 (**a**) Preoperative view of a 68-year-old woman with two previous pregnancies, seven scars from previous surgery, excessive skin, and diastasis of the rectoabdominal muscles. (**b**) Postoperative view 16 months after anchor lipoabdominoplasty

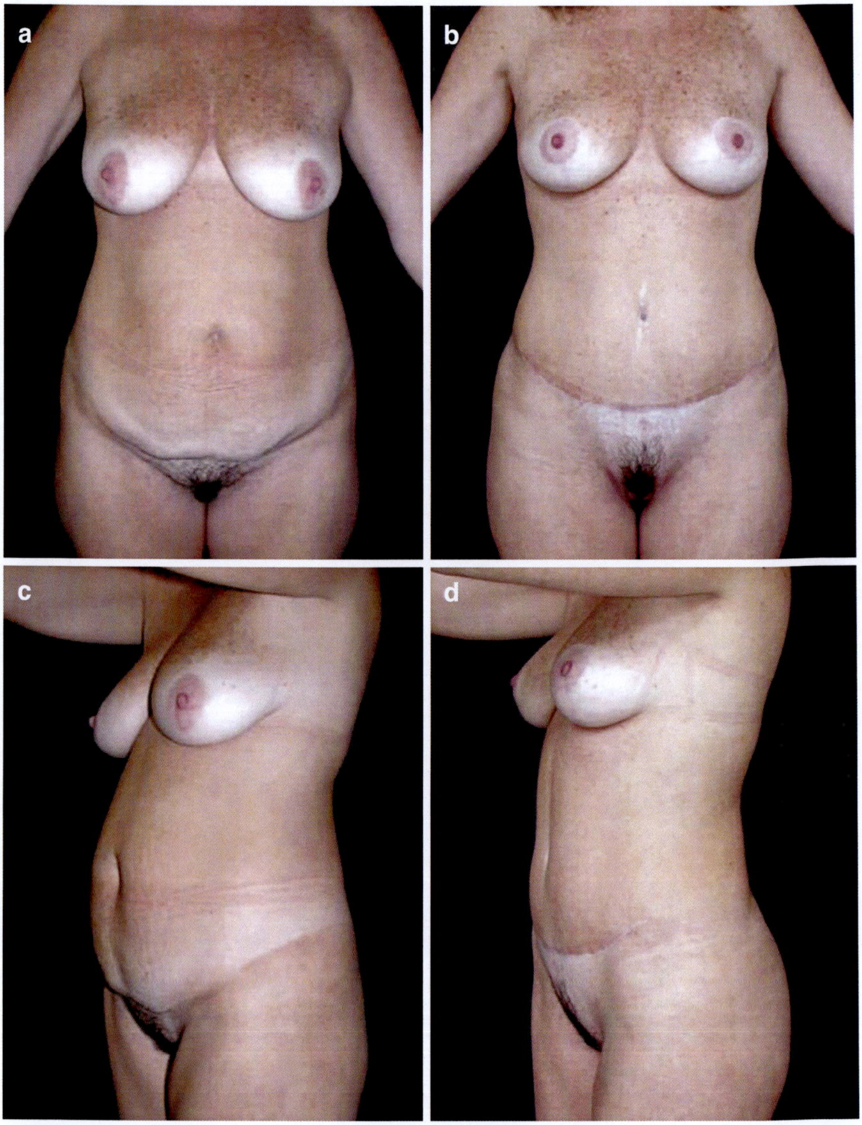

Fig. 9.13 (**a, c**) Preoperative views of a 42-year-old woman with three previous pregnancies and 60-kg weight loss. (**b, d**) Postoperative views 1 year after lipoabdominoplasty, mastopexy, and lipoplasty of the waist

References

1. Callia W. Contribuição para o estudo da correção cirúrgico do abdome pêndulo e globoso—Técnica original [dissertation]. Faculty of the Medical University of São Paulo, 1965.
2. Illouz YG. Une nouvelle technique pour lês lipodystrophies localisées. *Rev Chir Esth Franc* 1980;April:6.
3. Hakme F. Technical details in the liposuction associated with abdominoplasty. *Rev Bras Cir* 1985;75:331.
4. Wilkinson TS, Swartz BE. Individual modification in body contour surgery: the limited abdominoplasty. *Plast Reconstr Surg* 1986;779–784.
5. Bozola AR, Psillakis JM. Abdominoplasty: a new concept and classification for treatment. *Plast Reconstr Surg* 1988;82:983–993.
6. Matarasso A. Abdominolipoplasty: A system of classification and treatment for combined abdominoplasty and suction assisted lipectomy. *Aesthetic Plast Surg* 1991;15:111–121.
7. Pitanguy I, Salgado F, Murakami R, Radwanski HW, Manad R Jr. Abdominoplasty: classification and surgical techniques. *Rev Bras Cir* 1995;85:23–44.
8. Matarasso A. Liposuction as an adjunct to a full abdominoplasty. *Plast Reconstr Surg* 1995;95:829–836.
9. Matarasso A. Liposuction as an adjunct to a full abdominoplasty revisited. *Plast Reconstr Surg* 2000;106:1197–1206.
10. Illouz YG. A new safe and aesthetic approach to suction abdominoplasty. *Aesthetic Plast Surg* 1992;16:237–245.
11. Shestak KC. Marriage abdominoplasty expands the miniabdominoplasty concept. *Plast Reconstr Surg* 1999;103:120–135.
12. Avelar JM. Uma nova técnica de abdominoplastia—sistema vascular fechado de retalho subdérmico dobrado sobre si memo combinado com lipoaspiração. *Ver Brás Cir* 1999;13:3–20.
13. Avelar JM. Abdominoplasty: a new technique without undermining and fat layer removal. *Arq Catarinense de Méd* 2000;29:147–149.
14. Corrêa MA. Videoendoscopic subcutaneous techniques for aesthetic and reconstructive plastic surgery. *Plast Reconstr Surg*. 1995;96(2):446–53. https://doi.org/10.1097/00006534-199508000-00030. PMID: 7624421.
15. Saldanha OR, De Souza Pinto EB, Matos WN Jr, Lucon RL, Magalhaes FF, Bello EML. Lipoabdominoplasty without undermining. *Aesthetic Surg J* 2001;21:518–526.
16. Saldanha OR. Lipoabdominoplasty with selective and safe undermining. *Aesthetic Plast Surg* 2003;27:322–327.
17. Souza Pinto EB, de Erazo IPJ, Muniz A C, Prado Filho FSA, Salazar GH. Superficial liposuction. *Aesthetic Plast Surg* 1996;20:111–122.
18. Taylor GI. The superiorly based rectus abdominis flap: predicting and enhancing its blood supply based on an anatomic and clinical study. *Plast Reconstr Surg* 1988;81:721.
19. Uebel CO. Miniabdominoplasty—a new approach for body contouring. Presented at the 9th Annual Congress of the International Society of Aesthetic Surgery, New York, October 1987.
20. Delerm A. Refinements in abdominoplasty with emphasis on reimplantation of the umbilicus. *Plast Reconstr Surg* 1982;70:632–637.
21. Marques A, Brenda E, Pereira MD, De Castro M, Abramo AC. Abdominoplasty with two fusiform plications. *Aesthetic Plast Surg* 1996;20:249–251.
22. Abramo A, Viola JC, Marques A. The H approach to abdominal muscle aponeurosis for the improvement of body contour. *Plast Reconstr Surg* 1990;86:1008–1013.
23. Matos WN Jr. Onfaloplastia em forma de estrela. *Arq Catarinense de Méd* 2000;29:147–149.
24. Baroudi R, Moraes M. A "bicycle-handbar" type of incision for primary and secondary abdominoplasty. *Aesthetic Plast Surg* 1995;17:307–320.
25. Cardoso De Castro C, Marica Branco Cupello A, Cintra H. Limited incisions in abdominoplasty. *Ann Plast Surg* 1987;19:436–447.
26. Rebelo C, Franco T. Abdominoplasty with inframammary scar. *Rev Bras Cir* 1972;62:249.
27. Carreirão S, Pitanguy I, Correa WE, Caldeira MC. Abdominoplastia vertical. Uma técnica a ser lembrada. *Ver Bras Cir* 1983;79:184–194.

Chapter 10
Medium Definition Lipoabdominoplasty: A Natural Evolution of High-Definition Techniques

Giuliano Borille and Luis Fernandez de Córdova

Abstract The technique presented is the result of reuniting two surgical techniques, both described by Brazilian authors, the lipoabdominoplasty and medium-definition liposuction.

The term medium definition was selected in order to differentiate this approach from high-definition liposculpture techniques associated with the use of external energy devices.

The four cornerstones of medium-definition liposuction are

1. absence of external energy, which allows a more superficial liposuction,
2. creation of thinner flaps to mimic the conditions of an athlete in what we call the athletic triad,
3. use of continuous compression of key areas of the skin by customized handcrafted pads,
4. prevention of umbilicus sagging.

The umbilical scar is a key aesthetic landmark of the anterior abdominal wall.

The aim of this chapter is to share the results of two popular body contouring techniques combined, Medium definition Liposuction & Abdominoplasty. Taking into consideration that liposuction may lead to the presence of loose skin, adding to

G. Borille
Division of Plastic, Aesthetic and Reconstructive Surgery, Clinica Borille, Porto Alegre, Brazil

L. F. de Córdova (✉)
Division of Plastic, Aesthetic and Reconstructive Surgery, Global Plastic Surgery, Mexico, Mexico

Division of Plastic, Aesthetic and Reconstructive Surgery, Instituto Superior de Ciencias da Saúde Carlos Chagas, Rio de, Janeiro, Brazil

J. M. Avelar, R. Cavalcanti Ribeiro (eds.), *Body Contouring*,
https://doi.org/10.1007/978-3-031-42802-9_10

the equation the removal of excess skin and subcutaneos tissue through an abdominoplasty, allows for a tightening effect to occur, improving the body contour and the aesthtetic of the abdominal wall.

Keywords Lipoabdominoplasty · Liposuction · Abdominoplasty · Muscular definition

Introduction

The technique presented in this chapter is the result of combining two techniques: medium-definition liposuction (MDLipo) and lipoabdominoplasty. Coincidentally, both techniques were described by Brazilian authors, abdominoplasty without undermining and fat layer removal by (Avelar 2000; Juarez and Illouz 1986; Ribeiro et al. 2016; Saldanha 2003; Avelar 1983) and MDLipo by Borille.

In order to present abdominal definition, there must be three elements at the same time that the authors refer to as the athletic triad:

1. Muscle hypertrophy
2. Small amount of subcutaneous fat
3. Tight skin

One of the technique specifics that differentiate MDLipo technique from other definition techniques is that it does not sculpt muscle anatomy in the subcutaneous fat, creating volumes based on adipose tissue.

Medium-definition liposuction can be considered a sequence for obtaining natural and defined results, from soft to high definition, with four exclusive cornerstones:

1. Absence of external energy from medical devices
2. Creation of thinner flaps than those created by the traditional liposuction approach (Fig. 10.1)
3. The use of continuous compression of key areas of the skin by customized handcrafted pads, producing well-controlled fibrosis
4. Prevention of umbilicus sagging after liposuction

Since this procedure is based almost entirely on thinner flaps and wider subcutaneous undermining, MD lipoabdominoplasty is not limited to a narrow central tunnel as previously described techniques.

The lack of external energy allows the surgeon to create thinner flaps and aspirate in more superficial planes, minimizing the risks in regard to flap survival due to burns or necrosis, that are present when using Vaser, laser, or radiofrequency. These thin flaps depend on the vascular subdermal plexus preservation to ensure their long-term viability. The nuances in pigmentation, flap survival, and aesthetic results secondary to vascular territories are the reason for the specific cannula design used (three holes, in line, one side of the tube) sparing the plexus from mechanic and thermic trauma (Fig. 10.2).

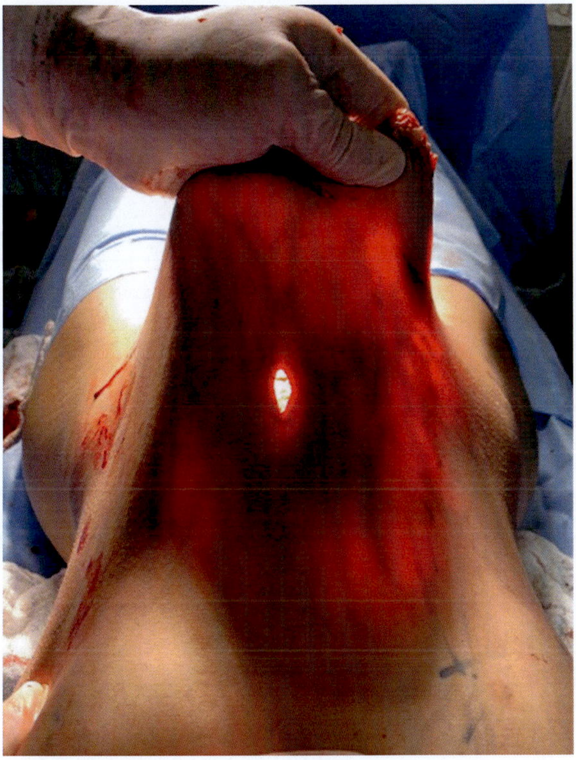

Fig. 10.1 Flap thickness evaluation by transluminescence

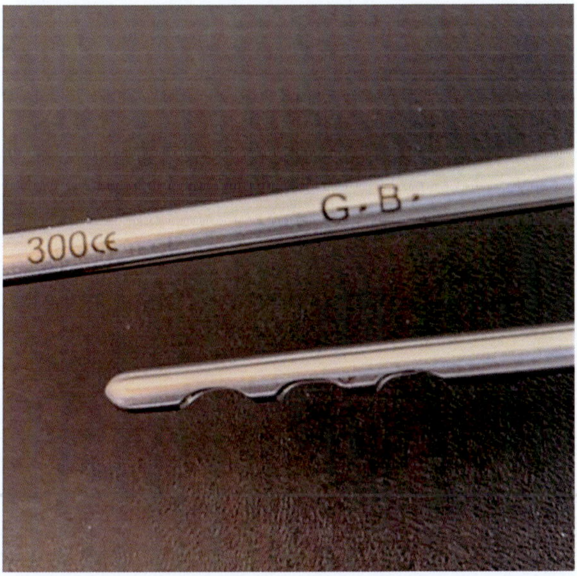

Fig. 10.2 Custom-made three holes, in line, one side of the tube cannulas to spare the plexus from mechanic and thermic trauma and ensure flap survival

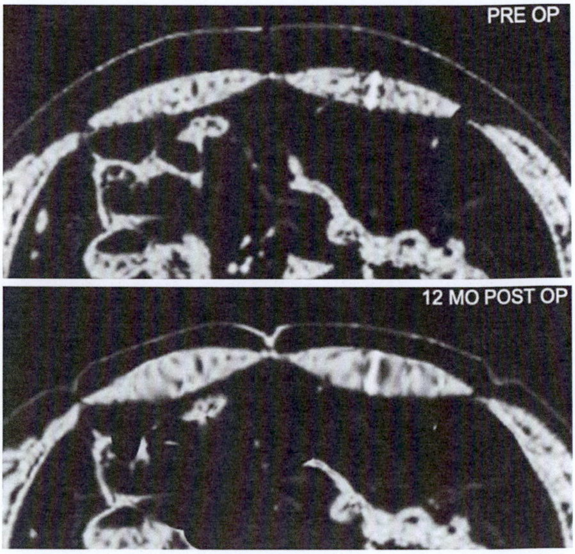

Fig. 10.3 Skin retraction and adhesion for muscular definition after 12 months PO MD lipoabdominoplasty

The instrument used during the procedure is as important as the customized handcrafted abdominal pads that will allow the skin to adhere to the deeper muscle anatomy through a process of well-controlled fibrosis production between the muscle transition and skin. This guided and controlled fibrosis aids in creating definition by exposing real muscular anatomy, hills and valleys, lights and shadows, replacing the role of external energy devices in skin retraction as shown in a 12 months postop abdominal CT scan (Fig. 10.3)

Patient Selection

Careful patient selection is critical to achieve ideal aesthetic results consistent with medium-definition abdominal etching liposuction. The patient should follow a consistent exercise and diet routine and must have an overall athletic look with a lack of abdominal definition due to muscular diastasis and the resultant muscular and skin sagging (Table 10.1).

Selection Criteria

1. Patients with hypertrophic and palpable rectus abdominis muscle under isometric contraction
2. Body fat index of 23% or less

Table 10.1 Similarities and differences between lipoabdominoplasty, from its first published description, and medium-definition lipoabdominoplasty (Avelar 2000; Juarez and Illouz 1986; Ribeiro et al. 2016; Saldanha 2003; Avelar 1983; Callia 1965; Illouz 1980; Hakme 1985; Avelar 1999; Wilkinson and Swartz 1986)

	Types of lipoabdominoplasty		
Characteristic	Original	Modified	Definition abdominoplasty
Lower abdomen	Superficial liposuction	Deep liposuction	Deep and superficial liposuction
Pubic liposuction	No	Yes	
Areas of liposuction	Inferior abdomen	Flanks or dorsum	Flanks and inferior abdomen
Type of liposuction	Conventional	Power-assisted	Conventional
Scarpa fascia	Complete preservation in inferior abdomen	Removal in the inferior abdomen	Removal in the inferior abdomen
Narrow undermine in midline	Yes	Yes	No
Mons & lipoplasty	No mons approach	Lipoplasty and mons lipolifting	No (Pubic dermolipectomy)
Pubic fixation	No	Yes	No (progressive adhesion sutures in abdominal flap

Skin Markings

Skin markings are guided by palpation of the muscular tendinous intersections of the rectus abdominis muscle, linea alba, and linea semilunaris. The patient's individual anatomy must be taken into account, because there are several different tendinous intersections between the abdominal muscles among patients. This is fundamental to prevent an artificial disconnection between the subcutaneous etched shape and the muscle layer in the deeper plane.

Infiltration

Less tumescent fluid is used compared to the regular wet or tumescent liposuction approach (700 cc solution in total containing saline 0.9% + adrenaline 1 mg/ml). Medium-definition liposuction is preferentially performed when the abdominal muscle outlines are still visible. This amount of tumescent fluid is sufficient to prevent distortions and postoperative swelling and still prevent bleeding.

Access Sites for Liposuction Cannulas

The sites of the incisions for the access of the liposuction cannulas are systematically and srategically planned to follow the skin markings and produce less visible scars.

Cannulas

Two regular cannulas (3.5 and 4 mm caliber) are used to perform the liposuction according to the location of abdominal fat levels. The cannulas are perforated on one side of the tube (3 in line perforation) as previously described.

Liposuction

The abdominal musculature is topographically visualized according to the skin markings guided by the palpation of the linea alba, the linea semilunaris, and the tendinous intersections of rectus abdominis muscle. These landmarks are enhanced with localized superficial liposuction to deepen the natural grooves or furrows, creating curves, light, and shadow effects on the skin (Fig. 10.4).

The authors start debulking the deeper layers of fat just above the abdominal muscles with 4 mm cannulas and continuing to the mid-lamellar layer and between muscle groups with 3.5 mm cannulas.

Superficial liposuction, to define the abdominal muscle that is outlined and marked, is then performed. Each treatment area undergoes liposuction by using a 3.5 mm cannula. It is very important to remove all the fat in the intersection areas, creating a delicate transition zone between the abdominal muscular intersections, to define the superficial anatomy landmarks. Creating smooth transition surfaces and avoiding sharp edges is key during this portion of medium-definition liposuction.

Abdominoplasty is performed, after liposuction, by an incision at the suprapubic area and tissue detachment up to the xiphoid process and lateral edges of the rectus muscle whenever necessary to achieve adequate tissue release with no tension nor retractions. After the abdominal flap undermining, a vertical plication is performed on the anterior rectus sheath, bringing the medial edges of the recti muscle together. An additional horizontal plication is made on the suprapubic region, at the end of the vertical plication (two layers with nylon 2-0 and Vicryl 1-0). After the plication, progressive adhesion sutures are used, taking superficial bites from the flap into the muscular wall.

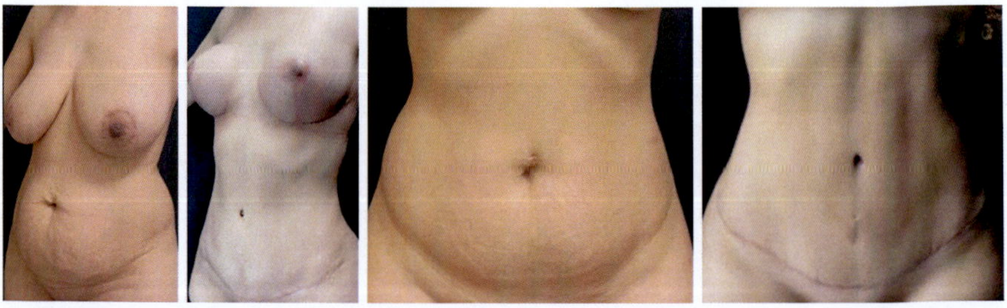

Fig. 10.4 Examples of pre- and post-op cases of MD lipoabdominoplasty

To prevent umbilicus sagging after liposuction, due to the upper abdomen skin losing tension and rolling over the umbilicus, creating a horizontalized shape even if excess skin surgically removed, we created an umbilicus suspension system using a temporary immobilization suture performed with a modified Reverdin's needle and 3-0 nylon suture.

Compression is of utmost importance. The authors place handcrafted pads, prepared in the operating room, to produce specific pressure points of contact between the skin and the underlying rectus abdominis fascia right under the traditional compression garment.

At 48 h post-op, patients remove and change the original compression pads for a new customized compression kit (pads and garment). Our recommendation is to use the pads and the garment for at least 1 month after surgery.

Discussion

A common concern when definition liposuction is performed is the pigmentation complications related to superficial liposuction; however, the author reports less than 1% of cases with dyschromia over the last 5 years.

Medium-definition lipoabdominoplasty aims to create a fit, natural look in selected patients who already have a regular exercise routine, muscular hypertrophy, and low body fat. The idea is to create an athletic and fit aesthetic look in patients who lack abdominal definition in relation to their whole body even under diet and exercise routines.

This approach is an alternative to definition techniques that need external energy devices resulting in a lower rate of seroma, dyschromia, and necrosis when compared with VAHDL cases.

Being the main source of vascular nutrition of the flap, knowledge of the characteristics of the subdermal plexus and its preservation, using the adequate cannulas, is critical for designing thin flaps. The subdermal or cutaneous plexus is considered to be the junction between the deep reticular portion of the dermis and the underlying subcutaneous fat tissue. The subdermal vessels have a kind of axiality, which plays an important role in the development of a thin flap. Several thin flaps in the abdominal region have been reported since Nakajima proposed the concept of thin flap in 1988. Furthermore, the author does not recommend the use of any type of external energy in these types of flaps, at risk of tissue damage and safety issues.

Using the proper approach, it is safe and feasible to produce thinner flaps than in previously described lipoabdominoplasty techniques, giving room for the surgeon to apply a handcrafted and individual dressing that connects the skin and the underlying subcutaneous tissue to the deeper muscle layer exposing the muscle definition.

The main idea is to reproduce the anatomical pattern of the "real six-pack" (muscle hypertrophy, small amount of subcutaneous fat, and tight skin) and mimic the physiology; therefore, we, plastic surgeons, do not stimulate the creation of a non-existing phenomenon in nature, which is a mass index of 25 or more with a muscular hypertrophic abdomen.

Conclusion

MD lipoabdominoplasty allows the correction of eventual muscle aponeurotic defects through suture plication and excess skin removal in order to produce a natural athletic look by ensuring the athletic triad is present.

References

Avelar JM. Abdominoplasty: A new technique without undermining and fat layer removal. Arq Catarinense Med. 2000;29:147–149.

Juarez M. A., Illouz, Y Lipoaspiraçao (1986) Ed. Hipócrates

Ribeiro RC, Matos WN Jr, Cruz PF. Modified lipoabdominoplasty: updating concepts. Plast Reconstr Surg. 2016;138:38e–47e.

Saldanha OR. Lipoabdominoplasty with selective and safe undermining. Aesthetic Plast Surg. 2003;27:322–327.

Avelar JM. Abdominoplasty: technical refinement and analysis of 130 cases in 8 years' follow-up. *Aesthetic Plast Surg*. 1983;7(4):205–212

Callia W. Contribuição para o estudo da correção cirúrgico do abdome pêndulo e globoso—Técnica original [dissertation]. Faculty of the Medical University of São Paulo, 1965.

Illouz YG. Une nouvelle technique pour lês lipodystrophies localisées. Rev Chir Esth Franc 1980; April: 6

Hakme F. Technical details in the liposuction associated with abdominoplasty. Rev Bras Cir 1985;75:331.

Avelar JM. Uma nova técnica de abdominoplastia—sistema vascular fechado de retalho subdérmico dobrado sobre si memo combinado com lipoaspiração. Ver Brás Cir 1999;13:3–20.

Wilkinson TS, Swartz BE. Individual modification in body contour surgery: the limited abdominoplasty. *Plast Reconstr Surg* 1986;779–784.

Chapter 11
MILA-Minimally Invasive Robotic and Endoscopic Lipo-Abdominoplasty

Marco Aurelio Faria-Correa

Abstract The author presents his insights concerning mini-abdominoplasty technique, introduces new concepts and reports his more than 30 years' experience in treating the functional and cosmetic deformities of the abdominal wall by using minimal incisions open methods and minimally invasive methods to treat rectus diastasis and lipodystrophy in patients without redundant skin. In 1989, he realized that:

- The rectus plication should not be limited to the lower abdomen but in its extension at all from the pubic bone to the xiphoid process.
- No skin resection when there was no flabbiness or redundant skin.
- Perform the entire procedure through the pre-existent scars, without adding longer scars.

In 1991, the author started research project adapting endoscopic methods to the subcutaneous territory and started doing endoscopic gasless subcutaneous rectus plication-endoscopic abdominoplasty to treat patients with no redundant skin and no previous scar. With approximately 300 cases done from 1991 to 2016, observing optimal functional and cosmetic results, in patients with more than 20 years' follow-up, it proved the efficacy and longevity of the endoscopic abdominoplasty method, giving to the author the enthusiasm for bringing the technique to the next level by introducing in plastic surgery the new emerging technology of robotic surgery, incorporating robotic da Vinci Surgical System in his practice to perform muscle-aponeurotic rectus plication-robotic abdominoplasty.

M. A. Faria-Correa (✉)
Singapore, Singapore
e-mail: drmarco@drmarco.com

J. M. Avelar, R. Cavalcanti Ribeiro (eds.), *Body Contouring*,
https://doi.org/10.1007/978-3-031-42802-9_11

Keywords Robotic plastic surgery · Robotic rectus plication · Robotic abdominoplasty · Rectus diastasis · Endoscopic rectus plication · Endoscopic abdominoplasty · Muscle-aponeurotic plication · Abdominal wall · Minimally invasive subcutaneous surgery · Subcutaneouscopic surgery

Introduction

We are seeing an increasing number of female and male patients presenting with small- and medium-sized abdominal deformities coming to our clinics asking for minimally invasive and scarless procedures that can effectively improve their core muscle and the aesthetic appearance of the abdomen (Faria Correa 2023). In many cases, the problem is not the cosmetic aspect of the skin, nor striae, nor the redundant folds of the skin, nor overweight nor abdominal lipodystrophy, but rectus diastasis (Figs. 11.1, 11.2, 11.3, 11.4, 11.5, 11.6, 11.7, 11.8, 11.9, 11.10 and 11.11). They complain that despite working hard at losing weight and having a strict and rigorous workout regime, they cannot get rid of that bulging stomach and/or the peri-umbilical deformity (sad belly button). The weakening of the muscle-aponeurotic abdominal wall due to congenital conditions, weight variation, ageing or pregnancy is a

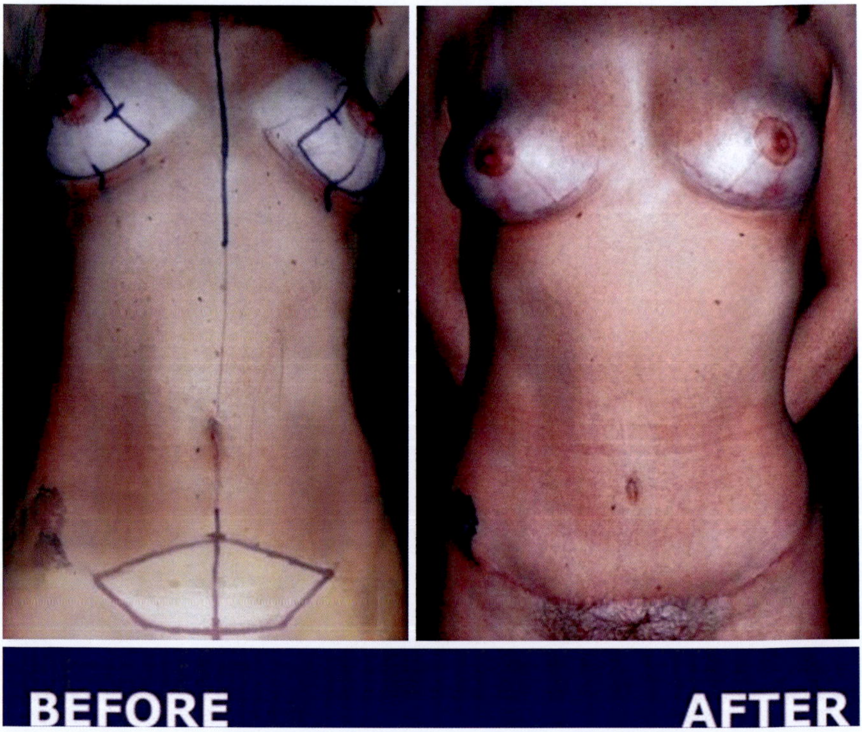

Fig. 11.1 Mini-abdominoplasty with mini-dermolipectomy done in 1986 caused an anatomical deformity by lowering the umbilicus position

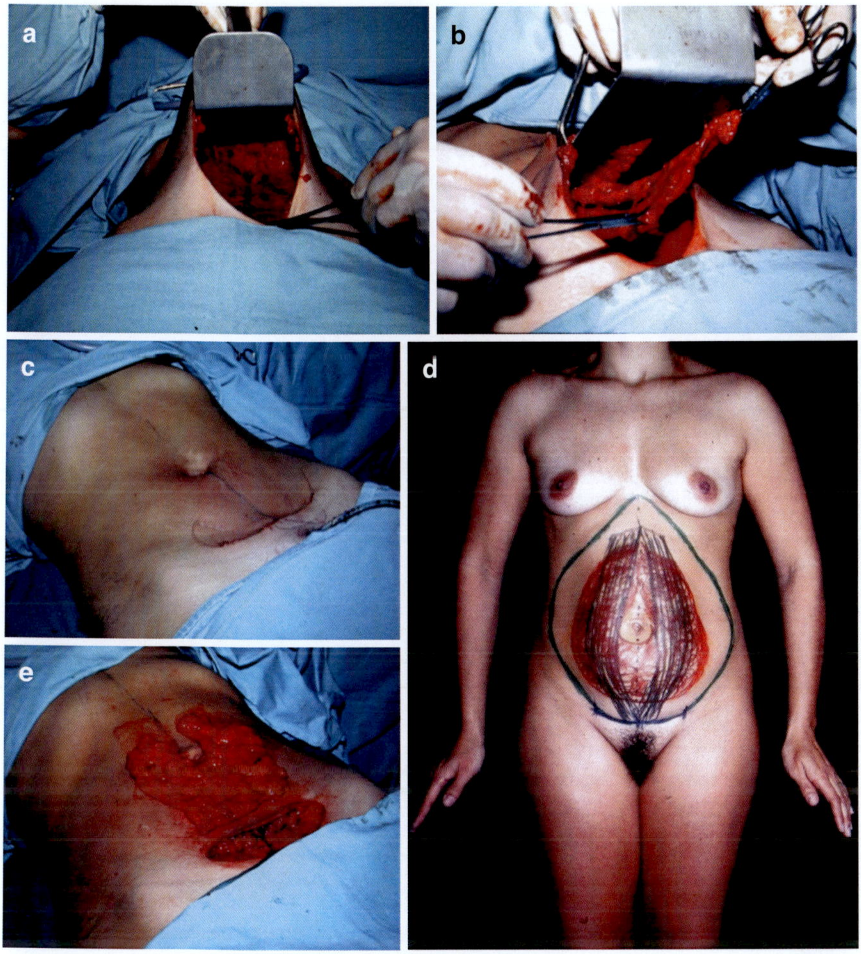

Fig. 11.2 Minimal scar abdominoplasty: xiphoid-pubic rectus plication, lipectomy, and no skin removal performing the whole procedure using the previous "C-section scar" with the aid of light source retractors. (**a**) Xiphoid-pubic rectus plication done. (**b**) Lipectomy being performed. (**c**) Closure of the previous C-section with no skin resection. (**d**) Pre-operative drawing/planning. (**e**) Adipose fat tissue excised and placed on top of the skin for demonstration

frequent cause of rectus diastasis and/or umbilical hernia that can alter the cosmetic aspect of the abdomen (Faria-Correa 2016; Nahas and Ferreira 2010). The rectus abdominal muscle plays an important role, not only in the cosmetic appearance of the abdomen but also in the stability of the spine. Depending on the degree of the rectus diastasis, it can lead to a vicious posture, spine problems, back pain, slipped disc, etc. Rectus plication can effectively restore function providing a balance between the anterior and posterior muscle of the abdominal wall and improve the cosmetic appearance of the abdomen (Faria-Correa 2016; Nahas et al. 2001). The long-term evaluation by ultrasonography and CT scan of the plication of the anterior rectus sheath (Nahas et al. 2004, 2011) as well as our long-term clinic follow-up (Fig. 11.6) as shown, the efficiency of the recti plication when properly performed.

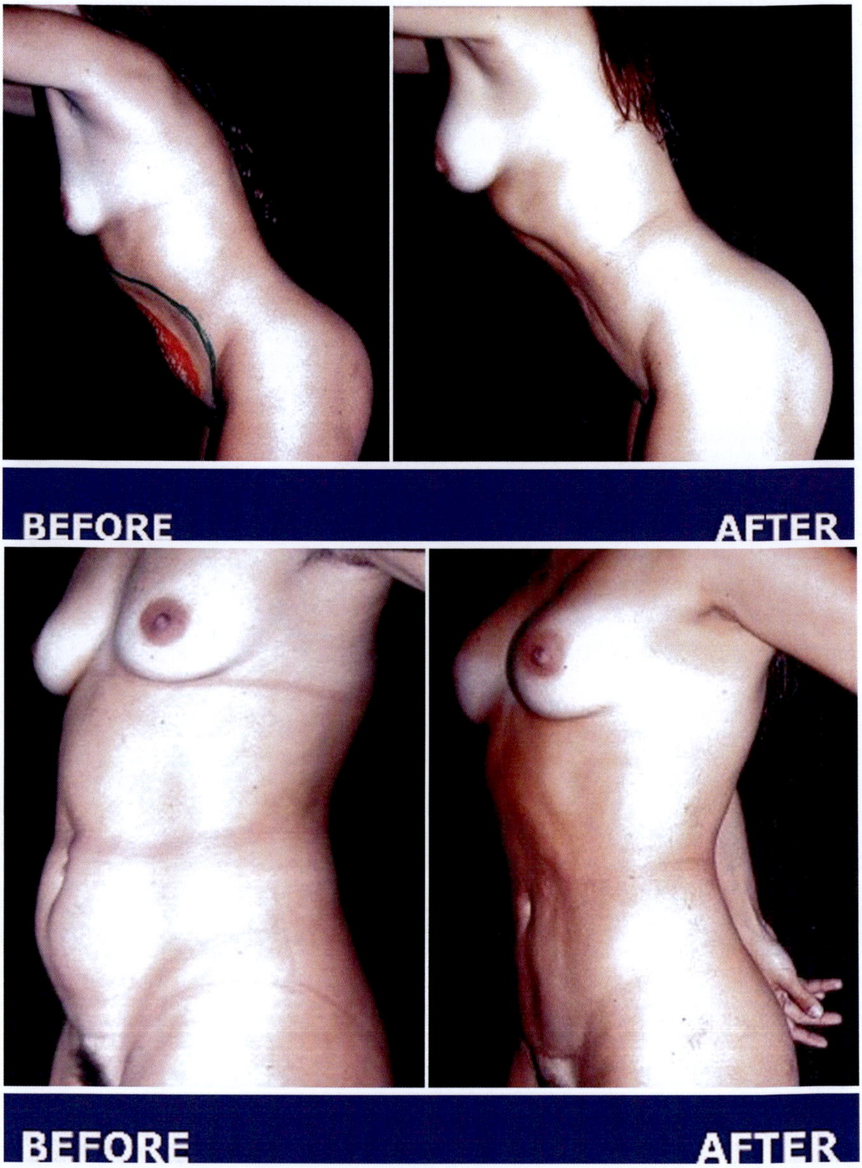

Fig. 11.3 Before and after minimal incision abdominoplasty

Evolution of the Thought

By analysing the results of mini-abdominoplasty in the treatment of small- and medium-sized abdominal deformities, I have drawn the following conclusions:

- Plication of the lower abdominal rectus may cause a protrusion of the upper abdomen; therefore, rectus plication from the pubis to the xiphoid process is required.

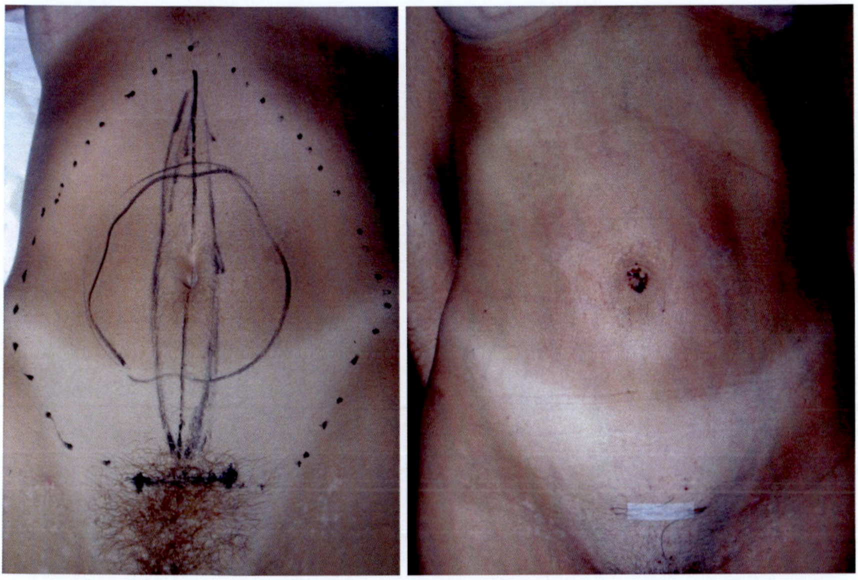

Fig. 11.4 Endoscopic abdominoplasty scars hidden inside the navel/umbilical area and inside the pubic hair-bearing area

- Small skin resections in the lower abdomen will not help in the flabbiness of the abdomen and may cause dog ears and/or long scars, so I recommend no skin resection and working through the smaller incision possible in patients presenting with good skin elasticity.
- The reposition of the umbilical scar below its original position may cause a distortion of the patient original anatomy, an unnatural and weird appearance, so I recommend reinserting it in its original site.

Evolution of the Method: *From the Light Source Retractors to Endoscopic and to Robotic Methods*

In 1989, I started performing mini-abdominoplasty without removing any skin, just using the previous C-section scar, with the aid of light source retractors freeing the umbilical scar, performing a xiphoid-pubic rectus plication and lipectomy and reinserting the umbilical scar in its original site (Figs. 11.2 and 11.3).

Minimal Scar Abdominoplasty Technique

The beautiful results achieved by effectively treating the cosmetics and functional deformities through minimal incisions, without adding new scars, but just by using the previous scars and even improving it, gave me the enthusiasm.

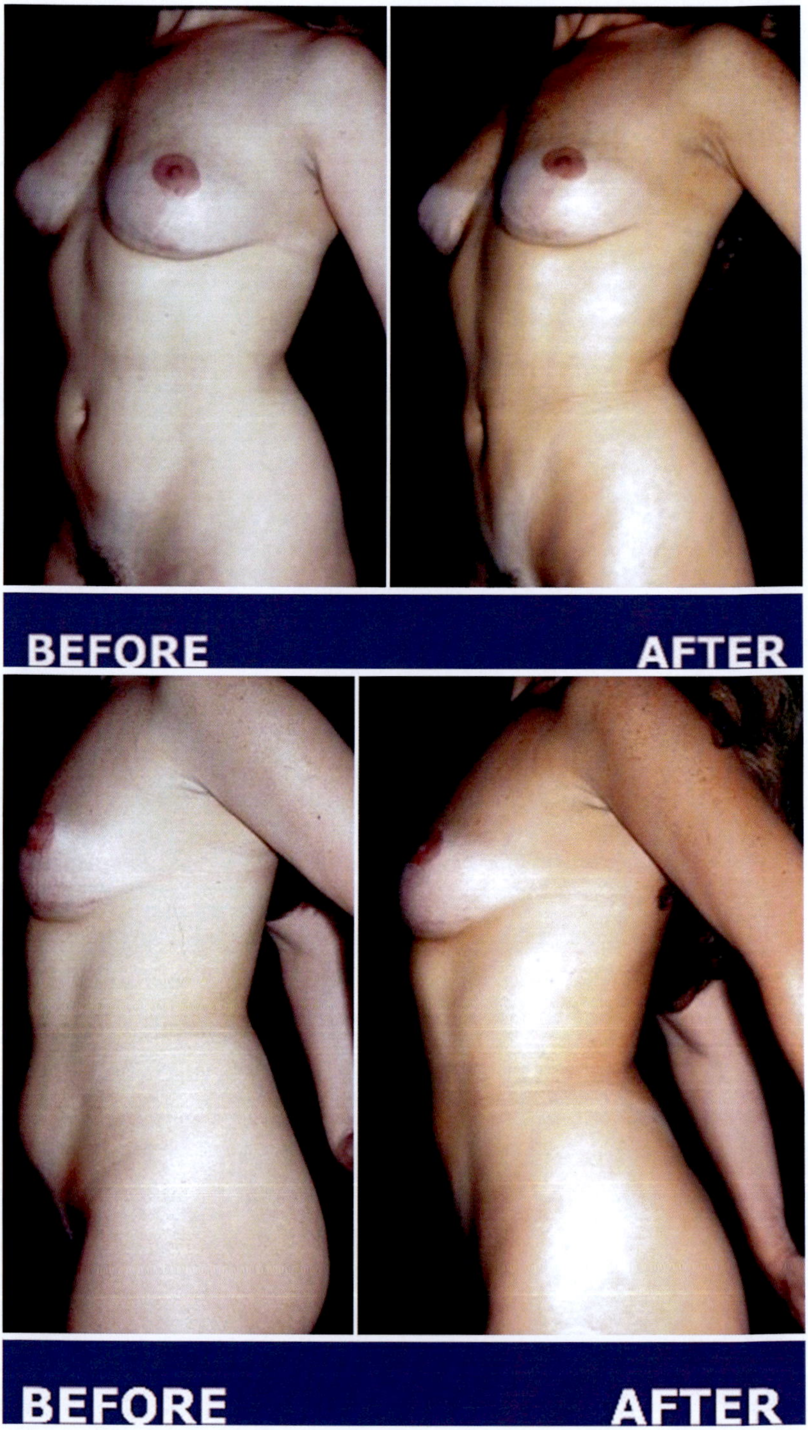

Fig. 11.5 Before and after endoscopic abdominoplasty

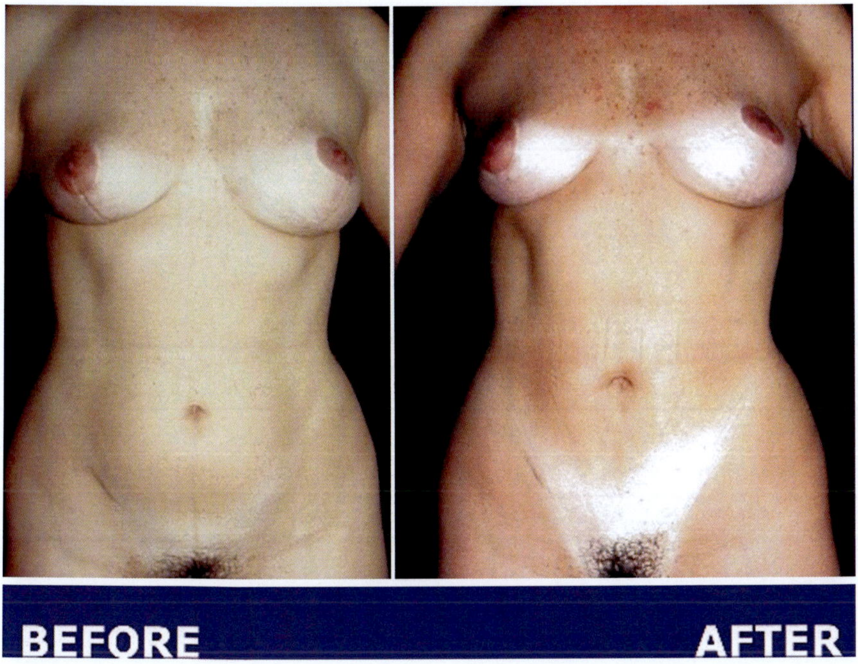

Fig. 11.5 (continued)

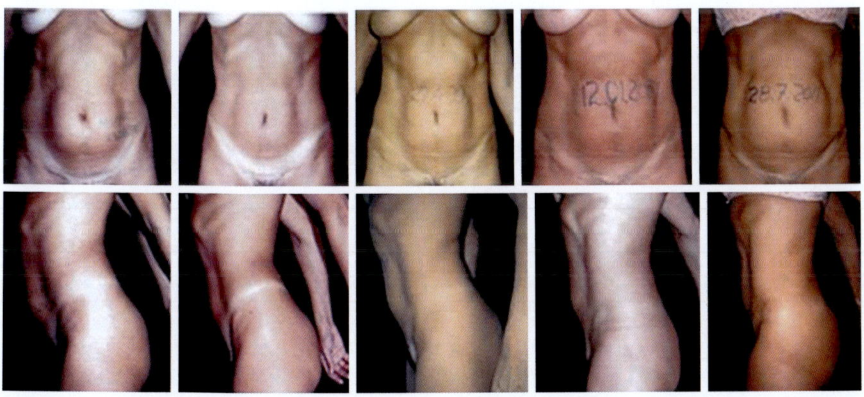

Fig. 11.6 Endoscopic abdominoplasty 20 years' follow-up showing the maintenance of the result of the rectus plication even after patient aging 20 years and put on 8 kg

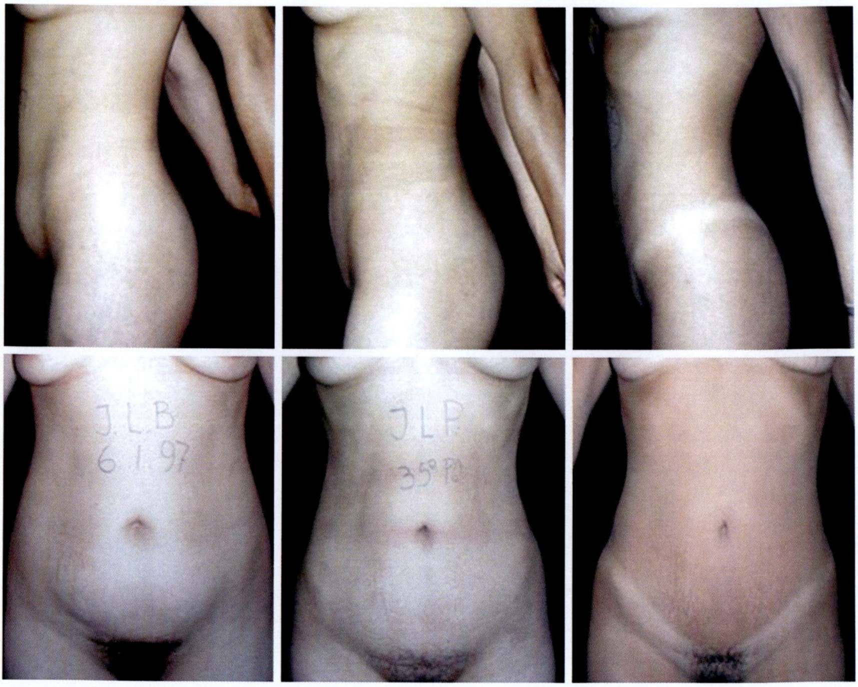

Fig. 11.7 Long-term follow-up of endoscopic abdominoplasty after 35 days showing a very fast recovery with minimal swelling. After 2 years, showing maintenance of the result of the rectus plication and fat plication

In 1991 came to me one patient without previous "C-section" asking me if I could treat her using a very small scar hidden inside her pubic hair-bearing area. Attentive to the emerging video-endoscopic method, that was so promising, allowing the surgeons working through very minimal incisions, I had the idea of using endoscopic methods in plastic surgery (Faria-Correa 1992a, 1994, 1995, 2008).

Then, at the University Hospital PUC Porto Alegre, I started a research project to adapt endoscopic methods to the subcutaneous territory for treating patients presenting with rectus diastasis and no redundant skin, working through incisions as small as 4 cm hidden in the pubic hair-bearing area and inside the umbilical area (Faria-Correa 1992a, b, 1994, 1995, 2008) (Fig. 11.4). Those days there was a concept that we should not use pressured gas in the subcutaneous to develop the optical cavity, the working space, due to the risk of gas embolism when cutting perforator veins during the flap dissection and also the risk of gas dispersion causing the subcutaneous emphysema. For circumventing those risks, I developed a set of instruments for gasless undermining of the abdominal flap, tenting the flap and stitching the muscle (Faria-Correa 1994, 1995, 2008) (Fig. 11.12).

Attentive to the development of new instruments, machines and methods in surgery that can facilitate and improve our task and result and with more than 20 years of follow-up showing the effectiveness of the technique and the beauty of restoring

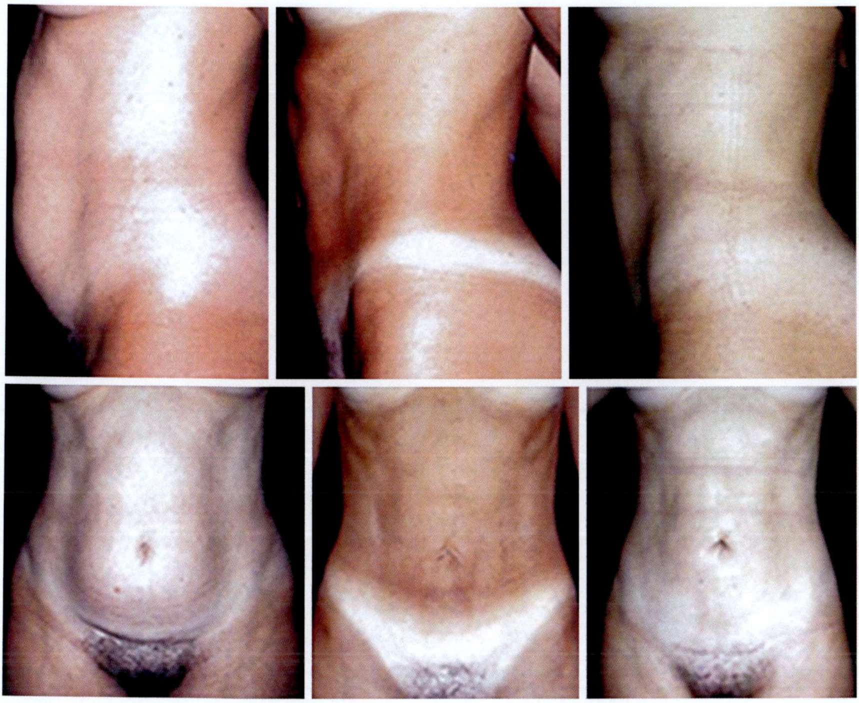

Fig. 11.8 The before photo showing patient had abdominal deformities after delivering twins and 8 kg overweight. 1-year follow-up after patient cut down 8 kg. After 5 years post-op, patient put back 5 kg. We observe the long-term maintenance of the result

the original anatomy leaving minimal and inconspicuous scars (Fig. 11.4), in 2013, I started studying and training robotic surgery with the enthusiasm of going for the next level, using the robotic da Vinci Surgery System to perform rectus plication in minimally invasive abdominoplasty (Faria-Correa 2016; Faria Correa 2023).

Robotic surgery is the "gold standard" of the minimally invasive surgery in many surgical fields. The robot high-definition three-dimensional view and the amplification of images give us a much better depth sensation of the surgical field than the 2D endoscopic view, and it is even better than our naked eyes. Laparoscopic instruments have a limited range of motion; the robot EndoWrist range of movements is comparable to the human wrist. The surgeon's hand tremor is transmitted through the rigid laparoscopic instrument, and this limitation makes delicate procedures more difficult (Lee et al. 2014; Morris 2005). The superb precision and stability of the robot arms, surgical field and instruments, all controlled by the surgeon seated at the console in a comfortable ergonomic position, without the need of coordinating camera and instrument movement with a surgical assistant, makes the surgery much easier, more precise and less stressful (Faria-Correa 2016).

In urology, robotic prostatectomy is such a solid application, presenting so many advantages over the open methods as well as over the endoscopic methods

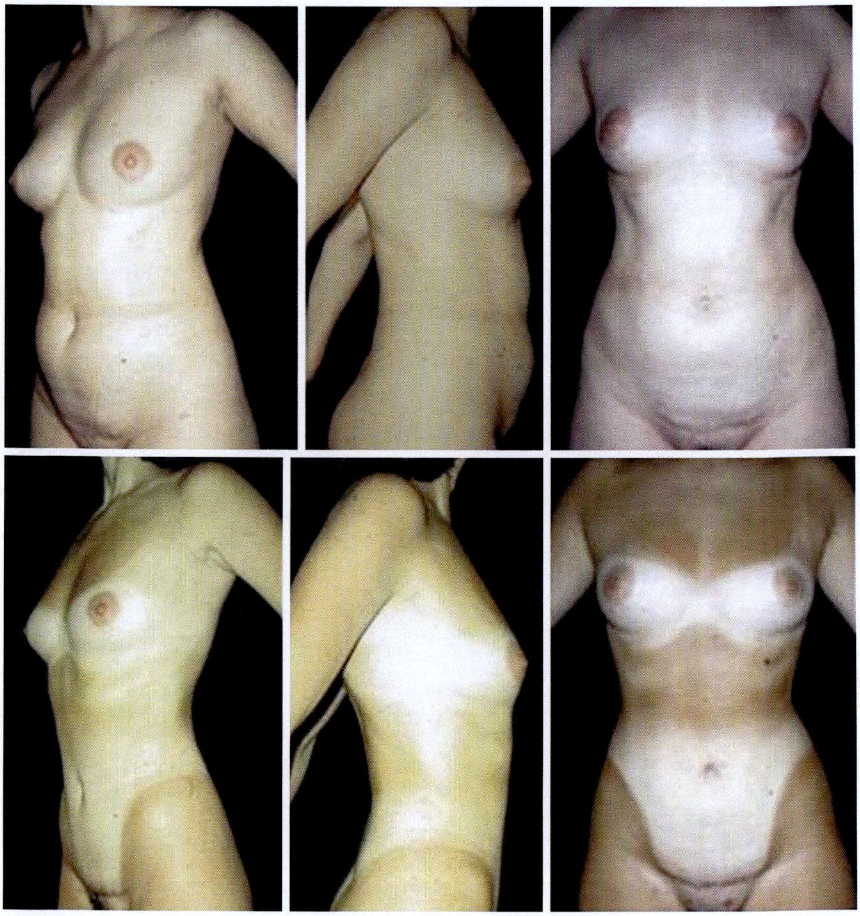

Fig. 11.9 Endoscopic abdominoplasty performed through C-section scar: before and after

(Lanfranco et al. 2004; Lee et al. 2014) that, if a patient has the chance to choose which methods to undergo, the best choice would be to go for robotics-assisted. In cardiothoracic surgery, the surgical robots are also proving to be the key in transforming technically challenging open procedures like mitral valve repair and heart revascularization into technically feasible, minimally invasive procedures. In any institution where robotics "da Vinci Surgical System" is available, the tendency for laparoscopic surgery (in gynaecology, colon-rectum surgery and general surgery) is being replaced by robotics-assisted surgery due to the many advantages that robotics-assisted surgery presents over laparoscopic method (Faria-Correa 2016).

In many surgical fields, robot is becoming a promising technology.

In reconstructive plastic surgery, it has already been used for the harvesting of latissimus dorsi in breast reconstruction, super microsurgery, hand surgery (Faria-Correa 2016; Selber 2009; Selber et al. 2012) and hair transplant.

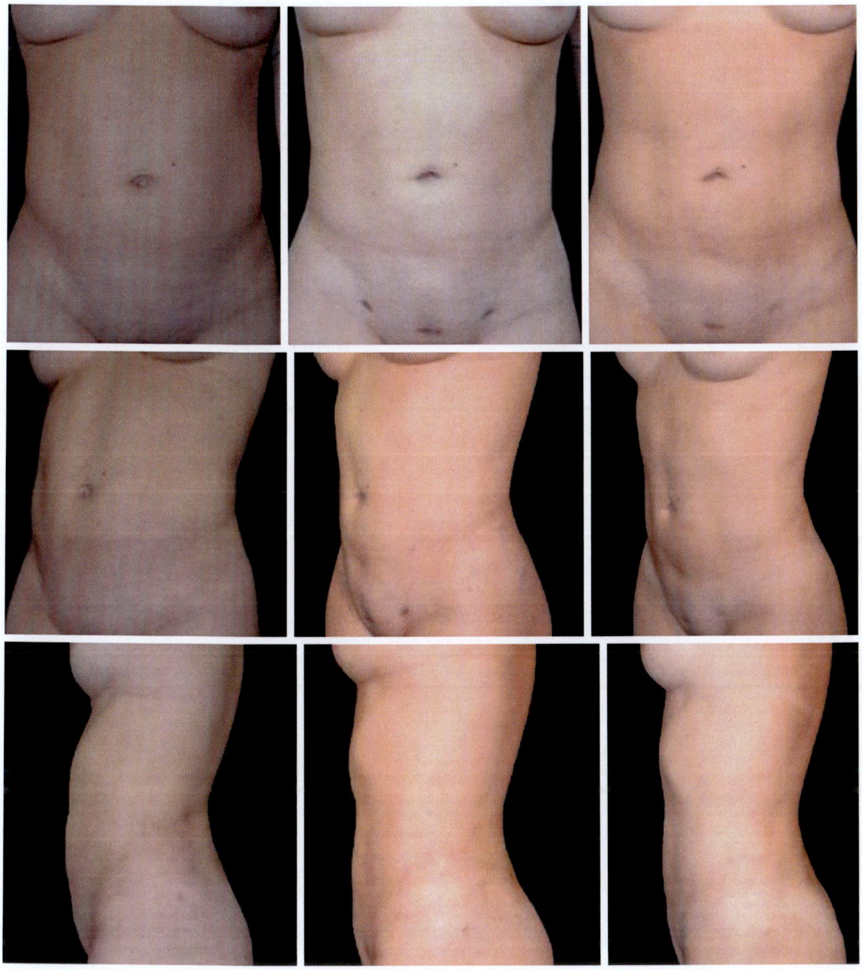

Fig. 11.10 Robotic abdominoplasty: before and after 3 months and 1 year. A 42-year-old very fit patient that after three pregnancies started to suffer from a moderate to severe degree of rectus diastasis that was causing her back pain and urinary issues (urgency to pass urine and leaking urine when coughing and practising sports). Patient refers tremendous improvement in her spine and urinary issues after repairing rectus diastasis. We can observe in the **frontal view** the *rd* all along the whole abdomen *before* and the improvement *after*. In the **profile view**, we observe an acute angulation of her spine and a bulging projection of her abdomen on the *before* view and a nice improvement *after*; in the **semi-profile** view, we can observe a global improvement of the function of her core muscles

So far I didn't find in the literature any report of other applications of robotics in aesthetic plastic surgery (Faria-Correa 2016).

As a cosmetic plastic surgeon, I feel it is very interesting that there is a fast-growing trend for the use of robot for performing trans-axillary robotic thyroidectomy and robot retro-auricular submandibular gland resection (Lee and Chung

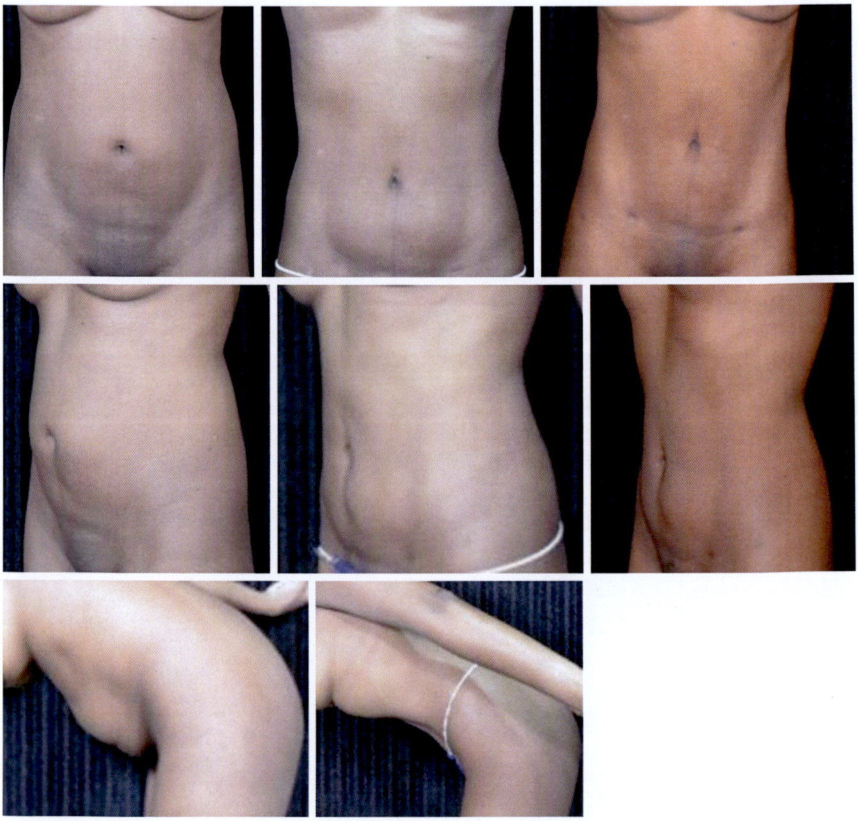

Fig. 11.11 Robotic abdominoplasty: BEFORE, AFTER 5 months, and AFTER 1 year. We can observe important improvement in her posture, a new definition of her core muscle, and in the hanging abdomen BEFORE and the new capacity of holding her abdominal viscera AFTER

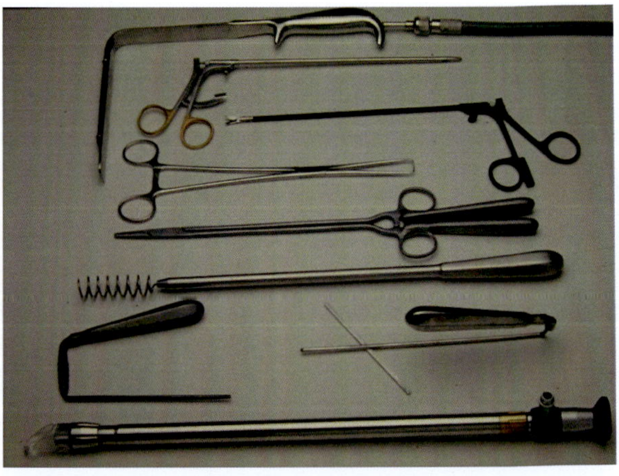

Fig. 11.12 Set of instruments developed by the author

2014; Mattei et al. 2014), procedures that are improved or tweaked to minimize visible scars or even relocate scars to other body areas that could be hidden. Yet little is done in the area of aesthetic plastic surgery, where scarring is of an important concern for patients (Faria-Correa 2016).

After completing my training and certification as a robotic surgeon, I designed retractors to perform a gasless muscle-aponeurotic rectus plication in the same fashion as I do endoscopic abdominoplasty. I performed my first case in April 2015, and since then up to now, 31 cases are done with no complication and very satisfactory results.

Surgical Robots: The equipment that I am using is the da Vinci Surgical System SI and XI. It consists of three components: the console where the surgeon sits to operate the robotic arms, the patient site robotic cart with three or four arms and the high-definition 3D vision system.

It is the surgeon that operates. The robot system does not have autonomy to do anything by its own, and every single movement is operated and controlled by the surgeon. Sitting at the console and using the joysticks, the surgeon drives the robot arms and EndoWrist instrument operating very precise miniaturized tools tools (Fig. 11.15). With the feet, the surgeon controls the camera, zoom-in zoom-out, monopolar and bipolar cut and cauterization, as well as switching use of the second and the third robot-working arms, without the need of coordinating the movements with an assistant (Faria-Correa 2016).

Surgical Technique

I use two different methods, the CO_2 method and the gasless method. In this chapter, I will describe the gasless method that is the direct evolution of the minimal scar abdominoplasty. It is the method that I recommend for the beginners.

Anaesthesia: For endoscopic abdominoplasty, epidural anaesthesia or general anaesthesia, and, for robotic abdominoplasty, general anaesthesia are my preference because after docking in the robotic arms, the patient should stay still, in a state where she could move as a reaction to pain or other stimuli. There is a so-called remote centre in the trocar that must stay in place to avoid tearing the skin. All the movements of the robot arms are around a fixed rotating point.

Infiltration: 500 mL of saline solution and 1 mL of epinephrine (1:500,000) is infiltrated at the area to be undermined in between the fat tissue and the muscular aponeurosis to facilitate dissection and reduce bleeding as well as in the incision sites.

Incisions: If the patient presents with previous scars from Caesarean sections or other abdominal surgery (Figs. 11.6, 11.7, 11.8 and 11.9), the surgeon assesses the need to repair the scars as well as the possibility of using them for access (Fig. 11.13) (Faria-Correa 1995, 2008).

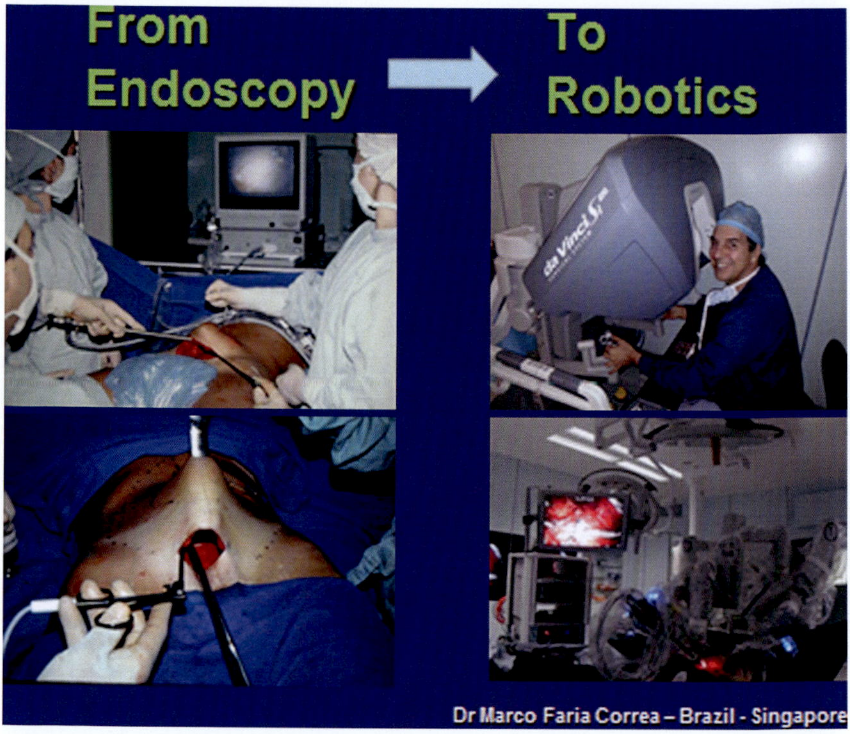

Fig. 11.13 Left-side endoscopic abdominoplasty: the patient and surgical team position with the video monitor and incisions. Right side showing doctor sitting at the console and operating the robotic arms

In endoscopic abdominoplasty technique, if there is no previous C-section scar, a 4 cm incision is made at the pubic hair-bearing area and another one inside the umbilical scar (Fig. 11.14).

In robotic abdominoplasty, I use two incisions of 0.7 cm at the bikini line 20 cm far from each other to avoid instrumental collision, one incision for the camera arm at the midline of the patient's abdomen, inside the pubic hair-bearing area at the pubic bone level, 3 cm above the vaginal furcula, measuring to 2 cm, and one "Y"-shaped incision made within the umbilical scar (Figs. 11.15 and 11.16). The umbilical port is used for the introduction of retractors for tenting the abdominal flap, for supplying sutures and gauze into the operative field and for the surgical assistant helping with laparoscopic instruments if necessary. Liposuction can be done using the same three incisions in cases of lipoabdominoplasty (Fig. 11.15).

The skin of the umbilical scar is detached from its stalk. If there is an umbilical or para-umbilical hernia to be repaired, I do it before proceeding for the rectus plication. The umbilical stalk is then transfixed using a 3-0 mono-nylon suture. The reinsertion of the umbilicus skin flaps is done after finishing the rectus plication, at its original site, deep inside the plication (Faria-Correa 2008). If there is redundant skin

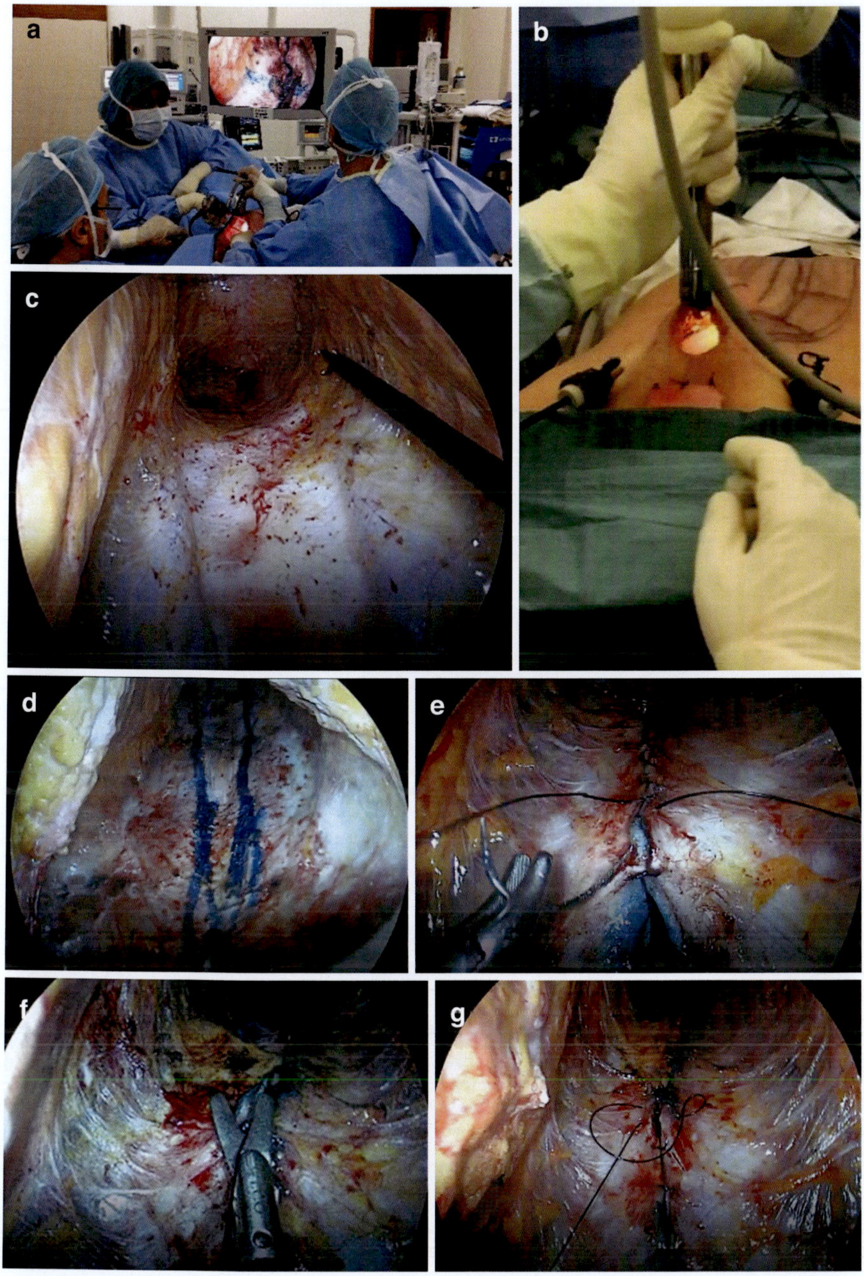

Fig. 11.14 Endoscopic abdominoplasty: (**a**) team positioning; (**b**) suprapubic incision; (**c**) dissection and identification of the rectus diastasis; (**d**) rectus abdominal muscle inner border demarcation; (**e**) first layer of plication using interrupted stitches; (**f**) cutting thread after stitching; (**g**) second layer of stitching, running suture using mono-nylon 2-0; (**h**) resulting scar hidden inside the pubic hair-bearing area

Fig. 11.14 (continued)

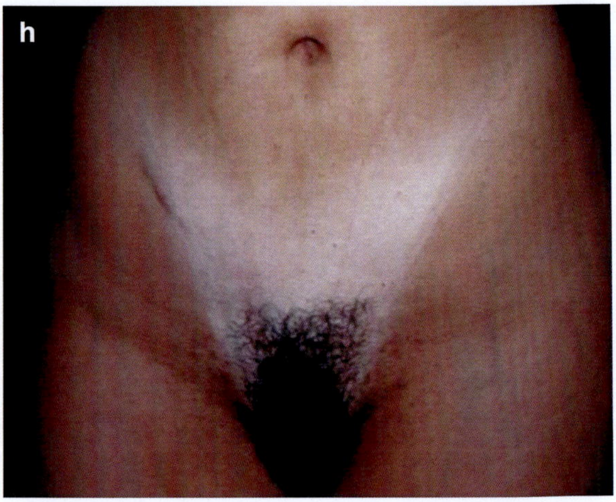

at the navel, a Y-shaped incision is made generating three or four triangular flaps (Faria-Correa 1995, 2008), and the closure of it will leave inconspicuous converging scars, following Avelar's original idea (Avelar 1976). By resecting part of these triangular flaps, we treat the redundant skin (Fig. 11.16) (Faria-Correa 1995, 2008, 2016).

Dissection and Elevation of the Abdominal Flap

In the gasless method, the undermining starts from the umbilicus progressing downwards through the midline towards the pubis and from the pubic incision upwards, or vice versa, to meet each other. The procedure begins with the use of traditional methods with conventional instruments as far as our eyes, fingers and instruments allow us to work safely and comfortably. With the aid of a 4 or 7 mm 30-degree endoscope, retractors and the "subcutaneous tomoscope" (Faria-Correa 2008) or electrocautery, we progress dissecting a tunnel from the pubic bone to the xiphoid process (Fig. 11.14), up to the outer borders of the rectus abdominal muscles to create the optical cavity. The undermining can be done endoscopically or with the aid of the robot system. If further undermining is necessary for a proper redistribution of the abdominal flap, we do a blunt dissection, creating tunnels, preserving vessels and nerves. Tunnelling preserves the sensitive innervation of the abdominal wall and provides faster recovery with earlier reduction of the oedema (Faria-Correa 2008) (Fig. 11.7). If there is any area that requires liposuction, the liposuction will be performed after the rectus plication. We aspirate only the deep surface of the derma-adipose flap. In the undermined areas, we use the cannula with the holes facing up. In the non-undermined areas, we use the cannula with the holes facing down in the traditional way, liposuction of the deep fat tissue area, creating tunnels preserving vessels creating a closed vascular system like described by Avelar (1999).

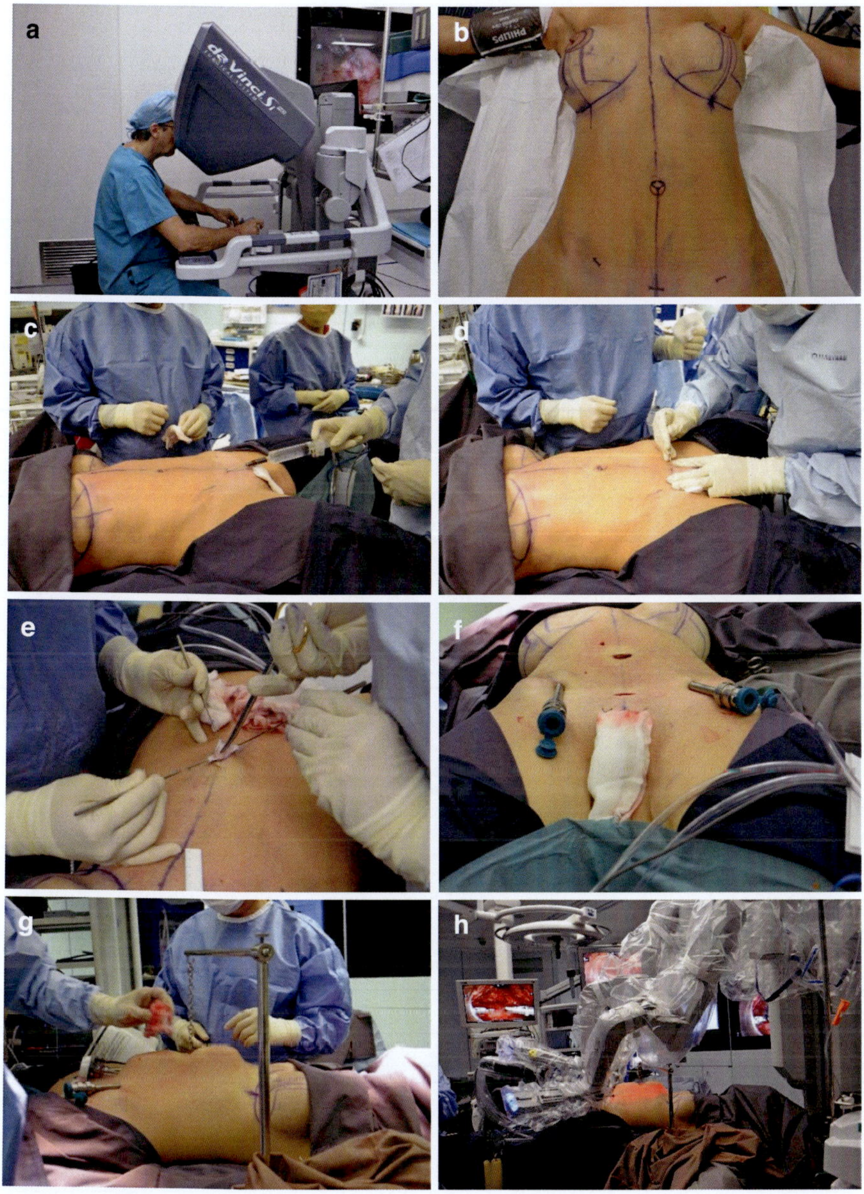

Fig. 11.15 Robotic abdominoplasty: (**a**) surgeon sitting at the console performing the rectus plication; (**b**) drawing the incisions; (**c**) infiltration of saline solution 1:500,000 adrenaline; (**d**) suprapubic incisions 0.7, 1.8, and 0.7 cm; (**e**) Y-shaped incision at the umbilicus; (**e**) Faria-Correa retractor tenting the flap to maintain the optical cavity in a gasless fashion; (**h**) robot arms positioned and the surgeon performing the rectus plication (**a**)

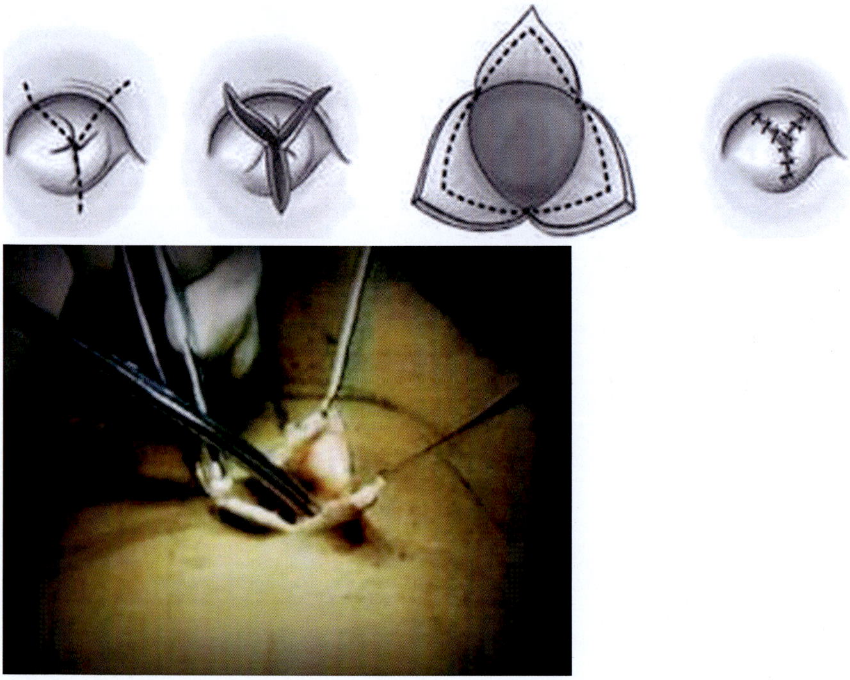

Fig. 11.16 The surgical sequence of umbilicoplasty technique is as follows: (1) Intraumbilical Y-shaped incision, (2) Three triangular flaps and a wide entrance port, (3) Partial resection of these flaps to treat flabbiness, (4) Closure leaving inconspicuous converging scars

Recti Plication

We identify the rectus diastasis (Figs. 11.14 and 11.17), and with a small cotton bud tinted with methylene blue, we demarcate the inner border of the rectus abdominal muscle aponeurosis to be plicated. Plication of the anterior rectus sheath is performed in two layers, the first layer using 2-0 or 3-0 nylon buried stiches 1.0 cm distant from each other and the second layer of two continuous sutures using V-Loc 00 nylon: one starting from the xiphoid process running till just above the umbilical stalk and another continuous running suture starting from just below the umbilical stalk to the pubic bone.

Supra-umbilical or peri-umbilical flabbiness is a frequent finding (Fig. 11.18). This deformity occurs during pregnancy when the abdominal muscles stretch and the subcutaneous fatty tissue attached to them is pulled away, creating a gap with skin flabbiness in the region. This subcutaneous fat gap is repaired by suturing the two edges of the fat tissue together with 4-0 Monocryl interrupted sutures. A small hole is left between the edges to permit these small triangular umbilical skin flaps to pass through it for the reinsertion into the umbilical stalk, which was previously secured by the spare suture mentioned earlier (Faria-Correa 2008).

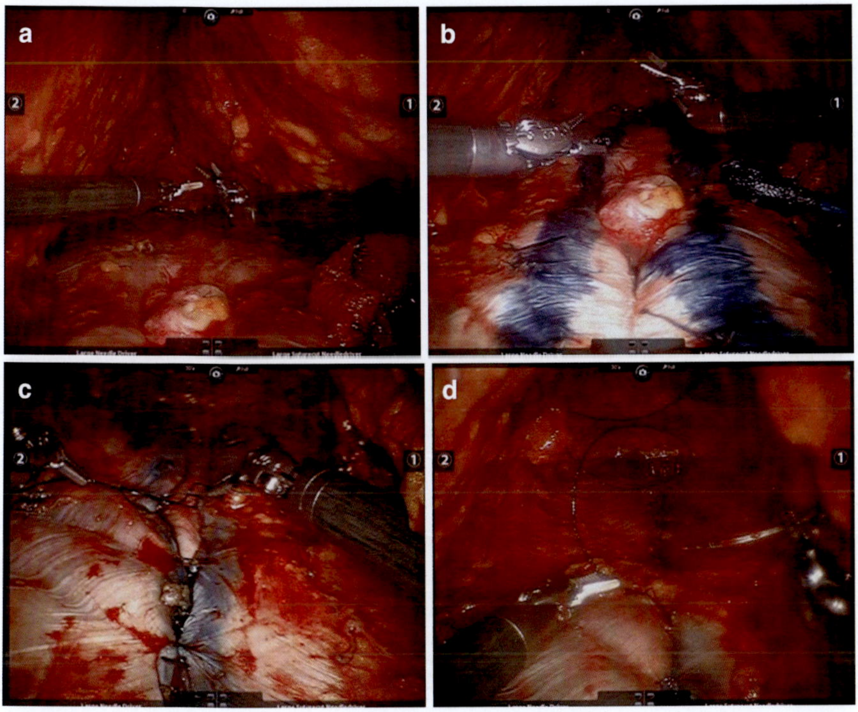

Fig. 11.17 Robot rectus aponeurotic plication. Surgeon's HD 3D view in the console. (**a**) Identify the rectus diastasis, (**b**) drawing the inner border of the rectus abdominis using a small cotton bud, (**c**) plication starts using 2-0 nylon interruptive stiches 1 cm distant from each other, (**d**) a second layer of plication by using a 2-0 V-Loc nylon running suture

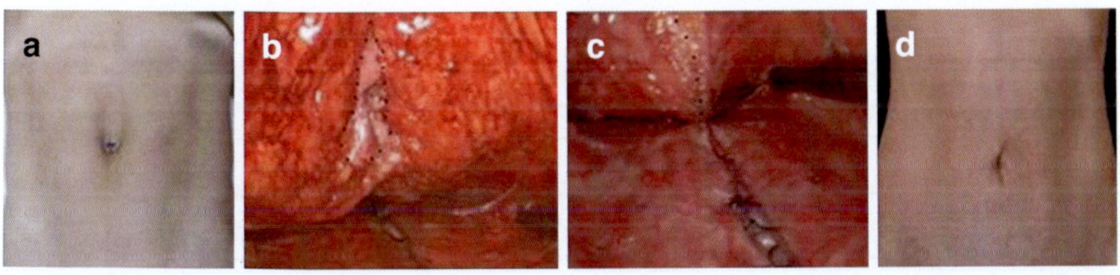

Fig. 11.18 (**a**) Pre-op showing the rectus and peri-umbilical fat diastasis, (**b**) intra-operative view of the repaired rectus diastasis and the mark of the edges of the subcutaneous fat gap to be repaired, (**c**) intra-op view of the rectus diastasis repaired and subcutaneous fat gap repaired, (**d**) immediate post-operation result

Results

I have done approximately 20 cases of minimal incision abdominoplasty from 1989 to 1992, approximately 300 cases of endoscopic abdominoplasty from 1992 to 2015, another 280 cases of endoscopic-assisted abdominoplasty and endoscopic abdominoplasty from 2015 till now (using both the CO_2 and the gasless methods) and 31 cases of robotic abdominoplasty from 2015 till now. I have many robotic abdominoplasty patients with up to 5 years of long-term follow-up (Figs. 11.10 and 11.11) and endoscopic abdominoplasty cases with up to 5- and 20-year follow-up (Figs. 11.6, 11.7 and 11.8). We can observe an important cosmetic improvement, a much flatter abdomen, an improvement in the posture and a natural reconstitution of the patient's original anatomy leaving minimal scars, and most of the patients inform an important improvement in quality of life by reducing their suffering of back pain and pelvic floor dysfunction.

The rectus plication has been shown to be effective and long-lasting in most of the cases when the plication method was done using two layers of stitching, the first layer interruptive stitches with nylon 00 and the second layer running stitches. It failed in a few patients that didn't respect the proper downtime and started exercises before 6 months.

I converted the minimally invasive abdominoplasty into a full abdominoplasty in about 20 cases. Some patients initially preferred to keep some degree of flabbiness or redundant skin rather than opting for a long scar from skin removal. However, as they gained weight and experienced increased flabbiness due to aging, they eventually requested skin removal.

Overall the results are very satisfactory when it is done in the right patients with no redundant skin and with realistic expectation and that don't want scars.

Complications

The complications in minimally invasive abdominoplasty, both endoscopic and robotic methods, are the same—seroma (Fig. 11.19) and haematoma. So far, in a total number of more than 600 cases in more than 32-year experience, I never had one case of infection and no skin necrosis, but I had some cases of skin surface irregularities due to the liposuction and cases of rectus diastasis failure because the patients started physical activities too early and are not following the recommendation of 6 months of no sports but only core muscle re-education exercises. We manage to reduce the incidence of seroma by reducing as much as possible the undermining area, creating a closed vascular system (Avelar 1999) and stitching the dermo-adipose flap to the muscle fascia, and suction drainage would have to be maintained minimal for 2 or 3 days or until the drainage over 24 h is less than 30 cc (Faria-Correa 1995, 2008).

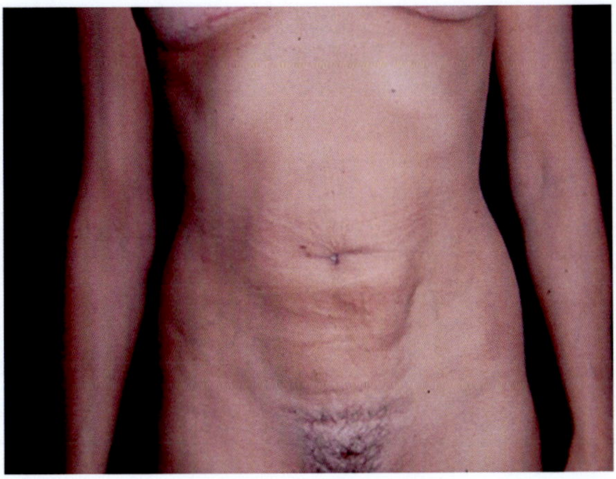

Fig. 11.19 Seroma

Discussion

A proper understanding of the patient concern, a correct diagnosis of the issues involved and a clear discussion with the patient about the surgical plan and the outcomes are paramount.

Treating patients with over-redundant folds of skin, flabbiness and skin damaged by striae is an easy task. We have no doubt in what to do. Our patients will be very happy to get a long scar to remove that ugly and redundant skin and get a new body contouring.

But the situation is not the same when it comes to the treatment of small- and medium-sized abdominal wall deformities. They ask for scarless minimally invasive procedures that can restore their original anatomy.

Post-gestational deformities are most of the time associated with rectus diastasis, the stretching of the linea alba, that causes a protrusion in the abdominal wall affecting the function of the core muscle, leading to medical and cosmetic issues. Rectus diastasis, most of the time, is not limited to the lower abdomen but extends towards the whole abdomen; that is why rectus plication from the pubis to the xiphoid is required for a proper functional and cosmetic result.

Many times, the skin is not the patient's concern. If the skin still presents with good elasticity with the capacity to retract and also presents with a nice cosmetic aspect, cutting a fuse of the skin in the lower abdomen will not help in treating small degree of flabbiness, but this will just create unnecessary scars and sometimes cause a lowering of the umbilicus positioning, distorting the patient's original anatomy, in nothing contributing to the beauty of the result.

Liposuction alone will not be enough if there is a rectus diastasis. Liposuction can be associated with rectus diastasis in very selected cases of real abdominal lipodystrophy.

Pregnancies can cause an imbalance of the core muscle. After repairing, reconstructing the linea alba, a physiotherapy work may be helpful to achieve the optimal result. We recommend a postural re-education with specialized physiotherapist to reinforce the core muscle, a proper wealthy lifestyle, maintaining the right weight.

Minimally invasive surgery presents many advantages compared to open methods like fast recovery, less pain, lower risk of infection and minimal scars that are our goals in cosmetic surgery. Plastic surgeons are not well trained in minimally invasive methods, and it will demand a lot of time, cost and dedication to develop skills in endoscopic surgery and robotic surgery. Robotic surgery also adds a cost for the patient, which makes it prohibitive for some patients to afford. In robotic surgery, an initial limitation is the loss of haptic feedback (force and tactile). Conventional endoscopy presents with a 2D image view, whereas the da Vinci system presents with a high-definition precise 3D image that compensates the loss of haptic feedback (Faria-Correa 2016).

But, even if minimally invasive methods present advantages over open methods, what I consider more important in this technique is *the new concept in mini-abdominoplasty*: do not remove skin; plication to be performed using non-absorbable stitches at least one layer of interruptive stitches and in the whole extension, from the pubis to the xiphoid; reinserting the umbilical scar in its original site; and liposuction when necessary. The use of minimally invasive technologies of endoscopic and robotic surgery is just a plus, to add the advantages of minimally invasive surgery and minimal scars (Figs. 11.4, 11.5, 11.10, 11.11 and 11.20).

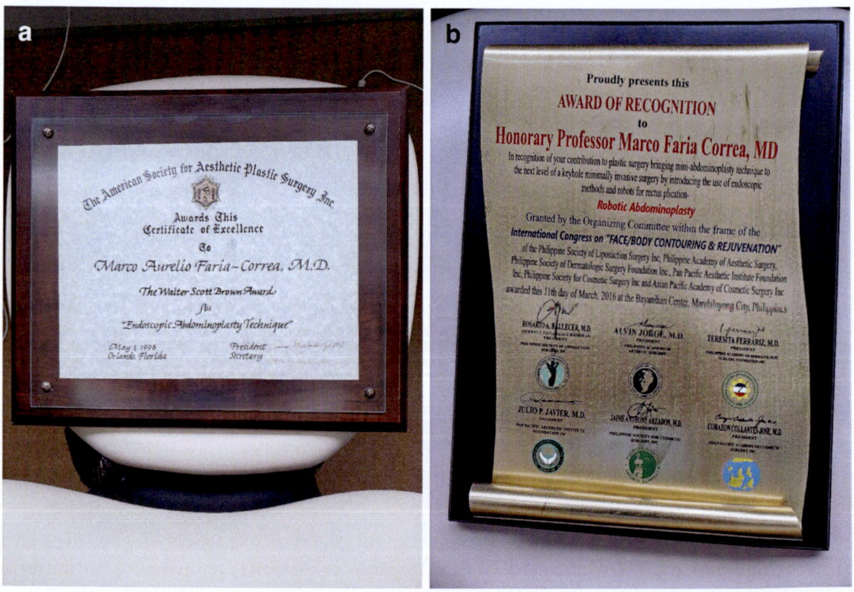
a
The American Society for Aesthetic Plastic Surgery Inc
Awards This
Certificate of Excellence
To
Marco Aurelio Faria-Correa, M.D.
The Walter Scott Brown Award
for
"Endoscopic Abdominoplasty Technique"
President
Secretary
b
Proudly presents this
AWARD OF RECOGNITION
to
Honorary Professor Marco Faria Correa, MD
Robotic Abdominoplasty
Granted by the Organizing Committee within the frame of the
International Congress on "FACE/BODY CONTOURING & REJUVENATION"

Fig. 11.20 (**a**)Award by "The American Society for Aesthetic Plastic Surgery Inc." in 1996 "Endoscopic Abdominoplasty Technique". (**b**) **Award of Recognition** in 2016 during the *International Congress on "FACE/BODY COUNTOURING & REJUVENATION"*: ***In recognition of my contribution to plastic surgery bringing mini-abdominoplasty technique to the next level of a keyhole minimally invasive surgery by introducing the use of endoscopic methods and robots for rectus plication – ROBOTIC ABDOMINOPLASTY***

Conclusion

We are living a new era in plastic surgery. We have learned a lot about the skin elasticity and capacity to retract. New technologies to help the skin to retract are available. Rectus diastasis so far still needs surgical treatment. Minimally invasive methods have shown many advantages over the conventional methods, and scars are one of the most important concerns in our cosmetic patients. Robotics in aesthetic plastic surgery is still at its infancy stage, but it is very promising considering its many advantages of minimally invasive surgery associated with high technology that helps us work through minimal scars with incisions at remote sites, leaving inconspicuous scars that are the hallmark of plastic surgery. Over the past 30 years, we are seeing an increasing number of female and male patients coming for the treatment of small- and medium-sized abdominal deformities. Many of them are presenting with rectus diastasis, with no redundant folds of the skin, with good skin elasticity and with or without abdominal lipodystrophy. They demand for scarless procedures that can effectively correct it. Liposuction alone will not be effective enough in many cases. The long-term evaluation of midline aponeurotic rectus plication, when properly performed, has proved its efficiency. Plastic surgeons are always looking for tools and instruments that can help us to better perform our procedures with more precision, efficacy, less trauma and faster recovery for our patients and leaving minimal scars. Since 1991, I started using endoscopic methods for the treatment of the described deformities. The efficacy of the method in patients with more than 20 years' follow-up gives me the enthusiasm of going for the next level. The "gold standard" of the minimal invasive video surgery is the use of robotic "da Vinci Surgery System" for the plication of the rectus diastasis. In many areas of application like urology, gynaecology, general surgery, neurosurgery and heart surgery, robot surgery has proved to have many advantages over conventional endoscopic methods due to the robot high-definition three-dimensional surgical view and amplification of images that makes it much more accurate than the 2D view provided by the conventional endoscopic methods, the superb precision and a much larger range of motion of the robot EndoWrist instruments that are comparable to the human wrist and the stability of the surgical field, camera and instruments, all controlled by the surgeon seated at the console in a comfortable position (Faria-Correa 2016). It is time to stop creating unnecessary scars and using minimally invasive methods in body contouring plastic surgery. It is time for robotics in plastic surgery.

References

Faria Correa M. Abstracts. Aesth Plast Surg 47 (Suppl 2), 251–562 (2023). https://doi.org/10.1007/s00266-023-03449-1

Avelar JM. Uma nova tecnica de abdominoplastia-sistema vascular fechado de retalho subdermico dobrado sobre si mesmo combinado com lipoaspiracao. Rev bras Cir, 1999; 88/89(1/6):3–20

Avelar JM. Umbilicoplastia-uma tecnica sem cicatriz externa. An do XIII Cong Bra de Cir Plast Porto Alegre, pp 81–82, 1976.

Faria-Correa MA. Abdominoplasty: the South America style. In Ramirez OM, Daniel RK, eds. Endoscopic Plastic Surgery. New York: Springer-Verlag, 1995.

Faria-Correa MA. Abdominoplastia videoendoscopica (subcutaneoscopica). In Atualizacao em Cirurgia Plastica Estetica e Reconstrutiva. Sao Paulo: Robe Editorial, 1994.

Faria-Correa MA Robotic Procedure for plication of the Muscle Aponeurotic Abdominal Wall. In New Concepts on Abdominoplasty and Further Applications. 11: 161–177 Springer 2016

Faria-Correa MA. Videoendoscopic abdominoplasty (subcutaneouscopy). Rev Soc Bras Cir Plast Est Reconstr 7:32–34, 1992a.

Faria-Correa MA. Videoendoscopic subcutaneous abdominoplasty. In Endoscopic Plastic Surgery 2nd edi. IV(16):559-586. Missouri: Quality Medical Publishing, Inc, 2008.

Faria-Correa MA. Videoendoscopy in plastic surgery: brief communication. Rev Soc Bras Cir Plast Est Reconstr 7:80–82, 1992b.

Lanfranco AR, Castellanos AE, Desai JP, Meyers WC.(2004) Robotic Surgery: A Current Perspective 239(1):14–21 doi: https://doi.org/10.1097/01.sla.0000103020.19595.7d

Lee HS, Kim D, Lee SY, Byeon HK, Kim WS, Hong HJ, Koh YW, Choi EC (2014). Robot – assisted versus endoscopic submandibular gland resection via retroauricular approach: a prospective nonrandomized study. British Journal Of Oral And Maxillofacial Surgery (2014) 52(2):179–184. doi: https://doi.org/10.1016/j.bjoms.2013.11.002

Lee J, Chung WY (2014). Robotic thyroidectomy and radical neck dissection using a gasless transaxillary approach. Robotics In General Surgery (2014) 24:269–270. doi:https://doi.org/10.1007/978-1-4614-8739-5_24

Mattei TA, Rodriguez AH, Sambhara D, Mendel Ehud (2014). Current state-of-the-art and future perspectives of robotic technology in neurosurgery (2014) 37(3):357–366; doi: https://doi.org/10.1007/s10143-014-0540-z

Morris B.(2005, September 25). Robotic surgery: Applications, limitations, and impact on surgical education. All about robotic surgery. Retrieved from http://www.allaboutroboticsurgery.com/avrasurgicalrobotics.html

Nahas FX, Augusto SM, Ghelfond C (2001). Suture materials for rectus diastasis: Nylon versus polydioxanone in the correction of rectus diastasis. Plastic And Reconstructive Surgery. The division of plastic surgery and radiology, hospital Jaragua. Sao Paulo, BR 107(3):700–706.

Nahas FX, Ferreira LM (2010). Concepts on correction of the musculoaponeurotic layer in abdominoplasty. Clin Plastic Surg (2010) 37:527–538. doi:https://doi.org/10.1016/j.cps.2010.03.001

Nahas FX, Ferreira LM, Augusto SM, Ghelfond C (2004). Correction of diastasis: long-term follow up of correction of rectus diastasis. Plastic And Reconstructive Surgery (2005) 115(6):1736–1741. doi:https://doi.org/10.1097/01.PRS.0000161675.55337.F1

Nahas FX, Ferreira LM, Ely PB, Ghelfond C (2011). Rectus diastasis corrected with absorbable suture: a long-term evaluation. Aesth Plast Surg(2011) 35:43–48. doi:https://doi.org/10.1007/s00266-010-9554-2

Selber JC. (2009). The role of robotics in plastic surgery. Quality Medical Publishing, Inc. Retrieved from http://www.plasticsurgerypulsenews.com/12/article_dtl.php?QnCategoryID=112&QnArticleID=236

Selber JC, Baumann DP, Holsinger FC (2012). Robotic latissimus dorsi flap for breast reconstruction. Plastic and reconstructive surgery 129(6):1305–12. doi: https://doi.org/10.1097/PRS.0b013e31824ecc0b

Chapter 12
Creation of a New Umbilicus During Abdominoplasty and Its Importance in Body Contouring

Juarez Moraes Avelar

Abstract A normal umbilicus is a scar in the geographical center of the abdomen in all human beings, as a result of the necrotic tissue that forms a few days after birth. Usually, it is a scar in the lowest part of a cavity with special skin around it. The scar is a result of necrosis in the central area of a suitable depression, and each one exhibits peculiar aesthetic behavior. Reproducing this anatomical region is a constant challenge to surgeons whenever they perform an operation on this region. When full abdominoplasty is performed, the plastic surgeon must be very concerned about the umbilicus because it is an important aesthetical reference point on the abdominal wall, and recreating it during an operation is a matter of art and skill.

Since the beginning of my activities, I have developed a personal method for avoiding leaving a circular scar around the umbilicus, to create a natural aesthetic appearance after full abdominoplasty. The main surgical principle of this method is to create three triangular skin flaps on the umbilicus, and another three cutaneous ones are cut out of the abdominal panniculus to be sutured in an alternating fashion with the flaps of the umbilicus. Another surgical principle is to suture the skin of the abdomen to depth to the umbilicus—instead of suturing the umbilicus to the skin of the abdominal panniculus. In addition, my method can be used for the correction of several deformities (congenital and acquired) in the umbilical region to create a natural umbilicus with outstanding results that improve the aesthetic appearance of the abdominal wall.

Keywords Umbilicus · Creation of an umbilicus · Importance of umbilicus · Location of the umbilicus · Abdominoplasty

J. M. Avelar (✉)
Brazilian Scientific Institute of Plastic and Reconstructive Surgery, São Paulo, Brazil

J. M. Avelar, R. Cavalcanti Ribeiro (eds.), *Body Contouring*,
https://doi.org/10.1007/978-3-031-42802-9_12

Introduction

The umbilicus—also known as the navel or the belly button—is the first scar on the human body, which is the final result after a natural necrotic phenomenon of the tissue cord that occurs a few days after birth. It is located in the central region of the abdominal wall, and it is an important reference point for the aesthetic appearance of the abdomen. The specific type of skin around the umbilical region resists surgery on this area. It is strategically located in the center of the abdomen and harmoniously balanced with the body, which is always noticed but not easily recreated during full abdominoplasty.

There are several situations that may damage the appearance of the navel, causing alterations to the umbilical region with physical and psychological repercussions, such as redundant skin, hernias (Fig. 12.1), diastasis in the rectus abdominalis (Fig. 12.2), unaesthetic surgical scars from previous operations (Fig. 12.3), absences in the umbilicus from previous operations (Fig. 12.4), deviations from the midline of the abdomen, flat surfaces (Fig. 12.3), burnt abdominal walls, and some other abnormalities that may disturb the normal anatomy of the umbilicus (Avelar 2016).

Among several anatomic alterations to the umbilical region, some may cause more-disruptive disturbances requiring local correction. First, several problems

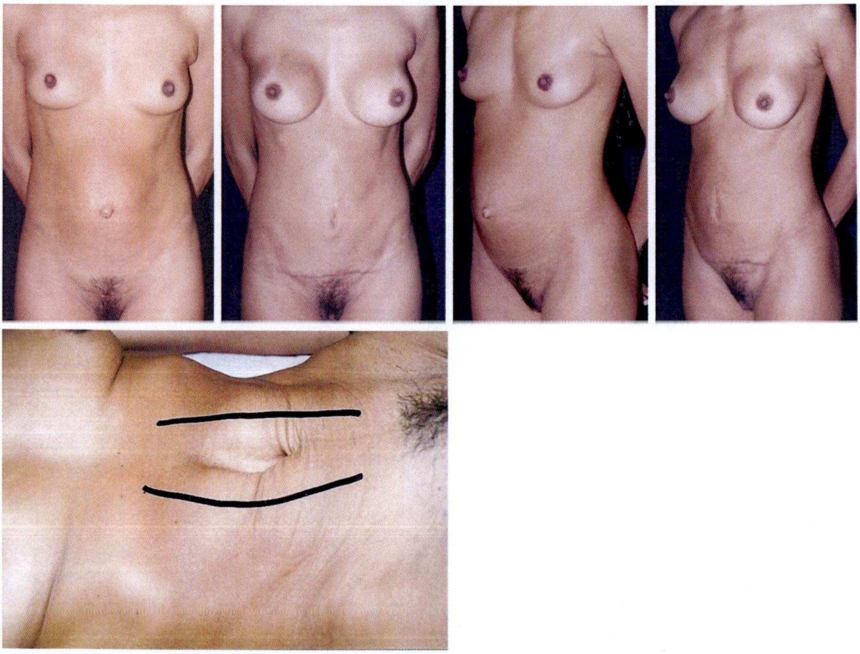

Fig. 12.1 Surgical correction of diastasis of the muscular abdominal wall through Callia's technique on lower abdominoplasty without reimplantation of the umbilicus combined with augmentation mastoplasty. Photos (**a, c**) preoperative of a 34-year-old patient; (**b, d**) post-operative photos combined with silastic implant; (**e**) preoperatory photo of the patient lying down showing severe diastasis of the umbilical region with patient making effort to elevate the torso trying to sit down

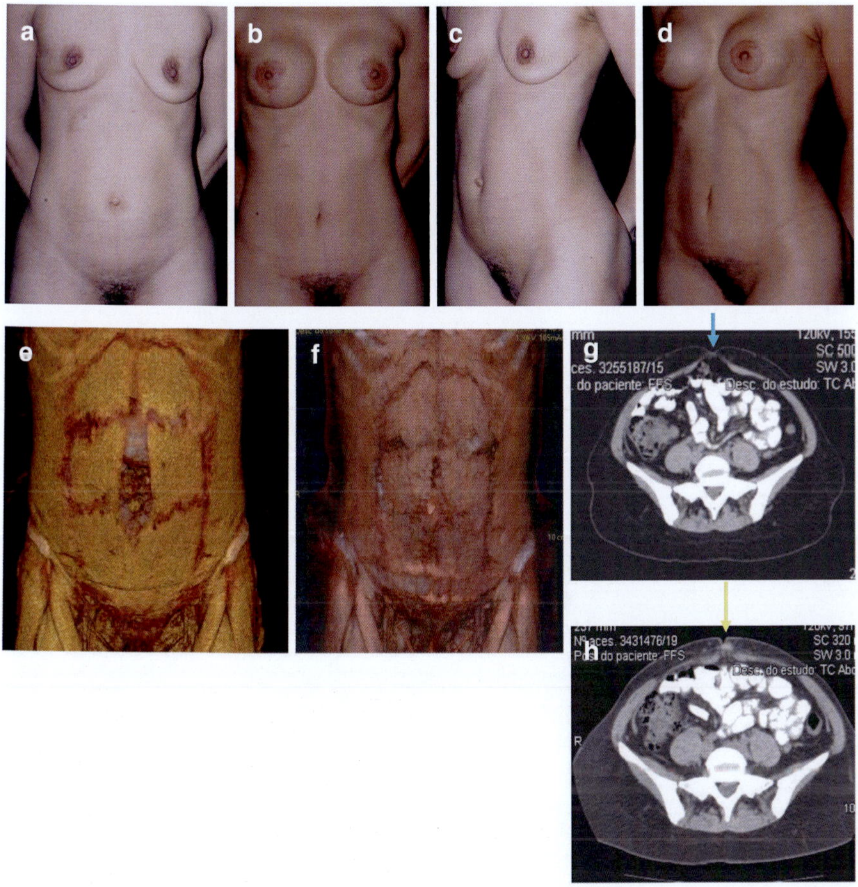

Fig. 12.2 Correction of diastasis of the muscular abdominal wall through Callia's technique without reimplantation of the umbilicus with lower abdominoplasty. Photos (**a, c**) preoperative of a 34-year-old patient; (**b, d**) post-operative photos combined with mastopexy with silastic implant; (**e**) computerized tomophagy before abdominoplasty presenting diastasis above the umbilicus on midline; (**f**) after surgery one can see correction of the diastasis by plication of muscular abdominal wall; (**g**) rotinaire tomography before abdominoplasty with diastasis indicated by arrow; (**h**) after operation with correction of diastasis with treatment of umbilical hernia

stem from the umbilicus and umbilical region, where severe alterations can be repaired through surgical treatment via appropriate techniques. So far, the most important have been those originating from previous surgeries trying to create a new umbilicus during full abdominoplasty (Figs. 12.3 and 12.4). For this purpose, I introduced new concepts (Fig. 12.5) (Avelar 1976a, b, 1979, 1983) to solve severe problems, such as the retraction and contraction of the scar around the new umbilicus after surgery, as reported by Grazer and Goldwyn (1977). They published an important survey in which they found a very high incidence of abnormalities as scars around the umbilicus with retraction and contraction.

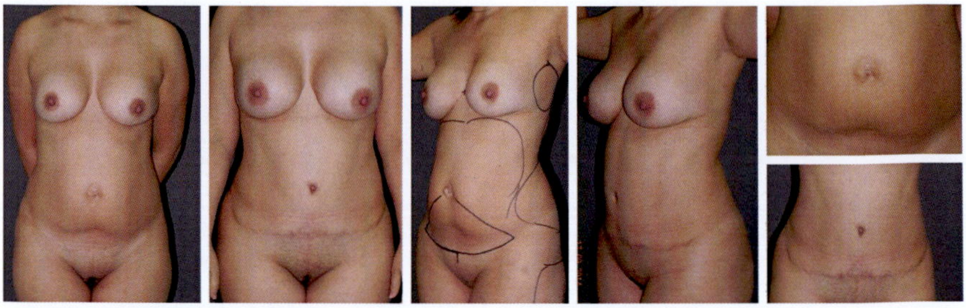

Fig. 12.3 Reparation of umbilicus region combined with secondary abdominoplasty in a 41-year-old patient underwent surgery elsewhere. Photo (**a**) patient presenting deep and unaesthetic surgical scar of the previous abdominoplasty and wide and flat umbilical region; (**b**) after secondary abdominoplasty with reparation of the umbilical and the supra pubic scar as well; (**c**) same patient in oblique left view with surgical demarcations; (**d**) 1 year after operation; (**e**) a close up of the unaesthetic scars on the umbilicus and supra pubic region; (**f**) photo in close showing the aesthetic appearance of the abdomen as well as the harmonious scar of the umbilicus

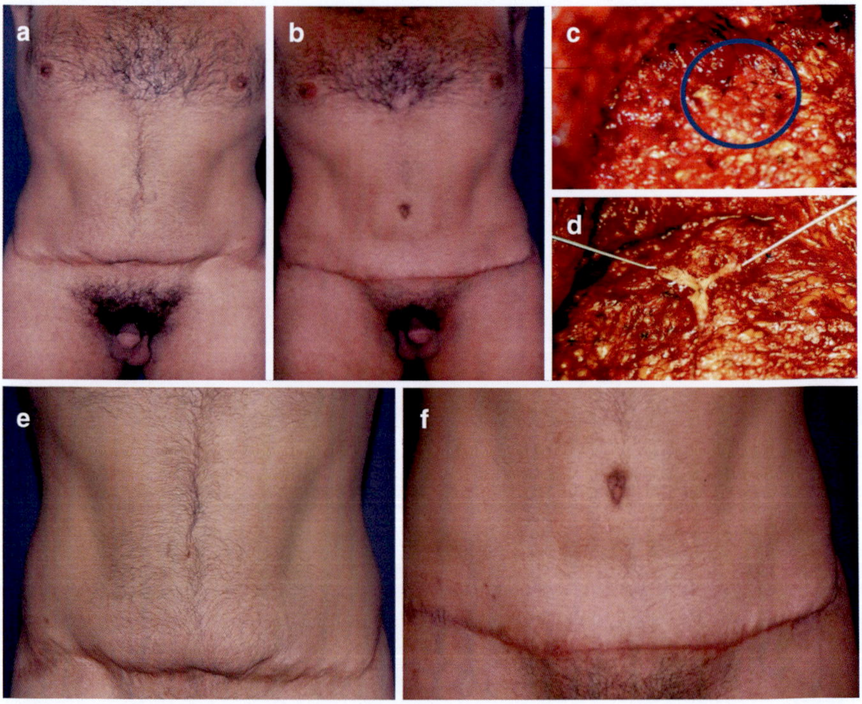

Fig. 12.4 Reconstruction of umbilicus after unsuccessful abdominoplasty in a 42-year-old male patient underwent elsewhere. Photo (**a**) patient presented unaesthetic surgical scar due to abdominoplasty and absence of the umbilicus; (**b**) after reconstruction with remnant skin of the umbilicus during am secondary abdominoplasty; (**c**) during surgery one can see an small segment of skin indicated by a circle; (**d**) it was possible to create three triangular flaps to be sutured to the new umbilical region; (**e, g**) photos in close showing unaesthetic appearance to the abdomen without umbilicus; (**f, h**) same patient after reconstruction of the umbilicus with three skin flaps on the umbilicus and other three created on abdominal wall similar to rotinaire operation during primary abdominoplasty

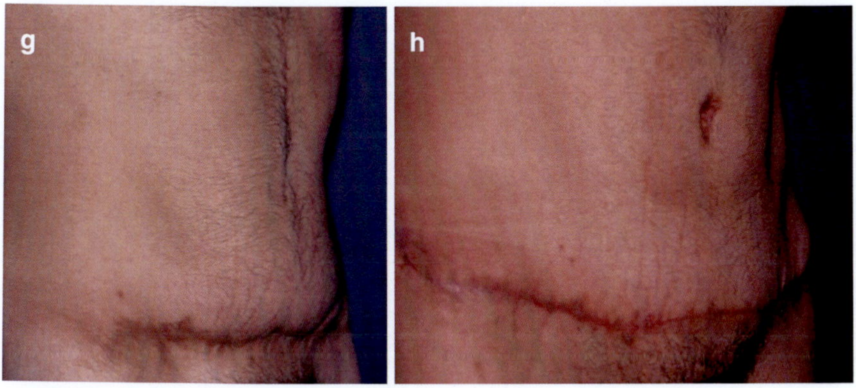

Fig. 12.4 (continued)

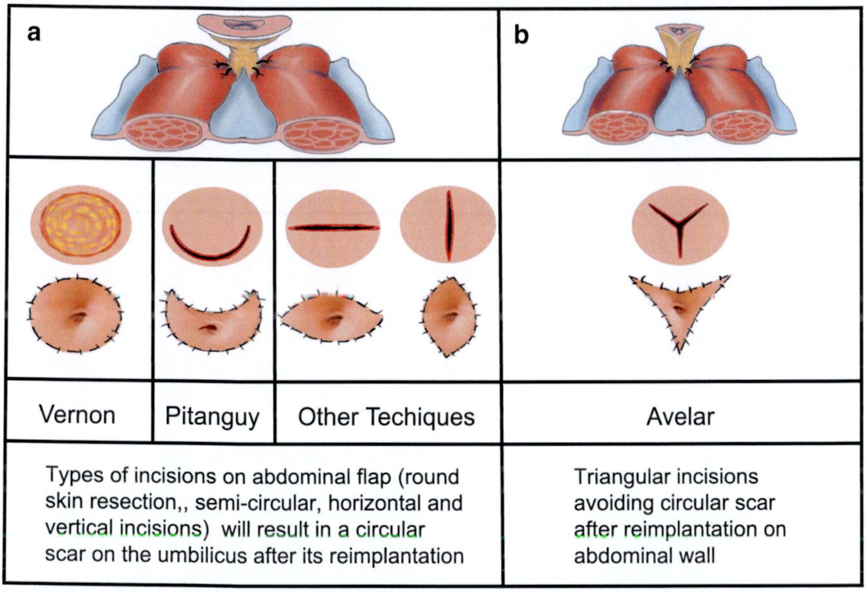

Fig. 12.5 Creation of the umbilicus during full lipoabdominoplasty. (**a**) When a circular incision is done around the umbilicus with reimplantation through circular incision with resection of a circle of skin, or semi-circular, horizontal or vertical incisions on the abdominal wall are done, the final scar will be always a circular one; (**b**) Avelar's technique is performed by triangular incisions around the umbilicus avoiding final circular scar around the umbilicus

Ever since I started my practice in 1974, I noticed that creation of a circular incision around the umbilical region during full abdominoplasty was the main cause of the unaesthetic surgical results. Looking for a solution, I developed a method (Avelar 1976a, b, 1978, 1979, 1983) in which instead of creating a circle around the new umbilical region, I introduced a star-shaped incision as a new surgical technique (Fig. 12.5).

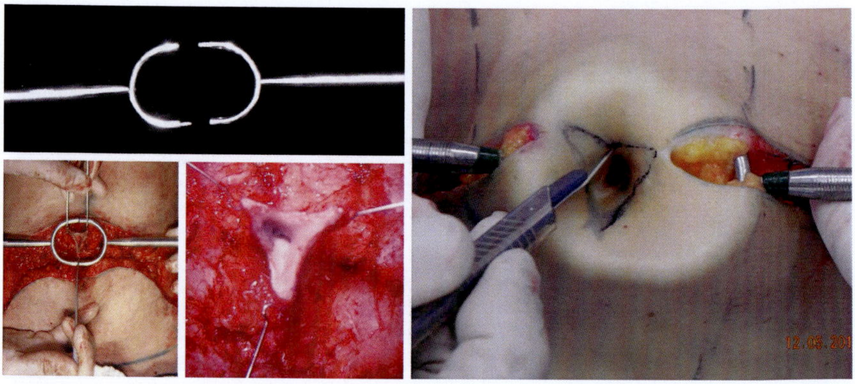

Fig. 12.6 Sequential photos of cutaneous incisions on umbilicus during full abdominoplasty, and lipoabdominoplasty as well, since the umbilicus is transposed and sutured to the abdominal wall. Photo (**a**) my double half semicircular instrument; (**b**) each segment is introduced on each side of the umbilicus in order to pull it upward to facilitate cutaneous incisions; (**c**) after incisions the umbilicus is in the center of the instrument; (**d**) close up of the cutaneous surface of the umbilicus with triangular shape

Method

The main surgical principles of the technique are to create three small triangular flaps on the umbilicus and another three on the cutaneous covering of the abdominal panniculus to be sutured in a one-by-one alternating fashion (Fig. 12.6).

Technique

The creation of a new umbilical region during full abdominoplasty is a routine procedure. All the panniculus below the umbilicus is resected, and its transposition is a matter of selecting the appropriate surgical approach, such as that introduced by Vernon (1957)—which removes a circle of skin on the abdominal flap, creating a circular scar around it (Fig. 12.5). Therefore, the reimplantation of the umbilicus on the abdomen wall opened up a new era in abdominoplasty. Several authors have published other procedures with vertical, horizontal, and semicircular incisions (Pitanguy 1967). No matter the type of incision that is performed on the abdominal wall, the final result will always be a circular scar around the transposed umbilicus (Fig. 12.5). Even when outstanding surgeons perform the operation, the final scar has not been satisfactory to most patients (Figs. 12.3 and 12.4).

A remarkable survey carried out by Grazer and Goldwyn (1977) on 10,540 abdominoplasties performed by plastic surgeons from several countries found that umbilical scar contractures occurred in 45% of the surgeries. According to that survey, 2% of the surgeons believe that some sort of retraction or contraction of the umbilical scar always occurs after abdominoplasty when transposition is performed. Ever since I started my practice in 1974, I paid special attention to creating a natural umbilical region during abdominoplasty in an attempt to solve some severe problems on the umbilicus associated with abdominoplasty. My original publications (Avelar 1976a, b, 1979) include descriptions of a new approach that avoids problems such as scars from retraction and contraction (Figs. 12.3 and 12.4).

Some of the surgical principles in my approach significantly diverge from those of other techniques:

1. The cutaneous incisions on the umbilicus are made by retracing the direction lines of the skin from outside to inside (Fig. 12.6b).
2. The final scars are similar to those of an atypical Z-plasty, which avoids unaesthetic appearance and scars from retraction and contraction.
3. The skin of the abdominal wall is pushed to its lowest depth in order for it to be sutured to the umbilicus (Fig. 12.7b, c).
4. The final appearance is a natural scar inside the surface of the cavity in the new umbilical region.
5. The final scars rest smoothly on the interior of the umbilical cavity (Fig. 12.7d.).

Over the years, the basic principles of the method have remained the same, but according to my observations, some technical details have been revised to improve the aesthetic results (Avelar 1983), even later on, when full lipoabdominoplasty is performed (Fig. 12.8) (Avelar 1999a, b, c). The technique is performed in two steps: first surgical demarcations and then the operation.

Surgical Demarcations

Before surgery meticulous demarcation is a mandatory step to creating a new umbilical region during full abdominoplasty because the umbilicus must be transposed preoperatively. When one performs full abdominoplasty or full lipoabdominoplasty, a new umbilical region must be created to rebuild the abdominal wall. Demarcations constitute a fundamental step and must follow surgical planning before any procedure in plastic surgery. For full lipoabdominoplasty, both steps are essential before the operation and must be carried out with the patient in a standing position and in a lying position. My preference is to demarcate all references points at the office on the day before surgery with the patient in a standing position and in a lying position in front of some mirrors so that they can follow my drawings. The demarcations on the umbilical region are also made according to my approach, published and presented at the Brazilian Congress of Plastic Surgery and the French Congress of Aesthetic Surgery (Fig. 12.6b, d) (Avelar 1976a, b). First, a circle of about 2 cm in diameter must be drawn around the umbilicus to delimit the umbilical area on the surface of the abdominal wall. Afterward, a star-shaped incision with three triangular flaps is made. One flap must be directed downward and other flaps directed obliquely upward to the right and to the left (Fig. 12.6b, d). On patients

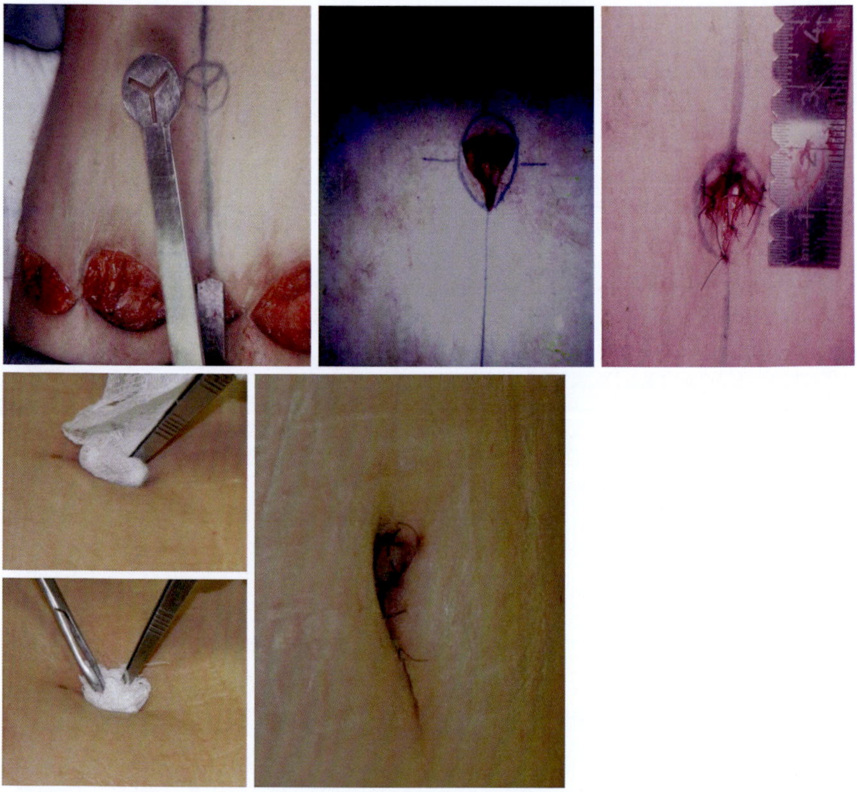

Fig. 12.7 Perioperative photos showing demarcation and creation of the new umbilical region during full abdominoplasty and lipoabdominoplasty using Avelar's surgical demarcator instrument. Photos (**a**) the inferior segment is placed on the umbilicus underneath the abdominal flap and the superior one lies on it and the new umbilical region is already demarcated inside of a circle; (**b**) cutaneous incisions were done creating three small triangular flaps inside the circle; (**c**) three skin flaps from the umbilicus are sutured alternatively with the other three from the abdominal wall; (**d, e**) local dressing is done with dry gauze inside the umbilicus; (**f**) the new umbilical region 1 week after surgery showing a natural depression of the umbilicus with rotation of the skin flaps from outside to inside (from surface to deep)

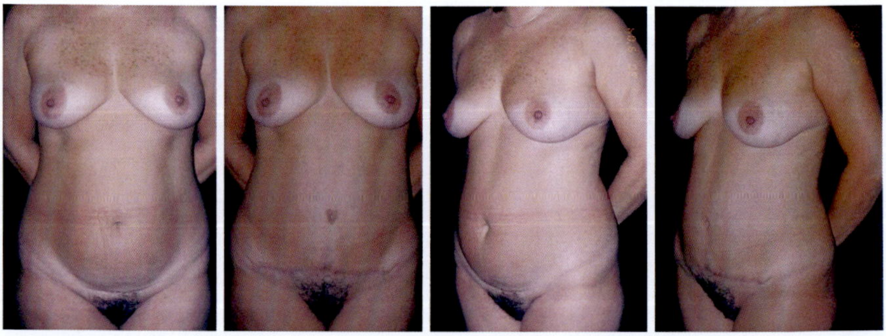

Fig. 12.8 Full lipoabdominoplasty performed on a 45-year-old patient with transposition of the umbilicus with Avelar's technique creating a natural umbilical region. Photos (**a, c**) preoperative views before surgery; photos (**b, d**) after surgery

who have undergone substantial weight loss or who present with excessive cutaneous flaccidity, the umbilical area shows some downward inclination. However, the umbilical region is always well identified thanks to its peculiar constitution of skin with a depression in the center.

The skin area of the abdomen to be resected is also demarcated before surgery. My preference is to follow Callia's (1965) technique and Sinder's (1975) techniques to leave the smallest possible final scar.

The Operation

The operation itself proceeds in several steps:

(a) Incisions into the umbilicus
(b) The transposition of the umbilicus
(c) Suturing the umbilicus
(d) Dressing

Full lipoabdominoplasty is a procedure of abdominoplasty without panniculus undermining in combination with the liposuction technique that must be performed at a hospital under an epidural or general anesthesia. Local infiltration with a special solution is carried out before liposuction and skin resection, which are fundamental procedures during the operation. A special solution is prepared: 1000 mL of serum plus 2 mg of epinephrine (1/1000), which makes the dilution 2/1.000.00. This solution allows surgeons to infiltrate the entire abdominal wall and the lateral sides of the torso. The infiltration is carried out on two levels: one on deep area below the fascia superficialis and on the area where skin resection will not be performed and one on the full thickness of the panniculus where skin resection will be performed.

Incisions into the Umbilicus

The operation starts in the umbilical region where cutaneous incisions are made following the star-shaped drawing inside the umbilicus, according to my demarcations (Fig. 12.9). Initially, two horizontal incisions are made on the right and left sides of the umbilicus, according to Sinder's technique. Afterward, following my new surgical instrument, which is two-in-one type of a double half circle that is to be articulated around the umbilical pedicle (Fig. 12.6a, b, c). Using this double half-circle instrument, the surgeon's assistant pulls the umbilical area upward. Such a maneuver is useful to elevate the cutaneous surface of the umbilical region away from the abdominal cavity to avoid accidentally perforating the internal abdominal organs. Unfortunately, this kind of complication has happened during surgery even when it was performed by well-qualified plastic surgeons. After cutaneous incisions have been made inside the umbilicus with a pair of scissors, the

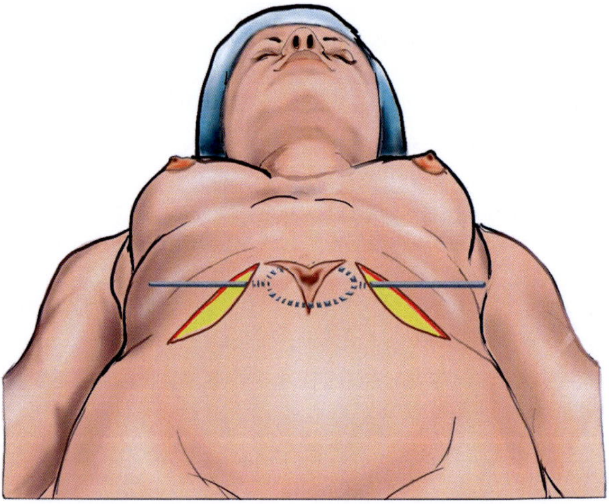

Fig. 12.9 Diagram from bottom showing full lipoabdominoplasty. Two cutaneous incisions are done on each side of the umbilicus to introduce my semicircular articulated instrument to lift the umbilical area in order to incise triangular incisions around the umbilicus to avoid accidental perforation of the abdominal cavity which may damage the internal viscera

pedicle is dissected downward until the aponeurosis of the musculoaponeurotic wall has been reached in order to isolate the umbilicus. At the end of this stage, the cutaneous surface of the umbilicus is now free, showing its triangular shape (Fig. 12.6c, d).

Afterward, liposuction is carried out on the deep layer of the panniculus, which is below the fascia superficialis, on the superior segment of the abdomen up to the costal rim, preserving the perforator vessels; a description of this procedure appears in Chap. X. According to Sinder's technique, the superior flap after liposuction on the lamellar layer is then pulled downward to evaluate whether it has reached the inferior border of the previous demarcations; a description of this part of the procedure appears in Chap. X. At this time, the operating table needs to be bent to conduction an evaluation. Once the evaluation has been completed, the surgical table is returned to the horizontal position, at which point liposuction is carried out on infraumbilical segment of the full thickness of the panniculus while preserving the perforator vessels and connective tissues. Afterward, the skin resection of the abdominal wall while tracing the demarcated area is performed. The subcutaneous tissue is held so that the knife does not damage the subdermal layer underneath, and consequently, no bleeding occurs.

When the patient presents with diastasis in the muscular rectus, it is a good indication that they need to undergo the reinforcement of the musculoaponeurotic structures (Figs. 12.1 and 12.2). I created a device (a dissector instrument) that is introduced in the umbilical area and moved upward on the midline through the connective tissue in order to expose the central border of the rectus abdominalis. The procedure for its plication is carried out on the midline with nonabsorbable material, making isolated stitches starting from 5 cm below the xiphoid process and up to the umbilical pedicle. Also, below the umbilicus, the aponeurosis is reinforced from the midline to the pubis.

The Transposition of the Umbilicus

Once again, the surgical table needs to be bent in order to facilitate the traction of the pulled-down abdominal flap. On the midline, a temporary stitch is applied to suture the inferior border of the upper panniculus to the border of the remaining panniculus in the suprapubic region (Fig. 12.10a). Then, the surgical table is returned to the horizontal position to demarcate the new umbilical area and the point corresponding to its projection on the cutaneous abdominal surface. The midline of the

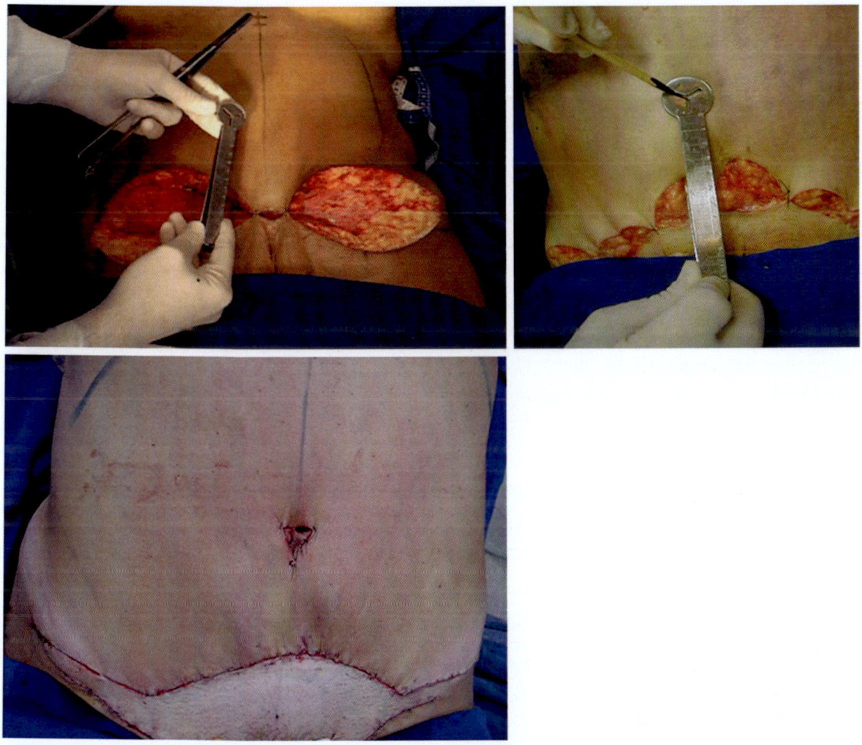

Fig. 12.10 Demarcation of the new location of the umbilicus on abdominal flap during full lipoabdominoplasty. Photo (**a**) my special instrument has two segments: one is placed on the umbilicus; (**b**) the superior segment is placed on abdominal flap to indicate the final location; (**c**) after cutaneous suture of the three flaps of the umbilicus with the three ones originating on the abdominal wall

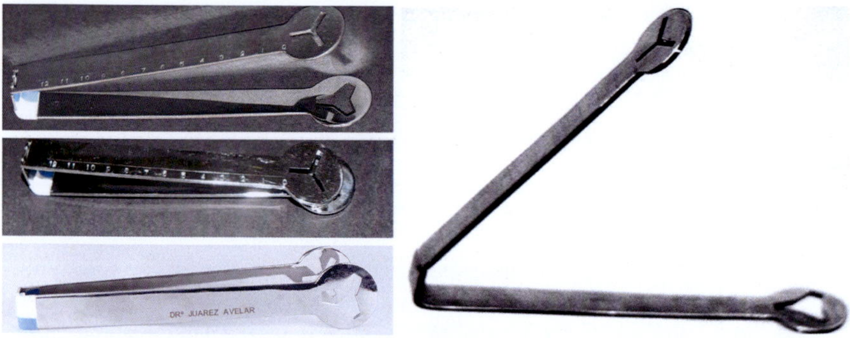

Fig. 12.11 Avelar's surgical instrument for demarcation of the new umbilical region on abdominal flap during full abdominoplasty and lipoabdominoplasty has two segments articulated between themselves: the superior one is 1 cm shorter than the inferior one. Photos (**a, b**) oblique views showing its position during demarcation; (**c**) posterior surface that one can see the lower segment; (**d**) the same surgical instrument with two segments in open position

abdominal wall must be drawn before surgery to establish the correct orientation for demarcating the new umbilicus at the aesthetic location on the abdomen. I created an appropriate surgical instrument, which acts as a marker and as a ruler (Fig. 12.11), that allows for achieving the exact position of the new umbilicus and for determining the appropriate distance from where the final scar will be. This instrument also protects the aponeurotic wall underneath and avoids damaging the intra-abdominal organs because it lies smoothly on the already-reinforced aponeurotic wall. According to my previous publications (Avelar 1983, 1985a, b, c), on later follow-up, the umbilicus is pulled upward by the upper abdominal segment. For this reason, the final position of the umbilicus is marked at least 1 cm lower than its projection on the abdominal flap (Fig. 12.11).

My instrument to determine the new umbilical area has two segments like a pair of forceps, where the upper one is 1 cm shorter than the inferior one so that the exact projection of the umbilicus can be marked postoperatively (Fig. 12.11). Usually, it is placed approximately 7 to 9 cm above the suprapubic incision. Very frequently, some patients present with a 2 to 4 cm increased elongation of that distance 1 year after surgery.

Suturing the Umbilicus

The umbilicus is then sutured with isolated stitches of 5-0 absorbable material. Following my technique, the tips of the three cutaneous flaps of the umbilicus are sutured between each small triangular skin flap created in the future umbilical region on the abdominal flap. In other techniques, the tips of the skin flaps of the abdominal wall are sutured between the cutaneous flaps of the umbilicus. Therefore, instead of leaving a circular scar around the umbilicus, which other techniques leave behind, the final scar after performing my technique is a "broken" line like an atypical multiple Z-plasty (Fig. 12.7b, c, f) (Avelar 1976a, b, 1979). The final scar has a triangular shape, which is very important to avoid scar retraction and even contracture.

Dressing

Dry gauze is placed inside the umbilical cavity and more gauze over it to maintain pressure on the umbilical area. Performing such a procedure keeps the flaps in their appropriate positions, avoiding scar-tissue contracture (Fig. 12.7d, e). The final scar has a triangular shape, which is important to achieve good aesthetical results without any scar-tissue contracture or retraction. The dressing is removed 5 to 6 days after surgery, at which time another dressing with dry gauze is placed inside the umbilicus, which should be changed every 10 days for at least 2 months. The final result of the umbilical region after abdominoplasty or lipoabdominoplasty always presents with a smooth scar around the umbilicus in harmony with the abdominal wall (Figs. 12.3, 12.4, and 12.8).

Complications

Since Vernon (1957) introduced the transposition of the umbilicus during abdominoplasty, such a procedure has become a mandatory step in all operations of full abdominoplasty and full lipoabdominoplasty, which may be considered one of the most important contributions to this field. Nevertheless, it also brought about many undesirable complications after operations for patients and surgeons, as reported by Grazer and Goldwyn (1977) in their important survey, in which they found very high incidences of abnormalities and scars around the umbilicus with retraction and contracture. Those complications motivated me to create my technique to solve some of them. In fact, when my procedure is properly performed, it avoids leaving a circular scar around the umbilicus. Because the skin around the inner aspect of the umbilicus is the result of the intussusceptions of the umbilical cord, the direction of the lines radiates from outside to inside.

Therefore, when a surgeon makes an incision into the skin, it should always follow that direction to avoid leaving scar tissue on the skin. If a circular incision is made around the umbilicus, it should be made in the opposite direction of the skin. In almost 40 years of practice employing my method on my patients, I have very seldom left such adverse scars after surgery. Only for one patient have I had to perform scar revision on the umbilicus, because she presented with very bad scaring in her suprapubic region. I have repaired and reconstructed the umbilicus of several patients secondarily to abdominoplasty (Figs. 12.3 and 12.4). In other methods described in the medical literature, the final result is a tendency to leave circular scars that may retract or contract (Fig. 12.5).

Discussion

Vernon's (1957) description was a remarkable scientific development in abdominoplasty. Afterward, many authors have devised other procedures either with vertical or horizontal incisions or with a semicircular incision (Pitanguy 1977), always resulting in leaving a circular scar around the transposed umbilicus (Fig. 12.5). Even when outstanding surgeons perform that operation, the final results have not been satisfactory. In a memorable survey reported by Grazer and Goldwyn (1977), they found very high incidences of abnormalities and scars around the umbilicus with retraction and contracture. According to the surgical principles of my technique, the final scar around the umbilicus is similar to that of an atypical Z-plasty (Avelar 1976a, b, 1979). In specific, three triangular flaps are created on the umbilicus, which are sutured to another three originating on the abdominal flap after the traction and resection of its excess (Figs. 12.6 and 12.7) (Avelar 1983). Since I developed and published my method, the creation of a new umbilical region has changed the surgical principles of abdominoplasty and lipoabdominoplasty.

One of the most important surgical principles of my technique is to push the skin of the abdominal wall to the deep structures of the musculoaponeurosis (Fig. 12.7). Such a technique is similar to that used on newborn children insofar as the necrosis of the umbilical cord is pulled from outside to the lowest depth. The final scar remains in the center of the umbilical cavity. As a consequence of this new aspect of my technique, the three small skin flaps created on the abdominal wall move in the direction of the already-sutured umbilicus close to the aponeurotic structures during the reinforcement procedure. Thus, the triangular flaps are sutured in an alternating fashion among the three triangular flaps created on the cutaneous surface of the umbilicus. Thanks to such movement of the skin flaps, a natural and smooth depression is created around the new umbilicus (Figs. 12.4, 12.7, and 12.8). In other methods described in the medical literature, the umbilicus is pulled from the depth to the surface of the abdominal wall, leaving a circular scar that may cause retraction and that frequently causes contracture.

There are descriptions creating four or five cutaneous flaps on the umbilicus. No matter how many flaps are created on the umbilical surface and on the cutaneous covering of the abdominal panniculus, the main surgical principle is to avoid leaving circular scars. To develop my method, I analyzed as many the geometric shapes as I could, and I determined that the most dissimilar one to the circle was a triangle. If another other shape with a greater number of cutaneous flaps is chosen, it will tend to approximate a circle. Such procedures are not new given that the basic principles are also fundamental to my 1976 method (Avelar 1976a, b).

In selected patients presenting with a very high location of the umbilicus and with flaccidity in the muscular abdominal wall, Callia's procedure (Fig. 12.12) ca be used to correct the diastasis without transposing the umbilicus, even without leaving a surgical scar around the umbilicus (Figs. 12.1, 12.2, and 12.13).

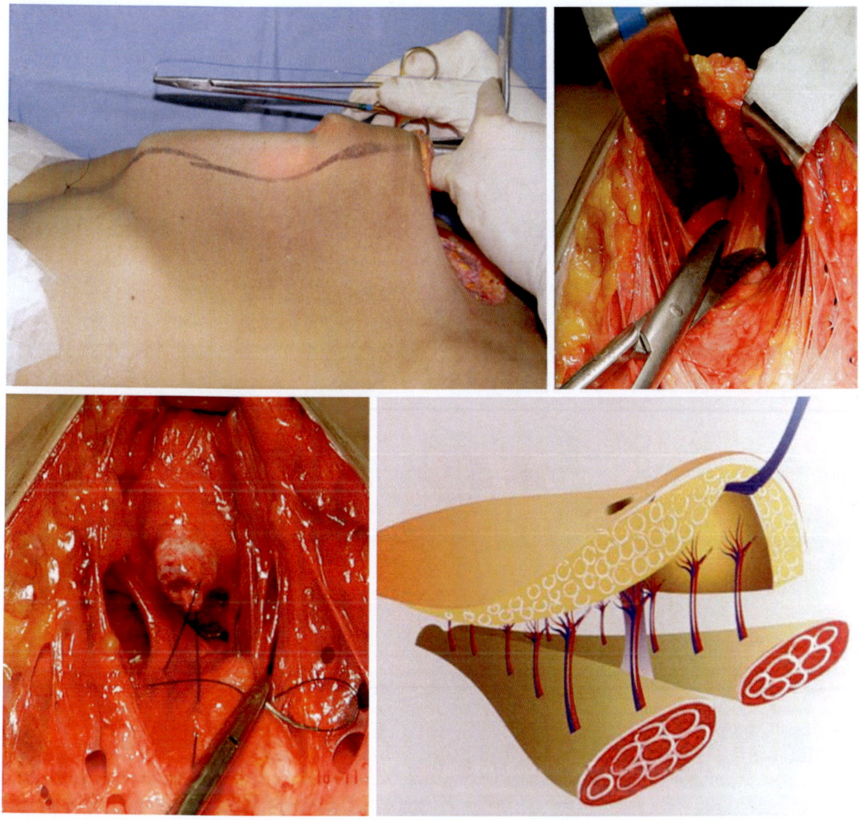

Fig. 12.12 Perioperative photos and diagram showing Callia's technique for abdominoplasty on atypical abdomen presenting high umbilicus on the abdominal wall. Photos (**a**) on profile view one can see the abdominal flap being pulled upwards through supra pubic incision; (**b**) section of the umbilical pedicle providing plication of the abdominal aponeurotic wall; (**c**) suture of the umbilical pedicle to muscular after reinforcement of the muscular wall; (**d**) diagram showing pulling upwards the abdominal flap exposing the perforator vessels and umbilical pedicle as well

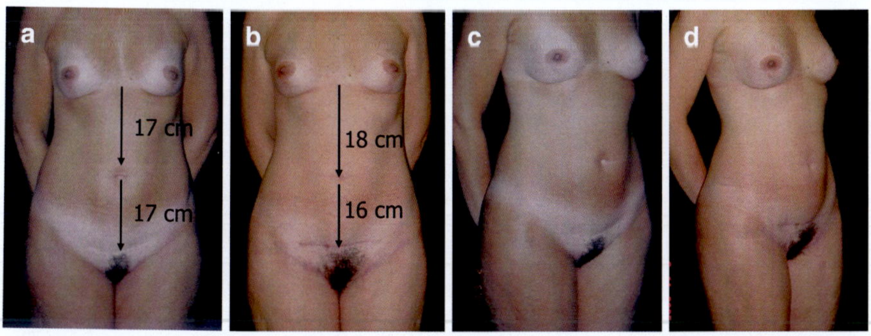

Fig. 12.13 Lower lipoabdominoplasty under Callia's technique with sectioning of the umbilical pedicle and its reimplantation combined with reinforcement of the muscular abdominal wall. Photo (**a, c**) before surgery in frontal view presenting 17 cm from xyphoid process to umbilicus and 17 cm from umbilicus to pubic region; (**b, d**) after surgery showing improvement of abdominal wall with sectioning of the umbilical pedicle with its fixation

Conclusion

Creating the new umbilical region during full lipoabdominoplasty is a mandatory procedure, and it is a constant challenge because it is located in the central area of the abdomen and always leaves scars around the umbilicus. By using my technique, good aesthetical results that avoid scar retraction and contracture can be achieved (Figs. 12.5, 12.6, and 12.7) (Avelar 1976a, b, 1979, 1983). Such unfavorable postoperative stigmata were reported by Grazer and Goldwyn (1977). According to previous evaluation, planning, and demarcation, the whole area of the cutaneous covering of the infraumbilical region is always resected. Cutaneous incisions into the umbilicus are made before skin resection (Fig. 12.9) (Avelar 2000a, b, c, d, e, f, g, 2001a, b, 2002a, b). When lower and upper lipoabdominoplasty is performed, the umbilicus is not transplanted, because the skin resection is limited to the suprapubic area or on submammary folds. The surgical principles of my method are new ones in that the final scar is not a circular one but rather are similar to those left after an atypical Z-plasty around the new umbilicus, creating a natural depression in the surface of the region in the center of the abdominal wall (Figs. 12.7 and 12.8).

References

Avelar JM (1976a) Umbilicoplasty – a technique without external scar (Umbilicoplastia – uma técnica sem cicatriz externa). 13rd Bras Cong of Plast Surg and First Brazilian Cong of Aesthetic Surgery. (13° Congresso Brasileiro de Cirurgia Plástica e 1° Congr Bras Cir Estética), Porto Alegre – RS (Brazil) 81–82

Avelar JM (1976b) Umbilicoplasty - A technique without external scar. Cahiers de Chirurgie Esthétique. Journees internationals de Chirurgie Esthetique. Vendredi 21 Paris (France) mai.

Avelar JM (1978) Abdominoplasty: Systematization of a technique without external umbilical scar. Aest Plast Surg 2:141

Avelar JM (1979) Umbilical scar – importance and technique for creating during abdominoplasty (Cicatriz umbilical – da sua importância e da técnica de confecção nas abdominoplastias) Rev Bras Cir 1(2):41–52

Avelar JM (1983) (Abdominoplasty: Technical Refinements and Analysis of 130 cases in 8 Years Follow-up). Aesth Plast Surg 7: 205–212

Avelar JM (1985a) Combined liposuction with traditional surgery in abdomen Lipodystrophy. XXIV Instructional Course of Aesth Plast Surg of ISAPS, Madrid.

Avelar JM (1985b) Fat-suction versus abdominoplasty. Aesthetic Plast Surg 9:265–276

Avelar JM (1985c) – Fat-Suction of the Submental and Submandibular Regions. Aesth Plast Surg 9:257–263

Avelar JM (1999a) A new technique for abdominoplasty – Closed vascular system of subdermal flap folded over itself combined to liposuction (Uma nova técnica de abdominoplastia – sistema vascular fechado de retalho subdérmico dobrado sobre si mesmo combinado com lipoaspiração). Rev Bras Cir 88/89, (1/6), 3–20. Nov–Dec

Avelar JM (1999b) New concepts for abdominoplasty (Novos conceitos para abdominoplastia). Paper presented at the 36th Congress of the Brazilian Society of Plastic Surgery. Rio de Janeiro

Avelar JM (1999c) Abdominoplasty: New concepts for a new technique (Abdominoplastia: Nuevos conceptos para una nueva técnica). XXVI Annual International Symposium of Aesthetic Plastic Surgery, Chairman: Prof. Jose Guerrerosantos - Puerto Vallarta, Jalisco - México. 10-13

Avelar JM (2000a) Abdominoplasty without detachment (Abdominoplastia sem descolamento). XX Jorn Paulista Cir Plast, São Paulo, Jun.

Avelar JM (2000b) Abdominoplasty with preservation of the Deep Vascular Sistem. (Abdominoplastia com preservação do sistema vascular profundo). Personal Comunication (Comunicação Pessoal). Monthly Meeting of the Brazilian Society of Plastic Surgery – Section of Rio Grande do Sul (Reunião Mensal da Sociedade Brasileira de Cirurgia Plástica do Rio Grande do Sul). May.

Avelar JM(2000c) Abdominoplasty: a new technique without undermining and fat layer removal (Abdominoplastia: uma nova técnica sem prejudicar e remoção da camada de gordura) Arq. Catarinense de Med 29: 147–9

Avelar JM (2000d) First Course of abdominoplasty (I Curso de abdominoplastia). Chairman: Prof. Willian Callia. Invited Professor: Dr. Juarez M. Avelar. Municipal Hospital. São Paulo, march

Avelar JM (2000e) Second Course of abdominoplasty (II Curso de abdominoplastia). Chairman: Prof. Juarez M. Avelar. Heart Hospital (Hospital do Coração). São Paulo, October

Avelar JM (2000f) A New Technique for Abdominoplasty Subdermal Flap Folded over Itself. XV ISAPS Congress, Tokyo

Avelar JM (2000g) Abdominoplasty: A New Technique Without Panniculus undermining and Without panniculus resection. 57th Instructional Course of ISAPS, Chairman: Lloyd Carlsen Montreal, Quebec, September.

Avelar JM (2001a) Abdominoplasty without lipectomy. Mini Course of ISAPS with Aesthetic Plastic Surgery Congress of Spain. Valladolid September.

Avelar JM (2001b) The new Abdominoplasty And Derived Technique. ISAPS and ASERF Annual Meeting. The Aesthetic Meeting. New York - September.

Avelar JM (2002a) Abdominoplasty Without Panniculus Undermining and Resection: Analysis and 3-Year Follow-up of 97 Consecutive Cases. Aesth Plast Surg 16–25

Avelar JM (2002b) Abdominoplasty. The Aesthetic Meeting of ISAPS, Istambul, Turkey September.

Avelar JM (2016) Creation of the New Umbilicus: My Technique on Abdominolipoplasty and Further Applications In: Avelar JM New Concepts on Abdominoplasty and Further Applications Springer, Heidelberg/New York, p 107

Callia WEP (1965) Contribution to the study of surgical correction of the pendulum abdomen and globus (Contribuição ao estudo de correção cirúrgica do abdomen pêndulo e globus). original art. Doctoral Thesis Fac Med USP, São Paulo - Brazil

Grazer FM, Goldwyn RM (1977) Abdominoplasty Assessed by Survey with Emphasis on Complications. Plast Recont Surg 59(4): 513–7

Pitanguy I (1967) Abdominal lipectomy: an approach to it through an analysis of 300 consecutive cases. Plast Reconstr Surg (40) 4:384–391

Pitanguy I (1977) Dermolipectomy of the Abdominal Wall, Thighs, Buttocks, and Upper Extremity. In: Converse JM, ed. Reconstructive Plast Surgery 2nd edition. Philadelphia: Saundrs, 3800–23

Sinder R (1975) Plastic Surgery of the abdomen - Técnica pessoal de abdominoplastia, com prévio deslocamento de retalho supraumbilical (antes da resseccão infraumbilical) e uso de retalho dermoadiposo, – VI International Congress of Plastic and Reconstructive Surgery, Paris (France) August

Vernon S (1957) Umbilical transplantation upward and abdominal contouring in lipectomy. Am J. Surg., 94: 490–492.

Chapter 13
Abdominoplasty (The Umbilical Lozenge Technique)

Marcelo de Oliveira e Silva

Abstract Obesity is a pandemic. The exponential increase in abdominal correction surgeries after important weight losses resulting from bariatric surgeries is a logical consequence. The umbilical scar reconstruction surgical time has a fundamental importance, and a lozenge-shaped navel contributes to the abdominal aesthetics. However, the literature shows that the neo-navel is something challenging in these surgeries, compromising the results and, sometimes, generating dissatisfaction on the surgeon's and the patient's perspective. Unaesthetic healing and stenosis due to scar contracture are common complaints when circular techniques are used and can be avoided using the lozenge technique. The most frequent complications related to omphaloplasty are post-necrosis effacement, stenosis due to circular retraction, enlargement of the circumference, lack of anatomical contours, and a rayed appearance due to the external suture marks.

Keywords Abdominoplasty · Bariatric surgery · Navel reconstruction · Dermolipectomy · Neo-omphaloplasty

Introduction

Obesity is a pandemic. The exponential increase in abdominal correction surgeries after important weight losses resulting from bariatric surgeries is a logical consequence. The umbilical scar reconstruction surgical time has a fundamental importance, and a lozenge-shaped navel contributes to the abdominal aesthetics. However, the literature shows that the neo-navel is something challenging in these surgeries, compromising the results and, sometimes, generating dissatisfaction on the surgeon's and the patient's perspective. Unaesthetic healing and stenosis due to scar contracture are common complaints when circular techniques are used and can be

M. de Oliveira e Silva (✉)
São Paulo, Brazil

J. M. Avelar, R. Cavalcanti Ribeiro (eds.), *Body Contouring*,
https://doi.org/10.1007/978-3-031-42802-9_13

avoided using the lozenge technique. The most frequent complications related to omphaloplasty are post-necrosis effacement, stenosis due to circular retraction, enlargement of the circumference, lack of anatomical contours, and a rayed appearance due to the external suture marks.

To avoid a stigmatizing appearance, the neo-navel should have the most natural and pleasant shape possible. The correct shape and positioning of the neo-navel are crucial to a satisfactory result. Above these aspects, among the most relevant points to a good aesthetic standard result are the navel size and the non-visible scars. There are several omphaloplasty techniques described in the literature, but there is no consensus as to the best technique for its execution.

The systematization of this surgical stage avoids excessive manipulation of the umbilical pedicle and reduces the surgical time spent in this step, minimizing the risk of necrosis by ischemia and improving the neo-navel's final aesthetic appearance, resulting in a patient's high satisfaction rate. The aim of this chapter is to describe omphaloplasty by the lozenge technique in abdominal dermolipectomy, demonstrating its technical details.

Prof. Ivo Pitanguy Abdominoplasty Surgical Technique

The classic technique described by Pitanguy simultaneously approaches the aesthetic and functional correction of the patient's abdomen, always obeying the same principles: the abdominal wall reinforcement, repair of eventration and herniations, excision of adipose tissue excess, and correction of skin deformities (scars or stretch marks).

After preparation of the anesthetic team and placement of surgical drapes, the midline of the abdomen is marked with a wire fixed to the xiphoid process and another 7 cm above the vaginal sternal notch. The incision is drawn keeping it low and following the inguinal pleat, curving upward on the sides. With the two long wires, the symmetry of the marking is verified, which must extend to a point located on an imaginary vertical line that passes over the anterosuperior iliac spines.

The navel is demarcated with a circular incision.

The transverse incision is performed by deepening the subcutaneous plane in a beveled manner, creating a discreet fat pad in the pubis. The detachment proceeds above the muscular fascia, meticulously performing hemostasis. The detachment will continue until the umbilical scar, where a circumferential incision allows to isolate the navel, leaving it inserted in the abdominal wall. The detachment continues superiorly until it reaches the xiphoid process, creating a tunnel to expose the sheaths of the rectus abdominis muscles. The lateral limits of the detachment are the costal margins (avoiding unnecessary lateral detachment).

The aponeurosis is reinforced from top to bottom, starting high enough to avoid prominence in the epigastrium. Two strong hooks are used to test the desired tension on the aponeurotic edges at the level of the navel. This anchorage must be performed checking the degree of diastasis, without excessive tension, with non-absorbable sutures and with inverted mattress stitches, that is, in X with the knot facing inward.

After diastasis correction, the anesthetist is asked to place the table slightly bent, elevating the patient's upper body by approximately 15°.

The upper flap is fixed to the suprapubic skin at the midline with a strong temporary suture. The lateral flaps are then pulled inferiorly. Pitanguy marking tweezers are used to determine the amount of tissue to be excised. The long sutures of the xiphoid process and above the vaginal notch serve to verify the symmetry of the marking and its position on the flap. With a firm countertraction of the auxiliary, the flap is excised, beveling the subcutaneous tissue in order to better accommodate the initial transverse incision.

The flaps are distributed with temporary sutures, compensating medially so as not to create "ears" (or "wrinkles") and decrease the final extension in the scar. The Pitanguy tweezer is again used to determine the position of the umbilicus in the midline.

The navel must be exteriorized through the appropriate circumferential incision. A straight incision of about 1–1.5 cm is made, since in the flap traction, it will become circular. A fat cone should be removed from the flap of this incision, allowing a better accommodation of the umbilical scar, thus creating a gentle periumbilical depression.

The final closure of the incisions is performed by planes. It is of paramount importance to redo the plan of Scarpa's aponeurosis, ensuring a firm plan of approximation. Drains are routinely exteriorized on the pubic region.

A compressive curative is applied using a plaster shield wrapped with cotton and bandage, allowing a firm and well-distributed compression. Umbilical curative must be done with gauze and spherical objects (e.g., marbles) to avoid stenosis.

The abdominal strap is placed the next day, and the patient is recommended to maintain a more curved posture, thus protecting the anchorage of the rectus abdominis muscles.

The Omphaloplasty Lozenge Technique in Abdominoplasty

In this technique, the preoperative marking of the suprapubic horizontal scar is made between 6 and 8 cm from the vaginal notch, during a superior traction maneuver of the prepubic region (Fig. 13.1). The marking is performed in bed, with the patient in an orthostatic position, and checked with the patient in the supine position, already in the operating room.

As prophylactic measures, cefazolin 2 g is administered, 30 min before the start of surgery, as directed by the hospital's infection control commission, and the pneumatic compression system is placed on the lower limbs over the previously worn compression stockings. The stockings are kept until the seventh postoperative day (Fig. 13.1).

Midline marking is performed with the patient in the supine position, connecting the xiphoid process to the vaginal notch. A uniform traction of the prepubic region into cranial direction, with the open hand in the region of the lower abdomen, gives the distance from the previously marked vaginal notch. At this point, starting from the midline, a horizontal marking of 6 cm is made on each side, with the aid of a compass. The horizontal and bilateral marking extends in an arcuate fashion, with the superior concavity toward the lower transverse fold of the abdomen, with the lateral limits of the

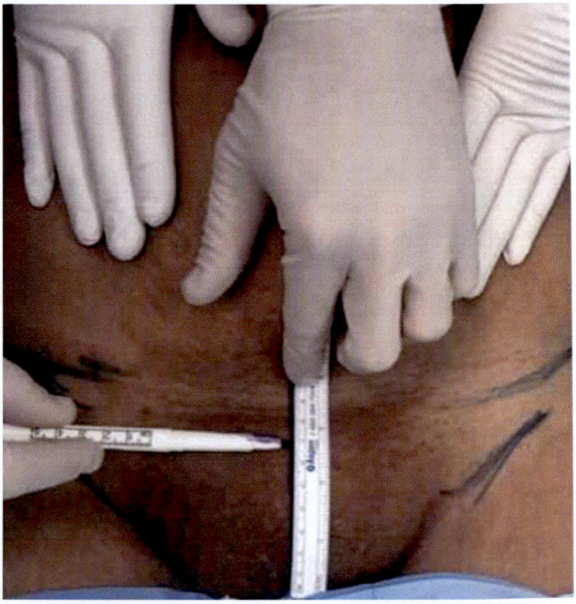

Fig. 13.1 The height incision's marking in abdominoplasty

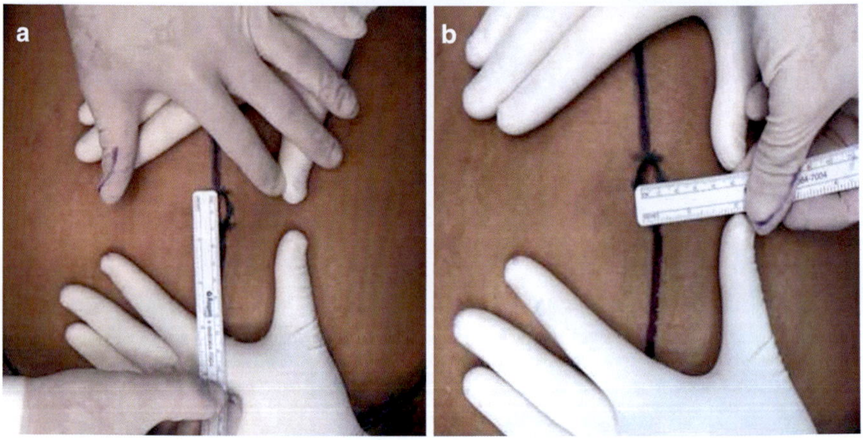

Fig. 13.2 (**a**) Vertical marking of umbilical incision's measure. (**b**) Horizontal marking of the umbilical incision's measure

anterosuperior iliac crests. Such marking can be extended later after compensation of the skin-fat flap, if necessary. The lozenge-shaped marking for the incision and release of the navel is made with the assistant surgeon distributing the skin in this region in an eccentric manner with both hands opened. The lozenge measurements are 1.4 cm, in the craniocaudal direction, and 1.0 cm, in the latero-lateral direction (Fig. 13.2a, b).

The first incision is made in the superficial lozenge-shaped marking in the periumbilical region, with a cold scalpel with blade no. 15. Then, in order to deepen the incision, in the same place, we used the no. 11 blade, and to finish the dissection and isolation of the umbilical shape, up to the aponeurotic plane, we used Metzenbaum scissors. Then, a horizontal suprapubic incision is made, and the skin-fat flap is detached, in a tunnel, up to the xiphoid process, allowing the plication of the rectus abdominis muscles. During this surgical stage, eventual ventral and umbilical hernias are corrected, without violating the umbilical stump skin.

The umbilical stump is fixed to the aponeurosis with four cardinal points, with 3-0 mononylon thread, preserving a distance between the skin and the aponeurosis of 0.5 cm (Fig. 13.3).

After resection of the excess skin-fat tissue from the detached flap, it is pulled and anchored, with temporary sutures, to the suprapubic flap, with 2-0 or 3-0 mononylon. Under the fixed flap, we digitally located the position of the umbilicus in the aponeurosis and marked the center of the location of the neo-navel, using the digital projection under the flap (Fig. 13.4).

The lozenge-shaped marking of 1.4 × 1.0 cm is repeated, and the lozenge center is defined by the previous digital maneuver (Fig. 13.5a, b).

A new incision, perpendicular into its full thickness, is made in the new lozenge-shape marked on the flap, to expose the umbilical stump fixed to the aponeurosis (Fig. 13.6).

Next, we mark the positioning of the upper flap in relation to the lower one, with a dermographic pen, and the temporary suture was removed, allowing the flap eversion. With this maneuver, we performed a lipectomy in the region of the lozenge, using Metzenbaum scissors, which contributes to reducing the tension in the umbilical scar, besides forming a depression in the peri-umbilical region, simulating the umbilical groove and, consequently, giving appearance of naturalness to the abdomen (Fig. 13.7).

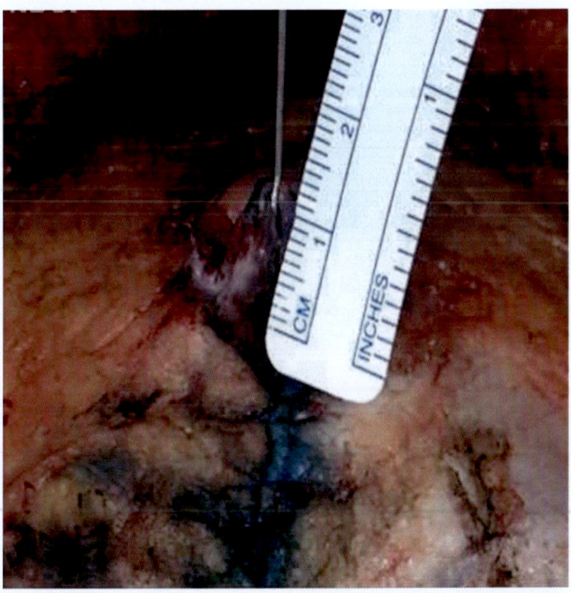

Fig. 13.3 The height of fixation of umbilical stump marking

Before the flap repositioning, we marked the upper and lower ends of the umbilical scar with two 4-0 mononylon threads. The two ends of the wires, with entry in the epidermis and exit in the subdermis of each end, are repaired with Halstead tweezers, at the lower end (straight), and curved, at the upper end (curve). Both are passed through the lozenge-shaped hole made to expose the umbilicus (Fig. 13.8a, b).

The wires repaired in the umbilical scar serve as a reference for the navel's position, avoiding twisting and facilitating the fixation of the umbilical stump in its

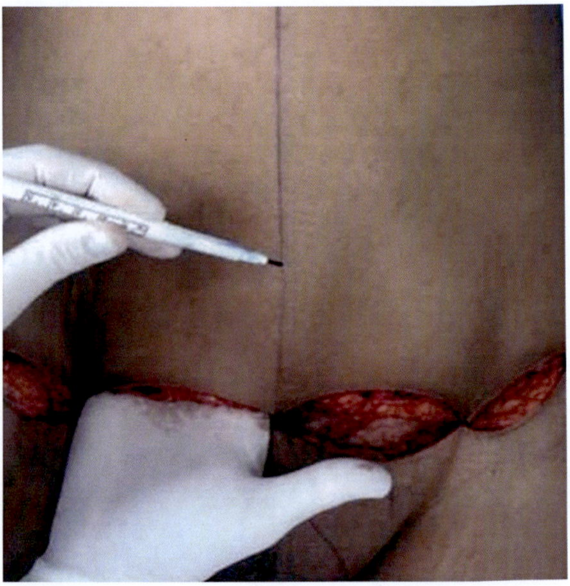

Fig. 13.4 The neo-navel marking

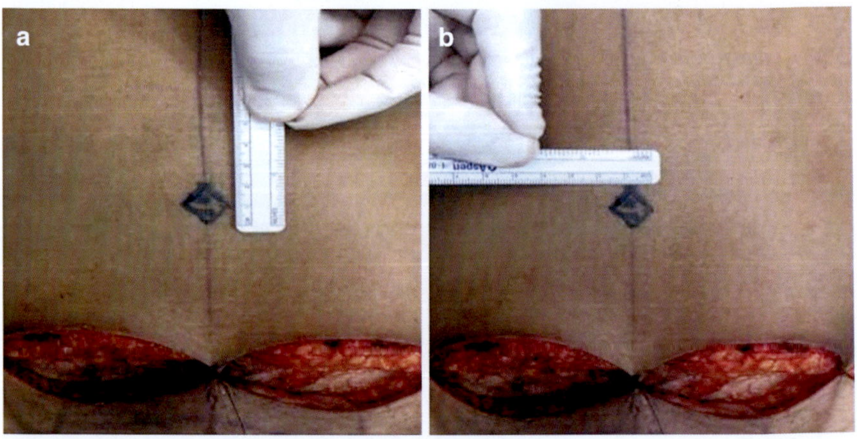

Fig. 13.5 (**a**) The neo-navel vertical measure marking. (**b**) The neo-navel horizontal measure marking

corresponding position in the flap. The four sides of the created lozenge-shaped hole are fixed with Gillies stitches, using 4-0 mononylon thread (Fig. 13.9).

The flap is repositioned according to the previous marking, and the closure is performed with sutures in layers, with absorbable thread 3.0 in two subdermal layers and with non-absorbable thread 3.0 in the intradermal layer. After closing the

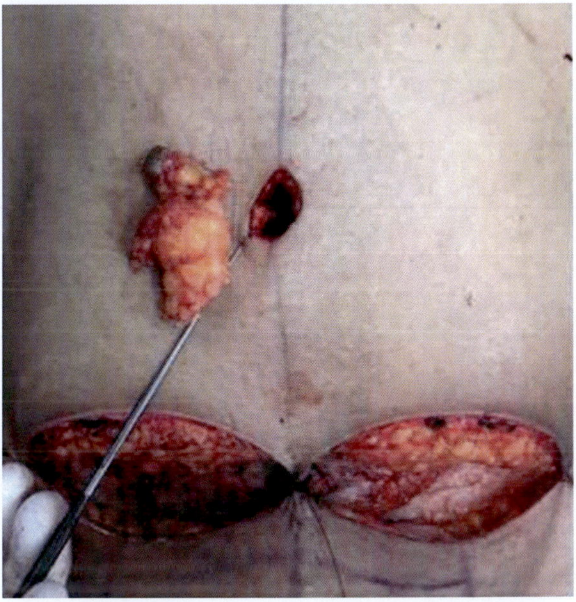

Fig. 13.6 The umbilical stump exposition throughout the flap

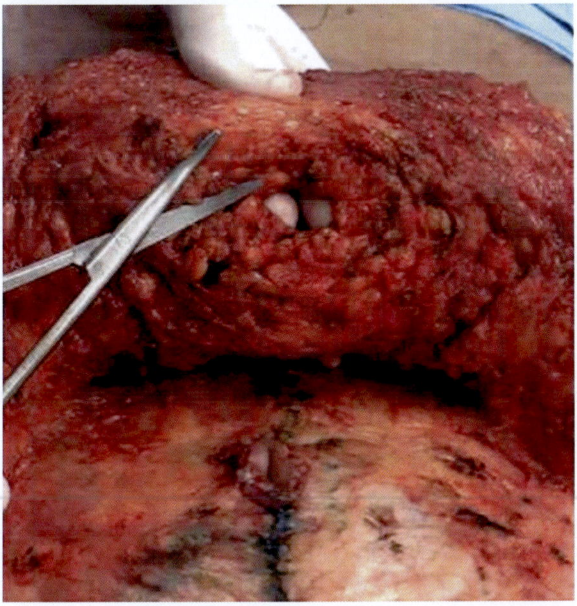

Fig. 13.7 Hemostasis and lipectomy to realize flap eversion

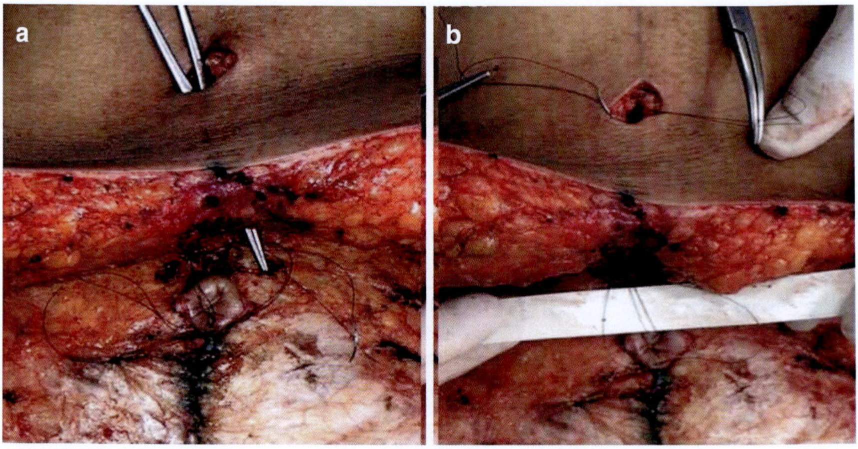

Fig. 13.8 (**a**) Mononylon 4-0 thread on the superior and inferior extremities of the umbilical stump, with epidermis entry and subdermis exit. (**b**) The repaired threads are passed through the flap hole

Fig. 13.9 The repaired threads are the reference of the navel's position in relation to the flap, facilitating the fixation of the umbilical stump in your corresponding position in the flap

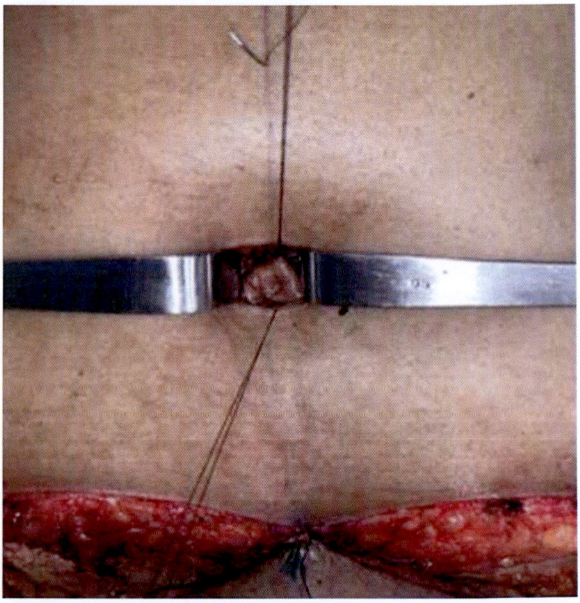

suprapubic incision, incisional VAC therapy is installed over the neo-navel and over the entire suture line (Figs. 13.10 and 13.11).

Patients are discharged from hospital 48 h after surgery. Incisional negative pressure therapy is withdrawn on the first outpatient visit (4 to 6 days after surgery). All patients are instructed in the same way regarding postoperative care and return to activities (Figs. 13.12, 13.13, 13.14, 13.15, 13.16, 13.17, 13.18, 13.19, 13.20, 13.21, 13.22, 13.23, 13.24, 13.25, 13.26, and 13.27).

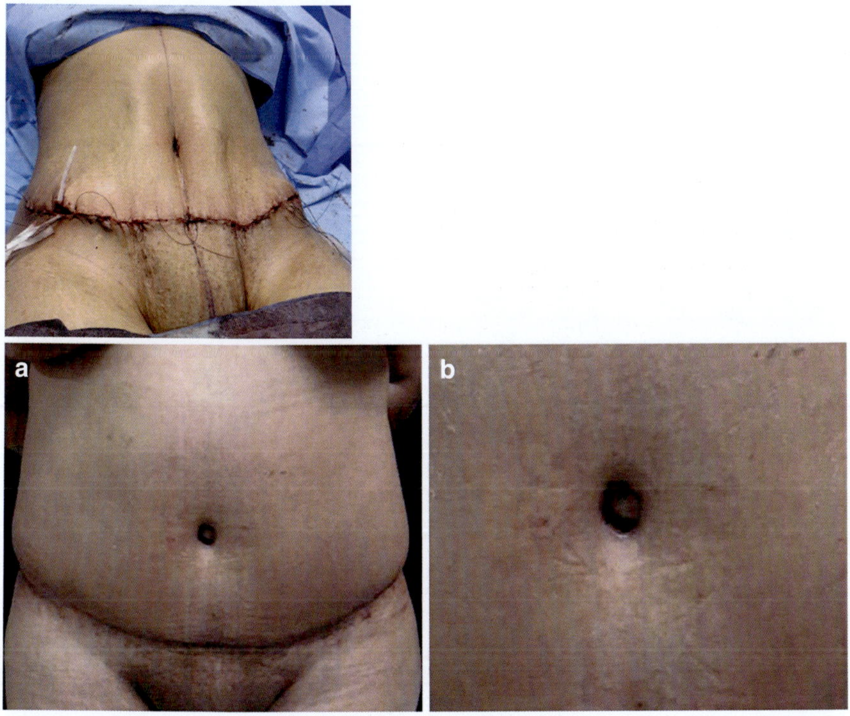

Fig. 13.10 Flap positioned and sutured by layers. (**a**) Case 01. (**b**) Case 01 (enlarged look of the neo-navel

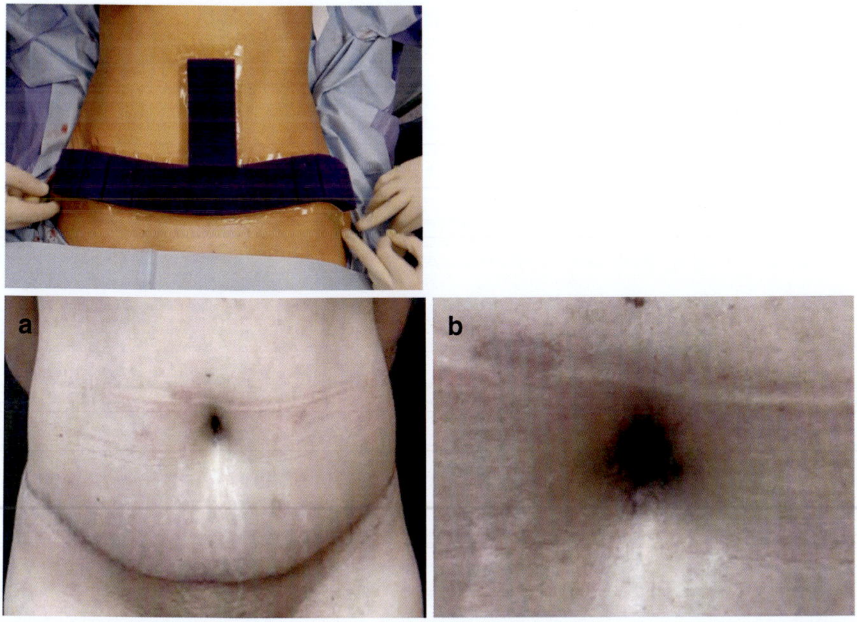

Fig. 13.11 Instalation of incisional VAC therapy. (**a**) Case 02. (**b**) Case 02 (enlarged look of the neo-navel)

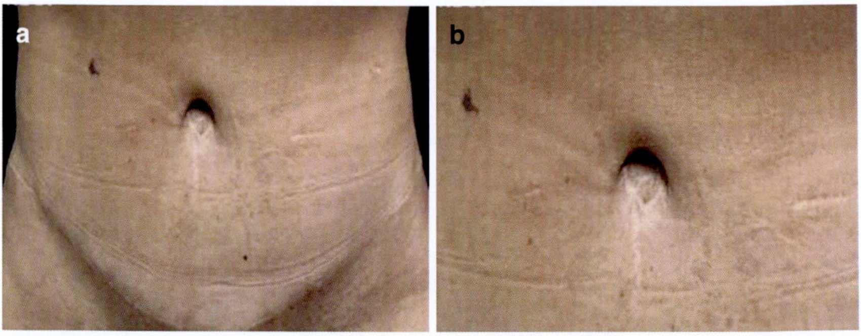

Fig. 13.12 (**a**) Case 03. (**b**) Case 03 (enlarged look of the neo-navel)

Fig. 13.13 Case 04 (enlarged look of the neo-navel)

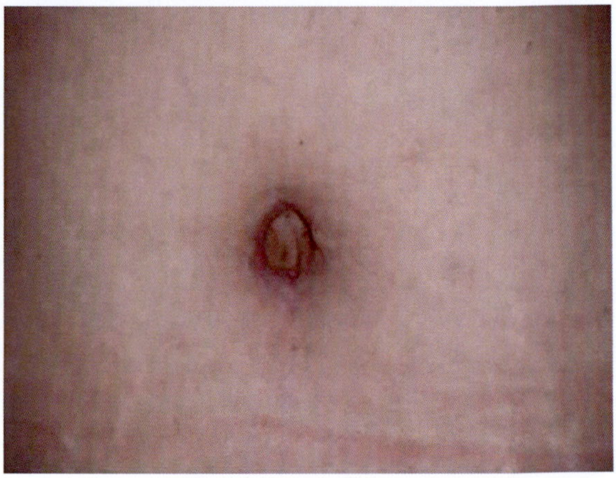

Fig. 13.14 Case 05 (enlarged look of the neo-navel)

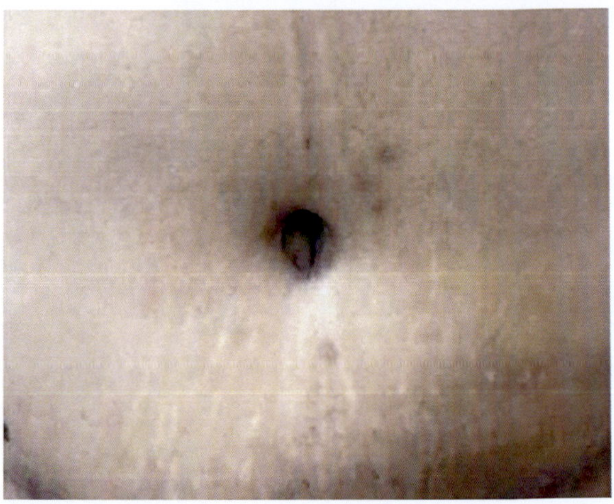

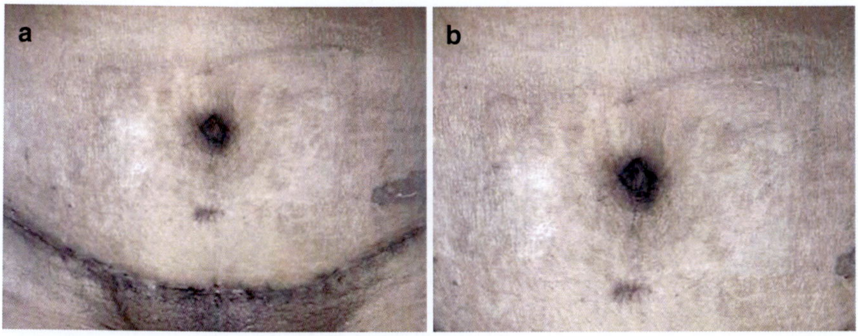

Fig. 13.15 (**a**) Case 06. (**b**) Case 06 (enlarged look of the neo-navel)

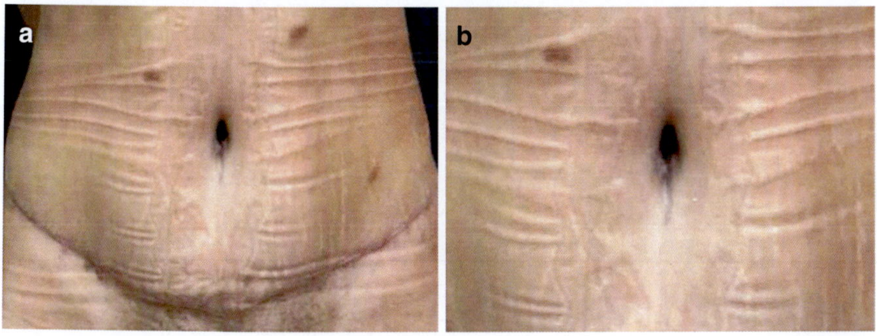

Fig. 13.16 (**a**) Case 07. (**b**) Case 07 (enlarged look of the neo-navel)

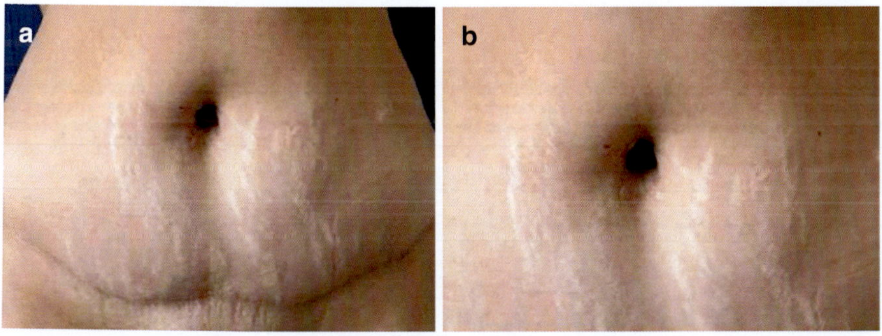

Fig. 13.17 (**a**) Case 08. (**b**) Case 08 (enlarged look of the neo-navel)

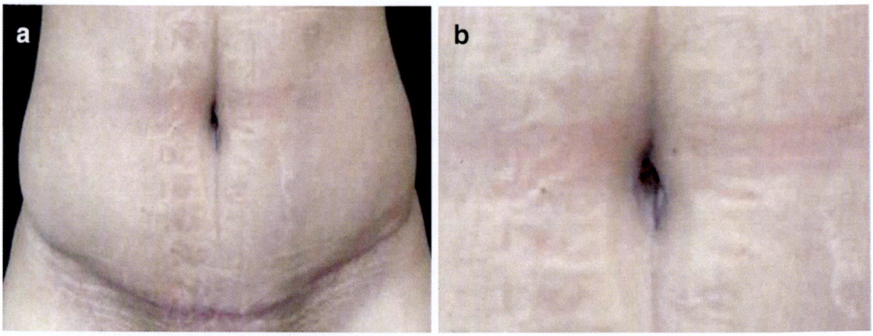

Fig. 13.18 (**a**) Case 09. (**b**) Case 09 (enlarged look of the neo-navel

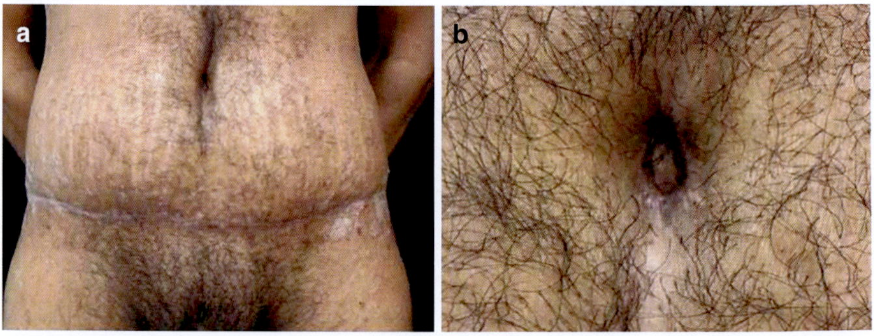

Fig. 13.19 (**a**) Case 10. (**b**) Case 10 (enlarged look of the neo-navel)

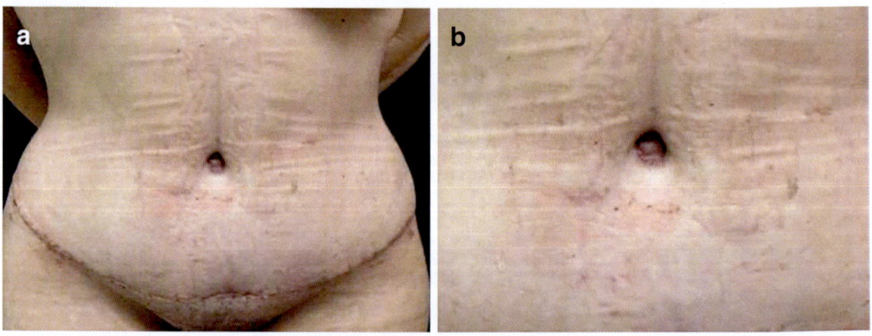

Fig. 13.20 (**a**) Case 11. (**b**) Case 11 (enlarged look of the neo-navel)

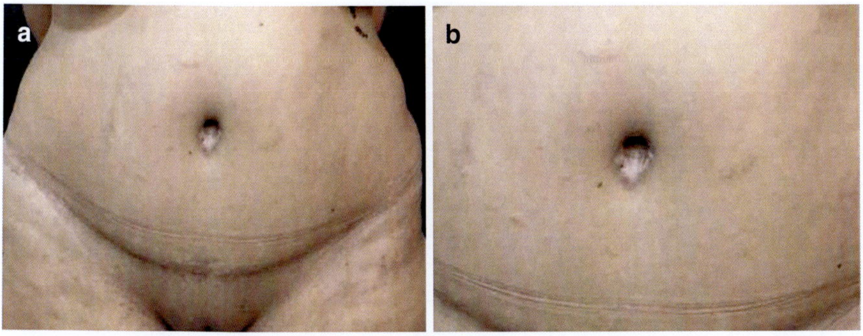

Fig. 13.21 (**a**) Case 12. (**b**) Case 12 (enlarged look of the neo-navel)

Fig. 13.22 Case 13 (enlarged look of the neo-navel)

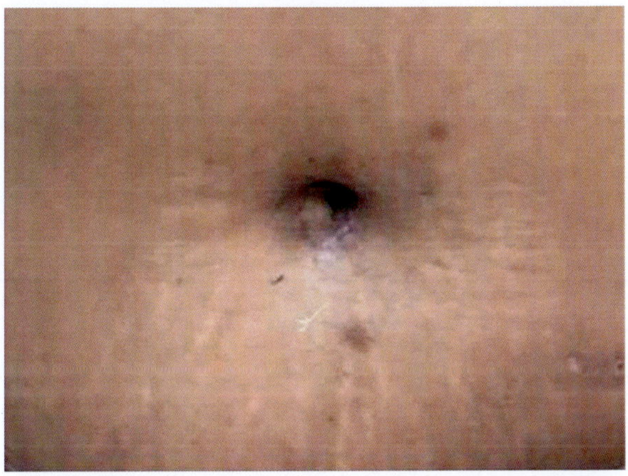

Fig. 13.23 Case 14 (enlarged look of the neo-navel)

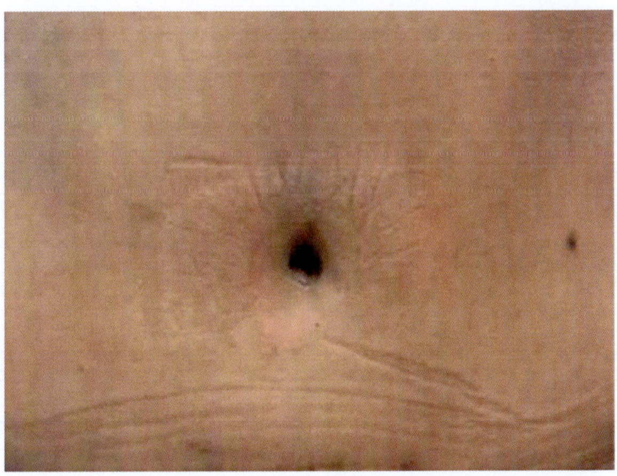

Fig. 13.24 Case 15 (enlarged look of the neo-navel)

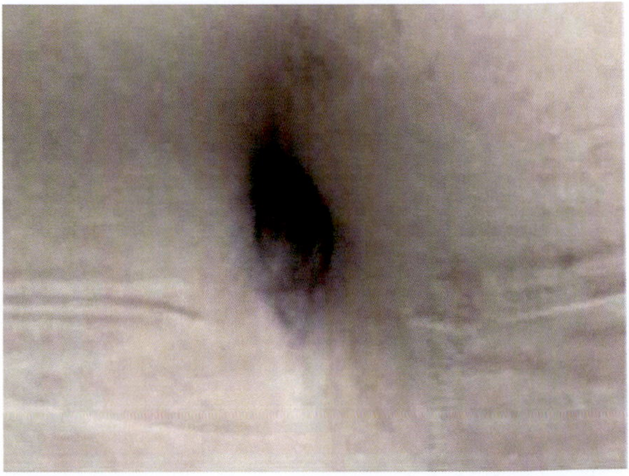

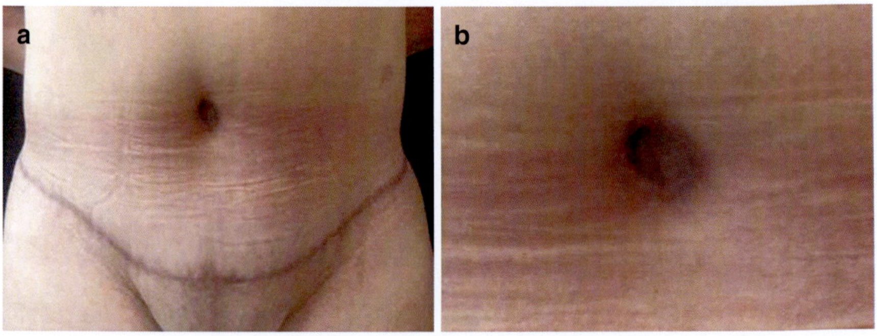

Fig. 13.25 (**a**) Case 16. (**b**) Case 16 (enlarged look of the neo-navel)

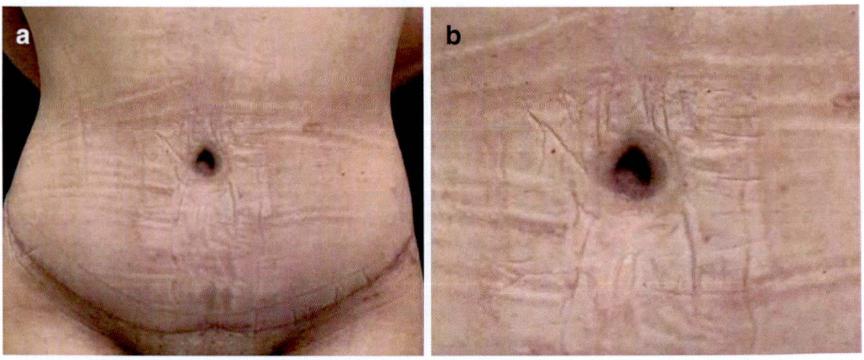

Fig. 13.26 (**a**) Case 17. (**b**) Case 17 (enlarged look of the neo-navel)

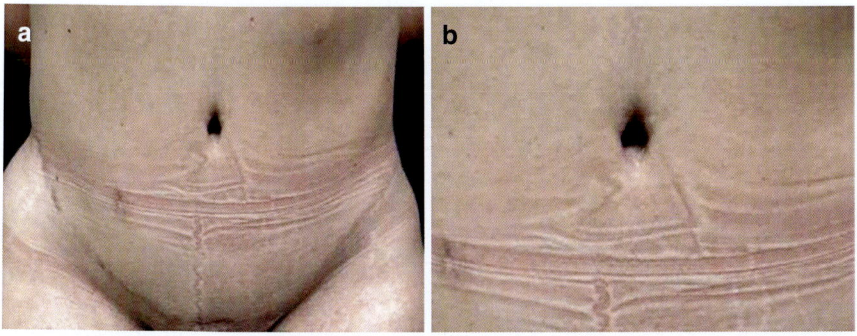

Fig. 13.27 (a) Case 18. (b) Case 18 (enlarged look of the neo-navel)

Results

During the postoperative period, patients were followed up with weekly outpatient visits.

All complications related to healing of the umbilical region during the study were recorded in the medical records (Table 13.1).

During the 6-month postoperative review consultation, each patient received a questionnaire to be answered outside the consultation, being returned to another surgeon in the team without identification, in order to avoid the partiality of the answers, informing, through this, their opinions about different aspects of the neo-navel. Regarding the questionnaire answered by the patients at the 6-month review visit, the shape of the neo-navel was classified as "Very satisfied" by 30 (100%) patients. The position of the navel was another evaluated characteristic, receiving as a classification "Very satisfied" by 30 (100%) patients. In relation to the general aspect, 24 (100%) patients opined as "Very satisfied," and another 6 (20%) opined as "Satisfied."

The aspects addressed in the questionnaire and the classification given to them by the patients themselves are shown in Table 13.2.

The 10 to 27 pictures illustrate some results of our series in which the lozenge omphaloplasty technique was used in horizontal abdominal dermolipectomies. Photos were taken by the author during the 6-month post-surgery review visit.

Table 13.1 Complications related to the umbilical region healing during the study

Dehiscence (total/partial)	0 (0%)
Wound infection	0 (0%)
Cutaneous necrosis	0 (0%)
Enlarged scar	1 (3.3%)
Keloid scar	0 (0%)
Hypertrophic scar	6 (20%)
Scar stenosis	0 (0%)

Table 13.2 Patient satisfaction questionnaire with the new navel

	Very satisfied	Satisfied	Indifferent	Unsatisfied
Shape	30 (100%)	0 (0%)	0 (0%)	0 (0%)
Position	30 (100%)	0 (0%)	0 (0%)	0 (0%)
General aspect	24 (80%)	6 (20%)	0 (0%)	0 (0%)

Discussion

Despite considerable advances in omphaloplasty techniques, we noticed that the scars generated are often still stigmatizing, compromising the result of abdominoplasty. In order to achieve natural results in this surgery, it is important that the new navel transmits an appearance similar to the original anatomy, with minimal visible scars and without stenosis (Furtado 2011). As described in the literature, this anatomy comprises a rounded or slightly elongated shape in the vertical direction, with a mean diameter of 1.2 to 1.8 cm, and variable depth depending on the thickness of the adipose tissue of the abdomen. Its position is in the midline, at a height that varies from 4 cm above to 2 cm below the horizontal line that passes through the anterosuperior iliac spines (Jaimovich et al. 1999; Ng 2010).

The technique presented is intended to reproduce these anatomical characteristics, using them in the vertical lozenge incision, in the release of the umbilical scar as in the skin-fat flap, in addition to the fixation of the umbilical stump 0.5 cm away from the skin to the aponeurosis so that the neo-navel has natural depth (Avelar 2016). In the studied series, this technique produced results with characteristics similar to those mentioned above.

Although the pathophysiology of hypertrophic scars has not yet been fully elucidated, the genetic factor is relevant and prevents its complete prevention (Lorenz and Sina Bari 2012). This explains the appearance of hypertrophic scars in six cases, as shown in Figs. 13.10, 13.13, 13.18, 13.22, 13.23, and 13.25. However, no cases of umbilical stenosis were identified among them. We attribute this fact to the fact that the diamond technique follows the idea of broken incisions proposed by Avelar (1979), reducing the incidence of stenosis resulting from circular incisions (Baroudi and Carvalho 1981).

The case shown in Fig. 13.21 was the only one in which lines of enlarged scars were identified in the umbilical region.

Some authors include in their techniques the degreasing of the abdominal wall around the navel for more natural results (Castro et al. 2014). In the described technique, lipectomy is also adopted and occurs under direct vision and in a controlled manner, with easy access to posterior hemostasis. This step contributes to reducing the tension in the scars, in addition to forming a depression in the abdomen in the umbilical region, which simulates the umbilical groove and gives the abdomen a natural appearance.

Furthermore, in a teaching service, involved in the training practice of plastic surgeons by residents, it is essential to routinely adopt a technique that is simple to perform, has well-defined steps, and can be transmitted in a didactic way, with a low incidence of postoperative complications, to facilitate learning and for all results to have a high-quality standard.

Skin healing is a known process. It is divided into three phases, which overlap and can last from 6 months to a year: inflammatory phase, proliferative phase, and maturation phase (Mélega et al. 2000). Based on this, this study involved the evaluation of scars in the sixth postoperative month.

For the evaluation of scars in general, subjective assessment scales, which are non-invasive and easy to handle, are considered clinically more useful. There are currently five scar assessment scales that use subjective parameters in an objective way: Vancouver Scar Scale (VSS), Manchester Scar Scale (MSS), Patient and Observer Scar Assessment Scale (POSAS), Visual Analogue Scale (VAS), and Stony Brook Scar Evaluation Scale (SBSES) (Fearmonti et al. 2010). However, these scales are more appropriate for comparative assessments or for the analysis of clinical results after a specific intervention for the scar treatment (Durani et al. 2009). In this study, we chose to use a method that enabled the assessment of the umbilical scar specifically, covering all its aspects.

These questionnaires were given to each patient during the 6-month postoperative review appointments to be answered in private. In this way, we avoided that patients' responses were influenced by their possible embarrassment for being in the presence of their surgeon. Returning the questionnaires without identification avoided the measurement bias by the author.

Although the evaluation of patients' satisfaction with the results of their surgeries is subjective and related to the expectations of each one of them, through the questionnaire used in this study, it was possible to obtain, in a simple and objective way, data which reflect that the technique used produced results that considerably pleased all patients involved in the study. When analyzing the questionnaires, we considered that the "Satisfied" classification given by six patients for the general appearance of the neo-navel is due to the fact that they are the same ones that evolved with hypertrophic scars, influencing the final result in these cases.

Conclusion

The lozenge omphaloplasty technique in abdominal dermolipectomy proved to be simple to perform and easy to learn, with a low incidence of postoperative complications, without cases of umbilical stenosis and with a high degree of patient satisfaction.

Appendix

Appendix 13.1 Study patient group characteristics

Age (years)	28–42	35 (media)
IMC (kg/m^2) in the surgery day	25.46–29.22	27.34 (media)
Gender	Women 28	Men 2
Previous bariatric surgery	Yes 18 (60%)	No 12 (40%)

References

Furtado IR. Onfaloplastia: técnica "infinito". Rev Bras Cir Plást. 2011;26(2):298–301
Jaimovich CA, Parra JFN, Pitanguy I. Semiologia da parede abdominal: seu valor no planejamento das abdominoplastias. Rev Soc Bras Cir Plást. 1999;14(3):21–50.
Ng JAA. Abdominoplastia: neo-onfaloplastia sem cicatriz e sem excisro de gordura. Rev Bras Cir Pl6st. 2010;25(3):499–503. DOI: https://doi.org/10.1590/S1983-51752010000300017
Avelar J. Creation of the new umbilicus: my technique on abdominoplasty and further applications. In: Avelar J, ed. New concepts on abdominoplasty and further applications. Switzerland: Springer International Publishing. 2016; p. 107–26
Lorenz P, Sina Bari A. Scar Prevention, treatment, and revision. In: Neligan PC, ed. Plastic Surgery. 3rd ed. Volume 1. Philadelphia: Elsevier Saunders; 2012. p. 297–318.
Avelar J. Cicatriz umbilical da sua importância e da técnica de confecção nas abdominoplastias. Rev Bras Cir. 1979;69(1–2) 41–52.
Baroudi R, Carvalho C. Neoumbilicoplastias. Um procedimiento ecletico em el transcurso de las abdominoplastias. Cir Plast Iberolatinoam. 1981;7(4) 391–401.
Castro DPR, Saldanha OR, Pinto EBS, Albuquerque FM, Moia SMS. Avaliação estética da cicatriz umbilical em duas técnicas de onfaloplastia. Rev Bras Cir Plást. 2014; 29(2):248–52
Mélega, J.; Viterbo, F. and Mendes, F. (2000). Cirurgia plástica. 1st ed. Grupo Gen - Guanabara Koogan.
Fearmonti R, Bond J, Erdmann D, Levinson H. A review of scar scales and scar measuring devices. Eplasty. 2010;10:e43.
Durani P, McGrouther DA, Ferguson MW. Current scales for assessing human scarring: a review. J Plast Reconstr Aesthet Surg. 2009;62(6):713–20. PMID: 19303834 DOI: https://doi.org/10.1016/j.bjps.2009.01.080

Further Reading

Silva Júnior V, Sousa FRS. Improvement on the neo-umbilicoplasty technique and review of the literature. Aesthetic Plast Surg. 2017;41(3):600–7. DOI: https://doi.org/10.1007/s00266-017-0847-6
Fantozzi F. Applications of anthropometry in torsoplastic surgery. Eur J Plast Surg. 2013;36:519–26. https://doi.org/10.1007/s00238-013-0854-z
Villegas FJ. A novel approach to abdominoplasty: TULUA modifications (transverse plication, no undermining, full liposuction, neoumbilicoplasty, and low transverse abdominal scar). Aesthetic Plast Surg. 2014;38(3):511–20. DOI: https://doi.org/10.1007/s00266-014-0304-8
Furtado IR, Nogueira CH, Lima Junior EM. Cirurgia plástica após a gastroplastia redutor: planejamento das cirurgias e técnicas. Rev Soc Bras Cir Plást. 2004;19(2):35–40
Rohrich RJ, Sorokin ES, Brown SA, Gibby DL. Is the umbilicus truly midline? Clinical and medicolegal implications. Plast Reconstr Surg. 2003;112(1):259–63. DOI: https://doi.org/10.1097/01.PRS.0000066367.41067.C2

D'Assumpção EA. Técnica Para Umbilicoplastia, Evitando-se um dos Principais Estigmas das Abdominoplastias. Rev Bras Cir Plást. 2005;20(3):160–6.
D'Assumpção EA. Complicações locais em abdominoplastias. Rev Bras Cir. 2002;92:21–8.
SchoellerT,WechselbergerG,OttoA,RainerC,SchwabeggerA,LilleS,etal.Newtechniqueforscarless umbilical reinsertion in abdominoplasty procedures. Plast Reconstr Surg. 1998;102(5):1720–3. PMID: 9774037 DOI:https://doi.org/10.1097/00006534-199810000-00064
Dias Filho AV, Valadão MGC, Guerra Filho TR, Moura RMG. Onfaloplastia: estudo comparativo de técnicas. Rev Bras Cir Plást. 2014;29(2):253–8
Avelar J. Abdominoplasty-Systematization of a technique without external umbilical scar. Aesthetic Plast Surg. 1978;2 (1):141–51. DOI: https://doi.org/10.1007/BF01577947
Mello DF, Yoshino H. Plicatura da base umbilical: proposta técnica para tratar protrusões e evitar estigmas pósabdominoplastia. Rev Bras Cir Plást. 2009;24(4):525–9.
Dogan T. Umbilicoplasty in abdominoplasty: a new approach. Ann Plast Surg. 2010;64(6):718–21. PMID: 20407366 DOI: https://doi.org/10.1097/SAP.b013e3181b02210
Lee MJ, Mustoe TA. Simplified technique for creating a youthful umbilicus in abdominoplasty. Plast Reconstr Surg. 2002;109(6):2136–40. DOI: https://doi.org/10.1097/00006534-200205000-00054
Del Toro, D.; Dedhia, R.; Tollefson, T.T. Advances in scar management: prevention and management of hypertrophic scars and keloids. *Curr Opin Otolaryngol Head Neck Surg.*, 2016 Aug; 24(4): 322–9.

Chapter 14
The Excision-Suture Tactic: A Quick and Low Bleeding Option for Tissue Resection

Ithamar Nogueira Stocchero, Gustavo Flosi Stocchero, Guilherme Flosi Stocchero, and Alexandre Siqueira Franco Fonseca

Abstract This tactic, which has been used for years, is aimed toward patients who present with skin laxity and, for various reasons, will greatly benefit from shorter surgical times. It is widely used in post-bariatric patients, being very useful for patients who do not object to having their issues addressed in steps, one at a time, often under local anesthesia.

Surgical technique: it involves precise marking of the skin, or skin/subcutaneous fat, to be removed. It is an unusual tactic, since the surgeon who incises is not the same who sutures, thus eliminating the step of changing positions. Both acts take place sequentially, which makes the end of the excision step almost coinciding with the end of the suture step.

Discussion: the greatest advantage offered by this option is to enable surgeries which would otherwise be more invasive, with greater risks of major bleeding and longer surgical time. Moreover, since this technique requires less complexity in operating room infrastructure, it may increase the job market, thus being a good alternative to be offered to patients.

Conclusion: when well-indicated, it is a great option for excess skin removal, provided that patients be well aware of what is proposed. This tactic permits convenient, frequently outpatient procedures that may offer fast recovery.

Keywords Quick suture · Quick tissue resection · Hemostatic suture · Post-bariatric surgery · Skin laxity correction

I. N. Stocchero (✉) · G. F. Stocchero · G. F. Stocchero · A. S. F. Fonseca
Centro Médico Viver Melhor, São Paulo, Brazil
e-mail: dr.ithamar@vivermelhor.com.br; gustavo@vivermelhor.com.br; guilherme@vivermelhor.com.br; dr.alexandre@vivermelhor.com.br

J. M. Avelar, R. Cavalcanti Ribeiro (eds.), *Body Contouring*,
https://doi.org/10.1007/978-3-031-42802-9_14

Introduction

The quest for excellence should guide all medical practice. However, in its own essence, medical practice involves recognizing its limitations, which can be translated in the famous saying “to cure sometimes, to relieve often, and to comfort always.” These words perfectly reflect our incapacities, which become evident according to the difficulty levels that we all face before the adversities of a period of time.

Sometimes, excellence lies within doing whatever is possible in the light of the present situation, always respecting the limits of the surgeon, the patient’s conditions, and the feasible techniques.

What the tactic herein presented aims is to expand the range of treatment options for patients whose health condition, lack of access to more complex care units, or lack of time or financial resources may all prevent them from getting more invasive procedures.

Undergoing a series of smaller, quicker surgeries in order to achieve acceptable results is better than having nothing at all.

The idea of this tactic first appeared in hair follicle harvesting for hair transplantation (Stocchero 2003). Since the scalp is prone to copious bleeding, the double act of resection and suture done by the same surgeon demands a counterproductive additional maneuver. If immediate suturing is performed right after incision, a precious amount of time is saved, which leads to lesser bleeding and a shorter surgical time.

Current Concepts

Obesity has become a major public health issue in the modern era. Due to its implications in morbidity, in the well-being of the population, and also for aesthetic reasons, it became the target of several therapies, such as specific medications, diets, exercise, and weight loss clinics, and, nowadays, with the great number of patients undergoing various types of bariatric surgeries, results have frequently become excellent.

The number of people who came to benefit from massive weight loss has resulted in patients who have recovered their health and their desire to live and to engage in communal activities and to live a life that is full. These people come from different levels, either related to their ambitions, their socioeconomic status, their moments of life, and even their health condition.

These patients present with a wide range of skin laxity, which may be present all over their bodies or only in certain areas, depending on their genetic characteristics, their age group, the type of obesity treatment, history of pregnancy, degree of weight loss, etc.—a myriad of possibilities.

Besides skin laxity, it is important to address the level of discomfort that each patient is experiencing. It may range from the absence of complaints up to severe depression. Within this array of situations, which sometimes is thin ice, it is the plastic surgeon's duty to perceive what is the best option for each patient. Success will come as a result of the level of satisfaction achieved, and not necessarily from the refinement of the technique employed.

Indications

Every time that a shorter surgical time and low bleeding are more important factors than technical refinement

For example, patients with low hemoglobin levels are excellent candidates.

There are also those who want a "one morning surgery," which may allow them to keep with their usual routine without the need for work leaves.

The tactic presented herein is not intended to compete with the traditional, renowned techniques used to address the well-known challenge of severe skin laxity, which results from massive weight loss. It is, in fact, an addition to those techniques, since it may be the necessary indication for the progressive correction of large areas of redundant skin throughout a body, which has often lost half of its weight and volume.

Its execution is reserved for linear resections, as this tactic is not adequate for contouring procedures with curved incisions. However, linear resections comprise most of the necessary surgical interventions for these patients, for example:

- Upper limbs: medial aspect of arms, dorsal aspect of wrists
- Dorsum: transverse torsoplasty, lateral excess skin
- Abdomen: vertical, transverse, or fleur-de-lis abdominoplasty
- Lower limbs: medial and lateral aspect of thighs, excess skin over the knees

Surgical Technique

Skin marking deserves special attention, since it will define the whole course of the procedure. Special care should be taken when using bimanual grasp of excess skin, since it will make all the difference in the result; in order to achieve the best aesthetically possible results, preoperative markings must be strictly followed during surgery (Figs. 14.1 and 14.2).

It is an unusual procedure, since the surgeon who incises is not the same who sutures. Practicing team synchronism is very important to obtain the desired result, because the excision-suture is a continuous act that requires full attention during the whole procedure.

There are two options for its execution:

1. Using horizontal mattress sutures, with relatively long passes of the needle, and placed close to the borders of the markings; a Reverdin needle may be useful in

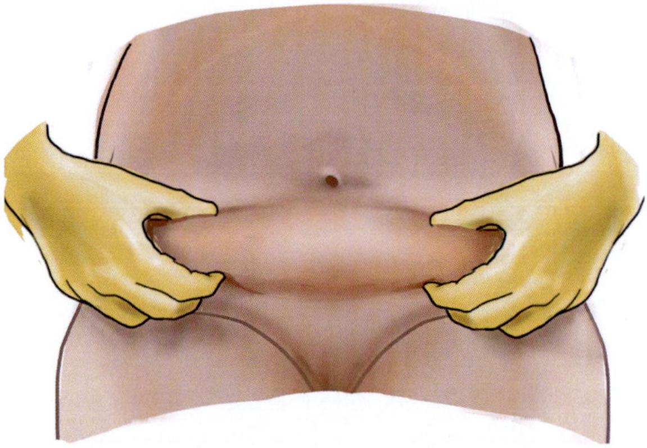

Fig. 14.1 Measuring the dermal-fat fold

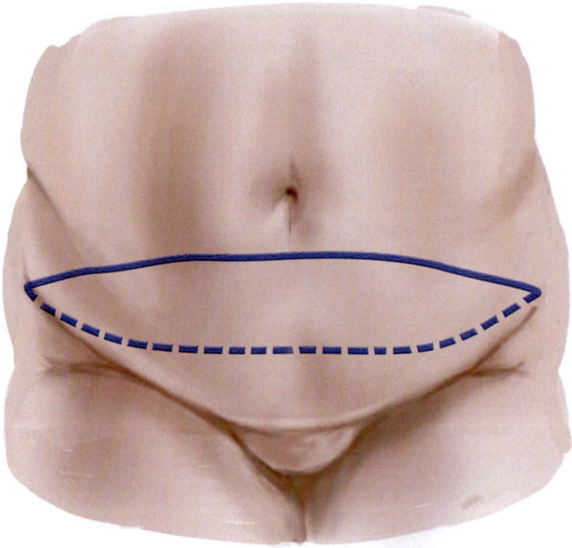

Fig. 14.2 Marking the dermal-fat fold

this step when the skin-subcutaneous fat fold is thicker (Fig. 14.3). This type of suture offers the advantage of lesser bleeding and tension during the excision-suture. Sutures may occasionally be left for 2 days, in cases where additional skin tension was produced, so that sutures may aid cutaneous expansion (Figs. 14.4 and 14.5).

2. Resection and suture without approximation sutures, which is well-indicated in cases with severe skin laxity (Figs. 14.6 and 14.7). If there is concern about skin tension, bolster sutures may be used in one of the wound edges, after anchoring the sutures to the dermis of the opposite edge; these sutures will be removed on the third postoperative day (Fig. 14.8).

When the tissue to be removed is quite thin, we will perform an essentially cutaneous excision, which is easy to work with. However, there are occasions when the

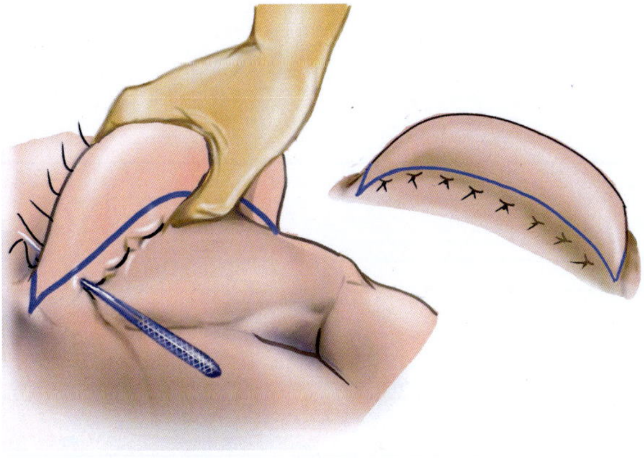

Fig. 14.3 Passing the horizontal mattress sutures and final aspect

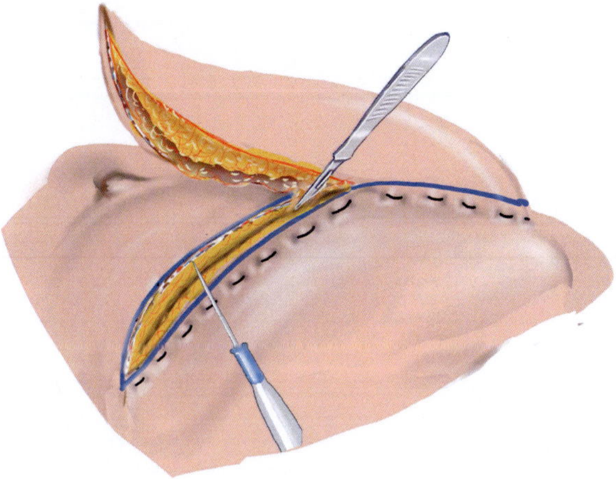

Fig. 14.4 Cauterization during the excision-suture with the horizontal mattress sutures

demarcated area of resection involves a certain amount of fat. It is advisable to use approximation sutures and suction excess fat right above the sutures, within the area to be incised and sutured (Fig. 14.9). Time should not be wasted on suctioning the entire flap, as it will be resected. It is enough to suction the base of the flap.

The sequence is the surgeon incises; if necessary, vessel cauterization is performed; and then the assistant surgeon sutures. In that manner, when the excision is completed, the closure will be practically finished.

Regarding the suture, there are situations in which agility is especially important (e.g., patients with hypertension, diabetes, or low hemoglobin levels). In such cases, a running mattress suture may be used while planning a future aesthetic revision when those health conditions are better controlled. This is a good option, especially after larger resections. Whenever possible, performing a running subcuticular suture will already yield a better result, combined with taping of the incisions, which will promote greater approximation of wound edges. Deep dermal sutures and staples are also an option (Figs. 14.10 and 14.11).

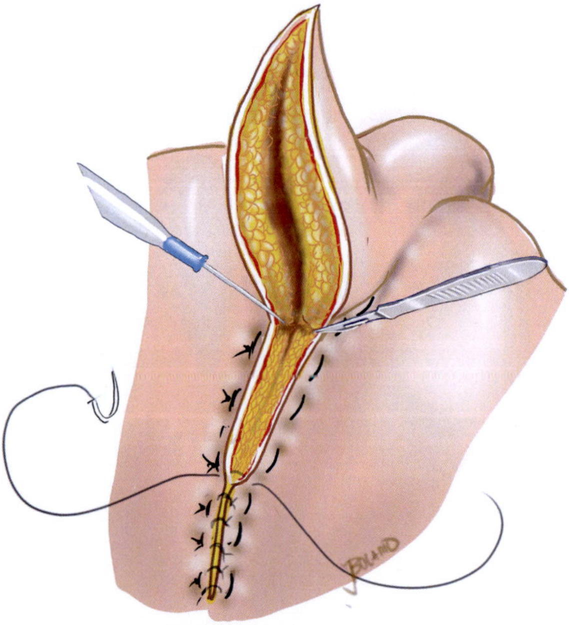

Fig. 14.5 Excision-suture with the horizontal mattress sutures

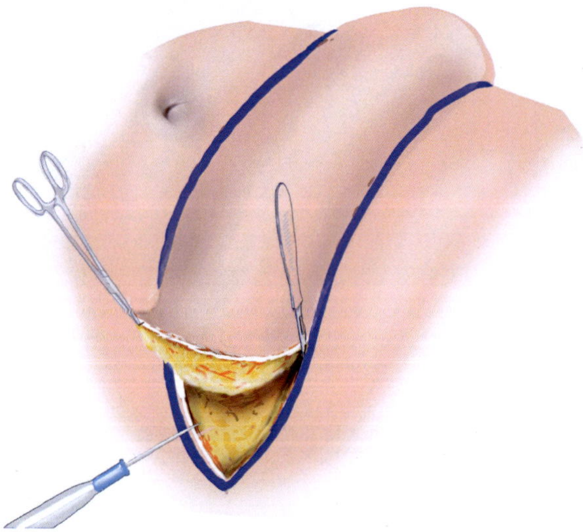

Fig. 14.6 Starting the excision-suture without the horizontal mattress sutures

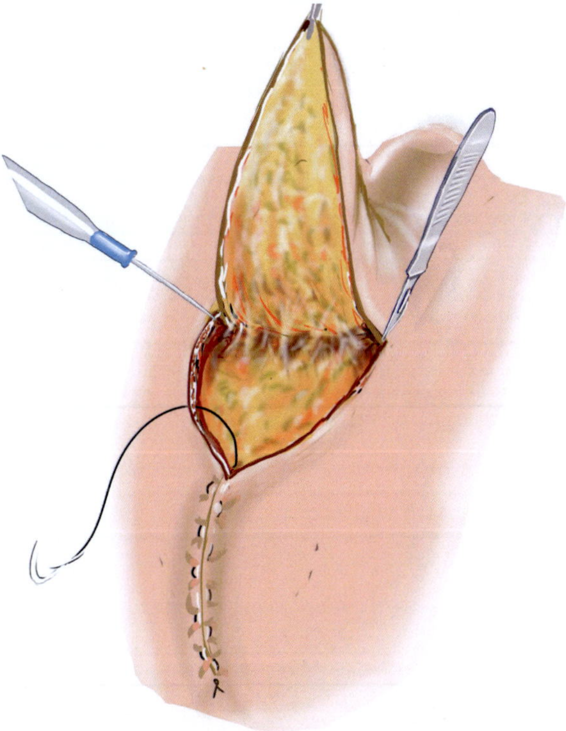

Fig. 14.7 Progression of the excision-suture without the horizontal mattress sutures

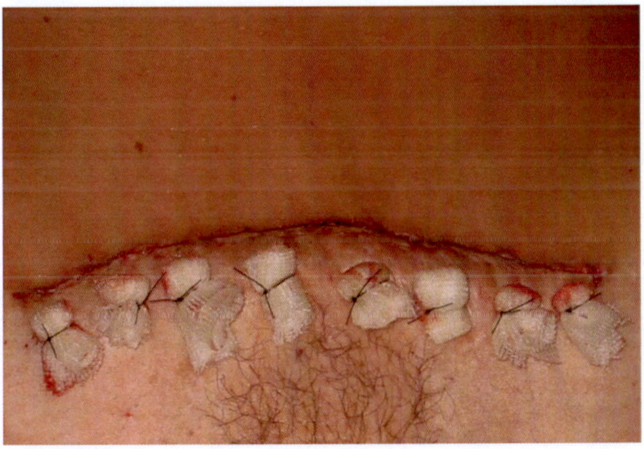

Fig. 14.8 Bolster sutures

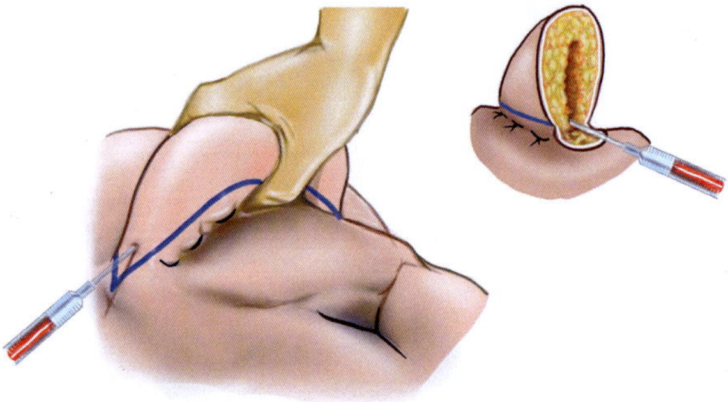

Fig. 14.9 Liposuction of the base of the flap

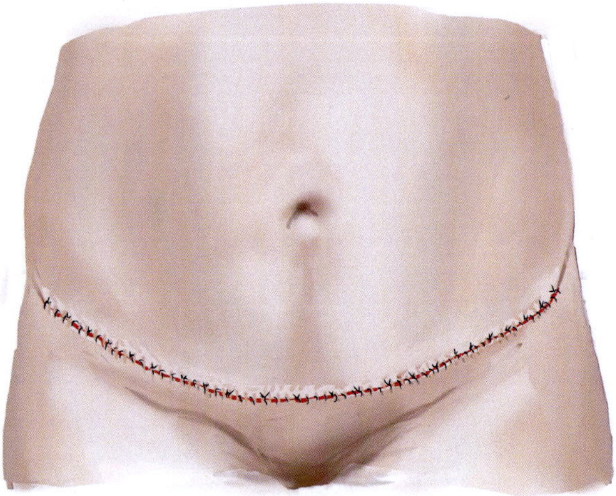

Fig. 14.10 Final aspect of the lower abdomen suture

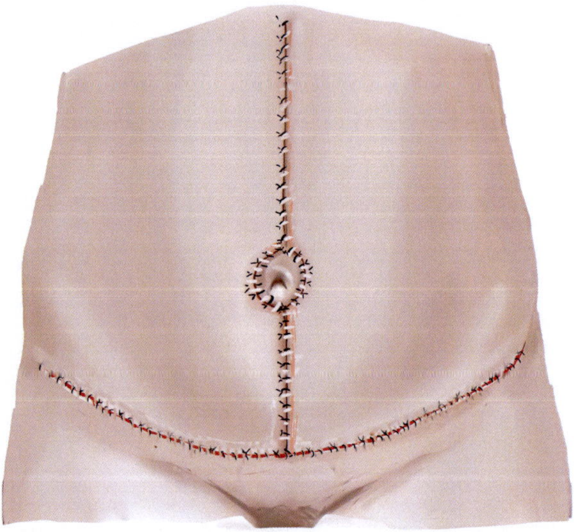

Fig. 14.11 Final aspect of the fleur-de-lis suture (diagram)

Results

Usually, results are very well accepted by patients who were adequately oriented in the preoperative consultations. In fact, results leave nothing to be desired when surgical planning was careful.

Case presented: a 54-year-old woman with hypertension, diabetes, obesity, breathing difficulties, abnormal gait, and a history of blood transfusion due to an ovarian tumor. She underwent oophorectomy combined with fleur-de-lis abdominoplasty, in which the excision-suture tactic was employed. Total surgical time, including a 7-kg monoblock resection of the surgical specimen, was 1 h and 40 min (Figs. 14.12 and 14.13).

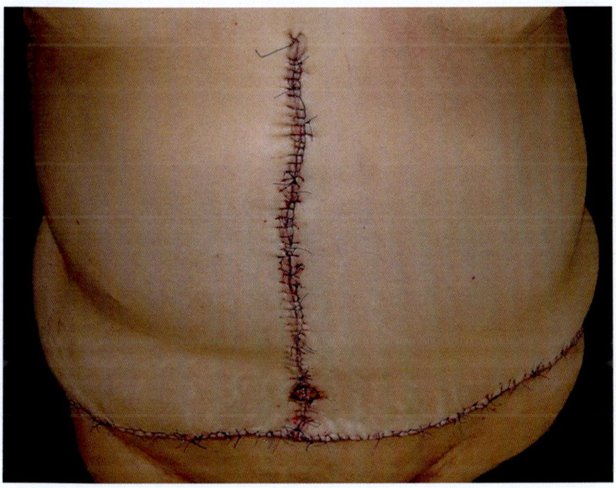

Fig. 14.12 Final aspect of the fleur-de-lis suture

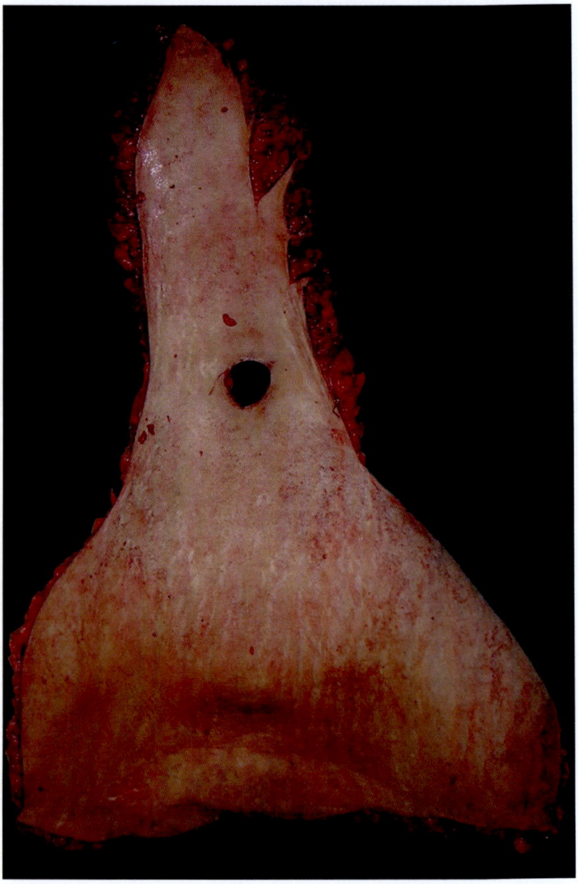

Fig. 14.13 Surgical specimen weighing 7 kg and measuring 70 × 50 cm

Complications

The most frequent complication is epidermolysis. Some small wound dehiscence may occur. Rarely, superficial ecchymosis in minimal areas may appear (Fig. 14.14).

Discussion

This hybrid manner of operating was conceived to save surgical time and to reduce bleeding. These are the prerequisites for its indication.

It is also fundamental to not expect refined remodeling in breast surgeries, nor use the technique with great undermining of tissues, since both these situations call for traditional, more complex techniques.

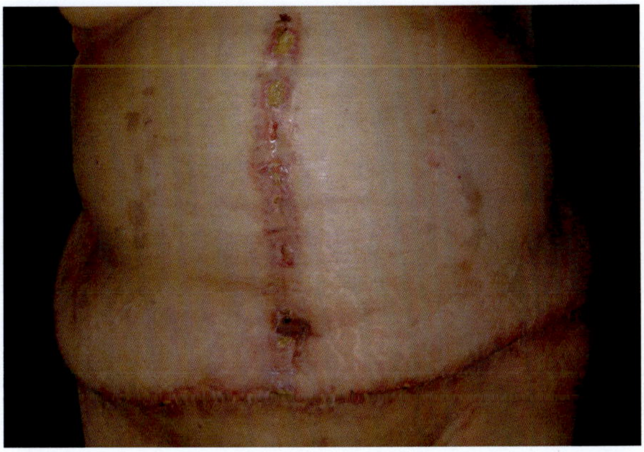

Fig. 14.14 Fleur-de-lis suture, 30 days PO

However, with correct training and engagement of the surgical team, excellent results may be achieved, which will expand the job market with these procedures as part of the range of options.

Key Points of the Chapter

Adequate indication for the surgery. Knowing that the patient has had the necessary level of understanding and clarification, especially when the primary objective of the procedure is aesthetic

In cases where indication for the surgery was based on health needs, it is always easier for the patient to accept a revision surgery at a later stage.

Tips for Better Results

Make the patient a partner in the quest for the best possible result.

Whenever possible, wait for the best time to perform the surgery, for example, until an additional weight loss may be achieved.

Be safe and honest when proposing the procedure. Make sure that all information was clarified and understood by the patient.

Reference

Stocchero IN (2003) The Ex-suture: a nonbleeding excision for hair transplantation, Plast Reconstr Surg; 111(5):1176.

Part III
Behavior of Breast Surgery Improving Body Contouring

Chapter 15
Reduction Mammoplasty with Lower Pedicle

Ricardo Cavalcanti Ribeiro, Aline Guimarães Gomes de Sousa, and Luis Fernandez de Córdova

Abstract Reducing mammoplasty with the use of an areolate lower pedicle is among the current techniques of breast reduction and, when well indicated, offers incalculable benefits for both the patient and the surgeon, due to the reduction of complications. The technique basically consists in the preparation of a dermo-adipose inferior pedicle flap containing the areola-papillary complex (CAP) to maintain its vascularization, therefore being considered a technique of choice in the treatment of large gigantomastias or mammary hypertrophy. Postoperative care is not very different from the guidelines given to patients submitted to other reduction mammoplasty techniques. Different studies have shown that there are no significant differences between reducing mammoplasty by other techniques and mammoplasty with lower pedicle elaboration, in terms of complications such as hematoma, seroma, necrosis, and infections. The authors indicate the technique mainly in young patients with reproductive expectations after surgery, due to the conservation of the glandular anatomy and the preservation of its continuity with the CAP.

Keywords Breast reduction · Lower pedicle · Breast hypertrophy · Gigantomastia

R. C. Ribeiro (✉)
Plastic and Reconstructive Surgery, Federal University of the State of Rio de Janeiro, Rio de Janeiro, Brazil
e-mail: rribeiro@centroin.net.br

A. G. G. de Sousa
Division of Plastic and Reconstructive Surgery, Casa de Portugal, Rio de Janeiro, Brazil

L. F. de Córdova
Carlos Chagas Institute, Rio de Janeiro, Brazil

Division of Plastic and Reconstructive, Surgery Global Plastic Surgery State of México, México

J. M. Avelar, R. Cavalcanti Ribeiro (eds.), *Body Contouring*,
https://doi.org/10.1007/978-3-031-42802-9_15

Synopsis

Reducing mammoplasty with the use of an areolate lower pedicle is among the current techniques of breast reduction and, when well indicated, offers incalculable benefits for both the patient and the surgeon, due to the reduction of complications. The technique basically consists in the preparation of a dermo-adipose inferior pedicle flap containing the nipple-areola complex (NAC) to maintain its vascularization, therefore being considered a technique of choice in the treatment of large gigantomastias or mammary hypertrophy. Postoperative care is not very different from the guidelines given to patients submitted to other reduction mammoplasty techniques. Different studies [1–33] have shown that there are no significant differences between reducing mammoplasty by other techniques and mammoplasty with lower pedicle elaboration, in terms of complications such as hematoma, seroma, necrosis, and infections. The authors indicate the technique mainly in young patients with reproductive expectations after surgery, due to the conservation of the glandular anatomy and the preservation of its continuity with the CAP.

Surgical Indication

The areolate flap is usually indicated in hypertrophy and gigantomastia, being very useful in these patients when they present a distance between point A and the areola of 8 cm or more, sometimes reaching 20 cm. In addition, due to the consistency of the breasts, present most often, more glandular component should be suspected than fat. In this situation, the risk of vascular complications increases when superior pedicle techniques are used, mainly due to the reduction of venous return. It is notorious that some authors in the mentioned situation prefer to opt for the autograft of the CAP, which may be dispensable with the lower dermo-adipose pedicle. Thus, the viability of the complex is protected, presenting low rates of vascular impairment.

Surgical Technique

After a thorough preoperative evaluation, the patient is marked standing and explained that the resulting scar will usually be shaped like an inverted T. Later, within the demarcation, the design of the lower pedicle is made with width ranging from 7 to 10 cm, which ensures the conservation of the vessels that feed it.

The authors prefer to perform the marking with the patient awake, rather than anesthetized, due to the ease of observation of breast dynamics in various positions (Fig. 15.1).

Under general anesthesia, the patient is positioned with open arms and may remain semised or not during surgery. The procedure begins with peri-areolar

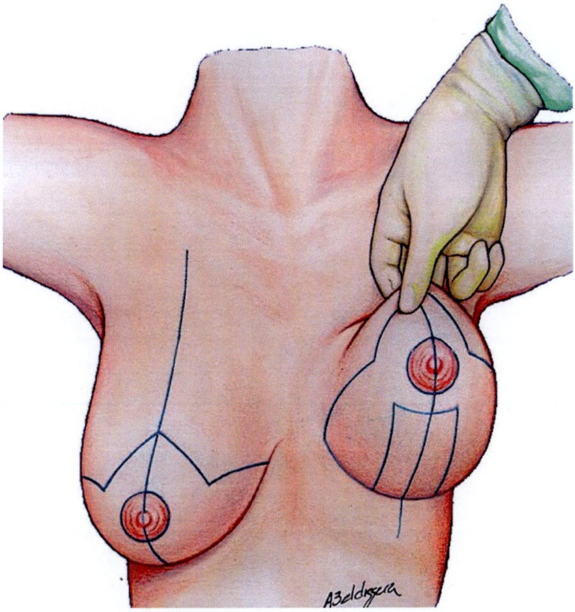

Fig. 15.1 Preoperative markings. Points A, B, and C are established and the flap is designed

decortication, as well as the entire lower cutaneous extension of the pedicle territory. A triangle-shaped upper segment formed by the AB, AC, and CB points is dissected to the muscular plane, fine-tuning the rest in the upper and lateral sectors (Fig. 15.2). This maneuver will result in exposure of the pectoralis major muscle. Once the muscle is exposed, excision of excess glandular and fatty tissue from the lower pole is performed and design of the neo-breast follows with a personalized pattern depending on each case (Fig. 15.3). Breast modeling is done through the union of the tissue that remains in the lower pedicle, partially dissected at its base in the proportion of 1:1 with equal or slightly greater width at its base. These points can be anchored to the muscle tissue of the pectoralis major, which confers stability to the flap and avoids repeated assemblies that cause more trauma to the tissues.

Finally, points A, B, and C are sutured, and the CAP is positioned with modeling and displacement of possible excess skin (Fig. 15.4). Strict control of hemostasis should be maintained to avoid hematomas or collections that may modify morphology or produce vascular compression with consequent suffering from the flap as well as from the CAP (Fig. 15.5).

The authors emphasize the use of suction drains and their maintenance until the drainage volume is less than 15 mL/day. The scar that will result in this surgery will be an inverted T, differentiating from other techniques by maintaining the late results, observing little movement of the ballast in the postoperative period.

The main disadvantage of this technique is the scar's length. Due to the width at the base of the breasts that most patients with breast hypertrophy, often

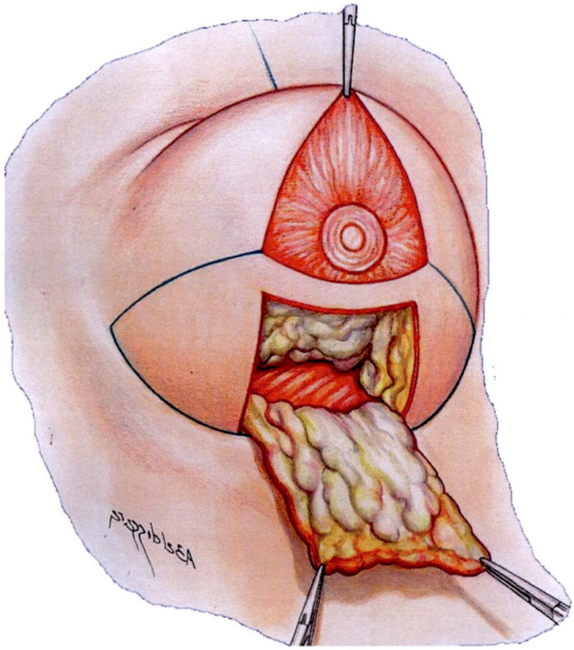

Fig. 15.2 After peri-areolar decortication, the breast is ready for excess glandular and fat tissue resection

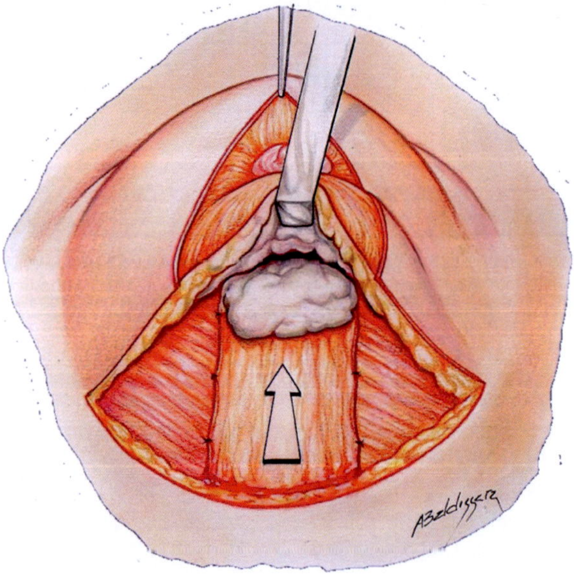

Fig. 15.3 Transoperative vision of the breast after fixation of dermal flaps in the pectoral fascia.

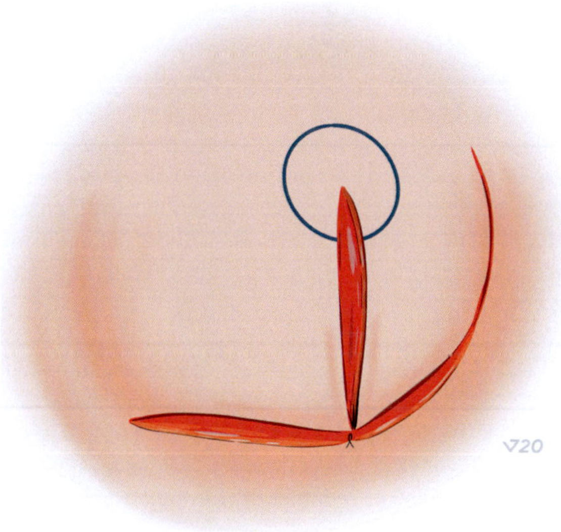

Fig. 15.4 After suturing points A, B, and C, the position of the CAP is decided and designed

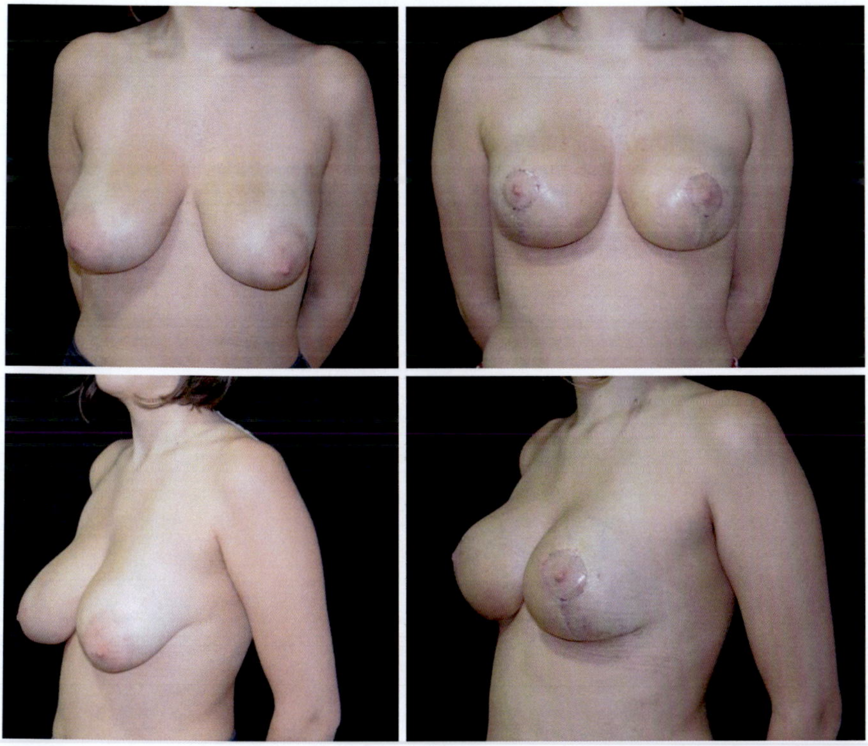

Fig. 15.5 Before and after pictures (21 days pot op)

gigantomastia, present, a reduced scar may not be an option and the aspect of the resulting scar should be taken into consideration and duiring consultation perform a cost-benefit analysis. There are refinements in this technique, as Hülya and Turmedem explain, which propose a modification consisting of the resection of a lower pedicle in pyramidal format by means of a dermal suspension technique to improve the long-term projection of the operated breast. During this refinement, the lateral dermal flaps are decorticated in the form of a triangle, as extension of the lower pedicle, and fixed on the fascia of the pectoralis major with important suspension of the pedicle, forming an internal support (inner bra), avoiding lateral displacement of the breast and a better projection, also improving the quality of the vertical scar, due to the lower tension required at the time of closure, and therefore, techniques that seek to achieve more limited scars could be justified. The authors made a modification to improve the contour of the breasts by developing a dermo-adipose flap with higher wings and removal of a dermo-adipose triangle at the junction of these with the lower pedicle (without compromising the base of the pedicle) to round the shape of the inner bra, giving more projection and stability to the dermal suspension.

This type of refinement does not increase the risks and/or complications trans- or postoperatively and has shown enormous acceptance and satisfaction on the part of patients, who seek not only to have a smaller breast but also to renew it.

Although the suspension by means of this new technique in the lower pedicle seems an ideal condition, the authors of the same state that there is no guarantee regarding the long-term suspension of the breasts, so they do not recommend it in the simple correction of ptosis, without breast reduction.

Other authors, such as Azad and Col., proposed block resection of excess breast tissue to avoid changes in the elaboration of the pedicle and ensure greater symmetry.

Postoperative Care

The authors recommend a series of postoperative care not very different from the guidelines given to patients undergoing reduction mammoplasty. In most cases, patients require hospitalization for 24–48 h. Drains are removed when the volume drained is less than 15 mL in 24 h.

Discharge is performed with specific instructions in writing and medicines for oral administration, such as an analgesic, an antibiotic for 7 days, and an anti-inflammatory for 4 days.

In general, the operated patient should not perform abduction movements with a rotational angle greater than 90° for an approximate period of 45 days, which will provide security until the scar fixation of the flap and avoid detachment of hemostatic clots that can cause late bruising. Stitches are usually removed in 12–15 days and we routinely apply micropore tape for 3–4 weeks.

Complications

Among the most frequent complications, the same as in all mammoplasty procedures, such as hematomas, seromas, fatty necrosis, partial necrosis of the CAP (usually due to technical error with section of vascularization or deep decortication of the skin), and hypertrophic or enlarged scars (in the case of excessive tension in the sutures or very heavy breasts in which the exaggerated reduction would compromise the vascularization of the flaps).

Different studies have shown that there are no significant differences between reducing mammoplasty by other techniques and mammoplasty with lower pedicle elaboration, in terms of complications such as hematoma, seroma, necrosis, and infections.

There is also no relationship between complications and the volume of the resected. However, there seems to be a direct relationship between suture dehiscence and resections greater than 1000 g in each breast, which may occur in the presence of undiagnosed subclinical infection; therefore, the incidence of this type of complication is highly limited when prophylactic antibiotic therapy is installed and maintained appropriately after surgery. Infections usually arise as a result of inadequate prophylaxis and, when they do occur, present as a severe condition with very unsatisfactory results from an aesthetic point of view. Therefore, prophylactic use of a first- or second-generation cephalosporin and its maintenance until the seventh postoperative day is recommended.

Another complication that occurs almost in a little with this type of technique and that has become the goal of several studies are the problems associated with breastfeeding after reducing mammoplasties, especially in young patients with severe hypertrophy or gigantomastia. Thus, it is currently considered in some countries as the surgical technique of choice for this type of patient.

Key points for reducing mammoplasty surgery with lower pedicle safe and successful
Adequate preoperative evaluation of the patient
Surgical indication with criteria for mammary hypertrophy or gigantomastia associated with pain or aesthetic complaints
Pre- and post-operative photographic record of the patient ALWAYS
Beware of section of vascularization or deep decortication of the skin
Care in the preparation of the lower pedicle
Prophylactic antibiotic therapy ALWAYS
Identify and treat complications early
Guidance and postoperative care

Conclusions

After more than 30 years of evolution of mammary reconstruction techniques, the use of a lower pedicle, became the technique of choice for the treatment of large gigantomastias or mammary hypertrophy. The authors indicate this technique mainly in young patients with reproductive expectations after surgery, due to the conservation of the glandular anatomy , thus avoiding the late complications associated with areola grafts used in the past and preserving lactation. These advances, together with the fact that they guarantee a lasting suspension, demonstrate the interest of current plastic surgeons in achieving a balance between the reality of the patient with this breast pathology and her aesthetic expectations, as well as maintaining their longings for personal fulfillment as having a victorious motherhood.

References

Rohrich RJ, Gosman AA, Brown SA, Tonadapu P, Foster B. Current preferences for breast reduction techniques: a survey of board-certified plastic surgeons 2002. Plast Reconstr Surg. 2004;114(7):1724–36.

Georgiade GS, Riefkohl RE, Georgiade NG. The inferior dermal-pyramidal type breast reduction: long-term evaluation. Ann Plast Surg. 1989;23(3):203–11.

Scott GR, Carson CL, Borah GL. Maximizing outcomes in breast reduction surgery: a review of 518 consecutive patients. Plast Reconstr Surg. 2005;116(6):1633–41.

Pérez-Macias JM. Long-lasting evolution of ptosis control after reduction mammaplasty using the hammock technique. Aesthetic Plast Surg. 2007;31(3):266–74.

Ribeiro L, Accorsi A Jr, Buss A, Marcal-Pessoa M. Creation and evolution of 30 years of the inferior pedicle in reduction mammaplasties. Plast Reconstr Surg. 2002;110(3):960–70.

Jurado J. Plásticas mamárias de redução baseadas em retalho dérmico vertical monopediculado. Anais XII Congresso Brasileiro de Cirurgia Plástica 1976;29.

Robbins TH. A reduction mammaplasty with the areola-nipple based on an inferior dermal pedicle. Plast Reconstr Surg. 1977;59(1):64–7.

Courtiss EH, Goldwyn RM. Reduction mammaplasty by the inferior pedicle technique. An alternative to free nipple and areola grafting for severe macromastia or extreme ptosis. Plast Reconstr Surg. 1977;59(4):500–7.

Calderon Ortega W, Arriagada Stuven J, Godoy Silanes M, Gomes SL. Anatomia y clinica de las mamoplastias de reducción según técnica del pedículo inferior. Rev Chil Cir. 1992;44(4):437–41.

Mandrekas AD, Zambacos GJ, Anastasopoulos A, Hapsas DA. Reduction mammaplasty with the inferior pedicle technique: early and late complications in 371 patients. Br J Plast Surg. 1996;49(7):442–6.

Wallace WH, Thompson WO, Smith RA, Barraza KR, Davidson SF, Thompson JT 2nd. Reduction mammaplasty using the inferior pedicle technique. Ann Plast Surg. 1998;40(3):235–40.

O'Grady KF, Thoma A, Dal Cin A. A comparison of complication rates in large and small inferior pedicle reduction mammaplasty. Plast Reconstr Surg. 2005;115(3):736–42.

Zambacos GJ, Mandrekas AD. Complication rates in inferior pedicle reduction mammaplasty. Plast Reconstr Surg. 2006;118(1):274–6.

Hunter JG, Ceydeli A. Correlation between complication rate and tissue resection volume in inferior pedicle reduction mammaplasty: A retrospective study. Aesthetic Surg J. 2006;26(2):153–6.

Nahabedian MY, Mofid MM. Viability and sensation of the nipple-areolar complex after reduction mammaplasty. Ann Plast Surg. 2002;49(1):24–32.
Pitanguy I, Salgado F, Radwansky HN. Reduções mamárias: técnicas pessoais sem descolamento cutâneo. In: Mélega JM, ed. Cirurgia plástica: fundamentos e arte. Cirurgia Estética. Rio de Janeiro: Médica e Científica; 2003. p. 477–84.
Schlenz I, Rigel S, Schemper M, Kuzbari R. Alteration of nipple and areola sensitivity by reduction mammaplasty: a prospective comparison of five techniques. Plast Reconstr Surg. 2005;115(3):743–51.
Ribeiro L. A new technique for reduction mammaplasty. Plast Reconstr Surg. 1975;55(3):330–4.
Georgiade NG, Serafin D, Morris R, Georgiade G. Reduction mammaplasty utilizing an inferior pedicle nipple-areolar flap. Ann Plast Surg. 1979;3(3):211–8.
Saldanha OR, Maloof RG, Dutra RT, Luz OAL, Saldanha Filho O, Saldanha CB. Mamaplastia redutora com implante de silicone. Rev Bras Cir Plást. 2010;25(2):317–24.
Bezerra FJF, Moura RMG, Silva Júnior VV. Mamoplastia redutora e simetrização de mama oposta em reconstrução mamária utilizando a técnica de pedículo inferior. Rev Bras Cir Plást. 2007;22(1):52–9.
Anger M, Schneider EJ, Souza CE, Nakayama LI. Mamoplastia redutora de pedículo inferior: sensibilidade aréolo-mamilar, indicações e resultados. Arq Catarin Med. 2001;30(3/4):32–7.
Souza AA, Faiwichow L, Ferreira AA, Simão TS, Pitol DN, Máximo FR. Avaliação das técnicas de mamoplastia quanto a sua influência tardia na distância do complexo areolopapilar ao sulco inframamário. Rev Bras Cir Plást. 2011;26(4):664–9.
Pacheco LMS, Pacheco AT, Batista KT. Mamoplastia redutora com pedículo medial: modificação na técnica de Skoog. Rev Bras Cir Plást. 2009;24(3):321–7.
Menderes A, Mola F, Vayvada H, Barutcu A. Evaluation of results from reduction mammaplasty: relief of symptoms and patient satisfaction. Aesthetic Plast Surg. 2005;29(2):83–7.
Arié G. Una nueva técnica de mastoplastia. Rev Latinoam Cir Plast. 1957;3(1):23–31.
Ariyan S. Reduction mammaplasty with the nipple-areola carried on a single, narrow inferior pedicle. Ann Plast Surg. 1980;5(3):167–77.
Castro CC, Salema RF, Ferreira VB, Gazola LA. Mamaplastia redutora pela técnica de pedículo dermogorduroso da base inferior. Rev Bras Cir. 1983;73(1):47–52.
Migliori MR, Muldowney JB. Breast reduction: the inferior pedicle as an axial pattern flap. Aesthet Surg J. 1997;17(1):55–7.
Castillo VMS, Hernández cmC. Incisiones mínimas para mastoplastias reductoras. Rev Cubana Cir. 2002;41(1):11–5.
Reis GMD. A técnica do pedículo de base inferior em mamaplastia redutora e mastopexia causa quistos? Rev Bras Cir Plást. 2006;21(2):73–6.
Plastic and Reconstructive Surgery, March 2003- 111 (3), page 1363.
Plastic and Reconstructive Surgery 107 (7) June 2002 page 2605

Chapter 16
Importance of Glandular and Dermoglandular Flaps for Breast Surgery

Carlos Oscar Uebel

Abstract We have many techniques for breast reduction and for mastopexies. Since Pitanguy presented his technique at the Second World Congress of IPRAS (International Plastic Reconstructive Aesthetic Surgery) in 1959 in London (Pitanguy 1959) and published his paper in 1967 in a peer-reviewed journal—the *British Journal of Plastic Surgery* (Pitanguy 1967)—many other papers appear in the literature, especially using dermoglandular flaps to enhance the volume and to fill out the upper pole of the breast. Skoog (Skoog 1971), Ribeiro (Ribeiro 1975), and Silveira Neto (Silveira Netto 1976) can be referred as introducers of this new approach. We have also started with two similar procedures that we want to discuss in this chapter—the superior glandular flap and the lateral dermoglandular rotation flap.

Introduction

We have many techniques for breast reduction and for mastopexies. Since Pitanguy presented his technique at the Second World Congress of IPRAS (International Plastic Reconstructive Aesthetic Surgery) in 1959 in London (Pitanguy 1962), and published his paper in 1967 in a peer-reviewed journal—the *British Journal of Plastic Surgery* (Pitanguy 1967)—many other papers appear in the literature, especially using dermoglandular flaps to enhance the volume and to fill out the upper pole of the breast. Skoog (Skoog 1971), Ribeiro (Ribeiro 1975), and Silveira Neto (Silveira Netto 1976)

C. O. Uebel (✉)
Division Plastic Surgery, PUCRS University, Porto Alegre, Brazil
e-mail: carlos@uebel.com.br

J. M. Avelar, R. Cavalcanti Ribeiro (eds.), *Body Contouring*,
https://doi.org/10.1007/978-3-031-42802-9_16

can be referred as introducers of this new approach. We have also started with two similar procedures that we want to discuss in this chapter—the superior glandular flap and the lateral dermoglandular rotation flap.

Method and Technique

Superior Pedicle Flap

This is a very simple procedure combined with the Pitanguy-Ariê technique (Ariê 1957) indicated for ptotic and medium breast hypertrophy. An ellipse of the skin is removed vertically reaching 2 cm above the inframammary sulcus or extended laterally as shown in Fig. 16.1a–c. A superior pedicle glandular flap is erased from below and rotated by itself into a tunnel undermined into the upper pole of the breast. This is a maneuver to fill out and to enhance the volume of the breast giving a good support as shown at postoperative 18 months (Figs. 16.2a–d and 16.3a–c). An intradermal suture is placed, and sterile strips are applied to protect the suture and are kept in place for 15 days. We can use the "L" technique published by Bozola (1990). Very often, in around 30%, we combine the procedure with abdominoplasty and other body contouring surgeries (Fig. 16.4a–c).

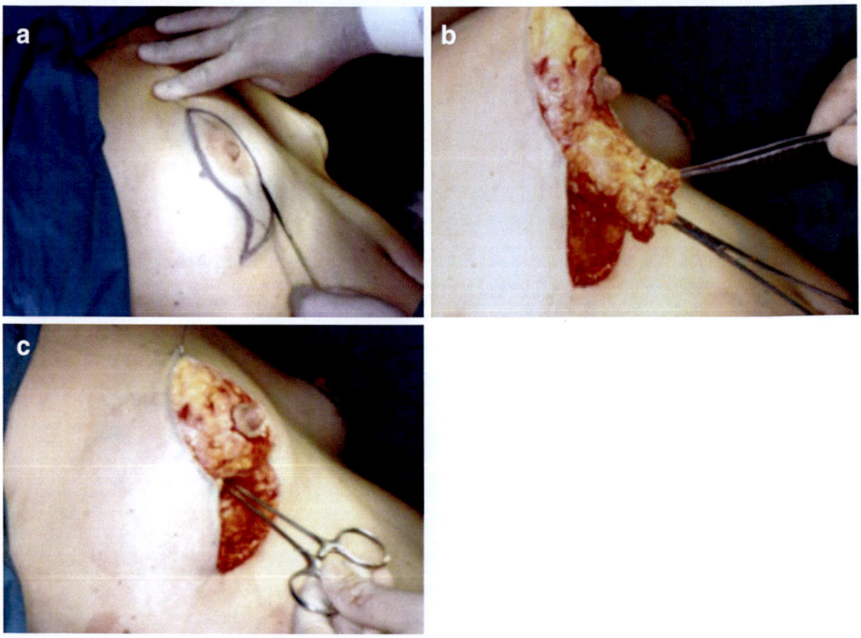

Fig. 16.1 (**a**, **b**, **c**) A superior pedicle glandular flap is erased and rotated by itself to fill out the upper breast pole

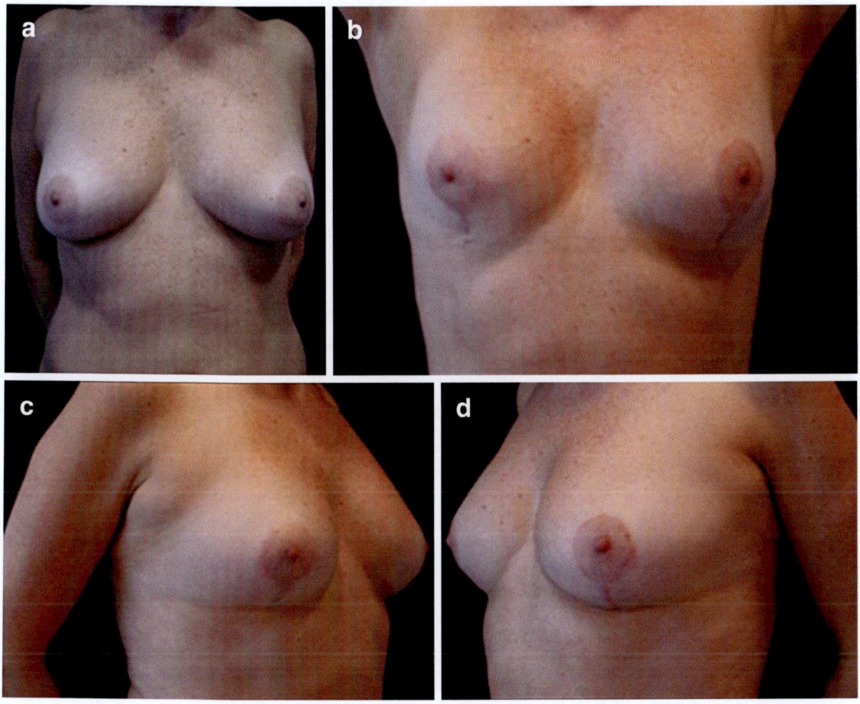

Fig. 16.2 (**a**, **b**, **c**, **d**) Postoperative 18 months with a fulfilling upper pole

Supralateral Dermoglandular Flap

The most common breast reduction technique still used in Brazil is the one described by Pitanguy in 1967. It consists of removing a keel-shaped portion of the breast tissue, which results in two lateral pillars that provide the necessary structure to raise the nipple-areola complex (NAC) in a very natural shape while maintaining good physiologic function. This technique is especially useful for patients with mild to moderate hypertrophic breasts (Fig. 16.5a–c).

However, for patients with larger breast hypertrophy, with or without asymmetry, it is significantly more challenging to raise the NAC, and the procedure may create some skin tension. For such patients, the techniques described by Skoog in 1971 (Skoog 1971) and Silveira Neto in 1976 (Silveira Netto 1976) and modified by the author in 1978 (Uebel and Uebel 1978; Uebel 2011; Uebel 2012) are very useful to be applied.

Technique

Points *A*, *B*, and *C* are marked with the patient in an upstanding position in the same fashion as in the Pitanguy technique. The **supralateral flap** is outlined (Fig. 16.6). The patient is given general anesthesia and sometimes epidural anesthesia through

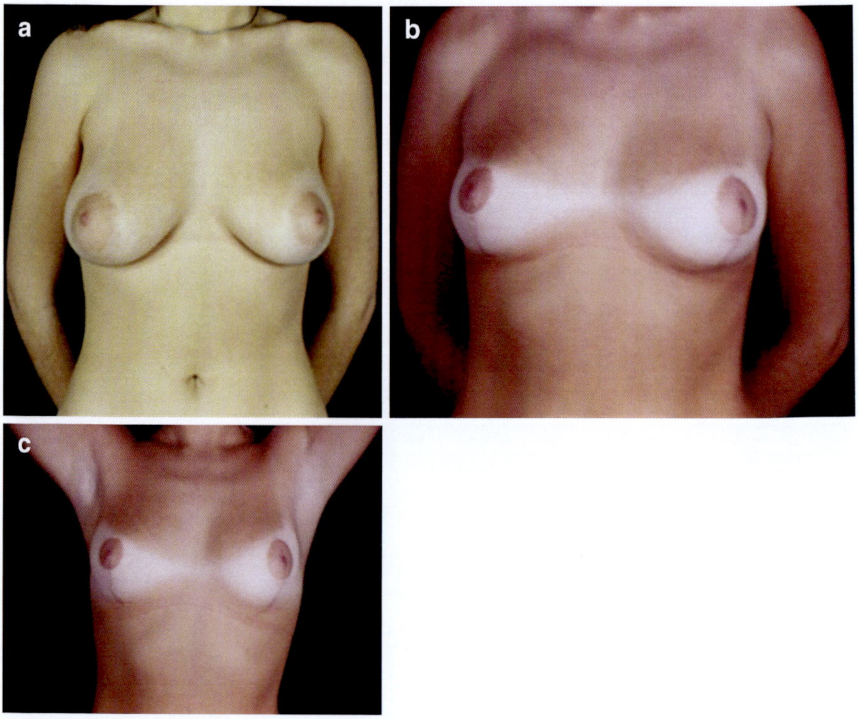

Fig. 16.3 (**a**, **b**, **c**) Ptotic breast with the Pitanguy-Ariê technique and superior pedicle flap to enhance the upper pole

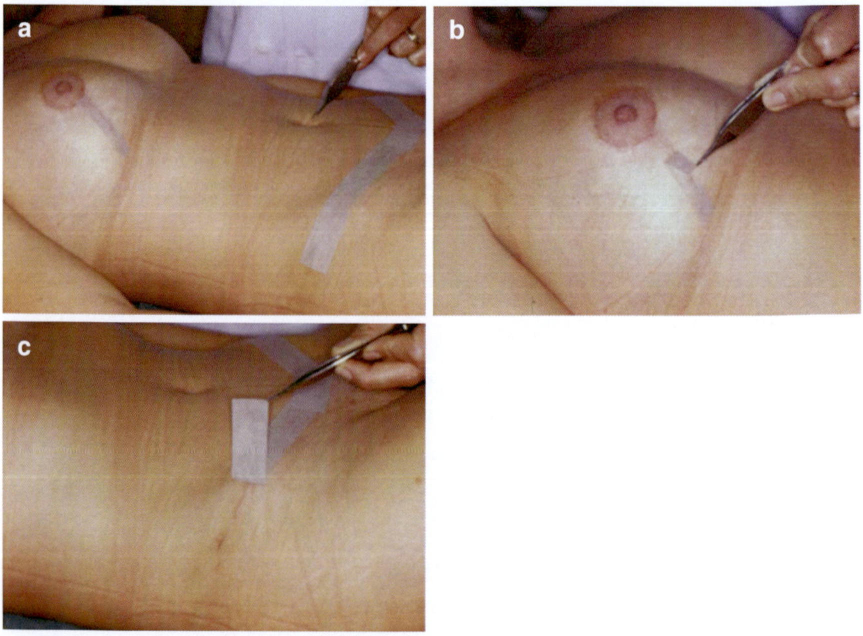

Fig. 16.4 (**a**, **b**, **c**) This technique can be combined frequently with abdominoplasty

a continuous-infusion catheter. To reduce intraoperative bleeding, a local infiltration of saline and epinephrine 1:200,000 is done. The dermoglandular flap is deepithelialized and prepared, together with the NAC; the flap is then ready to be relocated to its new site without excessive tension and with a good blood supply.

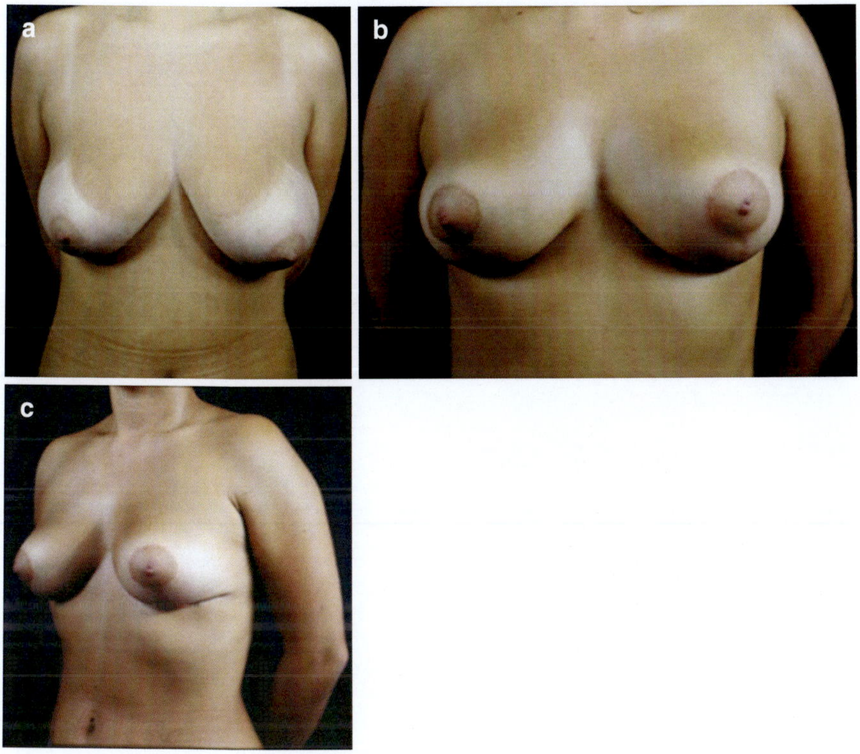

Fig. 16.5 (**a**, **b**, **c**) Medium breast hypertrophy treated with the Pitanguy technique

Fig. 16.6 The supralateral flap is outlined

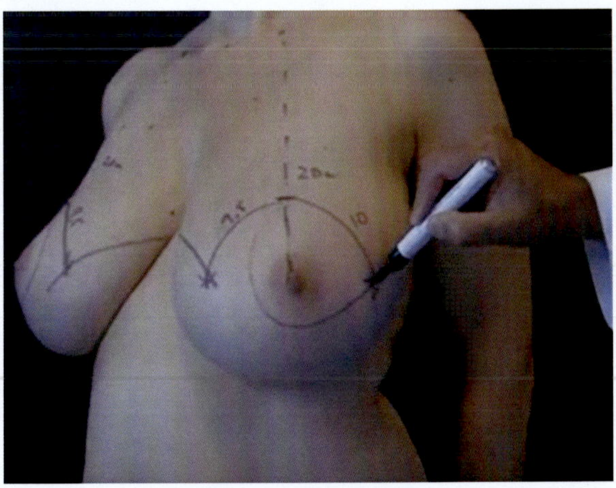

In 1971, Skoog published his nipple-areola-dermis flap rotation technique for severe hypertrophic breasts. However, this technique sometimes results in problems with vascular support and lactation. In 1976, and with the use of the same principles described by Skoog, Silveira Neto modified the technique by rotating an inner glandular flap which improved irrigation and lactation ability. In 1978, we published another variation of the technique outlining the **supralateral dermoglandular flap**. In addition to achieving good vascular support and function, this maneuver offers a better contouring to the upper pole of the breast and axillary regions (Figs. 16.7 and 16.8).

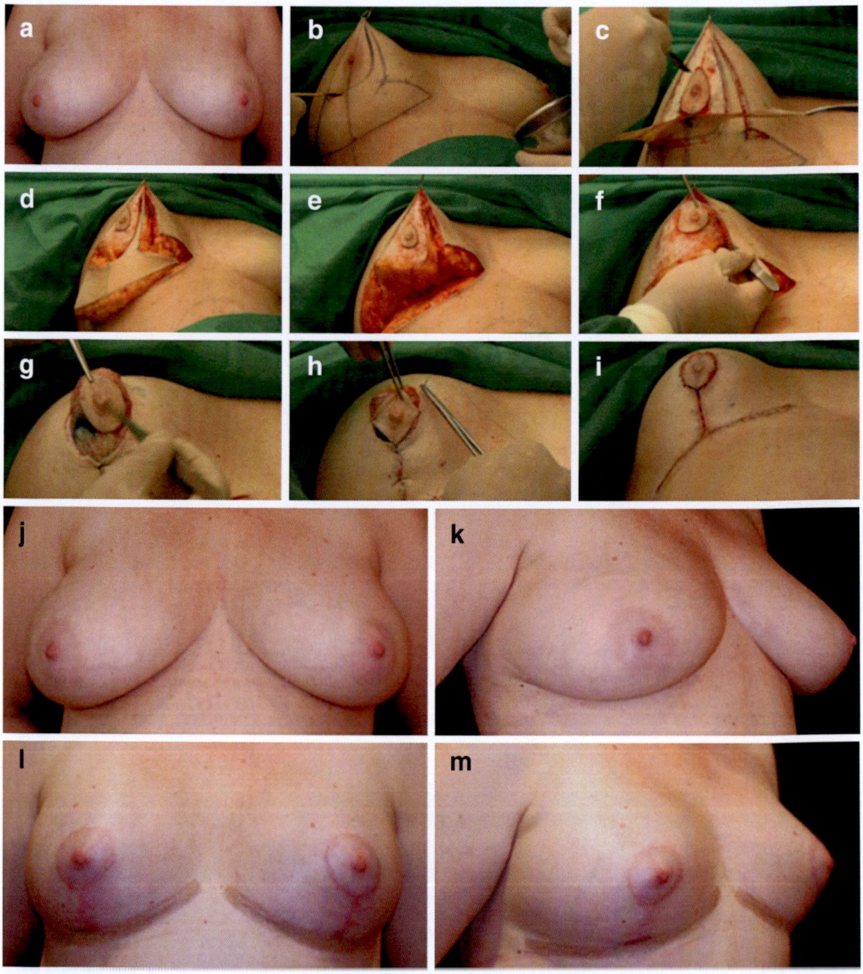

Fig. 16.7 (**a–m**) A 52-year-old patient with severe hypertrophy was treated with the **supralateral dermoglandular rotation flap** technique. She is shown 3 months postoperatively with improved breast contour, axillary reduction, and nipple-areola projection

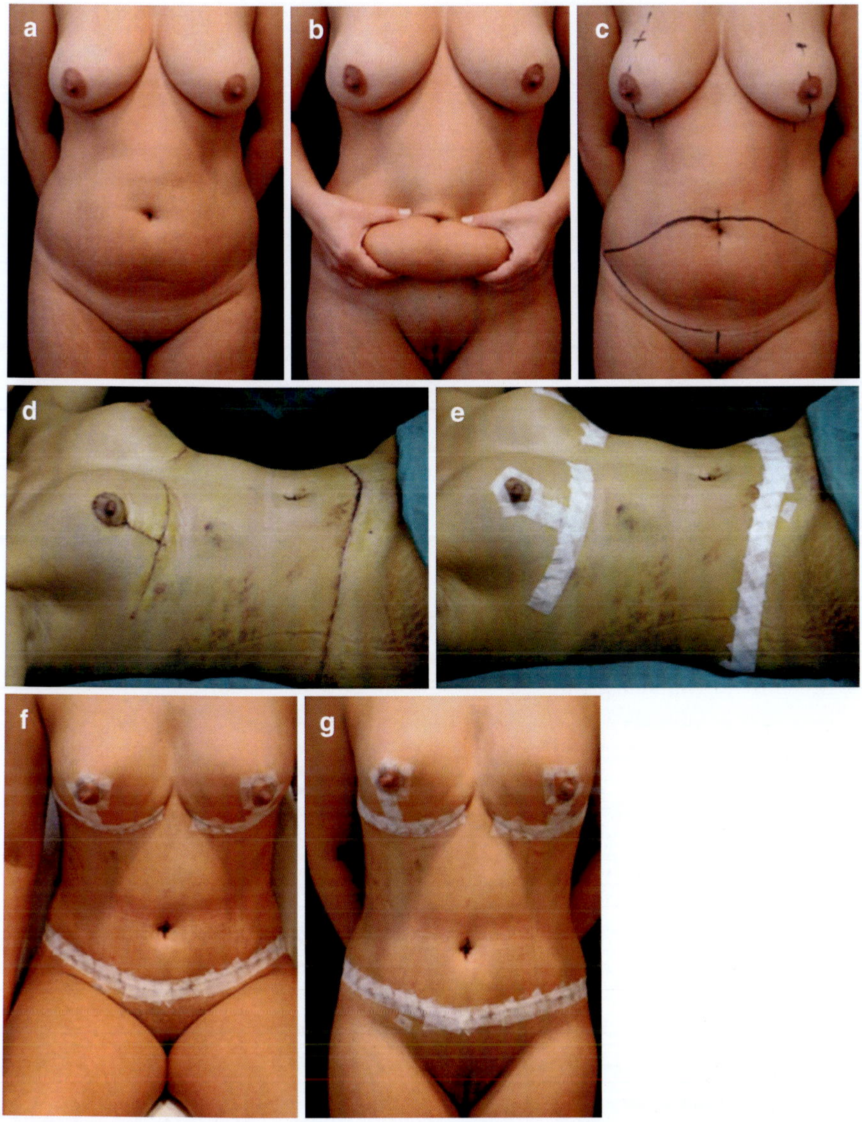

Fig. 16.8 (**a–j**) Very common association in a 42-year-old patient with breast hypertrophy and abdomen flaccidity. She underwent breast reduction with the **supralateral dermoglandular flap** and abdominoplasty. Two days postoperatively with sterile strips and 6 months postoperatively in sitting and standing positions

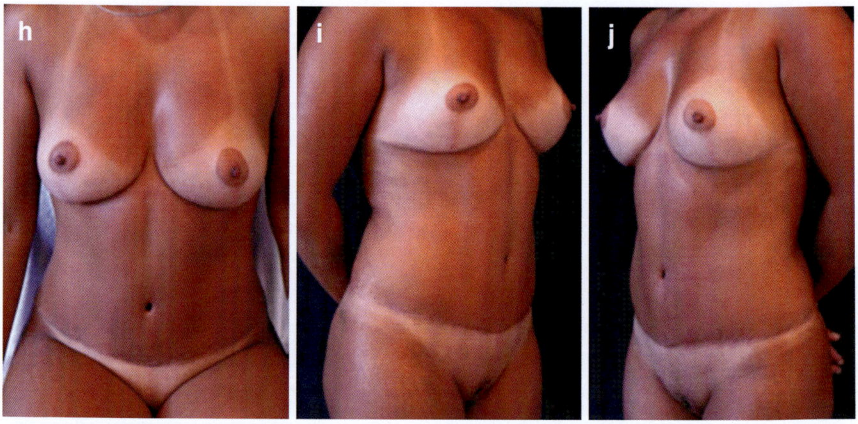

Fig. 16.8 (continued)

For patients with severe breast hypertrophy, with or without asymmetry, there is a bigger challenge to address when raising the NAC. In such cases, the technique of the **supralateral dermoglandular flap** is indicated to bring the NAC upward without any tension, thereby preserving the neurovascular supply and physiologic lactation function. Good sensitivity and a natural contour of the breast and axillary region can be achieved with this technique (Fig. 16.7).

The external **supralateral dermoglandular flap** is designed and deepithelialized, preserving the NAC. Resection is done en bloc, removing a complete piece of the mammary tissue reaching the pectoralis major fascia. The flap is rotated from the external site to upward to anchor the areola in the new position. Sutures of 4-0 nylon and 3-0 Monocryl are placed in all levels to close the glandular parenchyma. Intradermal sutures are placed, and sterile strips are applied. Sterile strips are maintained for more than 3 months (Fig. 16.8).

Conclusion

The definitive breast reduction technique continues to elude plastic surgeons. We have revisited the **superior pedicle flap** and the **supralateral dermoglandular flap**, both of which are important techniques to enhance breast contour and preserve the neurophysiologic function for breastfeeding. They are simple to execute and improve the axillary extension and the upper pole contour giving an excellent NAC projection and an outstanding patient satisfaction, as evidenced by a low revision rate. The operations should be an option when treating patients with medium-to-large breast hypertrophy.

References

Pitanguy I. Breast hypertrophy. In Transactions of the Second Congress of the International Society of Plastic Surgery. London: Livingstone, 1959-1960.

Pitanguy I. Surgical treatment of breast hypertrophy. Br J Plast Surg 20:78, 1967.

Skoog T. A technique of breast reduction transposition of the nipple on a cutaneous vascular pedicle. Acta Chir Scand 126:126, 1971.

Ribeiro L (1975) A new technique for reduction mammaplasty. Plast Reconstr Surg 55:330–334

Silveira Netto E (1976) In: Ely JF (ed) 13 Congresso Bras Cir Plástica. Mastoplastia redutora sectorial com pediculo areolar interno, pp. 13–15. Porto Alegre

Ariê G. Nova técnica em mamaplastia. Rev Latin Amer Cir Plast 3:28, 1957

Uebel CO. Uebel CO (1978) Breast reduction with the lateral dermo-glandular rotation flap. In: Annals of the XVth Brazilian congress of Plastic Surgery, Sao Paulo, SP

Uebel CO (2011) Breast reduction using the supralateral dermoglandular flap. IPRAS J 3:16–17

Uebel CO. Combined abdominal contouring and mastopexy. In Rubin JP, ed. Body Contouring and Liposuction. New York: Elsevier; 2012.

Pitanguy I (1962) A new technic of plastic surgery of the breast. Study of 245 consecutive cases and presentation of a personal technic. Ann Chir Plast 7:199–208

Bozola AR (1990) Breast reduction with short L scar. Plast Reconstr Surg 85:728–738

Chapter 17
Classification and Correction of Asymmetrical Breasts to Achieve a Balance in Body Contouring

Juarez Moraes Avelar, Marcelo Vaccari, and Jose Carlos Miranda

Abstract Asymmetry of the breast is quite frequent, causing an imbalance in the body after puberty when a great physical change occurs in female humans because of hormonal metabolic alterations. At such an age for female humans, the development of the breasts starts. Even in male humans, growth may occur as gynecomastia, which requires immediate treatment to avoid other consequences. Any alteration of the breasts can modify the body contouring, causing disharmony and imbalance to the whole body, which could lead to patient dissatisfaction. Consequently, any unwanted asymmetries in the breasts can be surgically repaired to achieve a balance between the breasts and with the chest, which improves body contouring.

There is a wide variety of breast asymmetries, and they need to be examined before surgical treatment aiming to achieve harmonious body contouring. There are two major types of asymmetries: congenital and acquired. A congenital asymmetry may appear without a chest deformity: bilateral hypertrophy, hypertrophy in the size of one breast and normal size for the other, hypertrophy in the size of one breast and hypomastia in the other, hypertrophy in the size one breast and ptosis in the other, bilateral hypomastia, hypomastia in one breast and normal size for the other, and asymmetrical breasts with bilateral ptoses. The following asymmetries appear with a chest deformity: bilateral hypertrophy, hypertrophy in the size one breast and normal size for the other, hypertrophy and hypomastia, bilateral hypomastia, and hypomastia and normal size. The following asymmetries appear without a nipple deformity: atelia and normal size, amastia and normal size, amastia and hypomastia, polythelia, and polymastia. The following asymmetries appear with a nipple deformity: atelia and normal size, amastia and normal size, amastia and hypomastia,

J. M. Avelar (✉)
Brazilian Scientific Institute of Plastic and Reconstructive Surgery, São Paulo, Brazil

M. Vaccari · J. C. Miranda
São Paulo, Brazil

J. M. Avelar, R. Cavalcanti Ribeiro (eds.), *Body Contouring*,
https://doi.org/10.1007/978-3-031-42802-9_17

polythelia, and polymastia. An acquired asymmetry may be the result of trauma (e.g., a burn or a human/animal bite) or iatrogenesis (e.g., after mastectomy for resection after breast cancer, secondary to augmentation mastoplasty, or secondary to reduction mastoplasty).

Keywords Breast · Asymmetry · Imbalance in the body · Hypertrophy · Hypomastia · Undeveloped breast

Introduction

The breasts of female humans undergo significant developments over a short period of time during puberty, due to complex hormonal alterations. Just after birth, the breasts may have minimal size because of hormonal influences from the mother at 1 to 2 weeks (Pitanguy 1961; Avelar 1989). Afterward, they remain as is in a latency stage, but after a short period of time, several physical changes occur, giving shape to the adolescent female body and acting as symbol of femininity. During adolescence, young girls' bodies undergo profound anatomical alterations to the body's silhouette, and when the breasts exhibit asymmetry, this can result in body-image disharmony and an imbalance in body contouring.

In addition, the appearance of asymmetric breasts may develop physical alterations on the vertebral column of the spine and torso (Fig. 17.1), with severe repercussions on the respiratory system caused by an imbalance in the chest, according to Pitanguy (1967). Therefore, its correction is a matter of physical reparation to achieve harmony in the body and avoid negative repercussions on wellbeing of the patient (Fig. 17.2). The treatment is essentially a surgical approach that frequently consists of mammary reduction in one side and a silastic inclusion in the other, which makes achieving a balance in the chest even more difficult (Fig. 17.3) (Pitanguy 1959). Until recently, when both breasts presented noticeable hypertrophies with severe asymmetry in adulthood, reduction mastoplasty can be performed for the resection of the excess breast tissue (Figs. 17.4 and 17.5). Even at such an age, the presence of adipose tissue may cause a similar asymmetry that demands careful management to achieve balance after the operation (Avelar 2000a). On the other hand, asymmetric breasts may present with bilateral hypomastia, which requires augmentation mastoplasty on both sides by using different sizes of breast implants.

In addition to conducting an accurate physical examination, mammography is a useful preoperative exam to reveal any alterations in the glandular tissue and the proportions between mammary tissue and fat tissue. Because mammary

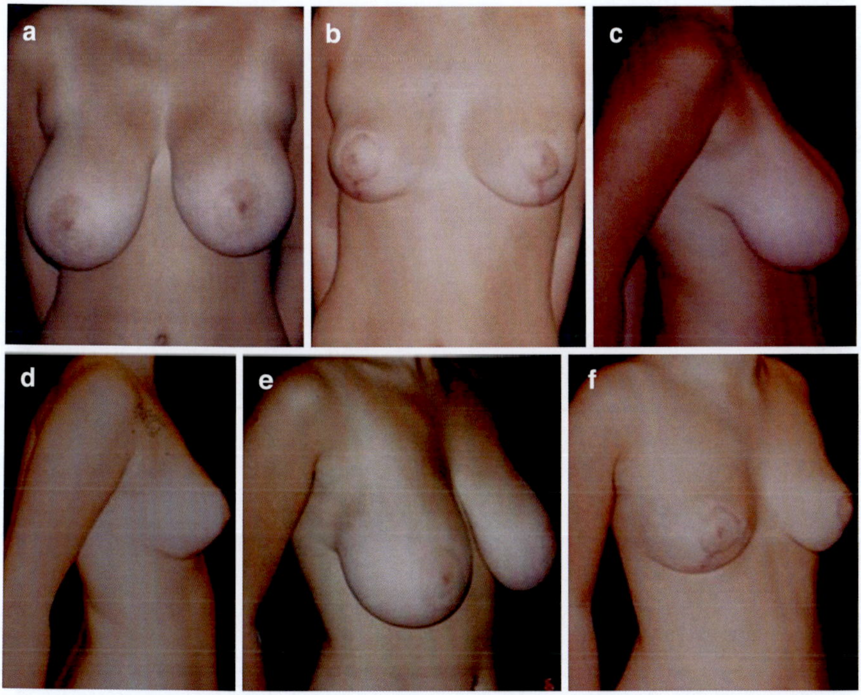

Fig. 17.1 A 21-year-old patient presenting bilateral hypertrophy with asymmetry of the breasts. Photos **a**, **c**, and **e**—preoperative showing the right breast larger than the left one presenting physical alteration on the chest with rotation forward of the shoulder; **b**, **d**, and **f**—the same patient 1 year after reduction mastoplasty with resection of 950 g on the right breast and 690 g on the left one. One can see correction of patient's posture

asymmetry is the most common, most patients present with some sort of difference in the size and shape of the breasts. Some abnormalities in the breasts that develop after mastoplasty may be due to the structural asymmetry of the tissues given that balance can be achieved through liposuction (Fig. 17.6) (Avelar 1986, 1989, 1993). Descriptions of the breasts and body contouring are necessary to safeguard plastic surgeons against malpractice lawsuits (Avelar 1980, 2000b, c). When a patient presents with some sort of asymmetry among their breasts and doesn't mention it to the surgeon, point it out to them before surgery is appropriate (Fig. 17.7). During consultation and before examination, surgeons may ask whether they notice any sort of asymmetry, though they rarely confirm it. However, during a physical examination, when patients stand in front of a mirror, most of them have some sort of abnormality.

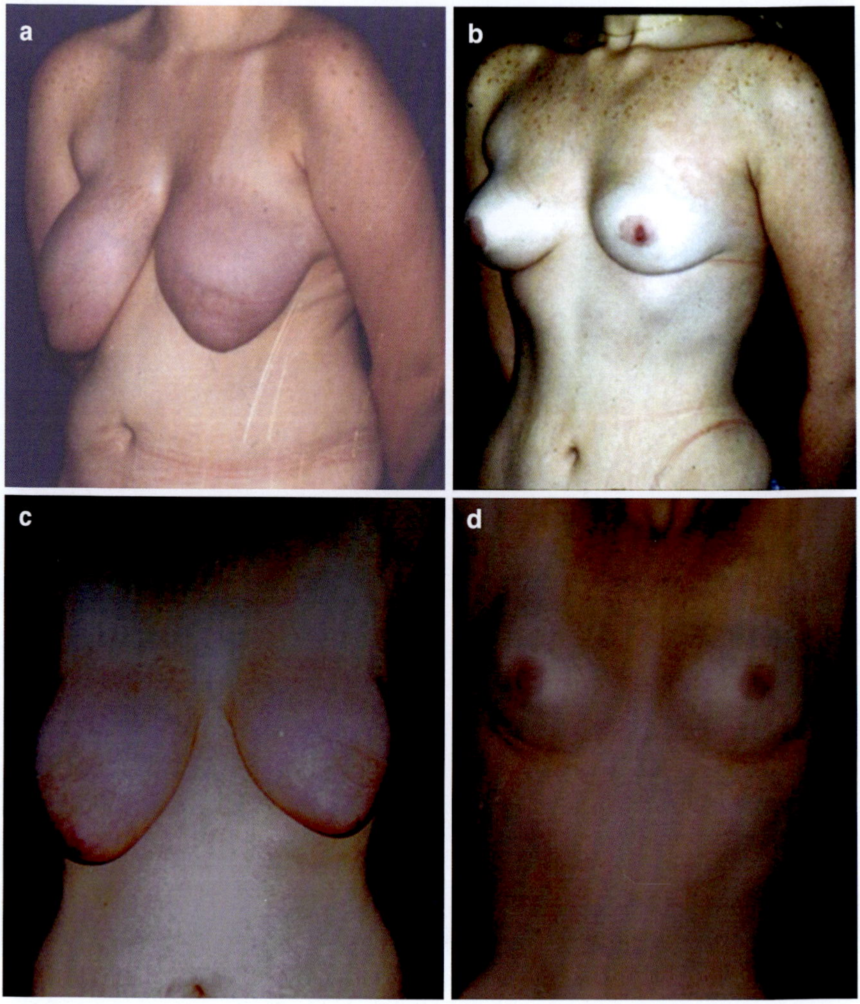

Fig. 17.2 Asymmetry of the breasts presenting severe bilateral hypertrophy in a 21-year-old patient. Photos **a** and **c**—preoperative photos showing physical alterations of the shoulder caused by breast hypertrophy; photos **b** and **d** after reduction mastoplasty with resection of 850 g on the right side and 640 g on the left side. Photos **c** and **d** with her arms up. After reduction mastoplasty with correction of asymmetry she loss weight with diet. Even she presents correction of the physical posture

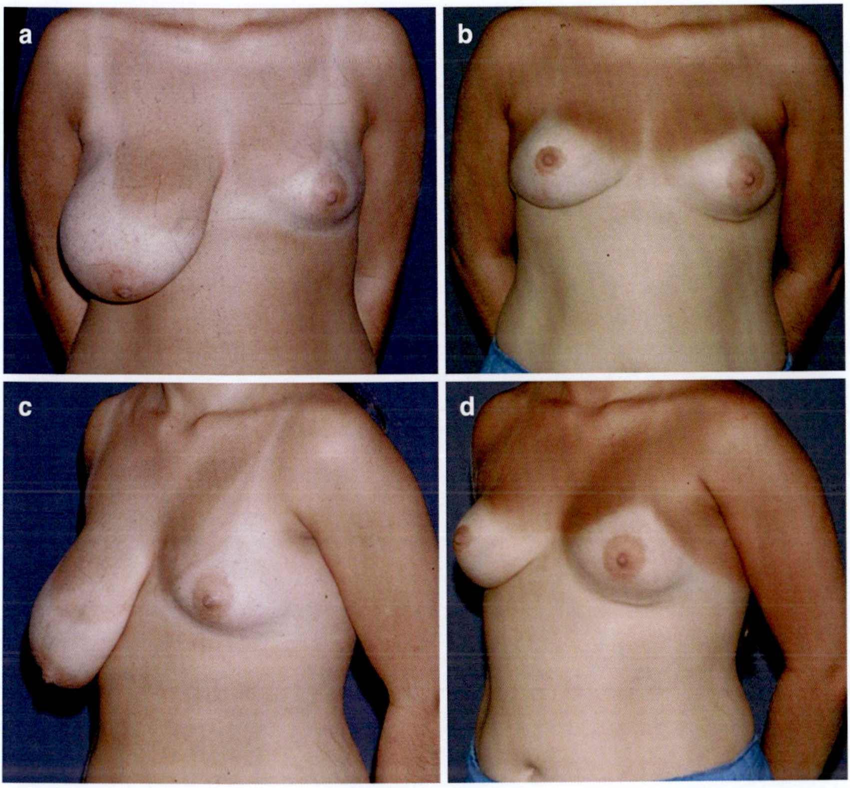

Fig. 17.3 Severe asymmetry of the breasts presenting hypertrophy and ptoses on the right side hyponasty on the left breast in a 19-year-old patient. Photos **a** and **c** – preoperative; photos **b** and **d**—1 year after reduction mastoplasty on the right side with resection of 500 g of mammary gland and silastic inclusion of 200 ml on the left side

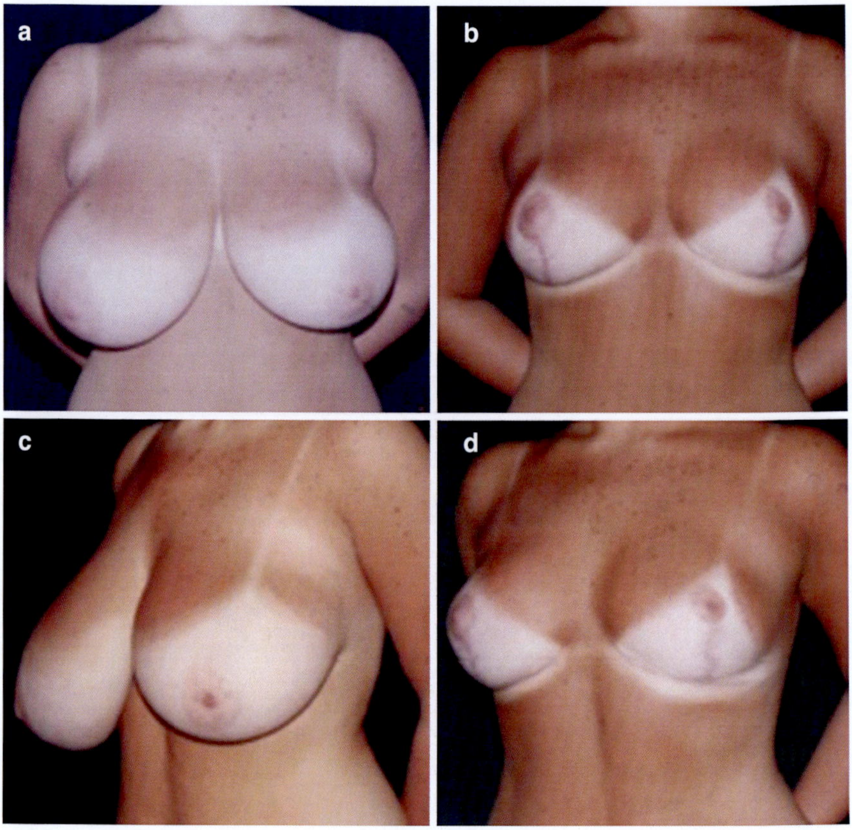

Fig. 17.4 Bilateral hypertrophy with severe asymmetric breasts on a 20-year-old patient. Photos **a** and **c**—preoperative; **b** and **d**—the same patient 9 months after reduction mastoplasty with resection of 850 g on the right breast and 380 g on left one

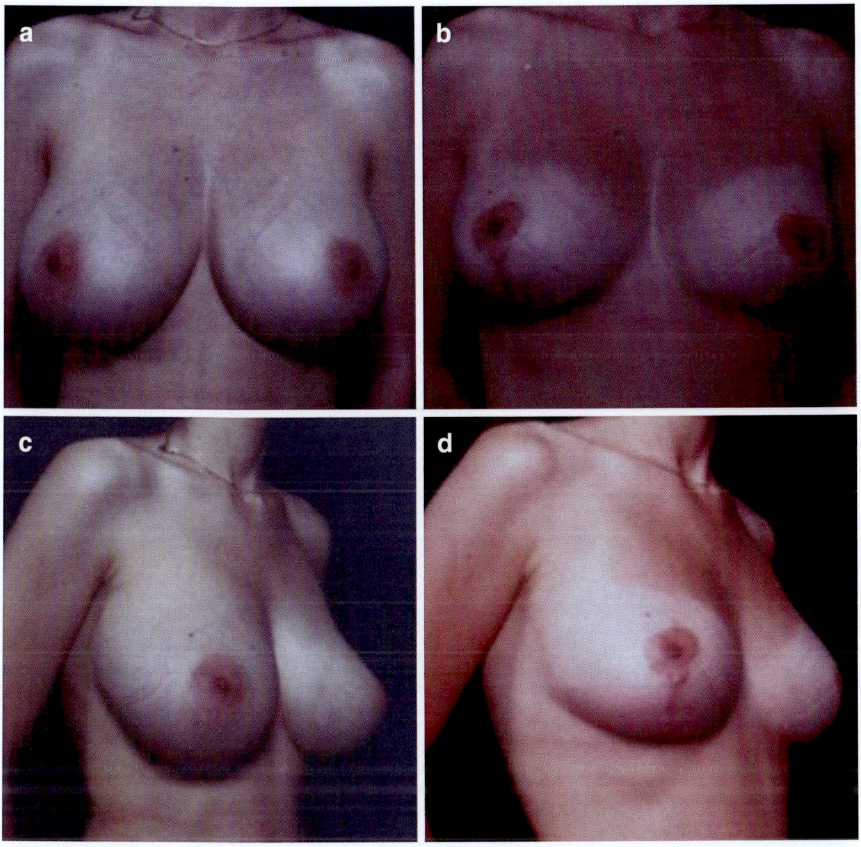

Fig. 17.5 Asymmetric breasts with bilateral hypertrophy. Photos **a** and **c**—preoperative; **b** and **d**—1 year after bilateral reduction Only with vertical approach without periareolar incisions with resection of 210 g on the right side and 150 g on left, with reparation of asymmetry .. -

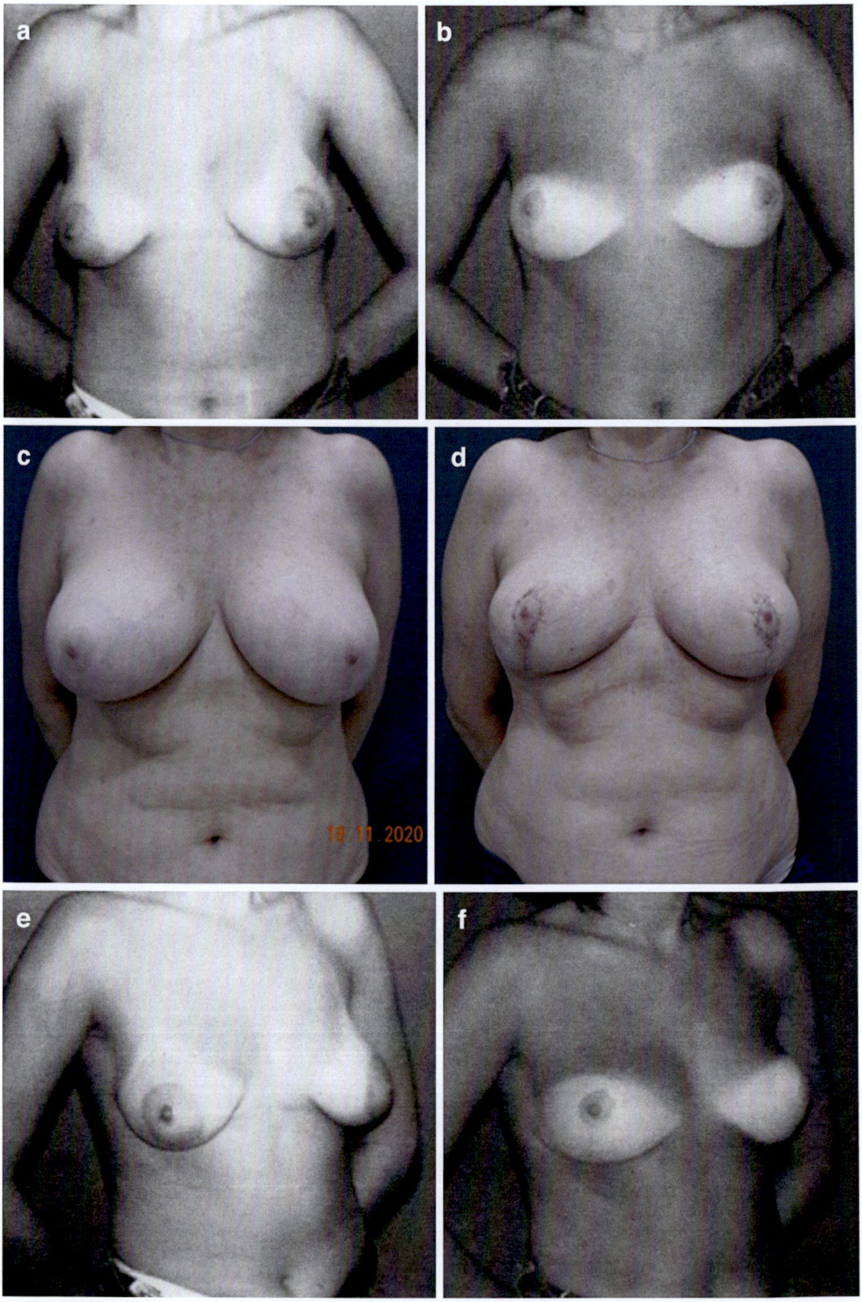

Fig. 17.6 Asymmetry of the breasts presents asymmetric mammary gland and cutaneous flaccidity as well. A 21-year-old patient complaint ptosis with asymmetry of the breasts (preoperative photos **a**, **e**); underwent mastopexy in 1977 (photos **b**, **f** after surgery); The same patient at age 64 years old presented asymmetry of the breasts with asymmetric hypertrophy (photos **c**, **g** before the second operation) underwent reduction mastoplasty in January 2021 (photos **d**, **h**) 6 months after surgery

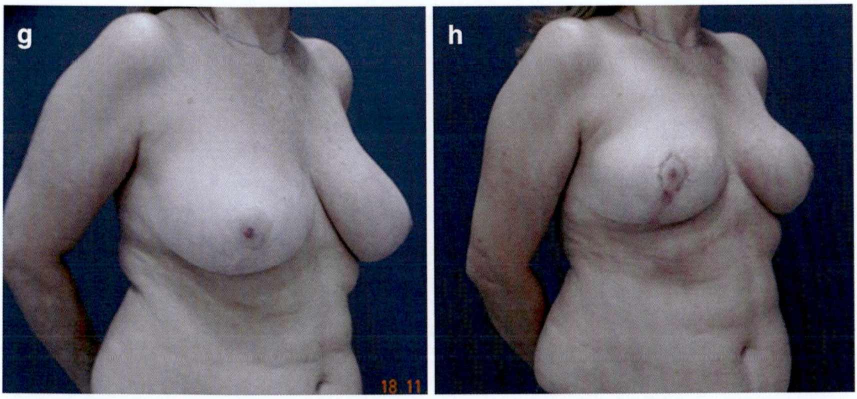

Fig. 17.6 (continued)

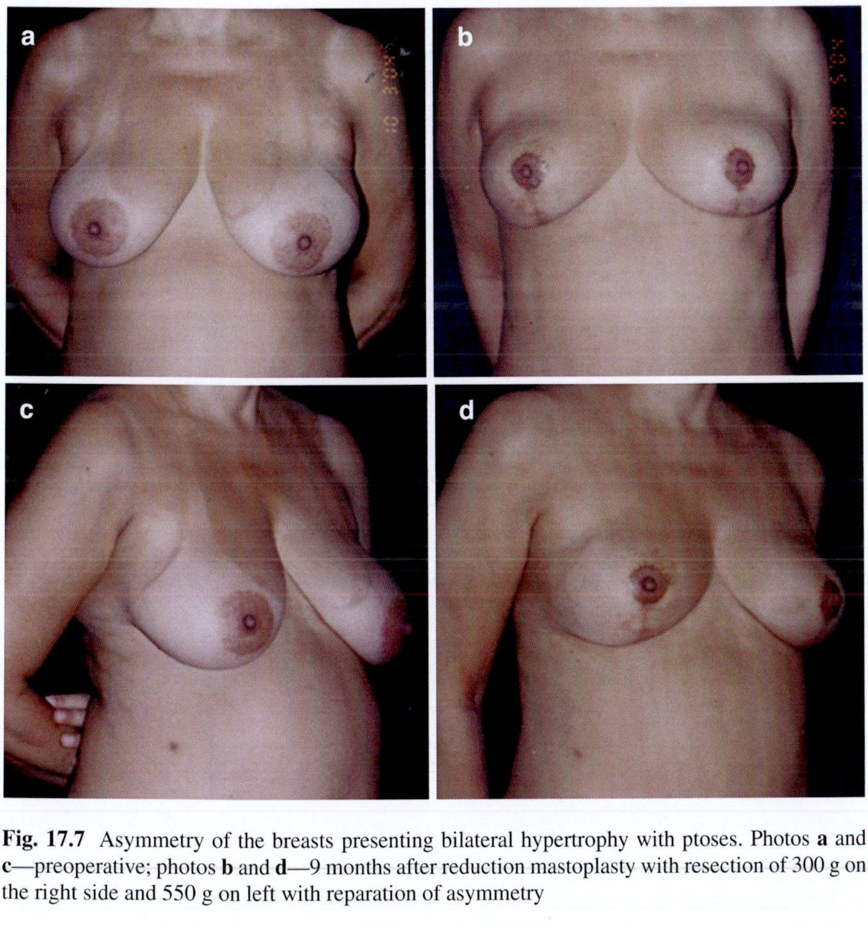

Fig. 17.7 Asymmetry of the breasts presenting bilateral hypertrophy with ptoses. Photos **a** and **c**—preoperative; photos **b** and **d**—9 months after reduction mastoplasty with resection of 300 g on the right side and 550 g on left with reparation of asymmetry

Classification of Breast Asymmetry

Mammary asymmetry has been reported since 1950, when Maliniac (1950) divided breast asymmetries into four categories: asymmetry with bilateral hypertrophy, hypertrophy on one side and amastia or hypomastia on the other, hypertrophy on one side and a normal size on the other, amastia or hypomastia on one side and normal breast size on the other. Pitanguy et al. (1973, 1977) referred to asymmetrical breasts and the physical repercussions to body contouring and to the respiratory system. Other authors have referred to this, such as Broadbent and Woolf (1978) and Sepúlveda (1981). Later, Juri (1989) presented a simplified classification of asymmetrical breasts, dividing them into only three grades. More recently, Jales (2004) and Karim et al. (2009) wrote reports on the asymmetry of the breasts and proposed specific classifications. Given that breast asymmetry is very common and is important in plastic surgery, it is divided (Avelar 1989, 2018a) into two major categories in accordance with what is helpful to know for surgical correction: congenital and acquired.

Congenital

(a) Without a chest deformity

1. Bilateral hypertrophy (Figs. 17.1, 17.2, 17.4 and 17.5).
2. Hypertrophy in one breast and normal size for the other.
3. Hypertrophy in one breast and hypomastia in the other (Fig. 17.3).
4. Hypertrophy in one breast and ptosis in the other.
5. Bilateral hypomastia.
6. Hypomastia in one breast and normal size for the other.
7. Asymmetrical breasts with bilateral ptosis (Fig. 17.8).

(b) With a chest deformity

1. Bilateral hypertrophy.
2. Hypertrophy and normal size.
3. Hypertrophy and hypomastia.
4. Bilateral hypomastia.
5. Hypomastia and normal size.

(c) Without nipple deformity

1. Atelia and normal size.
2. Amastia and normal size.
3. Amastia and hypomastia.
4. Polythelia.
5. Polymastia.

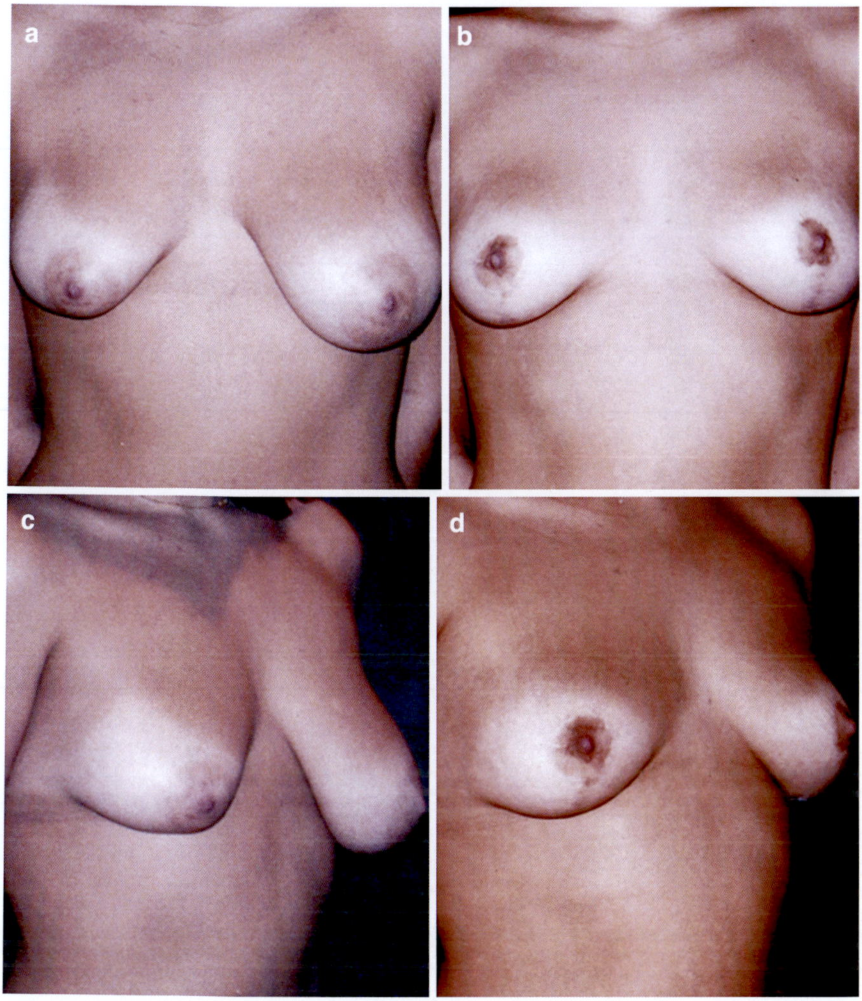

Fig. 17.8 Asymmetry of the breasts presenting severe ptoses with unilateral hypertrophy in a 19-year-old patient. Photos **a** and **c**—preoperative; photos **b** and **d** after reduction mastoplasty on the left side and mastopexy on right one

(d) With nipple deformity

1. Atelia and normal size.
2. Amastia and normal size.
3. Amastia and hypomastia.
4. Polythelia.
5. Polymastia.

Acquired

(a) Traumatic

1. Burns.
2. Human and animal bite.

(b) Iatrogenic

1. After mastectomy for resection of breast cancer.
2. Secondary to augmentation mastoplasty.
3. Secondary to reduction mastoplasty.

Method

Mastoplasty for the correction of asymmetrical breasts is always a challenge because during the operation, the surgeon must perform a one approach on one side and another on the other. It has been much more complex than a standard aesthetic

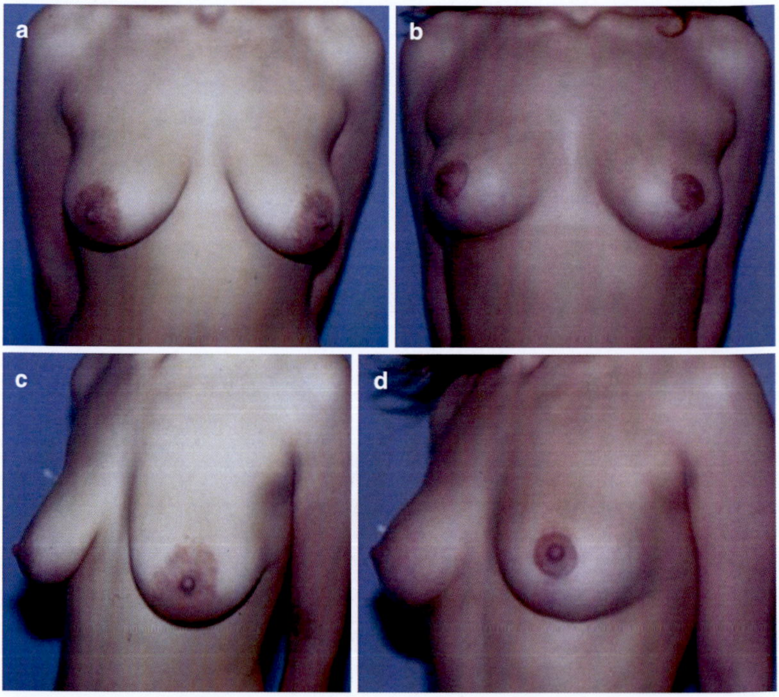

Fig. 17.9 Asymmetry of the breasts presenting asymmetric ptoses in a 21-year-old patient. Photos **a** and **c**—preoperative; photos **b** and **d** after bilateral mastopexy with inverted T and periareolar incision for reparation of asymmetric nipple-areolar complex

surgery because surgeons need to achieve an appropriate balance among both breasts and keep them in harmony with the chest to improve body contouring (Fig. 17.9).

Surgical Planning

Surgical planning is an essential step before any operation in plastic surgery, but for the correction of asymmetry in the breasts, it is even more important because of the different approaches necessary for this surgery. When a patient mentions an evident asymmetry between their two breasts, surgical planning will usually require two operations. A good example is when a patient presents with hypertrophy on one side and hypomastia on the other, in which case the surgical plan must include reduction mastoplasty on one breast and augmentation mastoplasty using an implant on the other (Fig. 17.3). However, when a patient presents with bilateral hypertrophy with noticeable asymmetry, surgical planning must be directed to reduce both sides for the reparation of the different sizes of the breasts (Figs. 17.1, 17.2, 17.4 and 17.5). Surgical planning for this surgery is much more complex because bilateral hypertrophic breasts featuring severe asymmetry may require specific procedures to achieve aesthetic bilateral balance (Figs. 17.1 and 17.4).

Surgical Demarcations

The surgeon should carry out premarking at their office or at the hospital before medication because at this time, the patient is awake and may follow the preliminary demarcation (Avelar 1989, 2018c). Also at this time, some references points are drawn on both breasts, as recommended by Erfon et al. (2018). In the case of mammary hypertrophy on one side, add a landmark for the reference points for reduction mastoplasty (Avelar 2018b). Depending on the abnormality in the opposite breast, appropriate premarkings are made. Nevertheless, when the patient is in operating room, the final surgical markings are made according to the surgeon's technique.

The Operation

In all cases of aesthetic breast surgery, the correction of deformities requires a previous clinical evaluation, meticulous surgical planning, and preliminary demarcations, as mentioned in the preceding subsection. In most cases of asymmetric breast ptosis, surgeons should create a medial dermogladular flap with a superior pedicle because it is versatile in remodeling the breasts (Figs. 17.10, 17.11 and 17.12) (Avelar 1980; Sinder 2018).

Asymmetry with breast hypertrophy on both sides requires bilateral reduction mastoplasty (Figs. 17.1, 17.2, 17.4 and 17.5). Although the purpose of this chapter is not to describe the operation, my preference is to perform breast reduction for the correction of asymmetry by using Pitanguy's technique because it is easy to adapt for each case of deformity (Figs. 17.13, 17.14 and 17.15) (Pitanguy 1959, 1961, 1967).

Also, the correction of asymmetry in a hypertrophic breast has been well described by Paulino Costa et al. (2018), Caldeira et al. (2018), and Martire Jr (2018); Matire used his versatile "L" mastoplasty technique.

When a patient presents with hypertrophy in only one breast, unilateral reduction mastoplasty must be performed. However, the most complex asymmetries feature hypomastia in one breast and hypertrophy in the other (Fig. 17.3). The surgical

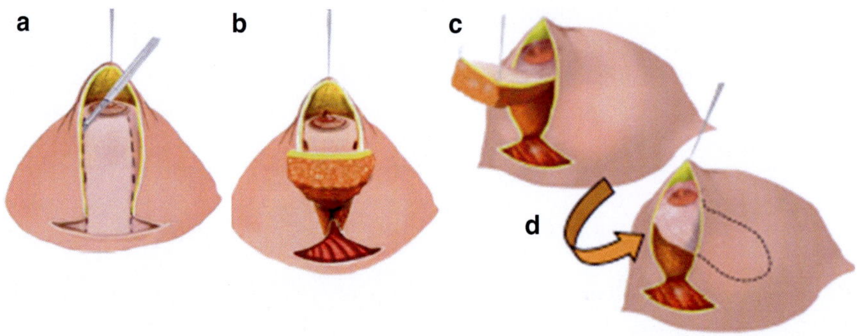

Fig. 17.10 Sequential diagrams to demonstrate mastopexy by creation of a medial glandular flap with superior pedicle (Avelar 1980). Drawing (**a**)—after resection of skin on inferior pole of the breast two parallel incisions are done; (**b**, **c**) the inferior pole of the glandular flap is pulled forward; (**d**) after backwards rotation, similar to a pendulum, it is sutured to the muscle on chest wall

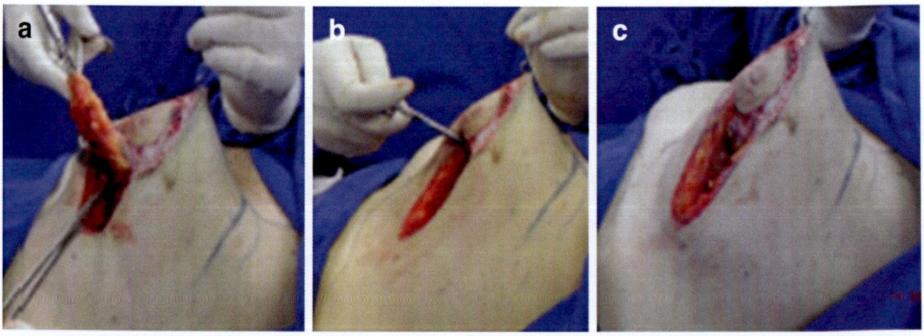

Fig. 17.11 Preoperative photos to demonstrate creation, rotation, and suture of the medial glandular flap with superior pedicle. Photo (**a**)—the mammary dermal flap is raised and pulled forward; (**b**) the flap is already rotated backward supported by borders; (**c**) after suture of the end of the dermal glandular flap to the muscle on the chest

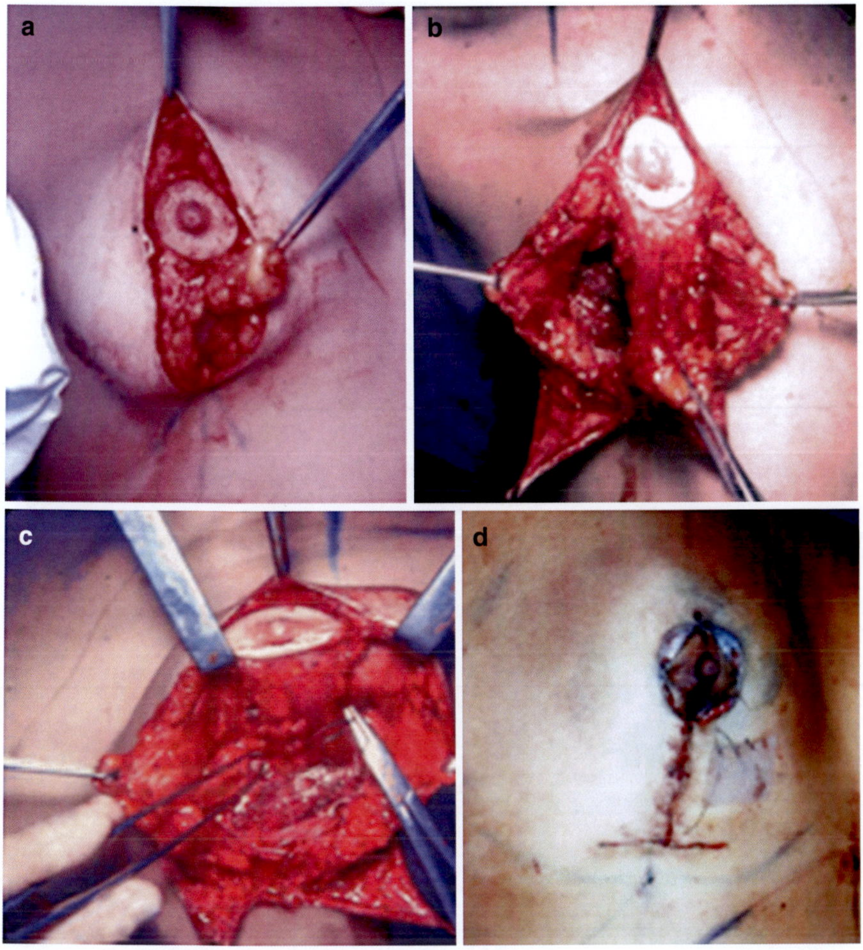

Fig. 17.12 Sequential photos during mastopexy with the creation of a medial dermal glandular flap with superior pedicle on the right breast. Photo (**a**) the mammary dermal flap is being incised; (**b**) the flap is pulled forward; (**c**) the flap is already rotated backward being saturated on the muscles of the chest wall; (**d**) the final suture of the cutaneous covering of the right breast

planning must be carried out with reduction mastoplasty on one side and augmentation mastoplasty on the opposite breast. Some patients have mentioned that since the age of 10 years, they have had a hyperdeveloped breast on one side and an underdeveloped breast on the other. The main purpose of surgery in this case is to correct the severe imbalance of the body contour, which can come with severe physical and psychological repercussions. There is very wide variation among breasts, nipples, and chest deformities according to the classification described above (Avelar 1989). Because of this immense variety of congenital anomalies, surgical planning is key to achieving balance between the breasts and with the chest (Avelar 2018c). The most frequent asymmetry of the breasts is ptosis associated with

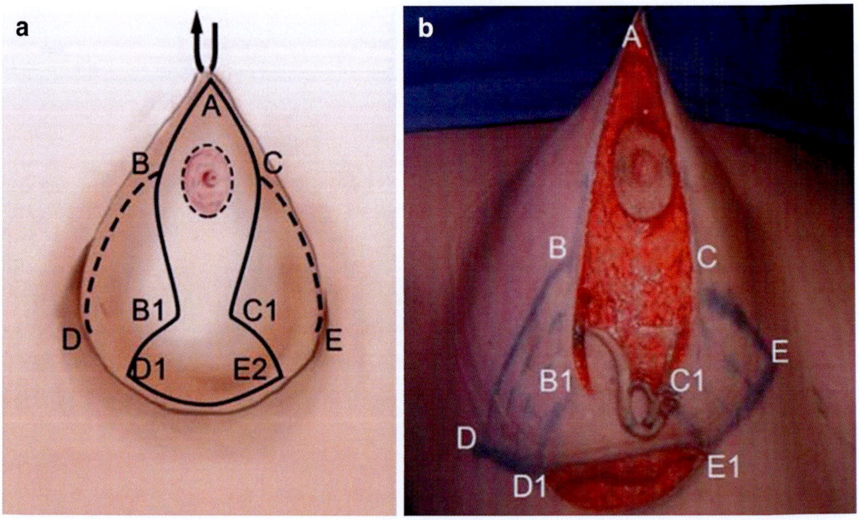

Fig. 17.13 Modifications on Pitanguy's technique to reduce the length of the horizontal scars on submammary fold during reduction mastoplasty. Scheme (**a**) and preoperative photo (**b**), demonstrate Avelar's contribution: points A,B, C, D, and E are demarcate according to original technique. Points A1, B1, C1, D1, and E1 are the references to reduce the scar

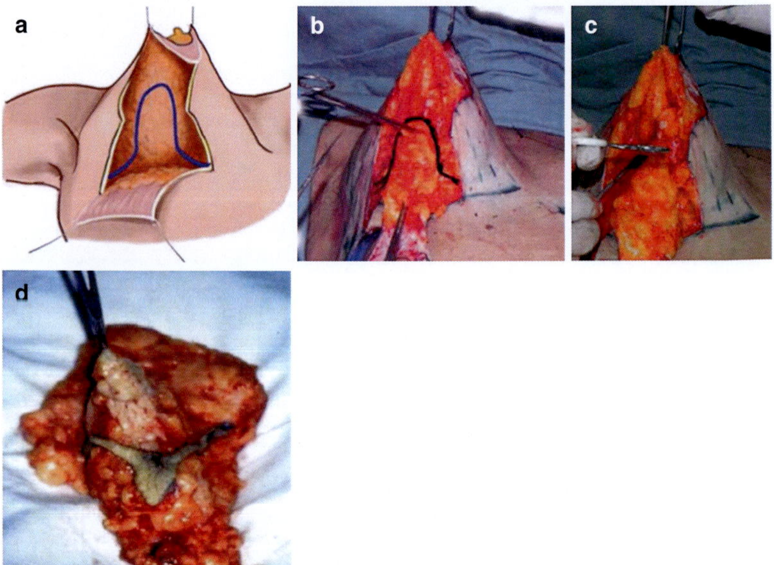

Fig. 17.14 Scheme and preoperative photos to demonstrate Pitanguy's technique for glandular resection during mastoplasty for correction of asymmetric breasts. Drawing (**a**) a medial segment is demarcated; (**b**) photos shows the amount of mammary tissue to be resected; (**c**) it is being resected with knife; (**d**) the segment already resected to demonstrate the shape of the glandular resected

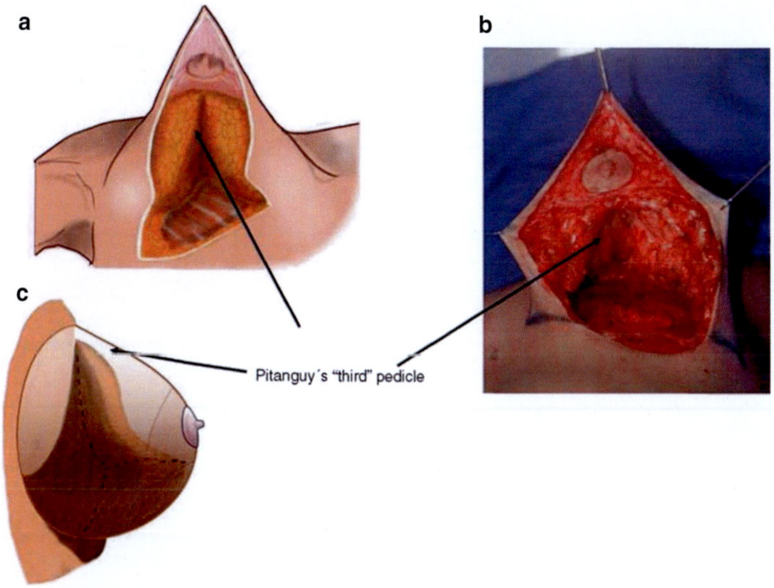

Fig. 17.15 Schemes and preoperative photo showing the creation of the "third" Pitanguy's pedicle during reduction mastoplasty with purpose to correct asymmetric breasts. Scheme (**a**) and photo (**b**) one can see the "third" pedicle from bottom; (**c**) scheme on profile view

flaccidity, which requires bilateral mastopexy with the removal of some of the mammary tissue to achieve a good balance between the two breasts (Figs. 17.6, 17.8 and 17.9). There are other congenital deformities, polymastia or polythelia, that become evident only during puberty, when the breasts start to develop. Patients bring up these abnormalities in consultation, but they are usually not aware of them unless they experience monthly alterations related to menstruation.

Acquired asymmetry of the breasts is a special field in which patients' normal organs incur damage, bringing imbalance to the body contour with physical and psychological repercussions. Deformities of the breast caused by burns to the chest are very common after accidents in infancy or adolescence (Avelar 2018a). As the mammary glands originate and develop from the dermis (Pitanguy et al. 1973), they may be damaged when the trauma impacts the chest wall. Surgeons must be very careful when a child presents with burns on their chest near the nipple–areolar complex (NAC).

During puberty, when physical development makes significant alterations to the body, the growing breast may show some asymmetry, which requires repair or reconstruction (Avelar 2018a). Just as some patients' ear deformities are caused by burns, some patients' breast abnormalities are caused by burns. Other traumas may also damage the breast, partially or totally. Human/animal bites are quite unusual causes, but when they occur, they may have severe consequences.

Nowadays, breast cancer is a substantial social and medical problem and is becoming more and more frequent. When unilateral or bilateral mastectomy is performed, severe wide deformities often occur. Neither the pathological conditions nor the treatment is within the scope of this chapter, except to demonstrate the imbalance of the body contours caused by mastectomy (Avelar 2018a). Therefore, in this chapter, the problem is limited to including one example of the causes of asymmetrical breasts.

Unsatisfactory Surgical Results

As the operation to repair asymmetrical breasts is performed, the most feared result is not achieving perfect bilateral harmony between the two sides because the anatomical mammary structures of each breast don't have a uniform constitution (Avelar 2000b, 2018d). Such a situation may be the main reason for litigation between patients and plastic surgeons. When the operation performed on one side is a reduction mastoplasty and on the other requires the implantation of a silicone prosthesis, achieving a high level of bilateral symmetry is quite difficult but possible (Figs. 17.3 and 17.8). Even when mastopexy is performed on both sides and when patients then have asymmetry, maintaining perfect symmetry is a constant challenge. Because there many patients with several kinds of asymmetries, each patient must be informed of the limits of the operation and those limited must be specified in the documents on informed consent (Avelar 2000a, b, c).

Discussion

The theme of breast asymmetry is important in the study of the pathological conditions of aesthetic breast surgery. Although it is recommended to delay surgical treatment until after puberty, quite often the problem originated at birth or during childhood (Figs. 17.3 and 17.8). Besides the asymmetric breasts presented in the classification in this chapter, tuberous breasts quite often exhibit deformities associated with asymmetry, as described by Ribeiro et al. (Ribeiro et al. 2018).

The asymmetry concerns not only the volume of breast tissue but also the mammary gland's structure, the thickness of the skin, the nipple–areola complex, and the thoracic wall (Figs. 17.6, 17.8 and 17.9) (Avelar 1989, 2000a, b, c). A broad classification of breast deformities has been presented, addressing the diverse pathological conditions and the appropriate age for surgery. Each patient must be treated according to the deformity in their breast(s). For this reason, clinical evaluation and surgical planning are crucial steps to carry out before the operation (Avelar 2018c).

Breast asymmetry is common and represents a problem for many patients (Avelar 2018a). Although most of them are looking for a mastoplasty procedure without any reference to some sort of asymmetry in their breasts, it may be solved during surgery. Even if they don't mention it before mastoplasty, any asymmetry after the operation may cause dissatisfaction (Avelar 2000a, b, 2018d). For this reason, adequate evaluation is crucial during consultation as surgery is planned and during surgical demarcation. However, the surgical technique isn't described in this chapter, because each deformity requires a specific approach to solve the asymmetry, but we did add a few words to state our preference for solving this problem. Since the beginning of our practice, we have sought to reduce the final scar on the submammary folds without causing any damage to the shape of the breasts. One should not insist on prioritizing small scars over the shape, harmony, and symmetry of the breasts. We employ Pitanguy's (1959) technique with our own contribution in order to obtain a short horizontal scar while adapting to the different sizes of asymmetric breasts.

Conclusions

From birth until puberty, the breasts remain in a latency stage. When a young patient presents with asymmetric nipples or breasts, the surgeon must inform their parent or guardian about the indication for surgical correction. Each deformity may be treated according to its specific problem. The most frequent abnormality is bilateral hypertrophy with asymmetry (Figs. 17.1, 17.2, 17.4 and 17.5). Therefore, surgical planning and surgical marking are essential to achieving good results with a good balance between the two breasts.

References

Avelar J (1980) Creation of a Dermal-Adipose-Glandular Flap with Superior Pedicle on Mastopexy with or without Silicone Prosthesis Inclusion (Criação de um Retalho Dermo-Adipose-Glandular com Pedículo Superior nas Mastopexias com ou sem Inclusão de Silicone). Brazilian Symposium on Breast Surgery organized by Psillakis and Avelar, Sponsored by Brazilian Society of Plastic Surgery – Regional São Paulo – August. São Paulo

Avelar J (1986) Reduction Mastoplasty Associated with Liposuction (Lipoaspiração Associada a Mastoplastia Redutora). In Liposuction (Lipoaspiração). Ed by Avelar JM and Illouz YG. Editora Hipócrates, São Paulo; 25-148-151

Avelar JM (1989) Breast asymmetry (Assimetria Mamária). In: Plastic Surgery in Infancy (Cirurgia Plástica na Infância). Ed. by Avelar JM, Ed. Hipocrates, vol 2. São Paulo, pp 413–418

Avelar JM (1993) Reduction Mastoplasty under local Anesthesia (Mastoplastia Redutora sob Anestesia Local). In: Loco-Regional Anesthesia on Aesthetic Surgery —(Anestesia Loco-Regional em Cirurgia Estética), ed. by Avelar JM vol 29. São Paulo, Editora Hipócrates, pp 244–260

Avelar JM (2000a) Body Asymmetry (Assimetria Corporal) in: Plastic Surgery – Obligation of Means Not Obligation of Results (Cirurgia Plástica Obrigação de Meio e não Obrigação de Fim ou de Resultado, ed. By Juarez M. Avelar, Ed. Hipócrates São Paulo 8-267-296

Avelar JM (2000b) Results in Plastic Surgery (Resultados em Cirurgia Plástica). in: Plastic Surgery – Obligation of Means Not Obligation of Results (Cirurgia Plástica Obrigação de

Meio e não Obrigação de Fim ou de Resultado, ed. by Juarez M. Avelar, Ed. Hipócrates São Paulo 10-335-379.
Avelar JM (2000c) Individuality. In: Plastic Surgery – Obligation of Means Not Obligation of Results (Cirurgia Plástica Obrigação de Meio e não Obrigação de Fim ou de Resultado, ed. by Juarez M. Avelar, Ed. Hipócrates São Paulo 8-237-266
Avelar JM (2018a) Asymmetrical Breasts: A Challenge for Aesthetic Repair. In: BREAST SURGERY-Aesthetic Approaches. Ed. By Juarez M. Avelar. Ed. Springer Verlag, 43:531-548.
Avelar JM (2018b) Importance of Pitanguy's Technique for the Evolution of Aesthetic Breast Surgery. In: BREAST SURGERY-Aesthetic Approaches. Ed. By Juarez M. Avelar. Ed. Springer Verlag, 1:3-22.
Avelar JM (2018c) Clinical Evaluation and Surgical Planning for Aesthetic Breast Surgery. In: BREAST SURGERY-Aesthetic Approaches. Ed. By Juarez M. Avelar. Ed. Springer Verlag, 3:33-45.
Avelar JM (2018d) Secondary Mastoplasty for Repair of Unfavorable Results. In: BREAST SURGERY-Aesthetic Approaches. Ed. By Juarez M. Avelar. Ed. Springer Verlag, pag. 507-520.
Broadbent TR, Woolf RM (1978) Unsatisfactory results in augmentation mammaplasty—chest and breast asymmetry. Aesth Plast Surg 2(3):251–269. https://doi.org/10.1007/BF01577958
Caldeira AML, Gómez SE, Rios MAT and Pautrat WM (2018) Pectoralis Major Muscle Flap: A Support Approach to Mammaplasty, Personal Technique: in BREAST SURGERY –Aesthetic Approaches, ed. by Juarez M Avelar, Ed. Springer, 11:175-189
Erfon J, Rodrigues CMM and Teles G (2018) Reduction Mammaplasty in a Single Central Block. In BREAST SURGERY –Aesthetic Approaches, ed. by Juarez M Avelar, Ed. Springer, 8:139-147
Jales RM (2004) Ultrassonografic Anatomy of the breast (Anatomia ultrassonográfica da mama). Faculdade de Ciências Médicas. http://www.fcm.unicamp.br/drpixel/pt-br/metodos-de-imagem/anatomia-ultrassonogr%C3%A1fica-da-mama
Juri L (1989) Mammary Asymmetry: A Brief Classification. Buenos Aries Argentina. Aesthet Plast Surg 13(1):47–53. https://doi.org/10.1007/BF01570325#page-1
Karim KE-L, Ashraf Maher F, Ahmed Mabrouk AW, Abd-Al-Aziz Hanafy A-A-A (2009) A management-based classification for breast asymmetries. Egypt J Plast Reconstr Surg 33(1):95–100. http://www.esprs.org/Content/Journals/331_16.pdf
Martire L Jr (2018) Martire's Technique for "L" Mastoplasty. In: BREAST SURGERY-Aesthetic Approaches, ed. by Juarez M Avelar, Ed. Springer, 31: 393-405
Maliniac JW (1950) Asymmetrical breast deformities.Am Surg 1934:734
Paulino Costa M, Barreiro GC and Teixeira NH (2018) Reduction Mastoplasty with Prismatic Resection on a Trapezoid Base for Median Hypertrophic Breasts and Breasts with a Large Base. In: BREAST SURGERY-Aesthetic Approaches, ed. by Juarez M Avelar, Ed. Springer, 25: 331-336.
Pitanguy I (1959) Breast Hypertrophy. Transactions of the International Society of Plastic Surgeons. Second Congress, London E&S, Livingtone, Edinburgh
Pitanguy I (1961) Ecletic approaches to the problems on mastoplasty (Aproximação eclética ao problemas das mamaplastias). Rev Bras Cir 41:179-196.
Pitanguy I (1967) Surgical treatment of breast hypertrophy. Br J Plast Surg 20:78-86
Pitanguy I, Carreirão E, Garcia LC (1973) Transareolar incision to augmentation mammaplasty. (Incisão transareolar para mamoplastias de aumento). Rev Bras Cir 63(9/10):301
Pitanguy I, Viana GP, Daher M, Batti RB (1977) Extranumerous Breast (Mama extranumerária). Rev Bras Cir 67(7/8):273–278
Ribeiro RC, López LEF and Romay S (2018) Tuberous Breast. In: BREAST SURGERY-Aesthetic Approaches, ed. by Juarez M Avelar, Ed. Springer, 39:487- 492
Sepúlveda ACA (1981) Breast Asymmetry—Surgical Treatment (Tratamento das Assimetrias Mamarias). Rev Bras Cir 71(1):11–18
Sinder R (2018) History of Breast Reduction. In: BREAST SURGERY – Aesthetic Approaches, ed. by Juarez M Avelar, Ed. Springer, 6:77–117

Chapter 18
L-Shaped Scar for Reduction Mastoplasty

Lybio Martire Junior

Abstract In this chapter, the author presents the characteristics of "L"-shaped scar mastoplasty for reduction mastoplasty, showing that it is a procedure that can be used in all sizes of breasts and all degrees of breast ptosis, with advantages over other ways of performing mastoplasty. Since he has experience with his technique, the martire´s technique, for over thirty years and has performed all types of mammoplasty with it. Among the advantages of the technique shown are the projection and shape of the breast without using a silicone prosthesis, there is no risk of necrosis of the areola, and.

Keywords Mastoplasty · "L"-shaped scar · Martire's technique

A mastoplasty for breast reduction with an "L"-shaped scar is one among several, existing procedures in which it is possible to proceed with breast reduction.

It is important to note that there is no such thing as an "L" scar technique or a "T" scar technique or a vertical scar technique, but there are different techniques that can obtain scars with these shapes. The scar is the final result. Performing the mastoplasty may have different approaches according to each technique, from the marking and treating of the breast tissue to the assembly of the breast. Therefore, a certain technique may not be able to obtain the same result as another, even if the scars have the same format.

L. M. Junior (✉)
Plastic Surgery and Surgical Technique (Surgical Clinic) at Itajubá Medical School (FMIT), Itajubá, MG, Brazil

Brazilian Society of Plastic Surgery, São Paulo, Brazil

International College of Surgeons, Brazilian College of Surgeons, Brazilian Society of History of Medicine, The Medical Academy of São Paulo, Instituto Prof. Lybio Junior Plastic Surgery and Health, São Paulo, Brazil

J. M. Avelar, R. Cavalcanti Ribeiro (eds.), *Body Contouring*,
https://doi.org/10.1007/978-3-031-42802-9_18

There are many different techniques which result in an "L" scar. However, what they all have in common is the absence of the medial branch of the scar in the breast crease, which gives all of them similar characteristics and principles.

Once this concept is established, we will then explore in this chapter some characteristics that are present in reduction mammaplasties with an "L"-shaped scar, so that the reader can draw their own conclusions about the advantages it presents.

My experience with L-shaped scar reduction mastoplasty dates back to the 1980s. In 1988, I presented a study entitled "Care and Tactics in Mastoplasty in 'L'," in which I showed my technique for mastoplasty, at the eighth Jornada Carioca de Aesthetic Surgery, in Rio de Janeiro (Martire Jr 1988).

I presented the technique at other Brazilian and international plastic surgery congresses (Martire Jr 1990; Martire Jr 1991; Martire Jr 1994).

Since then, I have performed all mastoplasties with this technique with excellent results. It can be used to reduce all breast sizes and all degrees of breast ptosis (Martire Jr 2018).

Figure 18.1 shows the marking of our technique and the result right after we completed the surgery. In an L-shaped scar mastoplasty, it is important that the scar has a 90° angle.

The technique and the amount of breast tissue removed may vary depending on the type and volume of the breasts. However, it is always important to empty the medial and lateral poles of the manas in an L-shaped scar mastoplasty.

In our technique, these tissues are used as flaps in the assembly of the breasts that will be crossed to help shape and project the breasts.

A favorable feature of an L-shaped scar mastoplasty is, of course, the absence of a medial scar.

With the L technique, one can achieve a perfect shape with a minimal scar and avoid a medial scar toward the sternum (Meyer 1995).

Women like to show cleavage that can be more or less ample, so the absence of scarring on the medial part of the breasts is an important and advantageous condition for women (Figs. 18.2 and 18.3).

Another interesting feature in mastoplasty with an "L"-shaped scar is the ease of ascending the nipple-areola complex (NAC), because when assembling the breast,

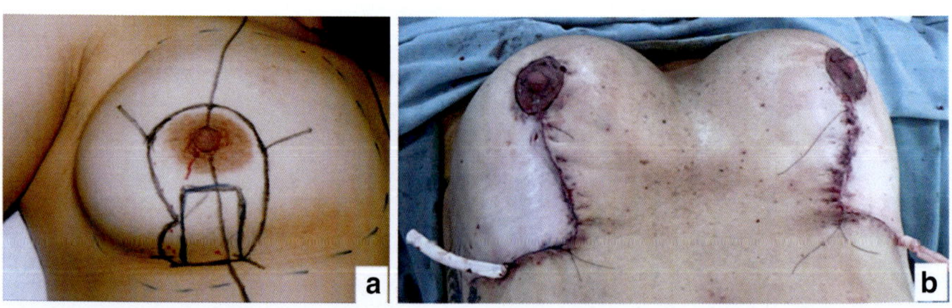

Fig. 18.1 (**a**) Marking of Martire's technique for mastoplasty with an "L"-shaped scar. (**b**) Immediate result at the end of the surgery; it can be observed that the scar is of small extension and the shape of the breasts is graceful with good projection, and there was no need for the use of silicone prosthesis

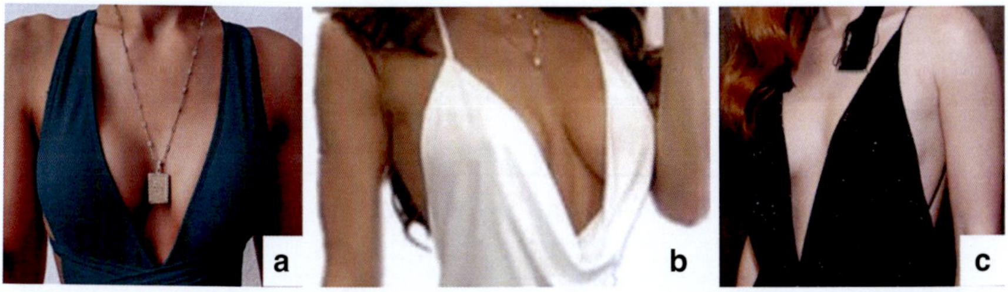

Fig. 18.2 (**a**, **b**, **c**) Types of female necklines that can expose the medial part of the breasts, showing that the absence of a medial scar after a mammoplasty is a considerable advantage

Fig. 18.3 The photo shows the space that could be used in a neckline without scarring in a patient who underwent mastoplasty with an "L"-shaped scar using Martire's technique

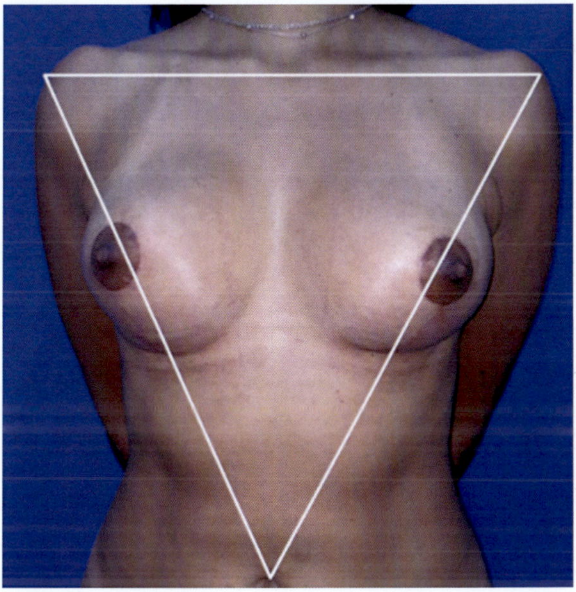

it undergoes rotation as the areola and the nipple rise naturally and very easily. The distance between the areola and the breast crease is not as important, the areola must be positioned at the apex of the breast cone simply (Fig. 18.4a–c).

Another important feature of the L-shaped scar mastoplasty is the abundant blood supply of the breast. The absence of a medial scar in the breast crease causes the medial skin flap to have a much greater blood supply, which makes the possibility of suffering necrosis of the areola or nipple practically null, because the base of the medial flap is much larger in a mastoplasty with an "L"-shaped scar (Fig. 18.5).

The mastoplasty with an "L"-shaped scar also allows for greater projection of the breasts; therefore, there is no need to include a silicone prosthesis to aid in the projection. The assembly projects the breasts satisfactorily, as they undergo rotation. In Martire's technique, the medial and lateral flaps used in the assembly further favor this feature (Martire Jr 2018) (Figs. 18.6, 18.7, and 18.8).

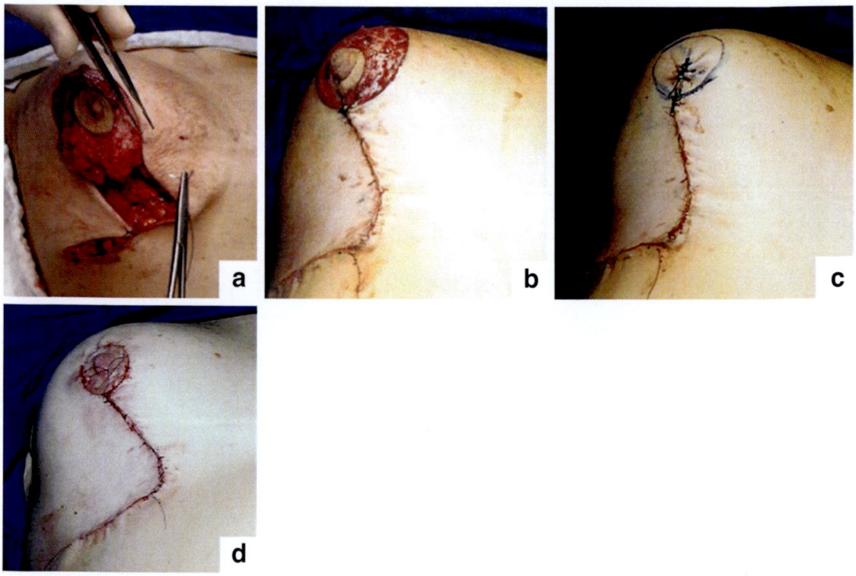

Fig. 18.4 The images (**a**, **b**) show the ease of rise of the nipple-areola complex. The image (**c**) shows that the distance from the nipple to the breast crease is not important, and the image (**d**) shows that the nipple is at the apex of the breast cone

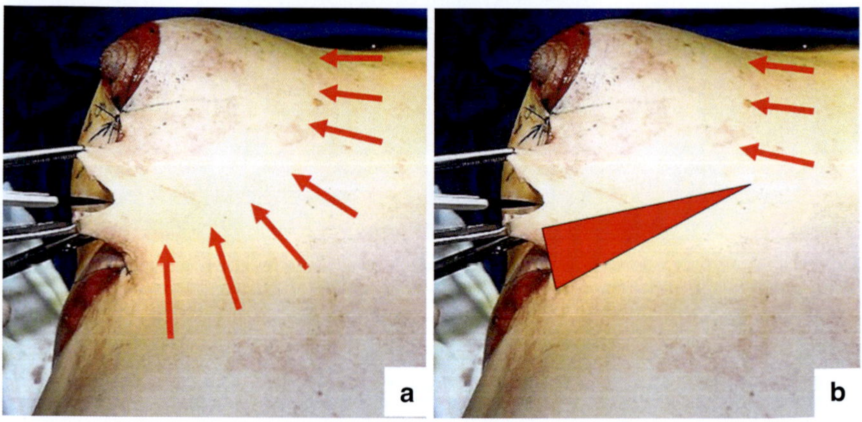

Fig. 18.5 The image (**a**) shows that the blood supply, represented by the arrows, is greater when there is no medial branch of the scar in the breast sulcus, decreasing the base of the skin flap, and the image (**b**) shows that the medial branch of the scar compromises blood supply at the base of the medial flap. This is why the chance of areola and nipple necrosis is practically null in an L-shaped scar mastoplasty (Martire 2016)

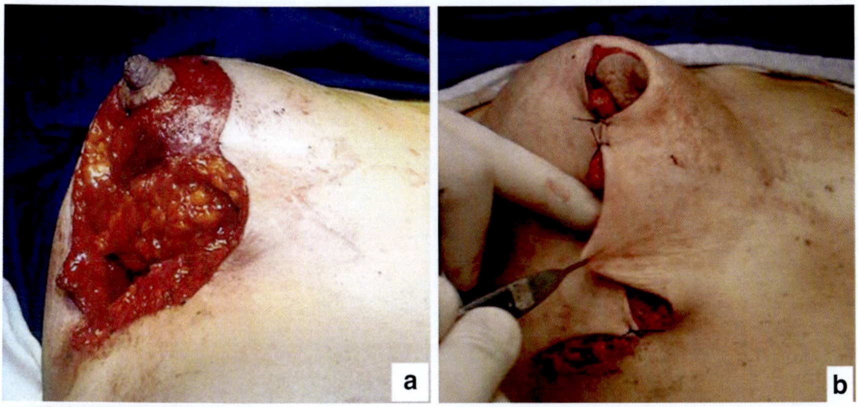

Fig. 18.6 The images (**a**, **b**) show that in a mastoplasty with an "L" scar, the breasts undergo greater projection, which favors the result without the need to include silicone implants to project it

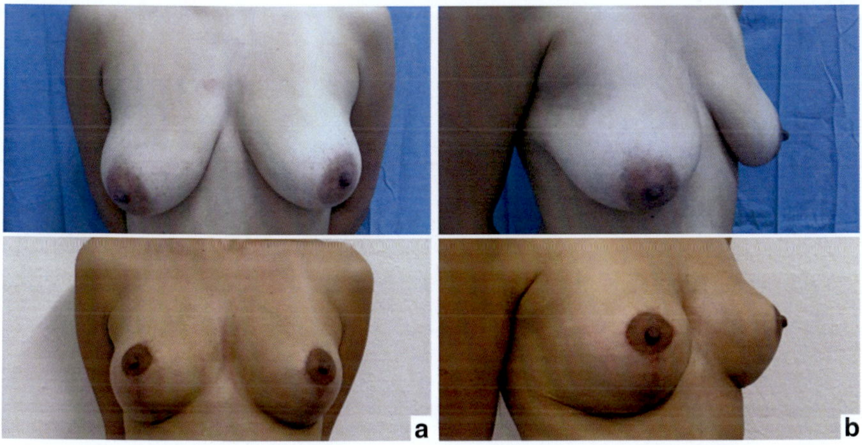

Fig. 18.7 The images (**a**, **b**) show the result of a mastoplasty with an "L"-shaped scar, using Martire's technique, with adequate projection without the need to use a silicone breast implant to project it

Another advantage of mastoplasty with an "L"-shaped scar is the possibility of correcting symmastia, that is, conditions in which the breasts are joined together in the sternal region. The treatment of the medial poles necessarily performed in an L-shaped scar mastoplasty promotes the correction and removal of the breasts naturally, without the medial scar (Martire 2016) (Fig. 18.9).

Another interesting application of mastoplasty with an "L"-shaped scar that proves to be very advantageous are cases in which there is breast dysmorphism. The intervention is performed on only one side, and the smaller scar on the operated breast is undoubtedly an advantage as can be seen in Fig. 18.10.

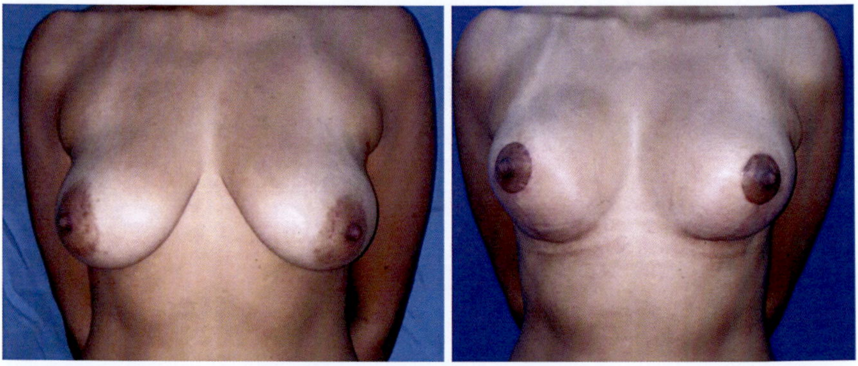

Fig. 18.8 The image shows the result of a mastoplasty with an "L"-shaped scar, using Martire's technique, to the left preoperatively and to the right postoperatively, with a 6-month evolution. One can see the proper projection of the breasts without the need to include a silicone prosthesis to project it

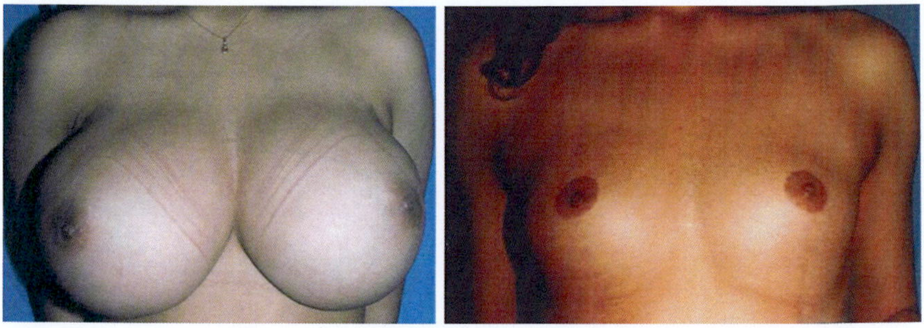

Fig. 18.9 The images show pre- and postoperative mastoplasty using Martire's technique, with 7 years of evolution, in a patient with symmastia, revealing that the mastoplasty with an "L"-shaped scar enables the correction of this condition without the medial branch of the breast crease scar, which is often joined in mammary surgery with an inverted "T"-shaped scar

The results of a mastoplasty with an "L"-shaped scar are very favorable and long-lasting, as can be seen in the patient operated on using Martire's technique, 26 years after the operation (Fig. 18.11).

It can be concluded, therefore, that the mastoplasty with an "L"-shaped scar is a safe procedure, which presents excellent results and can be used in any type of breast hypertrophy or ptosis with considerable advantages (Figs. 18.12, 18.13, and 18.14).

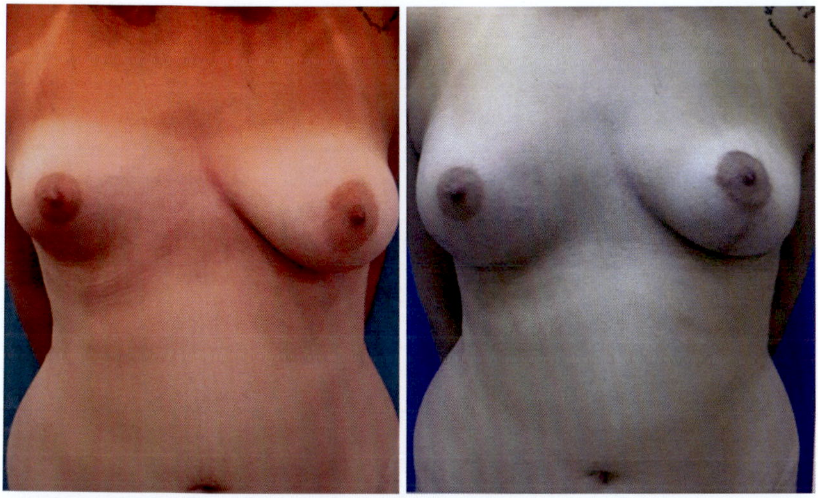

Fig. 18.10 The image shows the pre- and postoperative period, with a 1-year evolution, of a patient with breast dysmorphism in which a breast silicone was included in the right breast and a mastoplasty with an "L"-shaped scar using Martire's technique was performed in the left breast. The absence of the medial branch of the breast fold scar makes the breasts more similar and allows the use of cleavage

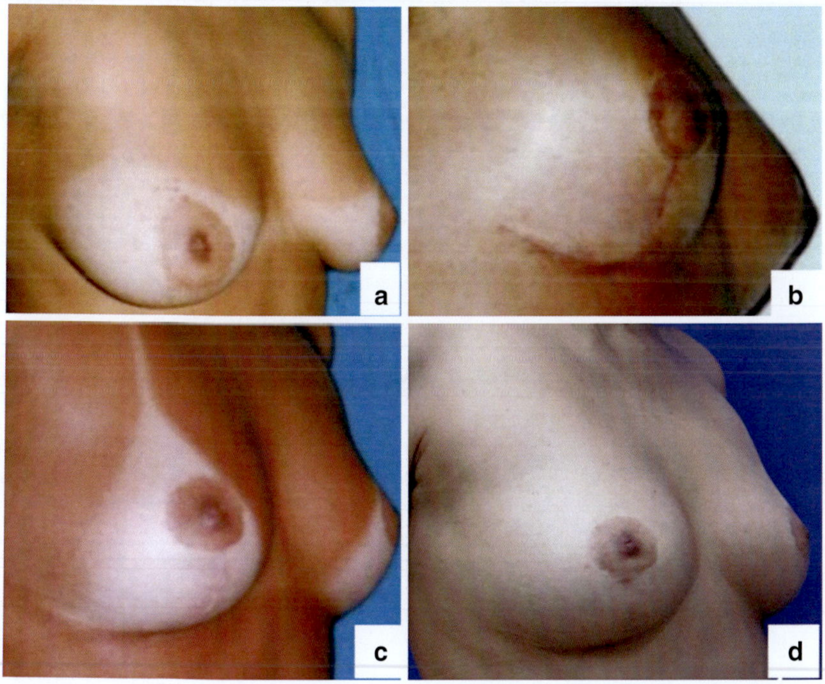

Fig. 18.11 The images show the durability of an L-shaped scar mastoplasty performed using Martire's technique. (**a**) Preoperative; (**b**) 30 days postoperatively; (**c**) 1-year postoperative period; (**d**) 26 years postoperatively

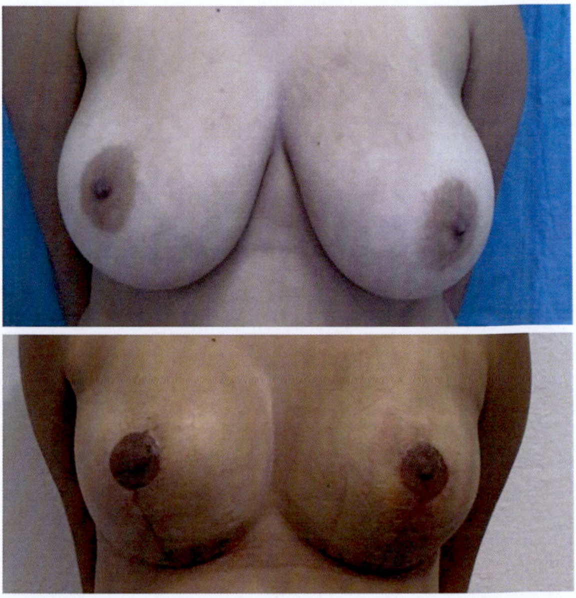

Fig. 18.12 The image shows a pre- and postoperative mastoplasty with an "L"-shaped scar performed using Martire's technique, with an evolution of 4 months

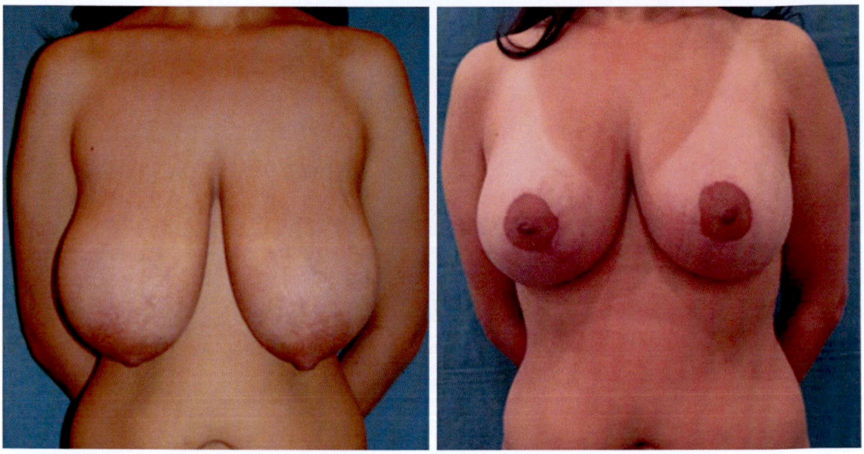

Fig. 18.13 The image shows a pre- and postoperative 1-year evolution of an L-shaped scar mastoplasty performed using Martire's technique

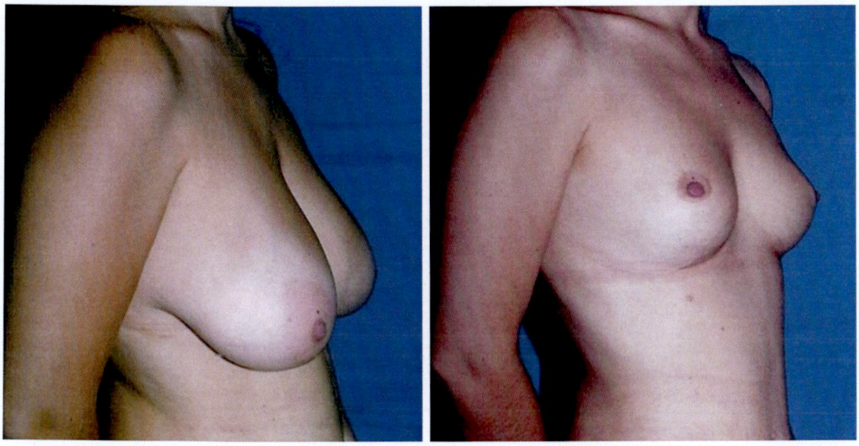

Fig. 18.14 The image shows a preoperative left and a right postoperative period with a 1-year evolution of mastoplasty with an "L" scar performed by Martire's technique

References

Martire Jr L (1988) Care and Tactics in "L" Mastoplasty, 8th Carioca Conference on Aesthetic Surgery, Rio de Janeiro, Brazil

Martire Jr L (1990) L-shaped mastoplasty – Our simple and objective systematization. 27th Brazilian Congress of Plastic Surgery, Rio de Janeiro, Brazil

Martire Jr L (1991) "L" Mastoplasty. Annals of the 28th Brazilian Congress of Plastic Surgery, Hotel Macksoud Plaza, São Paulo, Brazil

Martire Jr L (1994) Martire's technique for L mastoplasty. Annals of the X Congreso Iberolatino Americano de Cirugia Plastica, Viña del Mar, Chile

Meyer R (1995) "L" technique compared with others in mammaplasty reduction Aesthetic Plast Surg Nov-Dec 1995;19(6):541-8

Martire Jr L (2016) Mammaplasty - Personal 'L' Technique, A Procedure for All Types of Breasts. Annals of the X South Mineiro Congress of Plastic Surgery, Itajubá, Minas Gerais, Brazil

Martire Jr L. (2018) Martire's Technique for "L" Mastoplasty. In: Avelar J. (eds) Breast Surgery. Springer, Cham. https://doi.org/10.1007/978-3-319-54115-0_31

Chapter 19
Endoscopic Breast Reduction and Lifting

Marco Aurelio Faria-Correa

Abstract Various situations necessitate distinct approaches to breast reduction and lifting. Some patients have ideal breast size and good skin tone with minimal sagging or upper pole loss. Others exhibit slight breast asymmetry, content with one breast size while seeking reduction in the larger breast. They specifically request scarless surgery to achieve their goals, making endoscopic breast reduction and lifting an optimal technique for their needs.

Introduction

There is no one breast reduction and lifting technique that can attend all different situations. There are patients presenting with their ideal size of breast and good skin tone with minimal degree of ptosis or only the loss of the upper pole. There are also patients presenting with small degree of breast asymmetry, informing that they are happy with the size of the smaller breast, asking for reducing the larger breast, and requesting for scarless surgery that could help them to achieve their goals.

In 1991, the new concepts regarding skin elasticity were introduced into the field of plastic surgery by way of innovative techniques of liposuction and periareolar breast reduction (Avelar and Juarez-Illouz 1986; Peixoto 1980; Ribeiro 1989). These new concepts, which concern the capacity of the skin to retract, allowed the author to investigate the feasibility of applying endoscopic methods to subcutaneous tissue to avoid skin resection. The author began by modifying the mini-abdominoplasty technique and techniques for breast reduction and mastopexy—endoscopy was also used as an aid for flap harvesting and placement

M. A. Faria-Correa (✉)
Mount Elizabeth Novena Specialist Centre, Singapore, Singapore
e-mail: drmarco@drmarco.com

J. M. Avelar, R. Cavalcanti Ribeiro (eds.), *Body Contouring*,
https://doi.org/10.1007/978-3-031-42802-9_19

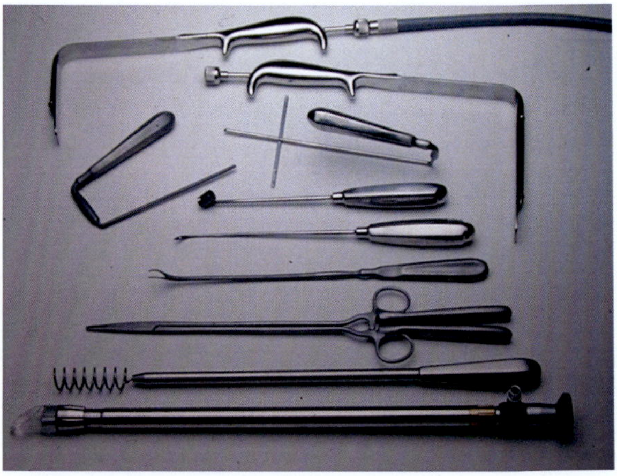

Fig. 19.1 Set of instruments developed by the author from superior to inferior: light source retractors; single and cross puncture elevators; transcutaneous suture set—guide, a modified Reverdin needle, and a fondue fork; a modified needle holder; "screw-suture"; "subcutaneous tomoscope"

of tissue expanders—and to develop promising research regarding axillary inguinal lymph node dissections (Faria-Correa 1992).

Video-endoscopic methods have been used in different surgical fields such as gynecology, orthopedics, and general surgery, where many advantages have been shown. There is less tissue trauma, lower rate of infection, and minimal scarring (Verbicaro 1993).

Laparoscopic procedures used pressurized CO_2 gas to create a space between the laparoscope and the tissue to allow visualization. In the subcutaneous tissue, however, pressurized gas is not recommended because of the risk of embolism. To circumvent this risk, the author developed the "subcutaneous tomoscope," which is an instrument that transfers into a transparent capsule the space needed for illumination and visualization. The optical cavity functions much the same way as a scuba diving mask does while serving as a blunt dissector because of its wedge-shaped capsule (Faria-Correa 1992). Specially designed retractors were developed to increase the necessary working space in addition to instruments such as special needle holders and needles (Fig. 19.1). All of these instruments were designed to work through minimal incisions.

With video endoscopy, delicate processes can be performed through minimal incisions that can be made at strategically placed and remote sites avoiding visible scars. This is an important goal in the field of aesthetic surgery where scars are undesirable and may sometimes compromise the final aesthetic result.

Material and Methods

Endoscopic versions for mastopexy and breast reduction were first performed in November 1992. Since then, the endoscopic technique has been used to treat 220 patients. The patients ranged in age from 14 to 62 years old. They presented with first- or second-degree ptosis with or without hypertrophy. Patients were selected on the basis of having good skin elasticity without significant excess skin. Breastfeeding and striae were not considered contraindications as long as the patient maintained good skin elasticity. Premature moderate ptosis recurrence was observed when the endoscopic technique was applied to patients presenting with skin flaccidity. An important application for this technique is in patients with a small degree of breast asymmetry, particularly in young patients. The larger breast can be reduced with no visible scar or loss of sensation to match the smaller, unoperated breast.

Technique

The traditional video-endoscopic system and the subcutaneous tomoscope, associated with endoscopic instruments, were used to create an optical space. Thus, monitor control could be used without CO_2 distension. Some instruments were modified, and new ones were developed creating a set of instruments that facilitate this procedure. Regular laparoscopic forceps and scissors connected to the electrocautery were used.

Positioning of the Patient and the Team

Proper positioning of both the patient and the surgical team is important for facilitating this procedure. The monitor is placed over the patient's head, and the anesthesiologist stays beside the patient's head. The surgeon works beside the patient. The surgical table must be adequate to allow change in the patient's positioning from supine to sitting.

Planning

In planning the mammoplasty, the breast must be observed as a three-dimensional structure (Figs. 19.2, 19.3, and 19.4). Working endoscopically and considering the three-dimensional breast volume as a cone, looking upward, the bottom of the cone can be seen (Fig. 19.5). The goal is to work on the base of the glandular cone. The first step is to plan the undermining of an enlarged area between the breast and the pectoralis fascia, thus creating a retromammary pocket. Both gland advancement (mastopexy) and breast tissue reduction are planned to proceed from the bottom of the cone. If only mastopexy is needed, the incisions are marked at the inframammary fold. If breast reduction is intended, the incisions must be placed a little above the fold.

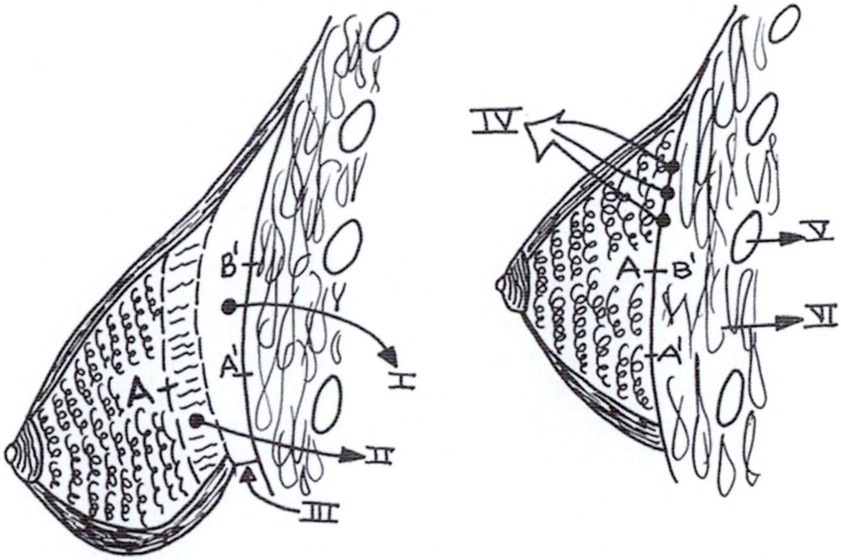

Fig. 19.2 Video-endoscopic breast reduction and mastopexy technique: A and A', level point; B′, upper position; I, retromammary pocket; II, tissue resection area; III, submammary sulcus incision; IV, sutures to fix the gland in its new position at the pectoralis fascia; V, ribs; VI, muscle

Fig. 19.3 Marking shows externally the breast tissue to be resected from the bases of the glandular cone

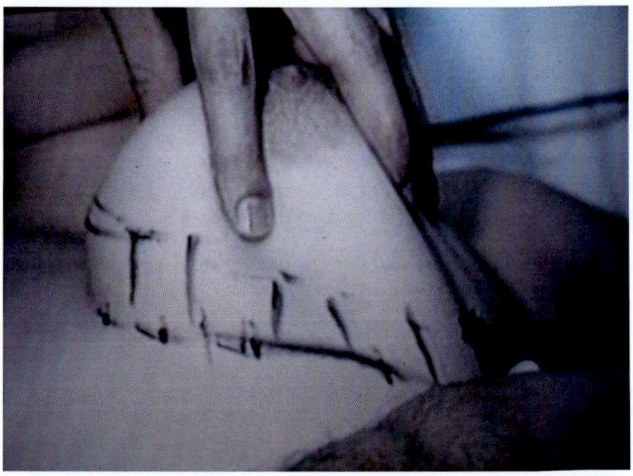

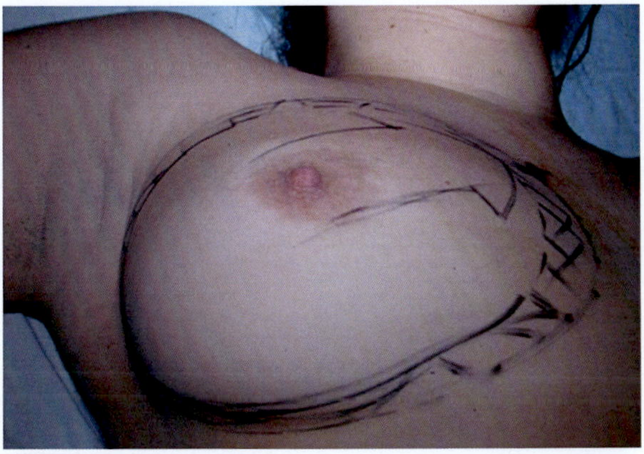

Fig. 19.4 Arrow shows the direction of the mastopexy toward upper medial position

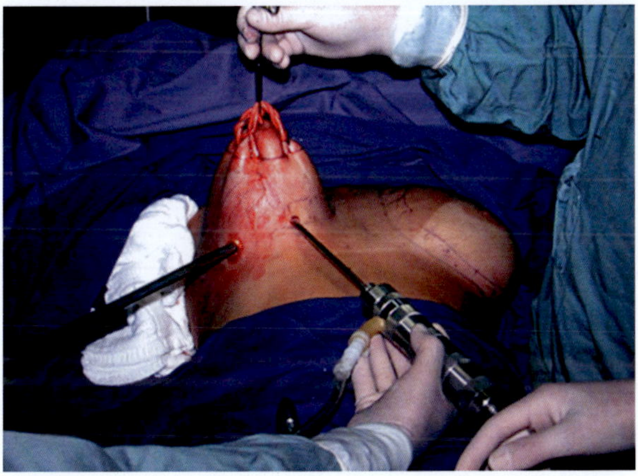

Fig. 19.5 Trans-operative view showing two small incisions (2 cm) at the submammary sulcus, through which the shaver and scope are introduced. Transcutaneous lifting sutures are used to maintain the optical cavity

Anesthesia and Infiltration

General, epidural, or local anesthesia can be used. To reduce bleeding, the process is begun by infiltration of epinephrine/saline solution (1:500,000). This is infiltrated at the base of the breast in the area to be undermined and inside the breast tissue.

Incisions

One or two incisions (1–2 cm) are made in the submammary sulcus. If necessary, a third incision can be made at the axilla to help tissue resection or suture placement.

Traditional open surgery is carried out in three dimensions; however, when working exclusively with monitor view, the third dimension is lost. This can be improved by simultaneously working through two different ports, such that we "triangulate" to a focal point. This provides us with a depth-of-field feeling in the operative area. The best performance is achieved with a triangulation of approximately 30–45° (Fig. 19.5).

Dissection

A retromammary pocket is created between the breast and the pectoralis fascia (Fig. 19.2). This undermining must be wide enough to allow the advancement of the ptotic gland from the lower lateral to the upper medial position on the chest wall. This also provides an ample area of internal scarring between the chest wall and the deep part of the breast tissue. This ample retromammary pocket is created with the aid of the tomoscope by blunt dissection under endoscopic control. The dissection area is similar to that where breast implants are placed. The bleeding is controlled endoscopically by the use of laparoscopic forceps connected to the electrocautery maneuvering them under monitor view. The dissection of the retromammary pocket is completed by using laparoscopic scissors connected to the electrocautery. The use of pressurized gases to create and maintain the work space is avoided. The optical cavity can be provided with the aid of specially designed, long, and thin elevators and retractors that are introduced through the work ports. An external lift can be used by placing sutures through the anterior portion of the cone of the breast (Fig. 19.5).

Breast Tissue Resection

The tissue resection is performed at the base of the gland under endoscopic control, preserving the anterior cone and glandular ducts. A video arthroscopic shaver can be used to reduce the breast. The shaver works as a punching aspirator. There are two cannulas, one rolling inside of the other (Fig. 19.6); both are equipped with windows through which the breast tissue is aspirated and resected. Some breast glands may be too rigid; therefore, its tissue cannot be resected by this punching aspirator. Thus, the procedure is performed by the use of a knife, scissors, electrocautery, or laser. This type of breast is the one that is seen on mammography presenting with a large amount of white fibrous tissue.

By resecting only the base of the breast cone, the functions and sensation are preserved. This is a physiological mammoplasty. The axillary pole and bottom of the mammary cone are resected. There is no resection of even small amounts at the

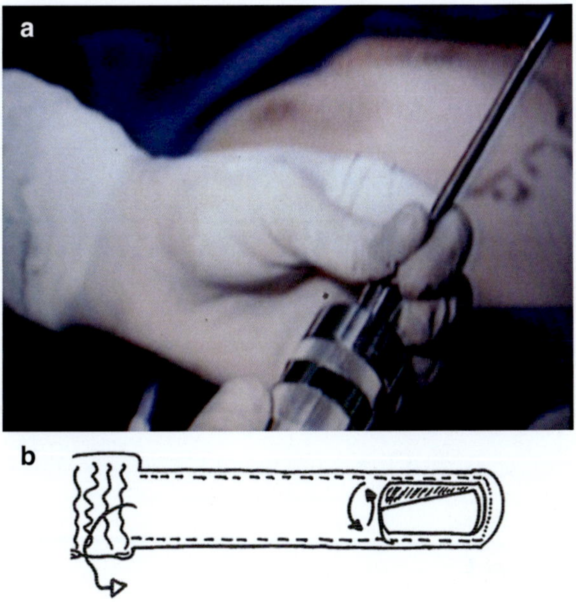

Fig. 19.6 (**a**) Shaver—a video arthroscopic instrument, originally employed to resect meniscus and debride fibrotic tissue inside the knee, used to carry out breast reduction. (**b**) Shaver instrument cannula. There are two cannulas, one rolling inside the other, and a punching aspirator

upper pole of the gland. Working endoscopically, the internal breast volume can be felt externally by hand palpation. By properly planning the tissue resection, the breast is modeled and sculptured into its new shape.

Breast Lifting Fixation

After obtaining adequate hemostasis, the next step is to lift and fix the gland into its new position (Fig. 19.7). Sutures are used to position the mammary gland and fix it to the pectoralis fascia. Suturing can be performed with laparoscopic needle holders. As many sutures as needed are placed to help in positioning the breast so that it is held in place during the maturation of the internal cicatrix, which ultimately fixes the breast permanently in position. Patients with good skin quality are good candidates for this procedure and gain an aesthetic advantage with the repositioning of the gland, as this recreates an upper pole to the breast.

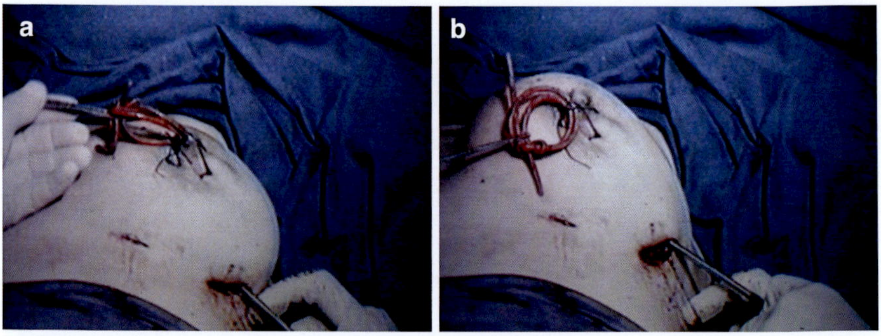

Fig. 19.7 (**a**, **b**) Grasping and testing the right position for placing the sutures

Dressings and Postoperative Care

Suction drains are used during the first 12 h and then removed. A micropore tape dressing (Fig. 19.8) helps to reposition the gland in its new site. This dressing is maintained for 20 days for a long-term support. Continuous use of a supporting bra is recommended for at least 3 months thereafter and as long as possible throughout the patient's life.

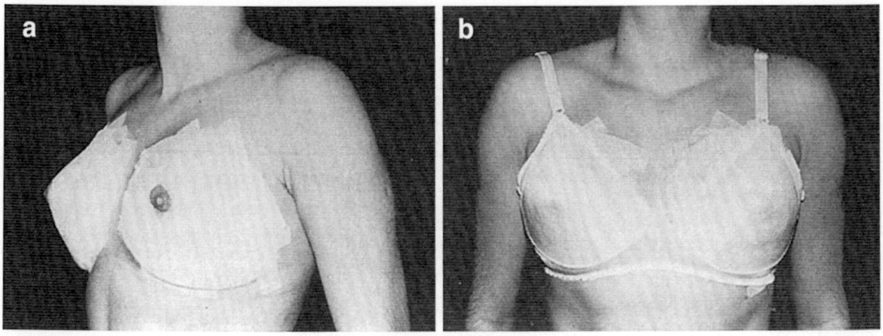

Fig. 19.8 (a, b) Micropore modulator dressing and drainage

Complications

Among the 220 cases, 5 cases of hematoma have been observed in patients in whom no drains were used, and 25 patients had early ptosis recurrence because of poor skin elasticity.

Discussion

The endoscopic breast reduction and mastopexy techniques preserve the breast function and sensation with minimal scars (Figs. 19.9 and 19.10) (Faria-Correa 1993, 1994a, b, c, d, e, f, 1995a, c, d, 2000). An important goal is to treat mammary asymmetry without using prostheses or adding long scars to the breast as opposed to the traditional procedures.

The breast is an anatomic structure that grows perpendicularly from the chest. The effects of gravity pull the breast down whether the patient is old or young or operated on or not. The maintenance of a long-term good result depends not only on the technique used by the author but also on the skin elasticity for retraction. Successful long-term follow-up relies on breast weight and precautions taken by the patient, such as the use of a steadfast modulator bra especially during the practice of sports.

In patients whose skin does not have the capacity to retract, the results are transitory as in usual mastopexies. Nevertheless, the characteristics of this minimally invasive technique that have been attracting patients' interest are the lack of visible scars and the maintenance of sensitivity and function.

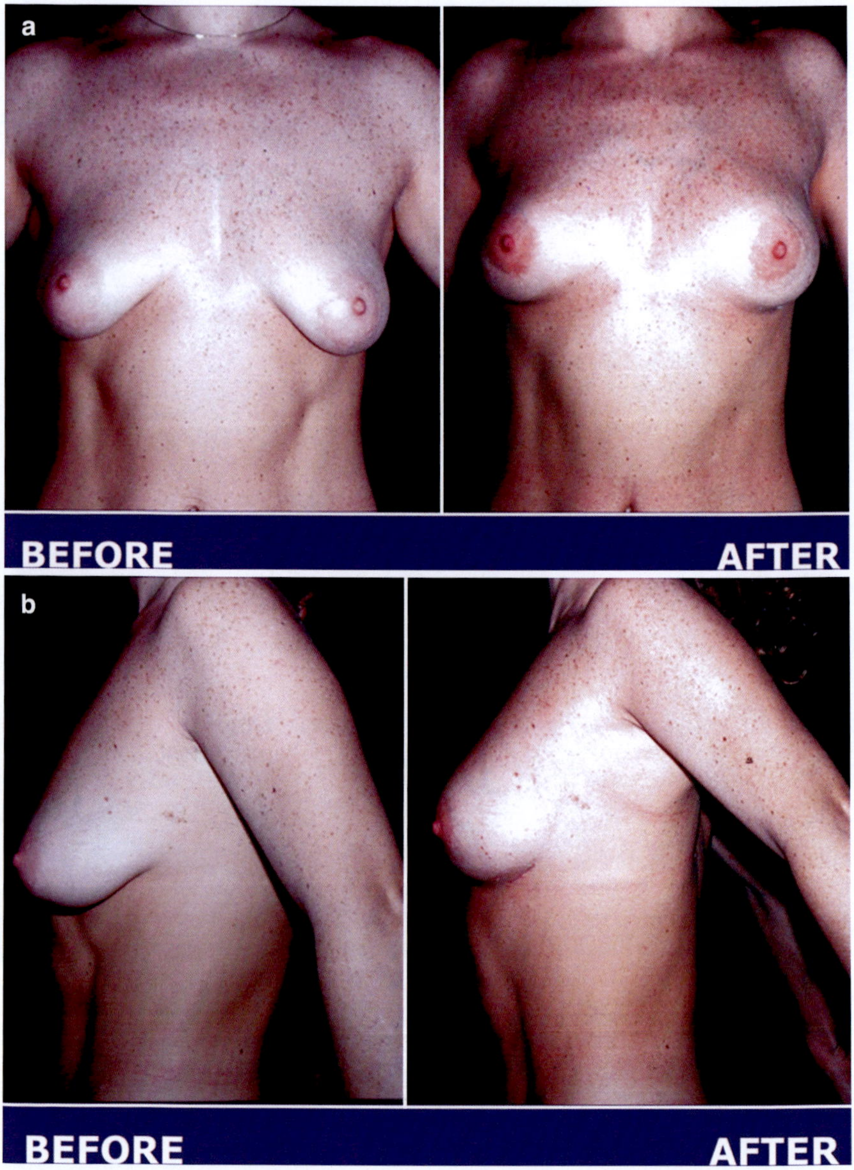

Fig. 19.9 (**a**1,2) Preoperative 32-year-old patient, who breastfed two children, presenting with breast ptosis, moderate amount of striae, and moderate degree of flabbiness. (**b**1,2) Eight months after endoscopic breast lift

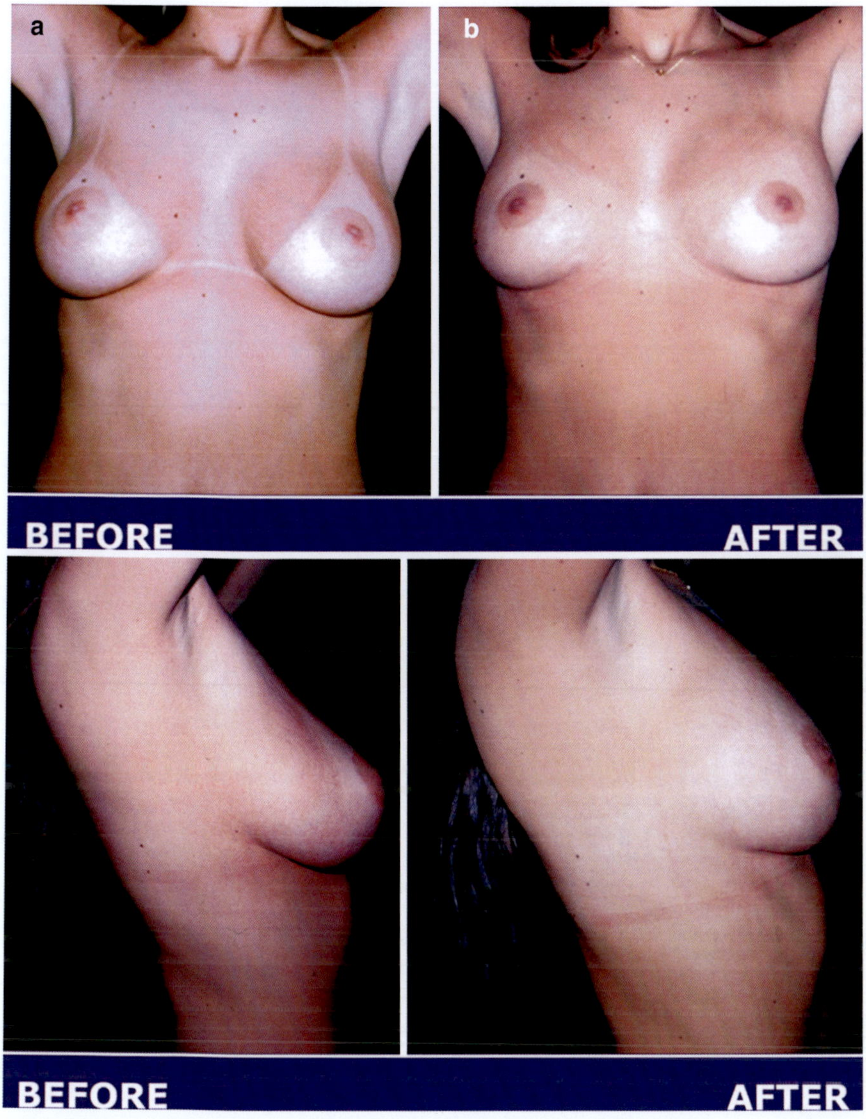

Fig. 19.10 (**a**1, 3) Preoperative 20-year-old patient with good skin elasticity, no striae, breast hypertrophy, and ptosis. (**b**1–3) Two years after video-endoscopic breast reduction and lift (120 g each breast), showing a nice upper pole, good skin retraction, no function or sensation damage, and no visible scars

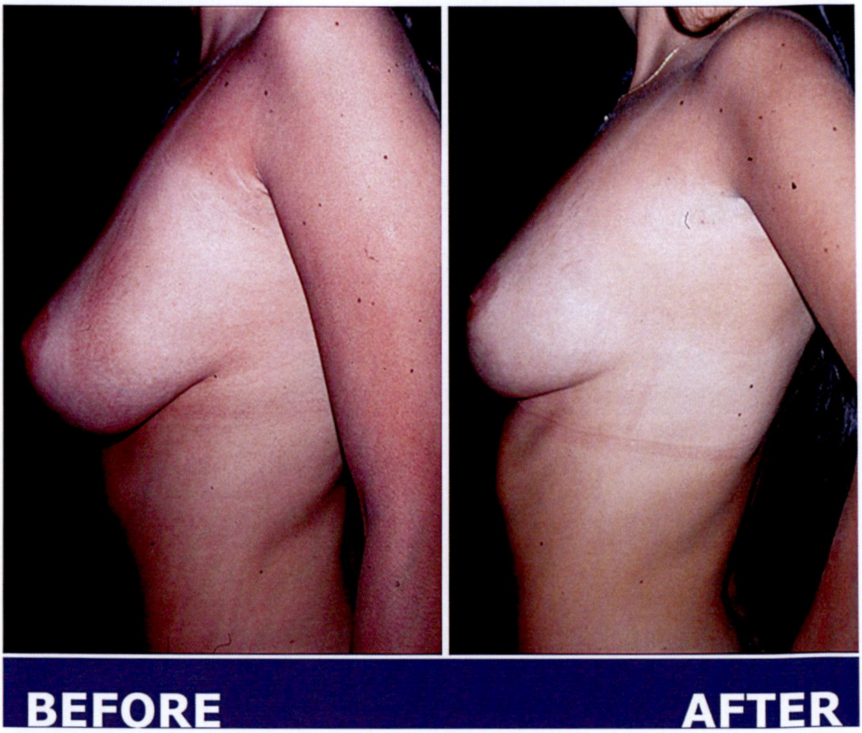

Fig. 19.10 (continued)

Conclusions

The results of 30 years' follow-up in 220 patients permit us to recommend its use in first-degree ptosis and breast reductions in younger patients. The technical procedure presented shows its utmost effectiveness and best aesthetic results in young patients who present with a small amount of hypertrophy or asymmetry, but with good skin elasticity, and who do not have significant excess skin. The author believes that the use of these endoscopic techniques is a new trend in plastic surgery when properly applied.

References

Avelar M, Juarez-Illouz YG: Lipoaspiraco. Hipocrates 1986;3: 320
Faria-Correa MA: Videoendoscopy in Plastic surgery: Brief communication – A videocirurgia na cururgia plastica: Rev Soc Bras de Cir Plastica Est Reconstr 1992; 7: 80-81
Faria-Correa MA: Endoscopic abdominoplasty, mastopexy and breast reduction. Clin Surg 1995a; 22 (4): 723-745

Faria-Correa MA: Endoscopic mammoplasty. World J Plast Surg 1995c; 1: 118- 119
Faria-Correa MA: Videoendoscopic subcutaneous techniques for aesthetic and reconstructive plastic surgery. Plast Reconstr Surg 1995d; 96 (2): 446-453
Faria-Correa MA: Mamoplastia por endoscopia. Rev Cirurg Plas Ibero Latino-Americana 1994a ; 20: 121-127
Faria-Correa MA: Mamoplastia Videodndoscopica Arquivos Catarinenses Med 1994b; 23: 116-118
Faria-Correa MA: Mamoplastia videoendoscopica e abdominoplastia videoendoscopica (subcutaneoscopica). In Tournieux AAB (ed), Atualizacao em Cirurgia Plastica Estetica. Sao Paulo, SP, Robe 1993: 411-418
Faria-Correa MA: Mammoplastia por endoscopia. J Cirurg Plast Ibero-Latino-Americana 1994c;20 (2): 121-127
Faria-Correa MA: Mammoplastia videoendoscopica. Rev Soc Bras Med Estet 1994d; 4; 33-36
Faria-Correa MA: Endoscopic mammoplasty. In: Transactions of the 7th Asian Congress of Plastic and Reconstructive Surgery, Bangkok, Holistic 1994e
Faria-Correa MA: Mamoplastia videoendoscopica. In: Tournieux AAB (ed), Atualizacao em Circugia Plastica Estetica e Reconstructiiva. Sao Paulo, Robe, SP 1994f
Faria-Correa MA: Reducao e pexia mamaria por videoendoscopia. In: Saltz 9 (ed), Cirugia da Mama-Esttica e Reconstructiva de Ricardo Ribeiro. Livaria e Editora Revinter 2000, pp 319-327
Peixoto G: Reduction Mammoplasty. A personal technique. Plast Reconst Surg 1980;65(2):217-226
Ribeiro L: Circurgia Plastica da Mama. Rio de Janeiro, Medsi 1989
Verbicaro E: Historico. In: Cruz 0 (ed). Manual de Cirurgia Videoendoscopica. Rio De Janeiro, Revinter 1993

Chapter 20
The Sting Technique: A New Procedure for the Correction of the Hypoplastic Lower Breast Poles

Gianluca Campiglio

Abstract Correction of hypoplastic lower breast poles is a difficult challenge during an augmentation mammoplasty. Many techniques have been described in the past such as rotation of glandular flaps and release of contracted superficial fascia with or without sessions of fat injections. Starting from the experience in the treatment of post-burn keloids and hypertrophic scars using big angiographic sharp needles (18 G), a new surgical technique ("sting technique") based on multiple percutaneous full-thickness puncturing of the hypoplastic interior quadrants of the breast is presented. This maneuver acts by breaking the cutaneous and subcutaneous restrictions that prevent a satisfying expansion of the lower pole and can lead to a double bubble deformity when the original inframammary fold is particularly tight. Preliminary results in patients with high inframammary fold (IMF) and short areola-IMF distance are encouraging even if longer follow-up and larger series can help to understand better in the future the real potentialities and limits of the sting technique. No major complications such as hematoma, infection, or permanent scarring have been observed in the patient treated so far.

Keywords Breast augmentation · Breast implant · Tuberous breast · Breast malformation · Surgical treatment

G. Campiglio (✉)
Campiglio Plastic Surgery Center, Milan, Italy

J. M. Avelar, R. Cavalcanti Ribeiro (eds.), *Body Contouring*,
https://doi.org/10.1007/978-3-031-42802-9_20

Introduction

Breast augmentation is a very common procedure aimed to increase the volume and improve the shape of the breast. Independently from the surgical technique adopted and the type of prostheses implanted, results are usually very satisfying for both the surgeons and the patients.

Nevertheless, mild malformations requiring additional surgical maneuvers in order to obtain a nice shape and a natural appearance of the augmented breast can complicate this procedure. This is the case, for example, of small breast with a hypoplastic lower pole, a high inframammary fold, and a short distance from the areola. This condition belongs to the large family of the tuberous breasts, initially described by Rees and Aston for small breasts characterized by a reduction in both vertical and horizontal diameters with glandular herniation behind a huge nipple-areolar complex (Rees and Aston 1976) and then expanded to include also tubular breast, nipple-areolar complex herniation, constricted breast, lower pole hypoplasia, narrow base breast, and snoopy deformity.

The exact prevalence of tuberous breast is a contentious issue. Some authors claim that it affects almost three fourths of the female population (Brown and Somogyi 2015), while others suggest that it is under a tenth (Dos Santos and Ruiz-Castilla 2021). This estimation is further complicated by the fact that less severe forms might go unrecognized to both patients and surgeons. DeLuca-Pytell reported an 88.8% incidence of these malformations in patients requiring a mammoplasty due to breast asymmetry (DeLuca-Pytell et al. 2005). Recently, Klinger et al. reviewed the incidence in aesthetic augmentation mammoplasty and also proposed a new terminology for all these breast anomalies introducing the concept of stenotic breast (Klinger et al. 2017). The authors distinguished *vertical stenosis* (upper position of the real inframammary fold with different grades of glandular development and ptosis) and *vertical-horizontal stenosis* (upper position of the real inframammary fold and a constricted breast base with different grades of glandular development and ptosis). Eight different presentations, from minor deformities to real tuberous breasts, can be the result of the combination of the type of stenosis, position of the inframammary fold, development of the gland, and grade of ptosis. In all these combinations, the common feature is the hypoplastic lower pole that needs an appropriate expansion in order to have a nice and round shape.

The use of needles to release retracted tissue is well known and quite popular in plastic surgery. Subcision, also called as subcutaneous incisionless surgery, a term coined by Orentreich and Orentreich in 1995 (Orentreich and Orentreich 1995), describes a minor surgical procedure for treating depressed scars and wrinkles using a tri-beveled hypodermic needle inserted through a puncture in the skin surface (hence, "incisionless" surgery), and its sharp edges maneuvered under the defect to make subcuticular cuts. The principle of this procedure is to break the fibrotic strands that tether the skin to the underlying subcutaneous tissue with a gentle back and forth movement of the needle. The depression is lifted by the releasing action of the procedure, and very often a thin layer of hyaluronic acid or of micro-fat is also injected in the new dead space in order to prevent or delay a recurrence of the aesthetic defect. Although subcision is most often used to treat wrinkle and acne scars, it may also help reduce scars caused by other conditions, like cellulitis, chicken pox, or surgery as in the case of caesarean scars.

Klinger et al. in 2008 were the first to describe the use of sharp needles in autologous fat grafting for the treatment of patients affected by burn scars, subsequently demonstrating its safety and versatility in overcoming the resistance of fibrotic tissues (Klinger et al. 2008).

Later Dr. Rigotti described the "Rigottomy technique," which is a subcutaneous release (subcision) of the contracted breast tissue with big needles creating multiple tiny 2 mm cavities to be filled of autologous fat (Khouri et al. 2014).

In this chapter, the preliminary results obtained using a new surgical technique named "sting technique" are presented. This technique is similar to the Rigottomy but at the same time differs for two relevant aspects: (1) it is a percutaneous and not subcutaneous release (subcision) of the stenotic tissue (in this way not only the gland but also the skin envelope is expanded) and (2) fat is not injected at the end of the needle treatment. The "sting technique" can be used in typical tuberous breasts together with other fundamental maneuvers such as areola reduction and reshaping of the glandular parenchyma or during an augmentation mammoplasty when the inframammary fold is high and the inferior breast pole is contracted.

Surgical Technique

A periareolar or inframammary approach is used to create a dual plane subpectoral or subfascial pocket for a round implant. After checking the hemostasis, the pocket is completely filled with gauzes soaked in antibiotic solution (clindamycin 600 mg diluted in 100 cc saline) containing 500 mg of tranexamic acid. This creates a soft mound against which to perform the "sting maneuver" that is the expansion of the constricted lower pole of the breast puncturing it many times with an 18 Gauge needle (Fig. 20.1). Each prick penetrates all the skin and the underlying tissue (fascia and gland) up to the gauzes inside the pocket. The distance between each hole measures few millimeters. The punctures of the sting technique can extend along all the inferior pole, from the nipple to the new inframammary fold when all the inferior pole has to be expanded (Fig. 20.2). When the maneuver is aimed to weaken a tight inframammary fold and prevent a double bubble deformity, puncturing is limited to a wide cutaneous strip between the old and the new inframammary fold (Fig. 20.3). The sting technique can also be performed asymmetrically if you need a different reshaping on the two sides or can be used to expand only the lateral or

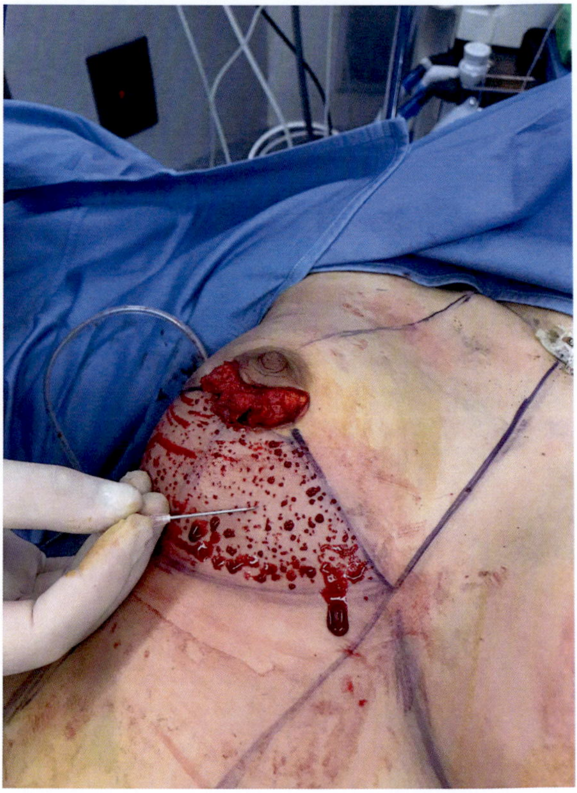

Fig. 20.1 Percutaneous full-thickness puncturing (sting technique) of the constricted lower breast pole using a sharp 18 G needle once the implant pocket is filled with gauzes

the medial quadrants of the breast if indicated. Puncturing creates a light bleeding that does not require any coagulation and stops spontaneously very soon. Subsequently, the gauzes inside the pocket are removed and substituted by the definitive implant. If indicated, a periareolar mastopexy is performed, but in most of the cases, the ptosis is only apparent. Once the inframammary fold is lowered and the implant positioned, the hanging breast is corrected. The subcutaneous tissue and skin are closed using re-absorbable sutures. The skin of the inferior breast pole is dressed with greasy gauzes and sterile gauzes.

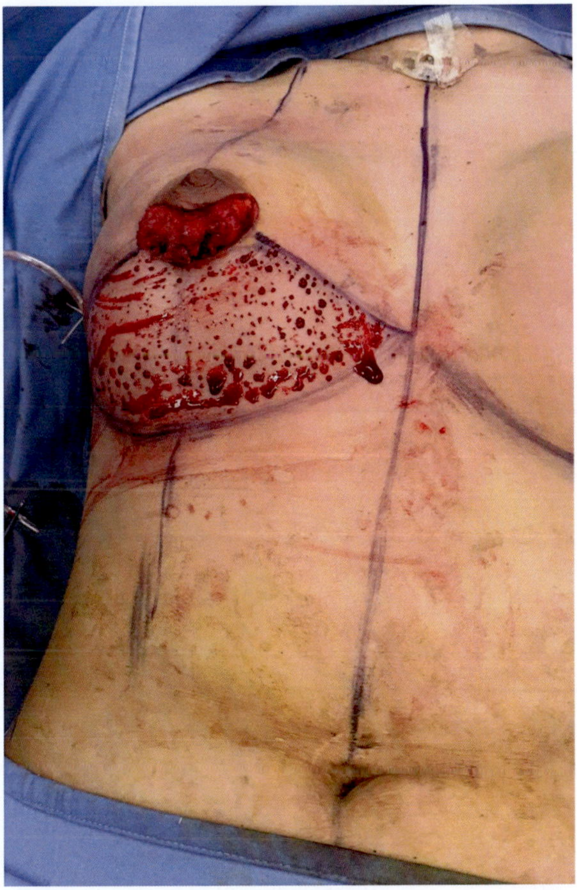

Fig. 20.2 The sting technique can be used to expand the entire inferior lower pole, from the areola to the new inframammary fold

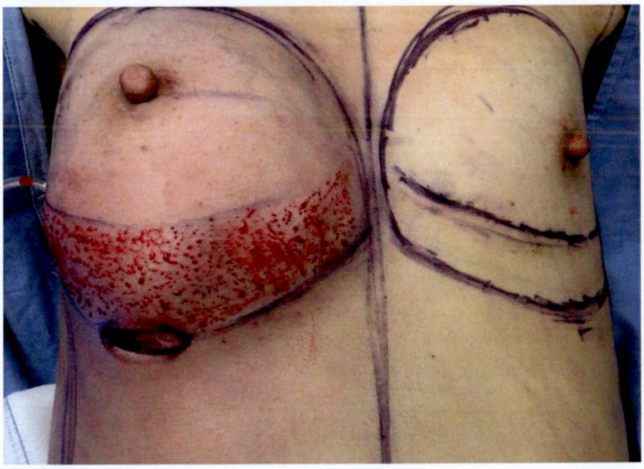

Fig. 20.3 In the case of high and tight inframammary fold, the double bubble deformity can be prevented by breaking the cutaneous and subcutaneous restrictions and puncturing a wide strip between the old (superior blue line) and the new (inferior blue line) inframammary fold

Postoperative Dressing

Dressing is removed after 48 h along with drains, when used. The patients are instructed to wear a sport bra for 4 weeks. The greasy gauzes on the treated area are left attached to the skin till when they spontaneously detach themselves. Healing of the punctured skin is usually completed in 7–10 days after the procedure (Fig. 20.4).

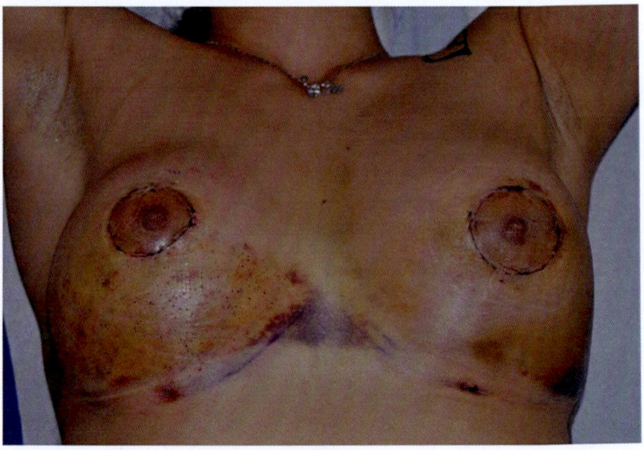

Fig. 20.4 Complete re-epithelialization usually occurs after 7–10 days without any scarring

Clinical Cases

A total of 30 patients affected by a high inframammary fold with a hypoplastic lower breast pole have been treated using the sting techniques. Age ranged from 21 to 35 years. Evaluation of the results was performed by three surgeons using preoperative and postoperative digital photographs with frontal, lateral, and bilateral oblique views for each patient. A questionnaire was used to evaluate each patient's satisfaction and graded from 0, extremely poor outcome, to 10, extremely satisfactory outcome. Categories used for the assessment by the surgeons and patients included lower pole shape, height and symmetry of the inframammary fold, breast volume, and breast symmetry (Figs. 20.5, 20.6, 20.7, 20.8, 20.9 and 20.10).

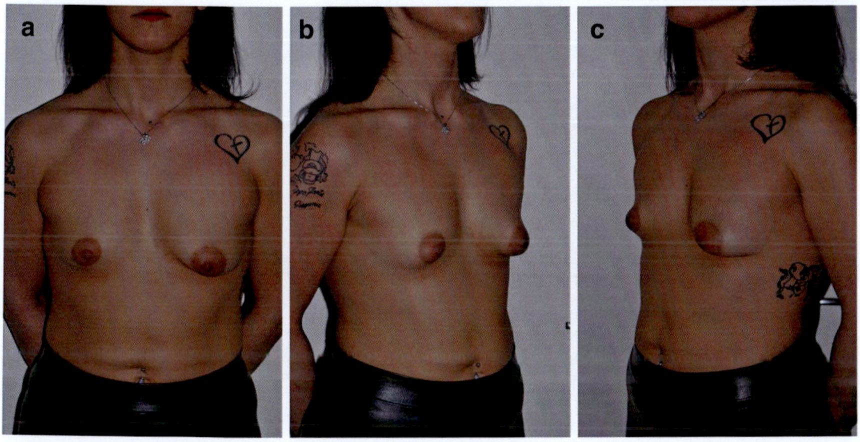

Fig. 20.5 Breast asymmetry with a smaller right gland complicated by a constricted lower pole. (**a**) Preoperative frontal view. (**b**) Preoperative three-quarter right view. (**c**) Preoperative three-quarter left view

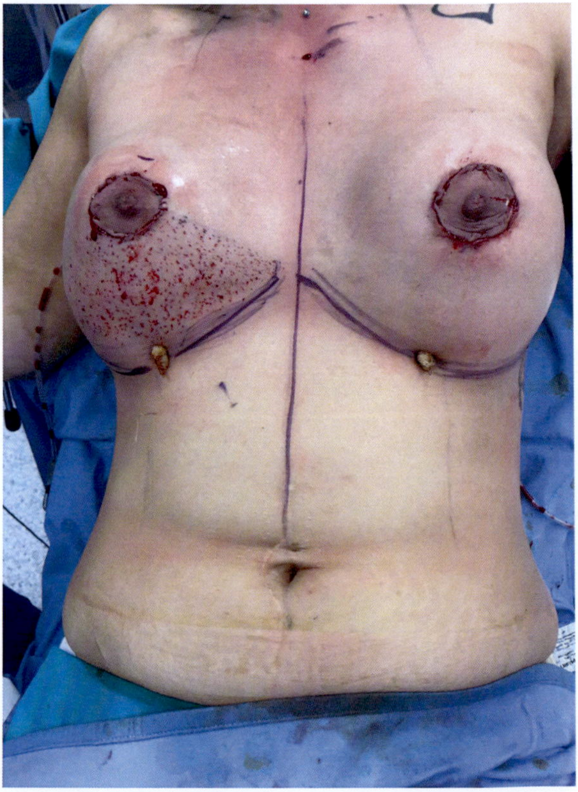

Fig. 20.6 Intraoperative view after expansion of the right lower breast pole using the sting technique from the areola to the new inframammary fold, augmentation with smooth round subpectoral implants (350 cc on the left and 375 on the right), and bilateral periareolar mastopexy

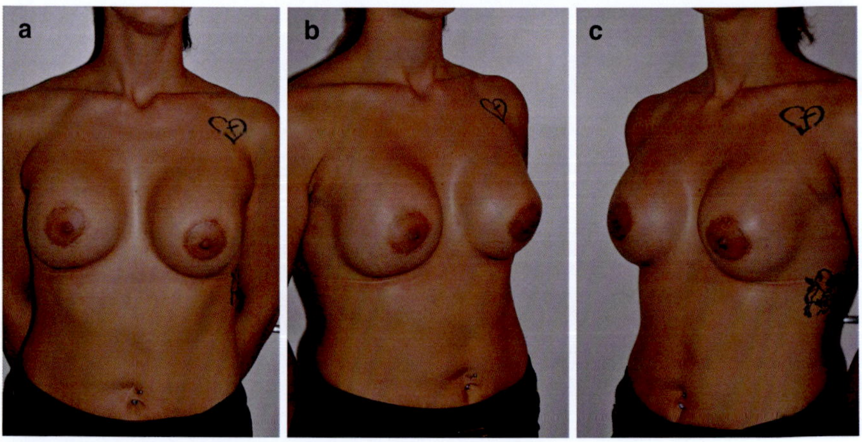

Fig. 20.7 (**a**) Postoperative frontal view. (**b**) Postoperative three-quarter right view. (**c**) Postoperative three-quarter left view

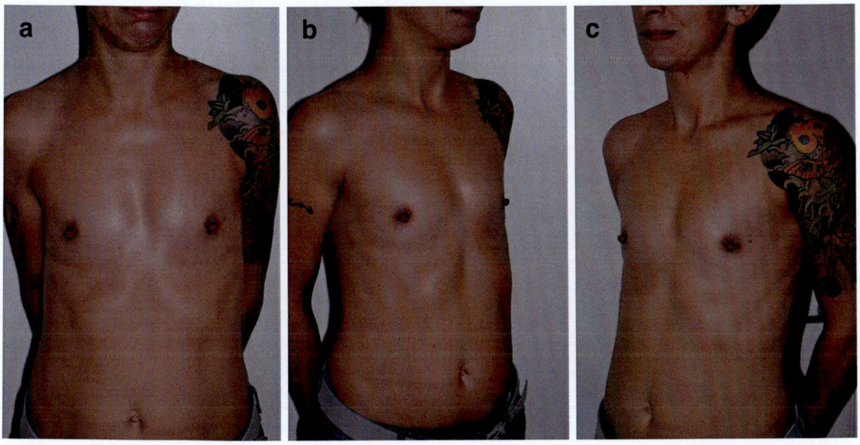

Fig. 20.8 Bilateral severe hypoplasia with tight inframammary fold and stiff inferolateral quadrant of the left breast. (**a**) Preoperative frontal view. (**b**) Preoperative three-quarter right view. (**c**) Preoperative three-quarter left view

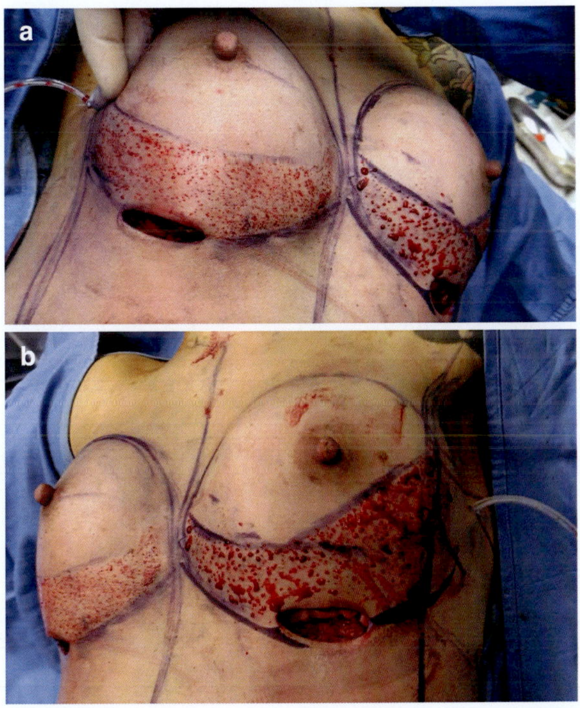

Fig. 20.9 Intraoperative view. Subpectoral dual plane round and smooth implant (350 cc). (**a**) Sting technique has been applied to a wide strip between the old and new inframammary fold in order to prevent a double bubble deformity. (**b**) The inferolateral quadrant of the left breast has been treated as well in order to expand it adequately after the placement of the implant

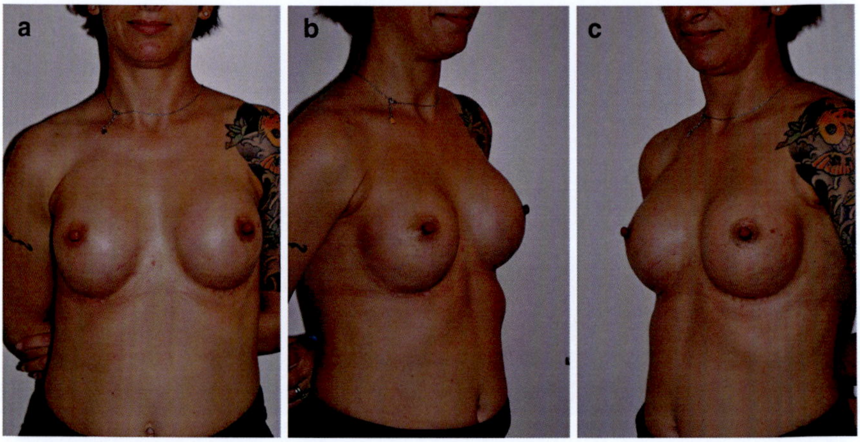

Fig. 20.10 (**a**) Postoperative frontal view. (**b**) Postoperative three-quarter right view. (**c**) Postoperative three-quarter left view

Results

Aesthetic results evaluated by the surgeons' group reported a mean aesthetical outcome of 7.7, whereas the ones of the patients reported a mean value of 8.5.

Complications

In two cases, the aesthetic result needed a revision consisting in a fat graft in order to improve the roundness of the lower pole. In seven cases, a subcutaneous blood effusion, due to the punctures of the skin, was observed. This complication never presented as a true hematoma and therefore did not require an additional drainage. After 7–10 days, it disappeared spontaneously and never led to other serious consequence such as skin retraction.

In two patients with darker skin (Fitzpatrick III), the small holes produced by the needle left pigmented spots that required the use of hydroquinone cream 4% for 2 months and then completely disappeared.

Any serious complication such as permanent scarring or infection was observed in this series of patients.

Conclusion

Hypoplastic lower pole with a high inframammary fold and short distance from the areola can complicate an augmentation mammoplasty. This condition belongs to the great family of the tuberous breasts. A key point for a successful result is the lowering of the inframammary fold so that an adequate volume of the prosthesis is located below the nipple, thus avoiding a high-riding implant deformity. Many surgical techniques have been described in the past to treat these features such as the use of inferior rotation of glandular flaps (Puckett and Concannon 1990) and the releasing of the superficial fascia alone or followed by fat grafting of the lower part of the breast (Servaes et al. 2010) (Oroz-Torres et al. 2014). Positioning of the new fold is determined by the position of the contralateral non-pathological side. If there is bilateral deformity, the fold is placed at a location that 55% of the breast volume is below the areola and the remaining 45% above it. Nevertheless, subcutaneous dissection in the inferior quadrants can be difficult due to the resistance of the skin and of the underlying fascia superficialis. Regardless of the severity of the deformity and the technique adopted, placement of either breast tissue or an implant in the new fold is necessary to maintain its new location. According to Pardo, if an implant is used, the inframammary fold should be placed 2 cm more inferiorly to allow for subsequent contraction (Pardo et al. 1999). In the case that the inframammary fold is adequately lowered but the constricted lower pole is not expanded, the tight crease of the original fold can indent the implant transversely, dividing it into two and creating a second "bubble" beneath the breast (double bubble deformity). Moreover, if the poorly treated constricted lower pole is combined with large breast implants, the risk of this iatrogenic deformity may increase further.

The use of big needles instead of blunt cannulas to inject fat has been firstly reported by Klinger et al. in 2008 (Klinger et al. 2008). They adopted sharp needle (18 G angiographic needles) to overcome the great resistance of the fibrotic tissue of severe post-burn hypertrophic scars and keloids. Sharp angiographic cannulas allow performing a highly precise technique making possible to lay a constant amount of fat at the dermal-hypodermal junction. Postoperative histologic examination of scar tissue showed new collagen deposition, neovascularization, and dermal hyperplasia. Clinically, the 6 months follow-up demonstrated a significant improvement of the skin texture, softness, and thickness. This positive effect was due to the regenerative properties of the adipose-derived stem cells (ADSC) but also to the mechanical breakage of the contracted collagen fibers by the sharp tip of the big needles. In another paper, the same group proved the safety of the procedure treating a large series of post-burn scars with fat delivered in this way (Maione et al. 2015). Complication rate was very low and mostly related to the use of needle such as bruising, swelling or transient numbness, hematoma, seroma, and infections. The most feared complication was intravascular fat injection, but it was easily avoided adopting a retrograde injection method. Caviggioli et al. subsequently demonstrated the versatility of the technique extending the application of the procedure to other types of scar and fibrotic tissue (Caviggioli et al. 2012). Other advantages of using sharp needles are that a skin incision with a scalpel for cannula access is not needed, thus minimizing the patient discomfort and avoiding a new scars. Angiographic sharp needles are also easily available, disposable, and low-cost devices.

A similar technique to treat contracted tissue or scar in the breast has been subsequently described by Khouri and named "Rigottomy" after its inventor Dr. Rigotti (Khouri et al. 2014). In this article, an innovative application of the sharp needles to prepare the optimal bed for fat micrograft during autologous breast enhancement is described. Indeed, if scarred or contracted tissue is present, the use of blunt cannulas is not able to deposit thin multiple fat layers and can lead to the formation of larger cavities that would not be a good graft to recipient interface. Exactly as in the post-burn scars, adopting sharp 18-gauge needles can break the hard fibrous architecture of the recipient sites and allows the creation of multiple tiny nicks. These microcavities are subsequently filled by fat particles that can survive by diffusion until neovascularization occurs. Being the purpose of Rigottomy to create the optimal bed for the subcutaneous fat grafting, the skin does not need to be punctured several times as in the sting technique but ideally only a couple just enough to introduce the needle under the skin and create the many subcutaneous microcavities (subcision).

The sting technique differs from Klinger and Rigotti procedures as sharp needles are not used to create spaces for fat particles. Indeed, multiple full-thickness prickings are performed to break and release the cutaneous and subcutaneous (glandular and fascial) restrictions along the hypoplastic breast poles. Insertion of the implant, immediately after the pricking, maintains this tridimensional expansion until re-epithelialization completes the healing. As fat is not used, there are not the problems associated both with the difficulty of harvesting enough adipose tissue in patients who often are very slim and the uncertainty and unpredictability of taking the graft (Gutierrez-Ontalvilla et al. 2020).

Complications of sting technique are rare and self-resolving as the subcutaneous blood collection or requiring a simple treatment as the long-lasting markings in darker skin. Any case of hematoma, scarring, or infection has been observed.

Hypoplastic lower breast poles can complicate the outcome of a breast augmentation procedure. The results obtained using the "sting technique" in this group of patients are satisfying showing the creation of a nice, round, and regular contour of the constricted inferior quadrants. Nevertheless, longer follow-up and larger series are necessary in the future to understand better the real potentialities of the sting technique in these kinds of breast malformations and the eventual applications in other populations such as male to female transgender along with its limits and risks.

References

Rees TD, Aston S (1976) The tuberous breast Clin Plast Surg; 3:339–47

Brown MH, Somogyi (2015) Surgical strategy in the correction of tuberous breast Clin Plast Surg; 42:53–549

Dos Santos B, Ruiz-Castilla M (2021) Inferior pole expansion with lipofilling for tuberous breast surgery Clin Surg; 6:3287

DeLuca-Pytell D, Piazza R, Holding J (2005) The incidence of tuberous breast deformity in asymmetric and symmetric mammaplasty patients Plast Reconstr Surg; 116:1894–1899

Klinger M, Klinger F, Giannasi S, Veronesi A et al (2017): Stenotic Breast Malformation and Its Reconstructive Surgical Correction: A New Concept From Minor Deformity to Tuberous Breast Aesth Plast Surg; 41:1068

Orentreich DS, Orentreich N. (1995) Subcutaneous incisionless (subcision) surgery for the correction of depressed scars and wrinkles. Dermatol Surg; 21:543–9.

Klinger M, Marazzi M, Vigo D, Torre M. (2008) Fat injection for cases of severe burn outcomes: a new perspective of scar remodeling and reduction; Aesthetic Plast Surg. May; 32(3):465–9.

Khouri R, Rigotti G, Cardoso E, Biggs T (2014): Megavolume Autologous Fat Transfer: Part II. Practice and Techniques; Plast reconstr Surg, 133: 1369

Puckett C and Concannon M (1990): Augmenting the Narrow-Based Breast. The Unfurling Technique to Prevent the Double-Bubble Deformity Aesth. Plast. Surg. 14:15

Servaes M, Mahaudens P, Sinna R, Vanwijck R, Denoel C (2010) Advantages of the superior areolar approach for tuberous breast II and III correction with implants. Ann Chir Plast Esthet, 56:342

Oroz-Torres J, Pelay-Ruata MJ, Escolán-Gonzalvo N, Jordán-Palomar E. (2014) Correction of tuberous breasts using the unfolded subareolar gland flap Aesthetic Plast Surg 38:692.

Pardo A, Watier E, Georgieu N (1999) Tuberous breast syndrome: report on a series of 22 operated patients Ann Chir Plast Esth; 44:583:592

Maione L, Vinci V, Klinger M, Klinger FM, Caviggioli (2015) F. Autologous fat graft by needle: analysis of complications after 1000 patients. Ann Plast Surg; Mar;74(3):277–80

Caviggioli F, Forcellini D, Vinci V, Cornegliani G, Klinger F, Klinger (2012) M. Employment of needles: a different technique for fat placement. Plast Reconstr Surg; Aug;130(2):373e-374e.

Gutierrez-Ontalvilla P, Naidu N, Lopez Blanco E , Condiño Brito B , Ruiz-Valls A (2020) Autologous Fat Grafting with Percutaneous Fasciotomy and Reduction of the Nipple-Areolar Complex for the Correction of Tuberous Breast Deformity in Teenagers Aesth Plast Surg; 44:264

Chapter 21
Importance of Evaluation of the Breasts by Photos and Photometry Related with Body Contouring

Paulo Rogério Quieregatto do Espirito Santo, Thales Waltenior Trigo Jr, Miguel Sabino Neto, and Lydia Masako Ferreira

Abstract Photography is the method most frequently adopted by plastic surgeons for recording and planning surgeries. The way photographs are obtained directly affects such surgical programming, as well as the evaluation of surgical procedures (Quieregatto et al. 2014a, b, 2020a, b).

Introduction

Photography is the method most frequently adopted by plastic surgeons for recording and planning surgeries. The way photographs are obtained directly affects such surgical programming, as well as the evaluation of surgical procedures (Quieregatto et al. 2014a, b, 2020a, b).

Standardization is essential for comparing pre- and postoperative photos and allows correct surgical programming (Hochman et al. 2005; Quieregatto et al. 2014a, b).

Photographic equipment has evolved from machines with a negative that produced printed photographs to digital machines with image files playing the role of a negative, which has required our familiarization with this new type of device.

P. R. Q. do Espirito Santo (✉)
UNIFESP/EPM e Membro titular da SBCP, São Paulo, SP, Brazil
e-mail: contato@pauloquieregatto.com.br

T. W. Trigo Jr
Universidade Presbiteriana Mackenzie, São Paulo, SP, Brazil

M. S. Neto · L. M. Ferreira
DCP da EPM e Membro Titular da SBCP, São Paulo, SP, Brazil

J. M. Avelar, R. Cavalcanti Ribeiro (eds.), *Body Contouring*,
https://doi.org/10.1007/978-3-031-42802-9_21

In addition, some factors directly interfere in photography standardization, including the patient positioning, especially stance of the arms, angulation relative to the camera, illumination, type of image file, distance between the patient and the camera, type of lens, reference sites on the patient, ruler for software calibration, and type of software used to evaluate the digital images (Quieregatto et al. 2020a, b, 2014a, b, 2015).

According to Jakowenko (2009), image capturing using a digital camera is frequently carelessly performed, which may lead to inaccurate results.

Hochman et al. (2005) stated that image recording for scientific research can fulfill its purpose of scientific documentation, especially considering reproducibility, if conducted in a systematized and standardized form.

Using photography instead of obtaining linear measures directly on the individual has been considered an efficient breast evaluation method (Sacchini et al. 1991). According to Nechala et al. (1999), indirect anthropometry (evaluation of images) has advantages over direct anthropometry (measurement directly on the patient) such as minimized measurement errors, millimetric precision, possible measurements over time, comparison between pre- and postoperative periods, reduced discomfort to the patient, and shorter exposure for measurements.

The photographic records routinely used in our clinic differ from those for scientific documentation, considering that a detailed scientific analysis requires absolute numbers for millimetric comparison. A comparative analysis using pre- and postoperative photos not always needs to be millimetric. Such a difference must be understood since, in case a comparison of measures is necessary, adhesive labels at specific sites and a ruler for software calibration must be employed during measurements (Quieregatto et al. 2020a, b, 2014a, b).

In the current study, considering the differences between segments, a standardization technique was developed for breast photographs, which allows subsequent analysis of the obtained images in a scientific and objective manner. Such standardization will be exemplified here.

Photographic Standardization

Standardization of Patient Positioning

A template made of ethylene-vinyl acetate (EVA) was employed to standardize at 30 cm the distance between the medial edges of the feet and at 70 cm the distance between the volunteer and the background. The distance between the volunteer and the lens is 2.5 m (Fig. 21.1).

The patients were instructed to remain in anatomical position with eyes looking straight ahead (Frankfurt plane) while photographs were taken.

Framing and Delimiting Anthropometric and Anatomical Points

The mammary region was delimited by the gnathion transversal line on the top and by the navel inferior edge on the bottom (Fig. 21.2). The frontal plane was chosen for allowing evaluation of different types of breasts, regardless of their base width and lateral extension. Photos in oblique and lateral planes show some limitations, as described by Quieregatto et al. (2014a, b) (Fig. 21.3).

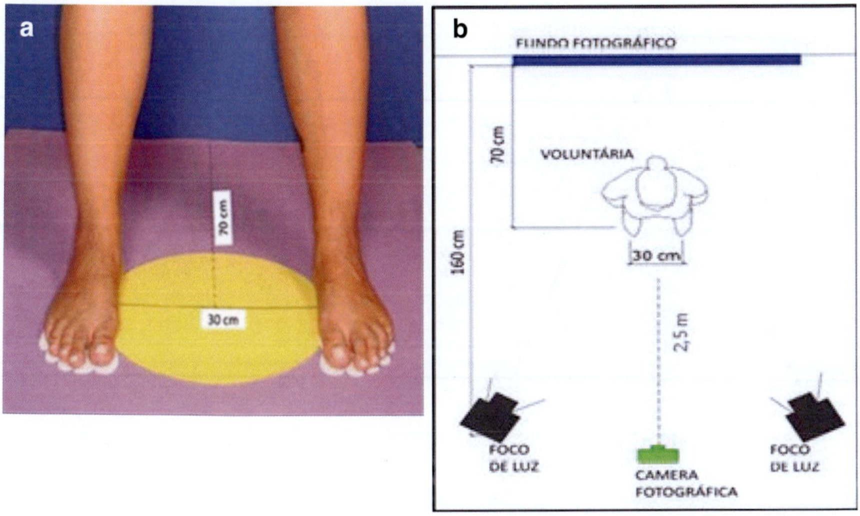

Fig. 21.1 (**a**) EVA template for positioning the feet. (**b**) Positioning and illumination of the photographic studio

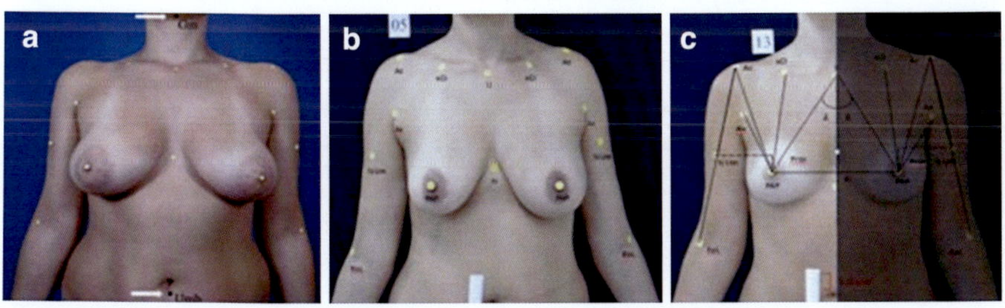

Fig. 21.2 (**a**) Photographic framing of the mammary region. (**b**) Marking of anthropometric and anatomical points with adhesive labels. (**c**) Segments that can be evaluated. Counterclockwise: **IJ** = center of the jugular notch; **xCl** = half the distance between IJ and acromion; **Ac** = lateral prominence of the acromion; **Ax** = proximal point of the anterior axillary line; **1/2 Um** = mean distance between Ac and EpL; **EpL** = anterior projection of the lateral epicondyle; **PAP** = center of the mammary papilla; **Xi** = basis of the xiphoid process; **Gn** = gnathion; **Umb** = inferior edge of the navel. Schematic representation of 17 segments formed by joining the adopted points, 8 line segments, and an angular measure for each hemibody

Adhesive labels of 0.6 cm diameter were used to evidence the central point. Eight points per hemibody were labeled, of which five are anthropometric: center of the jugular notch (IJ) and bottom of the xiphoid process (Xi), unilaterally, and center of the mammary papilla (PAP), acromion (Ac), and anterior projection of the lateral epicondyle (EpL), bilaterally. Other three anatomical points were adopted bilaterally: the point corresponding to half the distance between the center of the jugular notch and the acromion, named "x" point of the clavicle (xCl), the proximal point of the anterior axillary line (Ax), and the point corresponding to half the distance between the acromion and the lateral epicondyle, named mean point of the humerus (1/2 Um) (Fig. 21.2).

Joining one point to the other results in 15 line segments (Table 21.1).

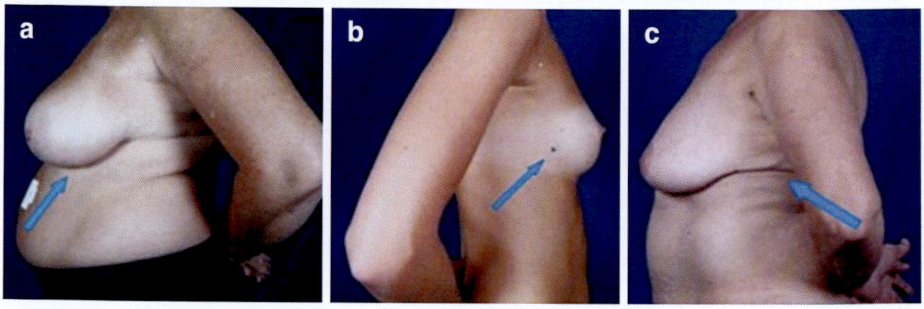

Fig. 21.3 (**a**) Impaired visualization of the median inferior point of the mammary groove. (**b**) Mammary groove of difficult definition. (**c**) Extension of the lateral point of the mammary groove

Table 21.1 Description of segments

Segment	Description
IJ-Xi	Center of the jugular notch to the bottom of the xiphoid process
IJ-PAP	Center of the jugular notch to the center of the mammary papilla
xCl-PAP	Half the distance between the center of the jugular notch and acromion to the center of the mammary papilla
Ac-PAP	Lateral prominence of the acromion to the center of the mammary papilla
Ax-PAP	Proximal point of the anterior axillary line to the center of the mammary papilla
LM-PAP	Anterior median line to the center of the mammary papilla
Ac-EpL	Lateral prominence of the acromion to the anterior projection of the lateral epicondyle
Ac-1/2 Um	Half the distance between the lateral prominence of the acromion to the anterior projection of the lateral epicondyle
Projection	Projection point on the breast, resultant of the mean distance between acromion and projection of the lateral epicondyle (1/2 um)
Â	Angle formed by segments IJ-xi (center of the jugular notch to the bottom of the xiphoid process) and IJ-PAP (center of the jugular notch to the center of the mammary papilla)

Photographic Equipment

The ideal photographic machine should allow the use of JPEG (Joint Photografic Experts Group) + *RAW* image files. A blue background provides the best contrast.

The mammary groove as a whole and its central point are not visible in the photo on the left. In the central photo, visualization of the final mammary groove in its most lateral portion is impaired, for patients with hypomastia. The photo on the right does not allow accurate definition of the lateral end of the mammary groove, for breasts showing extension of this point.

Discussion

All factors described above provide linear image capturing and consequently regular evaluation and recording of the necessary measures (Quieregatto et al. 2020a, b, 2014a, b).

As described for breasts, detailing is essential for each body segment so that patterns can be established to obtain regularity in photography (Quieregatto et al. 2020a, b).

The frontal plane was chosen since it allows evaluation of the largest number of patients. For cases of severe ptosis, in which the caudal position of the breast surpasses the navel, those framing limits should be extended.

Visualization of the mammary fold in frontal position and its lateral points is not possible for a certain number of patients; thus, they were not included in this study (Quieregatto et al. 2020a, b).

JPEG and RAW image files can be simultaneously captured with a semi-professional machine (Quieregatto et al. 2018a, b). Lens of 18 × 55 mm provided appropriate framing. A low-definition photographic machine may cause distortion of measures for scientific documentation (Quieregatto et al. 2014a, b).

The established focal distance was 2.5 meters between the lens and the patient, which resulted in more linear and parallel image with slight distortion.

To analyze these images, Adobe Photoshop CS8® is most recommended since it was the only software capable of analyzing images that were simultaneously obtained as JPEG and RAW files (Quieregatto et al. 2020a, b, 2018a, b).

It must be highlighted that the breast is subject to the interference of bone structures of the thorax; thus, evaluation based on photographs involves a specific moment. Changes in respiration and position of the arms and the spine affect the measures. These criteria must be considered especially when the photos under analysis were captured at different moments, e.g., evaluation of pre- and postoperative periods.

Conclusion

Photographs cannot be obtained indiscriminately. Standardization is required for an objective evaluation with parameters that fit both research purposes and daily practice.

Studies of other body segments must be conducted with the aim of developing photography patterns to be adopted by a larger number of surgeons either in their daily practice or in clinical research.

References

Hochman B, Nahas FX, Ferreira LM (2005) Photograph aplicada na pesquisa clínico-cirúrgica. Acta Cir Bras [serial online] 20(Suppl 2):19–25

Jakowenko J (2009) Clinical photography. J Telemed Telecare 15(1):7–22

Nechala P, Mahoney J, Farkas L (1999) Digital two-dimensional photogrammetry: a comparison of the three techniques of obtaining digital photographs. Plast Reconstr Surg 103(7):1819–25

Quieregatto PR, Sabino Neto M, Furtado F et al (2020a) JPEG and raw image files compared to direct measurement of the breast region. Acta Cir Bras 35(10): e202001008

Quieregatto PR, Machado AL, Ferrara S et al (2020b) Medidas da região mamária: antropometria direta ou indireta? *Rev Bras Cir Plast* 35(3):261–8

Quieregatto PR, Hochman B, Furtado F et al (2014a) Image analysis software versus direct anthropometry for breast measurements. Acta Cir Bras 29(10):688–95

Quieregatto PR, Hochman B, Ferrara SF et al (2014b) Anthropometry of the breast region: how to measure? Aesthetic Plast Surg 38(2):344–349

Quieregatto PR, Hochman B, Furtado F et al (2015) Photographs for anthropometric measurements of the breast region. Are there limitations? Acta Cir Bras 30(7):509–16

Quieregatto PR, Sabino Neto M, Furtado F et al (2018a) Conhecendo os tipos de arquivo de fotografia JPEG e RAW utilizados em pesquisa. Rev Bras Cir Plast 33(1):99–105

Quieregatto PR, Sabino Neto M, Furtado F et al (2018b) Medição das mamas com o Adobe Photoshop®. Rev Bras Cir Plast 33(1):106–13

Sacchini V, Luini A, Tana S et al (1991) Quantitative and qualitative cosmetic evaluation after conservative treatment for breast cancer. Eur J Cancer 27(11):1395–400

Chapter 22
Breast Anomalies: Diagnosis and Treatment

Ricardo Cavalcanti Ribeiro, Carlos José Ramírez Hanke, and Luis Fernandez de Córdova

Abstract Congenital and acquired breast asymmetries represent an enormous challenge during their treatment approach by the plastic surgeon, especially in pediatric patients. Another difficulty lies in the categorization of these deformities, which tends to be confusing. For this reason, a classification was extracted from the craniofacial literature and applied to pediatric breast anomalies. This classification system includes three categories, hyperplasias, deformities, and hypoplasias, thus providing a useful tool for decision-making regarding the conduct to be adopted according to the clinical finding.

In this chapter, we will address the diseases that predominantly generate asymmetries of the mammary gland.

Keywords Poland syndrome · Breast hyperplasia · Asymmetries · Hypoplasia · Athelia · Polythelia

R. C. Ribeiro (✉) · L. F. de Córdova
Plastic and Reconstructive Surgery, Federal University of the State of Rio de Janeiro, Rio de Janeiro, Brazil

Plastic and Reconstructive Surgery, Carlos Chagas Institute, Rio de Janeiro, Brazil

Division of Plastic and Reconstructive Surgery, Casa de Portugal Rio de Janeiro, Rio de Janeiro, Brazil

Division of Plastic and Reconstructive Surgery, Global Plastic Surgery, Mexico City, Mexico
e-mail: rribeiro@centroin.net.br

C. J. R. Hanke
Plastic and Reconstructive Surgery, Nürnberg, Germany
e-mail: info@nuernbergerklinik.de

J. M. Avelar, R. Cavalcanti Ribeiro (eds.), *Body Contouring*,
https://doi.org/10.1007/978-3-031-42802-9_22

According to the American Society for Aesthetic Plastic Surgery (ASAPS) (2011), individuals under 18 years old represent 2% of the aesthetic procedures in the United States. Although this percentage has remained constant over 10 years, there has been an increase in the total number of cosmetic procedures, due to greater demand each year. During 1996, 14,000 procedures/year were performed, increasing 14 times to 203,000/year by 2009.

Approximately 33,600 (26%) of the 125,400 cosmetic procedures in minors in 2010 were surgical, being breast augmentation (12%) and breast reduction (12%).

With an increasing demand of patients under the age of 18, there is a need to understand the specific aspects involved in the treatment of this age group.

Understanding body image in adolescent patients is essential because puberty is a period when the appearance of the body undergoes major changes that reflect on the adolescent and increase interest in the opinions of his peers.

Body image was first described by (Schilder 1934; Zuckerman and Abraham 2008), who theorized that a person's confidence is formed from a combination of general life satisfaction, body image, and self-esteem.

Recently, a Dutch study (Simis et al. 2000, 2001, 2002) sought to understand if the changes in attitudes exceeded the natural increase in the importance of body image in adolescent patients with cosmetic procedures when compared to patients without cosmetic procedures in the same age group. The study concluded that adolescents undergoing cosmetic procedures generated an improvement in body satisfaction and relief from physical, social, and psychological concerns related to appearance.

In general, adolescent candidates for cosmetic surgery were less confident in physical appearance and sex appeal than their age-matched controls, but were no different in overall self-confidence or mental health standards. More recent studies, also from the Netherlands, report that adolescent patients have a realistic view of their body, with parents and surgeons serving as control groups. It is worth mentioning that parents and adolescents had an equivalent assessment of psychological and social biases related to appearance.

From the surgeons' point of view, patients accepted for cosmetic surgery saw realistic flaws in themselves that correlated with their primary reason for seeking surgery. A study from the same group showed that patients accepted for cosmetic surgery were equally satisfied with their overall appearance compared to controls, but were more dissatisfied with a specific body part.

Hyperplastic Breast Abnormalities

Hyperplastic breast anomalies are characterized by excessive breast tissue and can be either symmetrical or asymmetrical.

Juvenile Breast Hypertrophy

Juvenile breast hypertrophy or hyperplasia (Fig. 22.1) is a rare condition of unknown etiology. Endocrinological studies are normal, and the patient shown exhibits normal body growth with the exception of breast tissue. The main goal of surgery is volume reduction with breast size symmetrization and repositioning of the nipple-areola complex (NAC) in the anatomically correct position (Simis et al. 2001; Malata et al. 1994; Schmidt 1998; Gilmore et al. 1996; Grossl 2000; Simmons et al. 2000; Sugai et al. 2002).

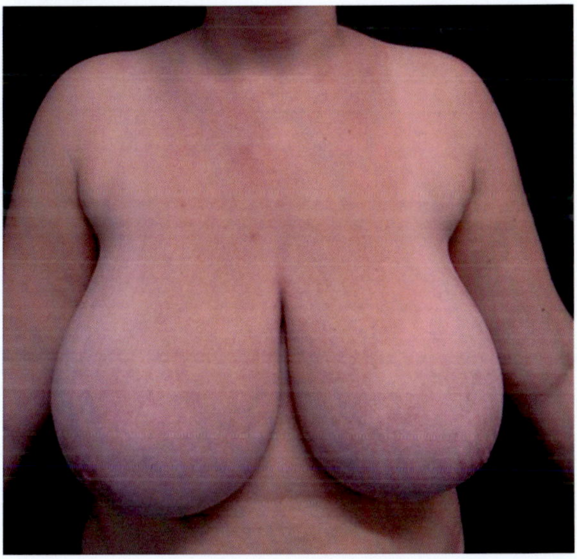

Fig. 22.1 Juvenile breast hypertrophy

Virginal Breast Hypertrophy

Prepubertal hypertrophy (which is usually bilateral) and virginal hypertrophy (which develops after menarche and which can be either unilateral or bilateral) (Fig. 22.2) are also treated with breast reduction techniques. Classification of asymmetry in hyperplasia includes unilateral hyperplasia, bilateral symmetrical hyperplasia, and a combination of hypertrophy and hypoplasia. Treatment involves a combination of reduction techniques (our preference is the inferior pedicle technique), which may require differential amounts of breast tissue resection to achieve symmetry. Surgery should be delayed until the end of puberty, when breast growth is complete; otherwise, revision surgery may be necessary due to continued breast growth.

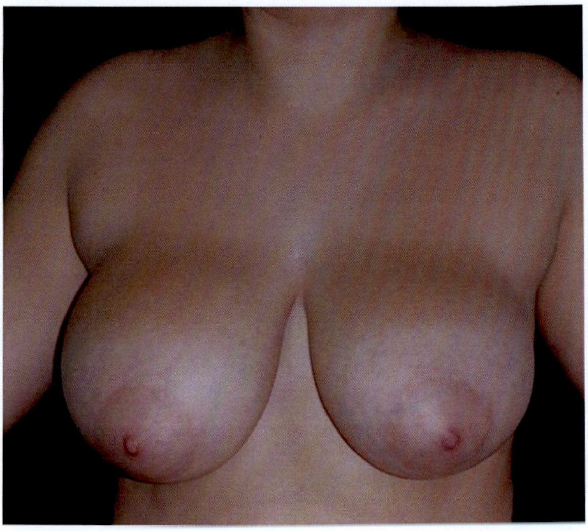

Fig. 22.2 Virginal hypertrophy

Polythelia

Polythelia, the presence of supernumerary nipples or nipple-areola complexes, is the most common anomaly of the pediatric breast and can occur in both genders. The condition usually occurs sporadically, but can be familial, and has been reported to have an incidence as high as 5.6%. Sporadic polythelia may be associated with kidney problems.

Polythelia can occur at any point along the embryonic milk line, from the axilla to the groin (Fig. 22.3). They are pigmented lesions within these embryonic lines that must be excised before puberty; after the onset of puberty in girls, resection may require a wider tissue excision because of the growth of glandular tissue. Cancerous degeneration of the accessory complex has been reported and provides additional justification for excision of these lesions. Elliptical excision of the nipple-areola complex is usually sufficient for removal (Sugai et al. 2002; Hsieh et al. 2001; Selamzde et al. 1999; Murphy et al. 2000; Lin et al. 2000; Smith et al. 1986; Rees and Aston 1976; Meara et al. 2000).

A particularly challenging problem can arise if multiple nipple-areola complexes occur in the breast. Magnetic resonance imaging may be needed to determine which nipple-areola complex is associated with glandular/ductal tissue.

Fig. 22.3 Polythelia

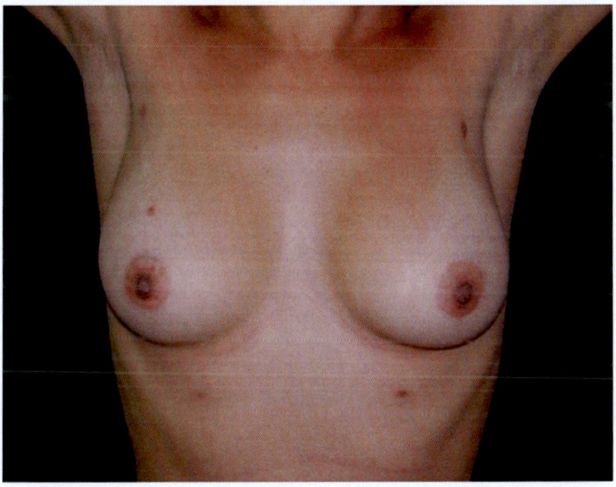

Polymastia

Polymastia is another anomaly that can occur anywhere along the embryonic milk line. The condition usually occurs sporadically, but familial cases have been reported; latent cases may become visible during puberty, pregnancy, or lactation. Polymastia can occur as an isolated finding or with a congenital renal syndrome.

Treatment requires removal of the anomalous accessory gland, with primary closure. Long-term follow-up should be indicated to the patient because of the possibility of developing cancer in any retained breast tissue.

Giant Fibroadenoma

Giant fibroadenomas are benign, discrete breast lesions that appear unilaterally during puberty and present rapid growth. The lesion is the result of the hypersensitivity of the breast tissue's reaction to normal sex hormone levels. The diagnosis is made by biopsy. Treatment involves breast reduction with conservative techniques. Intuitively, it may seem that a skin excision proportional to the excised tissue should be performed; however, that approach is too aggressive. Timing for surgery is dictated by the onset of fibroadenoma growth.

Iatrogenic Breast Abnormalities

One of the most common lesions of the pediatric breast is secondary to pleural drainage. The thoracotomy site develops a scar and a fibrous tract that ties the breast tissue to the costal wall, leading to a localized contour deformity. These patients require release of the fibrous tract to accommodate normal breast growth during puberty. No other intervention is usually necessary.

Girls who have undergone previous thoracotomy. In addition, they may have breast tissue adhered to the anterior chest wall because of the violation of the breast bud by the initial thoracotomy incision. It further results in breast hypoplasia. Scar tissue must be excised to free the breast.

Breast hypoplasia, which can be either segmental or total, requires breast reconstruction with implant placement. Pediatric breast tumors are usually benign and may rarely become malignant.

Breast Injury

The burned chest is a particularly difficult challenge for the plastic surgeon who treats pediatric patients. During puberty, breast growth may be compromised by a burn injury, if the development of the burned breast is inhibited by a constricting scar, acute tissue excision is recommended, and grafting should be done conservatively keeping in mind that the breast bud must be protected.

If the gland was not injured during the initial burn, breast growth will occur but may be hindered by scar contractures. Z-plasties and scar release from contractures and additionally skin grafts may be required to accommodate breast growth. Breast hypoplasia will result if the breast bud is injured during the initial burn. These patients will require breast reconstruction with tissue expanders, followed by placement of a submuscular implant.

If the contralateral breast has not been injured, it can be used as a source of reconstruction. NAC's reconstruction should be performed with skin graft flap techniques or with micropigmentation. It should be performed after complete breast reconstruction. Long-term follow-up of the patient is always necessary and aims to detect any subsequent changes.

Penetrating trauma to the breast presents a similar problem to those caused by thoracotomy. Correction requires release of the fibrous bonds between the gland wall followed by breast reconstruction using implants. Intervention during puberty is recommended when breast asymmetry increases with normal breast growth. Secondary surgeries are often necessary because the breast at the time of the initial operation has not reached its full growth.

Hypoplastic Breast

Athelia (absence of nipple), amastia (total absence of breasts and nipple), and amazia (absence of the mammary gland) are rare hypoplastic congenital anomalies of the breast.

According to Lin and colleagues, there are three groups of patients with amastia: those with bilateral absence of the breast secondary to congenital ectodermal defects, unilateral absence of the breast (a variant of Poland syndrome), and bilateral absence of the breast.

Amastia is associated with ectodermal birth defects, which affects both males and females; it is associated with changes in the skin and its appendages, teeth, and nails.

Bilateral absence of the breast may occur as an isolated abnormality or may be associated with other congenital anomalies of the palate and upper extremity. The defect can be sporadic or familial.

Breast volume reconstruction in patients with amastia can be performed with autologous tissues, including the transverse, the latissimus dorsi, and/or the rectus abdominis flap. The creation of the inframammary fold can be particularly difficult in these patients because of a lack of parameters. The breast can be created through tissue expansion and subsequent implant placement. Expansion should be done with caution due to possible damage to skin vascularization.

Breast hypoplasia (with intact NAC) can be unilateral or bilateral and requires reconstruction with implants in an attempt to improve breast symmetry. Treatment requires augmentation of a single breast in unilateral hypoplasia. In bilateral asymmetric hypoplasia, it may require a differential augmentation of the two breasts.

Tuberous breast (Fig. 22.4), a term first coined by Rees and Ashton, describes a hypoplastic deformity of the breast with reduced diameter, herniation of breast tissue through the areola, deficient skin envelope, and elevated inframammary crease.

Various classification systems have been developed to describe the tuberous breast. The three-layer system proposed by Meara et al. is the most used.

Worsening type I, II, and III deficiencies include progressive elevation of the inframammary fold, increasing skin scarcity, decreasing breast volume, and increasing ptosis. Unfavorable features for reconstruction with an implant include a short distance from the areola to the crease and a constriction of the base of the breast, making it difficult to accommodate implants. Division of breast tissue is often necessary to increase the base of the breast; however, an attractive result is difficult to obtain. More favorable features in a tuberous breast include a wider base, which adequately encompasses an implant, and compliance with the inframammary-nipple crease distance, allowing for simple release of the herniated breast tissue into the nipple-areola complex. The results in these cases are more favorable.

Fig. 22.4 Tuberous breast

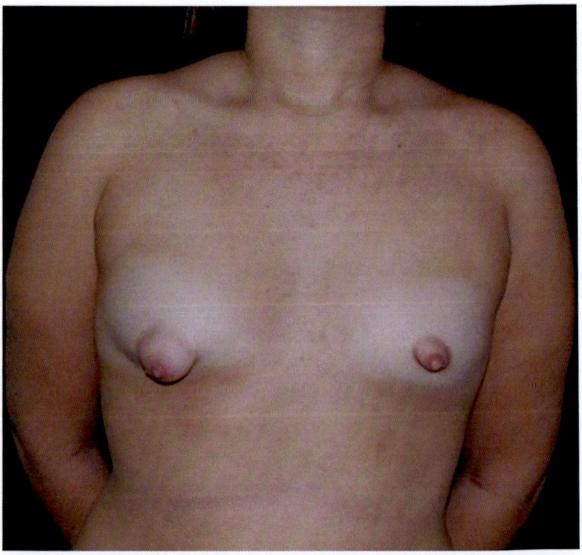

Poland Syndrome

Poland syndrome was first described by Alfred Poland in 1841. After performing an autopsy on a patient, Poland, who was an anatomy instructor at Guy's Hospital, observed the absence of the sternocostal portion of the pectoralis major muscle and malformations in the ipsilateral upper limb.

The etiology of Poland syndrome is still unknown. However, studies suggest that there may be a genetic influence or even that extrinsic factors, between the sixth and the eighth week of pregnancy, may interfere with the migration process of the pectoralis major muscle and the separation of the fingers that occurs in this period.

However, the manifestations of PS are more frequently observed in adolescence, progressing with breast hypoplasia, asymmetry of the nipple-areola complexes, and depression of the affected hemithorax. At this stage, these deformities generate a high degree of anxiety in patients with serious psychosocial repercussions. Therefore, it is common to search for medical advice to be made for merely aesthetic purposes. When the changes are restricted to the pectoralis major muscle and breast hypoplasia, cases are often diagnosed as breast asymmetry. Based on the above, the disease presents with a wide range of manifestations (Poland 1841; Larizza and Maghnie 1990; Beals and Crawford 1976; David and Winter 1985; Rasjad and Sutiaksa 1991; Marks et al. 1991; Ribeiro et al. 2009; Seyfer et al. 2010).

Regarding surgical options, Ribeiro and Seyfer propose different approaches depending on the degree of presentation of each case. Thus, in the mild form (first degree) of the disease (Fig. 22.5), the inclusion of breast implants is the best option in adult patients. In adolescents, on the other hand, due to breast growth, the inclusion of an expander prosthesis is prudent. In moderate cases (second degree), it may

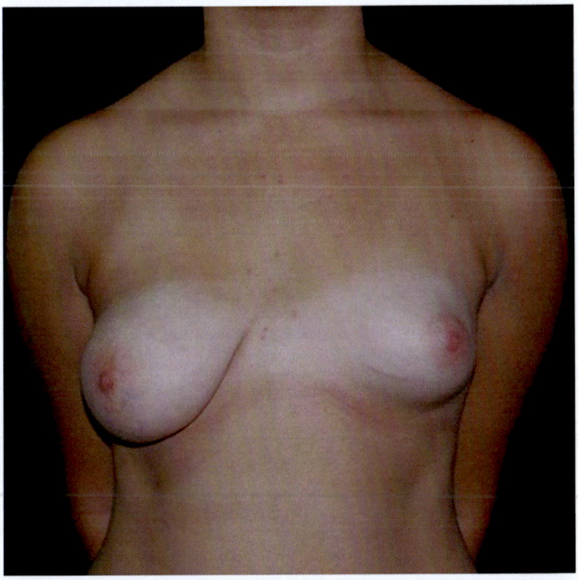

Fig. 22.5 Poland syndrome (I mild)

Table 22.1 Poland syndrome classification

Classification	Breast anomalies	Thoracic wall deformities	Ipsilateral arm alterations	Other congenital deformities
1 (mild)	Breast asymmetry	Absent	Absent	Absent
2 (moderate)	Hypomastia	Absent	Absent	Absent
3 (severe)	Amastia	Different deformities	Present	Present

be necessary to expand the tissue beforehand and then include customized or non-customized implants, with coverage of local flaps or even distant flaps. In very severe cases (third degree), the use of implants is always accompanied by a latissimus dorsi myocutaneous flap or another flap such as a microsurgical or pedicled rectus abdominis flap,either way, additional procedures in the contralateral breast, such as symmetrization and/or the nipple-areola complex are almost always needed. In Table 22.1, the authors summarized the deformities present in mild, moderate, and severe presentations of Poland syndrome.

References

American Society for Aesthetic Plastic Surgery. Cosmetic surgery national databank statistics: expanded data for 2010. Available at http://www.surgery.org. Accessed May 5, 2011.

Zuckerman D, Abraham A. Teenagers and cosmetic surgery: Focus on breast augmentation and liposuction. J Adolesc Health 2008; 43:318–324.

Schilder P. Localization of the body image (postural model of the body). Res Publ Assoc Nerv Ment Dis. 1934; 13:466–585.

Simis KJ, Hovius SE, de Beaufort ID, Verhulst FC, Koot HM. After plastic surgery: Adolescent-reported appearance ratings and appearance-related burdens in patient and general population groups. Plast Reconstr Surg. 2002; 109:9–17.

Simis KJ, Koot JM, Verhulst FC, Hovius SE. Assessing adolescents and young girls for plastic surgical intervention: Pre surgical appearance ratings and appearance-related burdens as reported by adolescents and young adults, parents and surgeons. Br J Plast Surg. 2000;53:593–600.

Simis KJ, Verhulst FC, Koot JM. Body image, psychosocial functioning, and personality: How different are adolescents and young adults applying for plastic surgery? J Child Psychol Psychiatry 2001;42:669–678.

Malata, C. M., Boot, J. C., Bradbury, E. T., Ramli, A. R., and Aharpe, D. T. Congenital breast asymmetry: Subjective and objective assessment. Br. J. Plast. Surg. 47: 95, 1994

Schmidt, H. Supernumerary nipples: Prevalence, size, sex and side predilection. A prospective clinical study. Eur. J. Pediatr. 157: 821, 1998.

Gilmore, H. T., Milroy, M., and Mello, B. J. Supernumerary nipples and accessory breast tissue. S.D.J. Med. 49: 149, 1996.

Grossl, N. A. Supernumerary breast tissue: Historical perspectives and clinical features. South. Med. J. 93:29, 2000.

Simmons, R. M., Cance, W. G., and Iacicca, M. V. A giant juvenile fibroadenoma in a 12-year-old girl: A case for breast conservation. Breast J. 6: 418, 2000.

Sugai, M., Murata, K., Kimura, N., Munakata, H., Hada, R., and Kamata, Y. Adenoma of the nipple in an adolescent. Breast Cancer 9: 254, 2002.

Hsieh, S. C., Chen, K. C., Chu, C. C., and Chou, J. M. Juvenile papillomatosis of the breast in a 9-year-old girl. Pediatr. Surg. Int. 17: 206, 2001.

Selamzde, M., Gidener, C., Koyuncuoglu, M., and Mevsim, A. Borderline phylloides tumor in an 11-year-old girl. Pediatr. Surg. Int. 15: 427, 1999.

Murphy, J. J., Morzaria, S., Gow, K. W., and Magee, J. F. Breast cancer in a 6-year-old child. J. Pediatr. Surg. 35: 765, 2000.

Lin, K.Y., Nguyen, D.B., and Williams, R.M. Complete breast absence revisited. Plast. Reconstr. Surg. 106: 98, 2000.

Smith, D. J., Palin, W. E., Katch, V., and Bennett, J. E. Surgical treatment of congenital breast asymmetry. Ann. Plast. Surg. 47: 92, 1986.

Rees, T. D., and Aston, S. The tuberous breast. Clin. Plast. Surg. 3: 339, 1976.

Meara, J.G., Kokker, A., Bartlett, G., Theile, R., Mutimer, K., and Holmes, A. D. Tuberous breast deformity: Principles and practice. Ann. Plast. Surg. 4S: 607, 2000.

Poland A. Deficiency of the pectoral muscles. Guy's Hospital Reports. 1841; 6:191.

Larizza D, Maghnie M. Poland's syndrome associated with growth hormone deficiency. J Med Genet. 1990; 27: 53-55.

Beals KR, Crawford S. Congenital absence of the pectoral muscle. Clin Orth Relat Res. 1976; 119:166-171.

David TJ, Winter RM. Familial absence of the pectoralis major, serratus anterior, and latissimus dorsi muscles. J Med Genet. 1985; 22: 390-392.

Rasjad C, Sutiaksa IGP. A case report of Poland's syndrome from Indonesia. Aust N Z J Surg. 1991; 61: 320-322.

Marks MW, Argenta LC, Izenberg PH, Louis GB. Management of the chest-wall deformity in male patients with Poland's syndrome. Plast Reconstr Surg. 1991; 87: 674-678.

Ribeiro, R.C., Saltz, R., Mangles, M.G.M., Koch, H. Clinical and radiographic classification of Poland's Syndrome—A proposal. Aesthetic Surgery Journal 2009 29: 494

Seyfer, A.E., Fox, J.P., Hamilton, C.G. Poland Syndrome: Evaluation and Treatment of the Chest Wall in 63 Patients. Plast Reconstruct Surg, 2010, 126(3):902-911

Chapter 23
Tuberous Breast

Ricardo Cavalcanti Ribeiro, Carolina Durán, and Luis Fernandez de Córdova

Abstract Tuberous breast syndrome refers to a deformity of the breast clinically presenting with hernia of the parenchyma through the nipple-areolar complex (NAC) and may involve varying degrees of breast hypoplasia; it was so named for its similarity with the tuberous roots of plants. This condition affects young women and can bring on serious disorders of self-esteem and psychosocial distress.

The deformity is characterized by hypoplasia, breast base constriction, inferior breast skin deficiency, superior malposition of the inframammary fold, areolar herniation, increased areolar diameter, and asymmetry. This series of morphologic alterations become evident at puberty with a wide spectrum of expression.

The term was first described in 1976 by Rees and Aston, and the exact incidence and prevalence are unknown, and the etiology is unclear, because of underdiagnosis and lack of clinical correlation in cases of breast asymmetry. Apparently, there is no

R. C. Ribeiro (✉)
Federal University of the State of Rio de Janeiro, Rio de Janeiro, Brazil

Division of Plastic and Reconstructive Surgery, Casa de Portugal Rio de Janeiro, Rio de Janeiro, Brazil

Plastic and Reconstructive Surgery, Carlos Chagas Institute, Rio de Janeiro, Brazil
e-mail: rribeiro@centroin.net.br

C. Durán
Division of Plastic and Reconstructive Surgery, Casa de Portugal Rio de Janeiro, Rio de Janeiro, Brazil

L. F. de Córdova
Division of Plastic and Reconstructive Surgery, Casa de Portugal Rio de Janeiro, Rio de Janeiro, Brazil

Plastic and Reconstructive Surgery, Carlos Chagas Institute, Rio de Janeiro, Brazil

Division of Plastic and Reconstructive Surgery, Global Plastic Surgery, México City, Mexico

J. M. Avelar, R. Cavalcanti Ribeiro (eds.), *Body Contouring*,
https://doi.org/10.1007/978-3-031-42802-9_23

family incidence, and the presence of a noxious stimulus early in pregnancy responsible for a failure in differentiation in a limited zone of the fetal thorax has not been established.

There are two hypotheses for this condition; one of them is the hormonal stimulus. It seems that the quality and quantity of the hormonal stimulus are not different from normal, but we know that it is in the lower quadrants which are the most affected that have less glandular tissue and less hormonal receptors.

The second hypothesis is an anomaly of the breast structures, which could be the abnormal superficial fascia, weakness of the periareolar supporting tissues, or a strong adherence between the dermis and the muscular plane at the lower quadrants of tubular breasts, which could restrict peripheral expansion of the breast, resulting in the tubular appearance due to forward tunnelization of breast tissue. Together, these theories describe how the superficial fascia thickening can cause constriction to the breast, combined with the absence of the superficial fascia under the areola predisposing to herniation.

Tuberous breast deformity presents itself in varying degrees, a classification for this degrees was first published by von Heimburg in 1996 describing four types: type I, hypoplasia of the medial lower quadrant; type II, hypoplasia of both lower quadrants with sufficient skin in the subareolar region; type III, hypoplasia of both lower quadrants with deficiency of skin in the subareolar region; and type IV, hypoplasia of all quadrants with severe breast constriction.

There are numerous surgical techniques to correct this condition, most of them aimed at redistributing volumes based on a combination of skin expansion and mammary gland remodeling. Prostheses and locoregional flaps can also be used to replace the missing volume. Fat grafting to the breast is another technique that has become popular. When combined with techniques such as external tissue expansion, the graft capacity ratio and recipient site vascularity increase, allowing for large graft volume.

Keywords Tuberous breast · Breast aesthetics · Hypoplastic breast

The term "tuberous breast" is used to define a syndrome consisting of a hypoplastic alteration of the breast, where there is a base of insufficient diameter for the glandular content, accompanied by a pseudo-herniation of the same through the areola, with a deficit of skin wrap and a poorly positioned inframammary crease, which is usually located above the desired location, thus giving the tubular appearance that identifies it (Ribeiro et al. 2018a, b). This entity is not recognized as a medical condition or actual disease but, apparently, has a strong association with other types of deformities, as elaborated in an article published by DeLuca-Pytell et al. This was a review of the incidence of tuberous breasts in 375 patients undergoing mammoplasty who only sometimes presented mammary asymmetry. It was performed through a retrospective preoperative analysis and presented interesting results, for example, that 80.1% of patients who underwent mammoplasty had mammary asymmetry, and of the patients with asymmetry, 80.8% had some type of tuberous breast, compared with only about 7% of patients with symmetrical breasts. This strong association can provide the etiology, which remains unknown, and the development of optimal techniques for treatment.

History

The concept of tuberous breasts has been studied as a change in breast morphology since the last century, although Longacre (1954) and Goulian (1971) had studied this breast alteration and proposed its treatment with the use of a dermoadipose pedicle to enlarge the breast base. It was only in 1976 that Rees and Aston described it as a "tuberous breast" for the first time. Several authors actively participated in search techniques for the correction of this abnormality, and so far, innovative techniques have been published with satisfactory results. Given that breasts identify a woman's femininity and that their function is not limited to breastfeeding and raising children and as they play a key role in sexual development and social acceptance, we can consider it important that the changes they reach are harmonious in appearance or they can otherwise cause unwanted psychological conduct with falling levels of self-esteem and stress of neurotic or bipolar disorders that could generate a progressive and destructive dissatisfaction with a woman's personal development.

Ribeiro et al. described a technique that uses an exclusive periareolar approach with horizontal incisions in the parenchyma and preparation of the inferior pedicle base, with resection of the medial and lateral extensions and fixing of the same in the chest wall, folding the pedicle base on itself. This technique enables correction of the shape of the breasts by filling the lower hypoplastic quadrants (Ribeiro et al. 2018a, b, c, 2002; Jurado 1976; Pitanguy 1984; Robbins 1977; Rohrich et al. 2004; Wallace et al. 1998).

In 2003, (Mandrekas et al. 2003) advocated a similar approach, but with a vertical incision in the parenchyma in a 6 o'clock semi-axis position and its separation into two pillars. Since 1983, the use of combined periareolar and inframammary incisions associated with breast implants has been described by Teimourian and Adham. Most patients with tuberous breast desire an increase in breast volume and improvement in shape, both of which are provided by this technique.

Since Coleman popularized lipofilling technique, it has become a recognized therapeutic tool for soft tissue augmentation. Khouri made a significant contribution with the introduction of external expansion to address the necessary capacity to graft ratio needed for successful outcomes. The number of sessions depends on the extent of the deformation, quality of the recipient site, and patients' adipose reserves. The presence of fibrous tissue in tuberous breasts makes fat grafting more difficult to perform; using external tissue expansion might prepare the recipient site by altering the fibrous aspect of the tissue, especially in the lower pole, which helps to accomplish the natural appearance and consistency of the breast.

Embryology and Anatomy

Embryologically, breast development begins from the ectoderm in the fifth week of intrauterine life, responsible for the close relations between the gland and the skin that becomes a real unit ensheathed by the mesenchyme. Between 10 and 14 weeks, the mammary buds of the thoracic region are surrounded by a layer of mesodermal tissue called the superficial fascia. Both glandular and nipple-areolar growth is complete at puberty, and the superficial fascia is the main structure responsible for forming conical breasts.

The formation of the mammary gland begins before sexual differentiation. The development of the mammary ridge or milk line, which is a surface spread of embryonic ventral ectoderm, extending from the axilla to the inguinal bilaterally, begins by the fifth week of embryonic life. The mammary crest, from which usually develops a single pair of mammary glands, disappears in human embryos at around the seventh week, persisting in only a small portion of the pectoral region. This involution of the milk crest is characteristic of the human species. Subsequently, there is invagination of the local ectoderm that will form the primary breast bud, which will give rise to 15 or 20 secondary branches. At first, these sprouts, consisting of ectodermal cells, are massive and branch out into the middle of the mesenchyme. In the third trimester of pregnancy, the ducts become tunneled, with a light appearance in their interior, open out into the mammary pits, which rise and form the nipple. The ramifications of the ducts end in a blind bottom, constituting lobular duct units or cellular terminals. Breast engorgement and secretion of colostrum, due to hormonal stimulation from the mother through the placenta, occur in approximately 80% of infants of both sexes. There is spontaneous regression of this phenomenon around the third or fourth week after birth, with the gradual elimination of hormones by the conceptus. Until the onset of puberty, the female breasts usually remain underdeveloped, starting development with ovarian stimulation that begins in this period. From then on, the development is glandular, together with the fat and connective tissue. During pregnancy, the development of the mammary glands is completed. Russo and Russo describe the development of the breasts, especially in their early years, to make the biological phenomena that govern the mammary epithelium comprehensible: nulliparous breasts consist of type I lobes, also called virgin lobes, because they are present before menarche. This type is the most undifferentiated. The lobes are formed of clusters of 6–11 ductules per lobe. Type II lobes are formed from the first; they have a more complex morphology and are formed by a larger number of ductular structures per lobe. Type III are characterized by having an average of 80 ductules or wells per lobe. They are often found in women on hormone therapy and during pregnancy. Type IV lobes are considered the ultimate expression of development and differentiation. They are found during pregnancy and lactation and, furthermore, are not noticed in nulliparous women in the post-puberty period. This differentiation diminishes the possibility of breast cancer—a pregnancy to term before the age of 24, according to those authors, reduces the relative risk (RR) of breast cancer development fourfold. Changes in breast morphology can be divided according to the time they are diagnosed into congenital and development and from the pathophysiological point of view and functional morphology. But many of these morphological changes can coexist with functional problems; thus, the authors consider the first classification more appropriate.

General Aspects

Clinical findings: Tuberous or tubular breasts are characterized as:

- Deficiency of glandular tissue plus elongation.
- Enlargement and swelling of the NAC.
- Constriction/herniation.
- Narrow base.
- Absence or poor lower pole.
- Association with other congenital breast diseases (Figs. 23.1, 23.2 and 23.3).

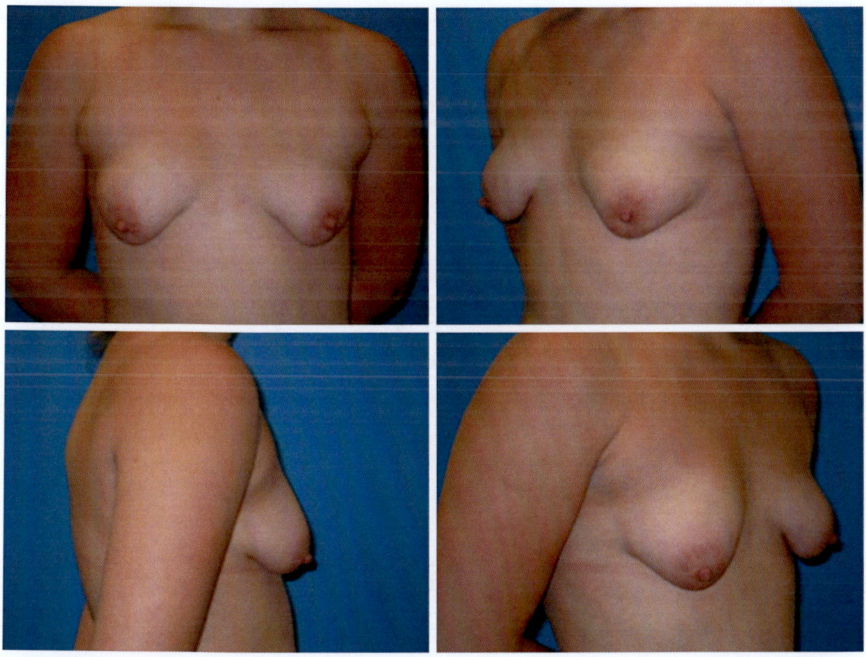

Fig. 23.1 Tuberous breast with asymmetry

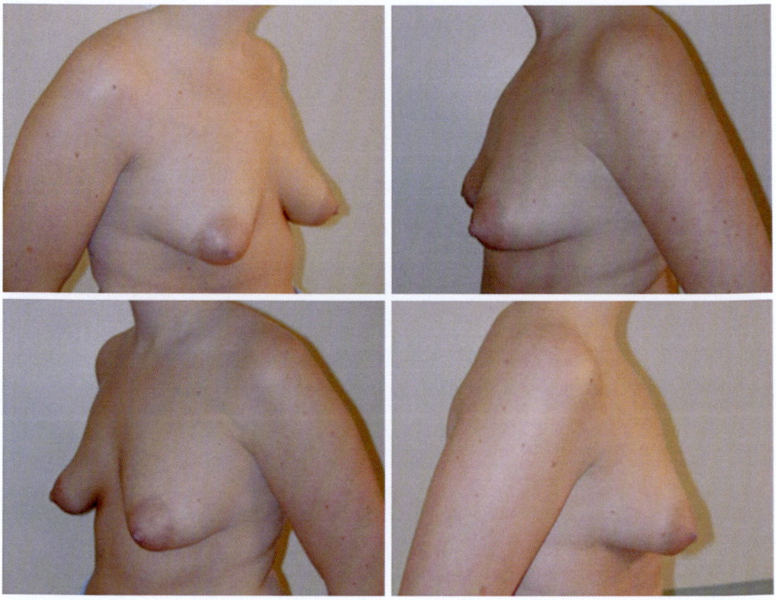

Fig. 23.2 Tuberous breast grade II

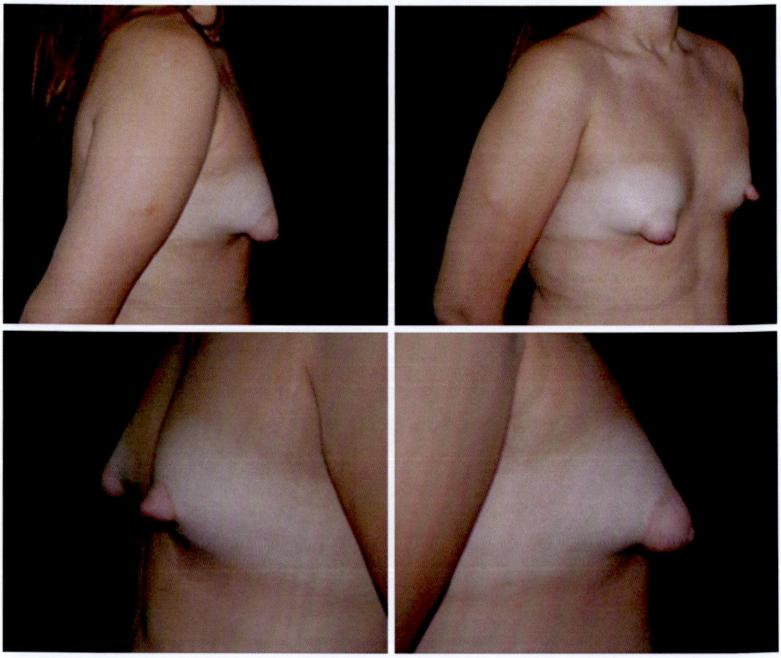

Fig. 23.3 Tuberous breast grade III with asymmetry

Classification

Morphologically, various proposals for tuberous breast classification have been described, one of which was advocated by Meara et al. (2000), which is most frequently used today. However, von Heimburg in 1996 presented a more refined version of this classification, which we consider adequate for academic purposes and is useful in comparing the postoperative results of procedures performed by different surgeons using different techniques to define the degree of correction of the defect. Based on this classification, the deformities can be classified into type I (hypoplasia of the medial lower quadrant), type II (hypoplasia of both lower quadrants), and type III (hypoplasia of the four quadrants with severe breast constriction). These types of breast shape deformities have in common a breast base anomaly that results in different degrees of clinical severity.

Grolleau et al. (1999) proposed another classification, which divides the breast into four quadrants and determines three degrees of deformity. Grade I corresponds to 56% of the cases. The lack of development is limited to the lower internal quadrant. The areola is deviated downward and inward, the volume of the breast being normal or hypertrophic. Grade II corresponds to 26% of the cases. The two lower quadrants are deficient in their development. In these cases, the areola is deviated looking downward. Grade III corresponds to 18% of the cases. All quadrants are affected and deficient, the mammary base is retracted, and the breast has a tuber or goat appearance.

Surgical Technique

With the patient in a semi-sitting position, a new areola is marked with the aid of 4–5 cm in diameter areola marker. The new submammary fold is marked, normally positioned 1.5–2 cm below the original.

The periareolar region is de-epithelialized in a donut fashion; the skin of the inferior half breast is incised and then undermined to pectoralis fascia (Fig. 23.4). Dissection continues down to new inframammary fold and then upward behind the breast parenchyma (glandular flaps Mandrekas/Ribeiro) (Fig. 23.5).

Division of the breast into two flaps is performed, one with a superior areolar pedicle and the other with an inferior pedicle, carefully releasing the medial and lateral extensions of the superior flap the subglandular pocket is created either for expanders or for permanent implants to be placed (Fig. 23.6).

The flaps must be handled carefully in order to avoid injuring the intercostal perforating vessels that supply the flaps.

The lateral and medial portions of the inferior pedicle are resected, ready to be inverted on itself to create the inferior pole of the breast and fixed with non-absorbable suture in the inferior part of the fascia of the pectoralis major muscle.

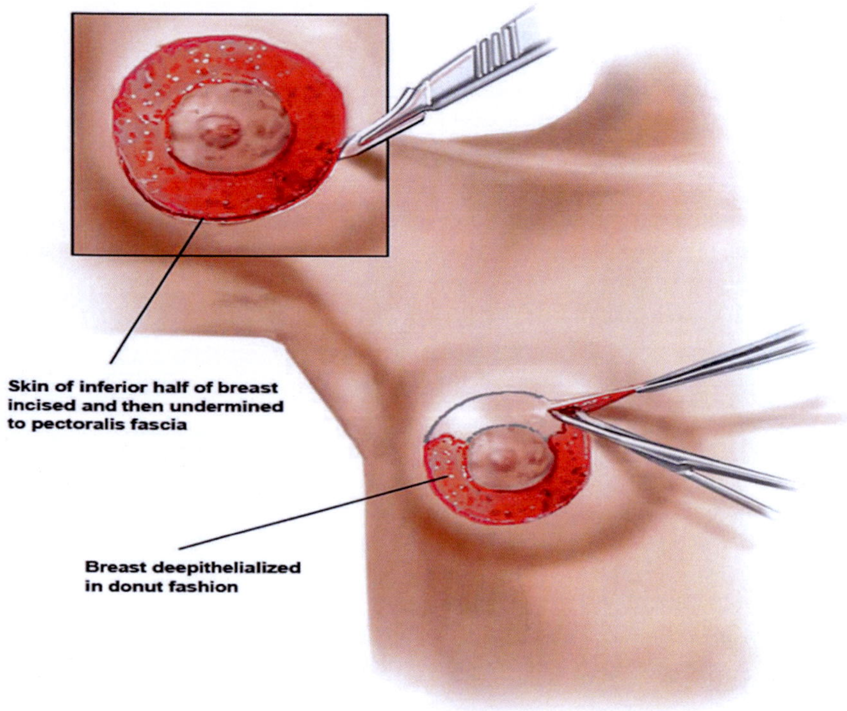

Fig. 23.4 De-epithelialization of the periareolar region

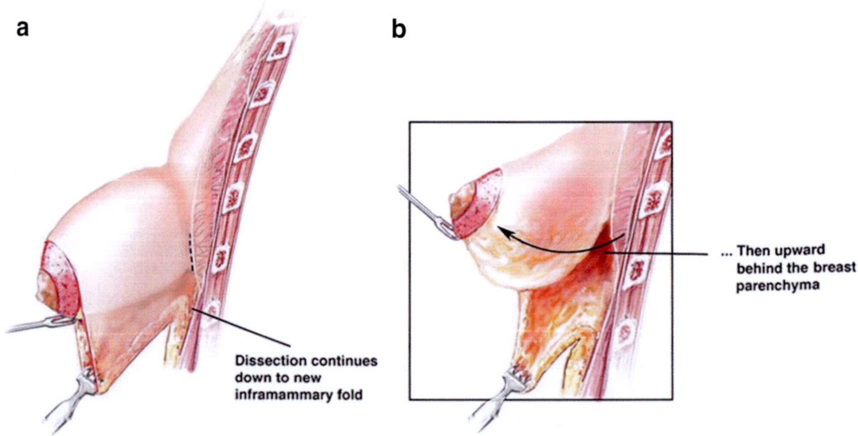

Fig. 23.5 Creation of new inframammary fold and Mandrekas/Ribeiro glandular flap

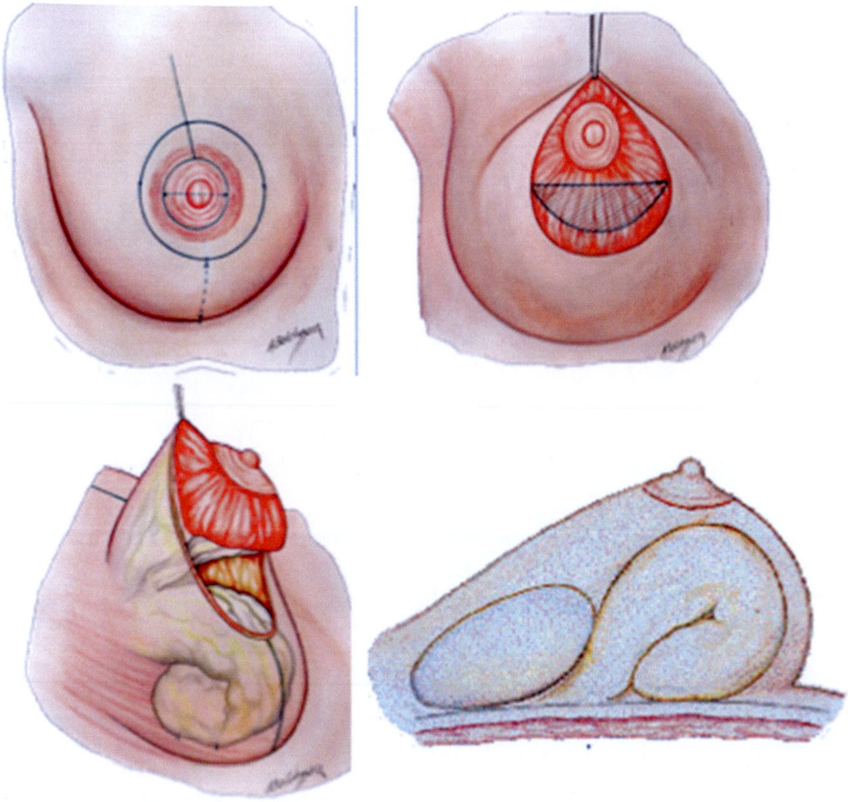

Fig. 23.6 Creation of pocket for flap repositioning

This inferior pedicle receives its vascularization through the fourth, fifth, and sixth intercostal arteries. The release of the constriction ring is performed, and the skin naturally slides over the pedicle, forming the base of the breast to be enlarged (Fig. 23.7).

The final suture of the areola is made with continuous round block stitches with non-absorbable 2–0 nylon thread. In certain situations, it may be necessary to suture with interrupted stitches with 5–0 or 6–0 nylon, and other threads may be used according to the surgeon's preference. Rigotomy may be performed to facilitate skin expansion (Fig. 23.8).

It is important to fix the breast with hypoallergenic adhesive tape for an approximate period of 15 days to model it.

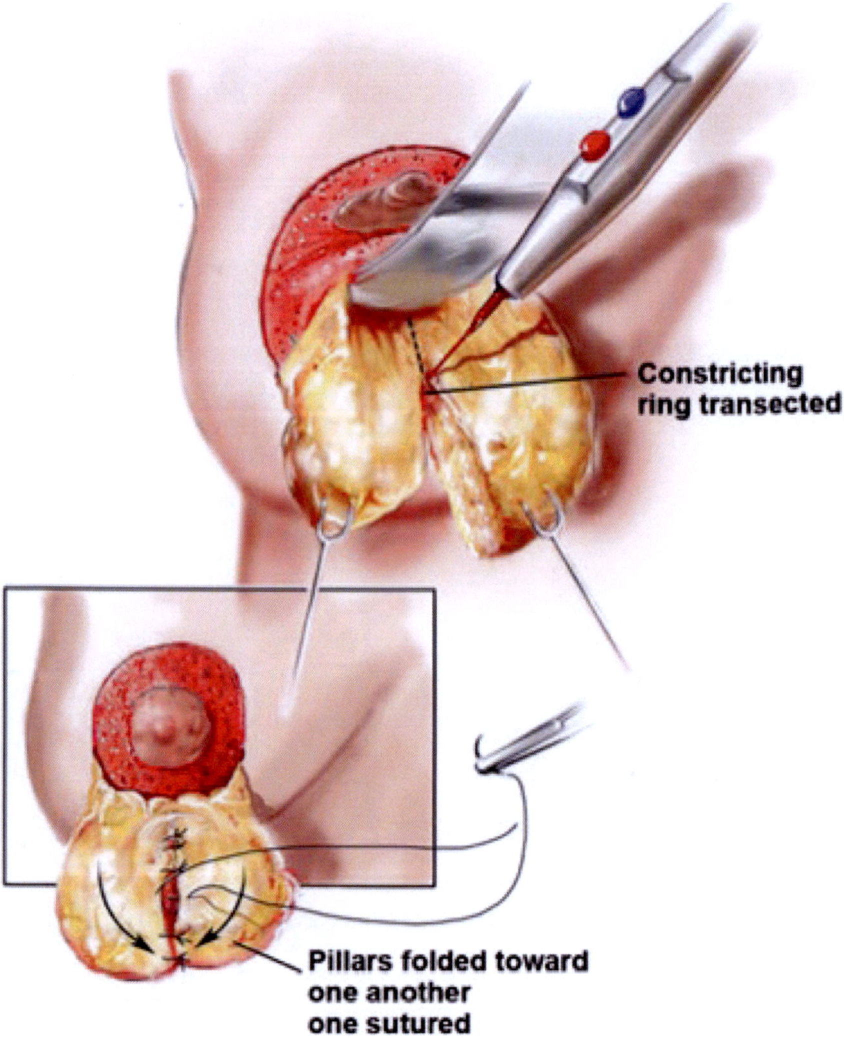

Fig. 23.7 Transection of constricting ring and reconstruction of breast pillars

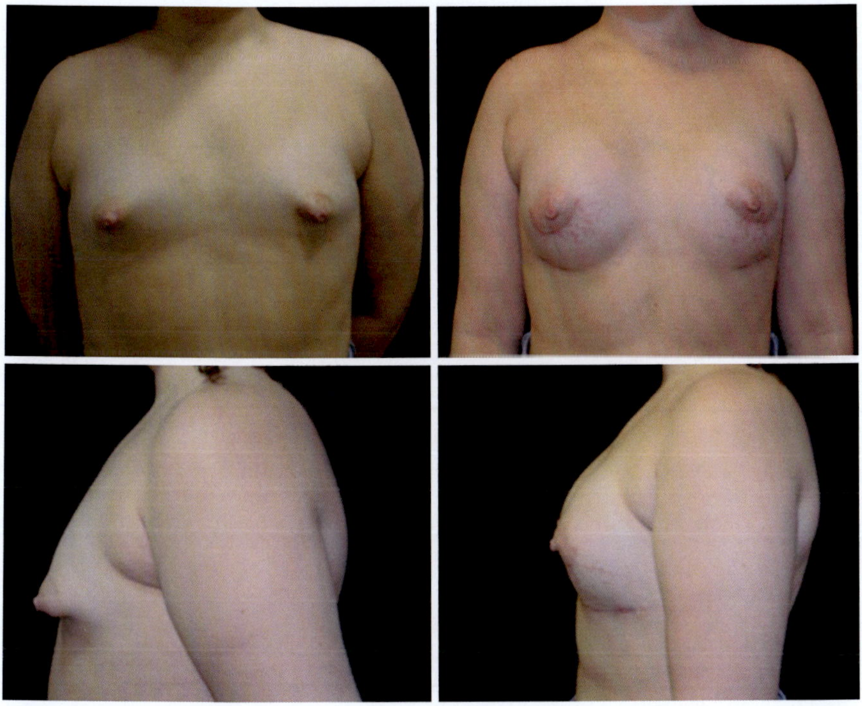

Fig. 23.8 Before and after pictures of a tuberous breast reconstruction with breast implants and rigotomy for skin expansion

Conclusions

Tuberous breast is a rare entity and difficult to treat, with numerous variations in its clinical presentation, which requires the individualization of each case to carry out a precise approach with the correct choice of technique to be used.

Thus, the treatment becomes even more complex in patients with marked breast asymmetry, which in many cases may require the combination of several surgical techniques and, sometimes, the performance of more than one surgical time to obtain better results.

Due to the diversity of clinical findings, there are different therapeutic possibilities, which can range from the placement of silicone implants, indicated when necessary, to the performance of glandular flaps in association with the techniques described above.

References

Ribeiro R.C., López L.E.F., Romay S. (2018a) Tuberous Breast. In: Avelar J. (eds) Breast Surgery. Springer, Cham. https://doi.org/10.1007/978-3-319-54115-0_39
Ribeiro R.C., Valderrama J.B., Mangles M.G.M. (2018b) Poland's Syndrome. In: Avelar J. (eds) Breast Surgery. Springer, Cham. https://doi.org/10.1007/978-3-319-54115-0_44
Jurado J (1976) Plásticas mamárias de redução baseadas em retalho dérmico vertical monopediculado. Anais XII Congresso Brasileiro de Cirurgia Plástica, vol 29
Pitanguy I (1984) Mamoplastia reductora con retallo superior em hipertrofia mamaria. Rev Bras Cir 74:265–284
Ribeiro L, Accorsi A Jr, Buss A, Marcal-Pessoa M (2002) Creation and evolution of 30 years of the inferior pedicle in reduction mammaplasties. Plast Reconstr Surg 110(3):960–970
Robbins TH (1977) A reduction mammaplasty with the areola nipple based on an inferior dermal pedicle. Plast Reconstr Surg 59(1):64–67
Rohrich RJ, Gosman AA, Brown SA, Tonadapu P, Foster B (2004) Current preferences for breast reduction techniques: a survey of board-certified plastic surgeons 2002. Plast Reconstr Surg 114(7):1724–1736
Wallace WH, Thompson WO, Smith RA, Barraza KR, Davidson SF, Thompson JT II. (1998) Reduction mammaplasty using the inferior pedicle technique. Ann Plast Surg 40(3):235–240
Ribeiro R.C., de Thuin R., de Figueiredo-e-Silva I.V., Rios M.T. (2018c) Aesthetic Approach to Breast Reconstruction. In: Avelar J. (eds) Breast Surgery. Springer, Cham. https://doi.org/10.1007/978-3-319-54115-0_46
Avelar J.M. (2018) Asymmetrical Breasts: A Challenge for Aesthetic Repair. In: Avelar J. (eds) Breast Surgery. Springer, Cham. https://doi.org/10.1007/978-3-319-54115-0_43
von Heimburg D, Exner K, Kruft S, Lemperle G. The tuberous breast deformity: Classification and treatment. Br J Plast Surg 1996;49:339–45
Longacre JJ. Correction of the hypoplastic breast with special reference to reconstruction of the "nipple type breast" with local dermofat pedicle flap. Plast Reconstr Surg 1954; 14: 431–41
Goulian D Jr. Dermal mastopexy. Plast Reconstr Surg. 1971 Feb;47(2):105–10. https://doi.org/10.1097/00006534-197102000-00001. PMID: 4925049.
Mandrekas AD, Zambacos GJ, Anastasopoulos A, Hapsas D, Lambrinaki N, Ioannidou-Mouzaka L. Aesthetic reconstruction of the tuberous breast deformity. Plast Reconstr Surg. 2003 Sep 15;112(4):1099–108; discussion 1109. https://doi.org/10.1097/01.PRS.0000076502.37081.28. PMID: 12973230
Meara JG, Kolker A, Bartlett G, Theile R, Mutimer K, Holmes AD. Tuberous breast deformity: principles and practice. Ann Plast Surg. 2000 Dec;45(6):607–11. https://doi.org/10.1097/00000637-200045060-00006. PMID: 11128758.
Grolleau JL, Lanfrey E, Lavigne B, Chavoin JP, Costagliola M. Breast base anomalies: treatment strategy for tuberous breasts, minor deformities, and asymmetry. Plast Reconstr Surg. 1999 Dec;104(7):2040–8. https://doi.org/10.1097/00006534-199912000-00014. PMID: 11149766.

Chapter 24
Aesthetic Approaches for Breast Reconstruction

Ricardo Cavalcanti Ribeiro, Ana Beatriz Arduini, and Luis Fernandez Cordova

Abstract Plastic surgery is indivisible, the binomial aesthetic and reconstructive plastic surgery raises its importance as both seek harmony, well-being and healing. We cannot dissociate them.

When talking about cosmetic breast surgery, we have many concepts, references, and techniques that can be applied and that were initially created for reconstructive purposes, for example oncoplastic surgery. Even though reconstructive surgery may seem more difficult, sometimes the aesthetic patient´s expectations represent a bigger challenge.

The idea of this chapter is to bring resources from reconstructive surgery to cosmetic surgery and broaden our horizons, always seeking not only the best result, but also observing the patient in a holistic and ethical way, aiming to balance body and spirit.

Knowledge of the anatomy of the cutaneous arteries and veins is fundamental to the design of skin flaps and incisions. In the last four decades, with the introduction

R. C. Ribeiro (✉)
Plastic and Reconstructive Surgery, Federal University of the State of Rio de Janeiro, Rio de Janeiro, Brazil

Plastic and Reconstructive Surgery, Carlos Chagas Institute, Rio de Janeiro, Brazil

Division of Plastic and Reconstructive Surgery, Casa de Portugal, Rio de Janeiro, Brazil
e-mail: rribeiro@centroin.net.br

A. B. Arduini
Plastic and Reconstructive Surgery, Carlos Chagas Institute, Rio de Janeiro, Brazil

L. F. Cordova
Plastic and Reconstructive Surgery, Carlos Chagas Institute, Rio de Janeiro, Brazil

Division of Plastic and Reconstructive Surgery, Casa de Portugal, Rio de Janeiro, Brazil

Division of Plastic and Reconstructive Surgery, Global Plastic Surgery, México City, Mexico

J. M. Avelar, R. Cavalcanti Ribeiro (eds.), *Body Contouring*,
https://doi.org/10.1007/978-3-031-42802-9_24

of the microsurgical free skin flap (Daniel and Taylor, *Plast Reconstr Surg*. 52:111, 1973; Taylor and Daniel. *Aust N Z J Surg*. 43:1, 1973), the revival of the musculocutaneous flap (McCraw et al. *Plast Reconstr Surg*. 60:341, 1977), the description of the fasciocutaneous flap (Cormack and Lamberty. *The Arterial Anatomy of Skin Flaps*. Church-Livingstone, Edinburgh, 1986; Ponten. *Br J Plast Surg*. 34:215, 1982), and the use of tissue expansion (Radovan. *Plast Reconstr Surg*. 69:195, 1982) and flap prefabrication (Baudet et al. Prefabricated free flap transfers. Presented at the 3rd Annual Meeting of the American Society for Reconstructive Microsurgery, San Antonio, Texas, September 12–13, 1987), that surgeons and anatomists have returned to the anatomic dissecting room to search and research the intricacies of the vascular pathways to and from the skin.

Keywords Breast aesthetics · Capsulectomy · Mammoplasty · Malposition

The concept of flaps and its variants become very important in what we seek to explain here, since they are techniques applied to mostly secondary mammaplasties. Knowledge of the anatomy of the cutaneous arteries and veins is fundamental to the design of skin flaps and incisions. In the last four decades, with the introduction of the microsurgical free skin flap (Daniel and Taylor 1973; Taylor and Daniel 1973), the revival of the musculocutaneous flap (McCraw et al. 1977), the description of the fasciocutaneous flap (Cormack and Lamberty 1986; Ponten 1982), and the use of tissue expansion (Radovan 1982) and flap prefabrication (Baudet et al. 1987), that surgeons and anatomists have returned to the anatomic dissecting room to search and research the intricacies of the vascular pathways to and from the skin. Once the patient has already undergone one or more aesthetic surgical approaches to the breast, due to surgical manipulation, resources in front of known flaps are becoming increasingly scarce.

It is clear that the primary objective of a surgery, whether augmentation or mastopexy, is to prevent complications and reduce reoperation rates, focusing on the avoidance of complications is an imperative, especially for an elective procedure. The same decisions and processes that reduce complications also predictably deliver superior aesthetic results. The modern breast augmentation prioritizes avoiding complications, reducing reoperations, and minimizing iatrogenic damage to breast tissue. The success of an operation can only be improved when objective endpoints are defined before surgery.

Breast implants are one of the top five procedures in plastic surgery; however, due to alterations such as capsular contracture, rippling, decrease of subcutaneous tissue thickness, rupture, malposition, among others, many cases will require plane and implant exchange (Ribeiro and Arduini n.d.).

Among the alternatives, we can mention our experience with capsule graft, mesh graft or even free tram.

Patient Selection

There must be an alignment of expectations towards the patient regarding the possible results, emphasizing that it is often a tertiary surgery onwards. The biggest challenges present themselves in the face of lack of tissue, thin and flaccid tissue, multiple approaches with the change of plans with loss of anatomy domicile, desire to increase the breast pocket with larger implants or an even greater challenge, mammoplasty with explant.

After aligning expectations in addition to a systematic assessment of the patient's health conditions such as body weight, patient height, and an estimate of breast volume requirements, we emphasize that the patient must be emotionally stable. Risk factors such as hypertension, diabetes, smoking, and obesity are not contraindications to reconstruction but may influence the choice of surgical technique and predispose a patient to complications in the donor area (Thorne et al. 2013).

Besides that, surgeons and patients tend to focus on the operation itself as the event that determines the surgical outcome, with preoperative discussion and postoperative management considered to be of secondary importance. Each step of a breast augmentation is no better than the one that preceded it: planning is dependent on patient education; the operative procedure is dependent upon the operative plan; recovery is dependent on the surgical procedure; and final patient satisfaction is the cumulative result of all of these steps. Most important of all is how perceptions of success after surgery were defined at the initial steps of education.

Capsular Contracture

Patients should be educated before surgery that it is normal to feel the capsule around the implant (Baker grade II), that the capsules on the two sides never develop equally, and that revision should only be considered for a Baker grade III (firm and distorted) or Baker grade IV (painful). Surgery is not indicated for a Baker II capsule because there is little likelihood of creating and maintaining a Baker I (no discernable capsule) (Thorne et al. 2013).

Capsular contracture is and has always been a leading cause of revisions (Thorne et al. 2013). As scar tissue thickens and tightens around the implant, the breast feels firmer, it looks becomes more spherical, the implant migrates, and the breast can be painful. Though patients may say, "my implants got hard," in fact, the implants are soft but constrained within a tightening envelope of their own tissue.

The main cause of capsular contracture is inflammation, which in turn can be caused by silicone gel bleed, glove talc, blood, tissue trauma, and bacteria. Current evidence supports Staphylococcus epidermidis biofilm as a significant cause of capsular contracture (Pajkos et al. 2003; Persichetti et al. 2011).

Faced with a scenario of Baker III or IV capsule contracture, when it becomes imperative to change the implant and often change the plane, we must consider the need for rearrangement and reinforcement of the breast pouch to receive the new

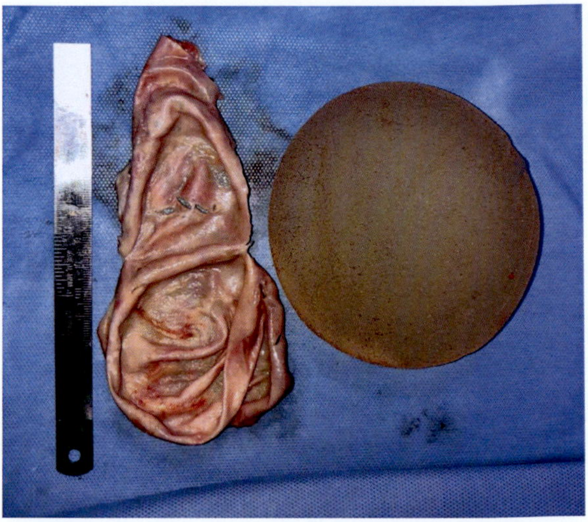

Fig. 24.1 Capsule and implant after total capsulectomy and breast implant removal

implant. Capsules with these characteristics: thick, fibrous, calcifications, granulomas and identified implant rupture or presence of seroma should be submitted to total capsulectomy (Fig. 24.1).

Malposition

Implant malposition creates some of the most severe deformities following breast augmentation. The appearance of the breast is determined by the amount and distribution of volume, in a container-content relationship, which in turn is determined by the position of the breast implant.

Over-dissection allows an implant to move out from its ideal position and incomplete dissection prevents an implant from settling in its ideal position. Even with a precise pocket, gradual migration from weight, pressure, and gravity can occur, particularly with chest wall deformities (Thorne et al. 2013) (Fig. 24.2). To avoid migration beyond the inframammary fold, the inferior cut edge of scarpa's fascia can be sewn to the muscle fascia, going back to anatomy as a "seat belt," in this way, some surgeons will routinely place such sutures with the inframammary incision.

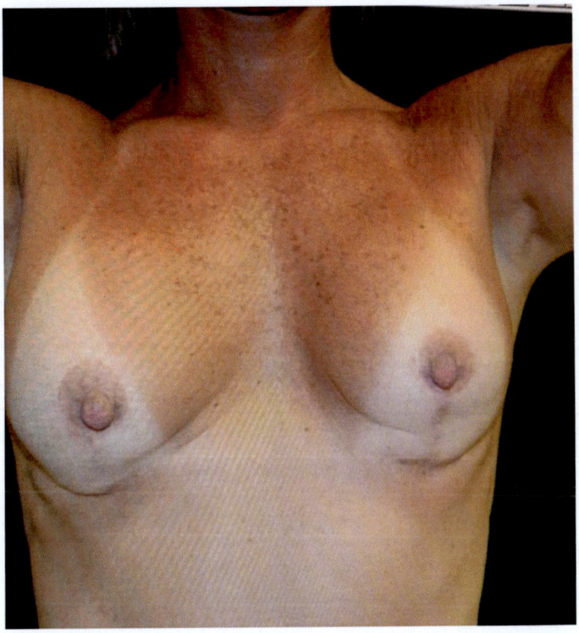

Fig. 24.2 Asymmetry in Inframammary fold due to implant malpostion

Size Exchange

Implant size change is usually avoided with proper patient education and selection. Weight fluctuations due to a new lifestyle, with the loss of breast tissue, associated or not with flaccidity and even after pregnancy, it is not uncommon for patients after these changes in the body, together with loss of the result in the breasts, to require replacement of implants, sometimes larger. We cannot rule out the social pressures to do so either (Fig. 24.3).

There are two major challenges here: the expansion of a store in the face of a restricted breast pocket, when the desire for a larger implant is desired, or the opposite, the desire to remodel the breast with a smaller implant or explant.

In the first case, we must educate the patient not to pay attention to a specific size, but that her desire will be contemplated as closely as her physical characteristics allow. In addition, we must emphasize the importance of tissue elasticity, if there are striations, sagging, positioning of the inframammary fold, excess medial detachment with risk of symmastia, or excessive lateral detachment with risk of lateralization of the breast, larger implants imply enlargement of the areola and nipple effacement (when not performed associated mastopexia) with displacement of the areola as well. Thus, often the need to enlarge the pocket to accommodate a larger prosthesis must be associated with the increase of some structures in order to reinforce them, as in the case of the pectoralis major, preserving it and allowing good containment of the implant, either in the submuscular plane or dual plane.

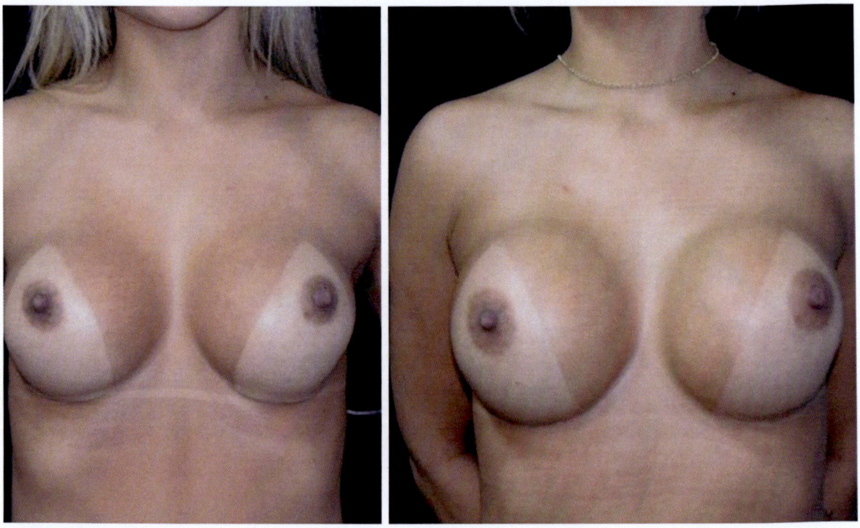

Fig. 24.3 Secondary Breast Augmentation 3 months postop

On the other hand, the change to a smaller implant causes less inconvenience in the sense of creating "more space," a new prosthesis can be included or not, associated with the remodeling of the mammary gland, with the subglandular or dual plane being preferred.

When the patient is well educated about contemplating her desire, along with her physical characteristics. Implant size is as much as patient's choice when she chooses to tell the surgeon to select the size that is best for her tissues as when she chooses to tell the surgeon a specific size.

Rippling

Rippling consists of the visible and/or palpable presence of ripples from the implant capsule. Rippling is probably the most distressing of all breast implant issues for patients (Thorne et al. 2013).

Breasts most prone to visible rippling are those with inadequate tissue coverage (e.g., when pinch thickness of the skin and subcutaneous tissue superior to the breast parenchyma is less than 2 cm) or when pinch thickness at the inframammary fold is less than 0.5 cm. Breasts with preexisting ptosis and those that are susceptible to postoperative ptosis are also prone to rippling. These situations should be identified preoperatively. No type of breast implant can compensate for inadequate tissue coverage, and deformities that occur are largely uncorrectable. Therefore, the priority at primary augmentation is to maximize coverage and avoid tissue damage.

All the factors mentioned above can coexist and lead to permanent tissue damage. Thus, thin, weakened, stretched, and damaged tissues are responsible for the occurrence, severity, and difficulty in correction of many of the common reasons for reoperation. The same minor malposition or capsular contracture which would not be visible under thick tissue and tight skin can be quite visible under damaged tissue. Rippling is rarely an issue with good tissue coverage but becomes one when tissue is thinned. Finally, any problem that requires correction is more problematic to correct when tissues are thinner or weaker.

Both the surgical act of dissecting a pocket for a breast implant and the long-standing presence of an implant can cause atrophy of breast tissue. Prudent implant selection and exacting surgical technique can help preserve tissue integrity and minimize long-term parenchymal atrophy (Fig. 24.4).

A breast implant that stretches the breast envelope as much as would lactation can be anticipated to permanently stretch and alter breast tissue. Highly projecting implants place more pressure per área than a wider implant of the same volume. If width is held constant, highly projecting implants can be nearly twice the volume and weight, thereby placing substantially greater pressure on the rib cage as well as the soft tissue. This causes parenchymal atrophy, thinning of subcutaneous tissues, thinning and stretching of skin, loss of skin elasticity, rib cage deformation, and loss of sensation (Thorne et al. 2013).

These tissue changes can result in rippling, skin stretch requiring mastopexy, and bizarre animation deformities (Thorne et al. 2013). Such problems are often not correctable, and attempts to mask them with highly cohesive implants, an acellular dermal matrix, and fat injections all result in imperfect corrections which are expensive and pose their own risks and drawbacks.

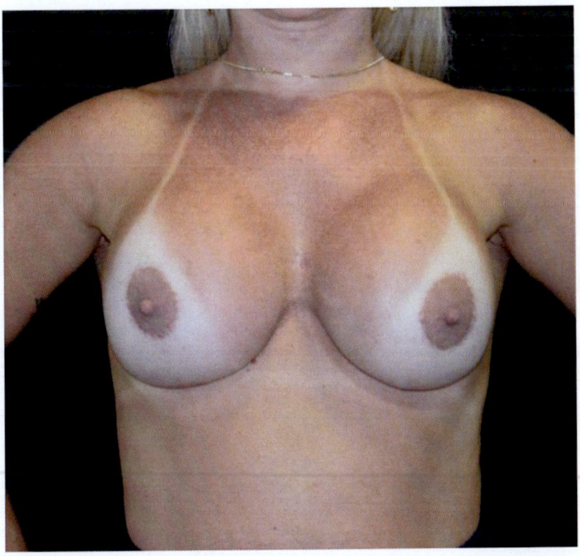

Fig. 24.4 Rippling

A worrying factor is when there is a very thin scratch, usually less than 5 mm, which results in serious complications of formation and various complications with local and systemic infection, which exists of breast tissue and tissue retraction. Thus, here are alternatives to the challenging cases and examples proposed above, demonstrating our experience with capsule graft, mesh or even free tram for selected.

Capsular Graft Technique

A breast implant capsule forms as a physiological response to the foreign material (Persichetti et al. 2014) and consists of fibrous connective tissue, mainly fibroblasts and collagen fibrils (Basseto et al. 2010). Previous reports have described their application as grafts or flaps (Yoo and Lee 2010; Gargano et al. 2002), considered as good material for reinforcement, especially to address breast implant-related problems in breast reconstruction (Persichetti et al. 2014).

The concept of this technique is to use a capsule with graft to replace the mesh or acellular dermal matrix (ADM) for secondary aesthetic breast procedures where some situations become a complex and challenging scenario, and also as a lower cost alternative. When replacement from the subglandular to submuscular plane is indicated, muscular reinforcement is mandatory. During the surgical application of this practice, it is important to take advantage of the breast pocket concept by adapting the skin envelope of the breast in order to reshape it (Baxter 2016).

To make use of this technique we must follow some criteria: thin tissue coverage, exchange of the implant by patient's request (older generation implants), malposition of implants, capsular contracture, and rippling. It is not recommended to perform this technique with patients affected by late or recurrent seroma and infection of the breast pocket were excluded. Intraoperative exclusion criteria applied for capsules with these characteristics: thick, fibrous, calcifications, granulomas and identified rupture of the implant or presence of seroma (Ribeiro and Arduini n.d.).

Surgical Technique

Starting from the incision previously proposed according to the surgical plan, a total capsulectomy is performed with en bloc resection of the implant and a rigorous hemostasis was conducted. Defatted capsule reverting and immersed in saline solution with a double antibiotic solution (1 g cefazolin +80 mg gentamicin). The new breast pocket was washed with saline solution, hydrogen peroxide and the same antibiotic solution (Ribeiro and Arduini n.d.).

It should be noted that re-approaches should, in most cases, be accompanied by replacement of the prosthesis due to the great chance of contamination of the old prosthesis, regardless of the size change or not.

Next, the implant's plane replaced from subglandular to submuscular due to thinning of the tissue, a piece of capsule graft sutured on edges of the pectoralmajor muscle with absorbable suture (Vylcril[R] 3–0) to expand the breast pocket, with the inner face of the capsule in direct contact with the implant. On the other hand, where the implant is placed in the subglandular plane because there is appropriate thickness of the tissue, the graft proposed for reinforcement in the prevention of deformities (Ribeiro and Arduini n.d.). With this technique, all the harvested capsular grafts were viable to obtain complete coverage of the breast contour deformities.

In this study, it was observed complete integration of the graft and better coverage of the implant, corrections of retractions and rippling, as well as tissue expansion in the subpectoral plane when the change of plane was performed. No complications or new episodes of contracture were observed and an aesthetic improvement and higher degree of satisfaction was reported by the patients.

The capsule graft seems to be an excellent coverage reinforcement mechanism in aesthetic breast revision using implants. Because the capsule is autologous tissue, there is no additional cost in contrast to the use of ADM or synthetic meshes (Neto and Gebrim 2019). Thus, the capsule graft does not generate rejection, it fully integrates with the patient's tissue, in addition to providing reinforcement of the structures in the above-mentioned tissues (Fig. 24.5).

Autologous material such as capsule graft or flaps and fat grafting can be useful in combination for recreating a stable breast implant pocket (Wessels et al. 2014; Bogdanov-Berezovsky et al. 2013) and still meet the criteria of suitable materials.

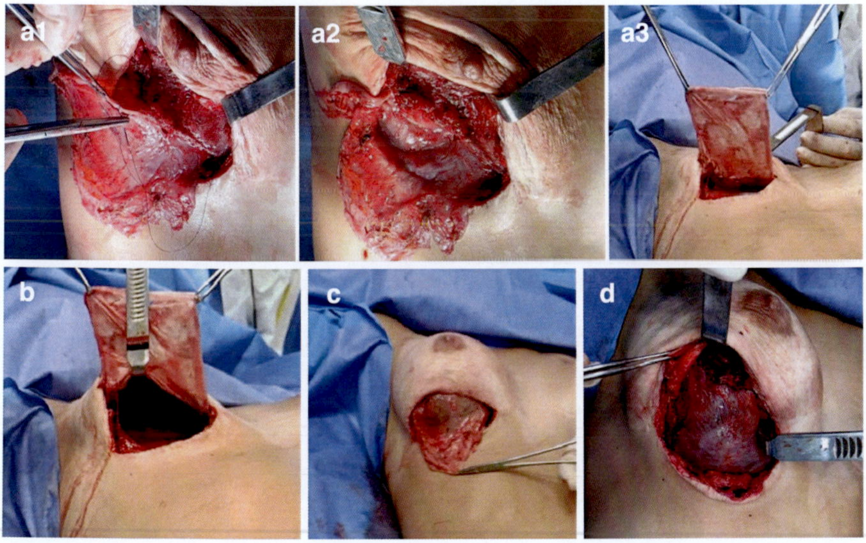

Fig. 24.5 Intraoperative view (**a1/a2/a3**) Capsule suture, (**b**) Newly created breast pocket; (**c**) Capsule reinforcement and implant replacement (**d**) Pocket closed

Mesh Graft

As shown with the capsule graft, the use of synthetic mesh also proved to be a viable and more economical alternative to reinforce the submuscular pocket and implant positioning, compared to the use of the acellular dermal matrix, due to the high cost. The difference in relation to the capsule graft is its quality, which must be discarded, following criteria such as: fibrotic and calcified capsule, silicone extravasation, contamination of the site, suspicion or diagnosis of BIA-ALCL. Given these scenarios, the use of synthetic mesh becomes a viable alternative (Fig. 24.6).

Complete coverage of the prosthesis by a submuscular pouch, in order to prevent implant exposure in the event of an eventual skin/wound dehiscence, has been shown to be quite effective and without significant changes in complications (Billon et al. 2019).

Synthetic meshes are non-biological materials that have been introduced and are available in absorbable materials: Vicryl® (Ethicon Inc., USA), SeraGyn® BR (Serag Wiessner, Germany) and TIGR® Matrix (Novus Scientific, Uppsala, Sweden); or partially absorbable: ULTRAPRO® (Ethicon Inc., USA) and TiLOOP® Bra (Pfm Medicalis, Germany).

The use of synthetic meshes in surgery has already been widely studied, proving to be a safe, biocompatible, hypoallergenic material with a low rate of complications (Gschwantler-Kaulich et al. 2018). Therefore, the use of these materials can be a good substitute for dermal matrices in surgeries.

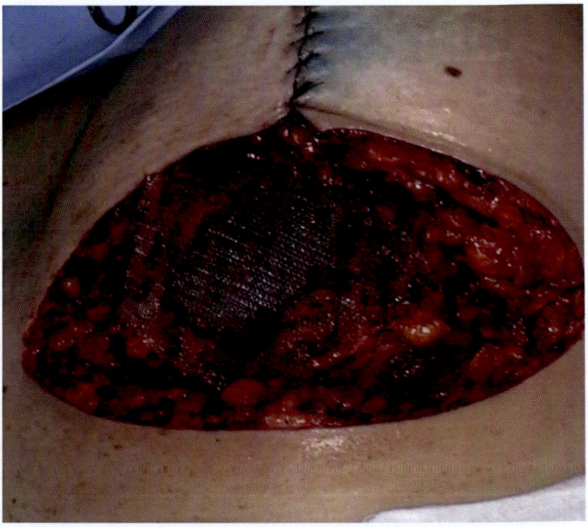

Fig. 24.6 Complete coverage of the implant in a synthetic mesh reinforced pocket

Surgical Technique

A pectoralis major submuscular pouch is dissected respecting a minimum of 1 cm of tissue thickness and of good quality. The inferomedial edge of the pectoral muscle (up to the second intercostal space) is elevated for placement of a silicone mold. The synthetic mesh (mesh) was sutured to this edge of the pectoral muscle, along its entire lower course up to the inframammary fold.

The size of the subpectoral pocket is calculated using the desired implant volume and the patient's anatomy. A mold of the desired implant volume is then inserted into the partial submuscular pocket to guide the size of the serratus anterior muscle fascia that will have to be lifted to accommodate the lateral portion of the implant, where the mesh will be sutured. After choosing the implant, it was introduced under the synthetic mesh, this material being fixed (with Vicryl® 2-0 suture thread) laterally at the level of the axillary line anterior to the dissected fascia of the serratus anterior muscle and up to the inframammary fold in the desired position. Two suction drains were placed, one in the submuscular pouch and the other in the subcutaneous tissue, through separate cutaneous accesses, followed by closure of the surgical wound in layers .

Studies with the placement of implants with full muscle coverage show complication rates of up to 40%, mainly in relation to poor implant positioning, asymmetry of the submammary crease and capsular contracture (Hansson et al. 2020). Therefore, the limitations of this technique are based on a restricted submuscular pocket, which prevents the placement of larger-volume implants and makes it difficult to create a natural breast and a defined submammary crease. The use of the mesh assists in the expansion of the pocket and better control of the positioning of the implant, as well as a greater expansion of the lower pole of the breast.

Conclusion

The only unequivocal endpoint assessing the quality of breast augmentation is the revision rate. Fortunately, the steps that reduce reoperations also create more beautiful breasts. The opposite of a malpositioned implant is an ideally situated implant; the opposite of a contracted capsule is a soft capsule, and so on.

The plastic surgeon's priority is to maximize preservation of tissue and prevent reoperation. This approach will simultaneously reduce her chances of facing the risks, costs, and emotional distress of another operation and maximize the likelihood of an optimal aesthetic result (Thorne et al. 2013).

The techniques mentioned above proved to be very effective in challenging scenarios such as secondary mammaplasties.

References

Daniel RK, Taylor GI. Distant transfer of an Island flap by microvascular anastomoses. *Plast Reconstr Surg*. 1973;52:111.

Taylor GI, Daniel RK. The free flap: composite tissue transfer by vascular anastomosis. *Aust N Z J Surg*. 1973;43:1.

McCraw JB, Dibbell DG, Carraway JH. Clinical definition of independent myocutaneous vascular territories. *Plast Reconstr Surg*. 1977;60:341.

Cormack GC, Lamberty BGH. *The Arterial Anatomy of Skin Flaps*. Edinburgh: Church-Livingstone; 1986.

Ponten B. The fasciocutaneous flap: its use in soft tissue defects of the lower leg. *Br J Plast Surg*. 1982;34:215.

Radovan C. Breast reconstruction after mastectomy using the temporary expander. *Plast Reconstr Surg*. 1982;69:195.

Baudet J, Rivet D, Martin D, Boileau R. Prefabricated free flap transfers. Presented at the 3rd Annual Meeting of the American Society for Reconstructive Microsurgery, San Antonio, Texas, September 12-13, 1987.

Ribeiro RC, Arduini AB. Capsular graft for secondary breast augmentation. ISAPS.NL:June20

Thorne, C. H., Chung, K. C., Gosain, A. K., Gurtner, G. C., Mehrara, B. J., Rubin, J. P., & Spear, S. L. (2013). *Grabb and Smith's plastic surgery: Seventh edition*. Wolters Kluwer Health Adis (ESP).

Pajkos A., Deva AK, Vickery K, Cope C, Chang L, Cossart YE. Detection of subclinical infection in significant breast implant capsules. *Plast Reconstr Surg*. 2003;111(5):1605-1611.

Persichetti P, Lombardo GAG, Marangi GF, Gherardi G, Dicuonzo G. Capsular contracture and genetic profile of ica genes among Staphylococcus epidermidis isolates from subclinical periprosthetic infections. *Plast Reconstr Surg*. 2011;127(4):1747-1748.

Persichetti P, Segreto F, Pendolino AL, Del Buono R, Marangi GF. Breast implant capsule flaps and grafts: a review of the literature. Aesthetic Plast Surg. 2014;38(3):540

Basseto F, Scarpa, Caccialanza E, Montesco MC, Magnani P (2010) Histological features of periprosthetic mammary capsules: silicone vs poliurethane. Aesth Plast Surg 34:481-485

Yoo G, Lee PK (2010) Capsular flaps for management of malpositioned implants after augmentation mammoplasty. Aesth Plast Surg 34:111-115

Gargano F, Moloney DM, Arnstein PM. Use of a capsular flap to prevent palpable wrinling of implants. *Br J Plast Surg*. 2002;55:269

Baxter RA. Internal bra: a unifying solution for reconstructive and aesthetic breast surgery issues. Plast Aesthet Res 2016;3:3-7

Neto MS, Gebrim LH. Capsular Flap for Implant Coverage in Breast Reconstruction Following Nipple-Sparing Mastectomy in Women With Previous Breast Augmentation. Plastic Surgery Case Studies. 2019. 5: 1-3.

Wessels L, Murphy S, Merten S. The capsular hammock flap for correction of breast implant ptosis. Aesthetic Plast Surg 2014;38:354-7

Bogdanov-Berezovsky A, Silberstein E, Shoham Y, Krieger Y. Capsular flap: new applications. Aesthetic Plast Surg 2013;37:395-7

Billon R, Hersant B, Bosc R, Meningaud JP. Acellular dermal matrix and synthetic mesh in implant-based immediate breast reconstruction: current concepts. Gynecol Obstet Fertil Senol. 2019;47(3):311-6. DOI: https://doi.org/10.1016/j.gofs.2019.01.010

Gschwantler-Kaulich D, Leser C, Salama M, Singer CF. Direct-to-implant breast reconstruction: higher complication rate vs cosmetic benefits. Breast J. 2018 24(6):957-64. https://doi.org/10.1111/tbj.13113

Hansson E, Burian P, Hallberg H. Comparison of inflammatory response and synovial metaplasia in immediate breast reconstruction with a synthetic and a biological mesh: a randomized controlled clinical trial. J Plast Surg Hand Surg. 2020;54(3):131-6. https://doi.org/10.1080/2000656X.2019.1704766

Chapter 25
Basic Science/Disease Process

Ricardo Cavalcanti Ribeiro, Luis Fernandez de Córdova, and Ana Beatriz Arduini

Abstract Reduction mammoplasty, as the central purpose of this chapter, aims to elucidate topics such as anatomy focused on plastic surgery, psychological aspects, safety in surgery, and, of course, the main techniques. Surgery for breast hypertrophy is one of the most performed in plastic surgery, and more than 100 techniques have been reported in the last century, aiming for a safer procedure, avoiding or at least decreasing complications, and obtaining breasts with natural shape, proportional volumes, long-lasting results, and minimal scars that challenge creative ability.

Keywords Basic science · Disease · Evolution

Reduction mammoplasty, as the central purpose of this chapter, aims to elucidate topics such as anatomy focused on plastic surgery, psychological aspects, safety in surgery, and, of course, the main techniques. Surgical treatment of breast hypertrophy is one of the most common surgical techniques performed in our field, with more than 100 techniques reported for reduction mammoplasty in the last century, we as plastic surgeons aim for a safer procedure, that avoids or at least decreases complications, and obtains natural shaped breasts with proportional volumes, long-lasting results, and reduced scars, which is a real challenge for our artistic creativity.

R. Cavalcanti Ribeiro (✉) · L. F. de Córdova
Plastic and Reconstructive Surgery, Federal University of the State of Rio de Janeiro, Rio de Janeiro, Brazil

Carlos Chagas Institute, Rio de Janeiro, Brazil

Plastic and Reconstructive Surgery, Global Plastic Surgery, Rio de Janeiro, Brazil
e-mail: rribeiro@centroin.net.br

A. B. Arduini
Plastic and Reconstructive Surgery, Mário Kroeff Hospital, Rio de Janeiro, Brazil

J. M. Avelar, R. Cavalcanti Ribeiro (eds.), *Body Contouring*,
https://doi.org/10.1007/978-3-031-42802-9_25

Etiology of breast hypertrophy is unknown, but it can be the result of an atypical response of the breast to circulating estrogens, causing breast tissue proliferation. There are hypertrophy and fibrotic changes of the fat tissue elements, but the glandular tissue remains with little change. Most women with breast hypertrophy have normal levels of estrogen circulation, as well as normal numbers of estrogen receptors in breast tissue. It usually starts at puberty or postpartum, and there is no evidence for hormonal therapy.

Virginal hypertrophy usually affects girls between 11 and 16 years, presented as a fast-growing breast reaching a degree of gigantism after menarche. This type of hypertrophy may be unilateral or bilateral, without evidences of hormonal changes.

Conceptually, we can classify breast hypertrophy according to the predicted volume, as shown in Table 25.1. There are varying definitions of what is an excessive breast tissue, such as when it exceeds approximately 3% of the total body weight. According to the literature, gigantomastia is considered when breast tissue removal is over than 1000 g from each breast, but this number can change depending on the references.

Breast are composed of mammary parenchyma, which contains glandular tissue divided into lobules, adipose tissue, Scarpa's fascia with its superficial and deep layers, Cooper's ligaments, Spence's tail, the nipple-areola complex (NAC), and lactiferous ducts, in addition to anatomical references. These elements add up to maintain the breast structure and give the final appearance of the breast.

In addition, another important parameter is the triple blood support—based on the perforating branches of the internal thoracic artery (60%), the lateral thoracic artery (30%), and the anterior and lateral perforating branches of the intercostal arteries (10%)—which is the main reference for making the flaps discussed in this chapter.

Thus, size, symmetry, proportion, and location of the breast, as well as its reference points on the chest wall, provide the aesthetics of the breasts in addition to well-defined signs of breast beauty such as conical shape with the areola at the apex.

It is necessary to have a precise knowledge of anatomy in order to choose the most suitable technique for each case.

Table 25.1 Classification of breast hypertrophy

Breast size	Breast volume (cm^3)
Ideal	250–300
Small hypertrophy	300–600
Moderate hypertrophy	600–800
Big hypertrophy	800–1000
Gigantomastia	>1000

Diagnosis/Patient Presentation

The breasts are a sign of femininity and a sexual organ of high importance for women. During the last decades, the expectations of women regarding the aesthetic and functional aspect of their breasts have increased significantly. In the case of women interested in having a breast reduction, besides a large spectrum of indications, the main motivations are function, form, and emotional issues related to self-esteem.

Generally, patients who are looking for this surgery have very specific symptoms, such as shoulder pain, headache, neck pain, shoulder groove (bra mark), kyphosis, inappropriate posture, intertriginous rash, and even neurological symptoms such as ulnar paresthesia. The compression of the brachial plexus between the coracoid process and the pectoralis minor due to the posture of bending the shoulders forward explains the paresthesia. On physical examination, in addition, we can find signs of fungal infection or even secondary bacterial infection in the inframammary folds.

We must analyze very well the psychical aspect, in which the women's self-confidence is usually affected, not only in self-image—they are not beautiful, socially accepted, and have difficulties finding partners or engaging in sexual activity—but also difficulties in finding suitable clothes, playing sports, and socializing, and sometimes making them with withdrawn personalities. If pathological disturbances have been suspected, a psychological consultation is suggested to determine the causes and treatment, if possible, prior to surgery.

Before venturing into this type of surgery, the plastic surgeon must be aware of the following factors that will influence the outcomes.

Breast Size

The choice of technique should be performed according to the degree of hypertrophy. No specific bra size should be promised.

Skin Type

While in younger women the skin is more tense and elastic, in multiparous women, older women, and those with the presence of stretch marks, the extension of the scar and the ability of the skin to retract will influence the outcome of the surgery.

Glandular Tissue Consistency

In younger women, the breast is generally more glandular; however, when they get older, a fat substitution is always observed. Thus, more compact result is obtained in young patients.

Height of the Nipple-Areola Complex

This aspect is fundamental in the choice of the vascular pedicle that will supply the areola. The distance from point "A" to the NAC determines the degree of ascent, and it can be performed through direct ascension, migration techniques, or graft. As much greater the distance to reach "A" point, more will be the risk of devascularization.

Breast and Chest Asymmetries

Several congenital or acquired factors can interfere with the "normal" shape of the breasts. Among the congenital anomalies are breast agenesis, Poland's syndrome, supernumerary gland, inverted nipple, Pectus excavatum and scoliosis. Another situation that must be looked for and evaluated, is tuberous breast. Therefore, the evaluation aims to define the parameters that will be modified with the surgery and clarify the types of asymmetry that cannot be corrected.

Previous Injuries or Scars

In order to identify previous aesthetic or reconstructive surgeries and exclude breast neoplasms, a careful investigation of what happened should be done, and, if possible, request the mastologist's evaluation. In addition, observe the presence of scar retractions due to burns among others and the quality of the scars and question whether there was any type of complication during the same.

Inframammary Fold and Degree of Ptosis

The degree of breast ptosis depends on the position of the NAC in relation to the IMF, according to Regnault´s classification of ptosis (Table 25.2).

Table 25.2 Regnault´s classification of ptosis

Complete or true ptosis	Grade I	NAC at the height of the inframammary fold and above the breast
	Grade II	NAC below the inframammary fold and above the breast contour
	Grade III	NAC below the inframammary fold and the contour of the breast
Partial ptosis	NAC above the inframammary fold and gland ptosis	
Pseudoptosis	NAC above the inframammary fold; loose, hypoplastic skin (e.g., marked weight loss after pregnancy)	

Imaging Exams

We routinely recommend performing at least one imaging study before the procedure, either to identify a benign or malignant condition that may interfere with the surgical schedule. For patients under 35 years, ultrasound is mandatory. On the other hand, high-resolution mammography is recommended for women over 35 years old. If there is family history for breast cancer or suspicious lesions, previous evaluation by the mastologist is required.

Photographs

At the first consultation, patients must be advised regarding differences between each breast and keep in mind that each breast's approach will be in an alternative way. Therefore, standardized photographs, preoperative and postoperative, with frontal, oblique, and profile views, are mandatory. The preference is for digital photography that offers the opportunity to show immediately the differences to the patient and later allows comparing and evaluating the results of the procedure.

Informed Consent Form

An exhaustive explanation of the procedure and the signing of informed consent terms regarding its limitations, risks, and complications are mandatory. The documents should be individualized for each patient. In Brazil, due to local laws, any resected surgical tissue must be sent for histopathological analysis.

Patient's expectations and understanding about the surgery and anesthesia must be clarified, as well as alerts regarding asymmetries, scar size, and unrealistic expectations. In addition, the procedure should be discouraged in cases of lactation, pregnancy, papillary discharge, palpable nodule, axillary and supraclavicular lymph nodes, skin and NAC lesions, and active infections. In these cases, surgery should be postponed until the diagnostic investigation and appropriate treatment are completed. The minimum age recommended is 18 years old.

Patient Selection

In the Brazilian context, we follow Pitanguy's principles and their variations, which include a wide variety of techniques for the most diverse breast characteristics. Therefore, the Inverted T pattern reduction mammoplasty is one of the most used techniques and has been improving continuously in order to minimize the scarring sequelae resulting from it.

There is a current tendency to seek reduced scars, in search of a higher aesthetic standard and in line with the increasing body exposure; however, it is very important to clarify to the patient that the best result cannot be sacrificed at the expense of a reduced scar.

In order to choose the best technique, besides the issues already mentioned, we must take into consideration gland texture, skin quality, the degree of breast hypertrophy and the estimation of fat and parenchyma volume. Anatomical landmarks and distances between structures such as the distance between the NAC and the sternal notch determine the necessary end position of the NAC and are of outmost importance in surgical planning. Thus, we propose the following algorithm:

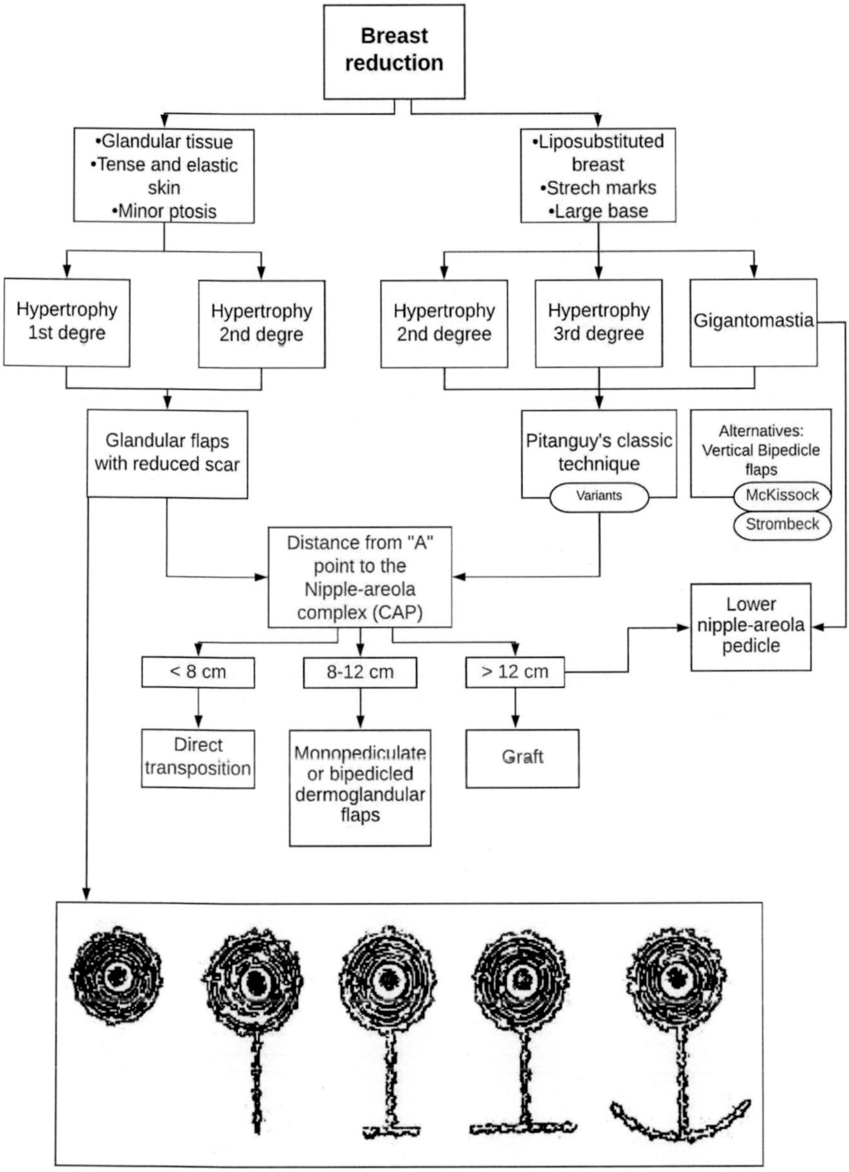

Once the criteria for choosing the technique are established, it is essential to carry out complementary exams and to evaluate the surgical and anesthetic risk, which has the following objectives:

- Detect new diseases that could interfere with the surgical and postoperative act.
- Assess known diseases.
- Determine if the patient can be submitted to the proposed procedure.
- Establish conducts that minimize morbidity and mortality.

We routinely request a complete blood count, coagulogram, blood glucose, urea, creatinine, chest X-rays (PA and profile), and EKG.

Treatment/Evidence-Based Surgical Technique

Marking:

- The preoperative marking in a T pattern breast reduction varies from author to author, but the geometric concept and principles proposed stay unchanged instruments as well may vary, but for academic purposes, we will describe our preference.
- Marking step by step with the patient standing up position, with the smaller breast as the main reference:
  - Hemiclavicular line: can vary from 5.5 to 7 cm and divides the breast into two equal parts.
  - "A" point: reflects the projection of the inframammary fold over the hemiclavicular line.
  - Extension of the sternal notch to "A" point that can vary depending on the patient's height between 18 and 22 cm. Note: We use this reference because geometrically it gives greater precision and symmetry to the marking.
  - Marking of the anterior axillary line, the inframammary fold, and the midsternal line.
  - "B" and "C" points: bi-digital handling through the pinching of the estimated skin and breast tissue, equidistant from the areola, forming a triangle with the "A" point.
    Note: In this marking time, verify the amplitude of the angle formed between these two points, under the principle that what matters is the tissue left and not the removed one. Usually this angle varies from 40 to 60° during this marking.
  - "D" and "E" points: marking at the medial and lateral limits in the inframammary fold, without going beyond the groove and keeping them equidistant from "B" and "C" points.
  - Joining the stitches: if there is excess skin, the design must be concave to the groove, and if there is excess gland, it must be convex.
  - Transfer the marking to the other breast by using wire or compass.

In addition to this standard markings, additional markings for the technique proposed may be performed, for example, an inferiorly based dermal pedicle nipple-areolar flap, resection areas, or liposuction areas, either of which may be indicated for a particular type of breast.

Once checked, the patient goes to the operating room, and anesthetic induction is performed, which we give preference to general anesthesia.

Surgical sequence:

- After the anesthetic procedure, followed by strict asepsis and placement of surgical fields, with the patient in the supine position at 0° and the shoulders abducted at 90°, the areola is marked under light tension with flat hands.
- Next, the infiltration, with a saline solution with adrenaline in a 1:200,000 dilution, makes at the breast marks. Infiltration of the breast base, parallel to the chest, can be performed.
  - Across tension performed by the assistant at the base of the breast, incisions are made around the areola of triangular shape.
  - De-epithelialization around the NAC in a triangular designed area, with preservation of the superficial vascular plexus until approximately 2 cm below the areola.
  - A hook is placed to hold at "A" point.
  - With the breast perpendicular to the chest wall, between "B" and "C" points, we amputate the base of the breast, according to the classic technique of the upper pedicle flap. In addition, a wedge or keel resection of the central excess of the mammary gland can be performed.
  - We do a medial approximation on the pillars with nylon 2-0 or 3-0 and its fixation to the pectoral fascia. This point will reflect the NAC's projection.
  - Pre-modeling of the breast through a suture between "B" and "C" points and the medial point of the inframammary fold, where we will observe the breast in a conical shape. This modeling must be reproduced in the contralateral breast.
  - Mark the final positioning of the NAC with areolotome between 5.5 and 7 cm above the IMF or where the apex of the cone is.
  - NAC final position is handled as a direct transposition, with dermoglandular flaps (monopediculate or bipedicled) or even as a graft.
  - Hemostasis is a dynamic process that occurs with each resection to avoid unnecessary blood loss.
  - Place and fix the suction drains on the horizontal scar.
  - Suture in three planes with inverted knot with 2-0, 3-0, and 4-0 nylon. Suture the NAC with Gillies stitch with 4-0 nylon and the intradermal closure with 3-0 monocryl sutures.

The dressing is of the closed compressive type, keeping the wound moist with antibiotic ointments for the first 48–72 h. Hospital discharge is 24 h.

Postoperative Care Protocol

The patient must follow a relative rest for 30 days, prevent carrying weight, and do domestic activities and gym activities during this period. From the fourth week onward, except in situations of complications, a patient is usually waiting to perform activities with moderate intensity, such as walking, and in the period of 60 days, she is released for activities with a load. In addition, the surgical bra should be routinely used for 30 days and an anti-thrombus socks for 7 days.

In most cases, suction drains are left at the horizontal portion of the Inverted T pattern scar, and these will remain until drainage is less than 30 ml per breast and are usually removed between 3 and 5 days postop.

Postoperative lymphatic drainage has a relative indication and brings benefits such as reducing pain, bruising, swelling, and preventing fibrosis, but without influence on the final result of the surgery.

In addition, antibiotic prophylaxis with first- or second-generation cephalosporins (cephalexin or cefuroxime) are routinely recommended, plus analgesics and anti inflammatory drugs for a minimum of 7 days. Other medications such as antiemetics and muscle relaxants are prescribed individually. Opioids are not necessary.

Prophylaxis of thromboembolism follows the recommendations of the Caprini scale. For all hospitalized patients pneumatic compression and early deambulation. When recommended, low molecular weight heparin 40 mg in a single dose, 12 h after the start of the procedure. We do not use heparin routinely for a prolonged period, except for cases of hemophilia or proven diseases.

Outcomes, Prognosis, and Complications

Complications are the same as those that can occur with other mammoplasty techniques. Breast reduction is considered a significant procedure, as it includes extensive dissections and resections, which increase the number of complications, and these vary by up to 10%.

Among the immediate complications, we can highlight seroma and hematoma, which are usually managed with immediate evacuation. Skin necrosis—mainly at the junction of the inverted T or NAC—is generally attributed to aggressive surgical manipulations and consequently poor perfusion of the flaps, further aggravated by postoperative edema and very tight sutures.

Signs of suffering from NAC are associated with ischemia due to excessive tension or venous congestion that leads to a change in perfusion, partial or total loss of this segment. It is important to note that excessive stress relief can be reversed for a period of 6 h, avoiding this complication.

Less frequently, steatonecrosis occurs due to circulatory disorders of the fat tissue, presenting with phlogistic signs and fluctuation and generally requiring drainage, in addition to strict dressing control.

Late complications are usually related to scarring, such as hypertrophy, enlargement, or keloid formation. The formation of epithelial cysts or a change in NAC sensitivity (hypo- or hyperesthesia) may also occur.

Prevention of complications:

- Use of the proper technique
- Delicacy with tissues during surgery
- Careful hemostasis
- Early drainage in the event of hematoma
- Absence of tension in the sutures
- Compression of scars

Pros and Cons

A versatile technique provides both the correction of hypertrophy and the improvement of ptosis. It serves both young breasts and older patients and has long-lasting results. The disadvantage is the size of the scar and possible handling to migrate the NAC, which may demonstrate technical difficulties depending on the surgeon's experience.

- Systematization of surgery.
- Good symmetry with natural breast shape.
- We can add other techniques such as inferior pedicle flaps to project the upper pole and flared bottom flap.
- Dermoglandular flap to rotate the NAC in severe ptosis.
- Low level of complications.

Marketing Aspects

This technique brings great functional and aesthetic satisfaction to the patients as it considerably improves pain complaints, poor posture, and above all psychological aspects, raises their self-confidence, and improves their social life.

Chapter 26
Gynecomasty

Luis Fernandez de Córdova and Ricardo Cavalcanti Ribeiro

Abstract Gynecomastia is a common and distressing benign enlargement of the breasts, affecting from 38% to 64% of the male population worldwide (Fruhstorfer and Malata, Br J Plast Surg 56:237–246, 2003); the incidence of bilateral gynecomastia also varies in the medical literature. This male thorax deformity of multifactorial etiology in most cases requires surgical treatment, being one of the most common plastic surgery procedures performed in men (https://www.isaps.org/wp-content/uploads/2020/12/Global-Survey-2019.pdf). The first record of this condition was made by the Egyptians depicting images of King Tutankhamen with gynecomastia (Daniels and Layer, ANZ J Surg 73:213–216, 2003).

Plastic surgeons as well as clinicians should not underestimate gynecomastia; although transient and benign by definition, it might have serious psychological consequences.

Palpable glandular tissue in the male breast presents itself through three peaks in the age distribution of gynecomastia occurring in neonates, pubertal boys, and elderly men, aiding also in the differentiation of physiologic or pathologic gynecomastia.

Keywords Gynecomastia · Pseudogynecomastia · Male thorax · Breast surgery

L. F. de Córdova
Carlos Chagas Institute, Rio de Janeiro, Brazil

Division of Plastic and Reconstructive Surgery, Casa de Portugal, Rio de Janeiro, Brazil

Division of Plastic and Reconstructive Surgery, Global Plastic Surgery State of México, México, Mexico

R. Cavalcanti Ribeiro (✉)
Plastic and Reconstructive Surgery, Federal University of the State of Rio de Janeiro, Rio de Janeiro, Brazil
e-mail: rribeiro@centroin.net.br

J. M. Avelar, R. Cavalcanti Ribeiro (eds.), *Body Contouring*,
https://doi.org/10.1007/978-3-031-42802-9_26

Introduction

Gynecomastia is a common and distressing benign enlargement of the breasts, affecting from 38% to 64% of the male population worldwide (Fruhstorfer and Malata 2003); the incidence of bilateral gynecomastia also varies in the medical literature. This male thorax deformity of multifactorial etiology in most cases requires surgical treatment, being one of the most common plastic surgery procedures performed in men (https://www.isaps.org/wp-content/uploads/2020/12/Global-Survey-2019.pdf). The first record of this condition was made by the Egyptians depicting images of King Tutankhamen with gynecomastia (Daniels and Layer 2003).

From an aesthetics point of view, the ideal male thorax is flat, firm, and muscular. The pectoralis major forms most of the muscle component of the chest, flat against the rib cage in its superior portion and convex at its inferior margin. The pectoralis major can be divided into clavicular, sternocostal, and abdominal portions. The convexity of the male chest is also due to a pectoral fat pad underneath the nipples; it is responsible for lipomastia, which is the enlargement of the male chest neither due to muscular hypertrophy nor a palpable glandular tissue disk under the nipple.

Palpable glandular tissue in the male breast presents itself through three peaks in the age distribution of gynecomastia occurring in neonates, pubertal boys, and elderly men, aiding also in the differentiation of physiologic or pathologic gynecomastia. Clinically, gynecomastia may present as subareolar breast tissue ranging from 0.5 to greater than 2cm, appearing at least 6 months after the onset of male secondary characteristics and typically regresses within 1 year. Multiple causes for pubertal gynecomastia have been suggested such as transient hormonal imbalance between estrogens and androgens; however, studies (Dunbar et al. 2005; Ersoz et al. 2002; LaFranchi et al. 1975) found conflicting results when comparing hormonal profiles between teenagers with and without gynecomastia. Elderly men will often develop gynecomastia as testosterone levels decline in plasma and peripheral aromatization increases (Table 26.1).

Table 26.1 Etiology of gynecomastia

Physiologic	Pathologic	Pharmalogic
Neonatal	Metabolic disorders*	Hormones
Pubertal	Endocrine disorders+	Psychoactive agentes
Elderly	Acquired hypogonadal states	Cardiovascular drugs
	Congenital hypogonadal states	Antiandrogens
	Hyperestrogenism	Cancer chemotherapeutics
		Antibiotics
		Antiulcer medications
		Drugs of abuse
		Metoclopramide
		Antiretrovirals

*Alcoholic cirrhosis, adrenal tumors, refeeding after a starvations state
+Thyroid disorders, adenal cortical hyperplasia

Plastic surgeons as well as clinicians should not underestimate gynecomastia; although transient and benign by definition, it might have serious psychological consequences.

Other disorders that can lead to masses in the male breast include the following: lipomas, hemangiomas, neurofibromas, lymphangiomas, dermoid cysts, and breast carcinoma distinguished from true gynecomastia due to eccentric breast enlargement.

Diagnosis/Patient Presentation

Several classifications exist for gynecomastia (Rohrich et al. 2003) considering different parameters such as degree of ptosis, type of tissue, size, skin redundancy, NAC's position, neither of which is universally accepted nor applicable to all cases. The lack of consensus in the classification of this condition limits the prospective comparison of successful treatment outcomes as well as the existence of an effective treatment algorithm for either medical or surgical treatment.

History and physical examination are the basis for the diagnosis of gynecomastia. Physicians must inquire about the duration of symptoms, if any, and presence of nipple discharge, skin changes, firm masses, presence of testicular masses, review patient's prescription and OTC medications as well as the use of alcohol and/or illicit recreational drugs.

Physical examination requires palpation of the breast tissue with assessment of consistency and symmetry.

Ultrasound is the imaging modality of choice for diagnosing gynecomastia by revealing hyperechoic fibroglandular tissue. A mammogram may be needed to exclude breast cancer. Other tests like chest X-rays, computerized tomography (CT) scans, and magnetic resonance imaging (MRI) scans may be recommended if tumors and pathologies of other organs are suspected to be the cause behind gynecomastia.

Grade I Gynecomastia

Grade I gynecomastia presents as a glandular enlargement with elastic skin and no inframammary fold, therefore liposuction is not required. The surgical approach recommended is the following: minimally invasive adenectomy through a semicircular periareolar incision followed by fixation of the NAC dermis to the fascia of the pectoralis major and either vertical mattress suture (Allgöwer type) or continuous intracutaneous suture (Fig. 26.1).

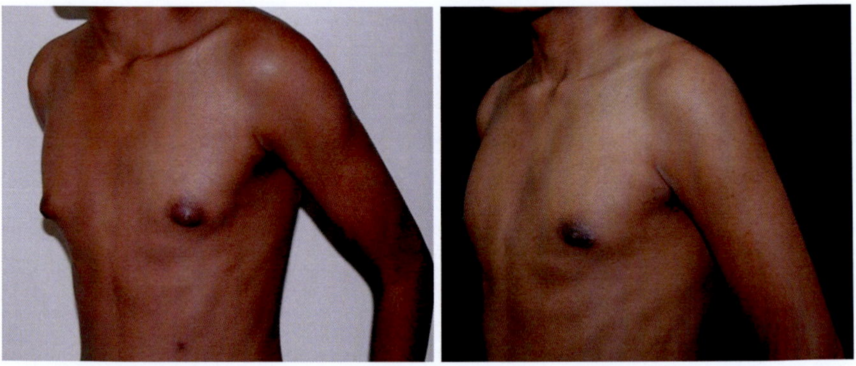

Fig. 26.1 Grade I gynecomastia: Before and after pictures (10 days Post Op). Technique used: simple adenectomy

Grade II Gynecomastia

Grade II gynecomastia is characterized by moderate hypertrophy of the structural components of the breast, glandular and fat tissue, (250–500 g). No excess skin is present and an inframmary fold appears. Surgery must act on both components, glandular and adipose tissue, ensuring that the skin loses the memory of the neo-inframammary fold. There is a first phase of vacuum- or power-assisted liposuction followed by minimally invasive adenectomy by means of a semicircular periareolar, intra-areolar, endoscopic, or pull-through incision.

Grade III Gynecomastia

Grade III gynecomastia (>500 g of breast tissue) presents excess adipose tissue, skin redundancy, inframammary fold, and grade II/III ptosis; this group can include male tuberous breast. Generally, skin sparing techniques doesn't suffice to offer a satisfying flattening of the thorax.

The surgery begins with liposuction to address the adipose tissue component of the gynecomastia followed by adenectomy. After the adenectomy is performed, periareolar deepithelialization takes place for NAC repositioning as well as reducing the areolar diameter. Always consider the contralateral side for symmetry and the reference canons for the male thorax. Closure carried out by round-block suturing and either vertical mattress suture (Allgöwer type) or continuous intracutaneous suture.

Pseudogynecomastia

Pseudogynecomastia (Fig. 26.2) patients present cutaneous and fat excess with different grades of ptosis, and lateral chest roll may or may not be present. Generally, these patients went through a massive weight loss. Surgical treatment will leave residual scars since the focal point of the treatment is skin resection by means of reduction mastoplasty. The magnitude of skin and fat excision is determined by push, grasp, and pinch tests after establishing a reasonable and stable weight.

Multiple techniques have been described for the treatment of pseudogynecomastia. Nowadays, the development of new techniques, focusing on aesthetic surgery and female breast surgery, makes it possible to solve severe cases of gynecomastia, such as the boomerang pattern correction of gynecomastia, which allows flattening of the torso from the axilla to the redundant skin around the areola. Refinement of the inferior pedicle may be achieved through vacuum- and/or power-assisted liposuction.

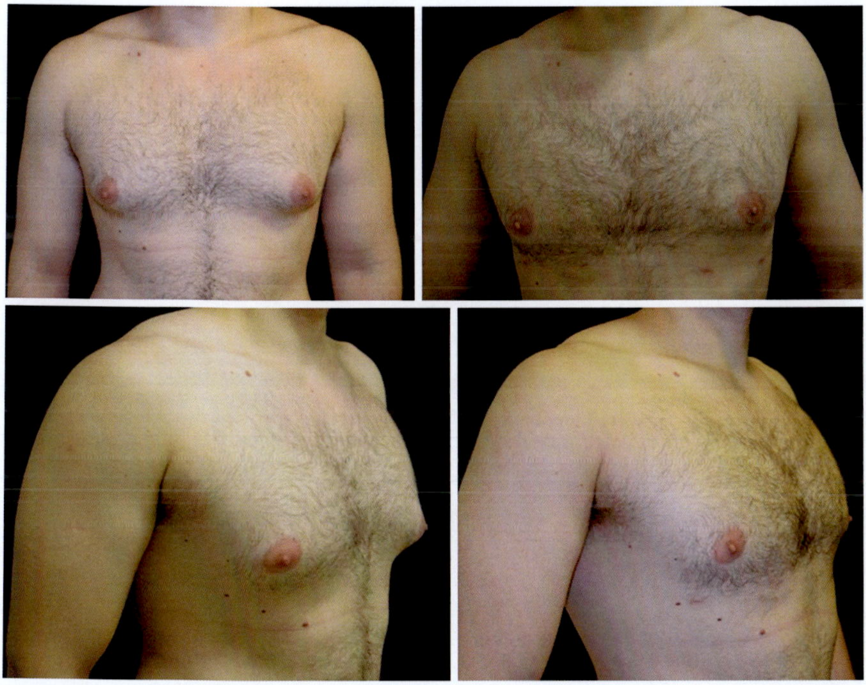

Fig. 26.2 Before and after pictures of pseudogynecomastia after liposuction

Treatment/Surgical Technique

Medical therapy, is described in the literature (Williams 1979; Andersen and Gram 1982) as most effective during the proliferation phase. Proliferation phase is characterized histologically by presenting ductal proliferation with epithelial hyperplasia, an increase in the stromal and periductal connective tissue, and an increase in vascularity and periductal edema.The end of the proliferation phase is defined by stromal hyalinization, dilation of the ducts, and a marked reduction in epithelial proliferation after a year of onset. The fibrotic tissue does not respond to medical therapies. If a trial period of medical therapy (danazol, clomiphene, testolactone, tamoxifen) is reported unsuccessful or if gynecomastia has been present for more than a year or if the etiology is not endocrine or drug related, the accepted standard treatment is the surgical removal of glandular tissue.

The objectives of the surgical treatment of gynecomastia are elimination of the inframammary fold and flattening of the male thoracic region, repositioning of the NAC, and removal of redundant skin. At least 25 surgical techniques can be traced in the literature.

The sequence of gynecomastia surgical treatment is as follows:

- Markings
- Anesthesia
- Antisepsis
- Infiltration of anesthetic-vasoconstricting solution
- Liposuction
- Minimally invasive adenectomy
- Correct positioning of the NAC (if applicable)
- Excision of redundant skin and fat (if applicable)
- Dressing

Markings in the sitting position using the aesthetic unit definitions of the male chest proposed by Caridi, R. (Fig. 26.1) and using anatomical references as follows: anterior median line, right and left midclavicular lines, right and left anterior and midaxillary lines, sternal notch, and NAC (Fig. 26.2).

Following anesthesia with the patient in the supine position, antisepsis first with chlorhexidine 2% with the sterile technique is performed. The next step is a new degermation of the area with 0.2% aqueous chlorhexidine solution, carried out by the surgical assistant, already duly attired.

The next step is the placement of sterile surgical drapes. The incisions are made, after infiltration of 0.5 ml of lidocaine (2%) with epinephrine with a surgical blade #11 with a mean longitude of 0.5 cm. In our practice, we perform the infiltration process using 60 cc syringes in a fan-shaped pattern monitoring skin turgor by continual palpation. After a 20 min window for the vasoconstrictor effect to begin, liposuction may begin.

Once we had achieved satisfactory flattening of the chest, by means of a semicircular intra-areolar incision, the adenectomy is performed. Fixation of the NAC dermis to the fascia of the pectoralis major followed by either vertical mattress suture (Allgöwer type) or continuous intracutaneous suture ends the surgery.

Massive Weight Loss Patient

Boomerang Pattern Correction

Boomerang pattern correction proposed by Hurwitz refers to the right angle elliptical skin excisions that drape each NAC removing redundant skin in both vertical and horizontal planes and correcting nipple position.

Postoperative Care Protocol

To achieve better results, complications must be minimized and NAC vascularization should be frequently monitored. Surgical vacuum drains are not placed routinely, unless otherwise indicated. A compression garment is placed at the conclusion of the surgery and maintained for 4–6 weeks.

References

Fruhstorfer BH, Malata CM. A systematic approach to the surgical treatment of gynaecomastia. Br J Plast Surg 2003;56:237–246

Daniels IR, Layer GT. How should gynaecomastia be managed? ANZ J Surg 2003; 73:213–216.

Dunbar B, Dundar N, Ecri T, Bober E, Büyükqebiz A. Leptin levels in boys with pubertal gynecomastia. J Pediatr Endocrinol Metab 2005; 18:929–93

Ersoz H, Önde ME, Terekeci H, et al. Causes of gynaecomastia in young adult males and factors associated with idiopathic gynaecomastia. Int J Androl 2002; 25:312 316.

LaFranchi SH, Parlow AF, Lippe BM, et al. Pubertal gynecomastia and transient elevation of serum estradiol level. Am J Dis Child 1975; 129: 927–931.

Rohrich, R., Ha, R., Kenkel, J., and Adams, W. P., Jr. Classifications and management of gynecomastia: defining the role of ultrasound-assisted liposuction. Plast Reconstr Surg 111: 909, 2003.

Williams MJ. Gynecomastia as a physical finding in normal men. J Clin Endocrinol Metab 1979; 48: 338-40

Andersen JA, Gram JB. Male breast at autopsy. Acta Pathol Microbiol Immunol Scand 1982; 90:91-7

Chapter 27
Importance of Mastoplasty Combined with Abdominoplasty Concerning Body Contouring

Paulo Roberto Becker-Amaral, Leonardo Possamai, and Luciana Carvalho da Cunha

Abstract In this chapter, we discuss patient evaluation, key safety points, useful techniques, and how to apply them. Data from the literature on complications highlight the need to carefully select patients, limit the duration and extent of surgery, and reduce the risk of adverse events via supportive measures and medication. A vigilant surgeon is a safe surgeon.

Introduction

Women seek combined liposuction, abdominoplasty, and mammoplasty when their body contours change because of their individual characteristics, pregnancy, lifestyle habits, or age. ISAPS 2019 reported that these surgeries accounted for 35% of all cosmetic procedures performed worldwide (International Society for Aesthetic Plastic Surgery 2019). This combination has been termed the "mommy makeover." Most patients prefer to undergo all surgeries contemporaneously, as this is practical and saves time and money. Combined abdominoplasty and breast augmentation was described by Rao in 1969 (Rao 1969); over the years, great efforts have been made to prioritize safety and ensure that the results are as good as when the surgeries are performed separately.

P. R. Becker-Amaral · L. Possamai (✉) · L. C. da Cunha
São Paulo, Brazil

J. M. Avelar, R. Cavalcanti Ribeiro (eds.), *Body Contouring*,
https://doi.org/10.1007/978-3-031-42802-9_27

Discussion

When a woman thinks about herself, a body image is formed internally, and this process may promote confidence or anxiety. Negative changes in female body contours can elicit emotional and behavioral responses that deeply compromise the quality of life. Patients with many defects attach equal importance to each defect and request liposuction, abdominoplasty, and mammoplasty to restore their bodies and, much more importantly, their feelings about themselves. Procedures performed in isolation may increase the level of dissatisfaction with the remaining defects. Pitanguy reported this phenomenon in patients exhibiting breast hypertrophy, ptosis, and abdominal flaccidity who opted for only one correction (Pitanguy and Ceravolo 1983). By contrast, combined surgery transforms the entire body in one session. Surgeons must decide whether combined procedures are viable in terms of safety and the quality of the results.

Preoperative Considerations

Preoperative consultations with the surgeon and anesthesiologist reveal the patient's complaints and expectations and allow her to become informed about the diagnosis, anesthesia, indicated surgeries, limitations, care, risks, scars, and costs. Photographs are taken to allow her to understand the planned surgery as well as the indications and limitations. The surgeon dispels myths regarding perfect symmetry, results that last forever, and scars that disappear.

Patient Selection

From an emotional viewpoint, good surgical candidates are those who evaluate themselves correctly and who can trust and establish a good relationship with their doctor. When patients intend to maintain the surgical results via diet and physical activity, they tend to be more satisfied in the long term (Rohrich et al. 2004). The following characteristics are associated with possible dissatisfaction despite a good anatomical result (Table 27.1) (Kaye and Gradinger 1984).

Table 27.1 Warning signs of potentially dissatisfied patients

Sensitivity to small "defects"
A belief that she is very important. A focus on detail, a demanding attitude, and great expectations
Depression, insecurity, indecisiveness
At least one prior operation with which she was dissatisfied
Criticism of colleagues of the surgeon (even good ones)
Development of a poor relationship with the doctor and the team

Clinical and Laboratory Evaluation

Anamnesis covers clinical conditions, previous and current pathologies, current medications, allergies, previous surgeries, lifestyle habits (alcohol, tobacco, or drug use), the gynecological and obstetric history (especially miscarriages), physical activity, any family history of pathologies, and follow-up by other specialists. Routine laboratory, cardiology, and other tests are scheduled.

Anatomical Evaluation

The body mass index (BMI), biotype, and muscle and fat masses are evaluated, particularly fat accumulations that may be removed by surgery. Overweight (BMI >28 kg/m^2) and obese patients tend to have higher rates of complications and poor results and are at higher risk of dissatisfaction, particularly if any emotional feature in Table 27.1 is present. An abdominal wall examination identifies flaccidity, excess skin and fat, diastasis of the straight abdominal muscles, any hernias, the position of the navel, and scars. Ultrasound evaluation of the abdominal wall can identify hernias that contraindicate liposuction. The breasts are evaluated in terms of shape, volume, sagging, stretch marks, symmetry, and scars. Mammography and breast ultrasound evaluation are routine, and magnetic resonance imaging is scheduled for breasts with implants over 10 years of age if rupture is clinically suspected. The areolae are evaluated in terms of their position, diameter, symmetry, and scars.

The Doctor-Patient Relationship

A good doctor-patient relationship is based on mutual feelings and is of major medical and legal importance. Postoperative problems can be better solved if they are supported by a good relationship, which should be established before surgery.

Informed Consent Form

The patient acknowledges the receipt of detailed information on the surgery and the alternatives, limitations, and risks and confirms that she participated in decision-making. The physician and patient sign the form, and the medical record contains data on the planned surgery and its evolution through discussion.

Key Security Points

Each doctor creates a personal safety mechanism and uses this to decide whether or not to perform the three procedures in one session. Pitanguy, in 1983, emphasized the importance of the surgeon's knowledge, correct patient evaluation, anesthetist competence, training of assistants, and an adequate surgical structure (Pitanguy and Ceravolo 1983). Smoking, obesity, diabetes, and an American Society of Anesthesiologists (ASA) class >2 may contraindicate the combination of procedures (Winocour et al. 2015). Age seems to be associated with more complications; the cutoff ranges from 53 to 60 years (Khavanin et al. 2015). The risk of complications is greatly affected by the duration and extent of surgery. A surgical time over 3 h appears to increase the risks of infection, hematoma, seroma, dehiscence, and necrosis, with a time over 4.5 h increasing these risks threefold (Hardy et al. 2014). Finally, liposuction should be performed conservatively when combined with abdominoplasty and mammoplasty. When procedures performed alone and with liposuction were compared, the latter procedures were associated with more venous thrombosis, pulmonary complications, and infection (Kaoutzanis 2017). The American Society of Plastic Surgeons considers that liposuction of over 5 L performed alone may trigger complications, although no "safe" volume is defined. If liposuction is combined with another procedure, an appropriate limit may be 3 L, depending on the extent of the associated procedure(s). If it is necessary to aspirate more fat, liposuction should be performed separately (Klein 1993). Table 27.2 lists important safety considerations.

Intraoperative Considerations

The team aims to achieve the optimal result in the shortest possible time. Resections ensure that sutures bring tissues together without excessive tension. General anesthesia and local infiltration (tumescent in liposuction areas) are established (the Klein technique) (Klein 1993). The first intravenous antibiotic injection is given at the time of anesthesia, followed by more injections, depending on the indications

Table 27.2 Key safety points

1. Patient under 60 years of age, ASA class ≤2, BMI <28 kg/m^2
2. Competent anesthesiologist
3. Limited surgical duration and extent
4. Adequate surgical structure
5. Good routines for surgeon and staff

Table 27.3 Intraoperative care

Antibiotic prophylaxis
Maintenance of oxygenation, body temperature, hydration, and arterial tension
Intermittent compression of the lower limbs
Careful patient positioning

and drug. To avoid perioperative hypothermia, dehydration, and hypotension, the body area exposed should be minimized, a thermal blanket should be used, and appropriate volumes of warm liquids should be infused intravenously. Intermittent compression of the lower limbs during surgery (and to the time of hospital discharge) reduces the risk of venous thrombosis. Although the principal surgeon is ultimately responsible for safety and the outcomes, the presence of two or three assistant surgeons who work simultaneously in different locations (establishing hemostasis and placing sutures) would reduce the surgical time; this is very helpful. Once anesthesia is established, the patient is placed in a prone position to allow liposuction of the back, flanks, and hips. As all areas are accessed simultaneously, the correction is optimal, especially if asymmetry is in play. As the muscles are relaxed, the change to the decubitus position must be performed very carefully (with the help of several people) to avoid orthopedic lesions. A pyramidal mattress protects the support points and prevents pain, paresthesia, and postoperative skin lesions. Table 27.3 summarizes the main features of care during and immediately after surgery.

Surgical Sequence

Back, Flank, and Thigh Liposuction

The crisscross technique is employed for liposuction, facilitating flap uniformity. Also, the cannula cannot burn a portal or create a depression around a portal. A pneumatic vibrolipoaspirator, 3-mm portals, and cannulae with six holes are used.

Lipoabdominoplasty and Abdominoplasty Without Liposuction

The Avelar technique is employed for lipoabdominoplasty. Liposuction is associated with minimal flap detachment (a safety feature), and umbilicoplasty avoids retraction and external scarring (Fig. 27.1) (Avelar 1978). If aspiration is not planned, any necessary detachment is performed. Adhesion points are created in the

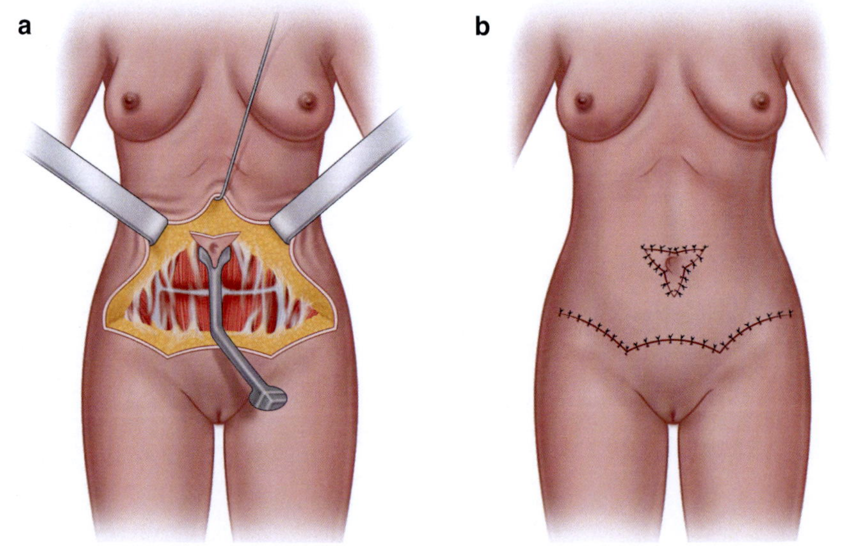

Fig. 27.1 The Avelar technique. (**a**) Liposuction is associated with minimal flap detachment. (**b**) Three-umbilical-flap technique, which results in a scar hidden inside the umbilicus

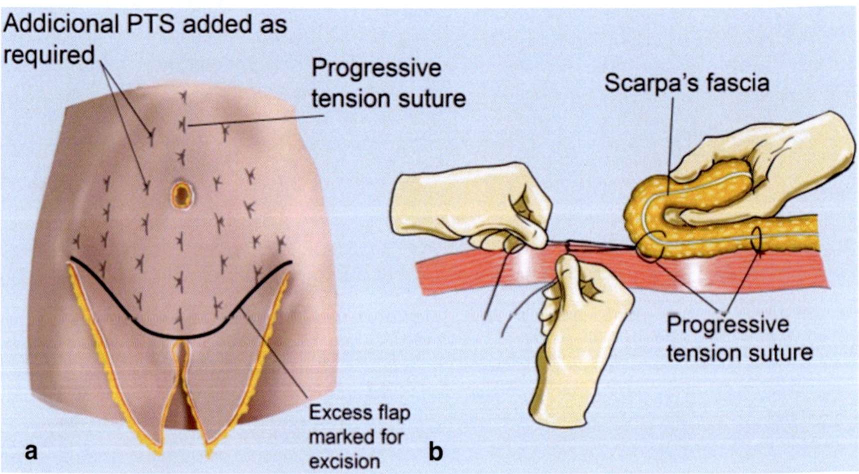

Fig. 27.2 Adhesion sutures in the abdominal wall. (**a**) Suture distribution in the abdominal wall. (**b**) The flap is pulled during suturing

detachment areas (the Baroudi technique); these facilitate flap migration and reduce the seroma incidence (Fig. 27.2) (Baroudi and Ferreira 1998).

In-block resections (Xavier et al. 2019) are very practical but must be carefully planned to avoid excessive resection. Usually, the flap surplus is estimated after traction and the creation of adhesion points. Before surgery (thus during planning), if low-level flaccidity affects the navel opening, the inferior incision is moved upward by 2 cm. Very low scars from previous surgeries are not treated. If the navel lies over 17 cm from the vulvar furcula, a small vertical scar can remain. The flap should not be tense.

Mammoplasty

Breast augmentation is performed via an inframammary incision, with implants generally placed in the retroglandular plane (sometimes the dual plane) but rarely in the retromuscular region. Preferred implants are round with a high profile and either coated with polyurethane or textured. Volumes above 300 mL are to be avoided. If asymmetry is evident, the maximum between-implant volume difference should be 50 mL. If this does not correct the asymmetry, tissue from the larger breast is resected. Mastopexies with augmentation are performed similarly, followed by adjustment of the gland and skin over the implant. If the target area is very flaccid, implants of volumes over 250 mL can be used in anticipation of the recurrence of ptosis. In mastopexies without augmentation, the breast consistency, shape, and position are corrected from the inside out; flaccid tissues are compacted by suturing without excessive tension. Whenever possible, the use of implants is avoided. Existing implants are removed via capsulotomy or capsulectomy and then replaced. Capsulotomies remove thin dystopic capsules and those exhibiting contracture up to Baker grade II. Capsulectomies are reserved for thick, calcified, or restricted capsules. Occasionally, we deploy Blake drains (bilateral or unilateral) and retain them until the daily drainage is less than 50 mL of clear liquid. When dealing with retromuscular capsules, the anterior leaflet is removed, and the posterior one is abandoned, because excision raises a risk of pneumothorax. The Pitanguy technique is used for reduction mammoplasties (Pitanguy 1967). If necessary, all three dimensions of the breast can undergo internal resection. Then, pillars are approximated and anchored to the thorax along the mid-breast line, remodeling and stabilizing the new breast. Internal flaps (Ribeiro et al. 2002) are sometimes required when assembling a new breast, but should not be under tension, because this raises a risk of steatonecrosis (especially in fatty breasts). The lower incisions of reduction mammoplasty and mastopexy are located near the inframammary fold and are sufficiently long to allow (optimal) skin finishes at the extremities. The areolar positions are defined after the breasts are set. A medially based areola flap is used (the Silveira-Neto technique (Silveira Neto 1976) when the areolae must migrate by up to 5 cm. In these cases, the flap can be thin or up to 2 cm thick and should rotate freely, thus without twisting or compression. The Robbins technique (Robbins 1987) is used to treat cases of grade III gigantomastia. The areolar flap features a 10-cm-thick inferior base when the areolae must migrate 10 cm or more. In breasts that have already undergone areolar mobilization, careful planning and execution are essential to ensure that areolar circulation is well maintained. After mastopexy and reduction mammoplasty, the skin should cover the surgical site adequately.

After abdominal procedures and mammoplasty, sutures are placed in several layers (separate stitches of Mononylon 4.0–5.0), and wound edges at the surface are approximated without tension (using a continuous suture of Monocryl 4.0). The umbilicus is closed using separate Mononylon 5.0 sutures.

Postoperative Considerations

Sutures are covered with two layers of gently applied microporous tape, and the patient is dressed in a soft compression girdle. Compression girdles are unnecessary and uncomfortable and increase the risk of venous thrombosis (Haidar and Nahas 2015). We recommend compulsory prophylactic analgesics for the first 3 days and then as needed. The patient should walk for 10 min every 2 h during the day for 10 days. The team remains in constant contact with the patient, and two check-ups weekly are performed for the first 2 weeks. Each patient is told to contact the team or to go to the hospital emergency room if she develops a fever (38 °C), pain, swelling other than what is expected, or dyspnea or chest pain.

Complications

A recent systematic review reported 5–14% risks of major complications such as death, hematoma, bowel loop perforation, deep vein thrombosis, pulmonary thromboembolism, myocardial infarction, necrosis of the abdominal flap greater than 5 cm, extrusion of the implant, necrosis, suture dehiscence, infection, and need for blood transfusion after the procedures described above (Michot et al. 2015). We agree that cardiac, pulmonary, and anesthesia-related risks must be considered, but the abovementioned risks are not statistically significant. Also, certain complications (such as the need for blood transfusion) are associated with the liposuction volume and not due to an association between lipoabdominoplasty and mammoplasty (Matarasso and Smith 2015). The most feared complication is deep vein thrombosis that precedes a fatal pulmonary thromboembolism (Keyes et al. 2018; Hatef et al. 2008) (Table 27.4).

Table 27.4 Measures preventing venous thrombosis

Evaluate any personal (e.g., abortion) or family history of venous thrombosis
Maintain body temperature, hydration, and blood pressure during surgery and perform intermittent lower limb compression
Limit the time and extent of surgery
Prescribe a soft compression shaper
Prescribe 40 mg/day of enoxaparin commencing at 12 h after the end of surgery for 10 days
Suspend hormones and oral contraceptives for 15 days prior to surgery
Encourage early ambulation for 10 min every 2 h during the day for 10 days

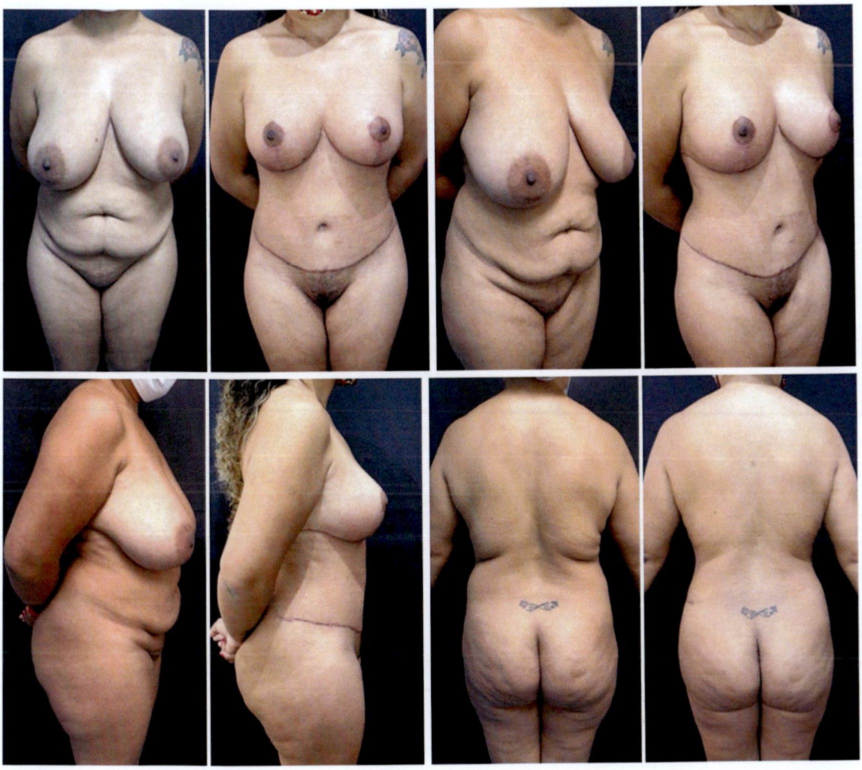

Fig. 27.3 A 38-year-old patient, with one previous pregnancy, BMI = 28 kg/m^2, and no comorbidity. Liposuction of the back, flanks, and abdomen, 2.5 L; lipoabdominoplasty, 1550 g; reduction mammoplasty, 1000 g. The results after 60 days

Results

We present the outcomes of two patients after the procedures described above (Figs. 27.3 and 27.4; Table 27.5).

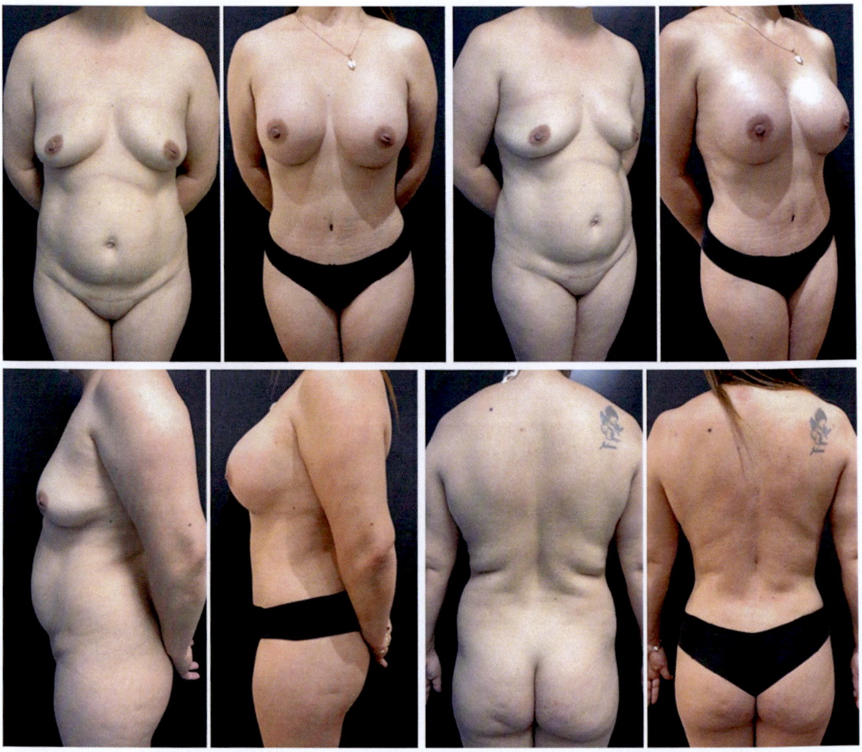

Fig. 27.4 A 35-year-old patient, with two previous pregnancies, BMI = 28 kg/m^2, no comorbidity, and a history of weight loss of 12 kg after dieting and physical activity. Liposuction of the back, flanks, and abdomen, 2.8 L; lipoabdominoplasty, 1900 g; augmentation mammoplasty with placement of textured implants 355 cc in volume (high profile). The results after 90 days

Table 27.5 Tips for optimizing safety and surgical results

1. Make careful diagnoses and review the indications
2. Select patients and know how to say "no"
3. Establish clear team routines
4. Operate in an appropriate surgical environment
5. Limit the extent of surgery
6. Be attentive to the patient postoperatively

References

International Society for Aesthetic Plastic Surgery. Statistics Report. 2019.

Rao YV (1969) Augmentation mammaplasty and abdominoplasty in one stage. Plast Reconstr Surg; 43(2):148—51.

Rohrich RJ, Broughton G, Horton B, et al (2004) The key to long-term success in liposuction: A guide for plastic surgeons and patients. Plast Reconstr Surg; 114:1945–1952

Kaye BL, Gradinger GP (1984) Symposium on Problems and Complications in Aesthetic Plastic Surgery of the Face. St. Louis, MO: CV Mosby

Pitanguy I, Ceravolo MP (1983) Our experience with combined-pro- cedures in aesthetic plastic surgery. Plast Reconstr Surg; 71(1):56—65

Winocour J, Gupta V, Ramirez JR et al (2015) Abdominoplasty: Risk Factors, Complication Rates, and Safety of Combined Procedures. Plast Reconstr Surg;136(5):597e 606e

Khavanin N, Jordan SW, Vieira BL et al (2015) Combining abdominal and cosmetic breast surgery does not increase short-term complication rates: a comparison of each individual procedure and pretreatment risk stratification tool. Aesthet Surg J; 35(8):999-1006

Hardy KL, Davis KE, Constantine RS (2014) The impact of operative time on complications after plastic surgery: a multivariate regression analysis of 1753 cases. Aesthet Surg J; 34(4):614-22

Kaoutzanis C (2017) Cosmetic Liposuction: Preoperative Risk Factors, Major Complication Rates, and Safety of Combined Procedures, *Aest Surg J; 37(6)680-694*

Klein J (1993) Tumescent technique for local anesthesia improves safety in large volume liposuction. Plast Reconstr Surg; 92(6):1085-100

Avelar JM (1978) Abdominoplasty: systematization of a technique without external umbilical scar. Aesthetic Plast Surg; 2:141-51

Baroudi R, Ferreira CA (1998) Seroma: how to avoid it and how to treat it. Aesth Surg J; 18(6):439-41

Xavier LB, et al (2019) Ronaldo Pontes's in Block Resection Abdominoplasty Technique. Int J Transplant & Plastic Surg; 3(2): 000135

Pitanguy I (1967) Surgical treatment of breast hypertrophy. Br J Plast Surg; 20:78-85

Ribeiro L, Accorsi A, Buss A et al (2002) Creation and evolution of 30 years of the inferior pedicle in reduction mammaplasties. Plast Reconstr Surg; 110(3):960-70.

Silveira Neto E (1976) Mastoplastia redutora setorial com pedículo areolar interno. In: Anais do XIII Congresso Brasileiro de Cirurgia Plástica e I Congresso Brasileiro de Cirurgia Estética

Robbins TH (1987) Reduction mammaplasty by the Robbins technique. Plast Reconstr Surg; 79(2):308-9

Haidar RB, Nahas FX (2015) Does the Use of Compression Garments Increase Venous Stasis in the Common Femoral Vein? Plastic and Reconstructive Surgery; 135(1)85-91

Michot A, Alet JM, Pélissier P et al (2015) Morbidity in combined-procedure associating abdominoplasty and breast surgery: A systematic review. Ann Chir Plast Esthet; S0294-1260(15)00131-4

Matarasso A, Smith DM (2015) Combined breast surgery and abdominoplasty: Strategies for success. Plast Reconstr Surg; 135:849e–860e

Keyes GR, Singer R, Iverson RE et al (2018) Incidence and predictors of venous thromboembolism in abdominoplasty. Aesthet Surg J; 38:162–173

Hatef DA, Kenkel JM, Nguyen MQ et al (2008) Thromboembolic risk assessment and the efficacy of enoxaparin prophylaxis in excisional body contouring surgery. *Plast Reconstr Surg;* 122:269–279

Chapter 28
Renuvion-Assisted Body Contouring Surgery

John Edwin Garcia Serna, Ricardo Cavalcanti Ribeiro, and Luis Fernandez de Córdova

Abstract Liposuction is one of the most frequently performed cosmetic surgery procedures worldwide (Markey, Clin Exp Dermatol 26:3–5, 2001), the second most commonly performed in the United States, and the most common procedure between the ages of 35 and 64 years (Wu et al., Cleve Clin J Med 87(6):367–375, 2020). Liposuction has rapidly evolved since the 1970s, when it was first described by Arpad and Giorgio Fischer, father and son, who developed the modern and popular technique of body contouring. It is currently widely used in clinical practice for many different aesthetic and reconstructive cases (Bellini et al., Ann Med Surg 24(August):53–60, 2017).

The aesthetics of the body is of great importance nowadays. Having a slim figure has become a primary goal for most people. Liposculpture cases have increased in recent years in an exorbitant way, in which bodies are subjected to transformations aiming to improve their appearance. Trying to have a slender figure is a notorious desire mostly for women, starting from an early age (García Cano, Tesis May:31–48, 2016).

Keywords Liposuction · Body contour · Power-assisted liposuction · Skin tightening

J. E. G. Serna
Plastic and Reconstructive Surgery, Clínica Corpus and Rostrum, Cali, Colombia

R. Cavalcanti Ribeiro (✉) · L. F. de Córdova
Plastic and Reconstructive Surgery, Federal University of the State of Rio de Janeiro, Rio de Janeiro, Brazil
e-mail: rribeiro@centroin.net.br

J. M. Avelar, R. Cavalcanti Ribeiro (eds.), *Body Contouring*,
https://doi.org/10.1007/978-3-031-42802-9_28

Liposculpture is an aesthetic surgical procedure that sculpts the body with the idea of giving it an attractive and stylized shape. It is one of the most frequently performed procedures worldwide (Markey 2001), the second most commonly performed in the United States, and the most common procedure between the ages of 35 and 64 years (Wu et al. 2020). It is important to emphasize that liposculpture is not a procedure for losing weight but for body contouring (Černauskis et al. 2020), eliminating localized fat deposits that do not respond to diet and exercise currently widely used in clinical practice for many different aesthetic and reconstructive cases (Bellini et al. 2017). After liposuction, the redundant skin, when present, will retract at some extent; when it does not readapt by itself to the new contour, surgical techniques with advanced energy technology such as *RENUVION* may be used.

RENUVION is the new treatment for maximum skin tightening based on the effect of ionized helium plasma, which allows heating of the tissues (heat on the tissue), applied in a minimally invasive procedure, combining the unique properties of cold helium plasma with radiofrequency energy deep into the tissue during application (Renuvion cosmetic tecnology 2018).

Most of the energy is delivered directly to the network of fibrous septa allowing a greater concentration of energy, a well-delimited area to be treated, and **up to 65% of** skin contraction, improving flaccidity in areas such as the abdomen, arms, back, thighs, face, and neck. **(It)** is an alternative for many people who do not want to undergo surgery due to undesirable scars. What makes this technology unique is that it can rapidly heat **(warm up)** subdermal tissues without leaving a burn injury. Helium plasma also **(has a long-term stimulation)** stimulates in the long term; during the following 6 to 9 months, the one session (will) keeps acting (settle) in the production of collagen and elastin, essential for tissue regeneration and skin tightening (Gentile 2018).

Preoperative Care

(The) Doctor-patient communication is of utmost importance. The **(patient's reasons/inquiries)** WHY of the patient must be understood thoroughly as well as the expectations linked to the procedure. We, as plastic surgeons, should make sure that only realistic expectations and attainable results are brought to **(into)** the conversation and try to understand the unique concept of beauty of each patient (Tabbal et al. 2013).

The overall health status of the patient is evaluated by four specialists (psychologist, anesthesiologist, internist, and plastic surgeon) through a complete medical history and a battery **(various)** of tests such as CBC, coagulation tests, pregnancy test, blood sugar, HIV, urinalysis, EKG, and BMI, among others.

Routine preoperative recommendations in our practice include the following:

- No medications before surgery : stop taking anti-inflammatories and anticoagulants from 1 to 7 days prior to surgery unless otherwise instructed, oral contraceptive pills or hormone replacement therapy should be suspended 2 months prior to surgery.

- No smoking, no drinking alcohol at least one month before the suregry.
- Full iquid diet for 2 days before the procedure.
- 12 H preop Fasting.

Surgical Technique

Markings must be done in front of a mirror, which allows **(allowing)** the patient to be an active participant in the process, and **(keeping a)** proper standing position **(posture)** and lateral decubitus (Figs. 28.1, 28.2, and 28.3).

The patient is transferred (**taken**) to the surgical area to take (**their**) vital signs, and venipuncture is performed to start prophylactic antibiotic therapy. The skin is surgically washed with iodinated solution with (**while**) the patient (**is**) in a standing position (**on their feet**).

The patient is placed on the operating (**surgical**) table in a sitting position under sedation, and the anesthesiologist proceeds to place the epidural anesthesia. Afterward, with the patient in supine position, we place intermittent pneumatic

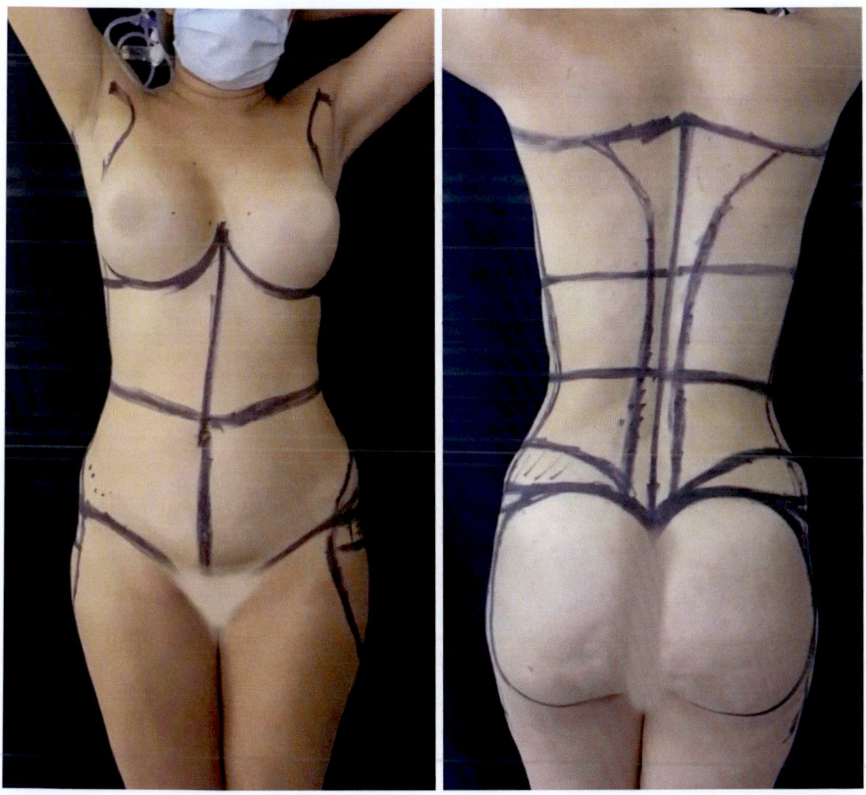

Fig. 28.1 Markings for surgery

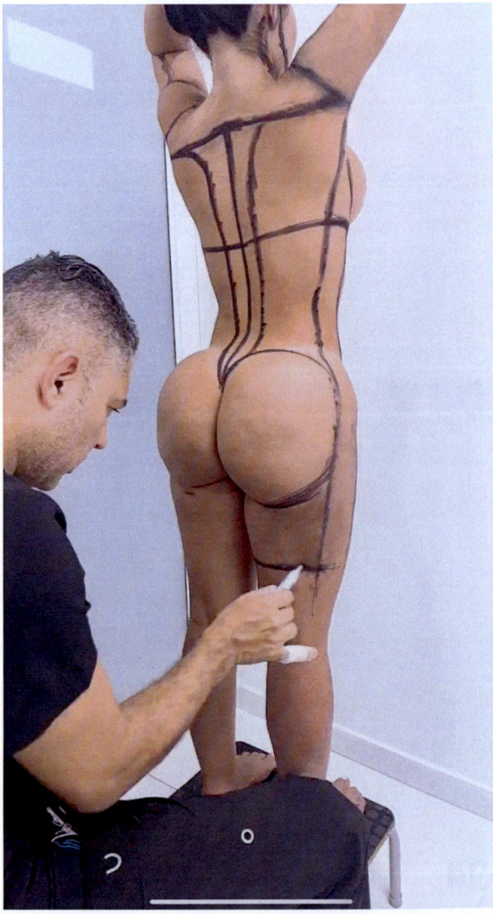

Fig. 28.2 Surgical marking in standing position

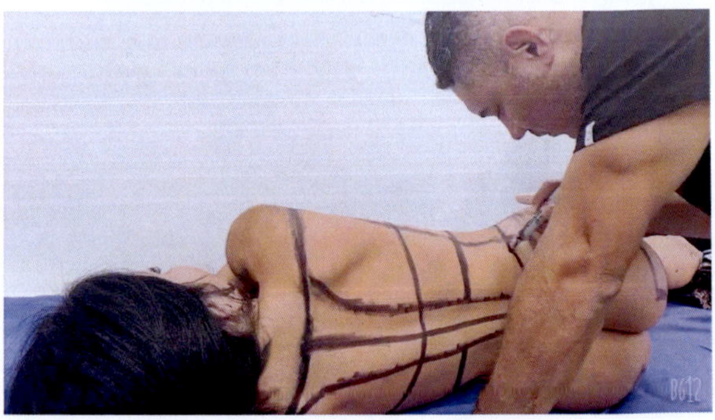

Fig. 28.3 Surgical marking in lateral decubitus

compression on the lower limbs and thermal insulation, urine output should be controlled with a Foley catheter introduced with aseptic technique, and sterile surgical fields are placed.

(The) Infiltration of tumescent solution through 0.04 cm incisions in the area of underwear **(on the underwear outline)** and skin grooves begins; with 1000 cc of SSN at 0.9% plus 1 cc of epinephrine, starting in the anterior region of the abdomen, thighs, and arms, we proceed to fix the skin protectors with silk sc24 and allow 15 min to pass for vasoconstriction to occur.

Liposuction of the infiltrated areas is carried out with ultrasound-assisted technology *(UAL) SONOCA*, a useful tool for the treatment of lipodystrophy, which can be beneficial in secondary cases due to its ability to break adhesions between the fascia and the dermis, which, in turn, reduces blood aspiration, emulsifies the tissue, and reduces considerably surgical time. It acts at a frequency of 2–3 MHz with the impulses that vary in terms of repetitions per second depending on the instrument; we use an intensity of 60 MHz and treat each quadrant for 30 s to maximum 1 min (**maximum**).

Next, power-assisted liposuction (PAL) of the emulsified tissue is performed. The most important parameter to consider is the cannula diameter. The most commonly used are 4 mm cannulas, and among them are the flat cannula, the Mercedes cannula, and the Vásquez cannula, which allow an easier passage through fat tissue layers and greater control for the surgeon to sculpt with precision small or large body areas (**with precision**) leaving no skin irregularities.

After traditional liposuction is performed, giving (**creating**) the desired contour to the body, the degree of flaccidity of the tissues in the treated areas is identified, followed by skin tightening with *RENUVION* helium plasma technology. The application protocol is respected: frequency, planes, vectors, and application time with an intensity of 80/20 for 15–20 min/quadrant. This advanced energy-based technology combines the unique properties of cold helium plasma with radiofrequency energy (Fig. 28.4). Its application must be by planes and vectors so that the energy is directed mainly to the tissue structures and the dermis (Fig. 28.5). Its distribution must be uniform. The helium plasma temperature should be maintained at 65 °C, for prolonged periods to maximize efficacy. At a temperature of 85 °C, the treatment time can be reduced. The higher the temperature, the lesser the time of helium plasma application. The frequency and duration is **(are)** a **(the)** surgeon's choice.

Positioning of the patient in lateral decubitus for 0.4 cm incisions to be made in (**the underwear outline area**) areas of underwear and skin grooves before repeating the process occurs. We systematically perform the Renuvion-Assisted Body Contouring Surgery in the following sequence: Infiltration, liposuction, and skin tightening covering the areas of the back, waist, arms, and thighs in the right side and then on the left side.

Once liposuction is over, we proceed (**with the lipo-injection**) to fat transfer to the gluteal region.

First, we position the patient in a prone position, and 0.4 cm incisions are made in (**the underwear outline area**) areas of underwear and skin folds in the gluteal region, one incision in the intergluteal region and two on each side of the gluteal region.

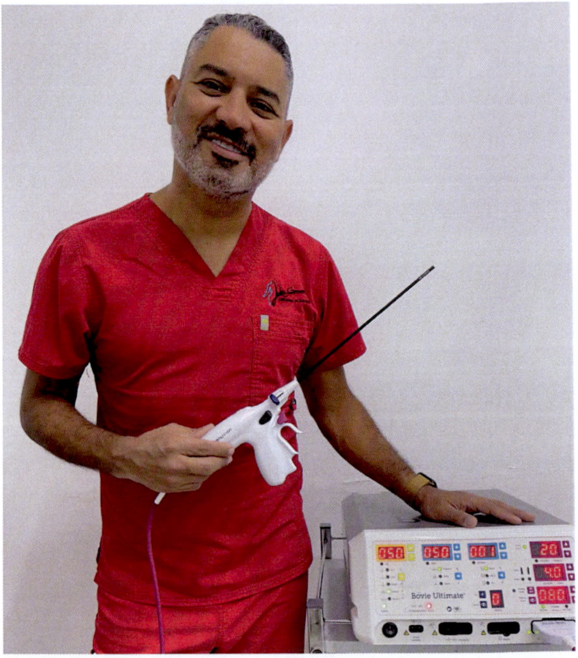

Fig. 28.4 Renuvion helium plasma technology

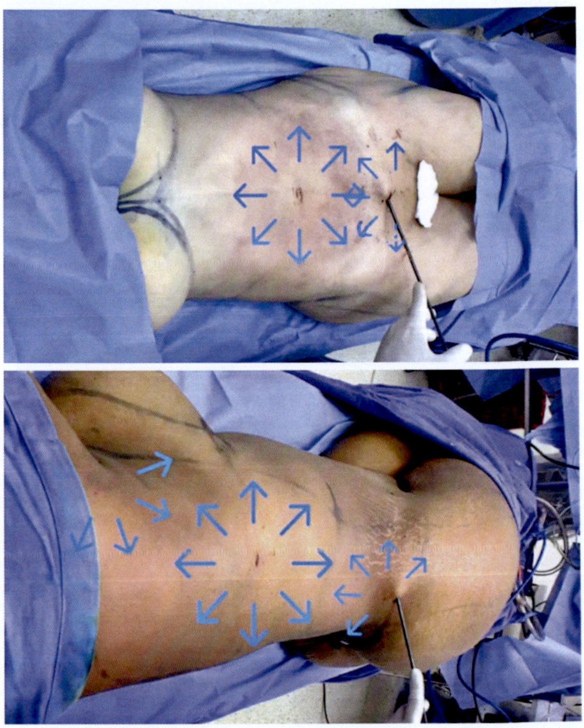

Fig. 28.5 Renuvion application by planes and vectors

1. Tumescent infiltration of the gluteal region.
2. UAL is performed at a frequency of 60 Hz for 30–45 s per gluteal quadrant.
3. Renuvion technology is applied for 7–10 min per gluteal region.

   (a) Renuvion application technique:

   Application planes
   Application vectors
   Application frequency
   Application time

4. Renuvion technology is applied for repolarization of the gluteal area (Fig. 28.6).
5. Fat graft is prepared (gentamicin 160 mg + clindamycin 600 mg is added to the previously decanted fat). Fat injection of the gluteal graft is performed at the level of **(over/on)** the subcutaneous cellular tissue. The volume will be defined according to the agreement made during the consultation with the surgeon.

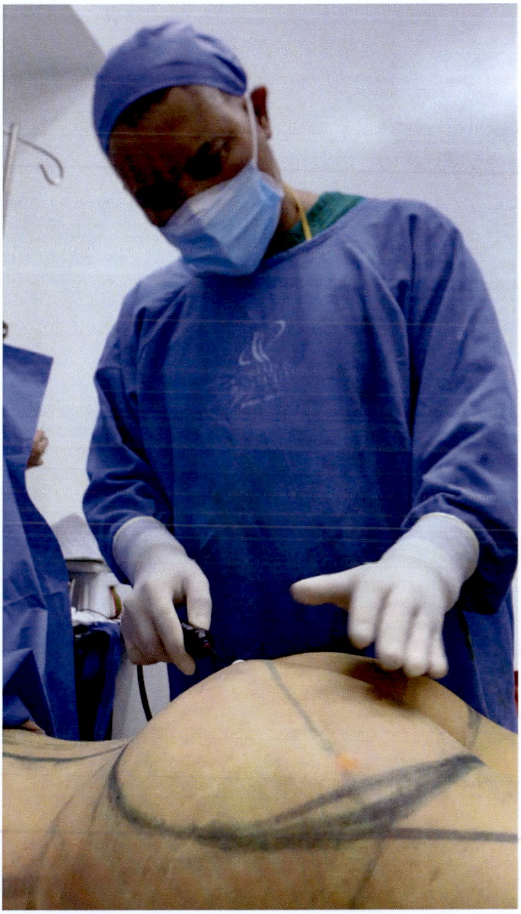

Fig. 28.6 Renuvion technology is applied for repolarization of the gluteal area

After occlusive dressing, the patient goes to a recovery room and will stay in the hospital for (one) a night.

Postoperative Care

Antibiotics, painkillers, and anti-inflammatories are prescribed. A cotton garment will be placed under the surgeon's orientation **(command/instructions)**, usually after the first follow-up **(appointment)**. Drainages and massages may begin the day after the surgery and must be performed by the recommended professional. We recommend to start the use of a rigid dressing/garment after the first postoperative week, and to change positions every 15 minutes; showering is allowed after 24 hours postop; restrict caloric intake is oriented and specific foods such as dairy, pork, seafood, and spicy foods; and drink plenty of fluids. Explain to the patient that red fluid output is normal and it may even moisten the garment. Orthostatic hypotension may occur, accompanied by symptoms such as blurred vision, paleness, dizziness, cold sweats, and palpitations that may resolve by lying down and raising the legs, and early ambulation should be stimulated and warning signs such as fever, abdominal pain, bleeding, vomiting, and excessive or difficult breathing **(must be)** reported to the surgeon.

Complications

Contour irregularities, seroma, hyperpigmentation, asymmetries, scar hypertrophy, skin necrosis, skin infection, post-surgical anemia.

Pros and Pearls

- UAL: decrease in blood loss, greater postoperative (**post-surgical**) skin retraction, and shorter recovery time.
- Correct diameter and cannula style: reduces bleeding due to less subcutaneous trauma.
- The use of helium plasma technology tightens the skin to the mold sculpted by the professional.
- Retraction of the skin in all vectors: minimizes and avoids unwanted scars.

- Decrease in the need of excision of excess of the skin (**skin excess**), obtaining doctor/patient satisfaction (**satisfactory**) results.
- Better aesthetic results with shorter surgical time, less surgical risk, decreased patient recovery time, and limited unwanted scarring.
- The use of vitamins, minerals, and supplements should be discontinued, and all non-essential agents before surgery can reduce the risk of a complication related to bleeding (Broughton 2nd et al. 2007).
- Informed consent requires that the patient (**must**) be informed of treatment risks, prognosis, and alternative treatments before consenting to treatment.
- Infiltration of several liters of wetting (**moisturizing**) solution.
- Always make two incisions in the skin, one for the entrance of the piece of helium plasma and another for the exit due to physical effect.
- Describe the use of the application of an assisted technology, and it does not depend on (**the**) results, but it depends on (**but the**) means, with a possible surgical time with a reduced scar.
- (Less than 10% chance of) Possible appearance of pneumothorax less than 10%, and its treatment is respiratory therapy and early ambulation.

This technique is reproducible with successful results.

Contraindications

Smoking is an important risk factor for wound healing complications.

Not leaving the patient hospitalized increases the risk of postoperative (**post-surgical**) complications.

Admitting patients who wish to undergo cosmetic surgery without meeting all the medical and psychological prerequisites (**pre-requirements**) can generate risks to the patient's health due to lack of information.

Comparative Photos Before and After (Figs. 28.7, 28.8, 28.9, 28.10, 28.11, and 28.12)

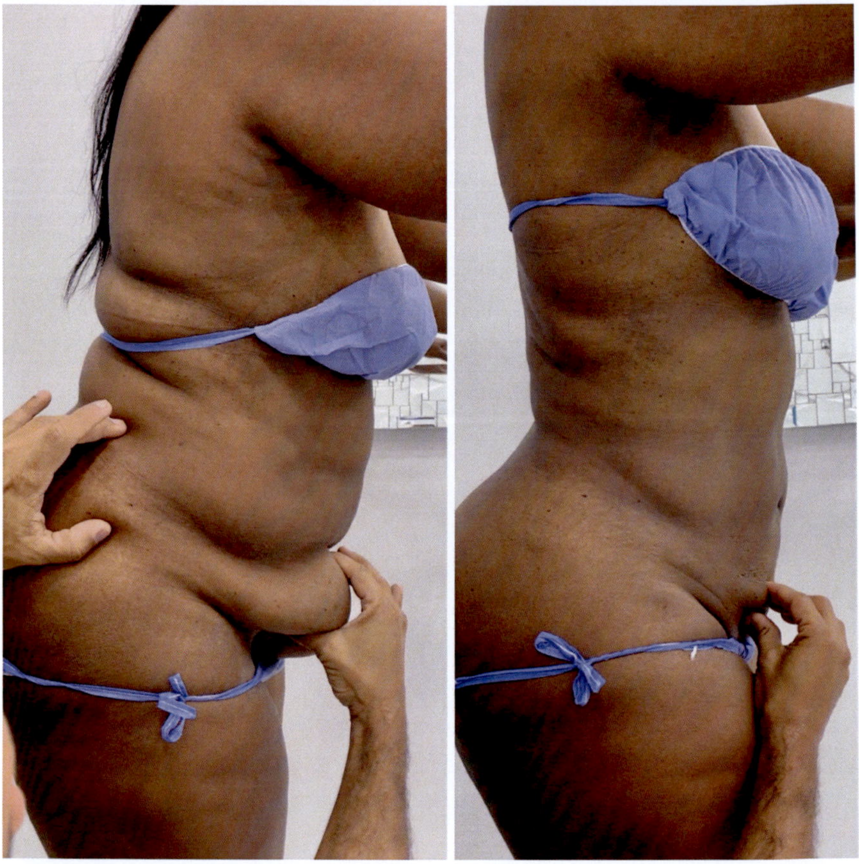

Fig. 28.7 Liposuction of the abdomen and retraction of the skin with Renuvion, pre-surgical and post-surgical 6 months

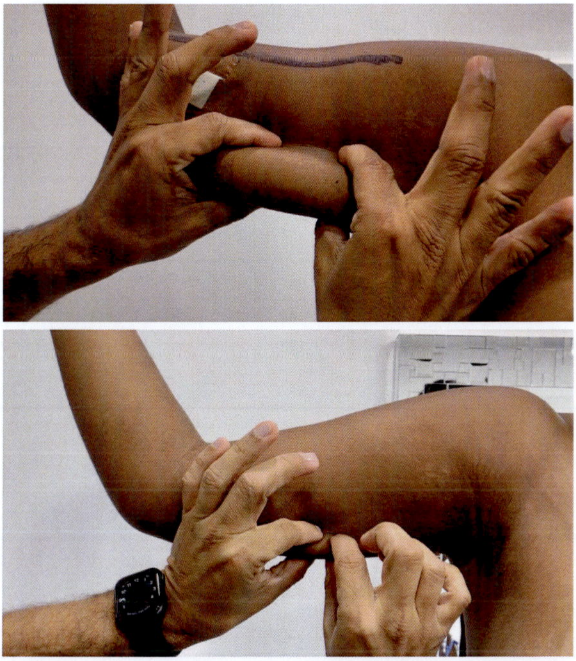

Fig. 28.8 Liposuction of the arms and retraction of the skin with Renuvion, pre-surgical and post-surgical 6 months

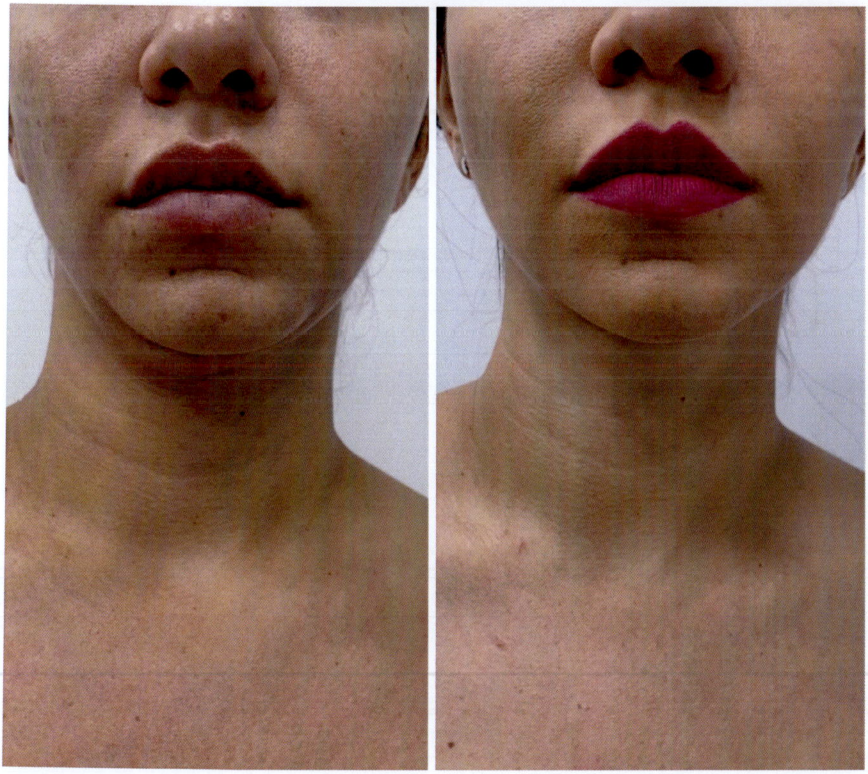

Fig. 28.9 Liposuction of the neck and retraction of the skin with Renuvion, pre-surgical and post-surgical 6 months

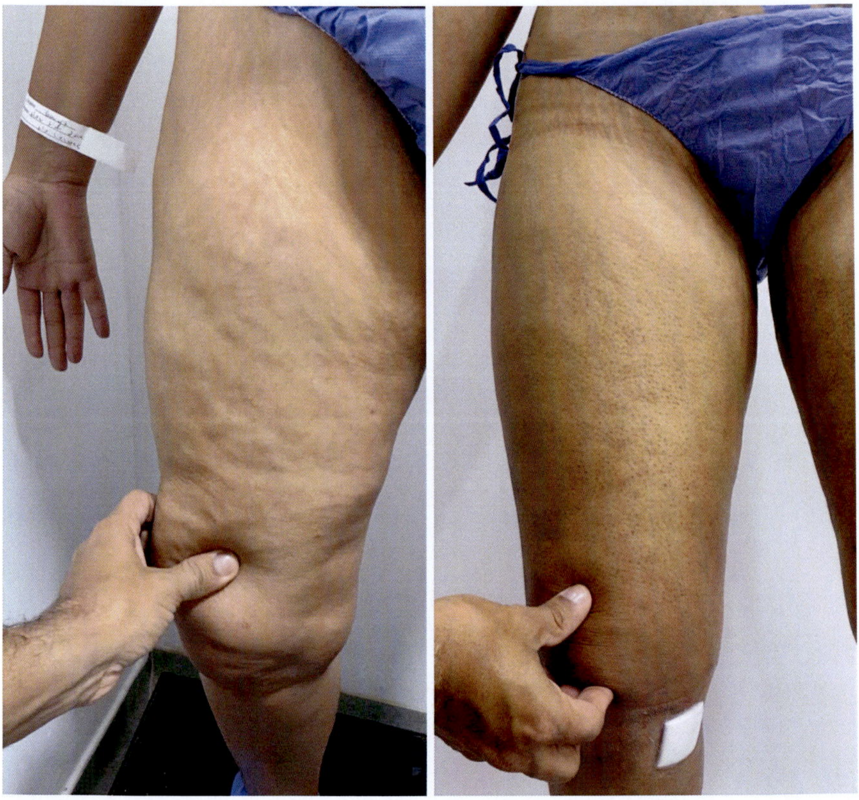

Fig. 28.10 Liposuction of the thighs and retraction of the skin with Renuvion, pre-surgical and post-surgical 6 months

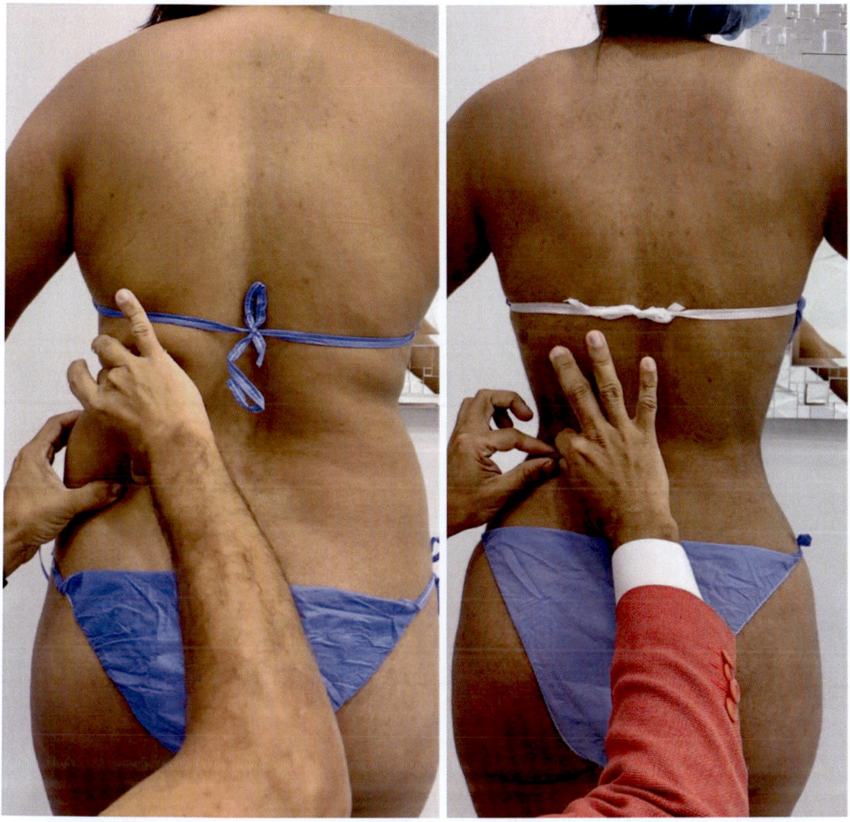

Fig. 28.11 Liposuction of the back and retraction of the skin with Renuvion, pre-surgical and post-surgical 6 months

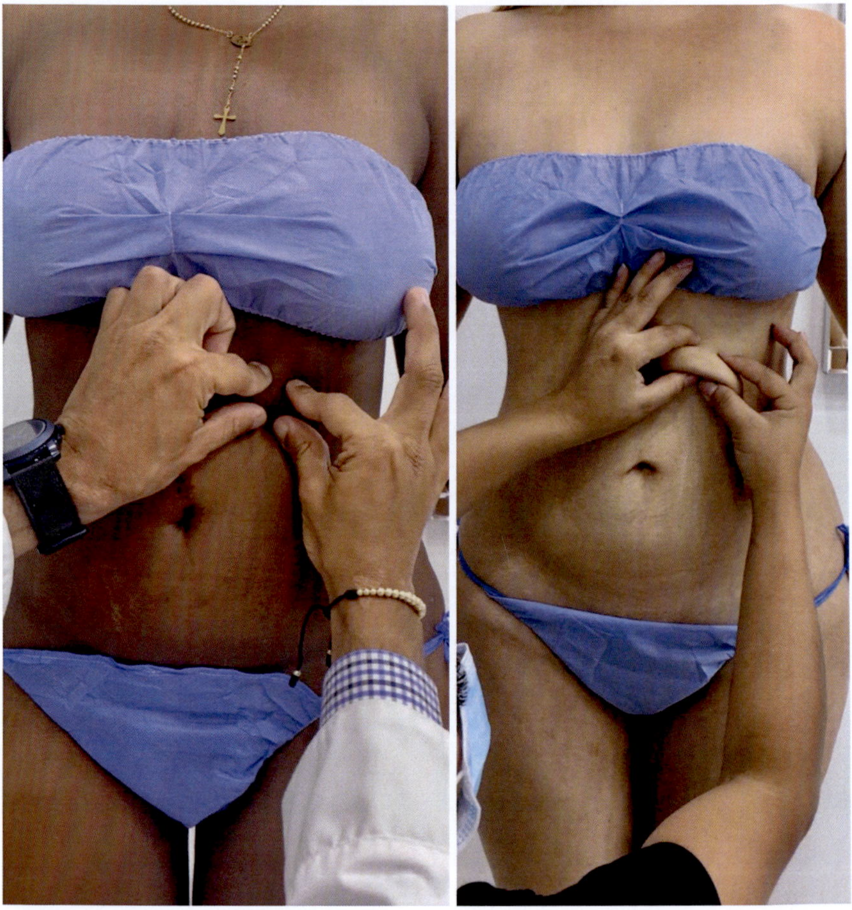

Fig. 28.12 Liposuction of the abdomen and retraction of the skin with Renuvion, post-surgical 6 months

References

A. C. Markey, St. John's Institute of Dermatology, St. Thomas' Hospital, London U. Liposuction in cosmetic dermatology. Vol. 26, Clinical and Experimental Dermatology. 2001. p. 3–5.

Wu S, Coombs DM, Gurunian R. Liposuction: Concepts, safety, and techniques in body-contouring surgery. Cleve Clin J Med. 2020 Jun;87(6):367–75.

Bellini E, Grieco MP, Raposio E. A journey through liposuction and liposculture: Review. Ann Med Surg. 2017;24(August):53–60.

Garcia cano Margarita. Subjetividades femeninas en las cirugias estéticas de la ciudad de cali. Tesis [Internet]. 2016;(May):31–48. Available from: http://bibliotecadigital.univalle.edu.co/bitstream/10893/9313/1/0534169-P-S-2016-1.pdf

Černauskis K, Kružyk S, Šukytė G, Venclauskas L, Sakalauskas M. Saugi liposukcija: klinikinis atvejis ir literatūros apžvalga. 2020;19:145–50.

Renuvion cosmetic tecnology. Renuvion cosmetic tecnology. 2018. p. 1–28.

Gentile RD. Plasma atmosférico frío (J-Plasma) y nuevas opciones para el contorno facial y el rejuvenecimiento de la piel del Rostro y cuello pesados. 2018;1(212):66–74.

Tabbal GN, Ahmad J, Lista F, Rohrich RJ. Advances in liposuction: Five key principles with emphasis on patient safety and outcomes. Plast Reconstr Surg. 2013;1(8):1–9.

Broughton G 2nd, Crosby MA, Coleman J, Rohrich RJ. Use of herbal supplements and vitamins in plastic surgery: a practical review. Plast Reconstr Surg. 2007 Mar;119(3):48e-66e.

Part IV
Importance of Liposuction Improving Body Contouring

Chapter 29
Critical Analysis and the Future of Liposuction for Body Contouring

Luiz S. Toledo

Abstract The date of 28 November 1980 is an especially important landmark for Brazilian plastic surgeons. It was then, in a small side room of a hotel in the city of Fortaleza, in the northeast of Brazil, that a French surgeon showed a technique with a 16 mm black-and-white film. The patient was an African woman with very large thighs. More than 40 years has passed since that first presentation. Liposuction underwent many changes. Many were only a change of name by the machine manufacturers for their marketing purposes. Some of the modifications were good and improved the technique, some were bad, and others were catastrophic. Soon we would see many doctors without plastic surgery training performing the technique, believing liposuction to be an easy procedure. It is not. It may be simple in theory, but it is not an easy surgery.

Introduction

The date of 28 November 1980 is an especially important landmark for Brazilian plastic surgeons. It was then, in a small side room of a hotel in the city of Fortaleza, in the northeast of Brazil, that a French surgeon showed a technique with a 16 mm black-and-white film. The patient was an African woman with very large thighs.

About 6 months before, I had helped my professor, Dr. William Callia, in São Paulo perform surgery to treat a similar problem, lipodystrophy, on a 16-year-old girl. The girl had a beautiful figure, but her thighs were thick and out of proportion to the rest of her body. She couldn't buy clothes that fit. Dr. Callia proposed a radical surgery, a dermolipectomy, making a vertical incision on the outside of the thighs,

L. S. Toledo (✉)
Dubai, United Arab Emirates

Lisbon, Portugal

J. M. Avelar, R. Cavalcanti Ribeiro (eds.), *Body Contouring*, https://doi.org/10.1007/978-3-031-42802-9_29

from the hips to the knees. He removed a fuse of fat about 50 cm long by 15 cm wide at the widest part, weighing more than 1 kg on each side. The scar, despite having been sutured with very fine threads and being practically invisible, remained forever. The result was good, and the girl was satisfied, as there was no other solution. But I already knew that I would never perform this technique.

When the French surgeon's film started, we were about 50 attendees in a small side room, while the other 500 were in the main room, watching other presentations of the Brazilian Congress of Plastic Surgery. It was a magical moment, in which all the plastic surgeons present were able to see for the first time Dr. Yves-Gèrard Illouz demonstrate a technique that would later become known as liposuction. When we watched fat being aspirated from the patient's thighs through a 1 cm incision, passing through a clear plastic tube, and being deposited in a glass vial, the audience could not believe what they were seeing. Here was the solution to a series of previously insoluble problems. Illouz was widely applauded and became the congress sensation, having to explain his technique several times. I felt I was witnessing a change in all fields of plastic surgery, which after that day splits into before and after liposuction.

More than 40 years has passed since that first presentation. Liposuction underwent many changes. Many were only a change of name by the machine manufacturers for their marketing purposes. Some of the modifications were good and improved the technique, some were bad, and others were catastrophic. Soon we would see many doctors without plastic surgery training performing the technique, believing liposuction to be an easy procedure. It is not. It may be simple in theory, but it is not an easy surgery. And I heard Illouz many times say in his heavy French-accented English "It is not easy to make simple!"

History

The first closed lipectomy was shown by Joseph Schrudde (Schrudde 1972), a German plastic surgeon in 1972 at the first ISAPS Congress in Rio de Janeiro. He used a curette to remove fat through a small incision. The technique caused many problems, such as delayed healing, seromas, and hematomas, and was abandoned. In Italy, in 1977 (Fischer and Fischer 1977), Arpad and Giorgio Fischer, father and son, devised what they called the planatome, a suction cannula with an internal cutting mechanism inside, connected to an aspirator. In 1975, Raymond Vilain (Vilain 1975) in France started using a curette to remove fat from the medial knee through a small incision. The next technique for the removal of excessive local deposits and subcutaneous fat using the curette was in 1978, by Ulrich "Uri" Kesselring and Rudolph "Rudy" Meyer from Switzerland (Kesselring and Meyer 1978). Bahman "Buck" Teimourian was the first American to use suction curettage in 1981 to remove excess fat for body contouring (Temourian and Fisher 1981). All these early attempts were unsuccessful, and it was only when Illouz developed the aspiration of fat with a blunt cannula that the technique became reproducible. Illouz's first publication was in 1980 in a French journal (Illouz 1980a).

Liposuction

I had witnessed something very important that would change many techniques. Realizing the impact of Illouz's discovery, I quickly bought the aspirator and cannulas, becoming one of the pioneers in the use of this technique in Brazil. At this time, I started working on the board of the Brazilian Society of Plastic Surgery, whose dynamic young president, Juarez Avelar, decided to organize symposia with live surgery, with Illouz (Illouz 1983a) and another pioneering French surgeon, Pierre Fournier (Fournier and Illouz 1984). In addition to helping organize the events, I took the opportunity to learn and discuss the details of the surgery with them both. But France would have even more surprises, with the fat grafting technique. In 1986, Juarez Avelar published together with Illouz the first Brazilian textbook on liposuction, emphasizing the pinch test to avoid abdominal perforation (Avelar 1986).

Illouz presented his technique for the first time in the United States at the end of 1982, at the ASPS Congress in Hawaii. The Americans were so impressed that they formed a "Blue Ribbon" Committee, with Simon Fredericks as president, to go to Paris, watch Illouz operate, and investigate the validity of the technique. Many members of this committee immediately bought the equipment in Paris and became advocates of the technique when they returned to the United States. A new society was formed by Gregory Hetter to teach liposuction to the American surgeons, the LSNA, the Lipoplasty Society of North America.

Nomenclature

Lipoplasty is the generic term for surgical correction of lipodystrophy. There are two types of lipoplasty: *Liposuction* is the surgical procedure in which fat excess is aspirated manually or mechanically with aesthetic purposes. *Liposculpture* is the aesthetic procedure to improve the facial and body contour through aspiration and injection of fat obtained from the same individual.

Anesthesia

Illouz in the early 1980s used local infiltration, a hypotonic solution alone or combined with epidural or general anesthesia (Illouz 1980b). In 1983, Fournier introduced the dry technique for lipoplasty, aspiration without any infiltration, under epidural or general anesthesia. The dry technique had no fluids injected into the tissues and resulted in 20–45% blood loss (Drake et al. 1991). Hetter was the first to add epinephrine to the Illouz formula in 1984 to decrease bleeding (Hetter 1984).

In January 1998, the ASAPS Lipoplasty Task Force showed the main factors that increase risk in lipoplasty. There was no mention of the potential problems caused by hypothermia, so we published a review of the effects of hypothermia during liposuction (Toledo et al. 2001). Hypothermia is responsible for a series of harmful effects to the patient, trembling and shivering, provoking an excessive consumption of oxygen, hypoxemia and intense discomfort, and significant alterations of hemostasis.

In 1984, Fournier had started using external cryoanesthesia (Fournier 1984), by placing ice bags on the skin surface, combined with sedation. In 1991, Fournier used internal cryoanesthesia (Fournier 1991), injecting the tumescent fluid at 4 °C. The use of a 4 °C solution aggravates the hypothermia normally associated with this procedure. Possible complications can be arrhythmia, heart attack and hypertension, prolongation of the effect of several anesthetic drugs, trembling and shivering, excessive consumption of oxygen, hypoxemia and intense discomfort, acidosis and hydro-electrolytic alterations, and alteration of coagulation. There is also evidence that intra-operative hypothermia is associated with the higher incidence of infection of the surgical wound. When we increased the temperature of infiltrated fluid to body temperature, we noticed an improvement in the safety of the procedure and a better postoperative recovery. Just by using a combination of tumescent technique with adrenaline at 37 °C, there is practically no bleeding. There is no need for hypothermia.

In 1987, Klein introduced the tumescent anesthesia (Klein 1987), with small doses of lidocaine, adrenaline, and saline. The tumescent technique produced a dramatic reduction in blood loss due to vasoconstriction of the area to be treated. In 1992, I felt the Klein formula was not strong enough to ensure a painless procedure, so I doubled the lidocaine. Since I injected most of the fat I aspirated, I changed saline to Ringer's lactate to better preserve the fat cells. I changed the formula to Ringer's lactate 500 ml, lidocaine 2% 20 ml, adrenaline 1:1000 1 ml, and sodium bicarbonate 3% 5 ml, injected at body temperature, in the proportion 1:1 (Toledo 1992a), i.e., 1 cc of fluid injected per 1 cc of aspirated fat, to avoid pulmonary edema and lidocaine overdoses. The tumescent state is reached when palpation shows a typical tension of the injected area. The injection at body temperature, circa 37 °C, avoids hypothermia and postoperative shivering. All measures that maintain physiologic temperature should be encouraged: the use of intravenous solutions warmed at 37 °C, the use of local infiltration fluids warmed at 37 °C, maintenance of the operating room temperature at acceptable levels, and the use of skin surface air warming systems intra-operatively and immediate postoperatively (Hohn et al. 1998). In 2001, we published our study on the effect of hypothermia on coagulation and its implications for infiltration in lipoplasty.

I always worked with an anesthesiologist present who would administer either sedation or general anesthesia, combined with the tumescence (Toledo 1990a). The patient is monitored, and the anesthesiologist starts the sedation with midazolam

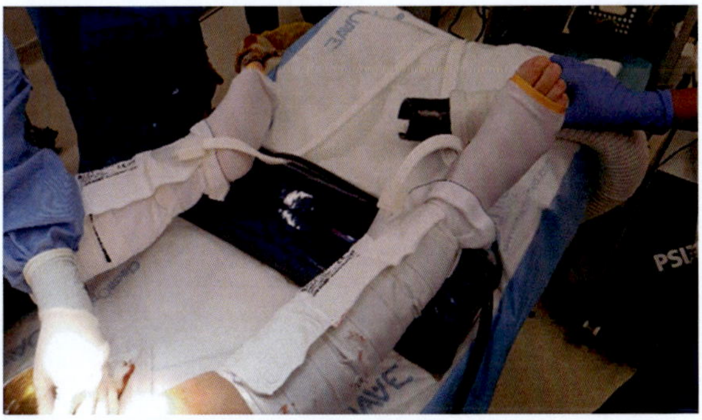

Fig. 29.1 DVT prevention with sequential compression boots and stockings

and fentanyl. Midazolam is used in the initial doses of 0.1 mg/kg IV up to a total dose of 0.3 mg/kg, according to the surgical procedure. Fentanyl is used at 50 μg/kg, slowly. Although the respiratory depression is very low with midazolam, it is necessary to have all the conditions to ventilate the patient, especially when fentanyl is utilized. Midazolam's action is antagonized with Lanexate (flumazenil) in variable doses from 0.2 to 1.0 mg IV. Propofol is used in sub-doses of 15–30 mcg/kg/min.

The advent of the tumescent technique increased the safety in lipoplasty, not only due to the decrease of peak plasma lidocaine concentrations and, consequently, drug toxicity but also to the reduction of blood loss. Studies show that for each 1000 ml of fat removed, 9.7 ml of whole blood was suctioned (Klein 1993). The tumescent technique is an exceptionally safe method of liposuction, which eliminates the necessity of blood transfusions. It is safer than liposuction under only general anesthesia, or epidural alone, and results in fewer complications (Hanke et al. 1995). To avoid the risk of DVT, we use sequential compression massaging boots intra-operatively (Fig. 29.1). Drug prevention of DVT is done with Fraxiparine (7500 UI/day) or Clexane (enoxaparin) (20–40 mg/day).

Instruments

Many companies produce aspirators today. Byron was one of the first companies in the United States and Richter in Brazil. Illouz's first cannulas were 1 cm gauge (Fig. 29.2), very thick for any refined work. We soon had cannulas of various lengths and gauges, according to the areas to be treated. The cannula tips, which initially were blunt, with one lateral hole started being modified. Grazer designed what he called the Mercedes tip, with three holes, and Hilton Becker designed a modification of the Mercedes, with a small "cage" at the tip, to aspirate fibrous tissue (Fig. 29.3). In 1988, I realized we needed an instrument to break the retinacula cutis and improve cellulite, release scars, and break fibrous adherences from previous liposuction. I designed the V-tip cannula, which became known as the Toledo cannula (Toledo 1992b). It was produced by many companies, in various lengths and gauges, depending on the area to be used (Fig. 29.4).

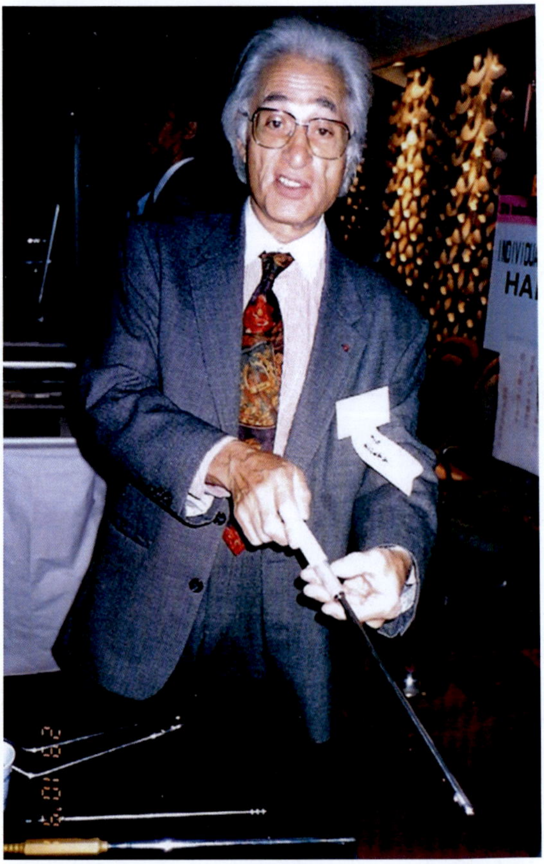

Fig. 29.2 Yves-Gèrard Illouz with one of the first liposuction 10 mm gauge cannulas

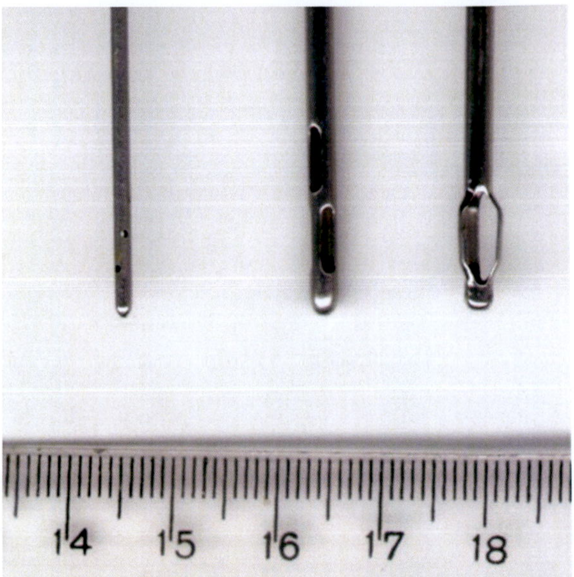

Fig. 29.3 Cannulas were modified. (Left) An anesthesia infiltration 3 mm gauge with multiple holes. (Center) A "pyramid tip" cannula with three holes. (Right) The Hilton Becker "basket" cannula to aspirate difficult fibrotic areas

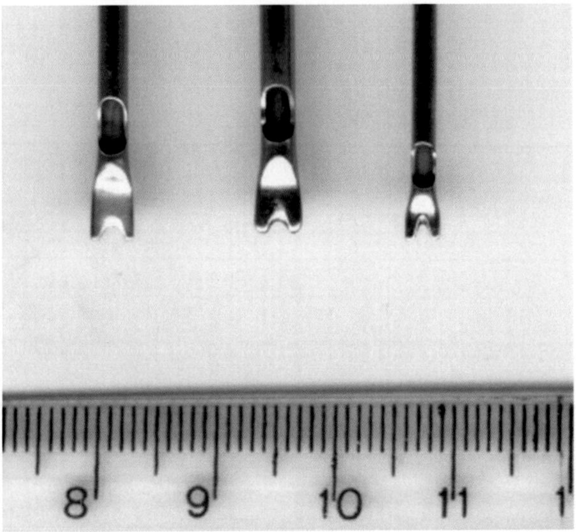

Fig. 29.4 The Toledo V-tip cannula to treat "cellulite" and scars and liposuction sequelae. The tips of the V are blunt, and the inside is cutting

Although working with the syringe was a simple and cheap method, many surgeons decided to continue using the aspirator. This posed a problem when aspirated fat had to be reinjected. It was easy with the syringe. You could just decant it for 10 min or centrifuge for 1 min at 1500 rpm. Together with Alberto Hodara, a plastic surgeon from Porto Alegre in Brazil, we designed a simple manual centrifuge to use with different size syringes, up to 60 ml (Fig. 29.5). I showed this simple device in my teaching courses, but soon it was forbidden to be used in the United States, because safety measures needed it to be totally covered. Today, I see many variations of that machine produced by many different international companies. But if you were using an aspirator to obtain fat, the only way to avoid fat contamination was to attach a sterile second vial to collect fat for reinjection. So, the industry kept producing new devices to aspirate, collect, decant, centrifuge, and inject fat.

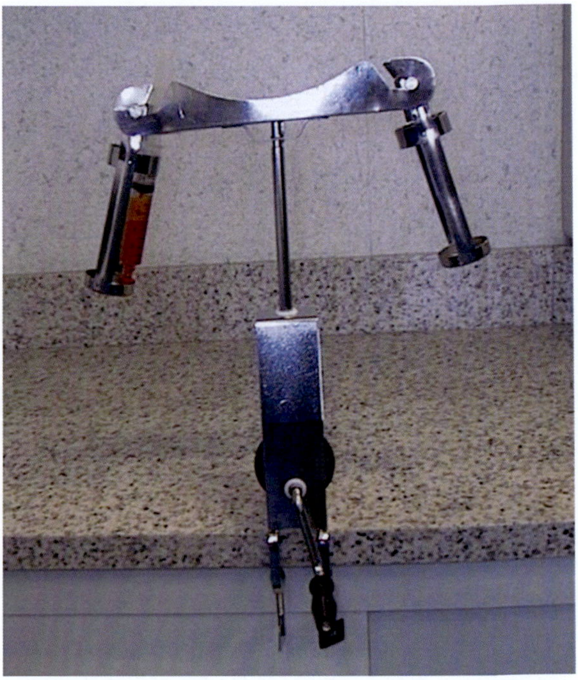

Fig. 29.5 The manual centrifuge. It can hold 10–60 ml syringes. It should be used at 1500 rpm for 1 minute to separate the fat from the anesthesia fluid without breaking the fat cell membrane

Fat Grafting

In 1983, Illouz (Illouz 1983b) and Fournier (Fournier 1985) began to graft the aspirated fat. Fournier called the new technique liposculpture. By aspirating and injecting fat, it was now possible to "sculpt" the patient's body. Between 1985 and 1986, I operated, with my associate Paulo Matsudo, over 200 cases of liposuction with fat grafting. Our results were presented in 1987 (Matsudo and Toledo 1987) and published in 1988 (Matsudo and Toledo 1988). We were aspirating and injecting fat from several areas of the body and face. We would also reduce breasts with a combination of liposuction and periareolar incision (Toledo and Matsudo 1989).

Syringe Liposculpture

Pierre Fournier demonstrated for the first time that it was possible to aspirate fat with a syringe (Fournier 1987). He discovered this by accident, when giving himself an injection and when he pulled the plunger, fat entered the syringe. In 1985, we were using only 10 ml syringes and 3 mm gauge cannulas to aspirate the neck and the face and reinjecting fat into depressions and folds. In 1988, the next step was to treat the whole body using 60 ml syringes to aspirate and inject fat. In the beginning, we used catheter tip syringes, which would often break at the tip, until we started using Toomey tip syringes, which solved this problem. I abandoned the use of the liposuction machine, and all my face and body contour work were performed using syringes (Toledo 1991a).

From 1988, I had been performing liposculpture with syringes only, aspirating and injecting fat, and it was in 1990 when Carson Lewis, one of the founding members of LSNA (Lipoplasty Society of North America), and Frederick Grazer, who organized courses for ASPS (American Society of Plastic Surgery), saw my lectures in a small meeting in Beverly Hills (Toledo 1990b) and invited me to give courses on the technique. Carson organized live surgery workshops in his La Jolla Clinic (Toledo 1991b) and Fred in his Newport Beach facility. These meetings were attended by plastic surgeons from all over the United States, and I started being called to organize body and facial contour teaching courses at the three important societies of plastic surgery, the ASPS (Toledo 1990c) (American Society of Plastic Surgery), ASAPS (Toledo 1990d) (American Society for Aesthetic Plastic Surgery), and LSNA (Lipoplasty Society of North America) (Toledo 1990e), which I did for over 15 years. LSNA organized two events every year back to back with the ASPS and ASAPS yearly congresses, with the sole purpose of teaching lipoplasty. LSNA ended up being absorbed by ASAPS.

Surgeons knew that it was perfectly possible to perform a full-body liposculpture using only syringes and a few cannulas. Soon I realized that the medical instruments' market was not pleased with this breakthrough. The industry needed to sell expensive machines. More and more companies were starting to sell aspirators with different names. Plastic surgeons were designing different cannulas and had their names connected to the technique.

When I moved to Dubai in 2005, my nurses were not used to my work with the syringe where they have to be extra attentive and busy changing syringes and cannulas and preparing fat for reinjection. I limited the use of syringes to small procedures and when fat injection was necessary.

Superficial Liposculpture

In 1989, I invited the Italian surgeon Marco Gasparotti to come to Brazil and lecture at the symposium I organized called RAPS, Recent Advances in Plastic Surgery (Gasparotti 1989). I had heard his technique was slightly different but had not yet seen him operate. For the sake of the program and the annals of the meeting, we decided to call Gasparotti's technique radical liposuction. Seeing him operate, I realized he was performing superficial liposuction. After the meeting, we established a long-term collaboration, he visited me a few times in São Paulo, and I would travel to Rome to see him operate. I combined his technique with syringe liposuction and started performing superficial syringe liposculpture (Toledo 1992c), aspirating and injecting fat. Illouz had just published his book *Body Sculpturing by Lipoplasty* (Illouz and DeVillers 1989), in which he was adamant that every liposuction should be deep, leaving at least a 1 cm layer of fat attached to the skin. He had published a body map, dividing the body into five areas, easy to treat, moderate, difficult, very difficult, and taboo, areas that should not be treated at all. This map is still a very good guide to young surgeons, starting with the procedure.

Working with Marco, we realized that it was possible to increase skin retraction by aspirating fat subdermally, very close to the skin. But it was important to aspirate in a uniform mode, to avoid irregularities and produce a good skin retraction. Together, Carson Lewis, Marco, and I published in 1993 with Springer-Verlag the book *Superficial Liposculpture – Manual of Technique* (Toledo et al. 1993), to lay the ground work and explain how we performed the technique. After the book was published, we were invited to do live courses in North America and Europe. Many surgeons heard about the idea and started performing superficial liposuction without the necessary training, and obviously many irregularities were created.

Power-Assisted Liposuction (PAL)

Liposuction can be a very strenuous operation. The in and out movements repeated for a few hours can be tiring and often even worse when treating secondary cases with fibrosis. The aspiration can be difficult at times and require special cannulas and instruments. Power-assisted liposuction (PAL) was developed to ease the movements of fat aspiration. The first machines used compressed air and would shake too much, eliminating any possibility of refinement. In 2015, I bought the German Moller Vibrasat (Fig. 29.6), the last generation of electric vibrating machines, which abolished the handpiece vibration (Fig. 29.7). Aspiration became easier and noiseless, which is very helpful in long procedures. It also has an integrated heating system for the local anesthesia, a pump for the anesthesia injection, a suction device, and a vibrating handpiece.

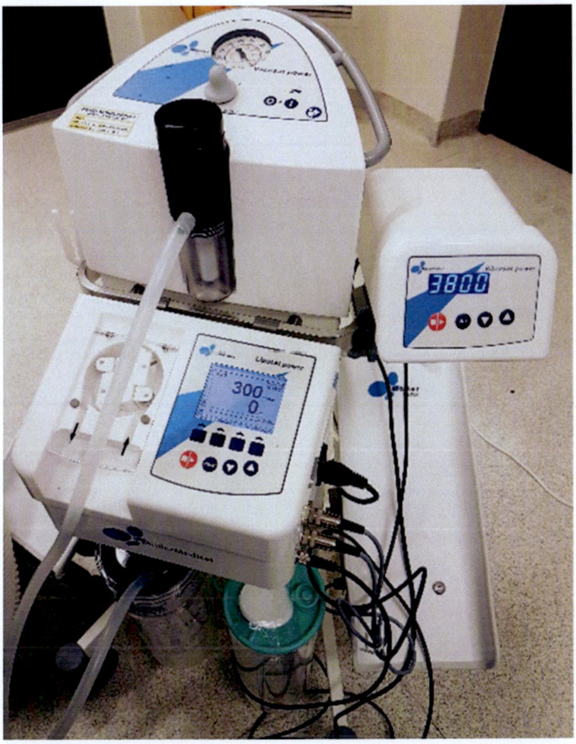

Fig. 29.6 The Moller Vibrasat PAL machine. It heats and infiltrates anesthesia and aspirates fat with vibration

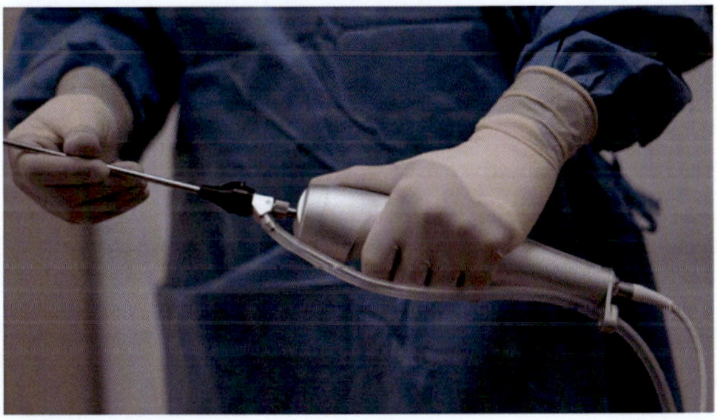

Fig. 29.7 The Moller Vibrasat handpiece is steady and allows for a refined liposuction

Internal Ultrasound-Assisted Liposuction (UAL)

In 1992, the first-generation internal ultrasound machines appeared in the market. The goal was to provoke an internal dermal "burning" and increase skin retraction. A Brazilian plastic surgeon from São José do Rio Preto came to my clinic to show me the ultrasound machine he had developed. He oversaw the procedure taking place, explaining that the ultrasound probe had to be constantly moved with in and out movements, never stopping in the same place to avoid burns and necrosis. The voluntary patient was a young girl with only a small lateral thigh adiposity, chosen to be the "perfect candidate" to demonstrate the technique. After the probe had been passed and the fat had "melted," I used the syringe to remove the excess fat. The patient went home but called me in the middle of the night saying her right thigh was much bigger than the left. I rushed her to the hospital where I aspirated about 500 ml from a hematoma. This was a hematoma from the lateral thigh, an area without any major vessels. I compressed the area, and the result finally and thankfully was not bad, but I immediately stopped using the device.

Ultrasound-assisted liposuction (UAL) had been shown by Klohen (Kloehn 1996) and popularized by Zocchi (Zocchi 1999). On my next trip to the United States, I realized ultrasound liposuction was now a big commercial hit with the launching of the second-generation Lysonix machine (Fig. 29.8). In order to be licensed to perform this technique, surgeons had to undergo a training course. The machine cost about US $40,000, and the company organized courses all over the country charging doctors US $2500 to get the needed certification. It was a money-making machine. This wave lasted for about 1 year. When reports of complications (Illouz 2014) started being published and shown in meetings, doctors stopped using the technique and tried to sell their machines. An Ultrasound-Assisted Lipoplasty Task Force was created (Fredericks 1999) to report on the safety and efficacy of this new lipoplasty procedure, which was soon abandoned.

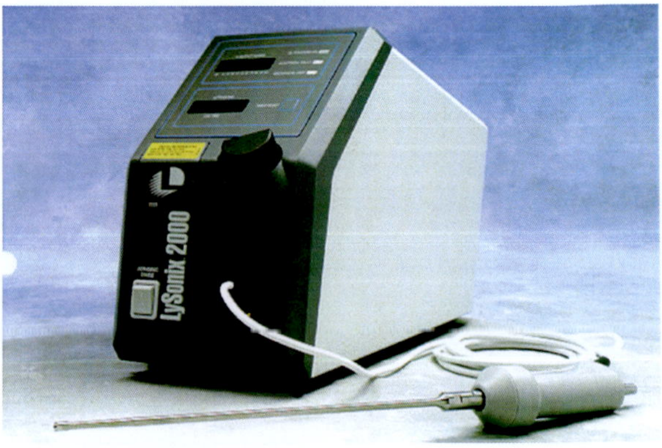

Fig. 29.8 The internal ultrasound was abandoned when reports of tissue burns and irregularities were published

The third-generation machine called Vibration Amplification of Sound Energy at Resonance (VASER) limited the power of the ultrasound energy and is less harmful to blood vessels, lymphatics, and nerves, but we still see irregularities, seromas, neural pain, and tissue burns. I have not seen the need to use these machines, but there is a media frenzy now, and doctors who do not use them are not considered up to date by prospective patients.

External Ultrasound-Assisted Liposuction (XUAL)

In 1997, I learned that we could use an external ultrasound device developed by Silberg (Silberg 1998) and the Wells Johnson Company to treat adiposities (Fig. 29.9). The idea was that the fat layer could be reduced just with the use of the external ultrasound with no need to perform an invasive treatment. I bought the machine and started using it in Brazil and quickly determined that results were better and more reliable if, after using the ultrasound, I aspirated the excess fat. I soon realized I was using the machine to justify the money I had spent and to be part of the "modern trend." The question was if the skin retraction was better with the use of the machine or not.

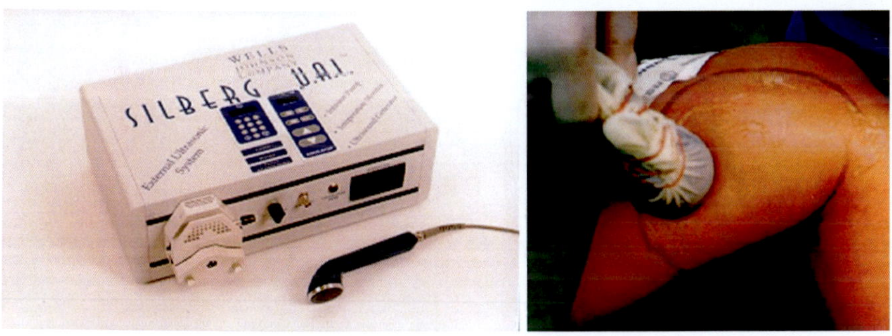

Fig. 29.9 The external ultrasound (XUAL) was used for a while, but also abandoned

Laser Liposuction

Internal laser was first used for lipoplasty in 1990 by Thomas Dressel from the United States. He used a Nd-YAG laser, with a glass fiber inside the cannula. The indications were for fibrotic and dense areas and for vascularized tissues. The cost of the equipment was too high, and the laser increased the complexity of the procedure. Results were the same as traditional lipoplasty. The method was abandoned.

In 2007, our hospital bought a Smartlipo laser machine (Fig. 29.10), and we used it for a few years. The main indication for me was when a patient asked if I was performing "laser lipo" and I could say that I was. I would use the machine and obtain the same results (Fig. 29.11).

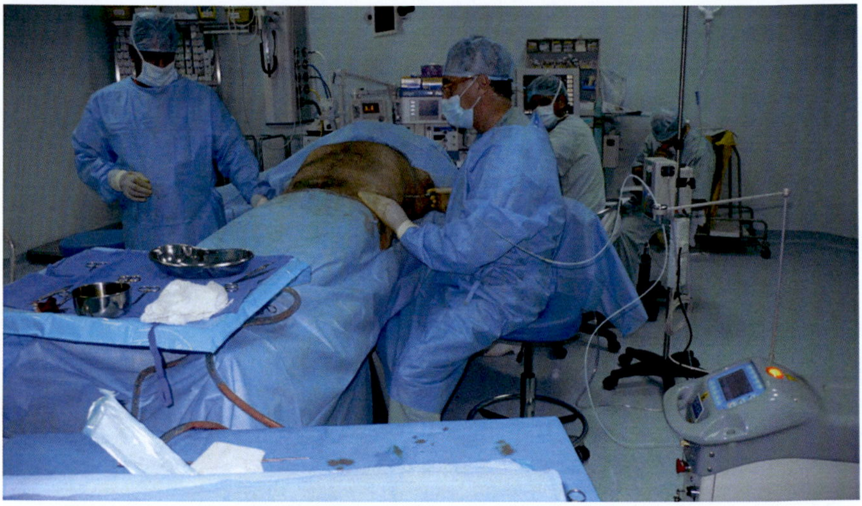

Fig. 29.10 I used the Smartlipo internal laser in areas that needed more skin retraction, but the result was similar to superficial liposuction

Fig. 29.11 The use of internal laser before aspiration of the neck

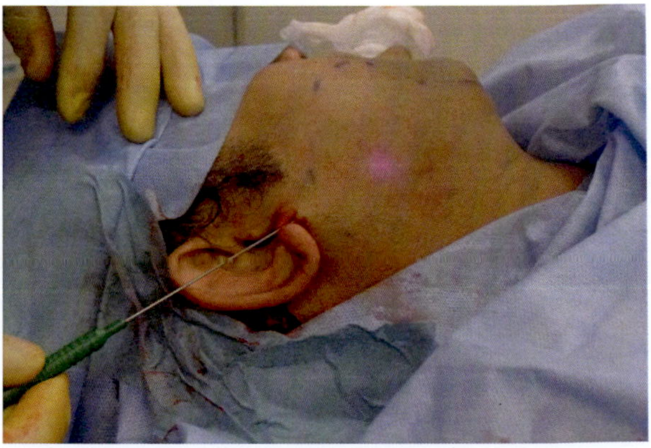

External Laser

I travelled a lot to many South American countries to lecture. In 2000, while in Cali, I met the Colombian plastic surgeon Rodrigo Neira, who was using an external laser to treat the fat before aspiration. Low-intensity laser therapy was normally used for postoperative and wound treatment at a potency of 50 mw at 660 nm. Neira had used it in 700 patients over 2 years to improve his liposuction results. I was organizing a meeting in Porto Alegre with Nelson Heller and invited him. He came, lectured, and performed demonstration surgeries (Toledo and Heller 2001).

I used the laser (Fig. 29.12), and in 2005, we wrote an article about our use of low level laser-assisted liposuction (Neira et al. 2006). Neira claimed the 4 L technique was an excellent adjuvant tool for the surgeon practicing liposculpture. His idea was that the low-level laser would create a transitory pore in the cell membrane of the adipocyte to move fat from inside the cell to the interstitial space outside without killing the cell. The technique had been performed successfully in in vitro and human adipose tissue cultures. The theory was to decrease the surgical trauma of liposuction by protecting and preparing tissues for the surgical trauma, modulating the inflammatory response to prevent short- and long-term side effects of surgery, and improving the quality and quantity of the healing process by accelerating recovery time, modulating secondary cicatrization, and preventing postoperative neuralgias.

The indications were to facilitate suctioning, shorten surgical time, decrease the risk of infection, decrease inflammation, improve skin retraction, and improve recovery. After using the external laser for a period of 6 months, I realized it did not facilitate suctioning or shortened surgical time. The laser probably decreased the risk of infection and inflammation, and recovery was slightly improved. But did it improve skin retraction? I could not find any clinical demonstration that retraction was any better.

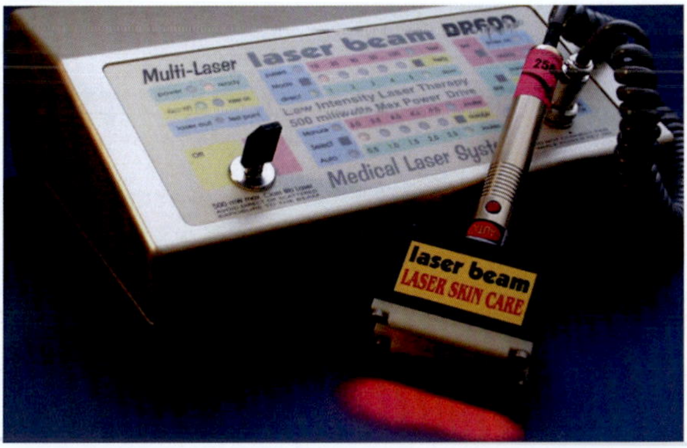

Fig. 29.12 The external laser was also used to provoke skin retraction after liposuction

J Plasma

This is another new name and new trend to try to improve skin retraction. A disposable device in inserted under the skin, which releases helium gas and radiofrequency (RF) to create a stream of energy. This energy generates heat to contract the skin while, at the same time, excess helium gas cools the treatment area. The idea is to contract the tissues just under the skin. Since the handpiece is expensive and disposable and its results are still not clear, we will have to wait for further research on the technique.

High Definition

Patients mostly wanted to get rid of excess fat, and a flat abdomen was what a high percentage of them were looking for, obtained by combining abdominoplasty with liposuction. In 1984, Jorge Psillakis published his modification of the traditional abdominoplasty (Psillakis 1984), adding contour and definition comparing the abdominal shape with the music instrument lyre. This was probably the first article written explaining an attempt to improve the anatomy accentuating the shape of the recti and obliquus muscles. His technique involved undermining the major oblique musculature to reduce the diameter of the waist and also reduce the diameter of the superior abdomen by resecting cartilage from the seventh and eighth ribs when the anterior projection was exaggerated.

In 2006, Gasparotti (Gasparotti 2006) used the term 3D in an article, and soon many other authors started using different names to describe their modifications, such as high definition (HD) and even 4D (!), adding another dimension to their procedures. I had been performing superficial liposculpture and observed that my female patients only wanted definition on the linea alba (patients joked about wanting a “Champagne groove”) and on the V shape formed by the oblique muscles (Toledo 1999) (Fig. 29.13).

The first presentation I watched about abdominal etching to create a six-pack effect was in the early 1990s by Larry Schlesinger, from Honolulu. He had many male body builder patients who wanted to accentuate the abdominal muscles, and he created the etching technique to produce a six-pack definition. There was a lot of criticism, and the consensus at the time was that this was not a technique for women, since it could masculinize the women’s body. In a later meeting, Larry showed a complication—a patient to whom he had created a six-pack had put on weight and was now overweight but still showing the six-pack design on his abdomen.

The combination of etching and high definition has become very popular recently. Some surgeons became specialists in creating “athletic” bodies, the shapes being created by areas of liposuction and fat injection creating the highs and lows, volumes, and depressions.

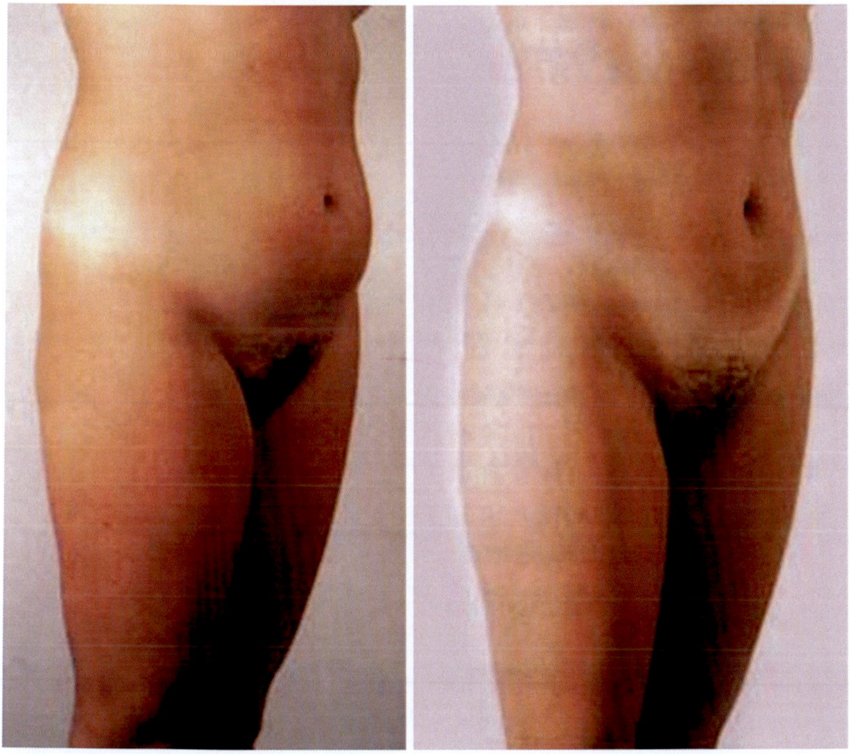

Fig. 29.13 Before and 6 months after superficial syringe liposuction of the abdomen and flanks with definition of the linea alba and oblique muscles

Noninvasive Body Contour

In 2013, I started using cryolipolysis (Toledo 2015) for local reduction of fat deposits to reshape body contours. I believe liposuction is the best, safest, and most reliable technique to remove localized fat when performed by qualified plastic surgeons. But there are patients who do not want a surgical procedure, are afraid of anesthesia, or simply do not have the money for it. With these patients in mind, I started using the Coolplas machine (Fig. 29.14). I knew there were other more expensive machines, which used expensive disposable parts for every treatment. The disposable gel pads of Coolplas are cheap cotton sheets saturated in a solution that protects the skin and ensures proper thermal coupling during a procedure.

Cryolipolysis is a noninvasive procedure to remove unwanted body fat by cooling the fat deposits and provoking subcutaneous fat reduction through cellular apoptosis. "Cellular apoptosis is a normal biological process whereby cells are eliminated as part of normal cell turnover. The injured cell enters an orderly, regulated process of gradual degradation and is absorbed by the body's immune system over time, usually 2 months. This reduces the subcutaneous fat tissue without damage to the

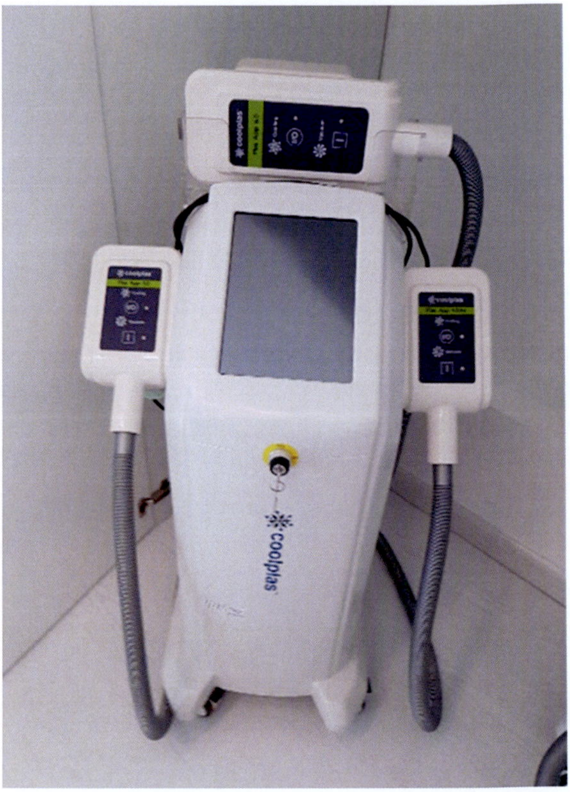

Fig. 29.14 The cryotherapy Coolplas machine. Non-surgical fat reduction

overlying skin." The procedure is simple and fast (45–60 min), and after the treatment, the patient can go back to normal activities. There is no downtime and no anesthesia, and it can be performed during a lunch break. The treatment can be repeated, if necessary, after 2 months. Cellular elimination through apoptosis is in contrast to cellular necrosis, or uncontrolled cell death, in which an acute injury to the cell leads to lysis of the cell. Cellular necrosis triggers an aggressive inflammatory response leading to fibrotic scar tissue formation, which is not observed with cellular apoptosis.

I had two machines in the office, and they worked very well. Patients were happy with the reduction of the fat deposits without having to undergo surgery. The reduction is uniform. It is not possible to "sculpt" the area to be treated as we can do with liposculpture. But these patients do not mind as they wanted a bulge reduction, and the Coolplas could achieve that in the majority of the cases. There are obviously more expensive machines, but this is a cost-effective treatment that has been well accepted by my patients (Fig. 29.15).

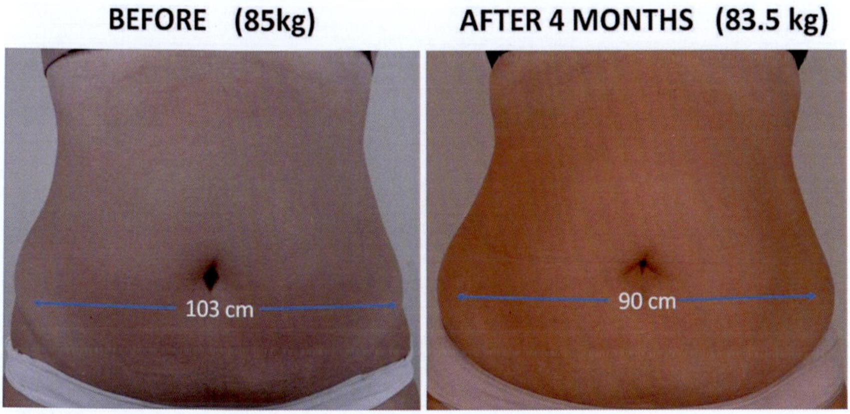

Fig. 29.15 A patient before and 4 months after two sessions of cryotherapy of the abdomen and flanks, with a reduction of 13 cm in the abdominal circumference

Pre- and Postoperative Treatments

In 1992, I understood that preoperative preparation and most importantly postoperative treatments helped to keep patients happy and involved in the process. I opened an aesthetic clinic behind my office with beauty therapists and physiotherapists, who would work with my patients pre- and postoperatively. One of the main treatments prescribed was the French massage therapy called manual lymphatic drainage (MLD), which was used before and after surgery (Fig. 29.16). Patients were advised to undergo five to ten sessions of MLD and would feel less pain and less swelling and bruising in the postoperative period. It was also a way of keeping an eye on my patients postoperatively and addressing any issues they might have immediately. Patients would also book skin treatments, advice on corsets, makeup, and exercise. Corsets should be used for 3–4 weeks postoperatively.

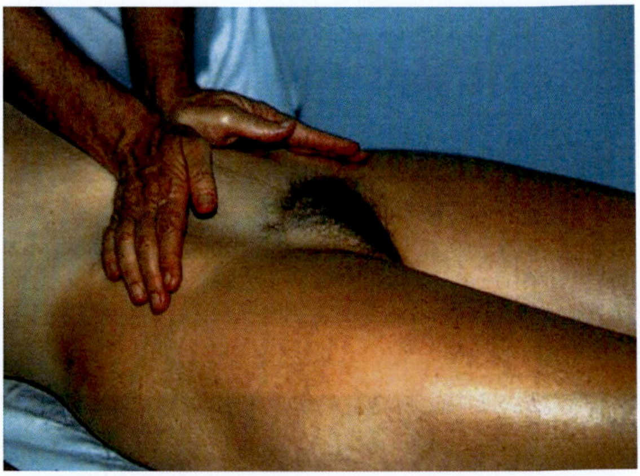

Fig. 29.16 Manual lymphatic drainage of the abdominal area post liposuction

Aesthetic Complications Treatment

Permanent color changes in the skin, uneven areas, and irregularities. Color changes in the skin may improve with time but are sometimes permanent. Uneven aspiration can be corrected with suction or injection of fat, fat shifting—dissection of the adjacent fat layers and redistribution of fat, mobilization of a fat graft, and subcision—by using the V-tip cannula to cut the adherences and inject or aspirate fat. And finally skin excess resection.

The Future of Liposuction

It is difficult to predict the future, especially after so many modifications have already been made to the original technique. We can expect more precise techniques to eliminate fat excess, new methods that allow for even skin retraction without tissue burns and irregularities, and techniques to improve skin quality. There is research continuing to evaluate the improved skin quality of patients who over the years have had facial fat injection for contour definition. We now have over 30 years of this practice to study the long-term effects of this fat replacement technique. Fat injection for breast augmentation, which was discouraged for many years, is now an acceptable method to augment the breast naturally as some patients are not comfortable with having the implants. Research will continue on how to eliminate fat excess without surgery. But while this does not happen, we can only rely on the good training of plastic surgeons in the available techniques. We have already witnessed one miracle in our lifetime. Will there be enough time for a second?

References

Schrudde J: Lipexeresis in the correction of local adiposity. Rio de Janeiro: Proceedings of the First Congress of the International Society of Aesthetic Plastic Surgery; 1972.

Fischer A, Fischer G. Revised technique for cellulitis fat reduction in riding breeches deformity. Bull Int Acad Cosm Surg. 1977;2:40–3.

Vilain R. Surgical correction of steatomeries. Clin Plast Surg. 1975;2:467–70.

Kesselring UK, Meyer R. A suction curette for removal of excessive local deposits of subcutaneous fat. Plast Reconstr Surg. 1978;62:305-6.

Temourian B, Fisher J B: Suction curettage to remove excess fat for body contouring, Plast Reconstr Surg 1981 Jul;68(1):50-8.

Illouz, YG: A New Method for Localized Lipodystrophies. La Revue de Chirurgie de Langue Française 19 (6) 1980a.

Illouz YG: Practical Liposuction Course. Hospital São Paulo, Andrews JM Service, Escola Paulista de Medicina, 1983a.

Fournier P, Illouz YG: Practical Liposuction Course. Hospital 9 de Julho, São Paulo, 1984.

Avelar JM (1986) Liposuction of Abdominal Wall. In Liposuction (Lipoaspiração). Ed. by Avelar JM. & Illouz YG. São Paulo (Brasil). Editora Hipócrates 27:158–176.

Illouz YG: A New Method for Localized Lipodystrophies. Rev Chir Esthet 4: 19 (6) 1980b.

Drake LA, Ceilley RI, Cornelison RL, et al. Guidelines of care for liposuction. Committee on Guidelines of Care. J Am Acad Dermatol. 1991;24:489–94.

Hetter GP. The effect of low-dose epinephrine on the hematocrit drop following lipolysis. Aesth Plast Surg 1984;8:19–21.

Toledo LS, Regatieri FL, Carneiro JD: The effect of hypothermia on coagulation and its implications for infiltration in lipoplasty: a review. Aesthet Surg J. 2001 Jan;21(1):40–4.

Fournier P: Cryoanesthesia and Cryolipoplasty. Presented at the Lipoplasty Society of North America – LSNA – Annual Meeting. Las Vegas NV, October 9th, 1984.

Fournier P: Cryoanesthesia and Cryolipoplasty. NeoCryoanesthesia and Neocryolipoplasty. In Liposculpture, the Syringe Technique. Arnette Blackwell. Paris 1991 p 165.

Klein JA: The Tumescent Technique for Liposuction Surgery. Am J Cosmetic Surg 4:263–267, 1987

Toledo LS: Superficial Syringe Liposculpture: A Personal Technique. *In* Annals of the 3rd International Symposium Recent Advances in Plastic Surgery – RAPS92 – March 14–15, 1992a, 170–175 Estadão, São Paulo, Brazil

Hohn L, Schweizer A, Kalangos A, Morel DR, Bednarkiewicz M, Licker M: Benefits of intraoperative skin surface warming in cardiac surgical patients. British Journal of Anaesthesia; 80: 318–323, 1998.

Toledo LS: Anesthesia. *In* Luiz Toledo – Refinements in Facial and Body Contouring. Lippincott-Raven, 1990a, p 51.

Klein JA: Tumescent technique for local anesthesia improves safety in large-volume liposuction. Plast Reconstr Surg 1993 Nov;92(6):1085–98; discussion 1099-100.

Hanke CW, Bernstein G, Bullock S: Safety of tumescent liposuction in 15,336 patients. National survey results. Dermatol Surg 1995 May;21(5):459–62.

Toledo LS: Equipment and Instrumentation. *In* Atlas of Suction Assisted Lipectomy in Body Contouring. Ed Frederick Grazer. Churchill Livingstone, 1992b, 23–25.

Illouz YG. Body contouring by lipolysis: a 5-year experience with over 3000 cases. Plast Reconstr Surg 1983b;72:591–7.

Fournier P. Microlipoextraction et Microlipoinjection. Rev. Chir. Esthet. 1985;10:40.

Matsudo PK, Toledo LS: Eighteen Month Experience of Injected Fat Grafting", presented at the IX Congress of the International Society of Aesthetic Plastic Surgery, Waldorf Astoria Hotel, New York, USA, October 11–14, 1987.

Matsudo PK, Toledo LS: "Experience of Injected Fat Grafting", Aesth Plast Surg 12:35–38, 1988.

Toledo LS, Matsudo PK: Mammoplasty using liposuction and Periareolar incision. Aesth Plast Surg 13:9–13, 1989

Fournier P. Body Sculpturing Through Syringe Liposuction and Autologous Fat Reinjection. Samuel Rolf International. US: 1987.

Toledo LS: Syringe liposculpture: A two-year experience. Aesth Plast Surg 15:321–326, 1991a.

Toledo LS: "Syringe Liposculpture" presented at the Symposium Recent Advances in Plastic Surgery, ASPER - The Beverly Hilton Hotel, Beverly Hills, CA, USA, 23–24 June 1990b.

Toledo LS: Practical Teaching Course on "Syringe Liposculpture". - La Jolla Surgicenter, La Jolla, CA, USA, April 22–23, 1991b.

Toledo LS: "Superficial Syringe Liposculpture" Presented at the 59th Congress of the American Society of Plastic Surgery – ASPRS * PSEF * ASMS, Boston, MA, USA, 21–25 Oct 1990c.

Toledo LS: "Fat Transplantation – Does it Work and Does it Last?" Panel at the Aesthetic Contouring of the Body PSEF/ASAPS Course, January 11–13, 1990d, Santa Barbara CA, USA.

Toledo LS: "Superficial Syringe Liposculpture" presented at the VIII Annual Scientific Meeting of the Lipoplasty Society of North America, LSNA, Boston, MA, USA, 20–21 October 1990e.

Gasparotti M: "Radical Liposuction", presented at the International Symposium Recent Advances in Plastic Surgery, Espaço Artefacto, São Paulo, SP, Brazil, 3–5 March, 1989.

Toledo LS: Superficial Syringe Liposculpture – A Personal Technique. In Annals of the International Symposium Recent Advances in Plastic Surgery – RAPS92 – March 14-15, 1992c. Ed. Luiz Sérgio Toledo, Estadão, 170–175.

Illouz YG, DeVillers YT (Eds). Body Sculpturing by Lipoplasty. Churchill Livingstone; Edinburgh: 1989. P. 29.

"Superficial Liposculpture – Manual of Technique," Luiz S Toledo, Carson M. Lewis, and Marco Gasparotti. Springer Verlag, New York, USA. April 1993.

Kloehn R. Liposuction with "Sonic Sculpture": six years' experience with more than 600 patients. Aesthet Surg J 1996;16:123–8.

Zocchi ML. Basic physics for ultrasound-assisted lipoplasty. Clin Plast Surg 1999;26:209–20.

Illouz YG: Liposuction – the evolution of the classical technique. pmfa news | APRIL/MAY 2014 | VOL 1 NO 4 | www.pmfanews.com

Fredericks S: Analysis and introduction of a technology: Ultrasound-assisted Lipoplasty Task Force. Clin Plast Surg. 1999 Apr; 26(2):187–204; vii.

Silberg B N: The technique of external ultrasound-assisted lipoplasty. Plast Reconstr Surg. 1998 Feb;101(2):552.

Toledo LS, Heller N: Simpósio Internacional de Inclusões em Cirurgia Plástica e Lipoplastia, Instituto Goethe, Porto Alegre – RS – Brasil – 07 e 08.12.2001

Neira R, Toledo LS et al: Low-Level Laser-Assisted Liposuction: The Neira 4 L Technique February 2006. Clin Plast Surg 33(1):117–27, vii

Psillakis JM: Plastic surgery of the abdomen with improvement in the body contour. Physiopathology and treatment of the aponeurotic musculature. Clin Plast Surg 1984 Jul;11(3):465–77.

Gasparotti, M: Three-Dimensional Superficial Liposculpture for Aged and Relaxed Skin. In Liposuction: Principles and Practice. Ed Melvin A. Shiffman, Alberto Di Giuseppe. Springer, 2006, 198–205.

Toledo LS: The Abdomen. *In* Refinements in Facial and Body Contouring. 1999 Lippincott-Raven, Philadelphia, p 178.

Toledo LS: "A New Fat Freezing Machine That Keeps the Office Busy" Presented at the – ASPS-Aesthetica 2015 Super Symposium – April 30 – May 2, 2015 – Las Vegas, NV

Chapter 30
Liposuction

Luis Fernandez de Córdova and Ricardo Cavalcanti Ribeiro

Abstract Precision liposuction slims and reshapes specific areas of the body by removing fat deposits, improving the body contours and proportion by removing excess in overweight patients, and revealing structures in patients with desirable weight. Back and gluteal regions are of difficult definition by diet and exercise only, making lipoplasty a popular and safe option to enhance their aesthetics.

Patient selection is as important as the surgical technique to achieve satisfactory results, and it is important to know the aesthetic considerations for male and women to prevent feminization or masculinization.

Physical examination and laboratory and imaging tests should be performed before liposuction, taking into consideration that best results are obtained in patients with a body mass index of 24 and lower.

The sequence of a liposuction surgery is as follows: markings, anesthesia, asepsis and antisepsis, infiltration of vasoconstricting solution, liposuction, and dressing.

Complications can be classified by the moment of presentation when they occur, i.e., perioperative and postoperative, and by the area or system(s) affected, i.e., local or systemic.

The accumulation of liquid in the lower back is the most common complication in our practice and presents during the first 7 days postop and is drained by needle aspiration. The final aesthetic result can be seen at 6 months, and as patients improve their activity level and make lifestyle changes, further changes may be noticed.

L. F. de Córdova
Department of Plastic and Reconstructive Surgery, Hospital Universitário Gaffrée e Guinle, Universidade Federal do Estado do Rio de Janeiro, Rio de Janeiro, Brazil

R. Cavalcanti Ribeiro (✉)
Plastic and Reconstructive Surgery, Federal University of the State of Rio de Janeiro, Rio de Janeiro, Brazil
e-mail: rribeiro@centroin.net.br

J. M. Avelar, R. Cavalcanti Ribeiro (eds.), *Body Contouring*,
https://doi.org/10.1007/978-3-031-42802-9_30

Keywords Liposuction · Body fat · Body contouring surgery · Brazilian butt lift

Introduction

Since first described by Illouz during the 1980s, precision liposuction slims and reshapes specific areas of the body by removing fat deposits, improving the body contours and proportion by removing excess in overweight patients, and revealing structures in patients with desirable weight [1–18]. Therefore, the surgeon is obliged to acquire a precise knowledge of osteology and myology for a satisfactory sculpting of the human body where instead of bronze, marble, wood, or metal, the sculpting substrate is fat. Back and gluteal regions are of difficult definition by diet and exercise only, making lipoplasty a popular and safe option to enhance their aesthetics.

We must take into consideration cultural aspects that could alter the expectations of the aesthetic patient, as it is the case of the Brazilian surgeons who popularized the "Brazilian butt lift."

It is helpful to classify patients on three types of lipodystrophy and skin redundancy:

1. Localized lipodystrophy: Generally younger patients with good skin tone.
2. Generalized lipodystrophy: Often patients with slightly diminished skin tone, some skin irregularities, and circumferential lipodystrophy throughout their trunk and extremities.
3. Skin redundancy and lipodystrophy: Patients with significant skin redundancy would benefit the most from excisional surgical techniques.

From William Sheldon [19], the American psychologist, we inherited the somatotypology system that describes three body types and is still widely used:

- Ectomorphs: they are typically thin and tall and have narrow shoulders, low body fat percentage, and high metabolism.
- Mesomorphs: they have medium bone structure with a solid torso and are muscular and lean with predisposition to gain weight if exercise is deficient or caloric intake is too high.
- Endomorphs: they gain weight easily requiring high-intensity exercise and dieting to become lean and have large bone structure and wide waist.

Liposuction has been utilized throughout the past and current century as a surgical solution for unwanted convexities due to exercise- and diet-resistant fatty deposits as described by Dolsky in (1987) [1].

Body mass index, calculated by dividing the body weight in kilograms by the height in meters squared, could be considered as an index of overall fat percentage with studies revealing that a BMI of 20 is considered optimally attractive in women and the goal of a "V"-shaped body with a low waist-to-chest ratio should be the aim for men.

When performing lipoplasty of the flanks, it is important to know the aesthetic considerations for male and women to prevent feminization or masculinization; males tend to be flatter inferiorly and posteriorly, while women exhibit fullness in these areas, whereas men have superior and lateral fullness, while women have not.

Diagnosis/Patient Presentation

Liposuction patients often present themselves with a variety of concerns, complaints, and expectations. As a general rule, aesthetic surgery, including liposuction, should be performed in healthy patients who maintain realistic goals. Patients committed to a positive lifestyle change involving a healthy diet and regular exercise or those who were already following a healthy lifestyle preoperatively and continued postoperatively experienced the best satisfaction scores.

During the initial evaluation, it is imperative for the plastic surgeon to translate the expectations of the patient into realistic results. Besides explaining the method, indications, and postoperative care, an informed consent should be signed, and photographs of the area to be treated must be taken. Problems can be avoided by taking into consideration that not every patient presenting for a consultation must be treated.

A proper physical examination should be performed including recording of height, weight, body mass index, circumferences of areas to be treated, asymmetries and surface irregularities, scars, associated cellulite, skin tone and laxity, presence of stretch marks, and muscle diastasis and/or hernias.

If the protrusion is due to subcutaneous fat and therefore theoretically easy to be removed by liposuction, it can be ascertained by a simple "pinch" test. The fat that the physician can pinch between two fingers is subcutaneous fat that can be removed by aspiration.

Physical examination should be paired with a psychological evaluation recording any symptoms of depression, anxiety disorders, or dysmorphophobia.

The following laboratory and imaging tests could be obtained before liposuction is performed (depending on the country and legal specifications for elective surgery):

- Coagulation (PTT, ProTime, INR)
- Complete blood count
- Creatinine, AST, ALT
- Glucose
- Lipid panel
- Electrolyte panel
- HIV
- Hep-C
- ECG
- Chest X-ray
- Abdominal wall ultrasound for hernia exclusion purposes

Taking clinical photographs requires the following simple rules (Fig. 30.1):

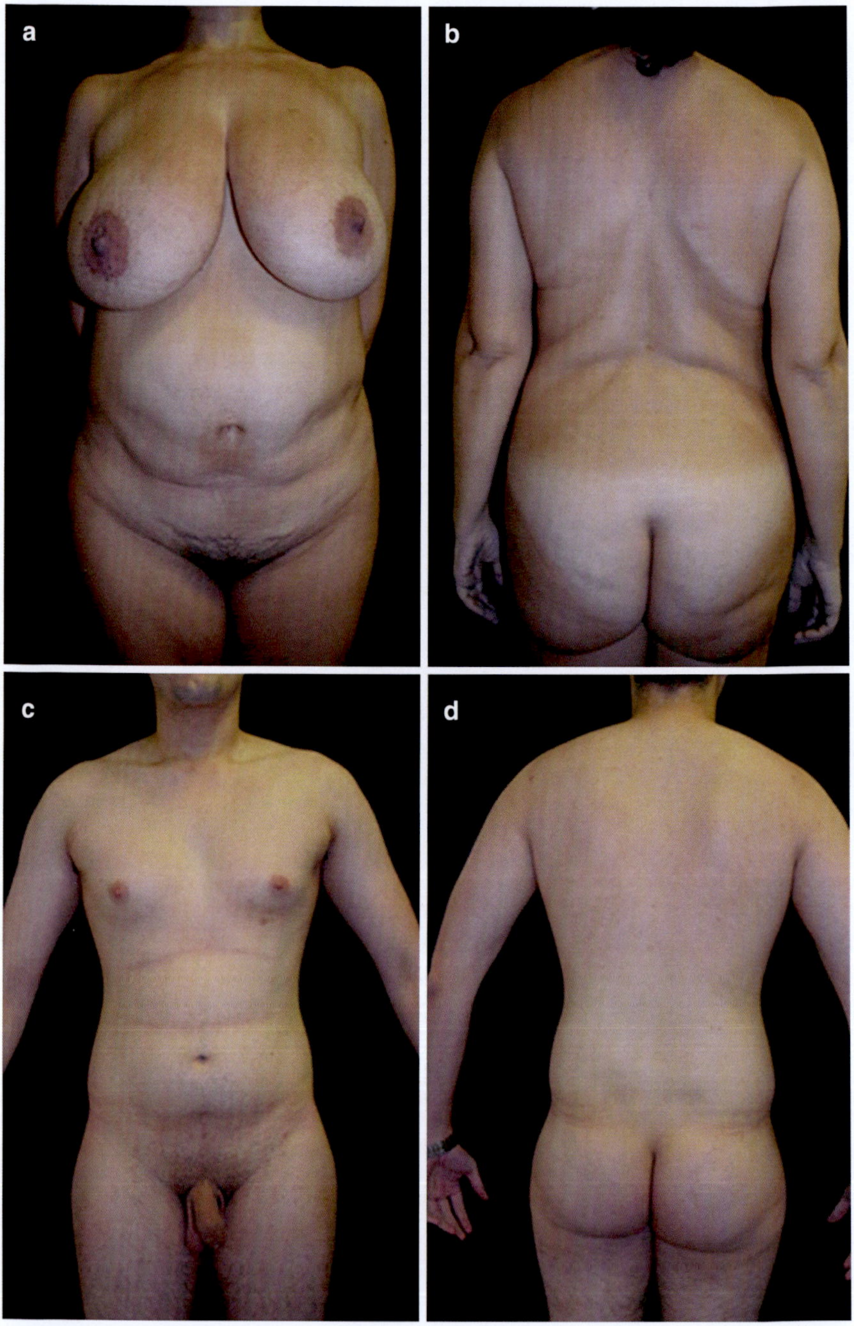

Fig. 30.1 Standardized preoperative pictures with frontal (**a**, **b**) and back (**c**, **d**) views. The suggested photographs in a clinical setting should include, besides anterior and posterior views, right and left profiles

- Use an appropriate backdrop and lighting light to medium blue or medium gray)
- Remove distractions (jewelry and clothing)
- Use controlled lighting
- Reduce cast shadows
- Record settings (the same camera settings should be used for every patient)
- Use consistent framing for each aesthetic unit

Look specifically for bleeding disorders, and it is imperative to know if the patient is under antiplatelet, anticoagulant, and/or contraceptive therapy as well as hormone replacement therapy.

Patient Selection

The range of indications for liposuction, initially developed for aesthetic procedures, has been extended for pathological tissue increase disorders such as benign symmetrical lipomatosis, adiposis dolorosa, gynecomastia, axillary hyperhidrosis, and mobilization of skin flaps, among others.

Ideal patients for liposuction are not obese, maintain a stable weight throughout time, and have incorporated the three key elements mentioned above into their perioperative regimen. Regularly, they present with localized or generalized lipodystrophy with good skin tone, no scars, and no stretch marks. Pregnant patients or those with morbid obesity, cardiopulmonary disease, body image perception issues, and wound healing anomalies should be excluded from liposuction.

The consultation should occur in a comfortable environment and in no rush; positive rapport and patient's trust in the surgeon are just as important as the qualifications of the surgeon. A patient who distrusts the surgeon or entered the operating room with doubts will be dissatisfied with the outcome regardless of the results.

If the patient smokes, they must stop smoking at least 2 weeks before the surgery and refrain from smoking at least 1 month postoperatively.

Nonessential medications should be excluded 3 weeks before surgery, including herbal remedies and supplements, since they are not regulated by the Food and Drug Administration and may add risk of complications, including bleeding or hypercoagulability.

In front of a full-length mirror, to allow an open dialogue between the patient and the physician, any areas of cellulite should be addressed as well as expected outcomes discussed in these areas.

Nowadays, anesthesia raises more concern on the patients than the surgery itself. It is up to the surgeon to determine the optimal surgical anaesthesia for each patient, as a general rule, to avoid epidural and spinal anesthesia in office-based procedures to reduce the risk of potential hypotension and volume overload. Small-volume liposuction can be performed with local anesthesia, with or without mild sedation, and large-volume liposuction or liposuction combined with other surgical procedure should be performed under general anesthesia.

There are four different terms used to describe the types of wetting solutions intended to reduce the blood loss during liposuction (Table 30.1).

Most wetting solutions utilize lidocaine as a local anesthetic, which raised the concern about toxicity. The traditional maximum dose of lidocaine with epinephrine is 7 mg/kg, but in a liposuction setting, various studies have reported safety of lidocaine concentrations from 35 to 55 mg/kg in volume cases. The signs and symptoms of lidocaine toxicity include from tinnitus, lightheadedness, and circumoral numbness to tremors, EKG alterations, seizures, and cardiopulmonary arrest.

Safety is a priority above cosmetic results. Many body contouring procedures require complex positioning. Improper pressure to neurovascular structures may lead to short- or long-term disability, and head positioning is extremely important in the prone position. The neck must be in a neutral position and stable when changing position intraoperatively to avoid carotid and/or vertebrobasilar arterial system dissection. Nerves across bony surfaces require appropriate angle and padding on the table to avoid compression and stretch. Avoid arm abduction greater than 90°. Pedal or calf compression devices should be applied. During the procedure, all areas not being treated should be covered by a forced warm air blanket, and wetting solutions should be warmed. In 2012, the consensus on liposuction in the Committee of Body Contouring Surgery of the Brazilian Society of Plastic Surgery concluded that the ideal volume to be aspirated safely goes from 5% to 7% of total body weight (Table 30.2).

Table 30.1 Techniques of lipoplasty may be divided into four types depending on the volume of solution infiltrated. The volume of infiltration is related to the estimated blood loss as percentage of volume aspirated being the superwet and tumescent techniques the safest [1-30]

Technique	Estimated blood loss as % of volume aspirated	Infiltrate	Volume aspirate
Dry	20–45	No infiltrate	To treatment endpoint
Wet	4–30	200–300 ml/area	To treatment endpoint
Superwet	1	1:1 ml infiltrate/aspirate	1 ml aspirate/infiltrate
Tumescent	1	Infiltrate to skin turgor	2–3 ml aspirate/ml

Table 30.2 Conclusions made in 2012 by the consensus on liposuction in the Committee of Body Contouring Surgery of the Brazilian Society of Plastic Surgery [31]

1. Is advanced age a contraindication	No
2. What are the absolute contraindications?	> ASA II, high risk for thrombosis
3. What is the most common anaesthesia used?+	Epidural
4. Is liposuction to be performed in dry conditions?	No
5. What is the proportion of injected physiological solution and adrenaline?	1:500 to 1:1000
6. What is the ideal volume to be aspirated?	5–7% of total body weight
7. What is the maximum acceptable volume of aspirate without the risk of complications?	4000 to 10,000 ml
8. Is the ICU used routinely in the postoperative period?	No
9. What analgesics are routinely used in the postoperative period?	Dipyrone, codeine and ketoprofen
10. Are compressive garments used?	Yes
11. What cannula diameter is used?	05-Feb
12. What is the preferred liposuction technique?	Superwet (1:1)

+ The authors prefer general anesthesia

Surgical Technique

No "orthodox" technique exists for liposuction, and each individual surgeon has a personal method and own technique reflecting artistic style and technical specifications.

The sequence of liposuction surgery is as follows:

- Markings
- Anesthesia
- Asepsis and antisepsis
- Infiltration of vasoconstricting solution
- Liposuction
- Dressing

Nowadays, there are multiple options of liposuction to perform such as suction-assisted liposuction (SAL), power-assisted liposuction (PAL), ultrasound-assisted liposuction (UAL), and laser-assisted liposuction (LAL). Since PAL, UAL, and LAL require a greater investment in technology and a greater learning curve, suction-assisted liposuction still remains the most common modality among plastic surgeons. The disadvantages of SAL include more physical work involved to break up and remove fat.

Power-assisted liposuction uses an externally powered cannula that oscillates at rates of 4000–6000 cycles/minute, which is the authors' preferred technique. In our daily routine, we choose the superwet technique using 0.9% saline solution or Ringer's lactate solution associated with adrenaline with different concentrations depending on the area to be treated as described in the following paragraphs.

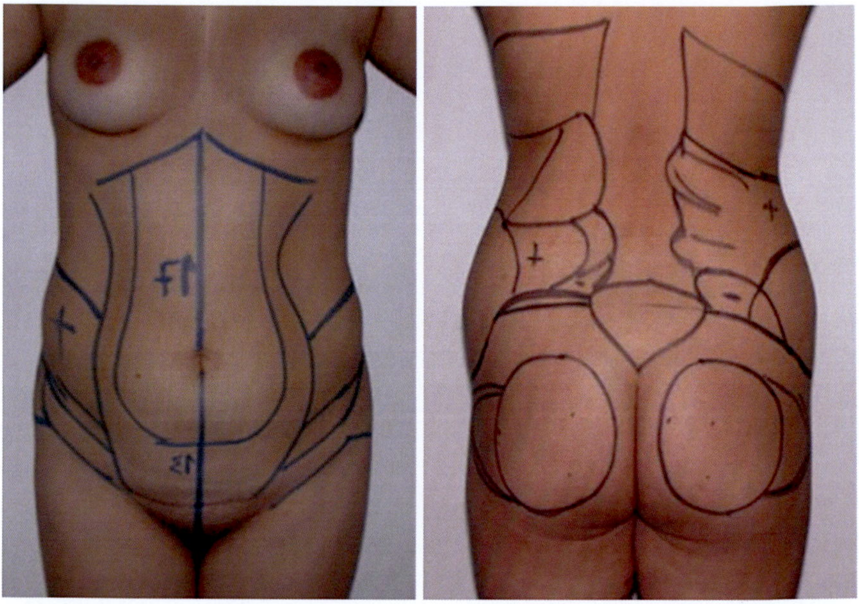

Fig. 30.2 Marking is performed prior to surgery in the erect position. The lines resemble the topographic map showing localized fat, focal depressions, and dimples

Markings are performed with the patient in the standing position using specific anatomical references as follows: the median longitudinal furrow, the iliac crest, the sacral triangle, the iliac line, and the supracristal plane (Fig. 30.2).

Following anesthesia, placement of a Foley catheter is to be done to closely monitor fluid output (minimum 0.5 ml/kg of body weight). Antisepsis first with 2% chlorhexidine with the sterile technique is performed. The next step is a new degermation of the area with 0.2% aqueous chlorhexidine solution, carried out by the surgical assistant, already duly attired.

The next step is the placement of sterile surgical drapes, where the areas to be liposuctioned are delimited. It is of utmost importance to choose access points that can treat multiple areas preventing incisions that could disrupt zones of adherence through the suctioning. If with the existing markings the access results are insufficient, do not hesitate in placing additional incisions. Asymmetric incisions may camouflage their appearance, therefore offering a better cosmetic result. The incisions are made, after infiltration of 0.5 ml of lidocaine (2%) with epinephrine with a surgical blade #11 with a mean longitude of 0.5 cm. For beginning plastic surgeons, we suggest following Hunstad's approach to specific regions of treatment (Table 30.3).

During a body contouring surgery, the patient should be positioned in four ways during the procedure when full lipoplasty is to be performed: prone position, supine position, left lateral decubitus, and right lateral decubitus. In our surgical practice, we chose to start by placing the patient in the prone position (Fig. 30.3).

With the patient properly prepared, the procedure can finally be started. First, we mark the incision areas with a sterile surgical pen for the infiltration procedures of the

Table 30.3 Recommendations of entry sites and patient position to treat different areas of the body [8, 13]

The Hunstad's approach to specific regions of treatment		
Location	Entry sites	Position
Abdomen	Groin, umbilicus, inframammary	Supine
Back	Bra-line, buttocks, axilla	Prone
Hip rolls	Buttocks	Prone/supine
Outer thigh	Gluteal crease, groin	Prone
Circumferential thigh	Groin, gluteal crease, knee	Prone/supine
Neck	Postauricular, submental	Supine
Arms	Axilla, elbow	Supine
Buttocks	Infragluteal, apical buttocks	Prone
Inner thigh	Groin, infragluteal	Prone/supine

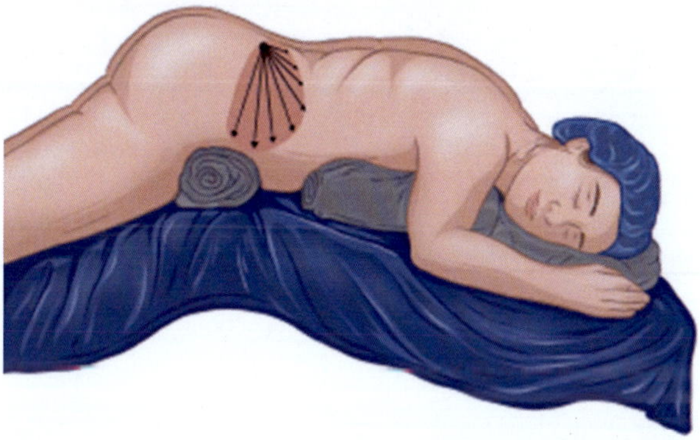

Fig. 30.3 The prone position for the patient gives access to all the posterior regions of the body making it possible to combine the technique with lipotransfer to the gluteal region. Safety recommendations such as the use of a thermic blanket and appropriate padding to rectify the surgical area and avoid intraoperative complications are to be considered and applied always

tumescent solution and subsequent access to the liposuction cannulas. In our clinical surgical practice, we observed that the scars from the incision areas do not present a great aesthetic concern to patients in the late postoperative period, which is not a major concern of the team, focusing on the final result of the procedure (Fig. 30.4).

As marking the incision areas, we always choose to look for transition areas between different areas to perform liposuction (thus facilitating access to larger areas) and also areas that have some aesthetic alteration (whether scars or stretch marks), thus avoiding new scars. The average longitude of the incisions is 0.5–1.0 cm, performed with a no. 11 scalpel blade, after applying intradermically 2% lidocaine. Afterward, the infiltration process of the previously prepared solution begins. It is emphasized here the importance of minimizing the time to prepare such a solution until its use in the surgical act, thus avoiding inactivation of adrenaline and also a possible contamination when being exposed after preparation (Table 30.4).

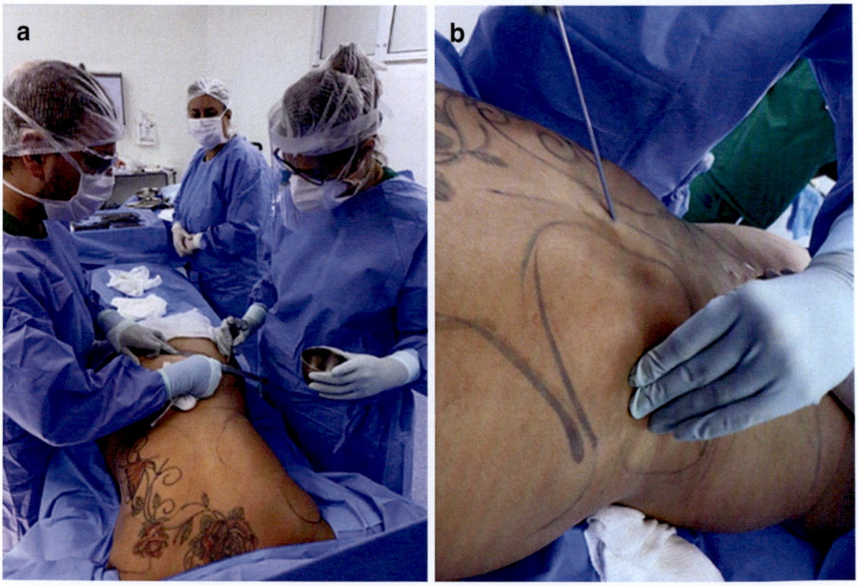

Fig. 30.4 (**a**) The infiltration is performed by zones/quadrants. Using reference points for incisions as the intersection of the iliac line and an inferior projection of the scapular line, the posterior axillary line, and the midvertebral line in the thoracic and lumbar regions. (**b**) With Klein cannulas attached to 60 ml syringes. With this resource, an equal infiltration is carried out in the different areas. At the end of the infiltration, we adopted as a rule the 20-minute wait for an effective action of the infiltrated solution, thus reducing the blood loss associated with the method, generating a faster recovery of the patient in the postoperative period and lower rates of complications. The red stars represent the localization of the incision

Table 30.4 Recommendations for volume infiltrated depending on the area to be treated

Area to be treated	Infiltration volume (ml)
Abdomen	1500 - 2000
Back	1500 - 2000
Neck	2000[a]
Gluteal region	
Arms	
Hips	

[a] When the infiltration volume is less than 1000 ml 1, the authors work with epinephrine in 0.5 mg/1000 dilution injected into 200 cc of 0.9% Ringer's lactate solution

There are a variety of infiltration systems, either manually or mechanical infiltration, which is an electrically operated pump system. In our practice, we perform the infiltration process using 60 cc syringes in a fan-shaped pattern. The deeper layers of subcutaneous adipose tissue are infiltrated first, to avoid build-up pressure close to the surface complicating the access to the whole thickness of adipose tissue to be treated. During infiltration, skin turgor is monitored by continual palpation. After a 20-min window for the vasoconstrictor effect to begin, liposuction may begin.

Depending on the legislation of each country and if office-based procedures are allowed, local anesthesia may be used for small-volume liposuction cases associated with or without mild sedation.

The process of liposuction requires that the surgeon's hands work in concert with the one hand denominated sensory hand and the other the motor hand. The sensory hand has several functions, being the most important to maintain the tip of the cannula between pinch manœuvre performed by the thumb and fingers, ensuring the surgeon not to penetrate any deeper tissues, and facilitating a safe and gentle liposuction by immobilizing the targeted fat making it possible to aspirate by preventing it to oscillate to and fro in unison with the cannula.

The motor hand provides the force and moves the cannula through the targeted subcutaneous fat. The authors prefer the PAL using cannulas of 3, 3.5, 4, and 5 mm progressively depending on the thickness of fat tissue in the area to be treated respecting the selected areas and avoiding, if possible, returning to areas that have already been liposuctioned. This measure prevents further blood loss, as it impedes the clotting process body to be interfered by a new passage of the cannula. The superficial layer is rarely treated aiming to avoid contour irregularities, vascular compromise, and the risk of hyperpigmentation. The cannulas with the wider diameters are used for the deeper planes, and cannulas with diameters 3.5 mm and smaller are used for contour refinement in our practice.

With the motor hand, the cannula is inserted, and the adipose tissue is broken loose from the fibrous stoma with multiple crisscross movements creating tunnels in the subcutaneous tissue. For the body, cannulas with lengths from 15 to 45 cm are preferred, whereas for the face and other delicate areas, diameters chosen go from 1 to 3 mm and 10 to 20 cm in length.

In our practice, we routinely take a blood sample and test for hemoglobin and hematocrit when performing combined procedures such as lipoabdominoplasty or large-volume liposuctions.

Once the lipoplasty is done, we use Nylon 5-0 to suture the incisions and apply a gauze dressing before placing the compression garment.

Postoperative Care Protocol

Body contouring procedures can result in significant fluid shifts, and the following formula mentioned by Rohrich et al. aids in fluid management for liposuction patients:

1. Replace losses from preoperative oral intake as needed.
2. Maintain fluid throughout the procedure and manage it based on vital signs and urine output.
3. Employ the superwet infiltration technique.

4. Administer crystalloid replacements 0.25 ml for each ml of lipoaspirate over 5 L.

In order to achieve better results and minimize complications after liposuction, a comprehensive postoperative protocol should be described aiming to:

- Identify and treat complications.
- Monitor and promote the healing process.
- Prevent and treat fibrosis or a pathologic scar process.

A compression garment is placed at the conclusion of the surgery, customized based on surgeon preference. Patients are encouraged to ambulate the day of the surgery, and sequential compression devices are placed on the patient until discharge. Showering is allowed 1 or 2 days postoperatively, and patients are instructed to keep the compression garment on 24 h/day during 4 weeks. Initial postoperative visits are scheduled weekly for the first month starting 4 days after hospital discharge. Return to activity can occur, depending on the procedure as early as 4 days or at 2 weeks. In our practice, we schedule visits at 7 days for suture removal, 15 days for first postop pictures, and 30, 60, and 90 days for final pictures (Fig. 30.5).

Volume changes and swelling may translate in an initial weight gain during the first days postop with edema peaking from 3 to 7 days after surgery. Patients should start to appreciate changes in their waist and contour by 2 weeks and at 6 weeks be able to perceive significant changes in their shape. The final aesthetic result can be seen at 6 months, and as patients improve their activity level and make lifestyle changes, further changes may be noticed.

Manual lymphatic drainage is encouraged to help manage the swelling and soften tissue induration due to fibrosis or fibrosclerosis, stimulate circulation and lymphatic flow, stimulate the immune system, and improve cellular nutrition and tissue recovery, often starting in the first 3–7 days after surgery.

Besides encouraging early ambulation to reduce venous stasis and help prevent thromboembolism, low molecular weight heparin should be considered if large volumes are removed or in patients who have combined surgical procedures. The incidence of deep venous thrombosis in liposuction has been reported at 1%, but a marked increase is demonstrated when combined with other surgeries such as abdominoplasty. Subcutaneous enoxaparin can be administered 1 hour after surgery without precipitating significant bleeding. The application of 40 mg per day for 6–11 days is recommended although the existing uncertainty of an optimal timing and duration of chemoprophylaxis. The Caprini Risk Assessment Module can be used as a guide for establishing a deep venous thrombosis prophylactic protocol (Table 30.5).

As a preventive measure for postoperative fevers and/or cellulitis, first-generation cephalosporins are administered perioperatively within 1 h of the incision and continued for 5 days, as well as dipyrone 500 mg 6/6 h and nimesulide 12/12 h for 3 days.

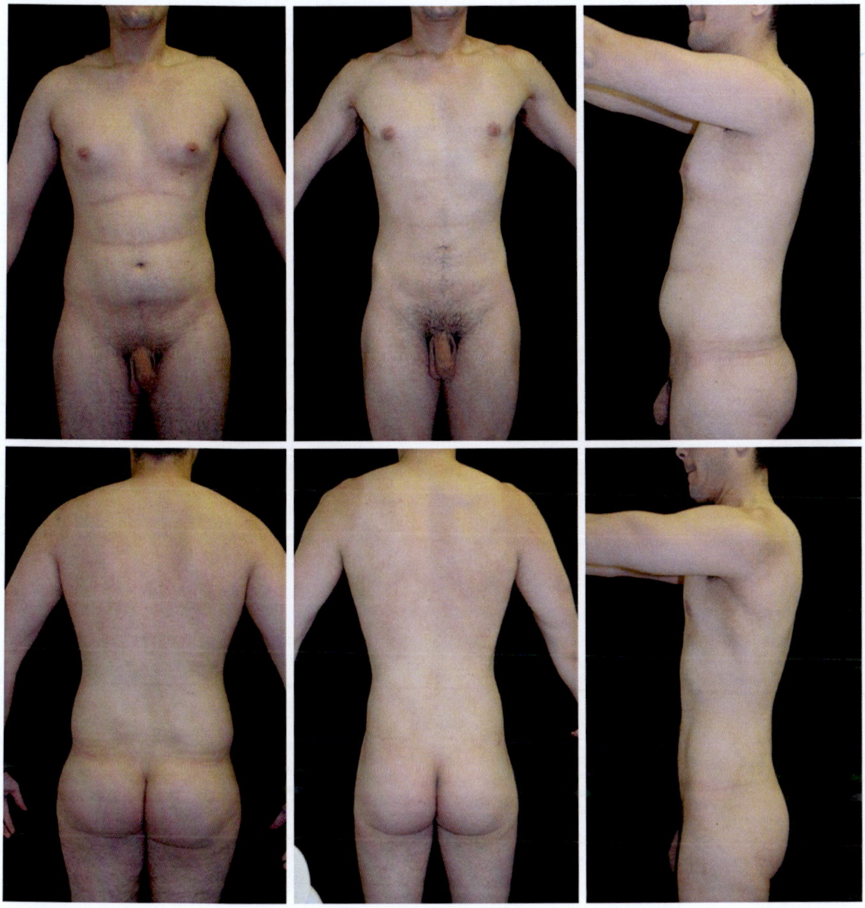

Fig. 30.5 21 days postoperative liposuction male patient

Table 30.5 Risk factors for venous thromboembolism based on the 2005 Caprini Risk Assessment Model and the measures to prevent thromboembolism in patients undergoing surgery under general anesthesia lasting more than 60 min [7-31]

1 point for each risk factor	2 points for each risk factor	3 points for each risk factor
Age 41–60 years	Age 60–74 years	Age over 75 years
Minors surgery planned	Malignancy (previous or present)	History of DVT/PE
History of prior surgery (<1 month)	Major surgery (>45 min)	Family history of thrombosis
Varicose veins	Patient confined to bed (>72 h)	Positive Factor V Leiden
History of inflammatory bowel disease	Central Venous access	Positive prothrombin 20210A
Swollen legs		Elevated serum homocysteine
Obesity		Positive Lupus anticoagulant
Sepsis (<1 month)		Elevated anticardiolipin antibodies
Abnormal pulmonary funcion		Heparin-induced thrombocytopenia
Other risk factors		Other congenital or acquired thrombophilia
For women only		
Oral contraceptives or HRT		
Pregnancy or postpartum (<1 month)		
History of unexplained stillborn infant, recurrent spontaneous abortion, premature birth with toxemia or growth-restricted infant		
2005 caprini RAM score	Recommendations	
3–6	Consider the option to use postoperative LMWH or unfractionated heparin	
3 or more	Consider the option to use mechanical prophylaxis throughout the duration of chemical prophylaxis for nonambulatory patients	
7 or more	Strongly Consider the option to use extended LMWH postoperative prophylaxis	

Discussion

Complications can be classified by when they occur, i.e., perioperative and postoperative, and by the area or system(s) affected, i.e., local or systemic. Local complications may be: insatisfactory results due to poor diagnostic and wrong liposuction indication, contour irregularities secondary to bad technique and skin hyperpigmentation when the vascular superficial plexus is compromised after liposuction in a superficial plane or untreated ecchymosis.

When it comes to systemic complications, hypovolemia or hypovolemic shock is of utmost importance although using the tumescent or superwet technique allows an almost bloodless surgical field. A bloody aspirate may be obtained in dense fibrotic areas such as the back, upper abdomen, or male breasts; if the aspirate is excessively bloody, avoid that region, or more tumescent fluid should be infiltrated. Preoperatively, patients should be advised not to take any medications, vitamins, or herbal supplements with antiplatelet effects for at least 7 days prior to the surgery.

Postoperative complications may occur in three different windows, being the perioperative period from 0 to 48 h, and can include anesthesia and cardiac complications, cannula trauma to the skin and/or internal organs, and volume-related anomalies from bleeding or fluid administration.

During the early postoperative period, from days 1 to 7, complications can include perforation, venous thromboembolism, infection, seroma, and skin necrosis. Several cases of intestinal perforation after liposuction have been reported causing peritonitis that may lead to sepsis and eventually death. Perforation can result from the cannula passing through a defect in the abdominal wall, an undiagnosed abdominal hernia, or careless movement of the cannula in vertical rather than a horizontal direction. Intraoperatively, the nondominant hand should always feel the tip of the cannula, or at the beginning of the learning curve, the use of pinch maneuver is encouraged. The use of an axillary incision for treatment of the upper back reduces the risk of intrathoracic penetration.

Classical clinical signs of DVT include Homan's sign, chest pain, shortness of breath, tachycardia, and lower extremity swelling. When properly diagnosed and treated, DVT/pulmonary embolism is an uncommon cause of death.

Infection is unusual following liposuction; however, wound infections including necrotizing fasciitis have been reported. Properly sterilized instruments and sterile technique help keep the incidence of infection at its lowest. Immunocompromised patients have an increased risk of infection, and if not excluded from consideration for lipoplasty, they should receive close monitorization in the perioperative period.

Necrosis may occur following aggressive superficial liposuction and is more likely if the patient at hand is a smoker. To minimize the incidence of necrosis, superficial maneuvers should be limited and excessive postoperative compression avoided.

Late complications include seroma, edema and ecchymosis, paresthesias, hyperpigmentation, and contour irregularities. A seroma is an abnormal collection of fluid as a result of trauma, burns, or friction. Seromas are more common in overweight or obese patients. The diagnosis could be made either clinically or through ultrasound examination and treated by drainage by needle aspiration followed by compression to avoid capsular formation. In our practice, we see seromas in the lower back during the first 7 days since we do not leave drains as a routine procedure.

Postoperative edema and ecchymosis occur in all patients. Prolonged edema may be present up to 3 months post-surgery and is treated with lymphatic massage and supportive care. The challenge with ecchymosis is the hemosiderin deposition that evolves to hyperpigmentation.

Table 30.6 Lipoplasty is one of the most popular aesthetic procedures worldwide; however, it involves risks and complications that should be avoided by following systematic protocols and select combined procedures when needed for better results [1-35]

Key points for safe and successful body contouring surgery
Adequate patient evaluation
Proper procedure indication
Do not try to "create new techniques"
Analyze pre- and postop pictures with the patient
Use of the superwet technique
Identify and treat complications
Always be aware of the location of the tip of your cannula
Know when to stop
Commitment to a positive lifestyle change

Paresthesias can occur in all forms of liposuction and are usually reversible during the first 10 weeks post-surgery, patients generally report recovery to be quicker with SAL than with UAL.

The most common late postoperative complication is contour irregularities, present in up to 20% of patients. Careful preoperative analysis, planning, and proper informed consent all help to minimize the risk of complaints due to contour irregularities. The treatment can be directed at re-injecting fat in the over-aspirated region or suctioning the adjacent areas in order to reduce the prominence and achieve a blending effect (Table 30.6).

Conclusions

Liposuction represents A versatile technique which provides, along with an adequate diagnosis and patient selection, the correction of body contouring, elimination of unwanted fat deposits and the improvement on the patient's self-esteem. Power-assisted liposuction is the authors' preferred approach, and has the following advantages:

- Less bruising, swelling, and trauma.
- Increased patient comfort and improved safety.
- Greater cell viability for autologous fat grafting and reinjection.
- Faster healing process because the connective tissue is not destroyed.
- Studies indicate that PAL produces high concentrations of adipose-derived stem cells, which hold great promise for a variety of medical therapies.
- PAL is not heat based, so patient burns are not a concern.

Technology-assisted liposuction needs expertise on conventional-assisted liposuction as well as investment from the plastic surgeon to buy the technology that most appeals to them.

Declaration of Conflicts of Interests The authors declare no potential conflicts of interest with respect to the research, authorship, and/or publication of this chapter.

Funding The authors received no financial support for the research, authorship, and/or publication of this chapter.

Level of Evidence V.

References

Dolsky RL, Newman J, Fetzek JR, Anderson RW. Liposuction history, techniques, and complications. Dermatol Clin 1987;5:313-33
Fischer A, Fischer G. Revised technique for cellulitis fat reduction in riding breeches deformity. Bull Int Acad Cosmet Surg 1977; 2: 40–1
Kesselring V, Meyer R. A suction curette for removal of excessive fat deposits of subcutaneous fat. Plast Reconstr Surg 1978; 62: 305–6
Teimourian B, Adham MN, Gulin S, Shapiro C. Suction lipectomy – a review of 200 patients over a six-year period and a study of the technique in cadavers. Ann Plast Surg 1983; 11: 93–8
Illouz Y. Body contouring by lipolysis: a 5-year experience with over 3000 cases. Plast Reconstr Surg 1983; 72: 511–24
Coleman WP III. The history of liposuction. Dermatol Clin 1990; 8: 381–3
Fournier P. Body Sculpturing Through Syringe Liposuction and Autologous Fat Re-injection. Corona Dee Mar, CA: Samuel Rolf International, 1987
Klein JA. The tumescent technique for liposuction surgery. Am J Cosmet Surg 1987; 4: 236–67
Sommer B, Sattler G. Vibration assisted liposuction (VAL) in tumescent local anesthesia (TLA). In Ring J, et al., eds. Skin and Environment – Perception and Protection. 10th EADV Congress, Munich, 2001. Bologna: Monduzzi Editore, 2001;
Sattler G, Sommer B. Tumescent liposuction in Germany: history and new trends and techniques. Dermatol Surg 1999; 25: 221–3
M. Zocchi, Ultrasonic liposculpturing, Aesth. Plast. Surg. 16 (1992) 287–298.
D. Apfelberg, Laser-assisted liposuction may benefit surgeons and patients, Clin. Laser Mon. 10 (1992) 259–264.
D. Apfelberg, S. Rosenthal, J. Hunstad, Progress report on multicenter study of laser-assisted liposuction, Aesth. Plast. Surg. 18 (1994) 259–264.
D. Apfelberg, et al., Results of multicentric study of laser-assisted liposuction, Clin. Plast. Surg. 23 (1996) 713–719.
Fodor PB, Vogt PA. Power-assisted lipoplasty (PAL): a clinical pilot study comparing PAL to traditional lipoplasty (TL). *Aesthet Plast Surg*. 1999;23:379–385.
Araco A, Gravante G, Araco F, Delogu D, Cervelli V. Comparison of power water-assisted and traditional liposuction: a prospective randomized trial of postoperative pain. *Aesthet Plast Surg*. 2007;31:259–265.
Man D, Meyer H. Water jet-assisted lipoplasty. *Aesthet Surg J*. 2007;27:342–346.
Sasaki GH. Water-assisted liposuction for body contouring and lipoharvesting: safety and efficacy in 41 consecutive patients. *Aesthet Surg J*. 2011;31:76–88.
Sheldon WH (1940) The varieties of human physique: an introduction to constitutional psychology by W.H. Sheldon with the collaboration of S.S. Stevens and W.B. Tucker. Harper, New York
Singh D, Young RK (1995) Body weight, waist to hip ratio, breast, and hips: roles in judgements of female attractiveness and desirability for relationships. Ethol Sociobiol 16:483–507
Toveé MJ, Cornelissen PL (1999) The mystery of human beauty. Nature 399(6733):215–216
Schider F (1957) An atlas of anatomy for artists. Dover Publications, New York
Rubins DK (1976) The human figure: an anatomy for artists. Penguin Books, New York

Simblet S, Davis J (2001) Anatomy for the artist. DK Publishing, New York
Rohrich RJ, Broughton 2nd G, Horton JB, et al. The key to long-term success in liposuction: A guide for plastic surgeons and patients. Plast Reconstr Surg. 2004;114: 1945–1952.
Iverson RE, Lynch DJ, ASPS Committee on Patient Safety. Practice advisory on liposuction. Plast Reconstr Surg. 2004;113(5):1478–1490.
Fodor PB. Wetting solutions in aspirative lipoplasty: a plea for safety in liposuction. Aesth Plast Surg. 1995;19:379–80.
Klein, J. A. Tumescent technique for regional anesthesia permits lidocaine doses of 35 mg/kg for liposuction. Dermatol Surg Oncol. 1990; 16(3):248–263
Ostad A, Kageyama N, Moy RL. Tumescent anesthesia with a lidocaine dose of 55 mg/kg is safe for liposuction. Dermatol Surg. 1997;22:921.
PDR. Physician's Desk Reference 2011. Montvale NJ: PDR Network; 2011:1084–1085.
Rev. Bras. Cir. Plást. 2017;32(3):454-466
Newall G, Ruiz-Razura A, Mentz HA, Patronella CK, Ibarra FR, Zarak A (2006) A retrospective study on the use of low-molecular-weight heparin for thromboembolism prophylaxis in large volume liposuction and body contouring procedures. Aesthetic Plast Surg 30(1):86–95
Reish RG, Damjanocic B, Colwell AS (2012) Deep venous thrombosis prophylaxis in body contouring: 105 consecutive patients. Ann Plast Surg 69(4): 412–414
Carson JL, Kelly MA, Duff A, et al: The clinical course of pulmonary embolism, N Engl J Med 326:1240-1245,1992
Douketis JD, Kearon C, Bates S, et al: Risk of fatal pulmonary embolism in patients with treated venous thromboembolism, JAMA 279:458-462,1998

Chapter 31
High-Definition Liposculpture: Critical Vision and Future Perspective

Felipe Massignan and Filipe Fuzinatto

Abstract The text objectively and simply talks about the technical foundations of high-precision three-dimensional surgeries. Scientific paradigms based on evidence and secular artistic concepts are explained. In addition, in a pleasant and summarized way, the preoperative marking is described, as well as the use of the technology adopted by the pioneers of the approach, associating with key points of the surgical sequence. It ends with a critical view, based on and experienced by the authors, adding to that the exercises of imagination compatible with the speed of technical advances in the area of aesthetic and reparative plastic surgery.

Keywords High-definition liposculpture · Three-dimensional anatomical relief · Ultrasonic technology

Introduction

Firstly, it is important to define the meaning of terms like **high-definition**, **hd lipo**, and **muscle marking**, in order to avoid inadequate meanings in surgical approach. Those are related to athletic humans exclusively. However, with that particularity, superficial anatomical relief is vast in detail in genres; and what expresses this abundance is the three-dimensionality concept.

As a definition, three-dimensional space is the one which has height, depth, and width and—in practice—indicates what is known as surface relief. The human body reflects light homogeneously (Schider 1957). When spotting the topography with predominance of shadows, one is faced with a slender fabric with null or concave

F. Massignan (✉) · F. Fuzinatto
São Paulo, Brazil

J. M. Avelar, R. Cavalcanti Ribeiro (eds.), *Body Contouring*,
https://doi.org/10.1007/978-3-031-42802-9_31

projection (Schider 1957). However, when viewing a light-reflecting area, it can be considered that the surface has projection and volume. The tonal progression extending from the shaded to the illuminated surface can be understood by the gradual increase in thickness and projection tissue, using the dark area as a starting point (Schider 1957; Massignan 2018).

Contemporary schools of plastic surgery adopt, as a safety rule, lamellar extraction for liposuction procedure (Avelar 1989; Pereira and Radwansky 1996). However, the three-dimensional body contour seeks to be reliable with the anatomical surfaces using multiple surgical strategies, as manipulating the lamellar layer, areolar layer, or both of them strategically, maintaining the current paradigm in safe (Avelar 1989; Hoyos and Millard 2007). As we can see, the challenge for the plastic surgeon is enormous, considering that he is trained from the beginning to follow evidence-based medicine practice. Thus, being humble to improve concepts such as the three dimensions from technical art becomes a promising starting point (Avelar 1989).

Liposuction as Sculpture

A large number of tools were inserted in procedures involving body contour surgeries but few proved their efficiency (Schider 1957; Jewell 2020). It is important to mention the third-generation ultrasound, produced since 2001, for example, and that 1 year after its launch with a pilot study of Jewell (Jewell et al. 2002) reached 2021 with Ali Juma (Juma et al. 2021), proving in dozens of articles its variability of positive statistics (Jewell 2020), among which decreased blood depletion by 36% (Nagy and Vanek Jr 2012), increased skin retraction by 53% compared to usual tools (Nagy and Vanek Jr 2012), the numerical increase of viable adipocytes after aspiration (Ince et al. 2019; Stosich and Mao 2007), and, in an unprecedented way, safety in surgical handling of the areolar layer (Massignan 2018; Hoyos and Millard 2007; Juma et al. 2021).

It can be inferred, therefore, that it is a device studied in several perspectives, for a long period, showing to be safe and, mainly, compatible with the technique (Massignan 2018; Jewell 2020; Rohrich et al. 1998). The negative points of this device shown by the guidelines are related to the long learning curve and the high cost of the equipment (Jewell 2020; Rohrich et al. 1998; Klein 1990).

Liposculpture, in those days, therefore, is based not only on a simple removal of fat but rather approaches which vary in strategies to respect the characteristics of the anatomical unit to be manipulated (Massignan 2018). Anatomical relief is vast in detail (Avelar 1989); therefore, the variations should be predefined with aspiration of the lamellar layer only or adipose collect with partial thicknesses of superficial and deep tissue or, still, aspiration of both following the histological characteristic of the topography to be carved (Avelar 1989; Cimino and Bond 1996; Berkenstein and Grotting 2000).

Surgical Technique

In order to achieve an aesthetically harmonic result, one must approach human anatomy with the "look of a sculptor." Although fat removal is part of the three-dimensional technique, this is not the main objective, as the focus is on revealing the musculoskeletal structures below the surface. The perception of static and dynamic anatomical alternation is essential (Massignan 2018; Hoyos and Millard 2007).

The skin is opaque for patterns of reflection and absorption of light in adult humans due to the gradual decrease in tissue thickness (Schider 1957; Jewell 2020). From the brightest point to the darkest, there is a tonal progression. The brightest region contains higher volume and projection, and the darkest is slender and deeper (Schider 1957).

Considering men, surgical reasoning is based on the premise that the musculature of the anterior thorax and upper limbs (pectoral upper, deltoid, and biceps) have higher volumes when compared to the anatomical units located caudally to these. That concept is fundamental for technical planning, as uniform volumetric proportions result in loss of balance (Schider 1957; Hoyos and Millard 2007). Lipografting, for that reason, is often performed in the pectoral and deltoid muscles (Hoyos and Millard 2007).

Considering women, the planning should be started from the cylindrical forms of the buttocks and breasts, as they are the angular anatomical centers with the other areas (Schider 1957; Massignan 2018; Hoyos and Millard 2007). Smaller muscles, obviously, have slender volumes, but they are adhering to harmonic balance. The rectus abdominal muscles are outlined by creating shadows in their contours. In those circumstances, the shape is related to the transitions and precise limits, being unnecessary volumetric increase (Hoyos and Millard 2007; Nagy and Vanek Jr 2012), since the perceptions of their edges are delicate and, in rare exceptions, hypertrophic.

The main anatomical landmarks of the human body, where the shadow areas are the sharpest, used as a "frame" to be carved (Fig. 31.1). The negative spaces neighboring them have two characteristics, which are as follows: its shaded color is less intense than the one mentioned above and the fabrics are thicker than those of the landmarks and slender than those of the adjacent topographies, which are characterized as positive spaces, because they have projection and reflect the light (Schider 1957; Massignan 2018; Hoyos and Millard 2007).

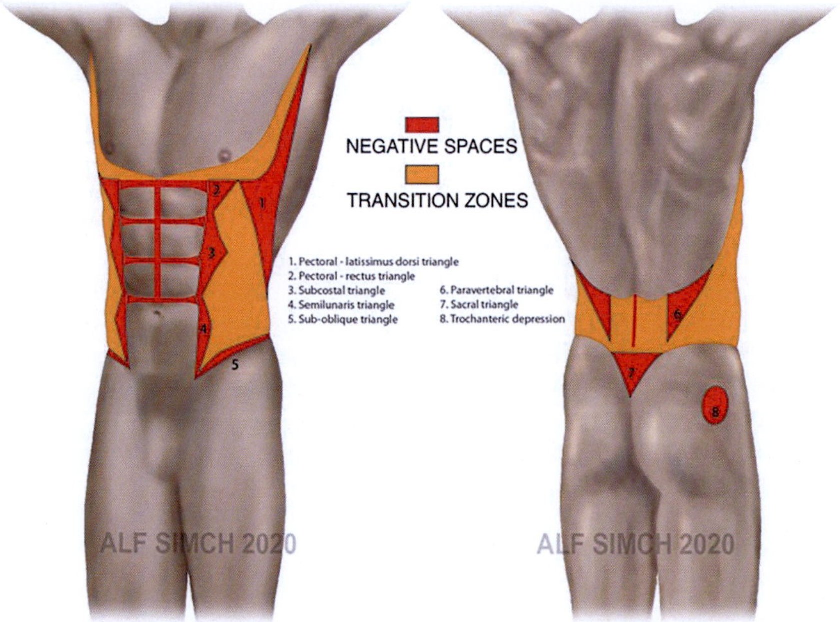

Fig. 31.1 Negative sapaces in men follow the numerical order above (Hoyos and Millard 2007)

Essential Surgical Approach, Infiltration, Emulsification, and Superficial and Deep Liposuction

1. Preoperative marking. In the preoperative marking, the areas of deep adipose tissue extraction are delimited in blue (Hoyos and Millard 2007) (Fig. 31.2). Next, the framework is made (Massignan 2018; Hoyos and Millard 2007), that is, the delimitation of anatomical landmarks (Fig. 31.3). After that, the delimitations of the negative spaces are made by interconnecting the entire areas.
2. Infiltration. Start with the deep layers, and after, approach the surface layers, with standard tumescent solution, with uniform distribution (Klein 1990). This movement will facilitate the correct handling of the lamellar and areolar layers. Ropivacaine solution 7.5% is used in a volume of 5 ml (appropriate to the body weight of each patient) in every 1000 ml of heated saline solution, associated with 1 ampoule of adrenaline and 250 mg of tranexamic acid (Massignan 2018).
3. Emulsification. Start emulsifying by the areolar layer, and then migrate toward the lamellar layer (Schider 1957; Rohrich et al. 1998). The sequence is important due to the gravitational characteristic of water protection. Succinctly the frequency of the ultrasonic device is on average 60–70% in the trunk and 50% in members in continuous mode (C) in the lamllar environment and 50% dispersion in VASER® (mode pulsatile V) in the areolar compartment (Massignan 2018; Hoyos and Millard 2007).

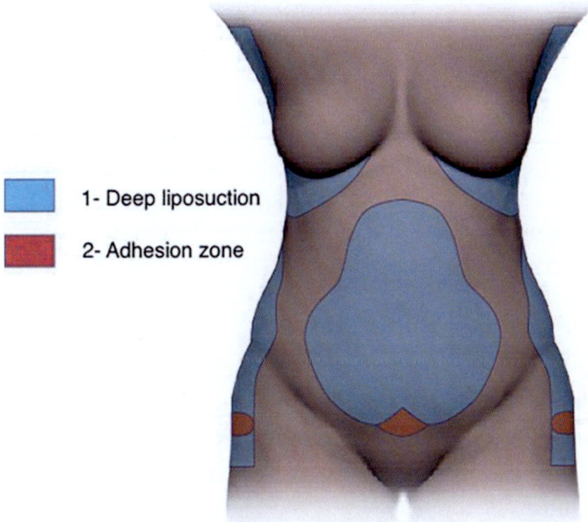

Fig. 31.2 Delimitation of deep fat tissue extraction areas

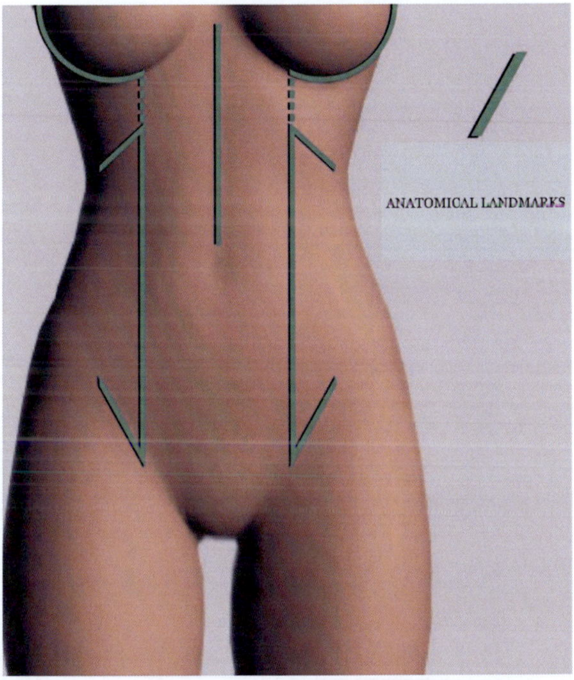

Fig. 31.3 Framing of the main anatomical lines

4. Deep extraction. The liposuction of emulsified tissue starts from the lamellar layer (deep) (Klein 1990). Follows from distal to proximal, with homogeneous fan-shaped movements. The surgeon's non-dominant hand remains flat and open by performing pressure movement perpendicular to the extraction point (Massignan 2018; Illouz 1992). The choice of the diameter of the cannulas and

their curvatures are selected according to the anatomical unit. During the approach of the lamellar layer, the extraction must be homogeneous (Juma et al. 2021; Rohrich et al. 1998; Illouz 1992).

5. Surface extraction. The liposuction in the emulsified compartment in the superficial planes of the subcutaneous cellular tissue (areolar) should be cautious and restricted in the marking areas for three-dimensional liposculpture (negative spaces) (Massignan 2018; Hoyos and Millard 2007). This care is very important to maintain the expected three-dimensional relief.

   The control of the cannula by the surgeon requires attention and precision in order to maintain parallel movement in relation to the skin plane; this prevents damage to superficial fascial planes, vascular interconnections (Camper, Scarpa), and subdermal plexus (Berkenstein and Grotting 2000). Cannulas should be selected according to their thickness (number 3) and curvatures respecting the anatomical unit to be carved.

6. Aspiration of negative spaces. Just as the artist sculpts and cuts the relief on an object of interest, strategically removing structural content to create three-dimensional shapes, the surgeon faithfully addresses subcutaneous cellular tissue in areas of transitions between the underlying muscle groups (Schider 1957). Negative spaces are the areas that both lamellar and areolar layers are handled in order to generate from them a deep relief effect (Massignan 2018; Hoyos and Millard 2007). And from them, a gradual tonal skin progression effect occurs in the negative spaces. This phenomenon can be understood with a gradual increase of tissue thickness begin in the shaded area until the topografy reflect light (Stosich and Mao 2007). This surgical maneuver is performed treating the region of interest from three skin accesses (Massignan 2018) (Fig. 31.4).

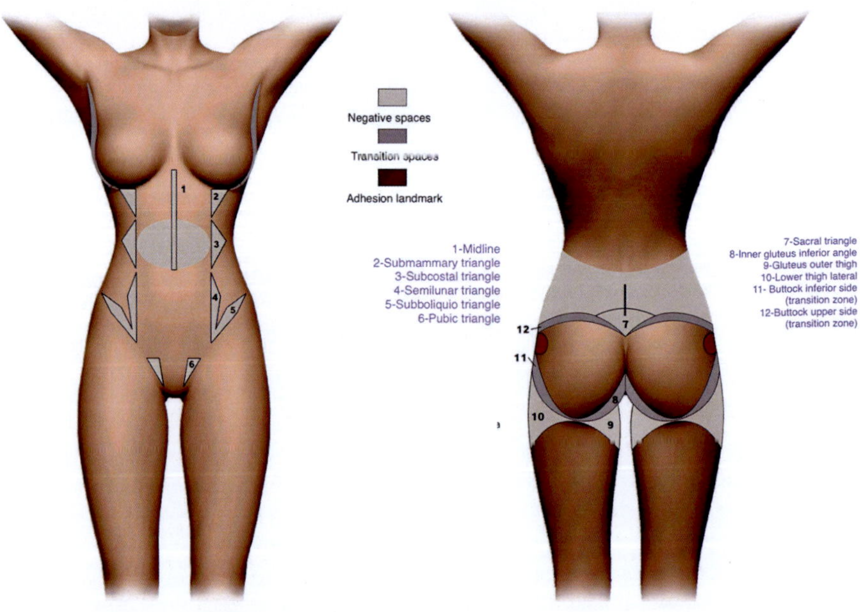

Fig. 31.4 Delimitation of negative spaces

Critical Vision

The learning curve seems to extend further and further as plastic surgeons delight in three-dimensional precision liposuction (Jewell et al. 2002; Rohrich et al. 1998). This point deserves special attention, because technical education must be improved at the same speed.

There is a growing progress in the surgical field and, consequently, its translation into results. Simultaneously, new obstacles arise, sometimes in search of even more refined standards, sometimes in the difficulty of keeping clear the foundations that shape this surgical variable to young professionals. Factors such as age, gender, surface tissue quality, and patient expectations will always be included in the context (Hoyos and Millard 2007).

Currently, the reliable anatomical relief is being reproduced in topographic extensions that extend from the posterior cervical region to the distal region of the lower limbs (Cimino and Bond 1996). Some topographies—due to their design—are still challenging to be sculpted, for example, the intersections of the with external oblique muscle, the geometric shapes formed in the movement of the scapulae, and the asymmetries of the deltoid muscle in mesomorphic patients.

The insertion of an artistic anatomy in the routines of plastic surgery (Massignan 2018), such as preoperative markings following precepts from centuries-old sculpture schools, and the proficient increase in surgical complexity and—consequently—the quality of the result offered to patients are considered enriching points in this field. Remember that the line between "beautiful" and "distorted" is tenuous (Massignan 2018). Therefore, the probability of inadequacies is predictable in young surgeons (Ince et al. 2019). Standardized algorithms would be a smart maturing formula for professionals and, in the same way, of protection in safety and quality of this new surgical line (Ince et al. 2019).

Future Perspectives

Body contour surgery is an area of plastic surgery that allows harmonic angulation between topographic units. Technological evolution is inserted to assist both in the aesthetic result and in patient safety.

The recent introduction of technologies such as radiofrequency devices (RF) (e.g., Renuvion®, BodyTite®, etc.) helps to improve the results of the procedure making pathologies such as fibrosis, cellulite, and "cutis marmorata" less complex in its treatment. Moreover, they decrease the rate of some complications (seroma, burns, bleeding, etc.). However, there is still insufficient research data for a definitive conclusion.

It is believed that the evolution will provide new horizons in the plastic surgery area. Art, technology, security, and tissue manipulation will be topics in development to the conceptual limit. In a futurology exercise, microinvasive surgery will be the next foundation of the set mentioned above, making possible the moment when fat removal will be performed in multiple sessions with minimal injury and morbidity to the patient, resulting in a gradual decrease in adipose deposits. Similarly, progressive body contour modeling will be millimeter, as well as sculptors carve marble or painters paint their canvases (Figs. 31.5, 31.6, 31.7, 31.8, 31.9, 31.10, and 31.11).

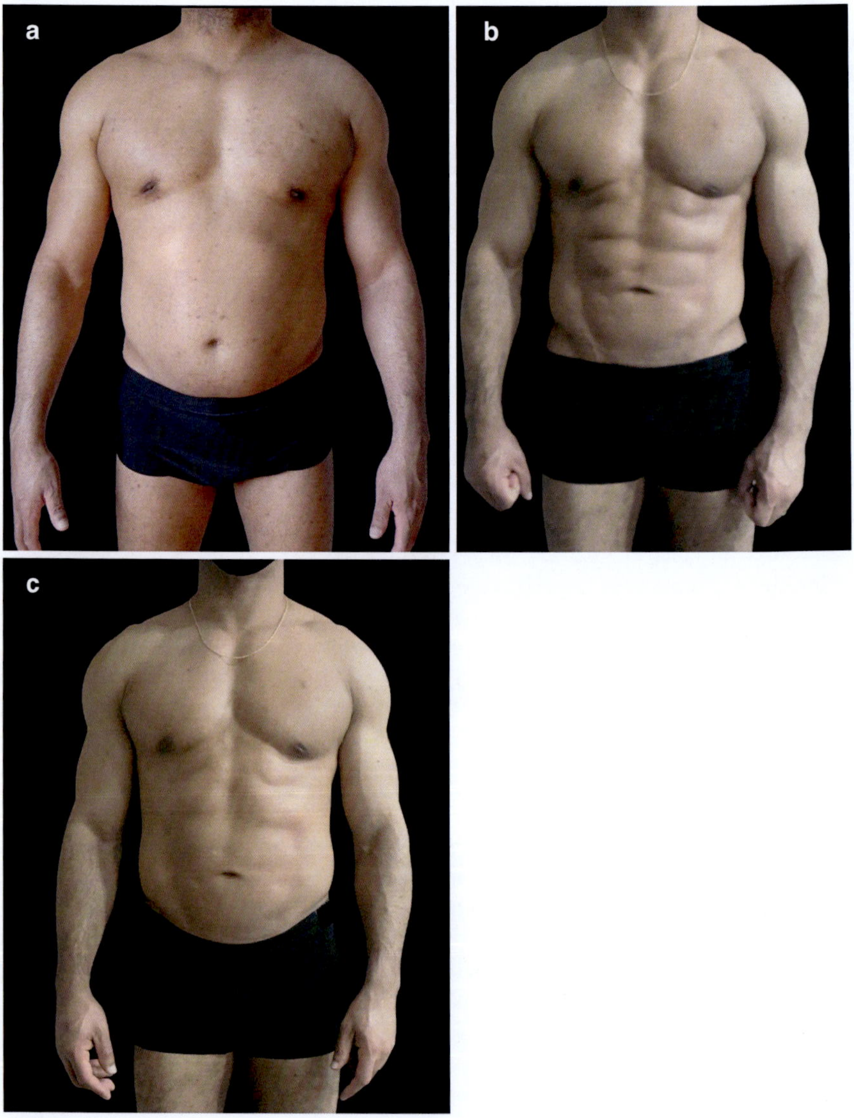

Fig. 31.5 A 43-year-old male patient, preoperative (**a**) and 1 year later in the postoperative period (**b**) with the muscle relaxed (static) and (**c**) with the muscle contracted (dynamic)

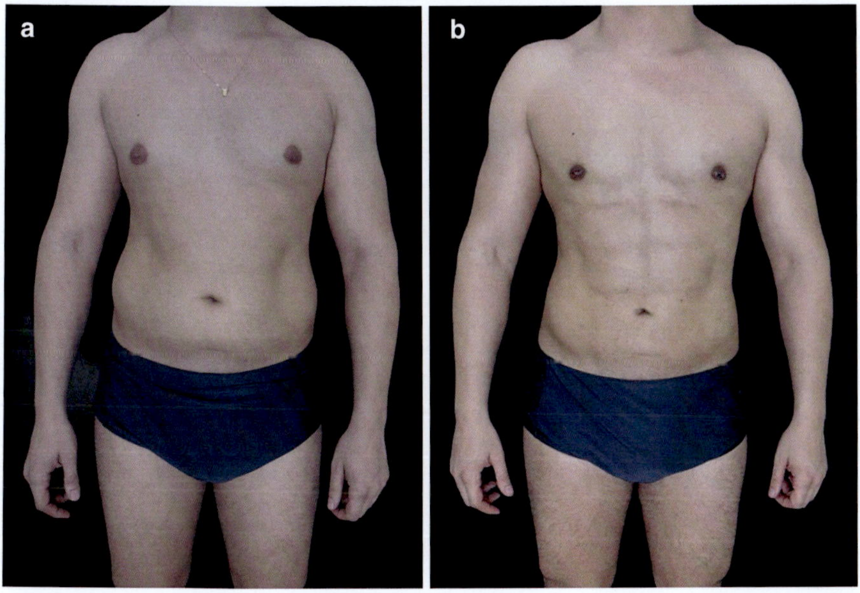

Fig. 31.6 A 26-year-old male patient with high-definition liposculpture preoperatively (**a**) and 4 months postoperatively (**b**)

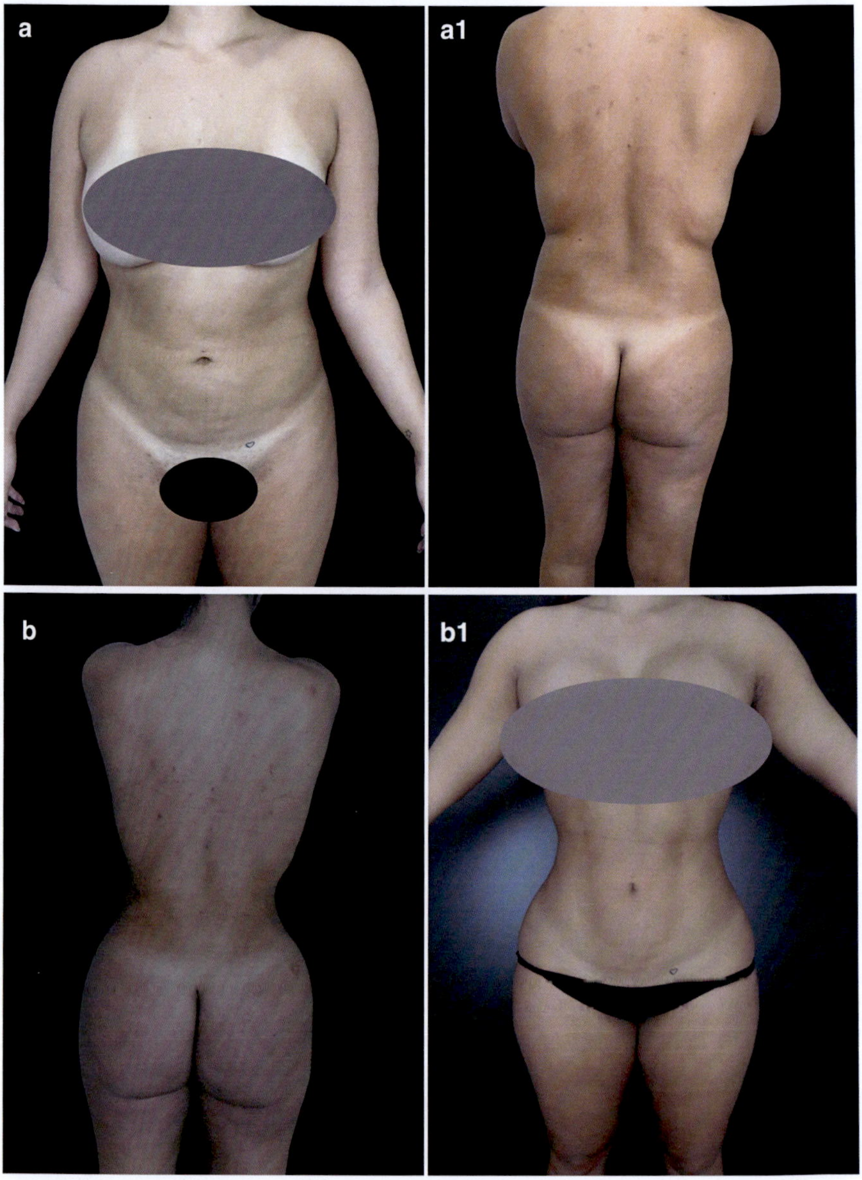

Fig. 31.7 A 25-year-old female patient with previous liposuction and overweight in the preoperative period of high-definition liposculpture. Preoperative (**a**, **a**.1) and 6 months postoperatively (**b**, **b**1)

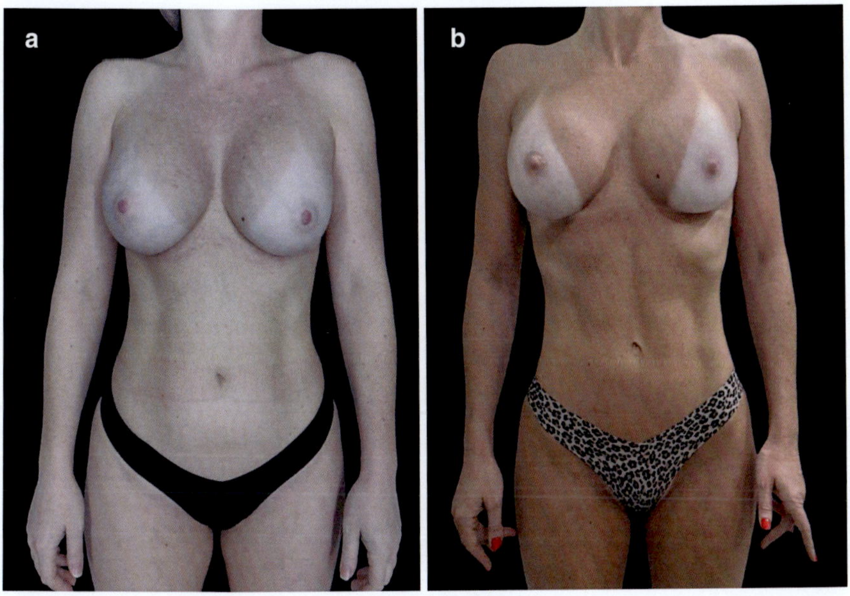

Fig. 31.8 A 36-year-old female patient with high-definition liposuction. Preoperative (**a**) and 1 year postoperatively (**b**)

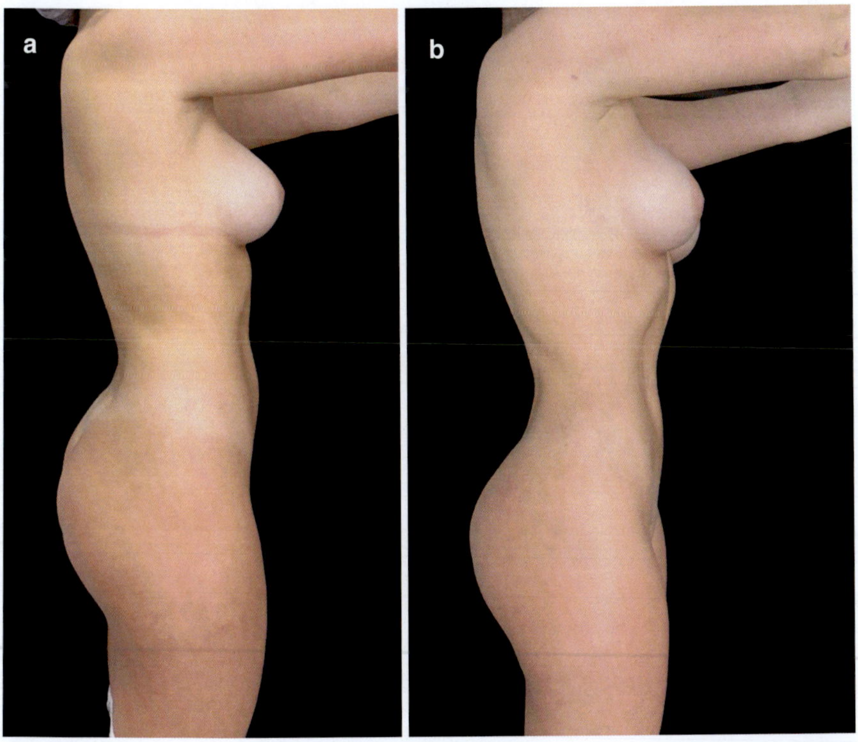

Fig. 31.9 A 23-year-old female patient with high-definition liposuction. Preoperative (**a**) and 6 months postoperatively (**b**) in profile position

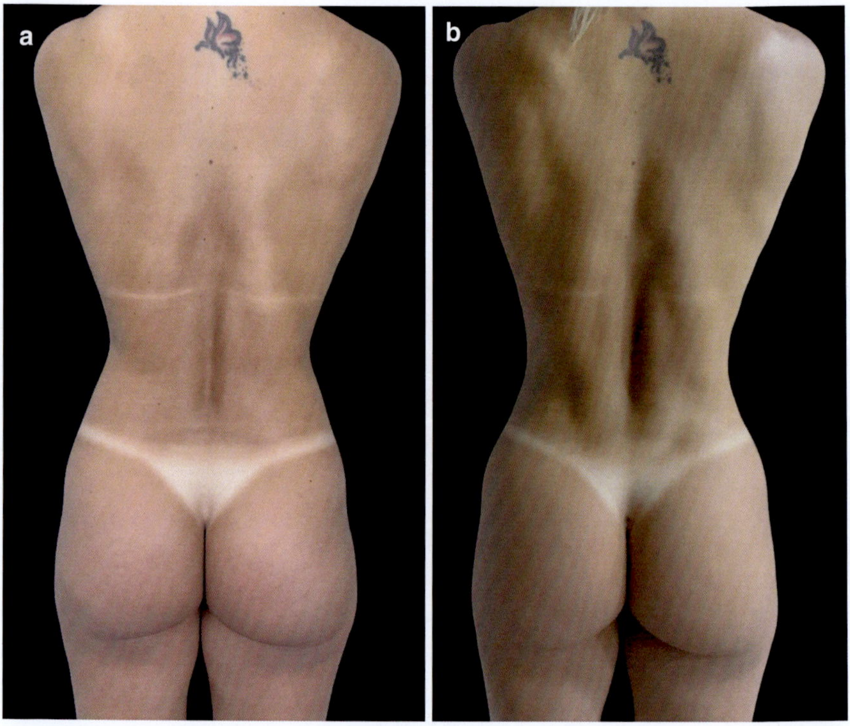

Fig. 31.10 A 33-year-old female patient with high-definition liposuction. Preoperative (**a**) and 6 months postoperatively (**b**) showing the three dimensionality of the back

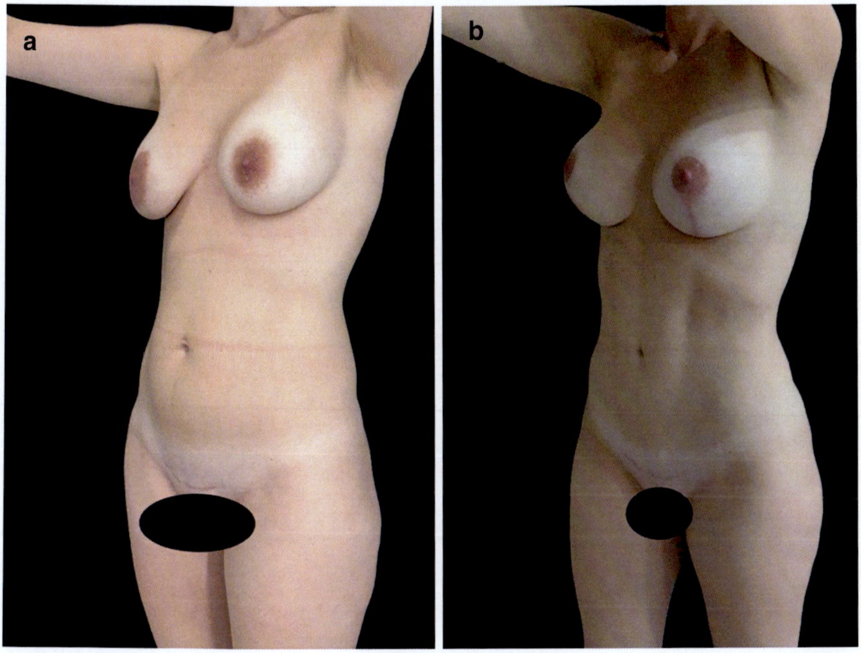

Fig. 31.11 A 39-year-old female patient with high-definition liposuction. Preoperative (**a**) and 1 year later postoperatively (**b**) showing a delicate abdominal relief

References

Schider, F. An Atlas of Anatomy for Artists. Dover Publications 1957; New York, N.Y.

Massignan, F. Safety Evolution Of "Vaser" in Body Contour Surgeries. 2018.

Avelar J (1989) Regional distribution and behavior of the subcutaneous tissue concerning selection and indication for liposuction. Aesthetic Plast Surg 3:155–165.

Pereira LH, Radwansky H. Fat grafting of the buttock and lower limbs. Aesthetic Plast Surg. 1996;20:409.

Hoyos AE, Millard JA. Vaser-assisted high definition lipoplasty. Aesthetic Surg J. 2007;27: 594-604.

Jewell, Mark L. Ultrasonic-Assisted Liposuction: Introduction and Historic Perspectives. In: Ultrasound-Assisted Liposuction: Current Concepts and Techniques. Garcia Jr. O. (Ed). Springer: LOCAL, ANO. 2020.

Jewell ML, Fodor PB, de Souza Pinto EB, Al Shammari MA (2002) Clinical application of VASER-assisted lipoplasty: a pilot clinical study. Aesthet Surg J 22(2):131–146.

The Safe Evolution of Liposuction into Liposculpture https://doi.org/10.5772/intechopen.9735. Ali Juma, Jamil Hayek and Simon Davies, 2021.

Nagy MW, Vanek PF Jr (2012) A multicenter, prospective, randomized, single- blind, controlled clinical trial comparing VASER-assisted lipoplasty and suction- assisted lipoplasty. Plast Reconstr Surg 129(4):681e–689e.

Bilsev Ince, Pembe Oltulu, Mehmet Emin Cem Yildirim, Majid Ismayilzade & Mehmet Dadaci (2019) Effects of aspiration time on immediate viability of adipocyte cell in ultrasound-assisted liposuction (UAL) and in traditional suction- assisted lipectomy (SAL), Journal of Plastic Surgery and Hand Surgery, 53:1, 14–19. https://doi.org/10.1080/2000656X.2018.1515770.

Adipose Tissue Engineering from Human Adult Stem Cells: Clinical Implications in Plastic and Reconstructive Surgery Michael S. Stosich, M.S. Jeremy J. Mao, D.D.S., Ph.D. New York, N.Y. Plast. Reconstr. Surg. 119: 71, 2007.

Rohrich RJ, Beran SJ, Kenkel JM, Adams WPJ, DiSpaltro F. Extending the role of liposuction in body contouring with ultrasound-assisted liposuction. Plast Reconstr Surg. 1998;101:1090–1102; discussion.

Klein JA. Tumescent technique for regional anesthesia permits lidocaine doses of 35 mg/kg for liposuction. J Dermatol Surg Oncol. 1990;16(3):248-263.

Cimino WW, Bond LJ. Physics of ultrasound surgery using tissue fragmentation: part I. Ultrasound Med Biol. 1996;22:89-100.

Berkenstein MS, Grotting JC. Ultrasound-assisted lipectomy using the solid probe: a retrospective review of 100 consecutive cases. Plast Reconstr Surg. 2000;105:2161–2174; discussion 2175.

Illouz YG. A new safe and aesthetic approach to suction abdominoplasty. Aesthetic Plast Surg. 1992;16(3):237-245.

Chapter 32
Numerical Methodology for Evaluation of Results in Liposuction

Ronan Horta de Almeida, André Villani Correa Mafra, Gnana Keith Marques de Araujo, and Huberth André Vieira Zuba

Abstract Liposuction was first described by Gerard Illouz in 1977. Its use to aspirate grease in the subcutaneous lamellar layer became the standard method to treat lipodystrophy. Illouz used the infiltrative technique with a subcutaneous infiltration of solution in the subcutaneous tissues before aspiration.

Introduction

Liposuction was first described by Gerard Illouz in 1977 (Souza Pinto et al. 2005; Toledo and Giovannetti 2003). Its use to aspirate grease in the subcutaneous lamellar layer became the standard method to treat lipodystrophy (Toledo and Giovannetti 2003; Coleman 2000; Pollack 1999; Illouz 1998, 2006; Hunstad and Aitken 2006).

R. H. de Almeida (✉) · A. V. C. Mafra
Preceptor of the Education and Training Center in Plastic Surgery, Mater Dei Hospital, Belo Horizonte, MG, Brazil

Brazilian Society of Plastic Surgery, São Paulo, Brazil

Mater Dei Hospital, Belo Horizonte, MG, Brazil
e-mail: ronan@ronanhorta.com.br

G. K. M. de Araujo
Brazilian Society of Plastic Surgery, São Paulo, Brazil

Mater Dei Hospital, Belo Horizonte, MG, Brazil

Faculty of Medicine, UFMG, Belo Horizonte, MG, Brazil

H. A. V. Zuba
Education and Training Center in Plastic Surgery, Mater Dei Hospital, Belo Horizonte, MG, Brazil

J. M. Avelar, R. Cavalcanti Ribeiro (eds.), *Body Contouring*,
https://doi.org/10.1007/978-3-031-42802-9_32

Illouz (1998) used the infiltrative technique with a subcutaneous infiltration of solution in the subcutaneous tissues before aspiration (Illouz 1998).

Liposuction became a consecrated method in the Brazilian plastic surgeon's therapeutical repertoire after the Brazilian congress in Fortaleza in 1980, when Illouz made its first presentation for the national community (Illouz 1998). Since 1980, some modifications have been proposed. In 1982, we had the advent of superficial liposuction. At the end of the 1980s, Zocchi introduced ultrasonic liposuction with unfavorable results, such as burning, difficulty in the control of edema, seroma, necrosis, and other complications, which discouraged the use of the new technique. Dr. Baroudi and Dr. Fournier reported that the dry technique reduced the surgical time and caused fewer distortions in the tissues but with a higher bleeding incidence. In the middle of the 1990s, Gross used oscillating devices to create his technique, so-called powered lipoplasty (Toledo and Giovannetti 2003).

However, the amplitude of areas to be treated sometimes makes it difficult to evaluate the perioperative results (Chang 2004). Translating the liposuction results into numbers yields a less-subjective demonstration.

Anatomic and Physiologic Considerations

Subcutaneous tissue is divided into two layers: the superficial areolar one and the lamellar or reticular one, located deeper. The two layers are separated by the fascia superficialis. The areolar layer contains voluminous turgid fat cells, while the lamellar one is formed by smaller, horizontally elongated cells with lower interior contents (Avelar and Illouz 1986; Duarte and Castellani 2002). The adipocytes in the lamellar layer are mainly responsible for the hypertrophy and increase in thickness in the fat tissue in that they are able to expand their original volume up to 100 times (Avelar and Illouz 1986; Duarte and Castellani 2002). Areolar adipocytes exhibit minor modifications.

Subcutaneous tissue presents noticeable differences in diverse corporal areas of obese individuals. Regions where skin is thicker and firm, such as the thorax, have greater development of the areolar layer with a thinner lamellar layer. Thus, we consider the cutaneous fold measure of this area a result reference for the areas submitted to liposuction.

Methods

The initial assessments of a patient, including a solid anamnesis, an evaluation of the patient's objectives and expectations, and a detailed physical examination, are fundamental. Whether the patient is suitable for liposuction surgery should be evaluated, checking comorbidities, smoking status, and nutritional status, among others. An ideal candidate for liposuction does not smoke and has a Body Mass Index (BMI) < 30, because they would use few medications and would have few comorbidities with good control. Patients who do not follow this pattern should receive a mistrial assessment with a risk stratification and an evaluation from the anesthesiologist to predict whether they are an eligible patient for surgical treatment (Mendez et al. 2019).

The surgeon is responsible for realistically reporting the results according to the patient's body. It is also important to inform the patient about the risks and complications and to educate them to prevent confusion and misunderstandings. Thus, the photographic record is an ally in the documentation and concrete evaluation of results after surgery. This record clarifies the level of outcome and the change undergone by the patient (Mendez et al. 2019).

Physical examination is another important part in surgical planning and predicting favorable and unfavorable results. The BMI calculation should be obtained upon examination. And having the patient stand in front of a mirror reveals six key elements: areas of concern for lipodystrophy and contour deformities, skin tone and skin quality, asymmetries, cellulite and dimpling, myofascial support and laxity, and zones of adherence (Mendez et al. 2019). In addition to these described above, another element that can help predict results is measuring skinfolds, as we will discuss in this chapter.

Complementary Techniques to Liposuction

Several devices on the market improve the liposuction technique by helping the surgeon perform their maneuvers or by enhancing the aesthetics of the surgical results. Collins (Collins and Moyer 2018) describes tumescent suction-assisted liposuction (SAL) with or without power assistance, laser-assisted liposuction (LAL), and ultrasound-assisted liposuction (UAL) as the most popular techniques (Collins and Moyer 2018).

The power-assisted liposuction technique provides reciprocating motion to the cannula, facilitates the removal of adipose tissue, and reduces operator fatigue (Chia et al. 2017). The laser-assisted liposuction technique promotes the coagulation of small blood vessels, the rupture of adipocytes, the reorganization of the reticular dermis, and the coagulation of collagen in fat tissues with various types of wavelengths (Chia et al. 2017). It has better results in the submental region, improving skin retraction. Studies have suggested that it may help decrease the overall operative blood loss in high-volume liposuction. The ultrasound-assisted liposuction technique uses sound energy at resonance with vibration. Its advantage is based on improving fat viability and retention in autologous fat transfer (Chia et al. 2017). There is evidence of benefits in the treatment of the dense glandular tissue in gynecomastia. Besides that, seroma rates are higher, and the benefits did not improve patient satisfaction, swelling, or bruising. Compared with the SAL technique, the results are controversial in terms of outcomes and long-term complications (Collins and Moyer 2018). Radiofrequency-assisted liposuction allows for the use of energy in the subcutaneous tissues without compromising the skin, aiding in tissue contraction. Studies have shown good results, with linear tissue contraction in the postoperative period (Chia et al. 2017). Finally, water-assisted liposuction uses pulsating solution jets with simultaneous aspiration. One study has shown better weight retention, less apoptosis, and greater angiogenesis (Chia et al. 2017).

The use of energy devices improves efficiency; however, they come with various complications, such as thermal injury, seroma, deformities, irregularities, and contractures. These may be associated with excessive use and the inexperience of the surgeon (Collins and Moyer 2018).

Method for the Thickness of the Cutaneous Fold

Using an adipometer or bidigital maneuver with a ruler, we measure the thickness of the cutaneous fold in the medium-axillary line between the nineth and tenth ribs (Fig. 32.1). We measure the areas to be treated by using the same methodology, and we show the differences to the patient. Anatomical guidance points for measuring the treatment areas are the linea alba above the umbilical of the superior abdomen, an imaginary line over the rectus abdominis muscles for the inferior abdomen, the iliac crests and their tubercles for the flanks, and the infrascapular area perpendicular to the latissimus dorsi muscle fibers for the dorsum. Another preoperative aspect observed is the presence of corporal contour asymmetries in the quantitative demonstration to the patient. We write down all the collected values in the patient's record for posterior comparison and then photograph the patient.

The patient is submitted to the preoperative delimitation of the area to be treated and is directed to liposuction via the humid or infiltrative technique with an infiltration of 0.9% sodium chloride solution and adrenaline at a concentration of 1/500,000, under peridural anesthesia and venous sedation performed by an anesthesiologist.

During the surgical procedure, the to-be-treated areas are repeatedly measured to determine via liposuction the dimensions of its cutaneous folds to the one collected in the thoracic region of reference. The ending of the surgery is determined by the equivalence of the values. This technique avoids both underaspiration and

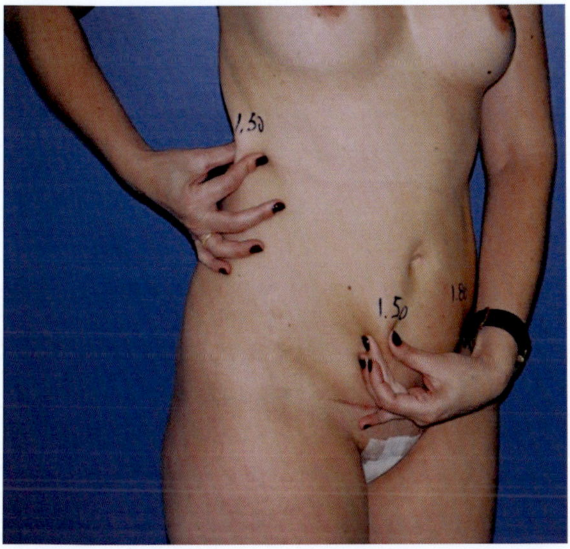

Fig. 32.1 Bidigital maneuver measure of the thickness of the cutaneous fold in the medium-axillary line and abdomen

overaspiration, thus reducing the risks of complications such as irregularities, nodules, and adherences. At one month after surgery, when approximately 80% of the edema has already regressed (Hunstad and Aitken 2006), the patient is again submitted to the measure of the cutaneous folds, and the values are compared against the preoperative data.

Results

Table 32.1 lists the preoperative and postoperative measurements in centimeters of the skinfolds of 20 patients. The mean measurements in centimeters of the skinfolds and the standard deviation for each patient were evaluated.

Table 32.1 Comparison between the standard measurements and the mean values in centimeters of the skinfolds analyzed in the study of liposuction, for each patient

	Preoperative period			Postoperative period (6 months)		
Patient	Standard[a] (cm)	Mean[b] (cm)	STDEV[c]	Standard[a] (cm)	Mean[b] (cm)	STDEV[c]
1	1.0	3.75	1.66	1.4	1.95	0.77
2	1.7	3.45	2.02	1.2	1.77	0.42
3	1.2	3.70	1.69	0.7	1.54	0.62
4	1.3	4.42	2.02	X	2.02	0.79
5	2.0	5.36	2.25	2.3	2.65	0.62
6	0.9	3.27	1.51	X	2.26	0.34
7	1.1	2.9	1.33	1.9	2.1	0.63
8	1.5	3.16	1.00	1.6	2.22	0.50
9	2.0	3.56	1.54	2.0	2.28	0.34
10	2.3	3.56	1.28	1.5	1.87	0.65
11	1.2	4.05	1.94	1.1	2.1	0.73
12	1.0	3.2	1.4	1.0	1.74	0.8
13	2	4.05	1.41	1.6	2.22	0.54
14	2.5	5	1.88	2	2.23	0.39
15	1.5	4.68	2.68	1.8	2.5	0.55
16	0.8	3.07	1.73	1	1.9	0.55
17	1.2	4.73	2.72	1	1.55	0.64
18	1.2	4.02	2.06	1.2	1.85	0.52
19	1.7	3.18	1.67	1.5	1.7	0.47
20	x	4.25	1.77	1	2	1
Mean//STDEV		386	0.69		2.02	0.29

[a] Standard: measured in centimeters from the skinfold corresponding to the medium-axillary line, between the ninth and tenth ribs

[b] Mean: arithmetic mean among all measurements, in centimeters, for each patient

[c] STDEV: standard deviation. The standard deviation is calculated by using the n-1 equation. Finally, x is the sample mean of the data studied (value 1, value 2, etc.), and n is the sample size.

This function uses the following formula: $\sqrt{\sum \frac{(x-\bar{x})^2}{(n-1)}}$

Discussion

Ilouz (Illouz 1998) reported that complications in liposuction are divided into two parts. The first one includes surgical and systemic alterations and complications that continue in the traditional technique (Illouz 1998). The second one includes unfavorable results and sequels, which are numerous and complex (Illouz 2006).

Patients want the best possible results from plastic surgery (Augustin et al. 1999). Subjective evaluations can lead to conflicting impressions between the surgeon and the patient. The use of a quantitative method for analysis makes a more-objective demonstration of the surgery results possible.

The method of measuring the skinfolds can be used during surgery to note thickness references for the abdominal and flank cutaneous folds after liposuction. Another advantage of the here-described method is its ease in demonstrating the eventual occurrence of ponderal gain with the increase in the subcutaneous tissue through the comparison of the measures in the immediate and late postoperative periods.

We have used this method in our service for the past 4 years with easy execution, at low cost, and with satisfactory results. The method is safer for plastic surgeons because it reduces conflicts and improves doctor–patient relationships (Figs. 32.2, 32.3, and 32.4).

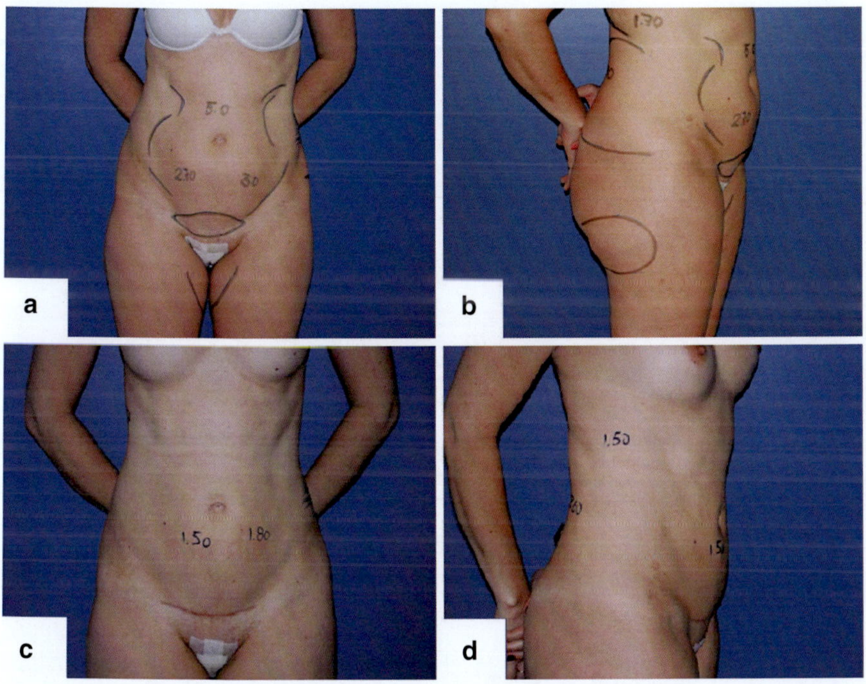

Fig. 32.2 (**a**) Treatment areas in the abdomen. Pleat measurements of the skin in the preoperative period. Front position (front view). (**b**) Treatment areas on the abdomen. Preoperative skinfold measurements (oblique view). (**c**) Treatment areas in the abdomen. Pleat measurements of the skin in the postoperative period. Front position (front view). (**d**) Treatment areas on the abdomen. Postoperative skinfold measurements (oblique view)

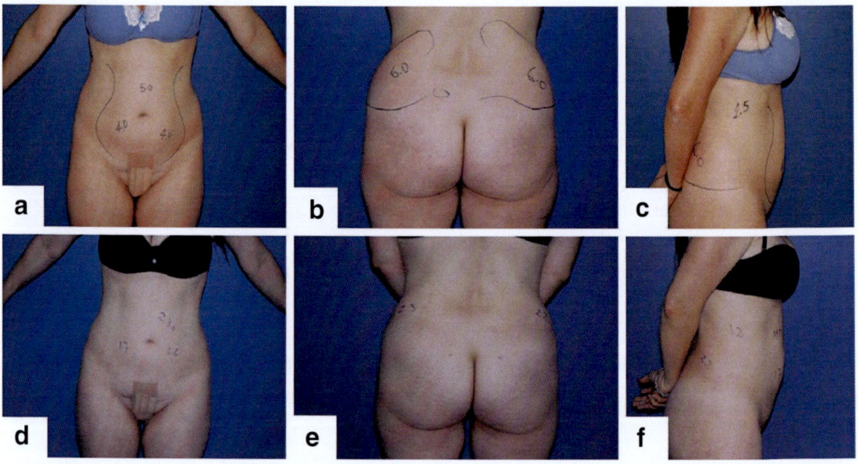

Fig. 32.3 (**a**) Treatment areas in the abdomen. Pleat measurements of the skin in the preoperative period. Front position (front view). (**b**) Treatment areas on the back. Preoperative skinfold measurements (rear view). (**c**) Treatment areas in the abdomen. Skinfold measurements in the preoperative period (profile view). (**d**) Treatment areas in the abdomen. Pleat measurements of the skin in the postoperative period. Front position (front view). (**e**) Treatment areas on the back. Postoperative skinfold measurements (rear view). (**f**) Treatment areas in the abdomen. Skinfold measurements in the postoperative period (profile view)

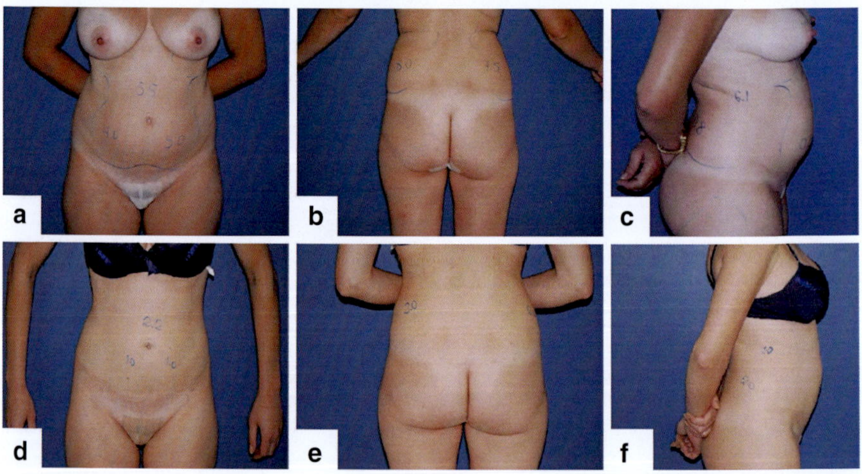

Fig. 32.4 (**a**) Treatment areas in the abdomen. Pleat measurements of the skin in the preoperative period. Front position (front view). (**b**) Treatment areas on the back. Preoperative skinfold measurements (rear view). (**c**) Treatment areas in the abdomen. Skinfold measurements in the preoperative period (profile view). (**d**) Treatment areas in the abdomen. Pleat measurements of the skin in the postoperative period. Front position (front view). (**e**) Treatment areas on the back. Postoperative skinfold measurements (rear view). (**f**) Treatment areas in the abdomen. Skinfold measurements in the postoperative period (profile view)

Summary

Liposuction is the standard method for lipodystrophy treatment. However, the amplitude of areas to be treated sometimes makes it difficult to evaluate the perioperative results. Measuring the skinfolds is anatomical work that allows for making pre-established mathematical comparisons for the patient. By applying this study method, surgeons can make more-objective demonstrations and exert a higher level of perioperative control over liposuction, which are associated with reducing patient complaints, asymmetries, and levels of hypocorrection in their respective treatment areas.

References

Souza Pinto EB, Abdalla PCSP, Maciel CM (2005). História da lipoaspiração. In: Carrerão S, Cardim V, Goldenberg D, eds. Cirurgia Plástica. São Paulo: Atheneu; cap.6.

Toledo LS, Giovannetti M (2003). Lipoaspiração e lipoenxertia nas deformidades do abdômen, dorso e flancos. In: Mélega JM, ed. Cirurgia Plástica: fundamentos e arte - cirurgia estética. Rio de Janeiro: Medsi. p.629-38.

Coleman WP (2000) 3rd. Powered liposuction. Dermatol Surg.; 26(4):315-8.

Pollack SV (1999). Liposuction of the abdomen. The basics. Dermatol Clin. 17(4):823-34.

Illouz YG (2006). Complications of liposuction. Clin Plast Surg. ;33(1): 129-63.

Illouz YG (1998). Lipesculpture et chirurgie de la silhouette. Chirurgie plastique reconstructrice et esthétique. Encycl Med Chir Edidions Scientifiques et Médicales. Paris: Elsevier. p.45-120.

Hunstad JP, Aitken ME (2006). Liposuction: techniques and guidelines. Clin Plast Surg. ;33(1):13-25.

Chang KN (2004). The use of intraoperative grid pattern markings in lipoplasty. Plast Reconstr Surg.;114(5):1292-7.

Avelar J, Illouz YG (1986) Anatomia cirúrgica e distribuição do tecido celular no organismo humano. In: Lipoaspiração. Rio de Janeiro:Hipocrates; p.45-57.

Duarte AC, Castellani FR (2002). Medidas antropométricas. In: Semiologia nutricional. São Paulo: Axcel Books do Brasil; p.34-57.

Mendez BM, Coleman JE, Kenkel JM (2019). Optimizing Patient Outcomes and Safety With Liposuction. Aesthet Surg J.; 39(1):66-82. doi: https://doi.org/10.1093/asj/sjy151.

Collins PS, Moyer KE (2018). Evidence-Based Practice in Liposuction. Ann Plast Surg.; 80 (6S Suppl 6): S403-S405. doi: https://doi.org/10.1097/SAP.0000000000001325.

Chia CT, Neinstein RM, Theodorou SJ (2017). Evidence-Based Medicine: Liposuction. Plast Reconstr Surg.; 139(1):267e-274e. doi: https://doi.org/10.1097/PRS.0000000000002859.

Augustin M, Zschocke I, Sommer B, Sattler G (1999). Sociodemographic profile and satisfaction with treatment of patients undergoing liposuction in tumescent local anesthesia. Dermatol Surg; 25(6):480-3.

Chapter 33
Laser Lipolysis: Skin Tightening in Lipoplasty Using HPL Dual Diode Laser

Moisés Wolfenson, Lydia Massako Ferreira, Joaquim Figueiredo, and Bruna Alves

Abstract **Background**: To present the changes in the dimension of the skin, obeying the safety parameters related to the energy accumulated in laser lipolysis procedures in different anatomical regions, using a double-wavelength diode laser device (924 and 975 nm).

Method: A prospective, cross-sectional case series study included 552 patients submitted to laser lipolysis for the treatment of facial and body contouring deformities between June 2008 and June 2019. Laser lipolysis was performed with a diode laser device with two independently controlled wavelengths, one of them operating at 924 nm and the other at 975 nm, using tips of three sizes according to suitability for small, medium, or large areas of treated adipose tissue. The measurements were compared using the Wilcoxon test, at a significance level of 0.05. The most important retractions occurred at the waist circumference, at the level of the umbilical scar—measured with a tape measure before and 90 days after the laser—and the second largest retraction at submental region: measured by parking meter in lines L2 and L3, before the application of double laser and after 90 days.

Results: In all these patients, there was significant skin retraction regardless of the surgical site (face, breast adiposity, arms, or waist), and the only complications that existed were erythema and edema that disappeared within 30 days after the laser.

Conclusion: The diode laser proved to be able to promote progressive and persistent skin retraction, obeying the proposed safety parameter.

Keywords Lipectomy/methods · Laser therapy · Plastic surgery

M. Wolfenson (✉)
Avenida Boa Viagem, Recife, PE, Brazil

L. M. Ferreira · J. Figueiredo · B. Alves
São Paulo, Brazil

J. M. Avelar, R. Cavalcanti Ribeiro (eds.), *Body Contouring*,
https://doi.org/10.1007/978-3-031-42802-9_33

Introduction

Almost all people have a body contour imperfection or deformity that causes discomfort or embarrassment. These deformities may result from normal and inevitable physiologic changes, such as those associated with repeated weight loss, localized fat deposits, and aging laxity. Other deformities may be associated with cosmetic failure of corrective procedures, such as conventional liposuction, plastic procedures, or augmentation lipoplasty.

Until recently, lipoplasty was commonly associated with postoperative complications, including bruising, decreased hematocrit resulting from significant blood loss, scarring caused by cannula insertion and friction with the skin that may be difficult or impossible to correct, or even sequelae such as changes in skin texture and skin waviness, among others (Triana et al. 2009). These complications were a challenge to plastic surgeons and served as a stimulus for the development of devices that allow partial or even total correction of skin deformities and body contour and that have become increasingly safe. At present, laser lipolysis may be performed using a dual-wavelength diode laser to facilitate liposuction by nonaggressive techniques.

The photothermal effect of laser irradiation on the hypodermis is used for heating fat cells, leading to membrane rupture, consequent release of intracellular lipase, and fat liquefaction, which facilitates liposuction. In addition, the heating of fibrous septa and reticular dermis causes tissue thinning, leading to an improved aesthetic result. The photothermal properties of the laser light may also be applied for cauterizing small blood vessels, decreasing at the surgical site.

Photothermal effects have been used in the development of devices for laser lipolysis operating at different wavelengths in the range of the absorption spectra of fat, water, and other chromophore associations. The dual-wavelength diode laser is one of the devices available for lipolysis. It operates at 924 nm, which is a wavelength specific for liquefying adipose tissue, and at 975 nm, which is a wavelength that acts on collagen and elastin fibers in the deep dermis. This system preserves the epidermis, thus eliminating most risks associated with its use.

The use of devices for laser lipolysis requires attention during the surgical procedure regarding the total energy transmitted by the laser to each region of the body, the so-called cumulative energy, for the best aesthetic result by the remodeling of fibrous conjunctive tissue. The control of the cumulative energy is essential to reduce risk of complications, such as necrosis, prolonged erythema, hyperchromic skin patches, secondary bacterial infection, and dyschromia.

This topic has been studied to determine the safety parameters for preventing treatment complications. The purpose of this study was to evaluate skin tightening after laser lipolysis using a dual-wavelength laser operating at 924 and 975 nm.

Even with excellent results in skin retractions on the face and body contouring with the use of laser, for cases of excessive flaccidity, we have rhytidectomy and abdominal dermolipectomy referred to as state of the art in our study.

Patients and Methods

This prospective, cross-sectional study was approved by the Institutional Research Ethics Committee and performed in accordance with Resolution 196/96 of the Brazilian National Health Council (Conselho Nacional de Saúde) and the Brazilian Ethical Review System on Research Involving Human Beings. Written informed consent was obtained from all patients before their inclusion in the study, and anonymity was ensured.

The study was conducted between June of 2008 and July of 2019. Participants were recruited from consecutive patients meeting the study criteria referred by the Plastic Surgery Outpatient Clinic of the Federal University of Pernambuco General Hospital to the Multi-Aesthetic Clinic (Clínica Multiplástica) in Recife, Brazil, and the study was sent and approved to the CEP of UFPE (Universidade Federal de Pernambuco).

Inclusion criteria were skin laxity after plastic surgery, sequelae after primary liposuction, submental adiposity, arm adiposity, gynecomastia, and laxity in the area around the umbilicus. Exclusion criteria were previous fat grafting, laxity after bariatric surgery with indication for plastic surgery, infection in general, diagnosis of autoimmune diseases, and cancer.

The study included 552 patients. All these patients are women who used laser lipolysis for the treatment of deformities of the face and body contour with a mean age of 53.4 years (between 35 and 62 years) and a body mass index ranging from 18.5 to 24.9 kg/m^2 and were included in the study and underwent laser lipolysis to correct contour deformities.

Laser lipolysis was performed using a dual-wavelength diode laser (SlimLipo, Palomar Medical Technologies, Burlington, Mass., licensed by the US Food and Drug Administration and by the Brazilian Health Surveillance Agency) operating at two wavelengths (924 and 975 nm) independently controlled for different output powers.

Three different tip lengths (80, 180, and 280 mm) were used, allowing treatment of small (submental region), medium (brachial region), and large (flank and abdominal regions) areas of adipose tissue. Before the procedure, 10 × 10 cm areas (100 cm^2) were marked on the skin with a bright green marker (Fig. 33.1).

The circumference of each treated body region was measured carefully at three time points (preoperatively, immediately after laser lipolysis, and on postoperative day 90). For the face, three lines (lines 1, 2, and 3) were measured at the three time points. Line 1 extended from the corner of the mouth (cheilion) to the lateral palpebral commissure (exocanthion) of the same side of the face; line 2 was constructed from the central part of the chin region (mental protuberance) to the inferior insertion of the earlobe (otobasion inferius); and line 3 connected the right otobasion inferius to the left otobasion inferius, passing through the submental area (Fig. 33.2).

Photographic documentation with standardized views, taken from the same distance with the same camera (Sony Cyber-shot DSC-P10, Sony, Tokyo, Japan), was also obtained from all patients at the three time points. A total energy dose of 5 kJ

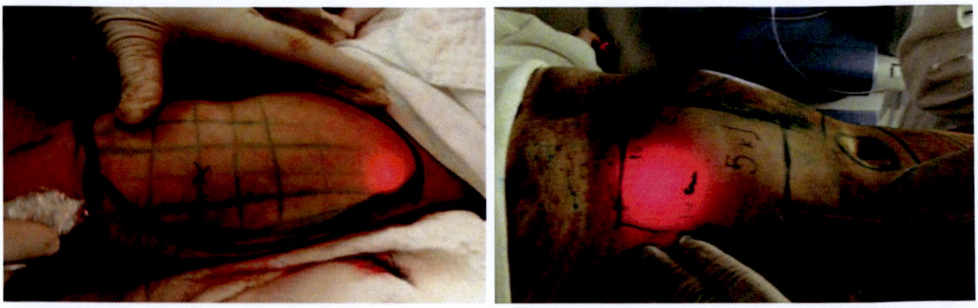

Fig. 33.1 Laser lipolysis performed in (above) the abdominal region showing one 10 × 10 cm skin area, with the diode laser programmed for a cumulative energy of 5 kJ, and (below) in a right arm marked with two 10 × 10 cm skin areas, with the diode laser programmed for a cumulative energy of 8 kJ

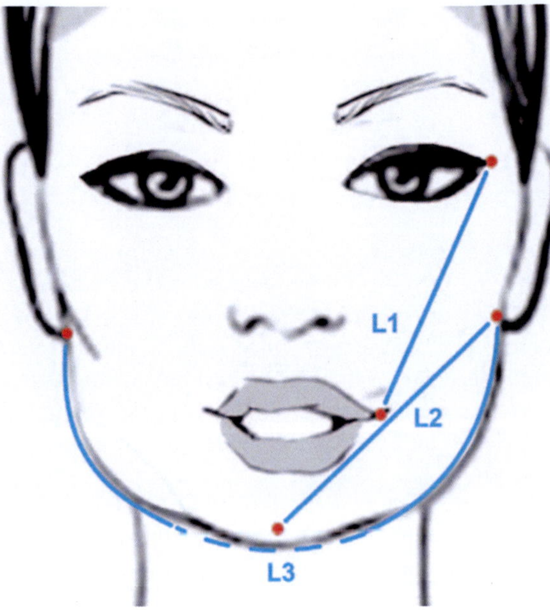

Fig. 33.2 Diagram showing the position of the lines used in measurements of the face performed preoperatively, immediately after laser lipolysis, and on postoperative day 90. *L* line

(5000 J) per 100 cm^2 skin area was used as a safety parameter to prevent treatment complications. The optimal cumulative energy, which is proportional to the contour deformity, was estimated based on the number of 10 × 10 cm skin areas within the treatment region. For example, a cumulative energy of 5 kJ would be delivered to a patient with a small brachial region (10 × 10 cm), whereas 15 kJ would be delivered to a patient with a large brachial region (10 × 30 cm), resulting in liquefaction of adipose tissue and skin tightening (Fig. 33.3).

In our sample, the patients were operated with a double diode HPL laser 924 and 975 nm, with high power and surgical laser. There were 552 female patients in 11 years, from June 2008 to June 2019. The mean age of patients is 53.4 years. 74.7%

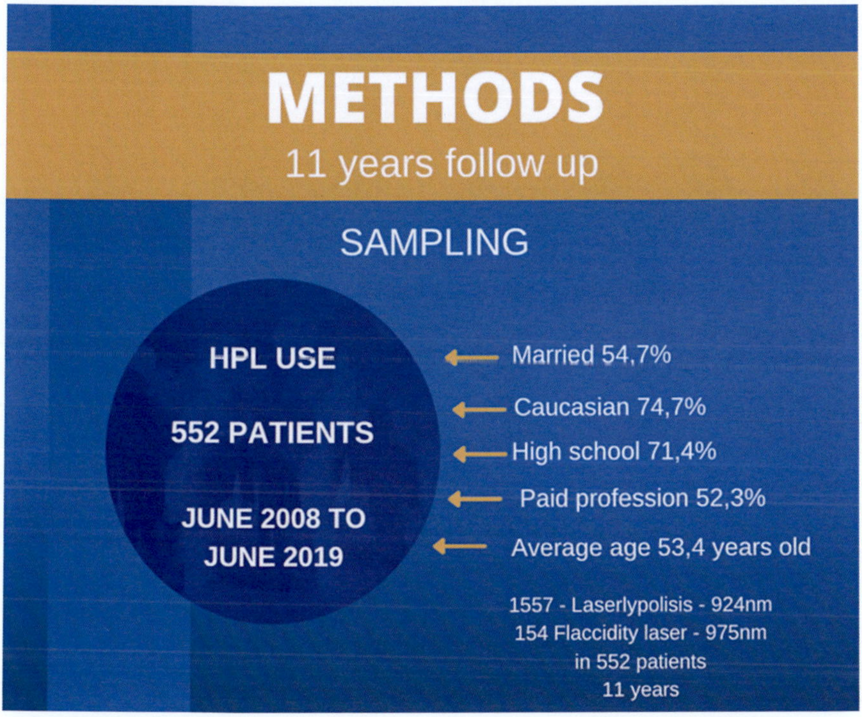

Fig. 33.3 Sampling of 552 patients, women, treated with double-wavelength diode laser—924 and 975 nm

are white and 54.7% married. In 154 patients, a laser with a wavelength of 924 nm was used to reduce sagging in the face.

Results

The distribution of the 552 patients who underwent laser lipolysis, according to the different treated body regions, is shown in Fig. 33.4. Laser lipolysis was mostly performed on the flank region, followed by the facial or submental region. Parameters such as cumulative energy, output power, and sequence of wavelengths used during laser lipolysis in the different regions of the body are listed in Table 33.1.

Measurements of the circumference of treated body regions taken preoperatively, immediately after laser lipolysis, and 90 days postoperatively are shown in Table 33.2. The results showed a progressive tightening of the skin over time at all treated sites.

Significant differences in circumference values were observed in all patients between preoperative and immediate postoperative measurements and between measurements from postoperative day 90 and both the preoperative and immediate

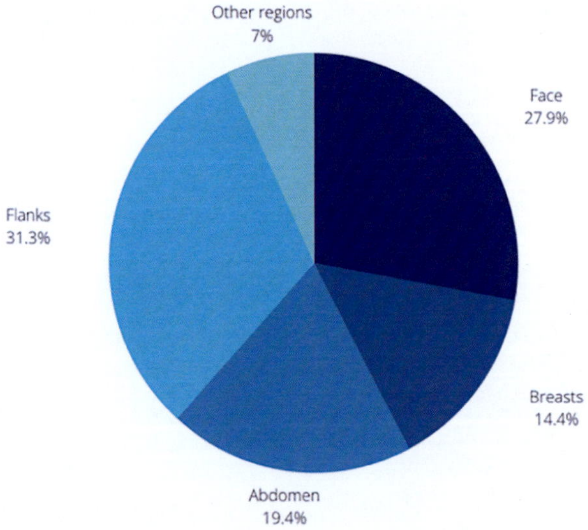

Fig. 33.4 Distribution of laser lipolysis procedures according to different body regions

Table 33.1 Parameters used in the different body regions

Body region	No. of squares (10 × 10 cm)	Cumulative Energy (kJ)	Output power (W)	Sequence of wavelengths
Face	1.4–1.6	7–8	14–16	Mixed
Arm	2	10	16–24	924 nm–mixed–975 nm
Breast	4–6	20–30	14	Mixed
Waist	12	60	24	Mixed

postoperative measurements, regardless of the body site involved ($p < 0.05$). Exceptionally, no significant differences were found between preoperative and immediate postoperative circumference measurements of the mid- and lower thirds of the left arm because skin tightening occurred late in five patients and was detected only 90 days after the surgical procedure.

Three months after laser lipolysis, the cutaneous and subcutaneous tissues appeared homogenous, the skin texture was very similar to normal skin on palpation, and a smoothing of the skin surface was observed visually, with marked improvement in adipose tissue distribution.

Photographic examples of results obtained with diode laser treatment, correcting laxity reduction with thermotherapy of face and body deformities, are shown in Figs. 33.5, 33.6, 33.7, 33.8, 33.9, and 33.10.

Table 33.2 Circumference of treated body regions at the three time points

Body regions/circumference (cm)	Preoperatively	Immediately postoperatively	90-day follow-up	*p*
Facial and submental regions				
Mean ± SD	30.00 ± 0.64	27.00 ± 0.39	23.50 ± 0.34	<0.001
95% CI	28.59–31.41	26.14–27.86	22.76–24.24	
Right aim				
Upper third				
Mean ± SD	36.43 ± 0.78	34.14 ± 0.67	32.14 ± 0.77	0.011
95% CI	34.51–38.34	32.50–35.78	30.26–34.03	
Mid third				
Mean ± SD	31.86 ± 0.86	30.43 ± 0.81	28.43 ± 0.68	0.26
95% CI	29.76–33.95	28.44–32.42	26.75–30.10	
Lower third				
Mean ± SD	29.14 ± 0.77	28.00 ± 0.69	26.14 ± 0.67	0.38
95% CI	27.26–31.03	26.31–29.69	24.50–27.78	
Left arm				
Upper third				
Mean ± SD	36.14 ± 0.99	33.64 ± 1.02	32.14 ± 0.86	0.016
95% CI	33.73–38.56	31.16–36.13	30.05–34.24	
Mid third				
Mean ± SD	31.29 ± 0.71	30.14 ± 0.80	28.57 ± 0.84	0.039
95% CI	29.54–33.03	28.19–32.10	26.51–30.63	
Lower third				
Mean ± SD	29.64 ± 0.47	29.43 ± 1.17	27.14 ± 0.86	0.018
95% CI	28.49–30.80	26.56–32.30	25.05–29.24	
Breast region				
Mean ± SD	121.11 ± 2.55	109.22 ± 2.27	99.00 – 2.09	0.008
95% CI	115.23–127.00	103.98–114.46	94.18–103.82	
Waist				
Mean ± SD	80.46 ± 2.41	74.46 ± 2.04	69.38 ± 1.88	0.001
95% CI	75.20–85.72	70.02–78.91	65.29–73.48	

Wilcoxon test ($p < 0.05$)

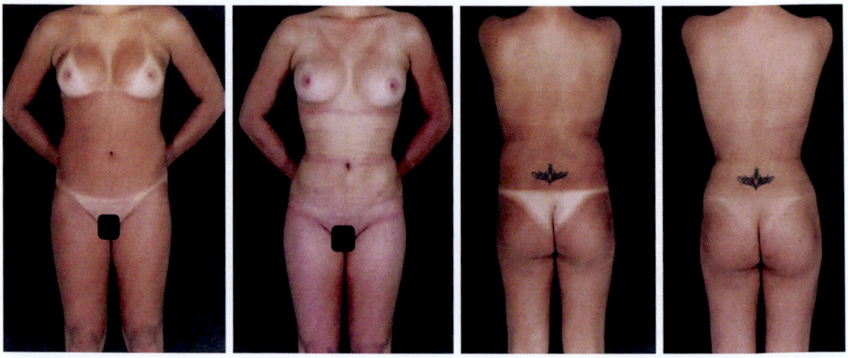

Fig. 33.5 Photographs of the same 41-year-old patient taken preoperatively (left) and 90 days postoperatively (right). The anterior views (above) show that no umbilical deformities were caused by laser lipolysis, and the posterior views (below) show the flank regions from which a lipoaspirate volume of 800 ml was removed with a cumulative energy of 30 kJ and a reduction in the waist region, corresponding to a decrease of 12 cm in the waist circumference with a total cumulative energy of 55 kJ

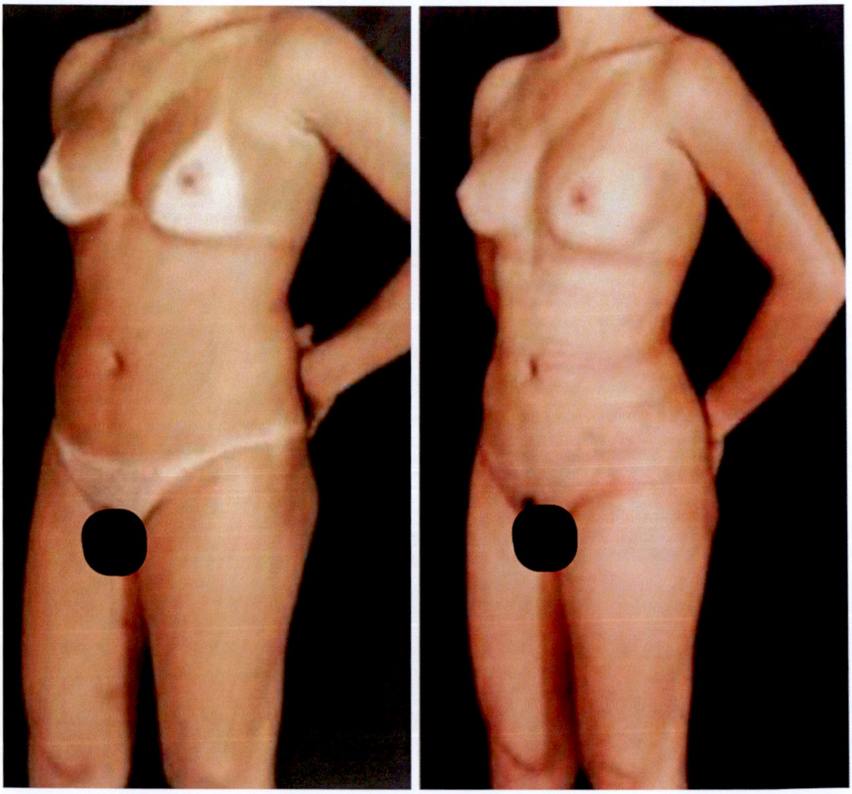

Fig. 33.6 Umbilical region. Preoperative and 90-day postoperative laser lipolysis, with removal of 800 g of adipose tissue with an accumulated energy of 30 kJ. The permanence of the belly button with its original shape is noted

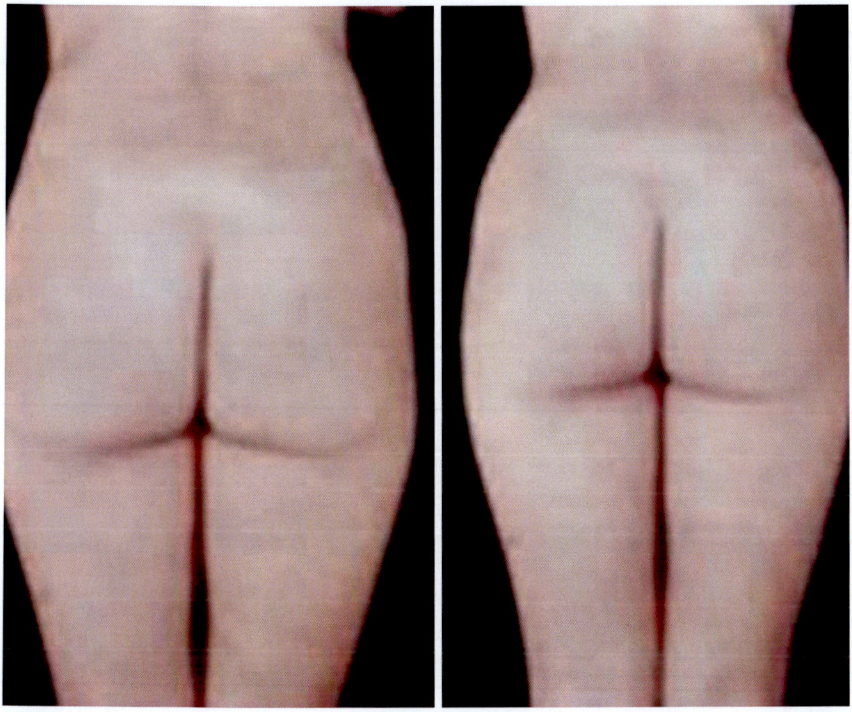

Fig. 33.7 Waist. Flank adiposity aspect in the preoperative and 90 days postoperative period. A reduction of approximately 10 cm is noted, with a total accumulated energy of 45 kJ

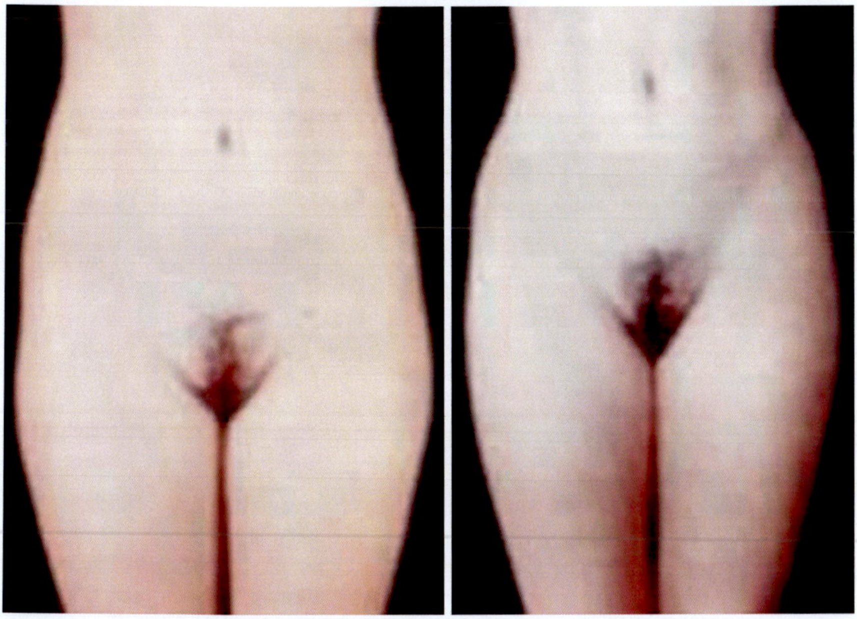

Fig. 33.8 Waist and umbilical region. Preoperative aspect: waist—prevention of a flaccid (sad) belly button, even with large removal of adipose tissue. Treatment in six areas of 10 cm², with a total accumulated energy of 30 kJ

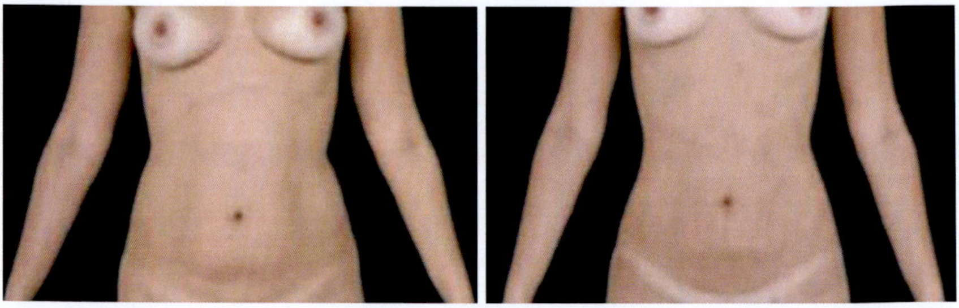

Fig. 33.9 Waist and umbilical region. Preoperative aspect: waist—prevention of a flaccid (sad) belly button, even with large removal of adipose tissue. Treatment in six areas of 10 cm^2, with a total accumulated energy of 30 kJ

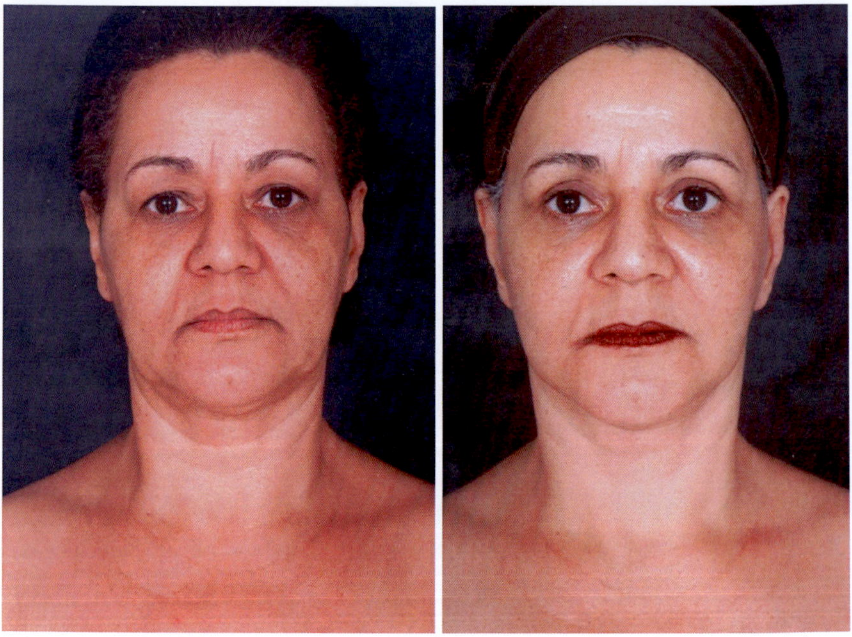

Fig. 33.10 Photographs (front views) showing the facial contour and submental region taken preoperatively (left) and 90 days postoperatively (right) of a 54-year-old patient. She underwent an upper blepharoplasty, and a lipoaspirate volume of 20 ml was removed with a cumulative energy of 9 kJ

Discussion

The significant tightening of the skin obtained in this study indicates that the use of a dual-wavelength diode laser (924–975 nm) allows remodeling of subcutaneous tissues and deep dermis. No complications (e.g., ecchymosis, prolonged erythema, anemia secondary to bleeding during surgery, or tissue necrosis) were observed, suggesting that laser lipolysis is a safe procedure. This may be attributed to both the characteristics of the device and the surgical technique.

The technical characteristics of the laser device were evaluated based on the 14 years of experience the authors have in working with various laser devices operating at different wavelengths, including continuous-wave lasers, pulsed and ultra-pulse carbon dioxide lasers, continuous and ultra-pulse erbium lasers, diode laser, and neodymium-doped yttrium aluminum garnet lasers. All these laser types provide good aesthetic results but may lead to postoperative complications (i.e., edema and erythema prolonged for up to 6 months), which have also been reported by several authors.

The diode laser used in the present study differs from other systems in that it operates at 975 nm, which is a wavelength that especially acts in the treatment of skin laxity. This system also allows the simultaneous use of two wavelengths (blend system), which stimulates tissue contraction in the deep dermis in a slow and progressive manner, reducing skin laxity at the same time that fat is liquefied, facilitating liposuction without ecchymosis formation. In addition, the dual-wavelength diode laser provides a better control of the output power by operating at two platforms (24 W and 40 W). The ability to control the output power has a direct impact on the aesthetic outcome, because the laser power delivered to the tissue is directly associated with both total cumulative energy and temperature rise at each treatment site.

Mordon et al., who developed the mathematical model explaining the relationships among output power, temperature, and cumulative energy, emphasized the need to determine the optimal cumulative energy as a function of the volume of adipose tissue to be removed by laser lipolysis.

The laser power and cumulative energy per treated area used in this study were determined based on experiments conducted by the authors, whose results were considered as a safety parameter by a consensus panel during the Advanced Fractional and Body Sculpting Symposium in New York, New York, in 2009. According to our experience, an optimal cumulative energy ranging from 3 to 5 kJ/100 cm^2 skin area is necessary for obtaining the best aesthetic outcome tailored to the patient.

The use of the optimal cumulative energy results in a moderate rise of temperature in the deep dermis, changing the sodium-potassium balance in the cell membrane, which allows the transport of extracellular fluid into the intracellular space. This increases the adipocyte volume, leading to the rupture of the membrane and release of lipases, which act in the adipose tissue, facilitating its aspiration.

At the same time, the optimal cumulative energy causes an increase in temperature that leads to connective tissue remodeling and cauterization of small blood vessels. A lower concentration of red blood cells was found in the sample obtained by laser lipolysis (A2) compared with that of a sample obtained by conventional liposuction (A1), indicating that laser lipolysis results in reduced blood loss compared with conventional liposuction. This agrees with the findings of a previous study.

The present study showed that a cumulative energy of 5 kJ/100 cm^2 skin area may be considered as an optimal energy because it led to a progressive tightening of the skin over time, without complications, such as ecchymosis, prolonged erythema, excessive bleeding, and skin dimples. The statement that the laser treatment resulted in a progressive tightening of the skin over time is supported by the fact that no significant difference in the circumference of the mid- and lower thirds of the left arm was found between preoperative and postoperative measurements, but a significant reduction was observed 90 days after the surgical procedure compared with previous time points. This indicates that laser lipolysis resulted in conjunctive tissue remodeling, according to the physiology of each patient.

Laser lipolysis was performed with a 2-mm-diameter cannula; a 280-mm-long laser tip was used to reach deep layers such as the lamellar fat, contributing to reduced temperature increases in the epidermis, which may lead to a superficial inflammatory process and synthesis of dermal elastic fibers that may result in skin dimples. The procedure resulted in a progressive skin tightening over time at all treated sites without complications that are usually associated with other lipoplasty techniques.

This may be attributed to both the characteristics of the laser system and the surgical procedure used in this study. Our results indicated that this technique stimulated collagen contraction, leading to dermal remodeling and reduction of skin laxity, when the safety parameter (i.e., cumulative energy of 5 kJ/100 cm^2 of skin area) was observed. To illustrate the photothermal effect of laser irradiation on skin flaccidity, laser irradiation (without fat aspiration) from a dual-wavelength laser diode was applied only in the left knee of a patient. Laser irradiation led to skin tightening, resulting in an improved aesthetic result.

In cases of a small contour deformity, in which the volume of fat to be removed is less than 200 ml, the laser may be applied without aspiration of the fat. Our years of experience have shown that for volumes greater than 200 ml, deposits of liquid fat may be formed, and although they can be removed, they may lead to postoperative complications, such as seroma formation and ecchymosis. Previous studies have compared the effects of laser lipolysis with those of conventional liposuction. Other studies have shown marked differences in treatment outcomes obtained with and without the use of laser during lipoplasty.

The use of a dual-wavelength diode laser has other advantages for both the patient and the surgeon, which have also been reported by Parlette and Kaminer. The authors Badin et al. (2002) "Laser lipolysis: Flaccidity under control" and Goldman et al. (2002) also described reduction of skin flaccidity with the use of laser. Laser lipolysis is performed under local anesthesia without the need for general anesthesia. Spinal anesthesia may eventually be used in the treatment of large areas. The surgical procedure requires 2–3 h of immediate postoperative rest, without the need for hospitalization, which leads to a rapid recovery (approximately 24–48 h), and the epidermis is preserved in all cases. Laser lipolysis with a dual-wavelength diode laser has a short learning curve for plastic surgeons already experienced in other laser systems.

Laser lipolysis is a cosmetic procedure that has attracted great attention throughout the world and that has the potential to radically change the paradigm of lipoplasty. The widespread dissemination of the results obtained with this procedure is essential to demonstrate its efficacy and safety when safety parameters are observed.

Conclusions

Laser lipolysis performed with a dual-wavelength diode laser, using a cumulative energy of 5 kJ/100 cm^2 of skin area as an optimum dose, was shown to be a safe treatment for correcting contour deformities in the facial, submental, breast, arm, and waist regions without the need for general anesthesia or hospitalization.

Patient Consent

Patient provided written consent for the use of patient's images.DisclosureNone of the authors has a financial interest in any of the products or devices mentioned in this article.

Clinical Question/Level of Evidence Therapeutic, IV.

References

Triana L, Triana C, Barbato C, Zambrano M. Liposuction: 5 years of experience in 26,259 patients using different devices. *Aesthet Surg J*. 2009;29:509–512.

Goldman A, Shavelzon DE, Blugerman GS. Laserlipolysis: Liposuction with Nd:YAG laser. *Rev Soc Bras Cir Plast*. 2002;17:17–26. 9.

Badin AZ, Moraes LM, Gondek L, Chiaratti MG, Canta L. Laser lipolysis: Flaccidity under control. *Aesthetic Plast Surg*. 2002;26:335–339.

Further Reading

Pozner JN, Goldberg DJ. Nonablative laser resurfacing: State of the art 2002. *Aesthet Surg J*. 2002;22:427–434.

Parlette EC, Kaminer ME. Laser-assisted liposuction: Here's the skinny. *Semin Cutan Med Surg*. 2008;27:259–263.

Mordon SR, Wassmer B, Reynaud JP, Zemmouri J. Mathematical modeling of laser lipolysis. *Biomed Eng Online*. 2008;7:10.

Ichikawa K, Miyasaka M, Aikawa Y. Subcutaneous laser treatment of axillary osmidrosis: A new technique. *Plast Reconstr Surg*. 2006;118:170–174.

Prado A, Andrades P, Danilla S, Leniz P, Castillo P, Gaete F. A prospective, randomized, double-blind, controlled clinical trial comparing laser-assisted lipoplasty with suction-assisted lipoplasty. *Plast Reconstr Surg*. 2006;118:1032–1045.

Badin AZ, Gondek LB, Garcia MJ, Valle LC, Flizikowski FB, de Noronha L. Analysis of laser lipolysis effects on human tissue samples obtained from liposuction. *Aesthetic Plast Surg*. 2005;29:281–286.

Weiss RA, Beasley K. Laser-assisted liposuction using a novel blend of lipid- and water-selective wavelengths. *Lasers Surg Med*. 2009;41:760–766.

Dornelles RFV, Silva AL, Missel J, Centurión P. Laser lipolysis with a 980-nm diode laser: Experience with 400 cases. *RevBras Cir Plast*. 2013;28:124–129.

Wassmer B, Zemmouri J, Rochon P, Mordon S. Comparative study of wavelengths for laser lipolysis. *Photomed Laser Surg*. 2010;28:185–188.

Wolfenson M, Cerqueira Norberto, F. Lipoplasty guided by ultrasound. *Rev Bras Cir Plast*. 2009;24:538–543.

Wolfenson M, dos Santos Filho FCN. Skin tightening in lipoplasty following security parameters for use of the diode laser with double wavelength 924 nm and 975 nm. Plastic and reconstructive surgery. 2012;130(1):235e-6e.

Wonfenson M, Ferreira LM. Uso do Laser no Brasil. Rio de Janeiro: I Ed, Dilivros editor. 2016. ISBN 978-85-8053-151-1

Wolfenson M, Hochman B, Ferreira LM. Laser lipolysis: skin tightening in lipoplasty using a diode laser. Plastic and reconstructive surgery. 2015;135(5):1369-77.

Wolfenson M, Santos Filho F.C.N. Cervicofacial Laxity Reduction With Thermotherapy With Diode Laser (975nm) - Chapter 43, Aesthetic Facial Surgery-Springer Nature Switzerland: Avelar JM, Editor. ISBN 978-3-030-57972-2; AG 2021.

Wolfenson M, Roncatti C, Alencar AH, Barros. T, Silva Neto JF, Santos Filho. F.C.N. Laserlipolysis: skin tightening and prevention of flabby umbilical region with lipoplasty following security parameters for use of diode laser with double wavelength 924 and 975 nm - Brazilian Journal of Plastic Surgery, 26 (2) Jan 2011.

Carpaneda CA, Ribeiro MT. Percentage of graft viability versus injected volume in adipose auto transplants. *Aesthetic Plast Surg*. 1994;18:17–19.

Illouz YG. Present results of fat injection. *Aesthetic Plast Surg*. 1988;12:175–181.

Mordon S, Eymard-Maurin AF,Wassmer B, Ringot J. Histologic evaluation of laser lipolysis: Pulsed 1064-nm Nd:YAG laser versus cw 980-nm diode laser. *Aesthet Surg J*. 2007;27:263–268.

Anderson RR, Farinelli W, Laubach H, et al. Selective photothermolysis of lipid-rich tissues: A free electron laser study. *Lasers Surg Med*. 2006;38:913–919.

Alexiades-Armenakas M. Combination laser-assisted liposuction and minimally invasive skin tightening with temperature feedback for treatment of the submentum and neck. *Dermatol Surg*. 2012;38:871–881.

Chapter 34
Liposuction: A Safer Approach in Four Stages

Arnaldo Lobo Miró and Julio Wilson Fernandes

Abstract The authors present practical guidelines for a safer liposuction, based on their extensive experience and recent multidisciplinary contributions. The physiology and clinical response to surgery are paramount to minimize all the risks and complication any liposuction may incur. Embracing anesthesiologist, vascular surgeon, and intensive care physician experiences in supporting the procedure, the authors summit a sound routine reproducible on the preoperative, transoperative, and postoperative periods of any liposuction.

Keywords Liposuction · Patient safety · Intraoperative complications · Postoperative complications

The liposuction procedure was first published by Yves-Gerard Illouz in 1980 (Illouz 1980). Beforehand, the technique was presented in Brazil in 1980 at the XVII Brazilian Congress of Plastic Surgery in Ceará, Fortaleza.

In 1986, the liposuction principles and its evolution were definitely established in Brazil after the iconic publication of Avelar and Illouz, enriched by many other experienced surgeons (Avelar and Illouz 1986).

Liposuction became the second most performed surgical procedure worldwide: in 2019, 639 liposuctions were performed every 24 h in Brazil, reaching 231,400 procedures per year, as surveyed by ISAPS—International Society of Aesthetic Plastic Surgery (ISAPS SURVEY 2019).

A. L. Miró (✉) · J. W. Fernandes
Private Practice, Curitiba, Brazil

Alumni Association of Professor Ivo Pitanguy, Rio de Janeiro, Brazil
e-mail: arnaldomiro@clinicamiro.com.br

J. M. Avelar, R. Cavalcanti Ribeiro (eds.), *Body Contouring*,
https://doi.org/10.1007/978-3-031-42802-9_34

Considering this extensive data, the expected number of complications such as infections, skin necrosis, seroma, hypovolemic shock, or even death became very noticeable. The mortality rate, surveyed in 2000 by ASAPS (American Society for Aesthetic Plastic Surgery) (Gomes 2003), was 19.1 for every 100,000 liposuctions, which revealed pulmonary thromboembolism as its main cause (Cupello et al. 2015).

The original Yves-Gérard Illouz's approach had a hypotonic solution with epinephrine and hyaluronidase infiltrated in the subcutaneous before the liposuction. This led his assistant Pierre Fournier to promote the "dry technique" (with no infiltration) for a while, before giving it up and embracing with enthusiasm the wet techniques. Nowadays, most advanced features lead to an easier detachment of the fat with less bleeding, less hand fatigue for the surgeon, the possibility of better skin retraction, and a less painful postoperative period.

Despite the laser-assisted liposuction, ultrasonic liposuction, vibroliposuction, water-assisted liposuction, and other approaches, the principle of skin retraction over a bed of hollow tunnels has been maintained over the years, with the same amazingly remarkable results and their unusual problems and complications. In other words, the equipment employed to perform a liposuction may change from surgeon to surgeon, but the body response and the surgical trauma it sustains remain chiefly the same.

The authors present over three decades of successful practice of liposuction in their private clinics, in a very practical guideline of four stages, as an invaluable safety protocol to any plastic surgeon, regardless of the equipment they may prefer in their daily quest for the optimum results. This progressive "ready to use" protocol is enriched by a relevant scientific background, interesting illustrations, and helpful supportive references.

Stage 1: Indicating Liposuction

As in any other surgical specialty, the correct perception of our patient's body, their needs, and expectations are the cornerstone to indicate the procedure.

It is important to reinforce that the best performed liposuction over a poorly selected patient can lead to a bad result and its uninvited consequences.

Your indications shall be:

Localized Lipodystrophy

It is the traditional, ideal indication in a slim or moderately overweight patient, with a very retractile skin (Fig. 34.1).

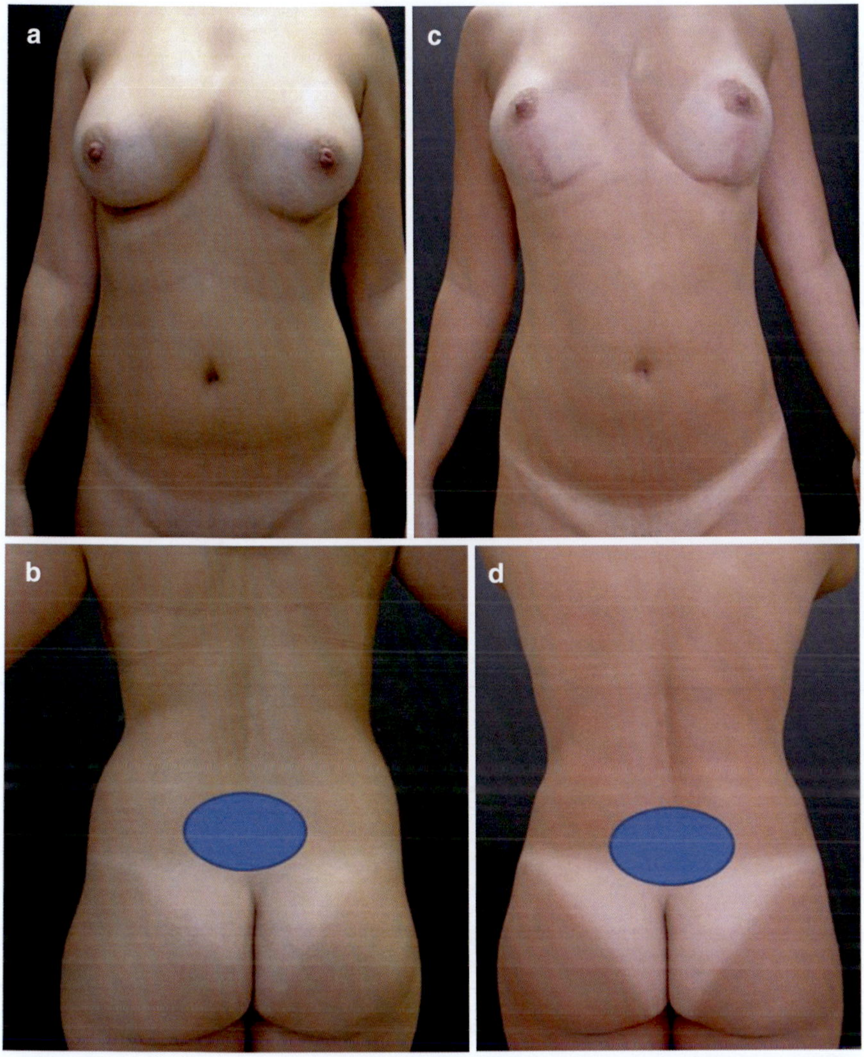

Fig. 34.1 A 29-year-old patient with lipodystrophy on the abdomen, flank, and back plus mammary hypertrophy. Underwent abdomen, flank, and back liposuction together with breast reduction. (**a**) Preoperative view. (**c**) Postoperative view. (**b**) Preoperative view (tattoos covered). (**d**) Postoperative view

Atypical Indication for Obese Patients

It is coadjuvant in the treatment of obesity for patients who accept the aesthetic limits of the procedure, having in their cases ephemeral results, without a lifestyle and nutrition change. Patients with previous failure in clinical treatment for obesity

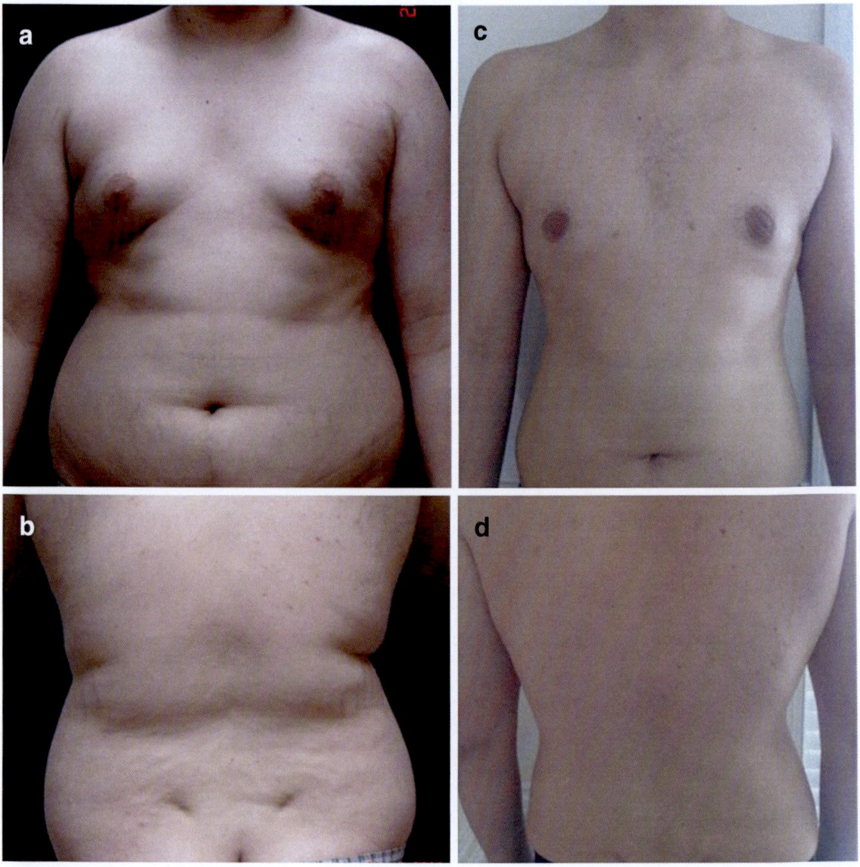

Fig. 34.2 (**a**) Preoperative view of a 118 kg obese patient subjected to adjuvant liposuction as a palliative treatment for obesity. (**c**) Postoperative view after liposuction of 4500 mL. (**b**) Preoperative view. (**d**) Postoperative view

and in need of additional motivation toward healthier habits may benefit from liposuction carefully indicated (Fig. 34.2).

A specific consent form is required before operating these patients besides antithromboembolism measures endorsed by a vascular surgeon.

Ancillary Procedure

Liposuction can extensively enhance the results in many aesthetic surgeries, from facelifts to breast cosmetic surgeries and full-body contour surgery. Even in reconstructive procedures, liposuction can be a great asset, thinning a thick skin flap, for instance (Figs. 34.3 and 34.4).

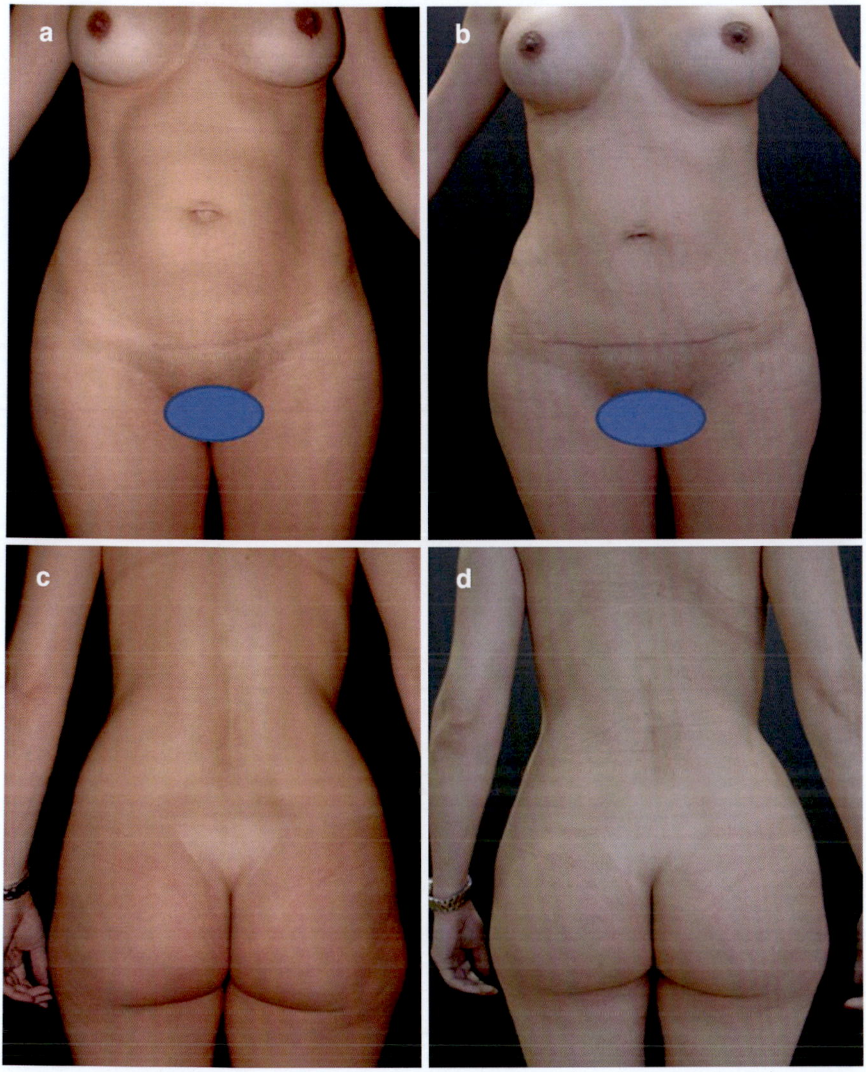

Fig. 34.3 A 28-year-old patient presenting with abdominal, flank, and back lipodystrophy with low abdominal laxity. Underwent abdominal, flank, and back liposuction, together with lower short scar abdominoplasty, preserving the umbilicus position. (**a**) Preoperative view. (**c**) Postoperative view. (**b**) Preoperative view . (**d**) Postoperative view

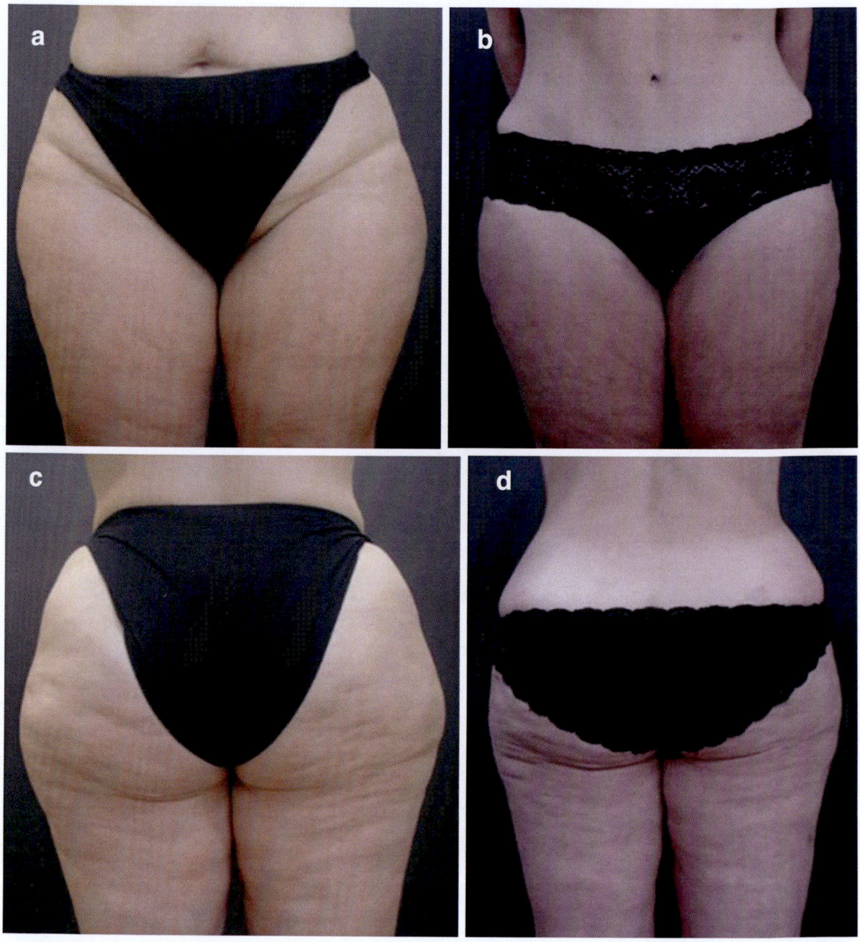

Fig. 34.4 A 43-year-old patient with trochanteric, upper inner thigh, and flank lipodystrophy. Underwent trochanteric, upper thigh, and flank liposuction together with traditional abdominoplasty. (**a**) Preoperative view. (**c**) Postoperative view. (**b**) Preoperative view. (**d**) Postoperative view

Atypical Indication

Liposuction may be indicated to patients who do not accept an abdominoplasty after considering its scar. Such results are unpredictable and paliative but may be surprising and preclude an abdominoplasty (Fig. 34.5).

The use of a specific consent form in this case is also required.

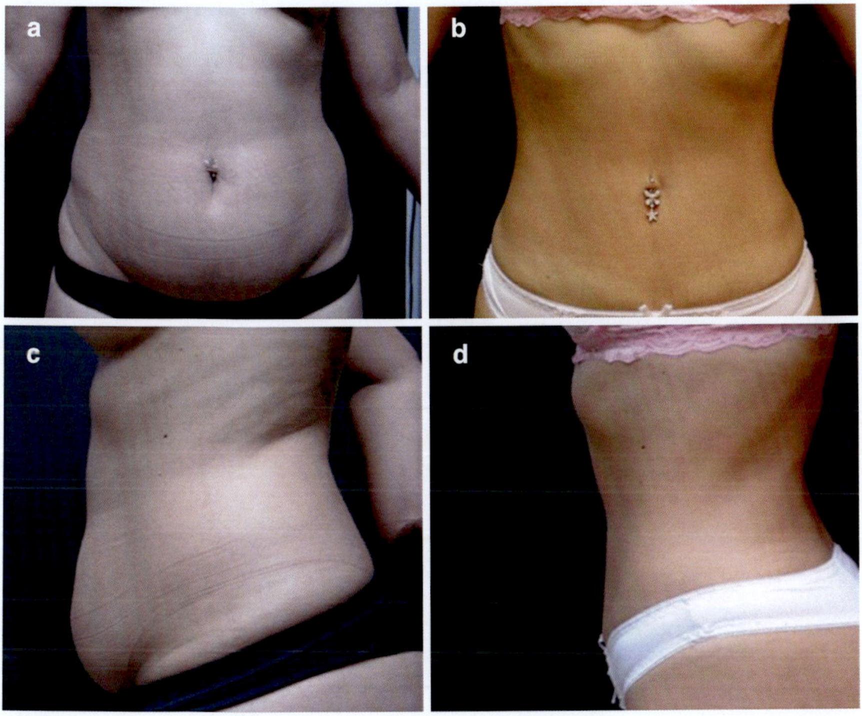

Fig. 34.5 (**a**) A 27-year-old patient with abdominal lipodystrophy associated with flaccidity, where an abdominoplasty could have been indicated. (**b**) Postoperative view after alternative liposuction, considering the patient did not accept the abdominoplasty previous indication and its scar. (**b**) Preoperative view. (**d**) Postoperative view

Lymphedema Treatment

Liposuction can be a great benefit addressing limbs affected by chronic lymphedema.

Lipoma Removal

Lipoma aspiration, avoiding scar, can be an interesting and effective indication, especially in patients with extensive multiple lipomas, as occurred in familial multiple lipomatosis and the Madelung disease (Chun-Ye et al. 2018). Previous ultrasound scanning is recommended.

Gynecomasty

It has been a consecrated approach to treat pseudogynecomastia with liposuction and the true gynecomastia by surgical excision (Webster incision or longer incisions if skin removal is necessary). In fact, in most cases, the two procedures are combined. Liposuction has changed this decision-making: employing larger "Mercedes" cannulas (5–6 mm) has made it possible to successfully remove mammary gland tissue in some true gynecomastia patients. Besides, when patients agree to a skin resection, if indicated, it can be delayed a few months, giving it a chance for the skin to retract, therefore having absence of scars or much shorter ones.

Stage 2: Preoperative Care (Fernandes et al. 2017)

Suspending Patient's Medication

- At least 15 days before surgery:
  - MAO inhibitor antidepressants
  - Anorexigenics
  - Estrogens (hormone replacement therapy)
  - Antiarrhythmics
  - Contraceptive pills, if possible
- At least 7 days before surgery:
  - Phytotherapic compounds: ginkgo biloba, ginseng, and ginger.
  - Vitamin E.
  - Antiplatelet agents (ASA): suspend only in cases of concomitance with other surgical procedures with a high likelihood of bleeding.
- On the day of surgery:
  - Oral hypoglycemic agents
    The following therapies are to be continued even on the day of surgery:
  - Antihypertensive drugs
  - Lipid-lowering drugs
  - Bronchodilators (inhaled beta agonists and leukotriene inhibitors)
  - Antidepressants other than MAO inhibitors
  - Anticonvulsant drugs
  - Anti-thyroid drugs

Smoking is always a drawback, especially for anesthesia and other concomitant extensive surgeries. Smokers can indeed undergo liposuction, but smoking interruption 2 months before any surgery or at least 24 h before is a remarkable clinical advantage.

Examinations

- Abdominal wall ultrasound scanning for most patients, especially with previous abdominal surgeries
- Blood count, coagulogram, fasting blood glucose, creatinine, beta human chorionic blood glucose, and beta human chorionic gonadotropin level evaluation
- Cardiological evaluation
- Anesthesiologic evaluation

Prevention of Thrombosis

Considering the thromboembolism and its associated pulmonary embolism are the most important mortality risk factors to be considered, we must analyze and foresee these possible complications as accurately as possible.

For this purpose, we use an algorithm classifying the degree of risk to be assumed.

The proposals published by Davison (Davison et al. 2004), Caprini (Caprini et al. 2001), and Sandri (Sandri 2005) J.L. are the best ones known; however, we prefer to adopt the protocol of the anesthesiologist Jorge Bayter Marin (Clinica El Pinar, Bucaramanga, Colombia) (Bayter 2007) because it is very practical and comprehensive.

Risk factors and their proportions	
Family history of venous thrombosis	2
Mobility impairment >72 h	2
History of fracture pelvis and long bones	1
Minor plastic surgery less than 2 h	1
Plastic surgeries between 2 and 5 h	2
Mayor surgeries (more than 5 h)	3
Minor liposuction (0–2 L)	1
Liposuction between (2–5 L)	2
Mayor liposuction (more than 5 L)	3
Smokers	1
Obesity–IMC 30–34	2
Obesity–IMC >34	3
Age–40–60	1
Age–60–70	2
Prior Thrombosis	3
Pregnancy or 1 month postpartum	1
Prior myocardial infarction	4
Prior venous surgery	2
Varicose veins (grade II)	1
Cancer or cancer treatment	2

Risk factors and their proportions	
Surgery combined with abdominoplasty	3
Travel more than 4h in 1 week	1
Oral contraceptive, hormone replacement	1

From the aforementioned risk assessment, the following algorithm is strictly applied to all our liposuction patients:

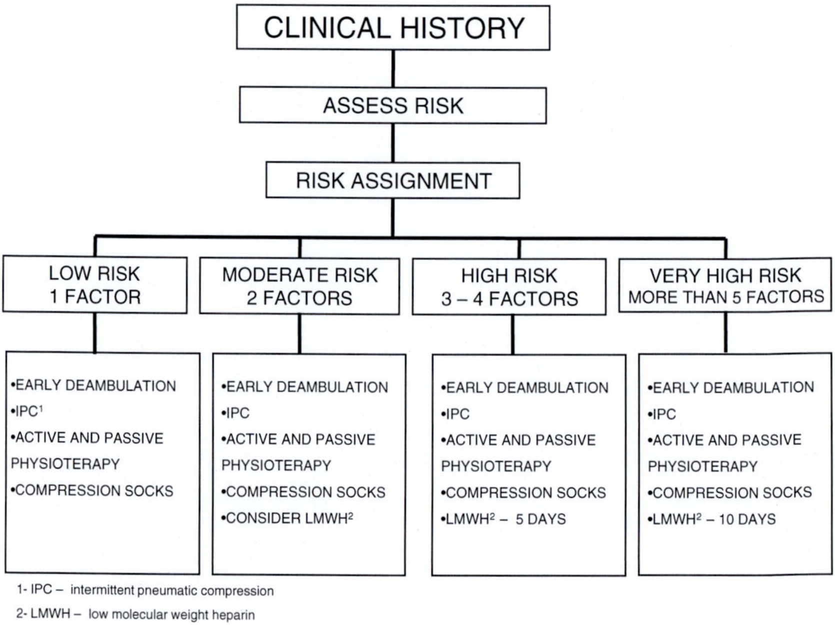

The enoxaparin will be administered only after the procedure, as described in Stage 4: Postoperative Care.

The evaluation by a vascular surgeon is fundamental for the following cases: patients with a history of DVT/PTE, patients with morbid obesity (BMI >59 kg/m^2), patients with acquired or hereditary thrombophilia (protein C or protein S deficiency, Leiden V factor, and antithrombin deficiency III), and carriers of inflammatory bowel diseases.

Stage 3: Transformative Approach, Surgical Room, and Key Points to Be Checked

The surgical team, as a routine, checks the surgical room temperature and the patient's warming system, a paramount concern in any extensive surgical procedure. The meticulous preparation of the infiltration to be used, the correct sterilization of the infiltration set/cannulas, and a quick briefing on patients' clinical conditions and medicines taken are a sound routine immediately before the anesthesia.

Anesthesia

The authors prefer epidural or general anesthesia and local anesthesia only to small areas, with an aspirate volume of approximately 200–500 mL, with particular attention to the immediate and late toxicity of lidocaine up to 14 h after infiltration.

Infiltration

The authors recommend saline solution administered at room temperature with one ampule of adrenaline in 500 mL of serum, respecting the maximum dose of 0.07 mg/kg, for example, five 1 mg ampules for a 70 kg patient.

A few considerations about infiltrations and lidocaine use, from our previous article on liposuction safety, are as follows:

Dry liposuction, which was recommended by Pierre Fournier and later abandoned, presented a blood loss of 20% to 45% of the aspirate. The superwet technique (Haeck et al. 2009), in which 1 to 2 mL of physiological solution with adrenaline is infiltrated for every 1 mL of aspirate, yields a blood loss of 1–2% of the aspirate and is the technique most commonly used in the clinical setting, and it is the authors' goal to be achieved by the end of the procedure.

The tumescent technique, proposed by Klein in 1985, infiltrates 3–4 mL of a solution containing 0.025–0.1% lidocaine and adrenaline (1:1,000,000) per mL of aspirate. The main criticism of this technique is that the firm consistency of the skin prevents the surgeon from "embracing the cannula" with the non-dominant hand. Failure to comply with this rule may lead to an inadvertent perforation of the abdominal wall, the pleura, or even the inferior lumbar triangle and severe damage to the internal organs. Another important aspect is that 70% of the infiltrate is transferred to the intravascular space in 2–10 h, and an excessive infiltrate leads to acute pulmonary edema (Fernandes et al. 2017).

Lidocaine is relatively lipid soluble and metabolized by the hepatic microsomal system. The binding of this drug to subcutaneous fat and the relatively poor vascularization under the skin delay its systemic absorption, and there is a risk of toxicity 6–14 h (or even 20 h) after drug administration if the maximum recommended doses are not respected. Even in adequate doses, it is important to remember that the excretion of lidocaine is decreased in liver diseases, during reduced hepatic flow caused by the associated adrenaline, in cases of hypoproteinemia, and during the use of medications, such as propranolol and cimetidine. When combined with adrenaline, the maximum safe dose of lidocaine for skin anesthesia is 7 mg/kg. Considering the effect of adrenaline, the low absorption of this lidocaine in the fat tissues, and the simultaneous aspiration, the dose of lidocaine was polemically increased to 35 mg/kg by some authors (Haeck et al. 2009). We do not agree or recommend such parameter and do not see any justification for the use of lidocaine in the liposuction infiltration under epidural or general anesthesia.

Change in Decubitus

In the prone position, the pressure gradients in the blood vessels are minimal because of the peripheral vasodilatation promoted by the spinal block if the legs remain essentially horizontal. For this reason, the possibility of severe hypotension or even cardiac arrest during changes in decubitus should always be considered. It must be done slowly and in stages. Use of alpha-1 adrenergic agonist (e.g., 1 mg of etilefrine, which may be prepared by diluting 1 mL of etilefrine from a 10 mg ampule in 10 mL of saline) intravenously before changing the decubitus may promote greater safety.

Maximum Volume to Be Aspirated

Despite this empirical background data, the authors support 5–7% of the body weight as the maximum volume to be aspirated. As an additional margin of safety, the authors consider the entire bottle aspirated volume and *not* only the upper fat fraction.

Stage 4: Postoperative Care

Discharge

Although subjective and lacking scientific evidence, patients subjected to liposuction may be discharged on the same day after 8 h of postoperative observation in the clinic or hospital. We consider to discharge them on the same day only in cases of liposuction of up to 5% of body weight using the superwet technique, a maximum aspirated volume of 4000 mL considering all the contents of the bottle, and absence of lidocaine use in the transoperative infiltration, besides the usual standard parameters for discharge of any surgical outpatient.

Electrolyte Replacement

For an aspirate equal to or less than the infiltrate, use 1 mL/kg/h of saline or Ringer's solution during fasting (usually 3 h). It can be replaced or supplemented orally with an isotonic solution if the patient does not have nausea. For aspirates higher than the infiltrate, the patient should receive that excess volume in Ringer or physiological solution intravenously. In aspirated volumes greater than 4000 mL, it is convenient to use a bladder catheter overnight in the clinic and maintain diuresis at 1 mL/kg/h.

Expected Clinical Parameters

For a safer postoperative period, a hemoglobin level of at least 9 g/dL, a diuresis of 1 mL/kg/h, and a systolic blood pressure of at least 90 mmHg are expected.

Blood and Blood Products

Transfusions are indicated considering the laboratory and clinical results of the patient in the postoperative period. It is indicated only in exceptional conditions. There is no indication for its routine prophylactic use, even as autotransfusion or reinfusion under the superwet technique (rigorously 1:1) in the absence of other concomitant surgeries and with a maximum aspirated volume of 5% of body weight. However, it can be used in liposuctions of 7% of body weight and in combination with other surgeries or considering the patient's clinical status regardless of the aspirated volume or technique used (wet, superwet, or tumescent). In patients without active bleeding and who are hemodynamically compensated, consider the following criteria (Carson and Kleinman) (Carson and Kleinman 2017):

Hemoglobin level <6 g/dL—Transfusion is always recommended.
Hemoglobin level of 6–7 g/dL—Transfusion is usually indicated.
Hemoglobin level of 7–8 g/dL—Transfusion is recommended in patients with cardiovascular disease or under conditions that do not respond to fluid replacement, including orthostatic hypotension, tachycardia, and myocardial ischemia.

In patients with active bleeding or comorbidities, in which anemia is determinant for clinical worsening, transfusion may be indicated even in patients with hemoglobin levels of 8–10 g/dL (Carson and Kleinman 2017). In cases of a high likelihood of extensive blood volume loss, autotransfusion or this alternative volemic replacement should be scheduled intraoperatively: some patients' blood should be stored in a special bag immediately before surgery (450 g) and kept in a cooler with ice. The patient receives saline and/or colloids throughout the procedure, and their blood is reinfused up to 5 h after the storage.

An interesting protocol to minimize blood transfusions after massive body contouring surgery and liposuction has been successfully proposed in Colombia (Bayter-Marin et al. 2021). However, considering the potential risks of any blood transfusion and the unavoidable physiologic changes the stored blood suffers (Fernandes et al. 2017), the authors argue the extensive use of blood products should not be a safeguard to over-extensive liposuction or any other aesthetic surgery.

Thrombosis Prevention (Fernandes et al. 2017)

In patients with no additional risk of DVT, enoxaparin sodium 40 mg should be used subcutaneously 6 h after epidural anesthesia or 8 h after spinal catheter removal (or immediately after surgery if general anesthesia was used). Intermittent compression boots should be used during and after surgery until discharge from the clinic and compression stockings during and after surgery for 30 days (except overnight at home) in the postoperative period. Ensure that the elastic stocking is placed correctly to prevent tourniquet compression by folds. It is essential to inform the patients and their relatives regarding the contraindication of daytime sleeping from the day after liposuction. For the patients who follow this recommendation and avoid the use of high-heeled shoes, the use of enoxaparin can be possibly interrupted in the day after liposuction.

For patients at a higher risk of developing DVT (history and/or the factors mentioned in stage 2 as "high risk" or "very high risk" groups), prevention recommendations should be provided on an individual basis, considering the evaluation and conduct of the vascular surgeon and the convenience of liposuction in these patients.

The authors strongly advise limiting the surgical associations to a single concomitant plastic surgery procedure with a maximum duration of 3 h and minimal blood loss whenever possible. The association of liposuctions with any gynecological, urological, or orthopedic surgeries is highly contraindicated (Cavalcanti et al. 2005).

Conclusion

The liposuction affords outstanding results, contributing to the physical, psychological, and social wellness of men and women. As one of the greatest plastic surgery contributions to medicine in the twentieth century, it must be performed by fully trained plastic surgeons under established safety protocols for its maximum safety. Regardless of the technical tools employed, liposuction requires an extensive understanding and commitment to the body response to surgery.

References

Illouz YG, (1980) Une nouvelle technique pour les lipodystrophies localisées. Rev. Chir Esth. Langue Franc, 6(9): Ap,1980.

Avelar JM, Illouz YG (1986) Lipoaspiração – Hipócrates Ed., São Paulo- Brasil.

ISAPS SURVEY (2019). Aesthetic/Cosmetic procedures.

Gomes RS (2003) Critérios de Segurança em lipoaspiração. ACM Arq Catarin Med 32(4):35-46.

Cupello AMB, Dornelas M, Aboudib Junior JH, et al (2015) Intercorrências e óbitos em lipoaspiração: pesquisa realizada pela comissão de lipoaspiração da SBCP. Rev. Bras. Cir. Plást.30(1):58-63.

Chun-Ye C, Qing-Qing F, Xiao-Feng et al (2018) Madelung's Disease: Lipectomy or Liposuction? BioMed Research International; 2018: Article ID 3975974. https://doi.org/10.1155/2018/3975974.

Fernandes JW, Miró A, Rocha AAS et al (2017) Practical criteria for a safer liposuction: a multidisciplinary approach, *Rev. Bras. Cir. Plást.; 2017;32(3):454-466*

Davison SP, Venturi ML, Attinger CE, et al (2004) Prevention of venous thromboembolism in the plastic surgery patient. Plast. Reconstr. Surg.114:43E-51E.

Caprini JA, Arcelus JI, Reyna JJ (2001) Effective risk stratification of surgical and nonsurgical patients for venous thromboembolic disease. Semin. Hematol 38:12-9.

Sandri JL (2005) Profilaxia do tromboembolismo em cirurgia plástica. In: Carreirão S, Cardim V, Goldenberg D, eds. Cirurgia Plastica – Sociedade Brasileira de Cirurgia Plastica. Atheneu, São Paulo; p. 119-25.

Bayter JE (2007), Protocolo Clinica El Pinar, Bucaramanga, Colombia

Haeck PC, Swanson JA, Gutowski KA et al (2009) ASPS Patient Safety Committee. Evidence-based patient safety advisory: liposuction, Plast Reconstr Surg.;124(4 Suppl):28S-44S. DOI: https://doi.org/10.1097/PRS.0b013e3181b52fcd

Carson JL, Kleinman S (2017) Indications and hemoglobin thresholds for red blood cell transfusion in the adult, UpToDate. https://www.uptodate.com/contents/indications-and-hemoglobin-thresholds-for-red-blood-celltransfusion-in-the-adult

Bayter-Marin JE, Cárdenas-Camarena L, Peña WE et al (2021) Patient Blood Management Strategies to Avoid Transfusions in Body Contouring Operations: Controlled Clinical Trial, Plast and Reconstr Surg.;147 (2):355-363. https://doi.org/10.1097/PRS.0000000000007524

Cavalcanti IL, Cantinho FA, Assad AR (2005) Anestesia para Cirurgia Plástica. Rio de Janeiro: SAERJ.

Chapter 35
Summary: Liposculpture

Ewaldo Bolivar de Souza Pinto

Abstract This present summary is intended to briefly present the knowledge expressed in the referenced book. In this perspective, it is worth mentioning that the statements hereinafter exposed are taken from the work *Lipomiosculptura* written by Dr. Ewaldo Bolivar; therefore, the statements will be based exclusively on the findings in the book. Therefore, the second chapter entitled Surgical Anatomy of the Skin states that "classical studies of human anatomy add little about the skin in surgical aspects in a systematic way [...], perhaps due to the restriction of procedures and techniques operatives" (Souza Pinto 2009). In this line, liposuction had a considerable evolution due to the improvement of methodologies and technological refinement. Consequently, it became necessary to recheck studies "relating to anatomical variations of the skin lining layers" (Souza Pinto 2009). This need for in-depth research is basically due to the behavior of the skin after the procedures, with variable retractability over time interfering directly in the desired result.

Keywords Aesthetic plastic surgery · Body contour · Lipoaspiration

Introduction

Basically, the skin is formed by three main layers, the apparent or superficial part called the epidermis, dermis, and hypodermis. The tissue that covers the body represents approximately 15% of the entire body weight of the human being, which presents several depressions and variations along its surface. Skin tone is due to several factors, including genetic-racial, regional, sexual, and thickness.

E. B. de Souza Pinto (✉)
São Paulo, Brazil

J. M. Avelar, R. Cavalcanti Ribeiro (eds.), *Body Contouring*, https://doi.org/10.1007/978-3-031-42802-9_35

The epithelium was studied by Anile, Chiarugi, and Rouvière who made a genetic description of the skin, which is composed of keratinized stratified squamous epithelium. The beginning of the epithelium is ectodermal that presents melanocytes from the 12th and 14th week of gestation.

The epidermis can still be divided into two layers. The first is deeper, also known as the germinal layer, which is separated from the thinnest part of the epidermis by the basement membrane. This layer is still able to be renewed between 20 and 30 days, and the thinnest element of the skin is usually sparse of granular and lucid layers of the epidermis; however, it still maintains the cornea to which it is limited.

The dermis is responsible for supporting the epidermis, which can reach a thickness of up to 3 mm at the feet. This thickness can vary a lot depending on the location on the body, and the literature summarized here points out that it can vary between 1 mm and 4 mm which are shaped to the epithelial cones; the dermal papillae are present in the dermis that present ripples along its entire length.

This undulating character of the dermal papillae may be responsible for the greater resistance of the skin, since, due to its undulating characteristic, it provides a larger contact area, which confers greater friction, in effect, greater resistance. Still watching the skin structure, it still has a bed of papillary (superficial) and reticular that is deeper.

This more superficial part, which is thicker, consists of loose connective tissue which is responsible for keeping the dermis and epidermis together. The papillary dermis, despite not following a rigid pattern of orientation throughout its extension, can still be observed a pattern of direction according to the region of the body, therefore being variable by region.

The reticular is composed of a dense connective tissue, which has collagen fibers with irregular orientation and arranged in blocks. However, the work reports that it was observed that the reticular has fibers arranged in directions that depend on the region of the body, as this is oriented according to the traction. The dermis in general is still composed of 78.85% of collagen in the papillary and 85.71% reticular, on average. These two layers have elastic characteristics that give the skin its retractable quality.

In this line, following the information collected throughout the chapter (referring to the cited authors), as well as the investigation based on studies with cadavers with less than 8 h of death, the author proposes a *classification of the arrangement of the dermal collagen fibers*, where they are organized second: fiber arrangement, density, and direction. Regarding the dermis, the presence of other components is also highlighted, such as lymphatic and blood vessels, hair, and sebaceous and sweat glands, in addition to nails.

Paying attention to the hypodermis, as mentioned above, this is the deepest layer of the skin which is made up of fat cells that are organized in lobes linked by vascular connective beams. Histologically, the cells that make up the hypodermis originate from undifferentiated mesenchymal cells, which would be characterized by many mitochondria and lipid inclusions insoluble in acetone and chloroform.

These fat cells are intended to store energy, and their thickness is quite variable, being related to the individual's nutrition and genetic characteristics. This fabric still has characteristics of protection against temperature variations and shocks (collisions). The dermis still has usual characteristics depending on the region of the human body.

For the neck, the dermis has two characteristics: the papillary dermis which has an average thickness of 0.08 nm and is homogeneous and dense with collagen and the reticular dermis that exhibits an average thickness of 1.8 nm. In the medial upper limb of the arm, the papillary dermis has a more homogeneous/denser and homogeneous/loose arrangement and, to a lesser extent, a heterogeneous/parallel arrangement.

In addition, in the upper part, the reticular dermis, has collagen disposition in a large part parallel and parallel/tangled in a small amount. Furthermore, the average percentage of collagen present in this segment can be up to 85% with an average thickness of 1.52 nm. For the regions of thorax, abdomen, and hip, it is of the papillary and reticular type.

For the papillary dermis, in 45% of cases it is homogeneous/dense and with a lower prevalence (5%) and homogeneous/compact with 81% collagen. For the reticular, the most common cases are the parallel type with an average thickness of 2.18 nm. For the dorsum and sacral region, the papillary dermis is largely homogeneous/dense with collagen from 76% to 77%, whereas for the reticular dermis, this is largely anarchic distribution with 97% collagen.

Regarding the medial surface of the thigh and knee, the most common papillary dermis is the homogeneous/dense one with an average of 76% collagen, and the reticular dermis presents the parallel type with 82% collagen. As for the culotte or trochanteric region, it is firm and thick with regularity throughout its contour. The papillary dermis of this region is commonly of the homogeneous/dense type with 80% collagen (on average), whereas to reticulate most of the cases it presents in parallel with 81% collagen on average.

The exposed ones regarding the structure and other characteristics of the skin are important for liposuction, since knowing about the arrangement of collagen fibers in the skin, future research regarding skin retraction and repositioning directly contribute to the efficiency of the procedure. In this direction, it is worth emphasizing the *liposuction and apparatus methods* (Chap. 5) of the work.

Methods

The present study is a discussion about the work *Lipomiosculptura* written by Dr. Ewaldo Bolivar. Therefore, the testimonies will be based exclusively on the findings of the book. For a deeper understanding of the topic, other studies were used for the theoretical basis of the topic and in the discussion.

Discussion

With the advent of new technologies in recent years, there is a continuous evolution in the knowledge and refinement of procedures that innovate in the implementation of equipment and methods, making liposuction increasingly efficient in its objectives. From the 1980s onward, the apparatus was disseminated in an accelerated way, providing surgeons with better conditions for their practice.

Therefore, *vacuum suction liposuction*, also known as conventional liposuction, involves the fragmentation of fat that is removed through cannulas and connecting tubes in a collector; this procedure has a vacuum pressure system (as indicated in the name). However, the course of fragmentation due to the vacuum system still lacks documentation/research with greater definition. But this process is possibly due to compressed air blows into the adipose tissue that force the fragmented entry of fat through the cannula (Souza et al. 1996; Souza Pinto et al. 2006).

The suction liposuction mechanism consists of a suction pump to which is connected to an electric motor, "a weak collector, a bottle with additional vacuum equipped with a mechanical valve system, a biological filter, an internal filter (against contaminants) and an exhaust filter" (Souza Pinto, 2009; Souza et al. 1996). In addition, the fat collector bottle has measurements in milliliters for fat removed; the capacity of the collector bottle still depends on the manufacturer.

An important bump comes from the vacuum pressure of the device, which is placed as crucial for its efficiency. The text also highlights that there is a need to observe all equipment components: *suction pump*, *weak collector*, *connection everything*, and *cannula*, among others; all components and the sum of their contributions make the equipment efficient presented. However, it is opportune to note the use of the equipment at high altitudes, as the fact that it loses suction capacity of approximately 1 inch of mercury per 1000 feet of altitude is mentioned.

Syringe liposuction was first developed by Fournier in 1985 for the removal and grafting of adipose tissue in a certain region of the body. For this purpose, needles, a trocar, or cannula was used to which it was mounted on a syringe. The procedure consisted of a mechanism that blocked the syringe plunger and, through a vacuum and manual maneuver, the suction of the adipose tissue was performed.

Among some advantages of this method is the ease of quantifying the volumes of aspirated fat and blood, less trauma, decreased dead space, lower rates of overcorrections and deformities, decreased edema, less pain after the process, greater control and precision, and lower cost, among others.

As for the disadvantages, it would be the increase in surgical time and the possibility of injury to large tendons. Indications for this procedure are for cases of small and medium volume, cellulite, fat grafting, and adiposities located in small regions, among others. However, there are still some contraindications, such as patients with excessive obesity, poor tissue tone, and systemic diseases.

The material used is easy to assemble and handle, the syringes can be made of plastic material with volumes ranging from 1 to 60 mL; this depends on where the procedure is being performed. For Brazil, the most common is the use of 10, 20, and

60 mL syringes for extraction and smaller volumes for grafting. As for the cannulas, small calibers are normally used, with variations in diameter and length. In fat grafting there is a preference for *flat* cannulas, due to their uniformity of fat distribution.

For the grafting of fat, stainless steel pistols are used to assist the application because the pistol mechanism facilitates the application of pressure with the least use of the surgeon's force, and, in addition, it also promotes greater control and precision.

Another highlight is the ultrasonic liposuction, which aims to add advantages to the limitations that other techniques have, such as vacuum liposuction. This methodology was not directly originated from liposuction, but from the diagnosis and treatment of cataracts and vascular and renal surgeries, among others.

Over time, the technique acquired new instruments and refinements, so in 1988, it was introduced. With the insertion of the method, manufacturers and other developers made efforts to improve ultrasonic devices capable of liquefying fat. From this perspective, sound waves can be identified as mechanical energy that is transferred from one point to another through matter, this type of wave needs a medium to propagate, and it occurs in solid, material, and gaseous media, among others.

Sound waves are said to be longitudinal waves; unlike transverse waves, sound waves have their propagation in the same direction as amplitude, therefore so-called longitudinal. Transverse waves (such as magnetic and electric fields) are defined as transverse as the propagation direction is different from its "amplitude sense," which forms an angle that is almost always perpendicular.

The movement in particles originating from waves (in this case, leaving aside all quantum effects for subatomic particles) causes the particle in question to acquire movement and, consequently, a kinetic energy that is partly dissipated through heat. The degree of agitation of these particles, therefore, defines the amount of heat it has: the greater the agitation, the greater the amount of heat generated by the particle.

It is also worth remembering that these definitions bring in essence a didactic explanation, and subatomic particles in this context do not behave as expected, that is, the degree of agitation is not due to waves, since in a quantum context, subatomic particles "never are quiet." Taking only this classical universe as a perspective, mechanical waves as an effect of energy transfer in a material medium promote oscillations that can have high or low frequency, therefore endowed with amplitude, distance, and resonance, among other effects and physical definitions.

Like classical sound waves, ultrasound also has the same properties, and they are longitudinal that propagate a wave (energy) in a material medium. The human being can hear waves between 20 and 20,000 Hz, for sound waves with frequencies lower than 20 Hz, they are called infrasound. As for sounds with a frequency higher than 20,000 Hz, they are defined as ultrasound which, due to its high frequency, cannot be perceived by the human ear.

Paying attention to the effects of ultrasound on liquids and tissues, this type of sound during the transfer of energy to the medium causes the liquid to create microbubbles that, when formed, also generate gases and vapors; this is because ultrasound has the cycles of compression and expansion (during energy transfer), causing these bubbles and gases to originate in liquids.

In this line, fabrics with large amounts of water or liquids also undergo a similar process. Fat, for example, has a much lower density compared to bone tissue; in fact, molecular cohesion is also lower and can be overcome by the effect that ultrasound has in this type of medium. The effects generated by ultrasound in this type of tissue are known as rarefaction. Because of the ultrasound on the cells, this in turn occurs the formation and collapse of micro-vesicles as a result of the vibration generated by the equipment, which is known as cavitation.

However, a series of events and conditions is necessary so that the desired effect can be achieved, in this case, the elimination of fat. For this, there must be good diffusion of gases in the tissues, the tissues must also contain nucleation sites that give rise to microbubbles, and a wave intensity is sufficient to exceed molecular cohesion, so that this occurs with the growth of bubbles with respect to density of the medium that shouldn't be so high.

As a result of the implosion of the microbubbles created by ultrasound inside the cells or in their contours, it causes greater agitation that consequently destroys the cell; therefore, it is necessary to pay attention to the effects of the procedure, which are thermal, cavitation, and micromechanics. Therefore, it is necessary to make brief elucidation about the interaction of adipose tissue with the components of ultrasound generating devices.

Ultrasound waves have some peculiarities for low-density tissues, such as fat. One of these is the fact that if the procedure is applied correctly, the fat can be dissipated, or, better said, liquefied, generating less trauma to the adjacent tissues.

Due to the weak intermolecular connections of the fat, it responds more intensely to the pressure drop caused by the waves, and the cavitation also occurs in an easier way. When adipocyte integrity is lost, its contents are expelled and the fatty acid is released, which forms a stable fat emulsion that can be removed by suction.

The loss of adipocyte integrity is basically associated with three factors: wave amplitude, tissue composition, and frequency. The amplitude of a wave, taking the case of transverse waves, can be understood (didactically) as the height that the wave reaches, and, for ultrasound, this can be between 40 and 130 μm. The end of the procedure must be carefully observed, in the first step the movement of the cannula is performed smoothly, where the perception of the body's resistance in the passage determines the end of the treatment, as well as the amount of blood.

Another step is the passage of the cannula repeatedly in the same places; this can generate burns in other tissues, not by the tip of the cannula on the tissues but by the propagation of waves that will have a greater thermal effect and, consequently, having the presence of burns. The lower resistance of the cannula in given regions is crucial to determine the procedure time and the emphasis regions of the procedure, thus not being necessary forced movements in attempts to reach regions of difficult access.

Ultrasonic liposuction equipment generally consists of a generator, connecting cables, vacuum suction pump, handpiece, activation control, probes and/or cannulas, and skin protectors. The electric generator normally follows a voltage pattern of 110 or 220 V, which normally has an on and off switch and amplitude, electrical, and mechanical indicators, in addition to another time indicator. The time indicator is of paramount importance, as it shows how much energy was applied in each anatomical region.

The connection cables are only conductors of electrical current originated by the generator, and these must be sterilizable, reusable, and of good length to facilitate handling. The activation control is normally done by means of a pedal, where the surgeon has full control of the device to turn it on and off, thus totally ceasing the applied power, which facilitates the surgeon in preventing burns.

The probes or cannulas are equipment responsible for transmitting energy to tissues; these in turn can be solid or hollow. For the solid probe, it does not have a suction device, unlike hollow probes, which are equipped with orifices that carry out suction during the process. The first ultrasonic liposuction devices used solid-type cannulas, but due to the low efficiency of the device compared to the methods already applied, it was not so widespread, forcing manufacturers and developers to make improvements that came through the second generation (cannula with suction holes).

Thus, hollow cannulas were able to perform the liposuction procedure at the same time as they performed the aspiration, which reduced the treatment time and, in this way, promoting an aspirated content that was very similar to that of liposuction already consolidated.

This new equipment brought some facilities, including the surgeon's greater ease and safety with the procedure, with greater tissue safety during energy release. A disadvantage of the solid cannula was the fact that it brought two phases to the procedure, the first was liposuction itself and the second was known as evacuation, which consisted of removing the material.

However, the standard procedure already performed removed approximately 70% of the emulsion during the process itself, and the rest was removed during evacuation. Solid type cannulas are more "powerful" compared to hollow ones, as they are made entirely of solid metallic material and transmit energy more efficiently, so it is pointed out that some authors prefer this type of cannula in procedures such as removal of cellulite, skin without elasticity, uneven surfaces, and secondary procedures.

Hollow-type cannulas still have some setbacks; the more traditional models have a shape with a smaller diameter lumen. In fact, they have a lower suction capacity of the emulsion. There are different shapes of cannula tip: square, rounded, flat, or curved shapes. However, perfectly rounded tips cause the energy distribution to maximize cavitation, thus decreasing thermal effects.

For the manufacture of cannulas, it is quite common that they are made of titanium because this type of metal provides less heat and transmits a greater amount of energy, thus making the cannulas and probes more efficient. Therefore, it is necessary to check the indications, limitations, complications, and special care.

The ultrasonic liposuction procedure is more efficient in fibrous areas of the body, such as the back, upper abdomen, and breast (male). It is necessary to consider the degree of obesity of the patient, for patients with mild obesity the procedure is also feasible; therefore, areas such as the knee, ankle, and calves are commonly avoided.

Another point of note for this textual section is the recommendation of not conducting concomitant subcutaneous tissue detachment in regions where there was treatment with ultrasonic aspiration. Therefore, it is recommended that infiltration with a tumescent solution is essential for the safety of the procedure, as the moist environment promotes more effective cavitation, in addition to preventing the prevalence of burns due to the moisture present.

The movements performed with the cannulas must be uninterrupted, that is, continuous movements that respect the resistance of the medium to disperse the effects of cavitation in the tissues, minimizing the possibility of increasing the temperature and possible injuries due to heat. During the procedure, the surgeon must be aware of the position of the cannula throughout its entire length, being recommended to use the nondominant hand to palpate the skin to gently feel the position of the tip of the cannula.

These and other precautions are intended to prevent accidents and unnecessary sequelae, the most common being burns, skin necrosis, seromas, and dysesthesia. Analyses performed in vitro and in vivo have already shown temporary functional loss and histological damage to the nerves, with demyelination of peripheral nerves. This type of problem is related to the number and frequency of steps with the extension of the nerve damage, with isolated cases of hyperpigmentation, infections, and bruises.

Therefore, to reduce the prevalence of these consequences, it is recommended to avoid long-term treatments; in medium and deep planes, it is necessary to keep the environment moist with continuous movement of the cannula. Another point is the application of at least 1 cm below the surface of the dermis, with limited application time per area of at least 1 min per 100 cc aspirated. Furthermore, the procedure cannot be performed with other procedures that compromise local vascularization.

At this juncture, the advantages and disadvantages of ultrasonic liposuction with the traditional one are the fact that the first appears to be less traumatizing for the patient regarding tissue damage adjacent to fat and greater preservation of vascular structures. In addition, due to the advantages of using the equipment, the surgeon applies less effort, which promotes greater attention to his practice.

There is also a more uniform body contour, with better skin retraction in obese, elderly, or gynecomastia patients. Another advantage to be highlighted is the fact that ultrasonic liposuction promoted faster recovery of skin perfusion compared to the traditional method using vacuum suction. Less postoperative pain, early return to work, less morbidity, less blood loss, lesser degree of ecchymosis, and edema are also highlighted in the literature and observed in cases, although there are controversies.

Liposuction using ultrasonic waves came as a traumatic methodology of mine to the tissue of patients; however, this has technical limitations because it presents complications due to burns, necrosis, and irregular scars. Because the technique presents good results and potential for improvement, the surgeons then dedicated themselves to developing a safer and more efficient apparatus, which could be applied with the reduction of the problems mentioned, in addition to the limitations of the application itself.

From this perspective, the third-generation ultrasonic liposuction emerged, which came with the *VASER* device that was developed by the company Sound Surgical Technologies. The device uses a low-energy, high-efficiency pulsed ultrasound technology that made the use of small-diameter, solid titanium cannulas available.

This new equipment uses only a quarter of the energy released by previous devices, and the pulsed technology allows for less heat generation, providing greater safety for the procedure. The acronym VASER stands for *Vibration Amplification of Sound Energy to Resonance* which represented a breakthrough for liposuction. The device consists of a precision system for infusion of liquid, hose for infusion, vials and collecting tubes, peristaltic infusion pump, aspirator with ventilation, amplifier, and cannulas with holes and solids.

The primary function of VASER probes was to improve fragmentation, which consisted of a longitudinal rod, a proximal end, a distal end, and an axis. This axis was part of the proximal to distal portion. The proximal termination of the longitudinal axis, on the other hand, had a connector for connecting the longitudinal axis to the power source.

In addition, the distal part of the shaft had a blunt projectile-shaped tip that could have between one and three grooves. These grooves redistributed the ultrasonic energy, which transferred the energy vibrations from the front of the tip to nearby regions. The groove walls provided the probe's distal contact area in planes perpendicular to the probe axis. Thus, there was a larger contact area for tissue fragmentation without the need to increase the diameter of the cannula.

The VASER probe was able to increase the fragmentation efficiency in different tissues; considering this more efficient fragmentation/emulsification process, the probes could have a smaller diameter with the same desired effect (if used with larger diameter cannulas). The diameter of VASER probes could be 2.2 mm for more sensitive regions and 2.9 mm for aspiration and refinement of small volumes of fat in soft or fibrous tissues. Probes with 3.7 mm were used for aspiration of medium and large volumes.

The indications for these devices are quite like previous devices that use ultrasonic liposuction, where there are promising results in fibrous tissue and superficial layers of fat. The equipment has also been applied in high definition liposculpture, especially those that want to improve the contour of the male abdominal muscles, in addition to the hip and perigluteal region of women.

There are some advantages of using this equipment when compared to the previous model: the 3–4 mm incisions, which are smaller than traditional ultrasonic liposuction, in addition to the lower tissue trauma rate, less bruising, and less pain. Postoperative period, greater degree of satisfaction, less blood loss, and reduced effort by the surgeon were reported.

Another fact is that the supernatant fat exceeds 85% of the total aspirated, and the aspirated histochemical analysis is around 70–90% cell disruption. Thus, no fatty acid release was found, which indicates that the remaining fatty tissue is not damaged. However, the learning curve for using the equipment together with the cost of the device is placed as the main disadvantages.

Complications with the use of the VASER equipment were lower compared to the previous methodology. Problems such as seroma, dysesthesias or hyperesthesias, access burns, distant burns, skin necrosis, cellulitis, and prolonged edema were cited as caused by poor execution and application of the technique, when the tip of the cannula traumatizes the dermis in a superficial application.

In view of the above comes the concept of vibroliposuction that was introduced with the technological refinement of the probes with the development of the *cellulosuctiontome* by Arpad and Giorgio Fischer. These cannulas had lamias inside them that made cuts through oscillatory movements that brought improvement in access to denser and fibrotic regions; however, as problems related to skin necrosis and burns are common, this type of instrument still needed improvements, which came through the knowledge of orthopedists and otolaryngologists who were the basis for the development of cannulas that vibrated at a frequency of 800–10,000 rotations/min, which allowed easy penetration and movement of the probe inside the adipose tissue with rapid removal of fat.

The advantages of this system compared to traditional liposuction are shorter surgical time, easier suction and fat extraction, greater volume of suction per minute, less surgeon fatigue, better performance in fibrous areas and in reinterventions, greater control in superficial liposuction, and better access to the umbilical, epigastric, and dorsal areas. Other advantages are for the treatment of superficial gynecomastia with 3 mm cannulas, which resulted in less skin contracting and reduced need for skin resection.

Patients also indicate less postoperative pain, lower incidence of edema and ecchymosis, greater skin contraction, and shorter healing and recovery time. Vibroliposuction has some advantages compared to the ultrasonic liposuction method, which does not have the inconveniences due to heat and cavitation. There is also the shortest operative time in vibroliposuction compared to conventional and ultrasonic liposuction. The equipment commonly used is the MicroAire, which has easier access to denser regions, areas of greater fibrosis, and secondary liposuctions with less evidence of ecchymosis.

However, the disadvantages are the cost of the equipment and the intensity of vibration in the surgeon's hand. There is still a prevalence (to a lesser degree) of seroma with the use of 3 mm probes, and, for cannulas with a larger diameter, there is the creation of subcutaneous tunnels that can acquire fluid accumulation.

Following developments in liposuction comes the *liposuction with laser* that was developed and introduced by Dressel in 1990 that currently make use of *laser neodymium YAG* (1.064 nm) or *laser diode* (635/980 nm). This technique can be applied through an optical fiber with a *laser* coupled to fine-caliber probes that are inserted into the tissue through small incisions.

The procedure consists of transferring the *laser* energy directly to the adipocytes, which, upon absorbing, expand and rupture. Energy absorption is accomplished through receptive chromophores, which produce enough heat to cause thermal injury. The application of the *laser* causes the rupture of the adipocyte membrane, which releases lipases responsible for the liquefaction of the tissues. After the fatty tissue undergoes this effect, it can be easily aspirated.

The indication is for the treatment of small regions, cases of moderate flaccidity, or areas subject to flaccidity already treated in other methods, in addition to regions with high vascularization such as the scapular region, wrists, and flanks. The most cited advantages are greater skin retraction, less edema, less intraoperative bleeding, wider and more uniform skin surface, and less effort by the surgeon.

The disadvantages are the high cost of the device, technical difficulties in maintenance, and a moderate learning curve. The prevalence of most common complications is cellulite, burns, seromas, paresthesias, asymmetries, hyperpigmentation, hematomas, bruises, and skin lesions.

Another method is water jet liposuction, which was developed with the objective of enhancing advantages and reducing inconveniences of tumescent infiltration. The water jet liposuction uses a fine jet, fan-shaped bleached at high pressure, the objective is to "soften" the fat cells while minimizing damage. The advantages of the method are less tissue trauma, no need for sedation and less infiltrated solution, less intraoperative edema, greater surgical precision, and more precise contours with less effort from the surgeon.

However, the equipment and its technologies are recent, which necessarily require further studies to better assess their performance and potential; the cost of the equipment is also something placed as a disadvantage for the acquisition of surgeons.

Thus, it is worth mentioning lipomyosculpture because the first half of the twentieth century made attempts to change the body contour in accordance with the concepts of beauty. Illouz was the one who introduced the concept of liposuction to become the best body contouring surgery option. For this, the morphohistology of the adipose tissue of the subcutaneous tissue, which is divided into two layers, must be briefly discussed.

First, the upper abdomen, irregular, elliptical, and rounded lobes are arranged in parallel with the epidermis. Thick and thin septa are arranged parallel to the lobes. The lower abdomen, on the other hand, consists of irregular, elliptical, and rounded lobes with a parallel arrangement with the epidermis. The lateral aspect of the thigh presents irregular (80%), elliptical (10%), and rounded (10%) lobes.

The inner surface of the thigh presents irregular (60%), elliptical (30%), and rounded (10%) lobes with a parallel arrangement with the dermis. The medial aspect of the thigh, on the other hand, has irregular lobes (90%) and elliptical (10%) with a parallel and perpendicular arrangement to the epidermis. The flank has irregular (70%), elliptical (20%), and rounded (10%) lobes arranged perpendicular to the epidermis.

The gluteal region has irregular (80%), elliptical (10%), and rounded (10%) lobes with an arrangement parallel to the epidermis. The sacral promontory has irregular (80%), elliptical (10%), and rounded (10%) lobes with an arrangement parallel to the epidermis. Finally, the submental region has irregular (90%) and elliptical (10%) lobes with a perpendicular arrangement to the epidermis with thick (40%) and thin (60%) septa and with a surrounding arrangement in relation to the lobes.

The most interesting muscle for lipomyosculpture is the platysma, which is in the subcutaneous tissue and originates within the subcutaneous tissue of the upper third of the chest and deltoid muscle, crossing laterally with the neck. The triceps and brachialis muscles that have a long, lateral, and medial portion.

The abdomen originates between the fifth and seventh costal cartilage and inserts into the upper margin of the pubis, between the pubic tubercle and symphysis. The external oblique originates from fleshy fingerings on the eight caudal ribs and free margin. It inserts into the outer lip of the iliac crest, the inguinal ligament, and the anterior lamina of the rectus abdominis sheath.

For the back there is the trapezius muscle and latissimus dorsi. The trapezius originates in the medial third of the superior nuchal line. The latissimus dorsi arises from the spinous processes of the thoracic vertebrae and the last lumbar vertebrae and sacral dorsal surface of the outer lip of the iliac crest through the fascia to columbary. Lipomyosculpture aims to sculpt the body contour so that the surface is based on the musculature.

Due to the beauty standard being based on the shape of the human body's musculature, lipomyosculpture respects the histological peculiarities in order to follow the direction of the muscle fibers, consequently seeking to sculpt the fat over the muscle. This technique also seeks to minimize some effects such as complications in the subcutaneous vasculonervous bundle that follows the same direction as the muscle fibers; therefore, it is easier to avoid injuries to it.

An important step for this procedure is the preoperative appointment, which is considered crucial for the success of the procedure. This, in turn, is performed with the patient in an erect and standing position, without the need to administer pre-anesthetics, which is done in front of the mirror with a three-dimensional face where the patient can follow the traces and indicate your opinions on regions that bother you the most (Hunstad and Repta 2008; Azevedo et al. 2012; Franco 2012).

In this line, it is recommended that the markings are made with an ink that is not soluble in water and made in different colors to identify the areas to be aspirated and drawn, in other words, for regions where liposuction and other colors for grafting must be applied (Figs. 35.1 and 35.2).

During this phase it is necessary to pay special attention to the knee, which must be conducted with the patient in a sitting position; this prevents it from being aspirated more than necessary. The antisepsis is performed with the patient in standing normally with a solution iodopovidone or chlorhexidine and then placed on a sterile field in the supine position with a bandage of the legs to prevent venous thrombosis.

The positioning of the patient in a comfortable and safe way is of paramount importance, and this must be done in a way to facilitate the handling and direction of the cannula. The most common positions are prone, supine, or right and left

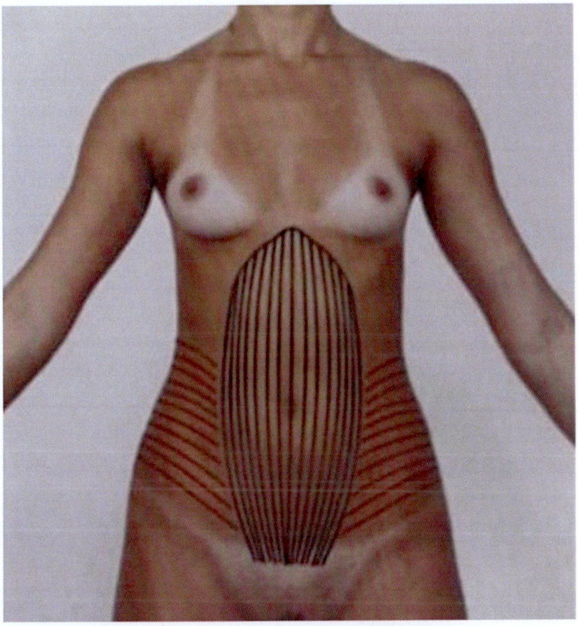

Fig. 35.1 Markings following the muscle fibers—frontal. Fonte: Souza Pinto (2009)

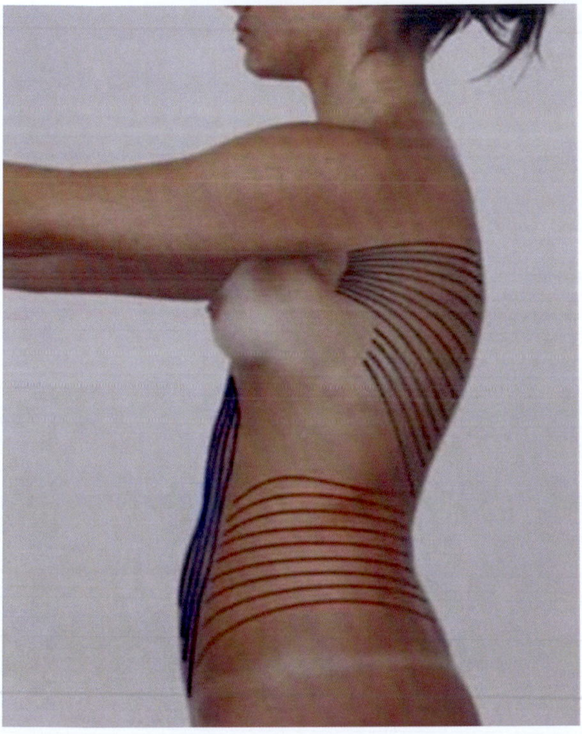

Fig. 35.2 Marking following muscle fibers—profile. Fonte: Souza Pinto (2009)

lateral decubitus. The incisions made are 5 mm, which must be in accordance with the perpendicular direction of the lines of force located in the peripheral area of the region to be treated. It is crucial to preserve a subcutaneous layer of fat of varying thickness to prevent excess flaccidity while also preserving the desired anatomy and contours.

Liposuction is always performed in the anatomical direction of the muscle fibers, and this part is essential in the lipomyosculpture technique, regardless of the procedure adopted: ultrasonic or vibroliposuction. Liposuction begins with the deepest layer of subcutaneous cellular tissue and, for the upper part, this is according to the specificities of the region.

In the submenu's region, a 3 mm cannula is used in the superficial layer, through a submental and median incision with guidance of the platysma muscle fibers. In Brazil, liposuction of the superficial layer is also performed with a 3 mm probe following the fibers of the triceps brachii with a proximal or distal incision.

In the upper abdomen, a 3 mm probe is used for conventional liposuction through an incision at the height of the xiphoid appendix with orientation of the rectus abdominis muscle. In the lower abdomen, the superficial layer becomes more compact and thicker than in the upper abdomen, thus using UAL and VL in the upper and superficial part with an incision at the level of the pubis, equidistant from the midline.

Finally comes the refinement test, which checks for irregularities in the superficial bed with a thin 3 mm probe that is slid through the skin in search of fat lobes that are caught between the fingers to be aspirated. The suture of the incisions is performed with 6-0 mononylon and covered with Micropore, in which the moderate compression belt is then placed 24 h after surgery, after bathing and changing the dressings; this is replaced with a duration of 30 up to 40 days (Figs. 35.3, 35.4, 35.5, 35.6, 35.7, 35.8, 35.9, and 35.10).

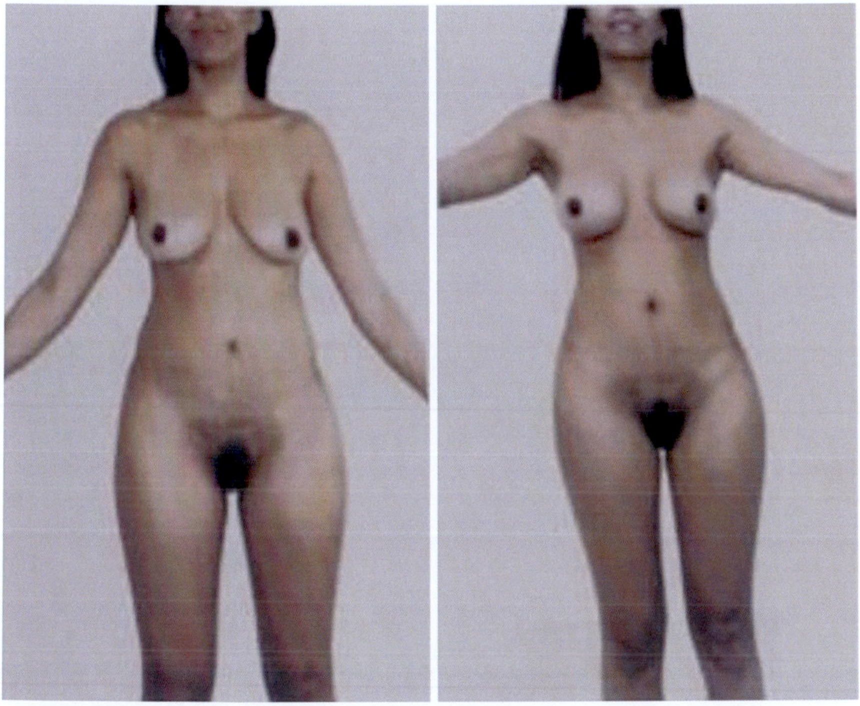

Fig. 35.3 Pre- and postoperative lipomyosculpture. Fonte: Souza Pinto (2009)

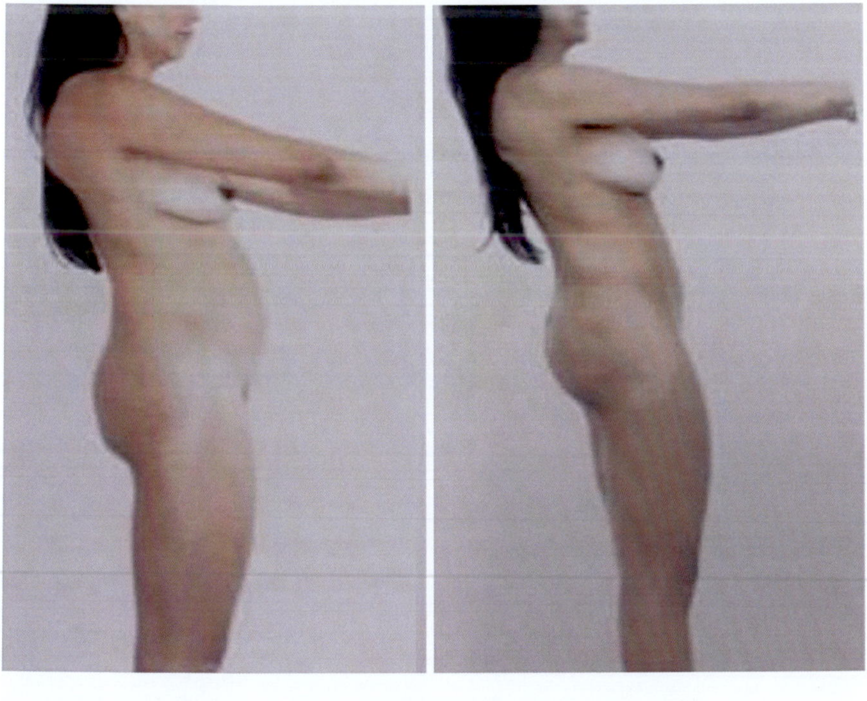

Fig. 35.4 Pre- and postoperative lipomyosculpture. Fonte: Souza Pinto (2009)

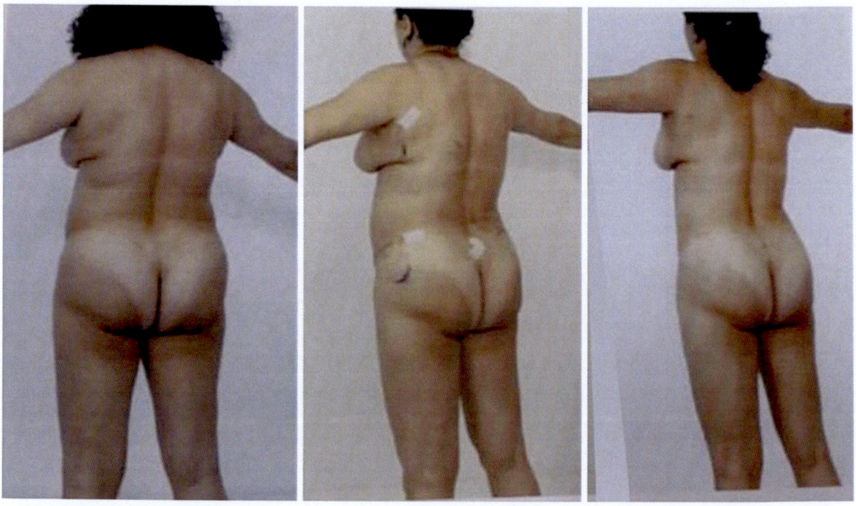

Fig. 35.5 Pre- and postoperative lipomyosculpture. Fonte: Souza Pinto (2009)

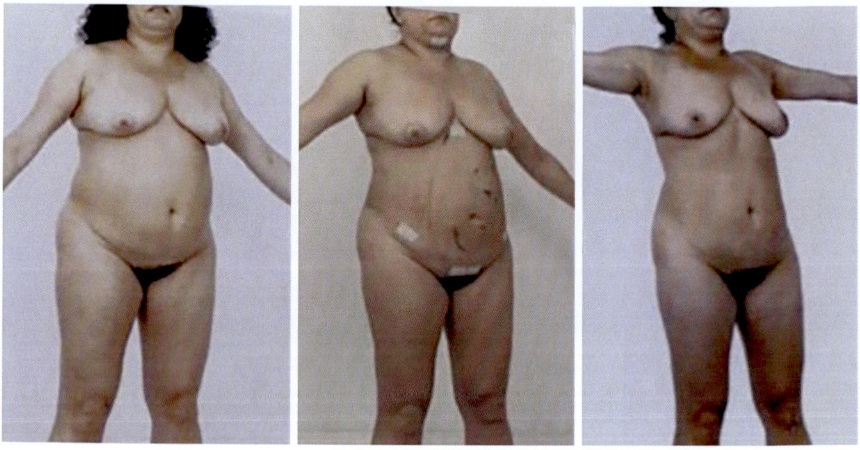

Fig. 35.6 Pre- and postoperative lipomyosculpture. Fonte: Souza Pinto (2009)

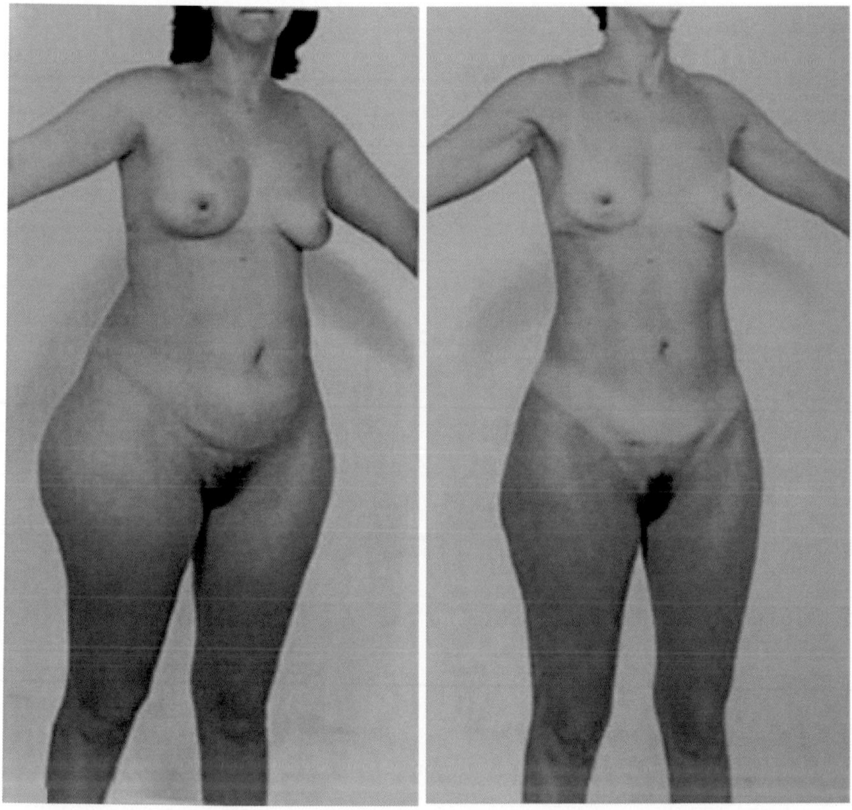

Fig. 35.7 Pre- and postoperative lipomyosculpture. Fonte: Souza Pinto (2009)

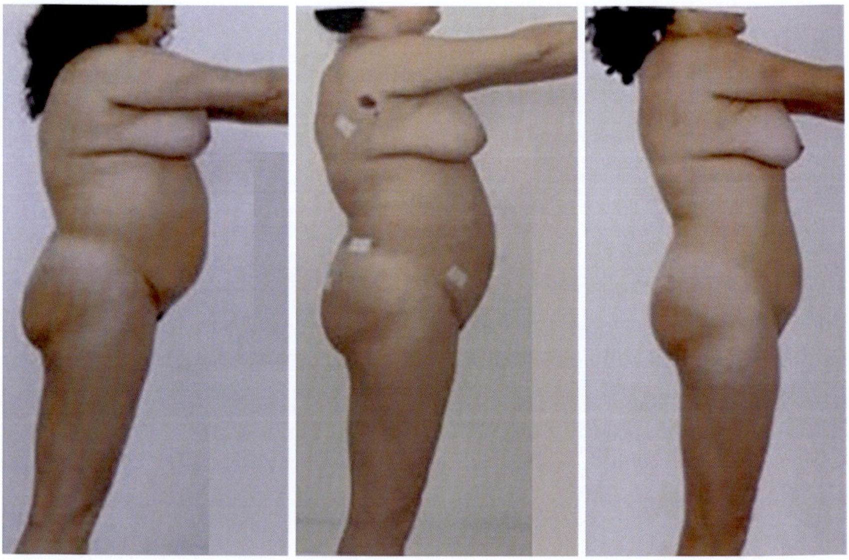

Fig. 35.8 Pre- and postoperative lipomyosculpture. Fonte: Souza Pinto (2009)

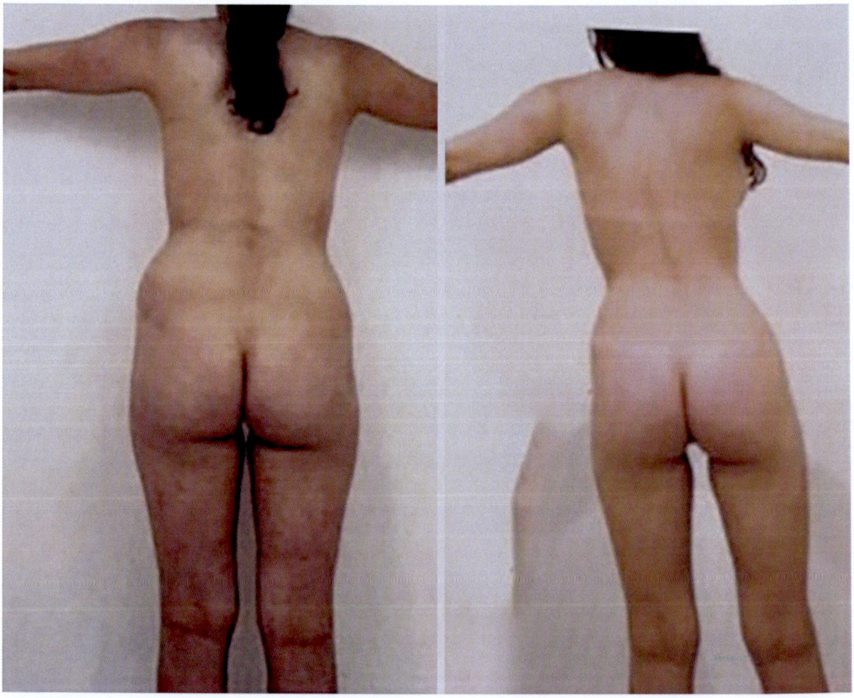

Fig. 35.9 Pre- and postoperative lipomyosculpture. Fonte: Souza Pinto (2009)

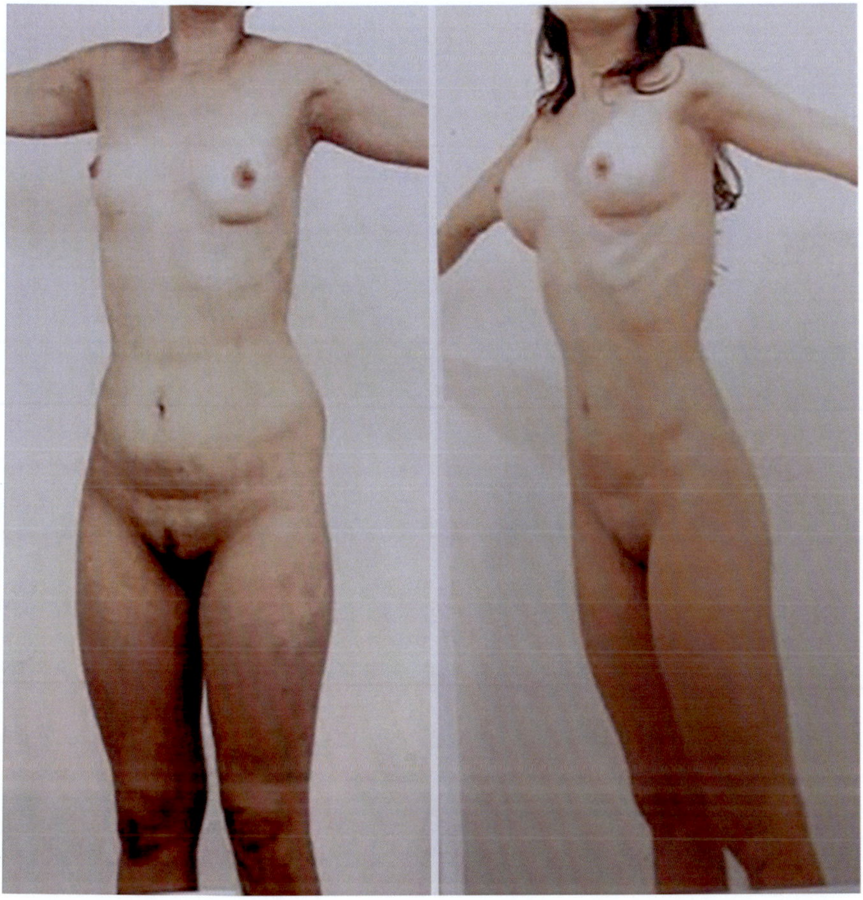

Fig. 35.10 Pre- and postoperative lipomyosculpture. Fonte: Souza Pinto (2009)

Conclusion

Liposuction has undergone considerable evolution due to the improvement of methodologies and technological refinement. in this context, it is extremely important to review studies related to the anatomical variations of the skin's covering layers. This need for deepening is basically due to the behavior of the skin after the procedures, with variable retractability over time, directly interfering with the desired result.

References

Azevedo DM, Gonçalves Junior P, Pereira J, Amoedo TB, Kuroyanagi FM, Cotes EF, Pinto EB, Saldanha OR. Augmentation gluteoplasty: experience at Dr. Ewaldo Bolivar de Souza Pinto Plastic Surgery Service. Revista Brasileira de Cirurgia Plástica. 2012;27:87–92.

Franco T. Augmentation gluteoplasty: experience at Dr. Ewaldo Bolivar de Souza Pinto Plastic Surgery Service. 2012.

Hunstad J, Repta R. Atlas of Abdominoplasty E-Book. Elsevier Health Sciences; 2008 Nov 28.

Souza Pinto EB, Abdala PC, Maciel CM, dos Santos FD, de Souza RP. Liposuction and VASER. Clinics in Plastic Surgery. 2006;33(1):107–15.

Souza Pinto EB, Erazo PJ, Prado Filho FS, Muniz AC, Salazar GH. Superficial liposuction. Aesthetic plastic surgery 1996;20(2):111–22.

Souza Pinto EB. Lipomioescultura, De Ewaldo Bolívar De Souza Pinto. Editora Dilivros, Edição 1ª Edição Em Português. 2009

Part V
Lipografting Improving Body Contouring

Chapter 36
Frag Fat: Fragmented Fat for Lipografting

Flavio Henrique Mendes and Fausto Viterbo

Abstract Body contour for massive weight loss (MWL) patients have become a common challenge, and plastic surgeons are facing important and conceptual shifts in order to handle the dramatic deformities, especially found in post-bariatric patients. Major deflation process presents a diverse and generalized pattern of body morphologic changes due to severe volume reduction and skin/superficial fascial system (SFS) disarrangement, which affects both upper and lower body, including the gluteal region.

Introduction

Body contour for massive weight loss (MWL) patients have become a common challenge, and plastic surgeons are facing important and conceptual shifts in order to handle the dramatic deformities, especially found in post-bariatric patients. Major deflation process presents a diverse and generalized pattern of body morphologic changes due to severe volume reduction and skin/superficial fascial system (SFS) disarrangement, which affects both upper and lower body, including the gluteal region (Mendes and Viterbo 2016a).

Although adipose tissue injection has made autologous lipografting an attractive and effective method to restore soft tissue and body contour (Condé-Green et al. 2016; Rosique and Rosique 2018), for many MWL patients, gluteal augmentation with autologous fat grafting is not an option because of the lack of donor sites. On

F. H. Mendes (✉) · F. Viterbo
São Paulo, Brazil
e-mail: mendesmd@fhmendes.com.br

J. M. Avelar, R. Cavalcanti Ribeiro (eds.), *Body Contouring*, https://doi.org/10.1007/978-3-031-42802-9_36

the other hand, surgical aprons resected during dermolipectomies contain loose adipose tissue that, although not best suitable for traditional liposuction, could be properly harvested and processed in order to establish an additional and new source of lipograft to be transferred to the buttocks and other areas. Those usually discarded materials hold precious adipose tissue, and efforts should target toward developing new processing techniques to make it possible to convert them into viable and injectable fat graft (Mendes and Viterbo 2021).

Keeping that in mind, we developed and tested a new fat fragmentation method in order to harvest and process great amounts of fine injectable lipograft from apronectomy specimens, willing to improve efficacy and to avoid possible limitations of traditional liposuction. As a new and revolutionary proposal, we established a scientific delineation to research different biologic aspects of such lipofragments, which included in vitro, in vivo, and clinical studies.

Gluteal Anatomy and MWL Deformities

According to Mendieta's classification, the gluteal region presents two distinct structures that influence overall contour: the *gluteal musculature* and the *gluteal frame* which comprises the bony framework, the subcutaneous fat, and the skin (Mendieta 2006). Morbid obesity causes generalized anatomical changes to the skin and subcutaneous layers. There is an overall increase in buttock dimensions (height and width), lengthening the inter-gluteal cleft and shortening the infra-gluteal fold. Bony framework and musculature may also be affected by weight disorders and influence gluteal aesthetics, but they cannot be targeted by surgical reshaping techniques.

Centeno described how gluteal aesthetic units and their relation to the frame should be considered to orient and determine which areas may benefit from reduction, augmentation, or lifting, according to patient's profile and aesthetic preferences (Centeno 2006). The sagging effect of gravity over the deflated frame structures makes it difficult to distinguish those units, as superficial fascial system becomes inefficient to sustain the skin and subcutaneous fat in straight contact to the deep muscular fascia. Although enhancing projection seems to be essential, it is important to evaluate the need for circumferential lipectomy to promote lifting and improve shape, before indicating any gluteal augmentation technique (Mendes and Viterbo 2021).

Skin Unlike most clinical comorbidities that regress after weight loss, literature has pointed that cutaneous disarrangement does not improve as well. The skin keeps loose, thin, non-pliable, and inelastic. Collagen structure is disorganized and damaged, with reduced fibroblasts at the papillary dermis and higher incidence of localized inflammation of the sebaceous glands. Elastin fibers are fragmented, with sparse scar evidence throughout the tissue. That poor skin quality may explain the higher wound-healing complication rates in those patients. Cutaneous disorders including collagen cross-link and structural disarrangement by defective biochemical signalization are probably some of the involved inhibiting mechanisms (Light et al. 2010).

Subcutaneous Fat The amount of adipose tissue also contributes to buttock projection and accounts for the different contour shapes. Fat distribution depends on both age and gender, as estrogen inhibits central deposition and stimulates it in gluteofemoral region, more than in other areas. Testosterone, in contrast, stimulates fat deposition in the abdominal region and inhibits it in the waist area. The volume of the buttocks may change, but usually the particular individual gluteal shape is maintained during obesity and tissue deflation. A great difference when evaluating the post-MWL buttock lies in the mobility and laxity of the subcutaneous layers, which makes the active physical examination crucial for surgical diagnosis toward lifting and projecting plannings (Mendes and Viterbo 2021).

Superficial Fascia System The superficial fascia system (SFS) is a constant structure, dividing superficial and deep fat compartments throughout nearly all the trunk and limbs. It is a connective tissue network that begins within the subdermal plane and continues down to the underlying muscle fascia, mainly composed of a single or many slender, horizontal membranous sheets divided by fluctuating amounts of fat with adjoining vertical or oblique fibrous septae. The architecture of the SFS may change with sex, adiposity, and body region, with the function to support and shape the fat of the trunk and extremities while adhering the skin to the underlying tissues. The irregular deep adherence characteristics of the overall system submitted to the action of gravity are responsible for the folds, creases, bulges, valleys, and other skin irregularities that ultimately determine body contour (Mendes and Viterbo 2016a). Large accumulations of fat in obese patients create a generalized mechanical stretching effect in the SFS. Meanwhile, weight loss causes massive fat reduction reflecting volumetric deflation of the subcutaneous layer without retraction of collagen fibers, which remain elongated and weak. Ultimately, SFS disability leads to significant looseness of the skin.

Buttocks Dynamics and Surgical Approach

Following massive deflation, patients experience generalized laxity with great mobility of the skin that directly impacts body contour. The zones of adherence promote a "selective limitation" in the mobility of skin coverage around the body (Aly 2006). This is the fundamental anatomic rule that defines body contour deformities in the MWL population, demanding a different approach, targeting the new bio-dynamics of the involved segments (Mendes and Viterbo 2016b). Figure 36.1 shows the clinical appearance and the distraction mechanism of the gluteal SFS during obesity and following MWL. Deflation and ptosis are the main concerns in the gluteal region. Orthostatic observation will show a decrease in buttock height and

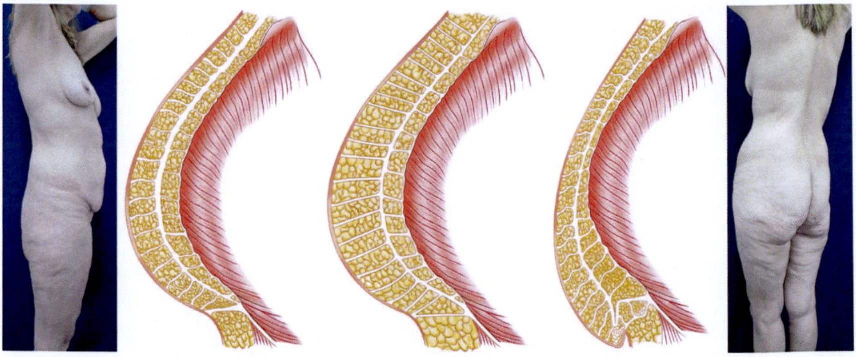

Fig. 36.1 Left and right: MWL gluteal contour—general deflation and ptosis. Center: SFS behavior—normal, obese and deflated

width, shortening of the inter-gluteal cleft, and lengthening of the infra-gluteal fold. Understanding the distinct physiopathology and tissue bio-dynamics is fundamental for diagnosis and surgical planning in these patients. Lower body contouring including gluteal reshaping usually demands surgical treatment of contiguous areas, such as the thighs, flanks, hips, back, and abdomen. Some patients like those with the classic "apple" somatotype may not require circumferential procedures to improve gluteal contour. On the other hand, those "pear" somatotype patients usually demand circumferential body lifting (CBL) to improve gluteal frame, even though it does not enhance buttocks volume. After the lifting procedure, if there is an important lack of gluteal projection, fat transfer, autologous flaps, and/or silicone implants may be indicated during the same procedure or at a later stage (Mendes and Viterbo 2021).

Considering the generalized pattern of MWL gluteal deformities, fat grafting allows full volume enhancement of the different buttock aesthetic units. Autologous flaps and silicone implants may help with localized gluteal projection; however, they are unable to restore deflated tissue and reshape the whole gluteal region. Better overall outcomes are obtained when fat grafting is widely transferred to the subcutaneous plane, with retro-injection maintaining the cannula parallel to the gluteal surface. Lateral and prone positions may be suitable for injection, depending on preoperative makings, the sequence for the circumferential approach, and surgeons' preference. In many cases, better contouring results come with the association of CBL and gluteal fat grafting, as long as it becomes possible to obtain enough amounts of viable lipograft. Being the only previously available harvesting technique (Fisher et al. 2013), traditional liposuction showed to be an aggressive, time-consuming, and quite inefficient option due to the specific deflated conditions of most MWL patients. In order to widely convert adipose tissue from circumferential dermolipectomies into injectable and viable lipograft, we started a scientific research to investigate and propose a new method for harvesting and processing adipose tissue through a specific fragmentation device.

Fragmented Fat X Lipoaspirate

We published our method to demonstrate the technique providing some initial data regarding quality and viability of the new *fragmented fat (frag fat)* in comparison to the *lipoaspirate*, which is already an established and accepted source of lipograft. In vitro and in vivo observations were designed to evaluate biologic standards that should possibly sustain human studies and further clinical applications (Mendes et al. 2019a, b).

One post-bariatric female patient, who underwent a fleur-de-lis abdominoplasty, had her infra-umbilical apron divided and submitted to liposuction (LA) and fat fragmentation (FF) under both dry (d) and tumescent (t) conditions (Fig. 36.2). All final sources of adipose graft were equally treated by centrifugation and then distributed for in vitro and in vivo studies. Each one of the four adipose tissue samples (FFd, FFt, Lad, and LAt) was grouped and distributed into 1ml syringes, labeled as a different "color" (blue, red, green, and black) to preserve blind manipulation during further experimental phases, until the results were finally ready to be registered and interpreted. Part of that material was sent to the in vitro preparations, while another part was immediately taken to the experimental lab, where each sample (FFd, LAd, FFt, and LAt) was subcutaneously retro-injected to different dorsum quadrants of ten Wistar rats. They were kept under standard environmental conditions and received daily subcutaneous injections of cyclosporine (2 mg/kg), in order to reduce immune reaction against the xenograft (Ferreira et al. 1995). After 6 weeks, all animals were euthanized and the retained dorsal grafts were surgically removed for a comparative evaluation of mass (Chyo JS-110 electronic balance) and volume (Archimedes' principle observation), as well as routine histological preparation for H&E and Masson's trichrome staining.

Fat Fragmentation Device The new fat fragmentator is a hand-driven stainless steel device (autoclavable), designed to receive fat trimmings by means of a feeding worm (auger) that progressively carries them through a horizontally mounted cylin-

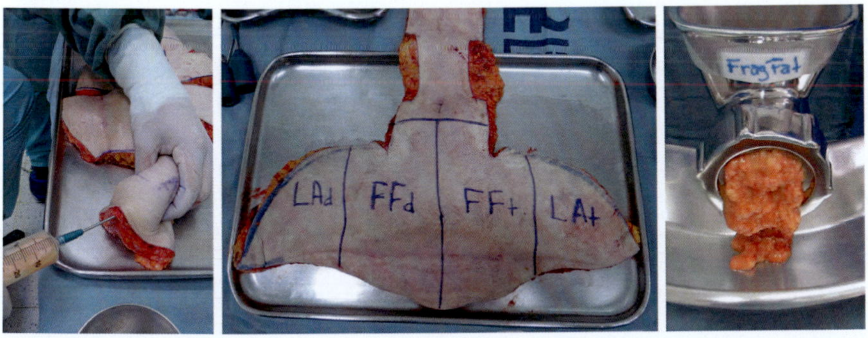

Fig. 36.2 Center: Fleur de lis abdominoplasty apron, divided into dry and tumescent halfs, both submitted to liposuction (LAd and LAt) and fat fragmentation (FFd and FFt). Left: Syringe liposuction. Right: Fat fragmentation

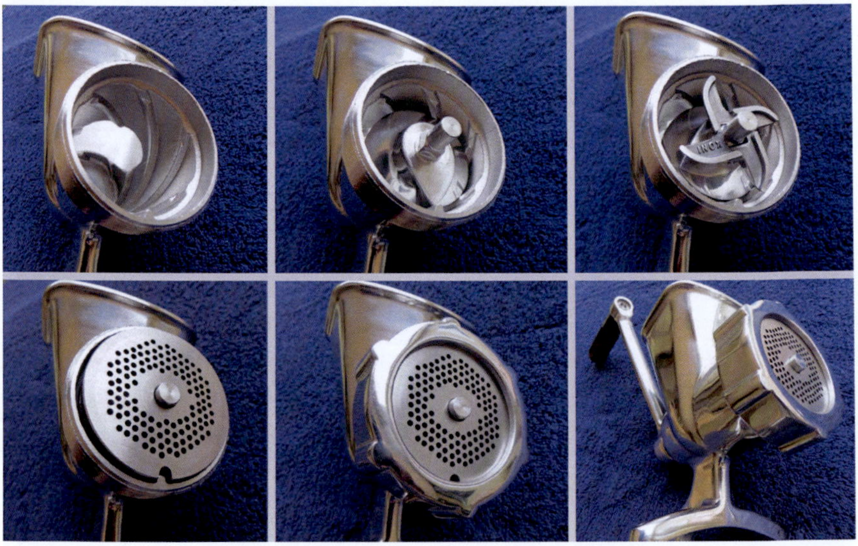

Fig. 36.3 Hand driven fat fragmentation device—assembling

der (barrel) into a distal cutting system consisting of rotating star-shaped knife and a stationary perforated disc (plate). As the skinless fat tissue is carried further by the rotating feeding auger and pushed in to the cutting system, it extrudes through the holes in the plate while being cut by the revolving star knife (Fig. 36.3). The degree of fat fragmentation is determined by the size of the holes in the perforated plate, providing the proper injectable consistency according to the internal diameter of different cannula sizes. We used 2 mm holes in the distal plate in order to obtain frag fat of similar sizing properties to the lipoaspirate harvested with a 2 mm cannula.

Histology, cell viability, and flow cytometry Blind analysis of both wet and dry groups of fragmented fat and lipoaspirate, including HE and CD34 immunocytostaining, showed similar histologic structural characteristics regarding tissue architecture and adipocyte integrity. Although there was a statistically significant difference regarding the number of lymphomononuclear cells among the samples, adipocyte viability did not differ significantly. Immunophenotyping of the samples by flow cytometry showed that both groups of frag fat and lipoaspirate had similar performances to the different markers used in this study. Table 36.1 describes this comparative analysis of cell autofluorescence by each marker on each preparation. Along the dry samples, frag fat (FFd) showed the highest autofluorescence level (11.91%) with the best performance for markers CD90 and CD105, obtaining a higher quantification of mesenchymal stem cells (Fig. 36.9). On the wet group, tumescent frag fat (FFt) showed a better performance for markers CD45, while

Table 36.1 Immunophenotyping of progenitor cells by flow cytometry with positive and negative markers (CD34, CD45, CD90 and CD105) and the mean fluorescence intensity in different samples (dry and tumescent Liposapirate and Frag Fat)

	Mean fluorescence intensity (%)						
	Ctl auto	Ctl ISO	CD45-FITC	CD34-PE	CD90-FITC	CD105-FITC	No. analyzed cells
FFD	6	11.91	52.98	51.81	92.22	69.09	11.095
FFT	5.07	6.64	84.12	57.67	55.98	65.42	20.000
LAD	2.61	3.4	61.39	63.78	51.52	37.23	20.000
LAT	6.09	4.21	56.14	78.33	70.67	68.68	20.000

tumescent lipoaspirate (LAt) was better for CD34 (Fig. 36.10). Trypan Blue test analysis showed no significant difference on cell viability between samples of frag fat and lipoaspirate, in both dry and wet groups.

Adipose-Derived Stem Cell Culture All the wet and dry samples of frag fat and lipoaspirate showed similar patterns of dish cultures, with regular expansion standards. The 72-h adhesion rate was found to be 25% for the FFd sample, which was significantly different from the others that showed a 10% rate. By the way, the confluence of 100% cells for the FFD sample happened earlier. Nevertheless, the final appearance of the fibroblastic cells did not differ among the samples. Figure 36.6 shows the dry frag fat culture plates at 15 and 30 days.

In Vivo Lipograft Analysis After 6 weeks, all rats were killed while their explanted xenografts were measured and used to compare biologic behavior of frag fat and lipoaspirate. Both "dry" (FFd X LAd) and "wet" (FFt X LAt) groups showed no statistically significant difference in their mass and volume retention (Fig. 36.11). Statistical treatment of the microscopic evaluation data on the retained fat grafts from the dry group (FFd and LAd) did not differ regarding inflammation, fibrosis, and neovascularization. Nevertheless, dry lipoaspirate showed significant higher grades for cell integrity and lower grades for cyst/vacuole formation when compared to dry fragmented fat. On the wet group (FFt and LAt), there was no significant difference for cell integrity, inflammation, and neovascularization, while tumescent fragmented fat showed significant lower cyst/vacuole formation and higher fibrosis in comparison to tumescent lipoaspirate (Table 36.2).

That preliminary study concluded that fat fragmentation widely converts dermolipectomy tissue into a new source of injectable lipograft with similar biologic characteristics of traditional handheld syringe lipoaspirate (Mendes et al. 2019a, b). Those results supported further investigations of frag fat in order to optimize the method toward clinical enhancement of fat grafting and possible regenerative applications.

Table 36.2 Histology data of retained grafts: Lipoaspirate X Frag Fat in both dry (LAd / FFd) and tumescent (LAt/FFt) groups

	Dry fragmented fat		Dry lipoaspirate		
	Mean	±SD	Mean	±SD	*p*
Cell integrity	1.8	0.63	3.0	0.94	0.0036
Cyst/vacuole	3.4	1,26	2.3	0.82	0.0333
Inflamation	2.7	0.67	2.3	0.82	0.2502
Fibrosis	2.1	0.74	1.9	0.74	0.5520
Neovascularization	2.1	0.88	2.2	1.03	0.8180
	Tum fragmented fat		**Tum lipoaspirate**		
	Mean	± SD	Mean	± SD	*p*
Cell integrity	2.3	1.16	3.4	1.26	0.0577
Cyst/vacuole	3.2	0.79	1.8	0.79	0.0009
Inflamation	2.3	0.67	2.3	0.95	1.000
Fibrosis	1.9	1.2	3.1	0.88	0.0197
Neovascularization	2.0	0.47	2.4	0.97	0.2603

Gluteal Frag Fat Augmentation

After our previous publications demonstrating in vivo as well as in vitro scientific validation for the new fragmented fat as a reliable source of injectable lipograft, we started our clinical application of the method for gluteal augmentation in MWL patients. We published our initial series of 20 consecutive post-bariatric female patients (Mendes and Viterbo 2022), who were submitted to gluteal frag fat grafting harvested from their surgically resected aprons.

Surgical Technique Preoperative skin markings are made on the day before surgery, according to individual indications and surgical plan. Patients have their gluteal regions symmetrically marked and divided into several zones (Cansancao 2016), which were designed to facilitate proper distribution of the available amounts of lipograft during prone and lateral positioning in the OR. Those undergoing circumferential dermolipectomies starting in the prone position have their posterior belt resected, and the skin is removed by an extra team who trims and sequentially fragments the fat tissue (Fig. 36.4, left). Although our previous research method had one group that used tumescent infiltration to the subcutaneous tissue before SAL and fat fragmentation, for clinical applications we indicate strictly dry fragmentation, which gives us pure adipose tissue without any other external components like saline, lidocaine, or adrenalin. No previous fat injections or further processing is done, and the plain fragmented adipose tissue is directly stored within 60-mL syringes for subcutaneous gluteal injection through a one distal hole 4mm cannula, immediately after posterior closure and before switching to the supine position (Fig. 36.4, upper right). On the other hand, patients whose first positioning starts supine, for initial anterior approach, have their aprons processed while fragmented fat is later transferred through sequential lateral positioning, evenly distributed according to the preoperative markings, with or without concomitant posterolateral

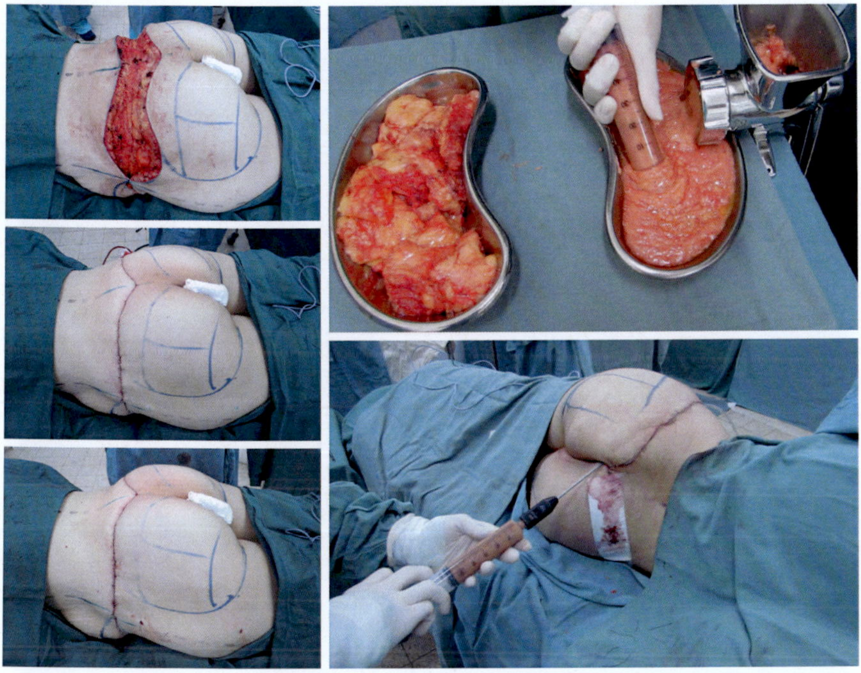

Fig. 36.4 Left: Prone gluteal frag fat transfer from concomitant posterior belt lipectomy. Upper Right: Fat trimmings submitted to fragmentation and storage in syringe for immediate gluteal grafting. Lower Right: Frag fat transfer in lateral position after anterior and ipsilateral belt resection

resections (Fig. 36.4, lower right). Standard pre- and postoperative photos and videos are taken in order to provide better comprehension of the results in terms of gluteal contour enhancement.

Surgical Outcome Three patients (15%) underwent circumferential belt lipectomy, 5 patients (25%) had the classic fleur-de-lis operation alone, and 12 patients (60%) had a combination of both belt lipectomy and fleur-de-lis abdominoplasty. No patient had associated gluteal flap or silicone implant during the procedure. Intravenous general anesthesia was performed in nine cases (45%), spinal blocks in four cases (20%), and a combination of both in seven patients (35%). Antibiotic prophylaxis was initiated intravenously in the operating room, 30 min before the incision, followed by a course of oral antibiotics after hospital discharge between 18 and 24 h after surgery. The average total volume grafted into the buttocks was 720 mL of fragmented fat (bilateral), ranging from 500 mL to 960 mL. Small spots of dehiscence along the suture lines were observed in four cases (20%). All were treated conservatively with local wound dressings, except in one patient who needed partial re-suturing of the vertical abdominal incision. No local gluteal complications were reported, such as seroma, infection, fat necrosis, or subcutaneous nodulations (Mendes and Viterbo 2022). Although postoperative results over 6–14 months of follow-up showed clear enhancement of body contouring, those who had associated circumferential lifts appeared to present better waist definition, lifting effect, and gluteal aesthetic contour results. Figures 36.5, 36.6, 36.7, 36.8, 36.9, 36.10, and 36.11 demonstrate several contouring outcomes of our MWL patient treated by injection of fragmented fat to the buttocks.

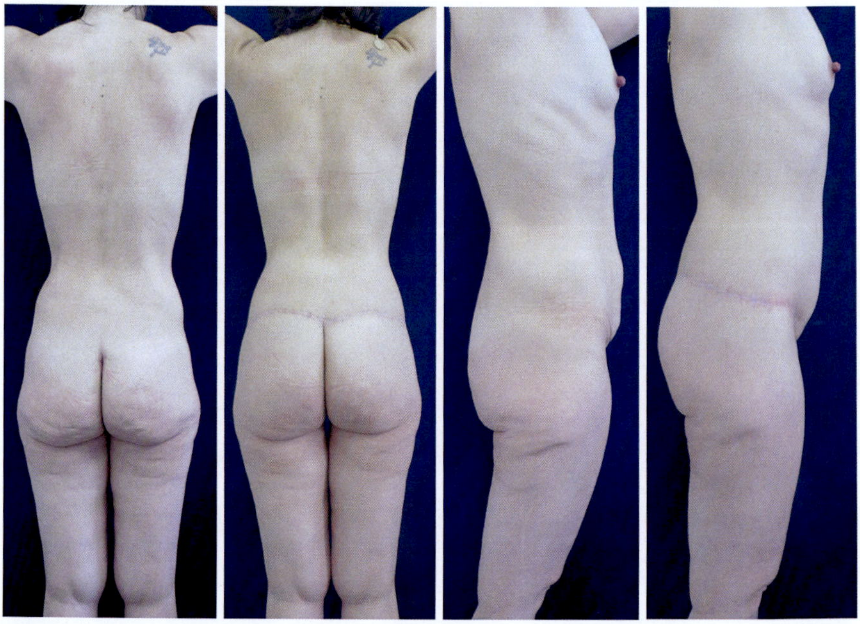

Fig. 36.5 Gluteal aspects of post bariatric 32-year-old woman who lost 55 kg and had a BMI of 23 kg/m^2. Pre and post operative result after 8 months of belt lipectomy with 250 ml of fragmented fat subcutaneously grafted to each buttock

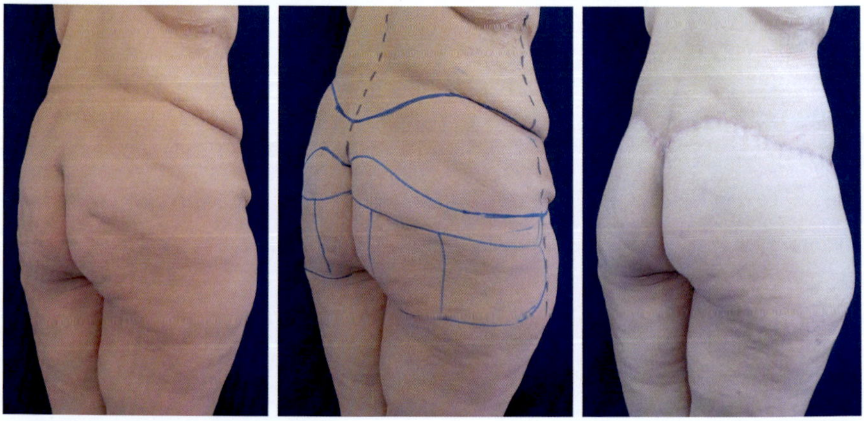

Fig. 36.6 Gluteal lifting and augmentation by circumferential belt lipectomy and fragmented fat transfer of 480 ml in each buttock. Pre (markings) and post-op result after 3 months

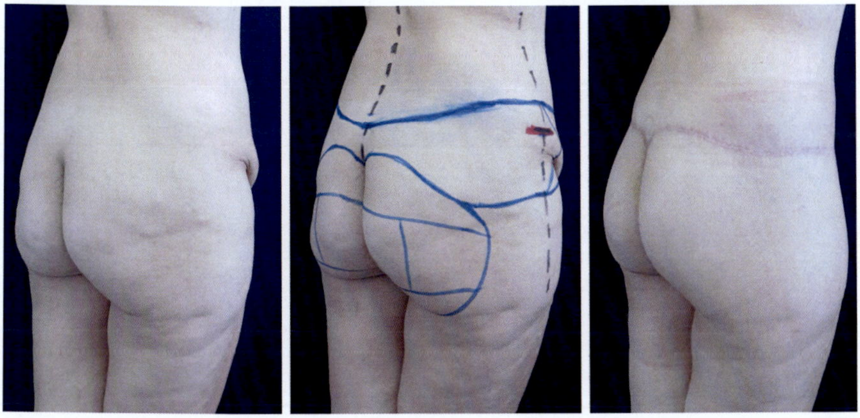

Fig. 36.7 Gluteal lifting and augmentation by circumferential belt lipectomy and fragmented fat transfer of 350 ml in each buttock. Pre (markings) and post-op result after 6 months

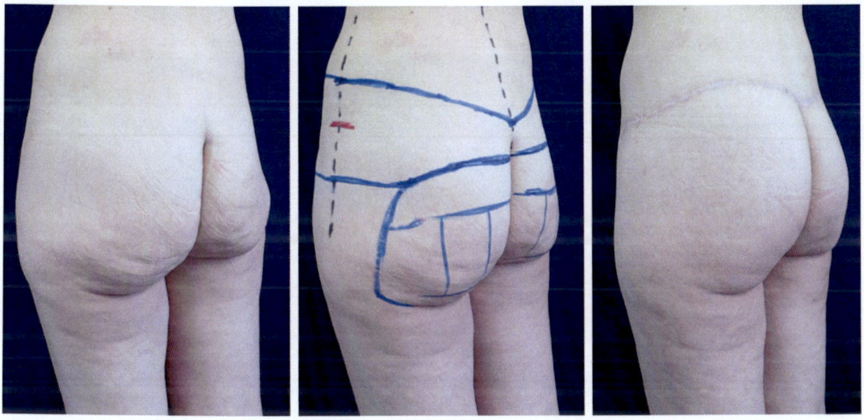

Fig. 36.8 32-year-old woman who lost 55 kg after bariatric surgery and came to a BMI of 23 kg/m^2. Pre (markings) and post operative result after 8 months of belt lipectomy with 500 ml of fragmented fat subcutaneously grafted to both buttocks

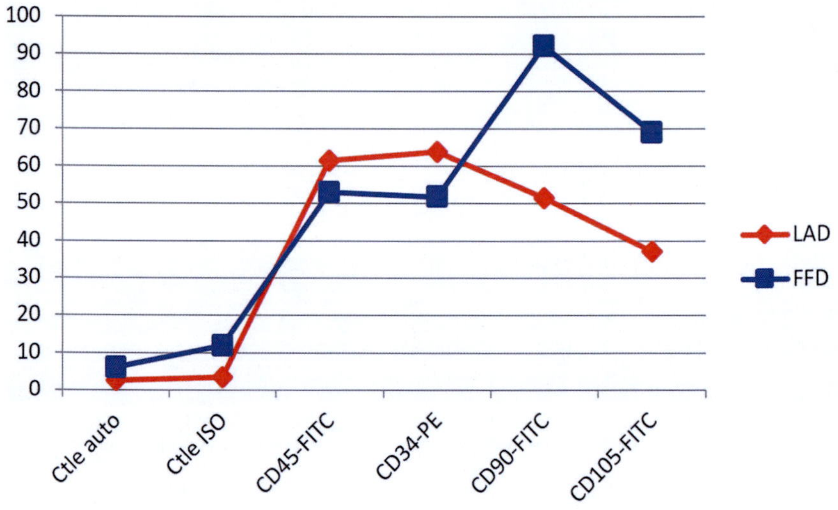

Fig. 36.9 Dry Group: Flow cytometry immunophenotyping comparing the samples of liposuction (LAd) and lipofragmentation (FFd)

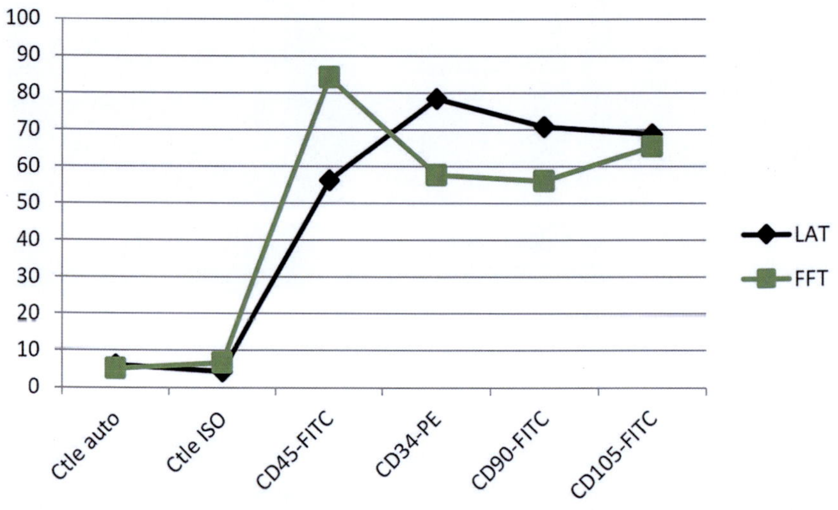

Fig. 36.10 Tumescent Group: Flow cytometry immunophenotyping comparing the samples of liposuction (LAt) and lipofragmentation (FFt)

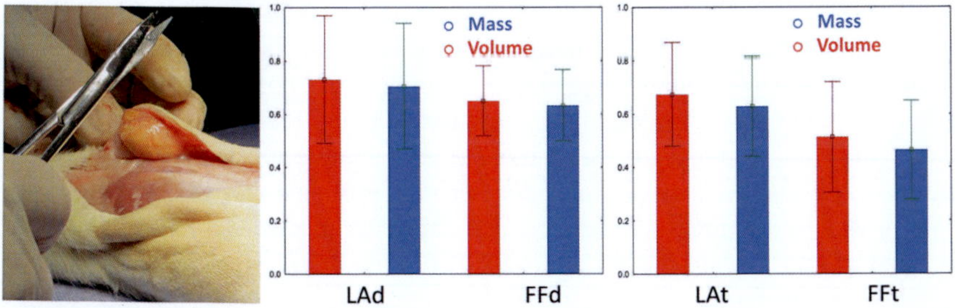

Fig. 36.11 Left: Detail of dorsal graft removal after 6 weeks. Center and right: mass and volume comparison of different retained grafts, in both dry group (LAd and FFd) and tumescent group (LAt and FFt)

Discussion

Since the very beginning, autogenous lipotransfer has shown to be an effective and useful technique for both aesthetic and reconstructive purposes; nevertheless, suction-assisted lipectomy (SAL) was the only accepted harvesting method and that has certainly restricted the range of indications, for different reasons (Bircoll and Novack 1987; Strong et al. 2015; Oranges et al. 2017). Most recently, we have introduced a new source of autogenous lipograft using a simple fragmentation device applied to process resected dermolipectomy specimens, with a small learning curve and very low cost (Mendes and Viterbo 2022). Our in vitro and in vivo observations showed that fragmented fat presented with very similar structural and biologic characteristics as those of the traditional syringe lipoaspirate (Mendes et al. 2019a; Mendes et al. 2019b).

Medical evidence of the dynamic and regenerative nature of fat grafts has emerged from different areas of plastic surgery, as well as from molecular and cell biology, including the possibility of direct transplantation of ADSCs along with their niche (fat niche), even without their isolation in culture, not only to enhance graft retention but also as different sources of cell therapies (Galie et al. 2008; Rigotti et al. 2007). An increasing body of evidence supports the location of matrix-related fibroblasts, fast response angioblasts, and a migrating monoblastic response within the perivascular scaffold, and the ability to readily procure adipose tissue fragments amenable to research is also a legitimate and promising approach (Mendes et al. 2019a). The mechanics involved in the fragmentation process probably incorporates more than just adipose cellular content but its collagenic scaffold structures as well. Flow cytometry with specific panel of surface markers along with dye exclusion cell viability test also helped to distinguish and confirm possible SVF populations on the fragmented fat without significant difference from the lipoaspirate material, showing that the new method did preserve and did not cause any significant damage to those important structures (Mendes et al. 2019b).

Post-bariatric patients usually present body contour deformities that often affect gluteal aesthetics due to a severe disarrangement of buttocks' frame with massive deflation and loss of normal projection. Circumferential body lifts may improve gluteal frame, but still major volume restoration is often necessary. Fat transfer has the ability to widely target and best promote general volume and projection enhancement; nevertheless, there may be such deflated and limiting donor area in that population, in which fat graft is less feasible and not easily harvested by SAL (Mendes and Viterbo 2021; Mendes and Viterbo 2022). Although in a small series, our lack of related complications and nice gluteal contouring results make fragmented fat transfer a promising approach for massive weight loss patients. In fact, not only the gluteal area may be addressed by frag fat transfer but also the breasts, face, and any other deflated areas demanding contour enhancement by lipofilling. More than that, not only MWL patients may benefit from this new technique, since fat fragmentation for regular patients should also meet several kinds of similar indications, in specific situations. It is very important to stress some strong aspects of this alternative augmentation technique which uses autogenous tissue, with low cost and small learning curve, does not increase surgical time, and avoids SAL surgical aggression. Being a new method for harvesting and processing of lipograft, we truly believe that fat fragmentation will rapidly account as a useful and outstanding approach for specific patients, either for aesthetic or regenerative purposes.

References

Mendes FH, Viterbo F. Abdominoplasty after massive weight loss. In: Avelar JM, editor. *New concepts on abdominoplasties and further applications.* Springer; 2016a; 23: 365-388.

Condé-Green A, Kotamarti V, Nini KT, et al. Fat Grafting for Gluteal Augmentation: A Systematic Review of the Literature and Meta-Analysis. *Plast Reconstr Surg.* 2016; 138: 437-446.

Rosique RG, Rosique MJF. Augmentation Gluteoplasty: A Brazilian Perspective. *Plast Reconstr Surg.* 2018; 142(4): 910-919.

Mendes FH, Viterbo F. Gluteal Augmentation in Post-Massive Weight Loss Patients. In: Cansanção A and Condé-Green A, eds. *Gluteal Fat Augmentation.* Springer; 2021, 31: 223-237.

Mendieta CG. Classification system for gluteal evaluation. *Clin Plast Surg.* 2006; 33: 333-346.

Centeno RF. Gluteal aesthetic unit classification: a tool to improve outcomes in body contouring. *Aesthet Surg J.* 2006; 26:200-208.

Light D, Arvanitis GM, Abramson D et al. Effect of weight loss after bariatric surgery on skin and extracellular matrix. *Plast Reconstr Surg.* 2010; 125: 343-351.

Aly AS. Belt lipectomy. In: Body contouring after massive weight loss. St Louis: Quality Medical; 2006. p. 71–145.

Mendes FH, Viterbo F, editors. Cirurgia Plastica Pós Bariátrica. Rio de Janeiro: DiLivros; 2016b.

Fisher C, Grahovac TL, Schafer M et al. Comparison of Harvest and Processing Techniques for Fat Grafting and Adipose Stem Cell Isolation. *Plast. Reconstr. Surg.* 2013; 132: 351 361.

Mendes FH, Viterbo F, Deffunne E, et al. Fragmented fat: a new method for harvesting and processing of lipograft. *J Plast Reconstr Aesthet Surg.* 2019a Jun;72(6):1030-1048.

Mendes FH, Viterbo F, Deffune E et al. Fat grafting: Lipofragmentation X Liposuction. *Rev Bras Cir Plást.* 2019b; 34(3): 368-377.

Ferreira LM ; Borsanyi JP, Bemhain P et al. Rat limb allotransplantation: Efficacy of subtherapeutic dose combination immunotherapy with cyclosporine and RS-61443. In Harii K ed: *Plastic Reconstructive and Aesthetic Surgery*. Kugler 1995; 2: 91-92.

Mendes FH and Viterbo F. Fragmented fat for MWL gluteal augmentation. *Plast Reconstr Surg*. 2022 Mar; In Press.

Cansancao AL. Brazilian buttocks: Fat grafting technique standardization. *Plast Reconstr Surg Glob Open* 2016;4(Suppl):29.

Bircoll M, Novack BH. Autologous fat transplantation employing liposuction techniques. *Ann Plast Surg*. 1987;18:327-329.

Strong AL, Cederna PS, Rubin JP, et al. The current state of fat grafting: a review of harvesting, processing, and injection techniques. *Plast Reconstr Surg*. 2015 Oct;136(4):897-912.

Oranges CM, Tremp M, di Summa PG, et al. Gluteal augmentation techniques: A comprehensive literature review. *Aesthet Surg J*. 2017;37:560–569.

Galie M, Pignatti M, Scambi I, et al. Comparison of different centrifugation protocols for the best yield of adipose-derived stromal cells from lipoaspirates. *Plast Reconstr Surg*. 122: 233e, 2008.

Rigotti G, Marchi A, Galie M et al. Clinical treatment of radiotherapy tissue damage by lipoaspirate transplant: a healing process mediated by adipose-derived adult stem cells. *Plast Reconstr Surg*. 119: 1409, discussion 1423, 2007.

Chapter 37
Behavior of Fat Tissue Transferred for Mastoplasty

Alberto Magno Lott Caldeira

Abstract Autologous fat grafting in plastic surgery has had important advances in recent decades, by showing a notable improvement and remodeling of the receptor zone. It was Neuber who in 1983 used an autologous fat graft to fill and improve the appearance of a sunken scar with good results, and in our experience, we have seen, without a doubt, that the use of autologous fat is a very useful tool for the plastic surgeon, easy to perform, with minimal predictable complications and with good results that last through the years.

Introduction

Autologous fat grafting in plastic surgery has had important advances in recent decades, by showing a notable improvement and remodeling of the receptor zone. It was Neuber who in 1983 used an autologous fat graft to fill and improve the appearance of a sunken scar with good results, and in our experience, we have seen, without a doubt, that the use of autologous fat is a very useful tool for the plastic surgeon, easy to perform, with minimal predictable complications and with good results that last through the years (Avelar 2018).

One notable surgeon who made improvements in the field during the mid-1990s was Sydney Coleman, who standardized the technique to make it reproducible and have predictable results (Pu et al. 2015). He stated that fat should be transferred in small quantities to the recipient tissues and deposited in multilayered tunnels using a retrograde technique, so that most of the injected adipocytes would be in close contact with well-vascularized tissues, increasing the survival

A. M. L. Caldeira (✉)
São Paulo, Brazil

J. M. Avelar, R. Cavalcanti Ribeiro (eds.), *Body Contouring*,
https://doi.org/10.1007/978-3-031-42802-9_37

rate of the fat transferred. It was imperative not to inject fat as a bolus, because it would form lakes of transferred adipose tissue without a good oxygen supply, which in the end would produce necrosis and reabsorption of most of the transfer (Bircoll 1987).

Without a doubt, we must mention the contribution made by Mel Bircoll MD, who in 1987 presented the first four cases published in the medical literature, where he conducted fat transfer to breast tissue in small amounts, establishing the principle that fat must be transferred in small tubular portions to improve their survival. In addition, in Brazil, Wilson Da Silveira Jacques M.D. in 1998 published in *The American Journal of Cosmetic Surgery* his cases with fat transfer to breast tissue with good results (Wilson Da Silveira 1998; Caldeira et al. 2016).

In augmentation and reconstructive mammoplasty, the behavior of the fatty tissue has shown excellent results; in the opinion of the author, we currently use a protocol established by our service that has produced interesting and above all long-lasting results.

Fat tissue transfer requires an interval of minimum between 4 and 6 months, corresponding to the period necessary to the development and maturation of new adipocytes. For the fat graft, we recommend the infiltration of the super-humid technique of the regions to be liposuctioned; we generally use as the main area fat donor the abdomen and dorsal region, although liposuction can be performed from any region of the body with lipodystrophy (Eto et al. 2009).

Composition of the Transferred Adipose Tissue

As is logical to analyze, the adipose tissue obtained from its donor zone not only contains adipose cells, in fact, thanks to immunohistochemical studies, the following composition has been evidenced (Suga et al. 2010a):

16% fat cells
30% stem cells
30% fibroblasts and muscle cells
15% endothelial cells
9% blood cells (Fig. 37.1)

But even more striking is the discovery of microscopic capillaries of less than 50 Um crossing the surface of the adipocyte and which is essential for the exchange of nutrients and oxygen and therefore its vitality.

However, at the time of obtaining the fat tissue by liposuction, some of these capillaries break, and therefore the adipocytes need, as in any graft, to start living by plasma imbibition until there is a capillary reorganization (Coleman and Saboeiro 2007).

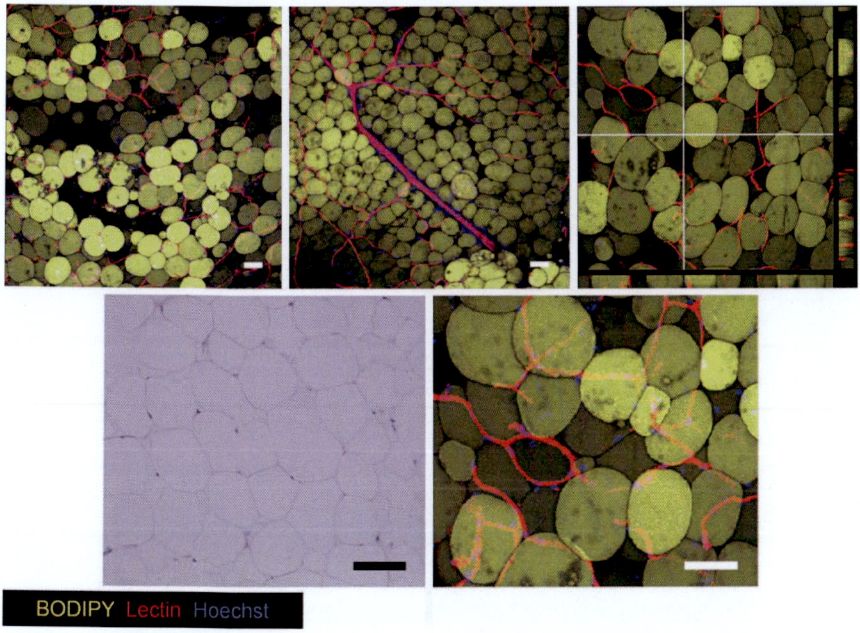

Fig. 37.1 Structure of living adipose tissue in whole-mount triple-stained images. Nonfixed aspirated and excised adipose tissues were stained with boron-dipyrromethene (adipocytes; *yellow*), lectin (endothelial cells; *red*), and Hoechst 33,342 (nuclei; *blue*) and investigated using a confocal microscope. There were many capillaries running alongside adipocytes in both aspirated and excised adipose tissues

It is important the fat to be transferred be placed in small quantities, like cylinders, to ensure the vitality of most of it, avoiding excessive volume in a single area (Cleveland et al. 2015).

Importance of the Ischemic Period of the Transferred Fat Tissue

When the fatty tissue is transferred to the receptor site, it suffers a moderate to severe ischemia; normally, cells such as some adipocytes or vascular cells are very sensitive to ischemia and suffer apoptosis and necrosis within the first 24 h. However, an important group of cells, SPC (stromal progenitor cells), seem to be resistant to periods of ischemia beyond 72 h, when the grafted tissue begins the revascularization phase, but above all, it should be noted that these cells are precisely stimulated by ischemia to be activated and fulfill the function of driving the regenerative changes that occur from the fourth day of fat grafting until approximately week 12 (Caldeira et al. 1988; Guerrerosantos 1996).

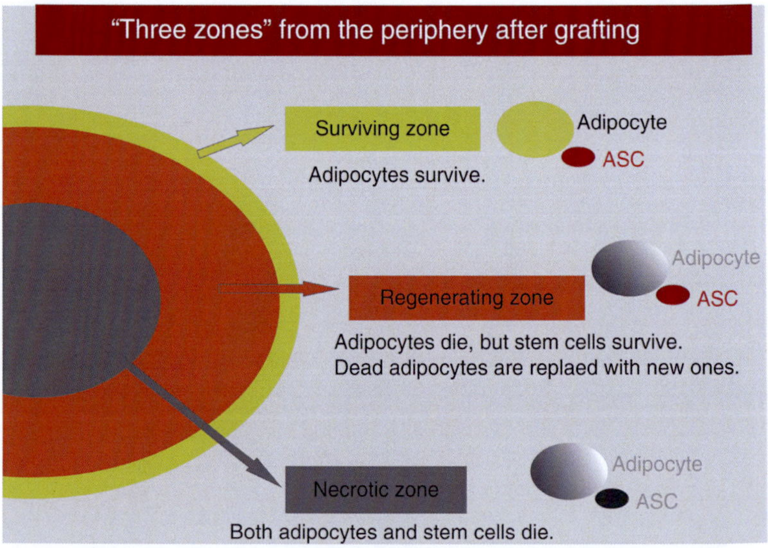

Fig. 37.2 Conclusive schema for three zones of the grafts. The most superficial zone is the "surviving zone," which is less than 300 μm thick. In the surviving zone, both adipocytes and stromal progenitor cells survive. The second zone is the "regenerating zone," the thickness of which varies depending on the microenvironmental conditions such as the vascularity of and attachment to the surrounding tissue. In this zone, adipocytes die as early as day 1, but stromal progenitor cells survive and provide new adipocytes to replace the dead ones. The most central zone is the "necrotic zone," where both adipocytes and stromal progenitor cells die, no regeneration is expected, and the dead space is absorbed or filled by scar formation (Reproduced with permission from Eto H, Kato H, Suga H et al. (2012) The fate of adipocytes after nonvascularized fat grafting: evidence of early death and replacement of adipocytes, Plast Reconstr Surg; 129(5):1081–92. https://doi.org/10.1097/PRS.0b013e31824a2b19

It is important to keep in mind that, when placing the transferred fat in the receptor site, if we imagine a kind of cylinder, we have an external wall that is in direct contact with the receptor bed and therefore has greater assured viability, an intermediate part that suffers ischemia and where the adipocytes die; however, SPC survive and promote the formation of new adipocytes, and finally a central zone, the one with less vitality because it is far from the periphery, which will die, will be absorbed and remodeled (Guerrerosantos 1996) (Figs. 37.2 and 37.3).

The body responds and fights ischemia to preserve the tissue transfer in the best way possible. It is ambiguous, but ischemia not only destroys endothelial cells and adipocytes but also regenerates them. Going into a more detailed way, two substances appear to be the most important for the survival of the transferred

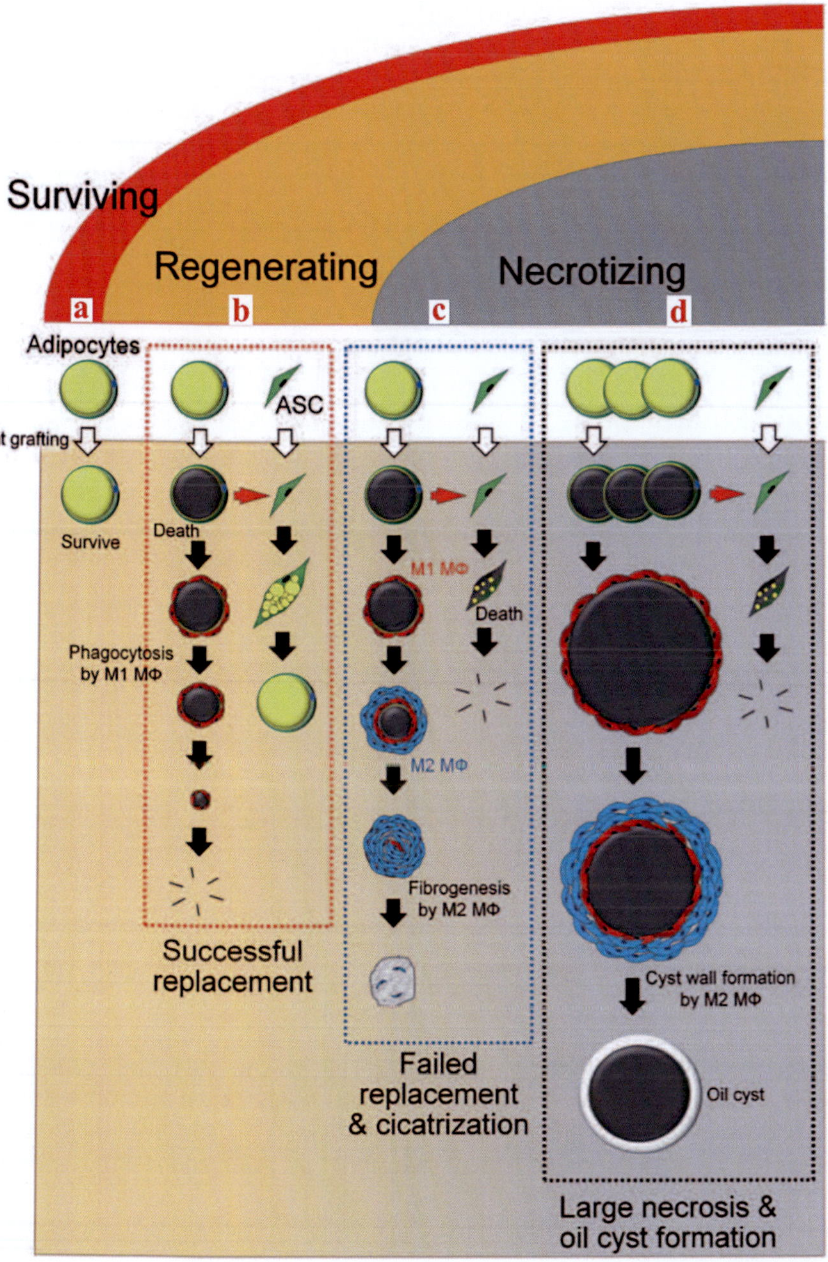

Fig. 37.3 Once the fat has been transferred, the following can occur: (**a**) the fat that is more in contact with the tissues has a greater probability of living. (**b**) Fat can disappear or be stimulated by SPC and generate new adipose tissue. (**c**) Type II macrophages are stimulated and lead to a healing and scar process. (**d**) Type II macrophages envelop the central portions of the transferred fat and form oily cysts that disappear over time

fat tissue against ischemia: the HIF-alpha (hypoxia-inducible factor) and FGF-2 (fibroblast growth factor) molecules produced by dying adipocytes that activate a more hypoxia-resistant cell lineage, the SPC. These types of cells can adequately resist hypoxia for 72 h or more, the time needed for angiogenesis to rebuild the capillary network around the tissue transfer. More importantly, when activated, they are transformed into new adipocytes (Suga et al. 2008; De Fillippo and Atala 2002).

Once again, although it is true that ischemia affects the central area, it is also relevant to mention that it is a determining and important factor to stimulate stem cells and their regeneration and production of new adipocytes.

Surgical Indications

We must conduct a complete evaluation of our patient in consultation. Measurements of the breasts, the thickness of the breast tissue, the measurement of the breast base, verify asymmetries of volume or shape, find out if the patient is in a weight loss regime, and taking history of hypertension, smoking, microangiopathies, or any pathology existing that affects microcirculation should be conducted.

Although any patient is eligible for this surgical procedure, we consider as ideal patients those patients with juvenile hypomastia who present some degree of fat, especially in the hypogastrium or flanks. In the same way, we consider ideal patients with large weight losses after which their breasts have become empty and flaccid and finally patients with breast asymmetries, tuberous breast, volume asymmetry, or who need a complement to their surgical procedure such as use implants or in conjunction with a mastopexy.

Surgical Technique

Liposuction is a low-cost and simple procedure with the advantage of using autologous fat to modify the body contour. However, because fat can be harvested from different body areas, survival rates have been reported to be highly variable from study to study, ranging from 30 to 95%. The difference in fat survival as it relates to various patient characteristics is broadly lacking and may play a significant role. Criteria such as donor-site choice, patient age, and body mass index may all be significant in their effect on fat survival (Yoshimura et al. 2009).

According to R. Rohrich, age affects adipocyte viability differently across anatomical regions. The lower abdomen appears to be a preferred source of adipocytes in younger patients, whereas the flank showed higher adipocyte viability in the older ones (Rohrich et al. 2006).

Liposuction is performed in the lower abdomen of young patients and in the flanks of older ones (Spear et al. 2005).

In our experience, we use the following protocol which has given us satisfactory results with high retention rates of the ideal fat transferred volume:

- Decantation of the fat is done using 60-mL syringes (Fig. 37.3).
- After decantation, transference of the fat to 10-mL syringes.
  The breast is marked into quadrants for easier fat distribution.
- 2-mm incisions are made in the center of the inframammary fold and at 12 o'clock on the areola (Fig. 37.4).
- Fat transfer is conducted using 1.7–1.9-mm blunt microcannulas.
- Layering the fat into different levels: subcutaneous, intraglandular, subglandular, and intramuscular (Fig. 37.5).
- Injection of the fat, according to Coleman's tunneling technique, in a retrograde fashion following fanning mode. Injecting 10 mL per tunnel, creating about 50 tunnels per breast depending on the amount of fat transfer.
- Dressing is applied.

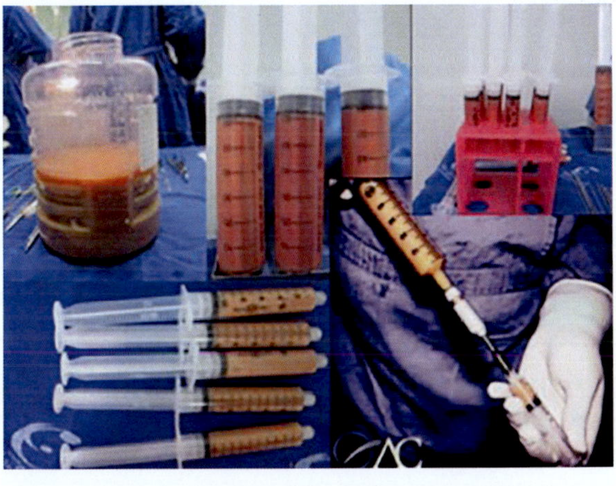

Fig. 37.4 Decantation of the fat and transfer to 10 mL syringes. Reproduced with permission from A. Caldeira's library

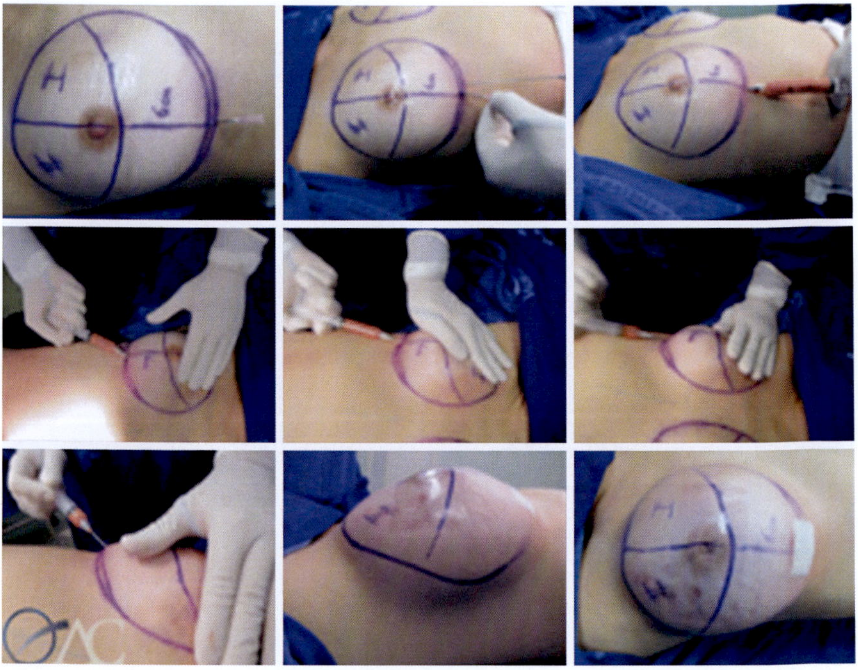

Fig. 37.5 Marking of the breast into quadrants and 2-mm incisions in the inframammary fold. Reproduced with permission from A. Caldeira's library

Complications

Fat tissue transfer in body reshaping surgery has proven over the years to be a safe procedure with low morbidity and whose complications do not represent great challenges for the surgeon.

Thus, it has been reported that hematomas may occur in a low percentage, temporary breast asymmetry as a result of differentiated edema, transient erythema, infection in a low percentage, and perhaps among the most common complications, the formation of oily cysts that remit spontaneously in the period of up to 1 year.

It is important to mention that there is no extensive fat necrosis since we are transferring small portions of fatty tissue, but there is the formation of cysts in those adipose cells that have suffered irreversible ischemia (Eto et al. 2012) (Fig. 37.6).

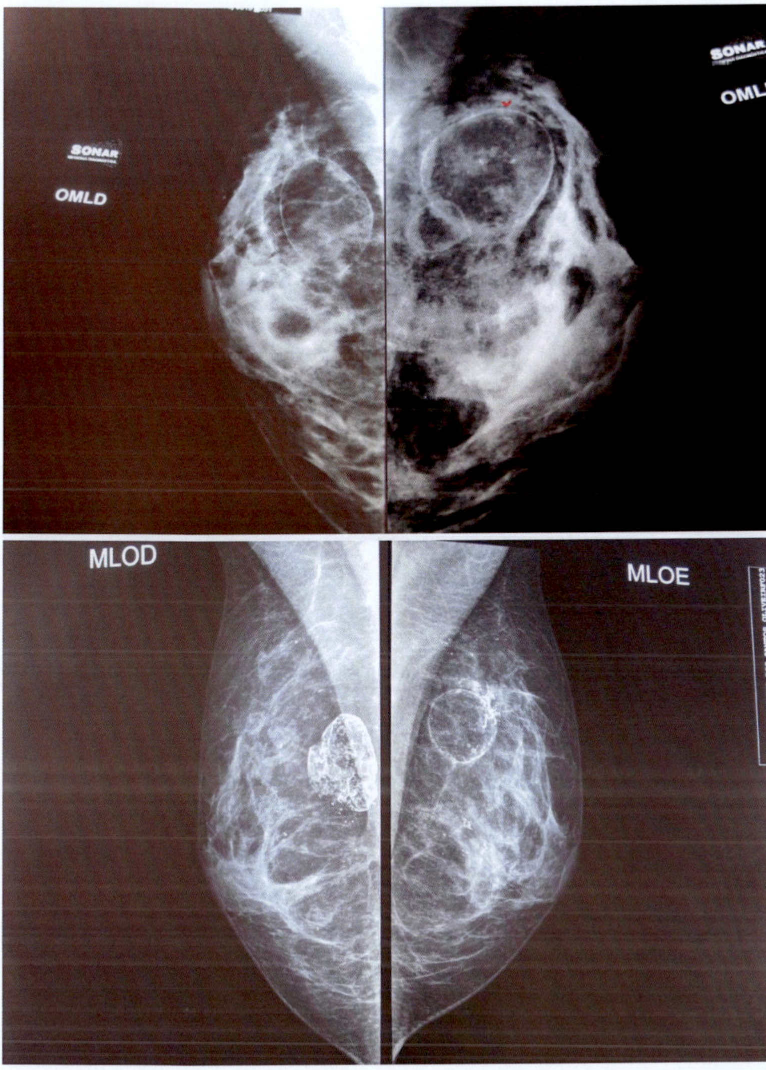

Fig. 37.6 Postoperative mammogram in the first year, showing a large oil cyst. Subsequently, at 3 and a half years, a control mammogram is performed, which shows involution of the oily cyst and decrease in size and content

Recommendations for a Successful Result

Recommendations for a successful procedure:

- The outcome of breast augmentation through fat transfer is related to the surgeon's level of expertise and the technique used.

- The technique must include all precautions to ensure that the maximum amount of fat survives:
  - Reducing the possibility of trauma to the harvest site.
  - Demonstrating correct refinement to the tissue.
  - Minimal fat manipulation.
  - Delivering droplets of fat through thin cannulas, never exceeding the 2-mm limit (Geissler et al. 2014).
  - Placement of small aliquots instead of large portions should be achieved.
  - Transferred fat should be placed in proximity to the patient's blood supply to increase fat survival rates and reduce both the implication of fat necrosis and calcification risk (Mineda et al. 2014).
  - A trained radiologist is necessary for reliable screening.

Results

We take advantage of the first surgery time to conduct fat tissue and transfer it in order to promote an increase in breast volume and improvement in the quality of the tissues circumscribed to the breast that allows to obtain a better result when the definitive remodeling surgery mammary is performed.

Fat transfer enables a comprehensive reshaping of the breasts, involving volumetric recomposition of breast tissue as well as the parenchymal, cutaneous, and muscular planes. This technique utilizes adipose tissue, carrying stem cells, to address both minor mammary deformities and major alterations. The key prerequisite for success lies in the ubiquitous presence of fat compartments, allowing for the achievement of this aesthetic goal. Therefore, we recommend its use always independent of the breast reconstruction technique, because it is the only way to rebuild the upper mammary pole in the short and long term. It is very important to know the nutritional status of patients who are going to have body contour surgery, with adequate replacement and correct balance to reduce as much as possible the surgical procedure risks (Suga et al. 2010b).

Presurgical laboratory evaluation determines this nutritional status and guides hematic replacement or trace elements above reference values if necessary. At our practice we have established a preoperative preparation protocol in all patients undergoing to large liposculptures with significant mobilization of aspirated fatty tissue. We have seen that this population of patients usually need replacement before any surgical procedure in order to maintain the homeostasis, decrease the inflammatory response, and prevent possible complications resulting from surgery. Although most surgeons today perform combined surgeries in these patients, there is no scientifically defined limits for number or extent of procedures to be conducted in a single operation. The aim of the procedures depends mainly of the experience and judgment of the surgeon.

We present the cases of three of our patients, in whom we performed mastopexy with augmentation mammoplasty using autologous fat transfer, with satisfactory results (Figs. 37.7, 37.8, and 37.9).

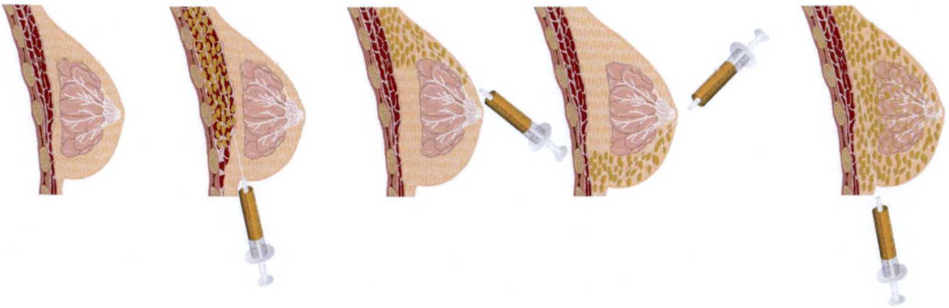

Fig. 37.7 Layering the fat into different levels. Reproduced with permission from A. Caldeira's library

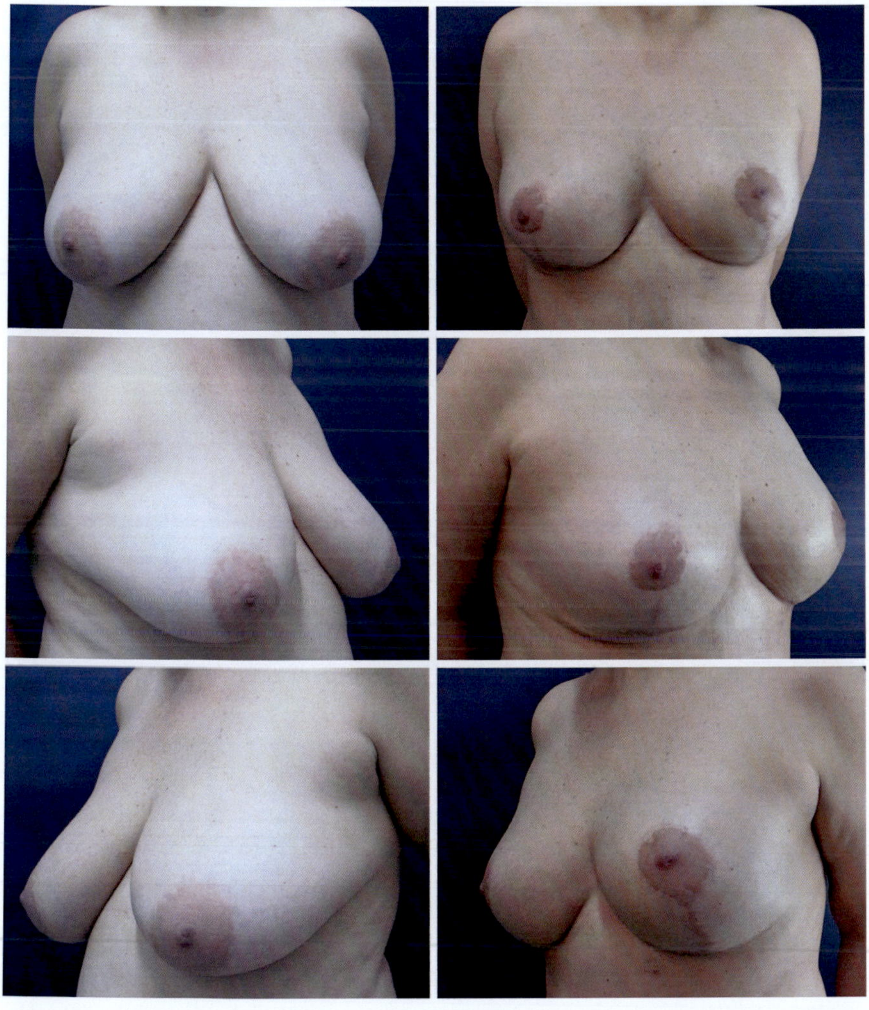

Fig. 37.8 A 43-year-old female patient with 20 kg weight loss who had liposuction + breast augmentation performed using autologous fat graft in 2015 who has undergone 200 ml of fat transfer for each breast. Photo: 9 months after surgery

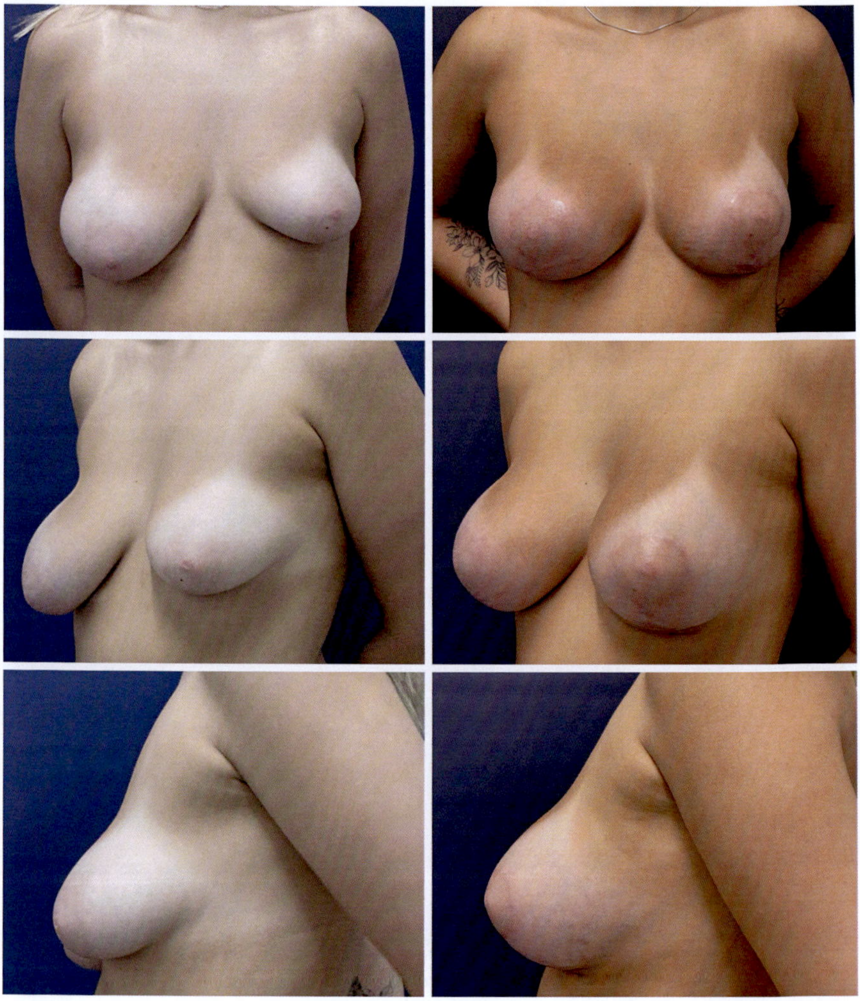

Fig. 37.9 A 19-year-old female patient who went under augmentation mammaplasty with 195 ml implants + mastopexy with triple-flap Caldeira's technique + breast fat graft: 80 ml right breast/90 ml left breast. Photo: 3 months after surgery

Discussion

The senior author's proposal, based on the use of fat grafting to the breast with adi pose derived and mesenchymal stromal cells, has demonstrated repair properties to replace damaged cells or missing, fill, and remodel deformities and, with that, promoted the volumetric increase of the breasts and the restructuring of adjacent tissues in the grafting area without the presence of additional scars, preserving the sensitivity and the lactiferous function of breasts, with significantly lasting, reliable, and safe results. Because of these observations, the breast augmentation in adolescent patients, or those who are at the end of the second or at the beginning third decade of life, should be performed primarily using fat tissue.

Our experience with autologous fat transfer for breast augmentation and remodeling began in 2008; it is 13 years to date with satisfactory, long-lasting results and minimal complications. We attribute a large part of our good results to the fundamental principle of the correct selection of our patients and to our protocol based on the use of recombinant human erythropoietin.

This glycoprotein has action on the hematopoietic system, being equally important are its effects on non-tissue hematopoietic where it plays an inhibitory role apoptosis and inflammation secondary to hypoxia, toxicity, or injury, in addition to being a potent inducer of angiogenesis with cardio and neuroprotective effects (Khouri et al. 2012).

Erythropoietin administered 6 days before the surgical procedure helps us raise the blood values of our patients and prepare them to better tolerate surgical stress.

More importantly, erythropoietin applied 6 days after the surgical procedure has been shown in vivo to promote the proliferation of these stem cells and the appearance of new adipocytes, which slowly reach a final result around 4–6 months, at which point which can be performed another breast augmentation procedure if desired and lipodystrophy areas are available.

The fat transferred to the breasts must be placed in all levels, from the muscular, the parenchymal, as well as in the breast fat tissue itself, since the transferred fat provides stem cells that are the most important cells due to their proliferative potential.

The importance and safety of the technique lie in the transfer of small amounts of fatty tissue in the form of cylinders, without trying to expand the tissue or depositing lakes of fat.

Although the tissue graft autologous fat offers several advantages, such as providing a moderate increase in volume, imperceptible scarring, and improved skin texture, without the complications associated with the use of foreign bodies, unpredictability and low tissue survival rate of the fat due to the partial volumetric loss of fat grafts are problems that still need to be addressed (Yoshimura et al. 2010).

We present here the evolution of our patient 1 year later by mammography control, where we can clearly see the apoptosis of breast tissue produced by the implant and how fat transfer improves breast tissue and reverses this process with a long-lasting result. In this way, fat transferred improves the quality of surrounding tissues as well as the quality of the skin (Fig. 37.10).

We also had the opportunity to treat a patient diagnosed with scleroderma, with breast involvement, irregularities, and the characteristic skin lesions, treated by fat transfer to the breast tissue, presenting an excellent evolution and an encouraging prognosis (Fig. 37.11).

We performed a control mammogram in the first postoperative year, finding the formation of oily cysts, which is the most common complication in the transfer of fat to the breast tissue, which does not need any type of aggressive intervention, it is

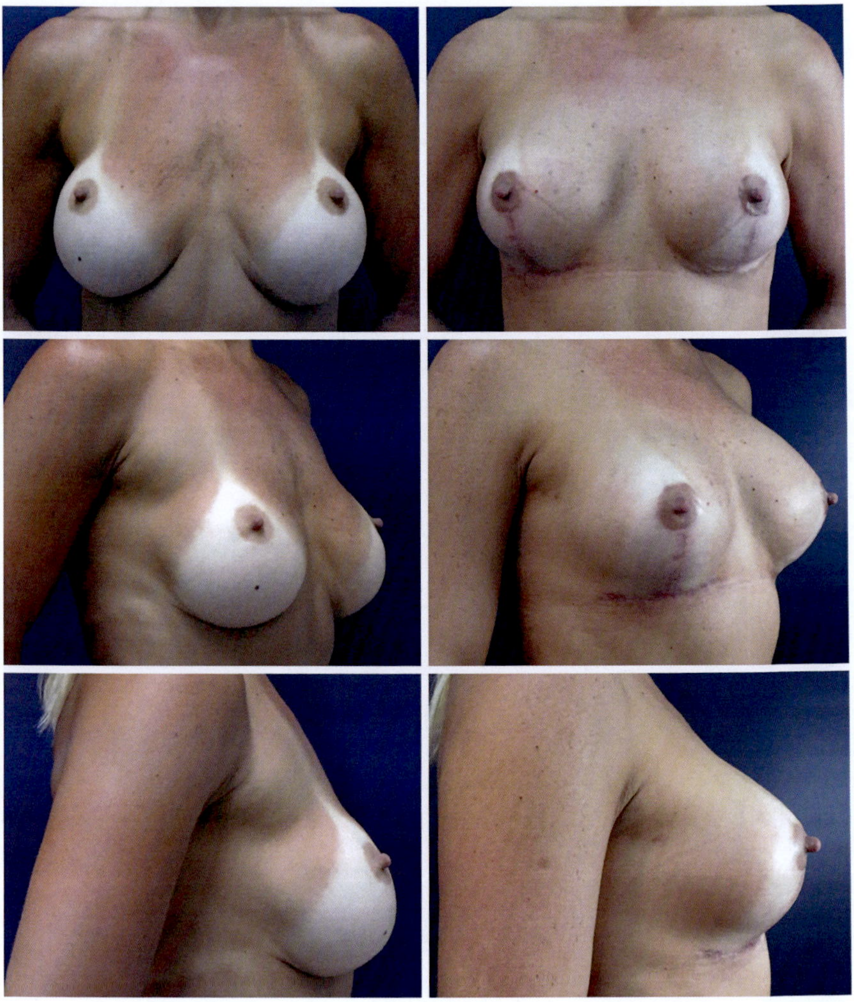

Fig. 37.10 A 44-year-old female patient under augmentation mammaplasty with 330 ml implants + mastopexy with triple-flap Caldeira's technique + correction of rippling caused by apoptosis of breast tissue by old implants with fat graft: 50 ml right breast/40 ml left breast. Photo: 3 months after surgery

enough to have expectant management, since the oily cysts regress over time until they disappear. If necessary, its content can be punctured and absorbed, and in the same maneuver the walls of the cyst can break and in this way the cyst is completely eliminated (Fig. 37.12).

An important fact to emphasize is that even when there may be a localized infection, stem cells act as inflammatory modulators, in such a way that they prevent the appearance of great edema. These cells remain inactive while the infection is resolved and subsequently continue to grow, with which the surgical result is not compromised (Parrish and Metzinger 2010).

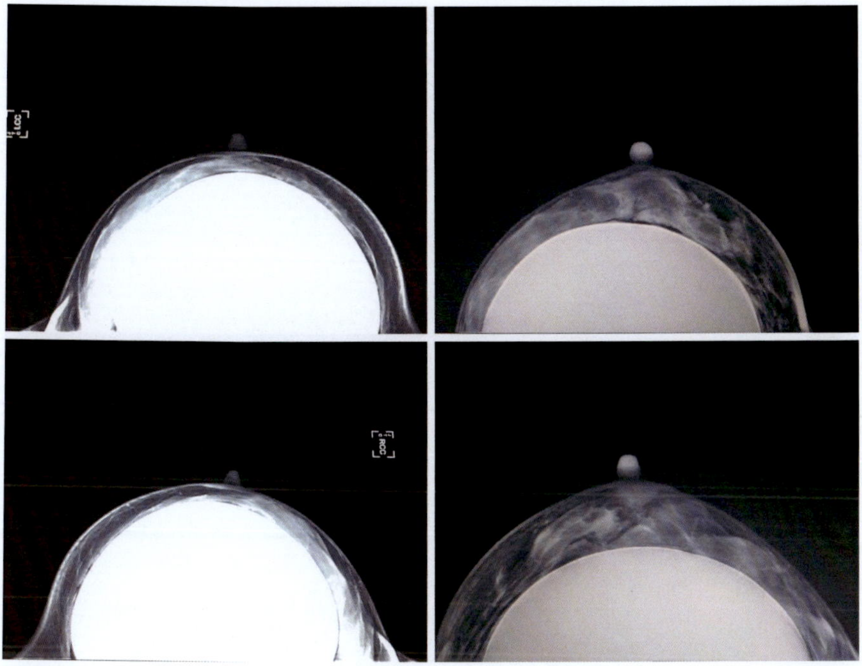

Fig. 37.11 Mammography 12 months later: correction of rippling caused by apoptosis of breast tissue. Image shows the apoptosis of breast tissue produced by the implant and how fat transfer improves breast tissue and reverses this process

Despite oncological and radiological concerns and efficacy, many surgeons believe that the benefits of fat transfer in the breast outweigh its risks, mainly because the behavior of cells mesenchymal in vitro may present differences in relation to that of mesenchymal cells in vivo (Bourne et al. 2016).

Effect of *N*-Acetylcysteine in Fat Transfer Survival

N-acetylcysteine is a widely known antioxidant that works by reducing oxygen free radicals using a sulfhydryl chemical group. It is established that during fat harvest, before the transfer, isolated cells are put under significant mechanical, ischemic, and oxidative stress, which results in cell injury and a reduced regeneration rate in the future. That is why in the last year, a research group was interested in determining whether *N*-acetylcysteine administered at the site of the harvest could improve long-term regeneration percentages (Gillis et al. 2015).

In addition to local factors, it allows an evident improvement in silhouette and body contour with treatment of areas of lipodystrophy. Breast augmentation by transfer of fat tissue is a safe and effective way to breast augmentation, a versatile process that can promote safe and satisfactory clinical and surgical results.

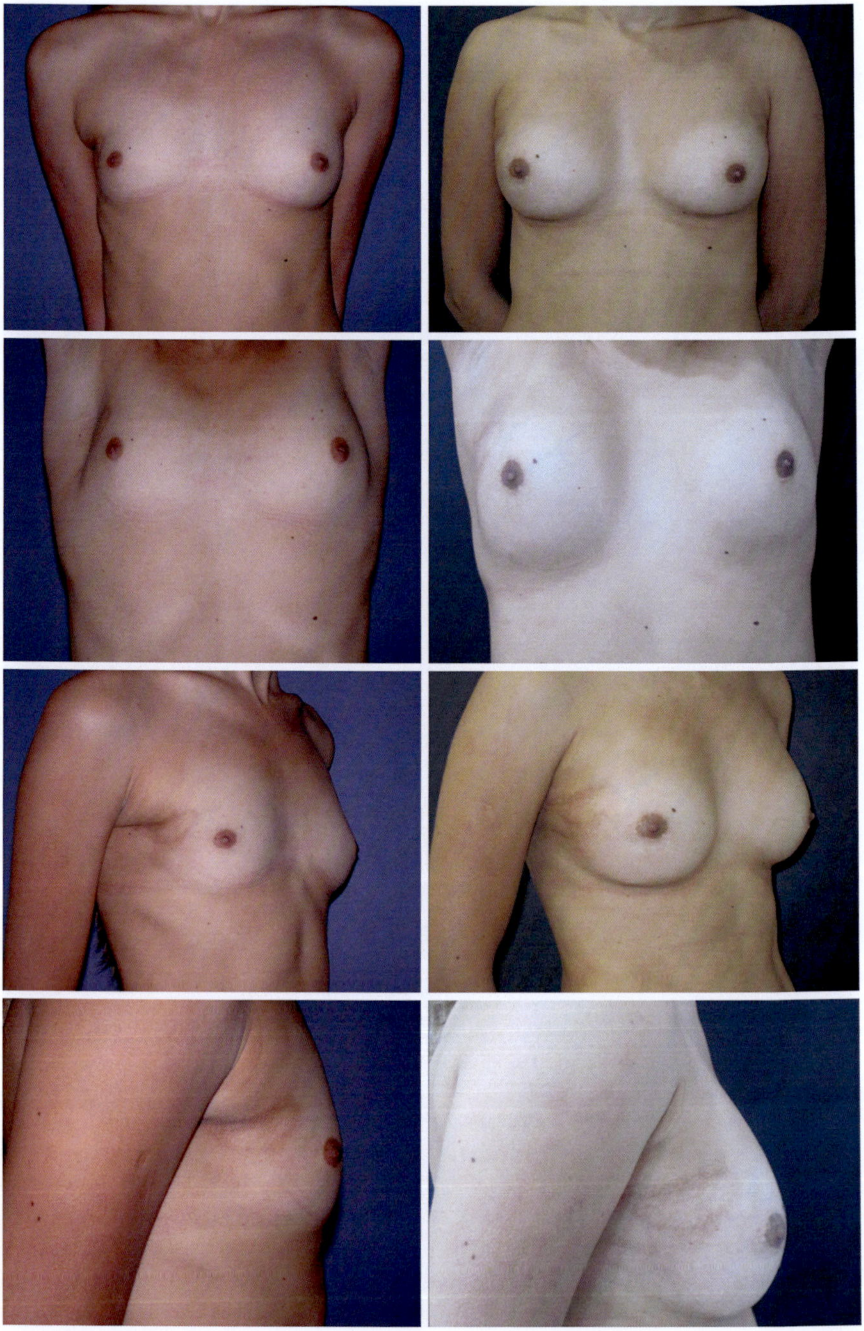

Fig. 37.12 A 19-year-old female patient diagnosed with scleroderma with breast involvement, retraction, and morphology alterations. Pre- and postoperative images are presented 6 years after her intervention with fat transfer showing a satisfactory and lasting result

References

J.M. Avelar (ed.), *Breast Surgery*. 2018. https://doi.org/10.1007/978-3-319-54115-0_48
Pu LL, Yoshimura K, Coleman SR (2015) Future perspectives of fat grafting. Clin Plast Surg 42(3):389–394. https://doi.org/10.1016/j.cps.2015.03.007
Bircoll M (1987) Cosmetic breast augmentation utilizing autologous fat and liposuction techniques. Plast Reconstr Surg 79(2):267–271
Wilson Da Silveira J (1998) The American Journal of Cosmetic Surgery, vol. 15, *n°2*
Caldeira A, Marrou W, Bromley M (2016) Fat transfer in augmentation mammography, a 3D volumetric evaluation. Oral presentation. ASAPS, Las Vegas
Eto H, Suga H, Matsumoto D et al (2009) Characterization of structure and cellular components of aspirated and excised adipose tissue. Plast Reconstr Surg 124(4):1087–1097. doi:https://doi.org/10.1097/PRS.0b013e3181b5a3f1
Suga H, Eto H, Aoi N et al (2010a) Adipose tissue remodeling under ischemia: death of adipocytes and activation of stem/progenitor cells. Plast Reconstr Surg 126(6):1911–1923. https://doi.org/10.1097/PRS.0b013e3181f4468b
Coleman SR, Saboeiro AP (2007) Fat grafting to the breast revisited: safety and efficacy. Plast Reconstr Surg 119(3):775–785
Cleveland E, Albano N, Hazen A (2015) Roll, spin, wash, or filter? Processing of lipoaspirate for autologous fat grafting: an updated, evidence-based review of the literature. Plast Reconstr Surg 136(4):706–713
Caldeira, A., Nieves, A., Maleombho, J., Arquero, S.P. Cirurgia do Rejuvenecimento Facial. Importância do Tratamento do Tecido Gorduroso. *Rev. Bras. Cir.* 1988; 78(6):375-392.
Guerrerosantos J (1996) Autologous fat grafting for body contouring. Clin Plast Surg 23(4):619–631
Suga H, Matsumoto D, Inoue K, Shigeura T, Eto H, Aoi N, Kato H, Abe H, Yoshimura K (2008) Numerical measurement of viable and nonviable adipocytes and other cellular components in aspirated fat tissue. Plast Reconstr Surg 122(1):103–114
De Fillippo RE, Atala A (2002) Stretch and growth: the molecular and physiological influences of tissue expansion. Plast Reconstr Surg 109(7):2450–2462
Yoshimura K, Shigeura T, Matsumoto D et al (2006) Characterization of freshly isolated and cultured cells derived from the fatty and fluid portions of liposuction aspirates. J Cell Physiol 208(1):64–76
Yoshimura K, Suga H, Eto H (2009) Adipose-derived stem/progenitor cells: roles in adipose tissue remodeling and potential use for soft tissue augmentation. Regen Med 4(2):265–273
Spear SL, Wilson HB. Lockwood T. (2005) Fat injection to correct contour deformities in the reconstructed breast. Plast Reconstruct Surg. 2005; 116:1300-5.
Eto H, Kato H, Suga H et al (2012) The fate of adipocytes after nonvascularized fat grafting: evidence of early death and replacement of adipocytes. Plast Reconstr Surg 129(5):1081–1092. doi:https://doi.org/10.1097/PRS.0b013e31824a2b19
Geissler PJ, Davis K, Roostaeian J et al (2014) Improving fat transfer viability: the role of aging, body mass index, and harvest site. Plast Reconstr Surg 134(2):227–232. doi:https://doi.org/10.1097/PRS.0000000000000398
Mineda K, Kuno S, Kato H et al (2014) Chronic inflammation and progressive calcification as a result of fat necrosis: the worst outcome in fat grafting. Plast Reconstr Surg 133(5):1064–1072. doi:https://doi.org/10.1097/PRS.0000000000000097
Suga H, Eto H, Aoi N et al (2010b) Adipose tissue remodeling under ischemia: death of adipocytes and activation of stem/progenitor cells. Plast Reconstr Surg 126(6):1911–1923. doi: https://doi.org/10.1097/PRS.0b013e3181f4468b
Khouri RK, Eisenmann-Klein M, Cardoso E, Cooley BC, Kacher D, Gombos E, Baker TJ (2012) Brava and autologous fat transfer is a safe and effective breast augmentation alternative: results of a 6-year, 81-patient, prospective multicenter study. Plast Reconstr Surg 129(5):1173–1187

Yoshimura K., Asano Y., Aoi N., Kurita M., Oshima Y., Sato K., Inoue K., Suga H., Eto H., Kato H., Harii K. (2010) Progenitor-enriched adipose tissue transplantation as rescue for breast implant complications. Breast J. 16(2):169-175.

Parrish J.N., Metzinger S.E. Autogenous fat grafting and breast augmentation: a review of the literature. *Aesth. Surg. J.* 2010;30(4):549-556.

Bourne D.A., James I.B., Wang S.S., Marra K.G., Rubin J.P. The architecture of fat grafting: what lies beneath the surface. *Plast. Reconstr. Surg.* 2016;137(3):1072-1079

Rohrich R.J., Gosmann A.A., Brown S.A., Reisch J. Mastopexy Preferences: A Survey of Board-Certified Plastic Surgeons. *Plast. Reconstr. Surg*. 2006;118(7):1631-1638.

Gillis J, Gebremeskel S, Phipps KD et al (2015) Effect of N-acetylcysteine on adipose-derived stem cell and autologous fat graft survival in a mouse model. Plast Reconstr Surg 136(2):179e–188e. https://doi.org/10.1097/PRS.0000000000001443

Chapter 38
Importance of Fat Grafting for Reparation of Unsatisfactory Results After Liposuction

Luiz Haroldo Pereira, Beatriz Nicaretta, and Aris Sterodimas

Abstract **Background**: Liposuction has evolved tremendously over the past three decades and is the most frequently performed aesthetic procedure. Although liposuction has been considered a safe surgical procedure, reports indicate that it can have significant sequelae. The increasing number of liposuction procedures, often performed by inadequately trained physicians, has led to a growing number of iatrogenic post-liposuction contour complications.

Methods: Fifty-five patients with post-liposuction depressions were operated during January 2017 and October 2019. Forty-one females and 14 male patients were included in this study group. Age distribution of patients ranged from 28 to 62 years, with a mean of 46.7 years. All the patients that were included in this study were candidates for autologous fat transplantation. Patients underwent the Stromal Enriched Lipograft technique for correction of their body liposuction sequelae.

Results: The total amount of clean adipose tissue transplanted varied from 20 to 150 ml. There were no cases of liponecrosis, which developed in the grafted area, and no liponecrotic lumps were palpated on postoperative evaluation on any operated cases. There were no cases of cellulitis at the donor or grafted area, no deep vein thrombosis, and no pulmonary embolism. There were no cases that needed additional session of fat grafting.

Conclusion: Liposuction continues to be a safe surgical procedure, but for maximum avoidance of complications, the surgeon should be mindful of all the factors

L. H. Pereira
LH Clinic, Rio de Janeiro, Brazil

B. Nicaretta · A. Sterodimas (✉)
Department of Plastic and Reconstructive Surgery, Metropolitan General Hospital, Athens, Greece
e-mail: aris@sterodimas.com

J. M. Avelar, R. Cavalcanti Ribeiro (eds.), *Body Contouring*,
https://doi.org/10.1007/978-3-031-42802-9_38

that could predispose to complications. Stromal Enriched Lipograft is a safe and effective technique that offers the possibility of finally fulfilling the key principle of replacing "like with like" as an aesthetic filler, without the drawbacks of the traditional autologous fat grafting technique.

Introduction

Liposuction has evolved tremendously over the past three decades since its introduction by Illouz (Illouz 1983). The abdominal area, the banana fold, and the sensuous triangle are difficult regions to work on and are responsible for serious local sequelae that are difficult to correct (Pereira and Sterodimas 2008a). Liposuction requires thoughtful planning and an artistic eye to achieve aesthetically pleasing postoperative results. Careful selection of patients, proper surgical technique, and diligent perioperative care of the patient help avoid contour irregularity sequelae. Outcome expectations should be based on realistic preoperative evaluation of the patient's age, skin elasticity, volume of fat to be removed, and area of liposuction (Sterodimas et al. 2012). The increasing number of liposuction procedures, often performed by inadequately trained physicians, has led to a growing number of iatrogenic post-liposuction contour complications. These are classified as major or minor according to the size of the area, the severity of the irregularity, the difficulty of the correction, and the visual impact. These complications include undercorrection, overcorrection, and irregular fat tissue removal with palpable and visible irregularities (Pereira and Sterodimas 2008b; Pereira et al. 2011). Human adipose tissue is an ideal source of autologous cells that is both plentiful and easily obtainable in large quantities through the simple surgical procedure of liposuction. Autologous fat transplantation is frequently used for a variety of cosmetic and reconstructive indications not limited to posttraumatic defects of the face and body, evolutional disorders such as hemifacial atrophy, sequelae of radiation therapy, and many aesthetic uses such as lip and facial augmentation and wrinkle therapy (Illouz 1986; Guerrerosantos et al. 2007; Bucky and Percec 2008; Phulpin et al. 2009; Sterodimas et al. 2008). In the past 20 years, the advances in techniques and instrumentation have produced results that make fat grafting a viable option for correcting liposuction sequelae (Coleman 2006; Pereira and Sterodimas 2009). Successful, three-dimensional repair of liposuction defects requires meticulous preoperative planning and optimizing the transplantation of adipose tissue. Modifications of lipo injection techniques to improve the survival rate for injected fat have been attempted in the last 20 years.

The role of adult stem cells in adipose tissue has gained much interest in the last decade (Sterodimas et al. 2009a, 2010, 2011). Lipoaspirate, an otherwise disposable by product of cosmetic surgery, has been shown to contain a putative population of stem cells, termed adipose-derived stem cells (ADSCs) that reside within the stromal-vascular fraction (SVF) in fat tissue which is thought to harbor cells that display extensive proliferative capacity and multilineage potential (Sterodimas et al. 2009b).

For cell-based therapies, an approach is to harvest SVF and give it back to the patient within a single surgical procedure, thereby avoiding lengthy and costly in vitro culturing steps. In Stromal Enriched Lipograft (SEL), freshly isolated SVF is attached to the aspirated fat, with the fat tissue acting as a living bioscaffold before transplantation (Sterodimas 2013a, b; Sterodimas et al. 2013). In this chapter we are presenting clinical results of patients with liposuction sequelae using the SEL for the correction of liposuction sequelae.

Patients and Methods

Fifty-five patients with post-liposuction depressions were operated during January 2017 and October 2019. Forty-one female and 14 male patients were included in this study group. Age distribution of patients ranged from 28 to 62 years, with a mean of 46.7 years. All the patients that were included in this study were candidates for autologous fat transplantation. Patients underwent the Stromal Enriched Lipograft technique for correction of their body liposuction sequelae.

Surgical Technique

Marking of the areas to be liposucted and fat grafted for the correction of liposuction sequelae is made while the patient is in standing position (Fig. 38.1). Preoperative sedation in the surgical suite is administered. Anesthesia consists of an epidural block and intravenous sedation. The patient is placed in prone position. After the injection of normal saline wetting solution containing 1:500,000 of adrenaline by a small bore cannula and waiting 15 min, a 20-cc syringe attached to a 3 mm blunt cannula is inserted through one small incision in the abdominal area. Fat is aspirated by using the syringe method (Fig. 38.2). A schematic representation of the Stromal Enriched Lipograft technique is shown in Fig. 38.3. The fatty tissue aspirated is treated in the following manner. First, the 2/3 of the aspirated fat is used in order to isolate the SVF. Digestion is done with 0.075% collagenase (Sigma, St. Louis, MO) in buffered saline and agitated for 30 min at 37 °C using the Automatic Cell Station produced by BSL, Seoul, Korea (Fig. 38.4). Separation of the SVF containing ADSCs is then done by using centrifugation at 1200 g for 15 min and washing the enzyme out. The SVF is located in the pellet derived from the centrifuged fat at the bottom of the lipoaspirate. The remaining 1/3 of the aspirated fat is treated in the following way: with the syringe held vertically with the open end down, the fat and fluid are separated. Mixing of the SVF containing ADSCs and the purified fat is finally done and transferred into 20 ml syringes for application (Fig. 38.5). This whole procedure is done inside the operating theatre, by two tissue engineers, automatically in a closed system, and the time required is about 55 min

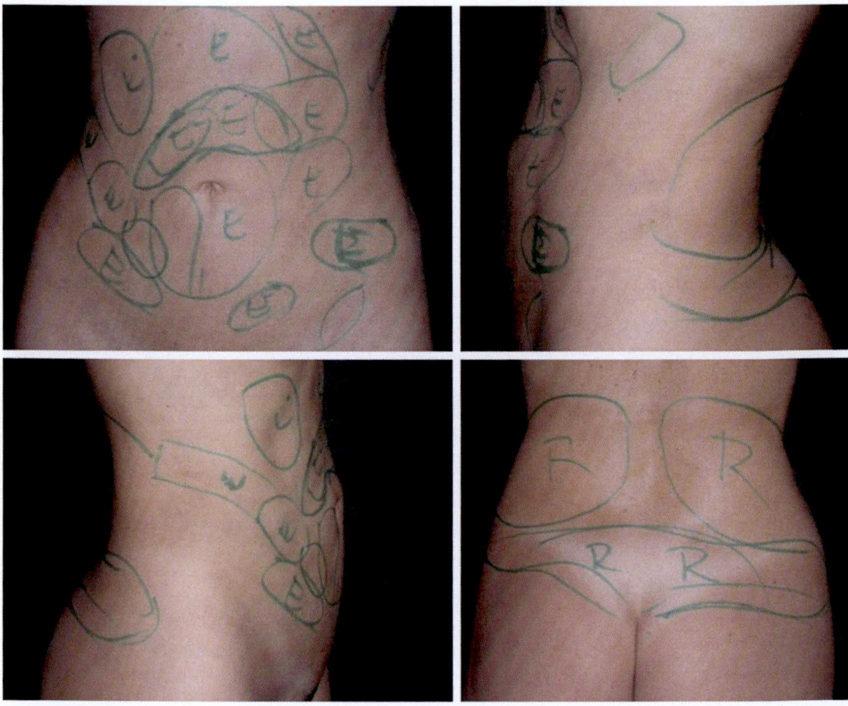

Fig. 38.1 Preoperative markings of liposuction and lipografting using the SEL technique

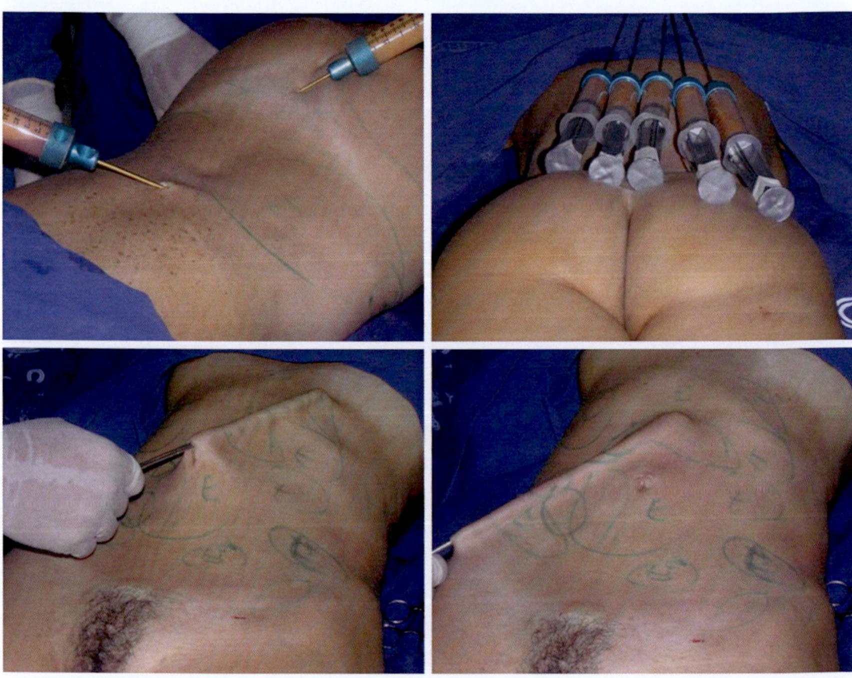

Fig. 38.2 Fat is aspirated using the syringe method

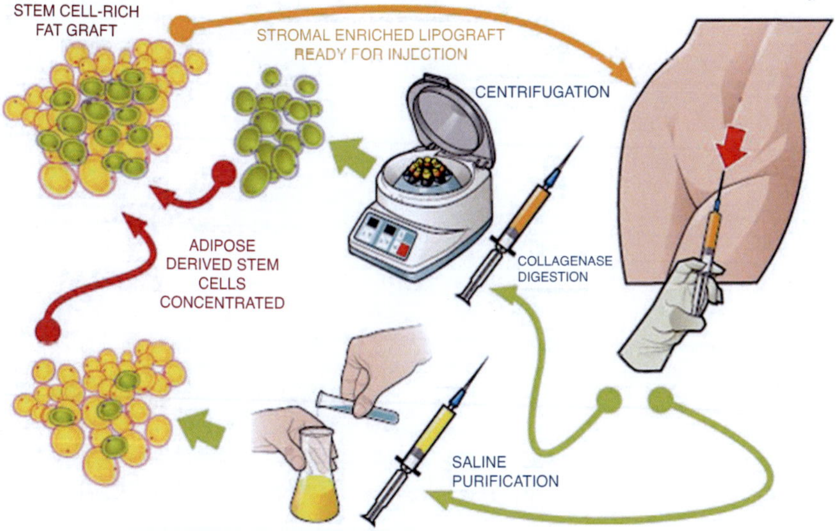

Fig. 38.3 Schematic representation of the Stromal Enriched Lipograft

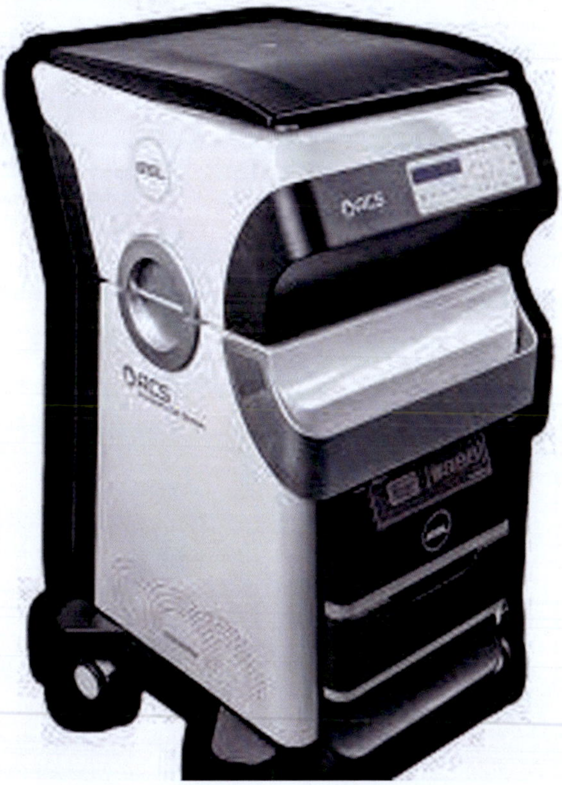

Fig. 38.4 The ACS equipment used for the SEL technique

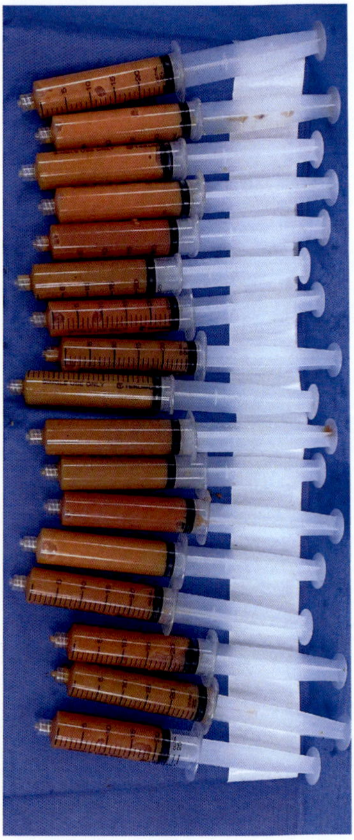

Fig. 38.5 Stromal enriched lipograft in 10 ml syringes to be used for liposuction sequelae correction

for hand rejuvenation. The adipose tissue graft enriched with SVF is inserted using the MAFT Gun, Dermato Plastica Beauty Co., Ltd., Kaohsiung, Taiwan. Fat droplets are delivered, while the MAFT-GUN™ is withdrawn. In a fan-shaped manner, numerous fat parcels (1/100 mL) can be consistently micro-transplanted by triggering the MAFT-GUN™. No pressure or molding of the transplanted fat is needed. A broad spectrum antibiotic, an analgesic, and an anti-inflammatory medication are prescribed during the following 3 postoperative days.

Results

The total amount of clean adipose tissue transplanted varied from 20 to 150 ml. There were no cases of liponecrosis, which developed in the grafted area, and no liponecrotic lumps were palpated on postoperative evaluation on any operated cases. There were no cases of cellulitis at the donor or grafted area, no deep vein thrombosis, and no pulmonary embolism. There were no cases that needed additional session of fat grafting.

Patient 1

This 36-year-old woman asked for treatment of her contour sequelae following liposuction in a different plastic surgery practice (Fig. 38.6a). She requested the least invasive procedure in order to correct the abdomen contour deformities. Stromal enriched lipograft was offered to her. 25 ml of SEL was inserted in the abdominal area and a mini abdominoplasty was performed. A photo was taken 14 months after the procedure (Fig. 38.6b).

Patient 2

This 45-year-old woman presented complaining of abdominal depressions following a liposuction procedure she had in a different institution (Fig. 38.7a). Stromal Enriched Lipograft was offered to her together with abdominoplasty. 32 ml of SEL was inserted in the abdominal area. Photos were taken 18 months after the procedure (Fig. 38.7b).

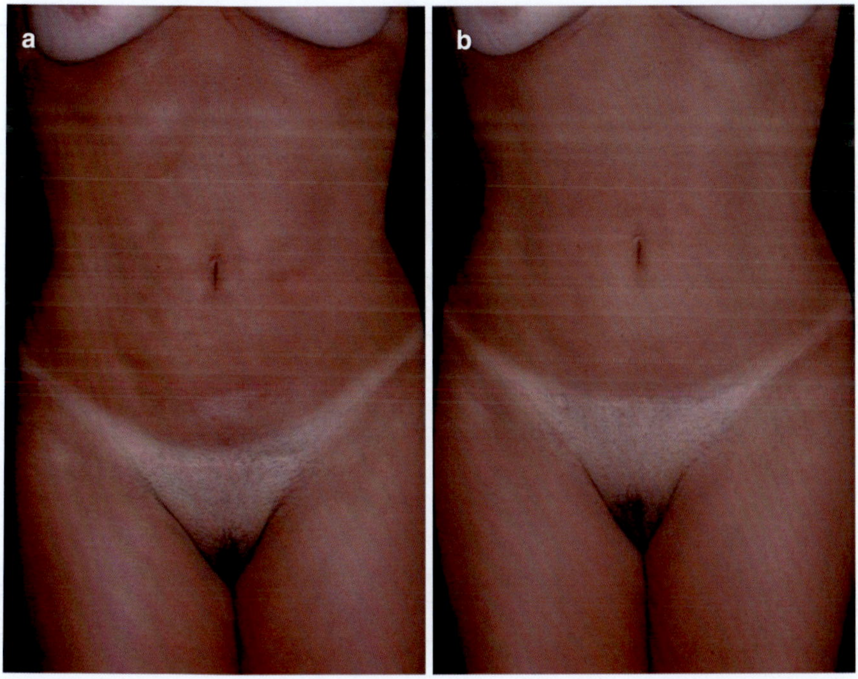

Fig. 38.6 (**a**) Preoperative photo of a 36-year-old woman requesting treatment of her contour sequelae following liposuction. (**b**) Postoperative photo 14 months after Stromal Enriched Lipograft and a mini abdominoplasty was performed

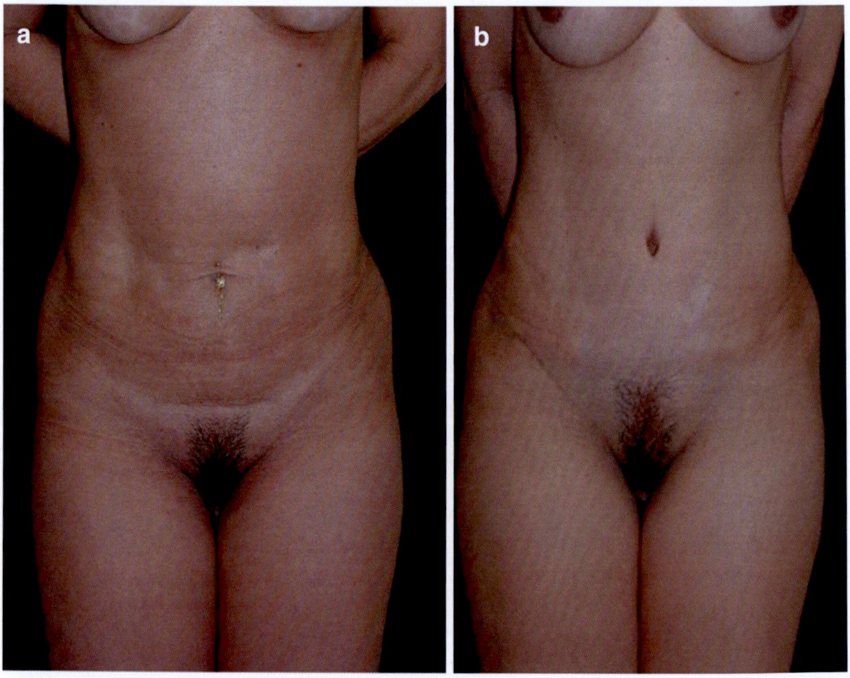

Fig. 38.7 (**a**, **b**) Preoperative photos of a 45-year-old woman complaining of abdominal depressions following a liposuction procedure. (**c**, **d**) Postoperative photos of a 45-year-old woman after Stromal Enriched Lipograft combined with abdominoplasty

Patient 3

This 47-year-old woman presented for correction of post-liposuction abdominal depressions (Fig. 38.8a). Stromal Enriched Lipograft was offered to her. 25 ml of SEL was inserted in the abdominal area. Postoperative photos were taken 22 months after the procedure (Fig. 38.8b).

Patient 4

This 35-year-old woman presented for correction of post-liposuction abdominal depressions and correction of her previous mini abdominoplasty. Stromal Enriched Lipograft was offered to her combined with abdominoplasty (Fig. 38.9a). Postoperative photos were taken 5 months after the procedure (Fig. 38.9b).

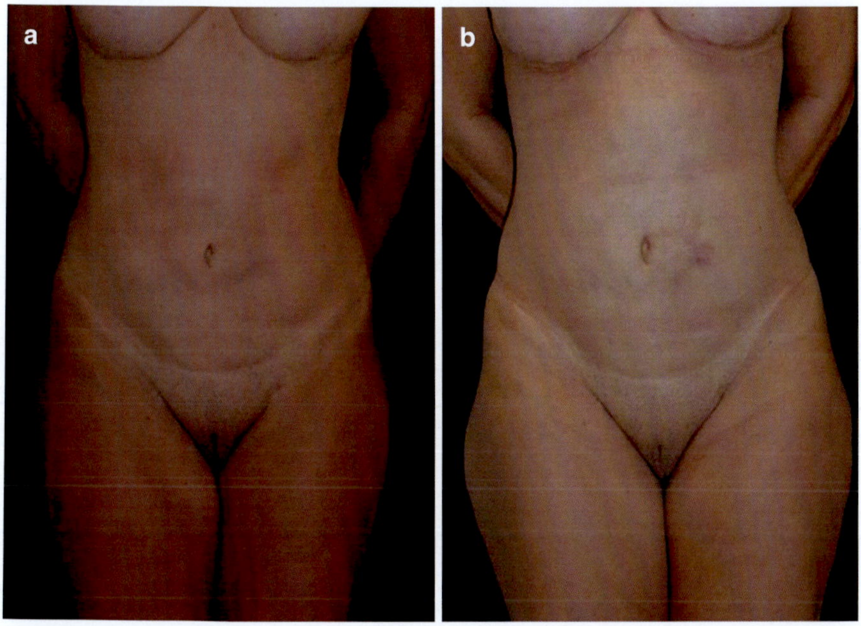

Fig. 38.8 (**a**) Preoperative photos of a 47-year-old woman complaining of abdominal depressions following a liposuction procedure. (**b**) Postoperative photos of a 47-year-old woman after Stromal Enriched Lipograft and scars revision in the abdominal area

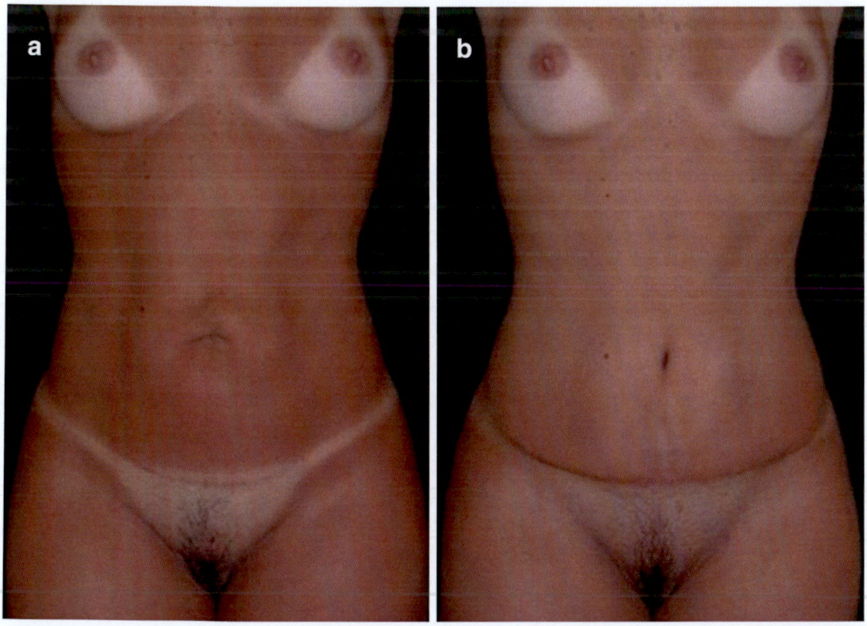

Fig. 38.9 (**a**) Preoperative photos of a 35-year-old woman complaining of abdominal depressions following a liposuction and mini abdominoplasty procedure. (**b**) Postoperative photos of a 35-year-old woman after Stromal Enriched Lipograft and abdominoplasty procedure

Discussion

True body sculpting with liposuction demands a three-dimensional artistic understanding of the anatomic and surgical adipose layers of the central trunk. This is essential to preventing complications from both ultrasound- and suction-assisted lipoplasty. The best results of liposuction are still obtained when treating moderate, localized fat deposits in a normal-weight patient that cannot be managed by diet and exercise. Physicians practicing liposuction surgery should have adequate training and experience in the field. This training and experience may be obtained in residency training, cosmetic surgery fellowship training, observational training programs, and CME-accredited postgraduate didactic and live surgical programs with trained credentialed surgeons experienced in liposuction techniques. The methods reported in the literature for the treatment of iatrogenic contour defects include liposuction for the area of protuberance, liposuction around the area of depression, and simultaneous fat grafting and dermolipectomy. Our experience with autologous fat transplantation used to treat various tissue defects has led us to apply this technique for the correction of iatrogenic post-liposuction abdominal tissue deformities (Pereira and Sterodimas 2008c; Haroldo Pereira and Sterodimas 2008a; Illouz and Sterodimas 2009).

Adipose tissue is believed to constitute an ideal source of uncultured stromal stem cells to be used for liposuction sequelae correction. The presence of adipose-derived stem cells has clinical implications for autologous fat transfer because adipose-derived stem cells may contribute to neoangiogenesis in the acute phase by acting as endothelial progenitor cells or angiogenic factor-releasing cells (Hamou et al. 2009; Mylotte et al. 2008a). Adipose-derived stem cells are known to secrete angiogenic factors such as vascular endothelial growth factor and hepatocyte growth factor (Kilroy et al. 2007). In vivo, ADSCs demonstrate the capacity to proliferate in response to a hypoxic insult remote from their resident niche, and this has been supported by in vitro studies showing increasing ADSC proliferation with greater degrees of hypoxia (Suga et al. 2009). ADSCs upregulate also their proneovascular activity in response to hypoxia and may harbor the capacity to home to ischemic tissue and function cooperatively with existing vasculature to promote angiogenesis (Thangarajah et al. 2009). ADSCs are thought to be more resistant to ischemia as is the case for bone marrow-derived mesenchymal stem cells, which can be functional for 72 h under ischemia (Mylotte et al. 2008b). In addition, they can affect long-term survival of transplanted adipose by acting as preadipocytes (Rehman et al. 2004).

The number of functional ADSCs is likely to be important for tissue repair and remodeling, and ADSCs differentiate into vascular endothelial cells which contribute to neoangiogenesis in the acute phase of transplantation (Kølle et al. 2013). A recent study has demonstrated no statistical differences in adipocyte viability among abdominal fat, thigh fat, flank fat, or knee fat donor sites (Ullmann et al. 2005). The abdomen though seems to be preferable to the hip/thigh region for harvesting adipose tissue when considering SVF cells for stem cell-based therapies in one-step surgical procedures (Jurgens et al. 2008).

An important consideration for harvesting and refinement in preparation for grafting is to respect and maintain the tissue architecture of living fat. Any mechanical or chemical insult that damages the fragile tissue architecture of fat will result in eventual necrosis of the injected fat (Pereira and Sterodimas 2010a). Based on this principle, the 1/3 of aspirated fat is treated as above described without the use of any chemical or mechanical procedure, and it is used as a natural scaffold. Recent reports have shown that mechanical centrifugation does not appear to enhance immediate fat tissue viability before implantation (Rohrich et al. 2004). Centrifugation, however, plays a beneficial role in concentrating SVF and adipose-derived stem cells although excessive centrifugation can destroy adipocytes and adipose-derived stem cells. The degree of adipocyte destruction differs among patients, but it has been shown that only minor differences exist in percentage of cell destruction between the different centrifugal forces (Kurita et al. 2008). In a previous study, it was found that centrifugation of aspirated fat at 1200 g decreases the fat volume by 30%, damaging 12% of the adipocytes and 0% of the ADSCs (Yoshimura et al. 2008). This has been confirmed by a recent study stating that cell survival rates are significantly lower when centrifugation forces of 1200 g are used for more than 5 min and of 3000 g when used for more than 1 min (Kim et al. 2009). The actual recommendation is 1200 g as an optimized centrifugal force among the tested centrifugal forces for obtaining good short- and long-term results in adipose transplantation. A recent study conducted in our department showed that the ADSC concentration is significantly higher in lipoaspirate that has been washed by saline compared to the decanted and centrifuged lipoaspirate samples. However, the pellet collected at the bottom of the centrifuged lipoaspirate sample showed the highest concentration of ADSCs. Based on this finding, the washed autologous fat (1/3 of lipoaspirate) is supercharged by the SVF isolated by centrifugation from the 2/3 of the remaining lipoaspirate. The SVF contains erythrocytes, leukocytes, ADSCs, vascular endothelial cells, and pericytes. It is important for the SVF to adhere on the purified fat before transplantation is done. This is achieved by gently mixing SVF and fat, which serves as a scaffold, before placing in the 1 ml syringes. The time needed in order to process the collected fat for SVF extraction is around 80–90 min. This is a limitation when compared to the time taken in order to perform the traditional fat grafting to the face.

The experience in our department with the traditional autologous fat grafting in treating various tissue defects has been published extensively (Haroldo Pereira and Sterodimas 2008b; Santana et al. 2010; Pereira and Sterodimas 2010b). The results of traditional autologous fat transplantation have been predictable and satisfying on the condition that the treatment is performed in stages with small quantities of adipose tissue fat injected in various treatment sessions (3–5 sessions). In this series of patients, only one treatment session produced aesthetically satisfactory results in patients who had liposuction sequelae.

There are cases where there is little or no fat reserve. This is common in young patients who have undergone extensive liposuction procedures. In those cases, the challenge for the surgeon is to obtain the maximum possible amount of fat without creating more contour defects. The authors recommend a minimum of 6 months before any revision surgery. This period is critical to allow swelling and edema to subside and to enable correct evaluation of the contour abdominal deformities.

Conclusion

Liposuction continues to be a safe surgical procedure, but for maximum avoidance of complications, the surgeon should be mindful of all the factors that could predispose to complications. With the overall acceptance of aesthetic surgery increasing as well as the number of patients undergoing liposuction, it is likely that plastic surgeons will see more patients requesting correction of liposuction sequalae in the future. Stromal Enriched Lipograft technique is a safe and effective technique that offers the possibility of finally fulfilling the key principle of replacing "like with like" as an aesthetic filler, without the drawbacks of the traditional autologous fat grafting technique.

References

Illouz YG (1983) Body contouring by lipolysis: a 5-year experience with over 3000 cases. Plast Reconstr Surg 72(5):591–597

Pereira LH, Sterodimas A (2008a) Correction for the iatrogenic form of banana fold and sensuous triangle deformity. Aesthetic Plast Surg 32(6):923–927

Sterodimas A, Boriani F, Magarakis E, Nicaretta B, Pereira LH, Illouz YG. Thirtyfour years of liposuction: past, present and future. Eur Rev Med Pharmacol Sci. 2012 Mar;16(3):393-406.

Pereira LH, Sterodimas A. Correction for the iatrogenic form of banana fold and sensuous triangle deformity. Aesthetic Plast Surg. 2008b Nov;32(6):923-7

Pereira LH, Nicaretta B, Sterodimas A. Correction of liposuction sequelae by autologous fat transplantation. Aesthetic Plast Surg. 2011 Dec;35(6):1000-8.

Illouz YG. The fat cell "graft": a new technique to fill depressions. Plast Reconstr Surg. 1986 Jul;78(1):122-3

Guerrerosantos J, Guerrerosantos F, Orozco J Classification and treatment of facial tissue atrophy in Parry-Romberg disease. Aesthetic Plast Surg. 2007 Sep-Oct;31(5):424-34

Bucky LP, Percec I. The science of autologous fat grafting: views on current and future approaches to neoadipogenesis. Aesthet Surg J. 2008 May-Jun;28(3):313-21; quiz 322-4

Phulpin B, Gangloff P, Tran N, Bravetti P, Merlin JL, Dolivet G. Rehabilitation of irradiated head and neck tissues by autologous fat transplantation. Plast Reconstr Surg. 2009 Apr;123(4):1187 97

Sterodimas A, Huanquipaco JC, de Souza Filho S, Bornia FA, Pitanguy I. Autologous fat transplantation for the treatment of Parry-Romberg syndrome. J Plast Reconstr Aesthet Surg. 2008 Aug 15.

Coleman SR. Facial augmentation with structural fat grafting. Clin Plast Surg. 2006 Oct;33(4):567-77.

Pereira LH, Sterodimas A.Macroscopic and microscopic proof of long-term survival of gluteal fat transplantation. Plast Reconstr Surg. 2009 Apr;123(4):162e-163e
Sterodimas A, De Faria J, Correa WE, Pitanguy I. Tissue engineering in plastic surgery: an up-to-date review of the current literature. Ann Plast Surg. 2009a Jan;62(1):97-103.
Sterodimas A, de Faria J, Nicaretta B, Boriani F. Autologous fat transplantation versus adipose-derived stem cell-enriched lipografts: a study. Aesthet Surg J. 2011 Aug;31(6):682-93.
Sterodimas A, de Faria J, Nicaretta B, Papadopoulos O, Papalambros E, Illouz YG.Cell-assisted lipotransfer. Aesthet Surg J. 2010 Jan;30(1):78-81.
Sterodimas A, De Faria J, Correa WE, Pitanguy I. Tissue engineering in plastic surgery: an up-to-date review of the current literature. Ann Plast Surg. 2009b Jan;62(1):97-103.
Sterodimas A. Stromal enriched lipograft for rhinoplasty refinement. Aesthet Surg J. 2013a May 1;33(4):612-4.
Sterodimas A. Kalodimou V, Nicaretta B Adipose Derived Stem Cells Characterization from Human Lipoaspirate: A Comparative Study Journal of Biomimetics, Biomaterials & Tissue Engineering 2013 Dec; 18:73-83
Sterodimas A Stromal Enriched Lipograft in Plastic & Reconstructive Surgery Prime J. 2013b Sep;31(6):24-45
Pereira LH, Sterodimas A (2008c) Free fat transplantation for the aesthetic correction of mild pectus excavatum. Aesth Plast Surg 32:393–396 209
Haroldo Pereira L, Sterodimas A (2008a) Aesthetic restoration of axillary contour deformity after lymph node dissection. J Plast Reconstr Aesthet Surg 61:231–232. Epub 2007 Nov 19
Illouz YG, Sterodimas A Autologous fat transplantation to the breast: a personal technique with 25 years of experience.. Aesthetic Plast Surg. 2009 Sep; 33(5):706-15
Hamou C, Callaghan MJ, Thangarajah H, Chang E, Chang EI, Grogan RH, Paterno J, Vial IN, Jazayeri L, Gurtner GC. Mesenchymal stem cells can participate in ischemic neovascularization. Plast Reconstr Surg. 2009 Feb;123(2 Suppl):45S-55S
Mylotte LA, Duffy AM, Murphy M, O'Brien T, Samali A, Barry F, Szegezdi E. Metabolic flexibility permits mesenchymal stem cell survival in an ischemic environment. Stem Cells 26(5), 1325–1336 (2008a)
Kilroy GE, Foster SJ, Wu X, et al. Cytokine profile of human adipose-derived stem cells: expression of angiogenic, hematopoietic, and pro-inflammatory factors. J Cell Physiol 2007; 212:702–9.
Suga H, Eto H, Shigeura T, Inoue K, Aoi N, Kato H, Nishimura S, Manabe I, Gonda K, Yoshimura K. IFATS collection: Fibroblast growth factor-2-induced hepatocyte growth factor secretion by adipose-derived stromal cells inhibits postinjury fibrogenesis through a c-Jun N-terminal kinase-dependent mechanism. Stem Cells. 2009 Jan;27(1):238-49.
Thangarajah H, Vial IN, Chang E, El-Ftesi S, Januszyk M, Chang EI, Paterno J, Neofytou E, Longaker MT, Gurtner GC. IFATS collection: Adipose stromal cells adopt a proangiogenic phenotype under the influence of hypoxia. Stem Cells. 2009 Jan;27(1):266-74.
Mylotte LA, Duffy AM, Murphy M, O'Brien T, Samali A, Barry F, Szegezdi E. Metabolic flexibility permits mesenchymal stem cell survival in an ischemic environment. Stem Cells 26(5), 1325–1336 (2008b)
Rehman, J., Traktuev, D., Li, J., et al. Secretion of angiogenic and antiapoptotic factors by human adipose stromal cells. Circulation 109: 1292, 2004
Kølle SF, Fischer-Nielsen A, Mathiasen AB, Elberg JJ Enrichment of autologous fat grafts with ex-vivo expanded adipose tissue-derived stem cells for graft survival: a randomised placebo-controlled trial. Lancet. 2013 Sep 28;382(9898):1113-20
Ullmann Y, Shoshani O, Fodor A, Ramon Y, Carmi N, Eldor L, Gilhar A. Searching for the favorable donor site for fat injection: in vivo study using the nude mice model. Dermatol Surg. 2005 Oct;31(10):1304-7.
Jurgens WJ, Oedayrajsingh-Varma MJ, Helder MN, Zandiehdoulabi B, Schouten TE, Kuik DJ, Ritt MJ, van Milligen FJ. Effect of tissue-harvesting site on yield of stem cells derived from adipose tissue: implications for cell-based therapies. Cell Tissue Res. 2008 Jun;332(3):415-26.

Pereira LH, Sterodimas A. Long-term fate of transplanted autologous fat in the face. J Plast Reconstr Aesthet Surg. 2010a Jan;63(1):e68-9.

Rohrich RJ, Sorokin ES, Brown SA. In search of improved fat transfer viability: a quantitative analysis of the role of centrifugation and harvest site. Plast Reconstr Surg. 2004 Jan;113(1):391-5; discussion 396-7

Kurita M, Matsumoto D, Shigeura T, Sato K, Gonda K, Harii K, Yoshimura K. Influences of centrifugation on cells and tissues in liposuction aspirates: optimized centrifugation for lipotransfer and cell isolation. Plast Reconstr Surg. 2008 Mar;121(3):1033-41; discussion 1042-3

Yoshimura K, Sato K, Aoi N, Kurita M, Hirohi T, Harii K. Cell-assisted lipotransfer for cosmetic breast augmentation: supportive use of adipose-derived stem/stromal cells. Aesthetic Plast Surg. 2008 Jan;32(1):48-55; discussion 56-7.

Kim IH, Yang JD, Lee DG, Chung HY, Cho BC. Evaluation of centrifugation technique and effect of epinephrine on fat cell viability in autologous fat injection. Aesthet Surg J. 2009 Jan-Feb;29(1):35-9

Haroldo Pereira L, Sterodimas A.Aesthetic restoration of axillary contour deformity after lymph node dissection. J Plast Reconstr Aesthet Surg. 2008b;61(2):231-2. Epub 2007 Nov 19

Santana KP, Pereira LH, Sabatovich O, Sterodimas A. Foreign-body granulomas caused by polymethylmethacrylate (PMMA) microspheres: successful correction by autologous fat transplantation. J Plast Reconstr Aesthet Surg. 2010 Feb;63(2):e139-41

Pereira LH, Sterodimas A. Autologous fat transplantation and delayed silicone implant insertion in a case of Mycobacterium avium breast infection Aesthetic Plast Surg. 2010b Feb;34(1):1-4.

Chapter 39
Liposculpture and Buttock Lipograft: Safety Aspects

Marcelo Paulo Vaccari-Mazzetti, Juarez Moraes Avelar, Ryane Schmidt Brock, and Thalita Galdino de Oliveira

Abstract Smooth body contouring is the aim of plastic surgery. To achieve the ideal gluteal contour the gluteal submuscular region, lipograft is the surgical technique with the best results for the maintenance of fat, but the risks of a fatal complication require the plastic surgeon to undergo adequate training in the technique to prevent (microscopic or macroscopic) fat embolisms and other complications. In this chapter, the collection and preparation of donor fat is detailed. The maintenance of the submuscular fat was studied for it. A preventive technique and the different fat embolisms are explained. Other complications, such as infection, asymmetry, and nerve damage, and how to prevent them are described.

Introduction

According to the Brazilian Society of Plastic Surgery and the American Society of Plastic and Reconstructive Surgery, liposuction is one of the most common aesthetic procedures done in Brazil and in the United States, secondly only to breast augmentation (American Society of Plastic Surgeons 2019; International Society of Aesthetic Plastic Surgery 2019; Sociedade Brasileira de Cirurgia Plástica 2019). The technique demands professional training and an appropriate physical structure to be performed with security. Liposuction is in such high demand because it improves the body contour with few scars. It can also use lipografts of autologous

M. P. Vaccari-Mazzetti (✉) · R. S. Brock · T. G. de Oliveira
Brazilian Society of Plastic Surgery, Face Defects Research and Study Center, São Paulo, Brazil

J. M. Avelar
Brazilian Scientific Institute of Plastic and Reconstructive Surgery, São Paulo, Brazil

J. M. Avelar, R. Cavalcanti Ribeiro (eds.), *Body Contouring*,
https://doi.org/10.1007/978-3-031-42802-9_39

adipose tissue to achieve better results on liposculpture. Buttock augmentation with submuscular lipografts is combined with subcutaneous lipografts to improve the body contour. The abdomen is the most common donor area to obtain the fat tissue that will comprise the lipografts (Avelar 1986a); however, the fat tissues collected from the dorsum, thigh, arm, and knee can also be used.

There are many techniques for performing the suction, and the fat from this suction can be used to improve the body contour or can be discarded. When the fat is used, the surgical procedure is usually called liposculpture (Harrison and Selvaggi 2007). Liposculpture is an important technique to improve the results of liposuction and requires expertise in the biology of lipografts. The donor site, the fat collection, the treatment of the fat, and the receiving site can change the results and determine the success or failure of the surgical procedure (Harrison and Selvaggi 2007).

The resultant shape of the buttocks is related to the volume of graft fat: Sometimes the amount of available fat is less than surgeons desire to improve the shape by making it round and full (Vaccari-Mazzetti and Brock 2016). Studies have shown that the best choice to manipulate fat is to purify fat cells and put these into the muscle to provide better vascular supply and improve the maintenance of the fat volume (Lewis 2004; Murillo 2004; Pu et al. 2008).

Using an appropriate and safe surgical technique is crucial to success in this surgery and avoids complications. With the right technique for aesthetic reconstructive surgery, the body contours of our patients can be improved to the satisfaction of both the patient and the plastic surgeon (Vaccari-Mazzetti and Brock 2016).

Nowadays, regenerative medicine and tissue engineering are commonly applied in all fields of medicine. Mesenchymal stem cells are already known for their multipotential regenerative activities (Fitzsimmons et al. 2018; Grambow et al. 2020). These stem cells were first described by Friedenstein et al. (1966, 1970), who discovered fibroblastic cells from the bone marrow of mice and guinea pigs. Caplan (1991) described their capacity to generate cartilage and adipose tissue, and Pittenger established that stromal cells from human bone marrow have multipotent regeneration activities (Pittenger et al. 1999).

The ideal butt is almost impossible to define (Avelar 1986c), but one ideal butt appears to be a Brazilian one (Pitanguy 1986), according to some studies that have shown different preferences for butt size in different coutries (Heidekrueger et al. 2017).

Technique

Anatomical and Image Studies

After conducting a series of anatomical studies (Fig. 39.1), we defined the emergence of the neurovascular ischiatic major branch between the medium and minor gluteus muscles, in the middle of two osseous structures, which was confirmed by image studies (Vaccari-Mazzetti and Brock 2016).

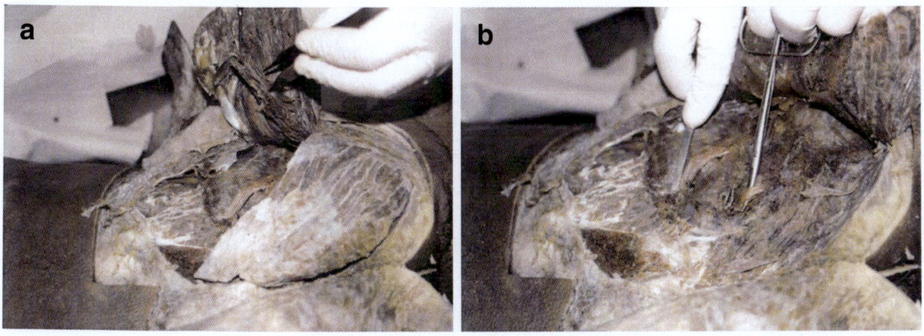

Fig. 39.1 Anatomical studies with (**a**) gluteus maximus batting and (**b**) exposure of neurovascular bundle

Other studies have illustrated the vascular branches in the deep and superior part of the gluteal muscles, the superior gluteal artery, and nerve exit sciatic foramen above the piriform muscle. They pass through the plane between the gluteus medius and the gluteus minimus. These muscles are supplied by this artery, and the vein has a parallel trajectory. The gluteal muscles contain three compartments with inelastic boundaries: the gluteus maximus, the gluteus medius–minimus, and the fascia lata tensor (Chamosa 2004; Vaccari-Mazzetti and Brock 2016). Most of critical neurovascular structures are in the gluteus medius–minimus compartment. The superior gluteal artery, vein, and nerve exit from above the piriformis muscle, and the inferior gluteal artery, vein, and nerve exit beneath the inferior edge of the piriformis and above the superior gemellus muscle to penetrate the maximus muscle (Chamosa 2004).

A pelvic magnetic resonance study was conducted on ten patients, after the exclusion of eight patients. All the patients' body weights increased at the end of the study, and the patients whose weight increased or decreased by more than 2 kg were excluded from the study. The exams were carried out without contrast, in a weighted sequence of T1, T2, and fat suppression, in the axial and sagittal planes, by using the open field Siemens Open Viva, 0.25 Tesla and signa contour GE 0.5 Tesla, with the patients in the prone position.

The magnetic resonance was performed for 7 days before the surgery and 7, 30, and 180 days after the surgery. The images had been analyzed via the fat-subtraction technique in all the resonance studies, which were performed in the axial (Fig. 39.2) and sagittal (Fig. 39.3) planes.

The measurements were taken by using four predetermined radiological lines: line 1 (anteroposterior)—femur posterior edge at the ischiatic tuberosity level and the gluteus muscle's posterior edge; line 2 (anteroposterior)—superior acetabulum posterior edge and the gluteus muscle's posterior margin; line 3 (latero-lateral)—the great axis at the tebrosity ischiatic level and the gluteus muscle; line 4 (latero-lateral)—the great axis at the superior acetabulum level and the gluteus muscle's lateral margin (Figs. 39.4 and 39.5).

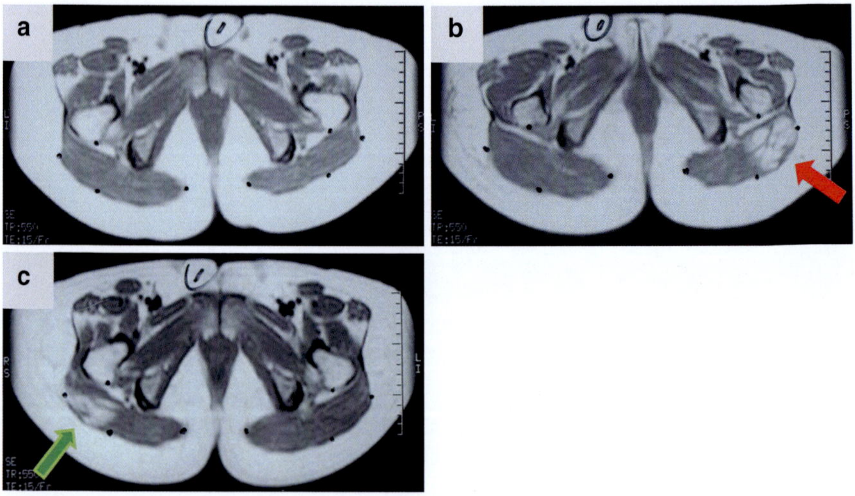

Fig. 39.2 Resonance magnetic axial images with black points used to make the measurements in (**a**) preoperative view, (**b**) 1-week post-operative with areas of fat inside the lateral part of the muscle, more evident left side marked with red arrow, (**c**) maintenance of fat after 6 months, more evident in the right side marked with green arrow

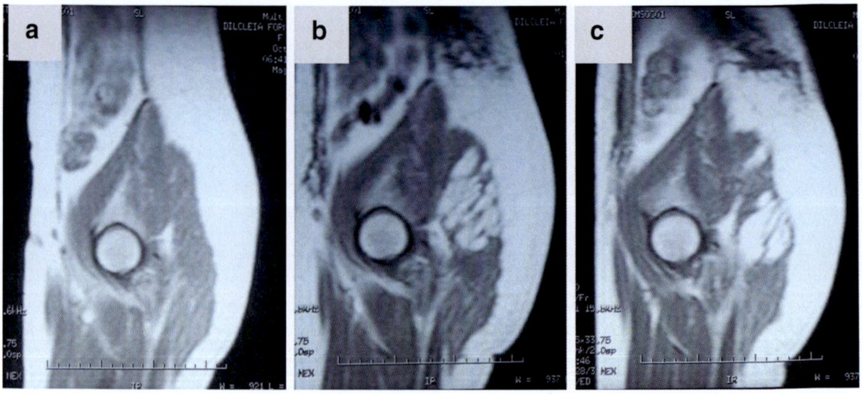

Fig. 39.3 (**a**) Resonance magnetic sagittal images in preoperative view, (**b**) 1-week post-operative with the areas of fat inside the superior part of the muscle, (**c**) maintenance of fat after 6 months

During lipograft injection, after this magnetic resonance image study was completed in two patients of our regular clinical series, we simultaneously performed ultrasonography on the gluteus so that we could identify the vital vessels and nervous structures. The lipografts were visible when they were injected into the muscle. The clinical evaluations of the patients showed gluteus augmentation and a decrease in the pelvic circumference in each case. Edema was present in each case: Two of them showed a substantial edema in the legs, so they were submitted to a duplex exam, which excluded vascular problems.

Follow - up	Radiological Measurements							
	Femur-Gluteus posterior margin		Acetabulum-Gluteus posterior margin		Sciatic tuberosity – gluteal edge		Superior Acetabulum – gluteal edge	
	RG	LG	RG	LG	RG	LG	RG	LG
Pre-operatory	5,9	5,3	5,9	6,1	9,2	9,7	8,5	9,5
1 week	6,6	6,7	6,9	7,0	11,0	10,6	11,1	10,1
6 months	7,0	6,1	7,0	6,8	8,6	9,6	8,8	8,8

Fig. 39.4 Radiological medium measurements in axial view of gluteal magnetic resonance. *RG*—right gluteus, *LG*—left gluteus

Follow - up	Radiological Measurements			
	Femur- posterior gluteal muscle margin		Fêmur-posterior gluteus margin	
	RG	LG	RG	LG
Pre operatory	7,4	7,6	10,2	10,2
1 week	8,9	8,1	12,3	12,0
6 months	6,5	7,0	9,0	9,0

Fig. 39.5 Radiological medium measurements in sagittal view of gluteal magnetic resonance. *RG*—right gluteus, *LG*—left gluteus

The clinical exams were carried out weekly and showed the complete removal of the edema within 4 to 8 weeks. Similar results were observed in our regular clinical series. At 6 months after the procedure, the results demonstrated that 90.4% of the measurements were maintained (indirectly indicative of fat volume) in the axial plane and 76.9% in the sagittal plane. Some patients showed a larger volume than the initial one, and that initially confused us, but now that we have posterior studies on adipose stem cell biology, we finally understand that the adipose cells multiply from stem cells after 3 months. For our calculations, all volume measurements higher than 100% were considered 100%.

After the radiological study, we were able to arrive at some conclusions so that we could safely perform gluteus submuscular lipografts while avoiding major complications. Knowing the lipograft areas (triangular areas) and the vectors of lipografting (safety vectors) are vital for safety reasons. Other aspects of surgical planning also helped us to perform a safe procedure (Vaccari-Mazzetti and Brock 2016).

In the initial cases in our clinical practice, before we had these radiological studies, safety triangles, and vectors, we had a case of a macroscopic fat embolism. Although the patient survived, we had to stop performing the procedure and had to look through scientific papers, anatomical studies, and radiological studies until we determined a safe method to perform submuscular lipografts again. After that, we performed more than 700 lipografts on patients without encountering a macroscopic fat embolism.

The Safety Triangles, Danger Triangles, and Safety Vectors of Lipoinjection

In anatomical and magnetic resonance studies, we observed two significant osseous landmarks: femoral acetabulum and ischiatic tuberosities.

The area where neurovascular structures arise contains three points: the end of the sacral area at the beginning of the intergluteus groove (1 cm below); the skin projection of the femoral acetabulum; and the ischiatic bone (tuberosity). It is characterized as a danger triangle and must be avoided during submuscular lipografting. While this triangle is dangerous, two other triangles, which are made in the lateral (with lateral border of the Gluteus) and medial positions (with intergluteal fold) to this one, mark relative safe areas to introduce submuscular lipografts (Fig. 39.6). In the superior triangle, the deeper muscular plane must be avoided because the gluteal

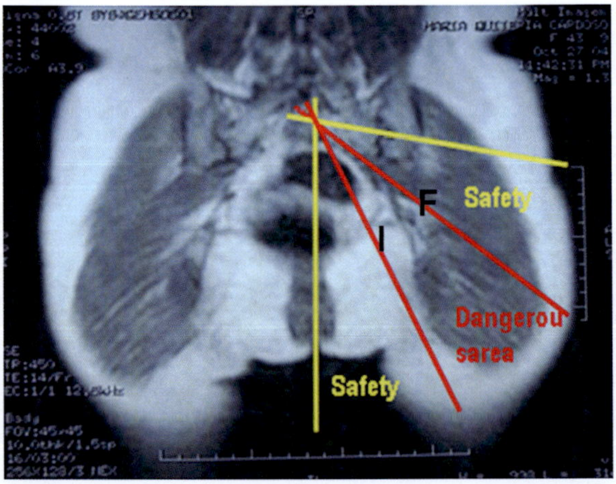

Fig. 39.6 Tomographic coronal image of the gluteal region, with two osseous landmarks: F (femur) and I (ischiatic bone), the dangerous triangle safety in red color, the two safety triangle in yellow color, superior triangle, in a superomedial position and other in an inferomedial position

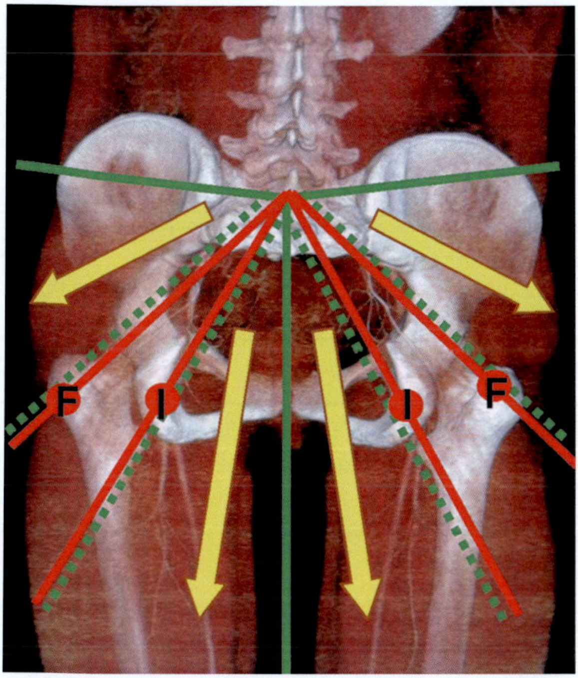

Fig. 39.7 The safety triangles identified by green lines and dots, the dangerous triangle identified by red lines, the red points to determine it: ischiatic tuberosity (I) and femoral projection (F). The safety vectors are in yellow

superior vein is present, very close to the bone. An important point in the level of safety of that triangle is the vector of lipoinjection. These vectors must be parallel to the great vessels, and we recommended the intergluteus groove hole for the injection canula as a starting point for performing submuscular lipograft injection (Fig. 39.7).

Treatment of Fat

The fat for lipografts is prepared with a sieve. All the removed fat is sieved, and this process turns a share of the liquid part of the fat with blood, such as oil, into a fat paste. After the production of this fat paste, it is conditioned in BD's 50 cc sterile syringes (Fig. 39.8), and it can be lipoinjected into patients no later than 40 min after collecting it from the body. However, ideally, the extracted fat should be collected, prepared into a fat paste after sieving it, and immediately injected into the patient (Vaccari-Mazzetti and Brock 2016).

The high pressure in the muscular compartment facilitates the penetration of microscopic fat (Chamosa 2004). High pressure can be detected when the fat

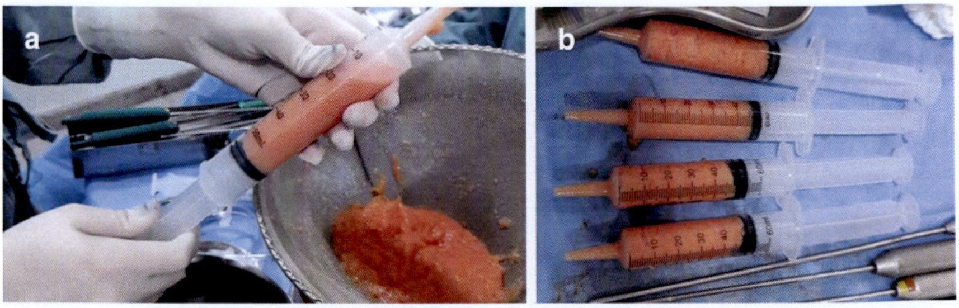

Fig. 39.8 Figure deomnstrate the ideal fat color of lipografts (**a**) fat paste in the sieve and into a syringe, (**b**) the syringes ready to be injected, the maximum time out of the body must be 40 min, the ideal is collect, prepare, and inject immediately

reflows by the canula. This will also serve as the clinical signal to stop the lipograft procedure in this location, but the canula must be left until the reflow has stopped.

Surgical Technique

General or peridural anesthesia is used; the operating room is prepared with a minimal ambient temperature of 24 °C, and the saline solution infusion is kept at 30 °C to avoid hypothermia. The legs are covered with a thermal coat (Warm Touch) to avoid the excessive loss of corporal temperature. The fluid reposition used is the Ringer's lactate solution, whose volume depends on the urinary volume and aspect (Vaccari-Mazzetti and Brock 2016).

When the patient is in the prone position, cushions are placed under the shoulders and the pelvis to improve lung airflow and avoid perforation. In the supine position, cushions are placed under the pelvic girdle and the patient is oriented at the correct angle to introduce the canula (parallel to the abdominal wall), which helps to avoid perforation (Fig. 39.9).

The wet technique is used in this liposuction procedure. The fluid injected into the subcutaneous tissue contains 1 L of Ringer's lactate solution, 20 mL of 2% lidocaine, and 3 ampoules of epinephrine. The same volume is used in the front and in the back of the patient (Vaccari-Mazzetti and Brock 2016). To liposuction, a number 4 modified Mercedes (five-hole) cannula connected to a vacuum aspirator is used. With it, the fat aspiration and fat collection are performed in a sterile, closed system.

The collected fat is submitted to the filter process with a stainless steel conical sieve immediately after the fat has become clear and macroscopic and is free of blood. It is stored in a 50 cc syringe (Fig. 39.8) to be injected later. Before fat injection, the danger triangle and the safety triangle are marked (Fig. 39.10).

The injection is carried out with a number 5 cannula, with three sequential holes, marked every 5 cm, deep into the muscle in the two safety triangles (latero-superior

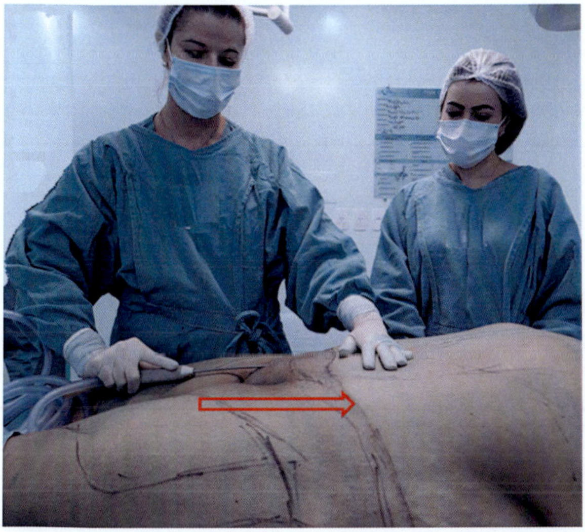

Fig. 39.9 Supine position with the cushions and correct angle to introduce the canula, parallel to the abdominal wall as showed as by the red arrow. The other hand of the surgeon must be over the canula to give more tactile information to the surgeon

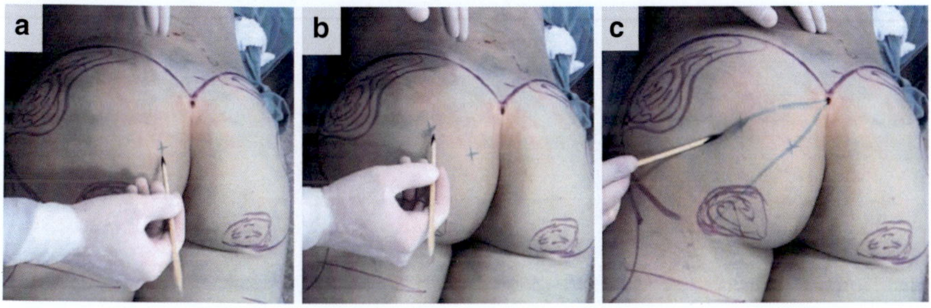

Fig. 39.10 The gluteal area is demarked before the surgery with the depressed areas and the dangerous triangle marking with bright green dye. (**a**) Sciatic point, (**b**) femoral point, (**c**) safety triangle

and medio-inferior). After this injection, aspirate and wait a few seconds to identify any possible minor vascular injuries; after that, softly press against the syringe used for fat graft retro-injection (Fig. 39.11). Do this several times in parts of the gluteus to fill in any depressed areas and/or to improve gluteus size. A subcutaneous lipografting should be performed in small, mashed tunnels by using a 2 or 2.5 mm microcannula with a round point. The gluteus contour (border) could be subcutaneously grafted to improve its roundness.

When the aspirated fat changes color to a red pattern, the collection period has finished, which marks the start of technical refinement with a superficial number 3 cannula connected to a lipoaspirator (Vaccari-Mazzetti and Brock 2016).

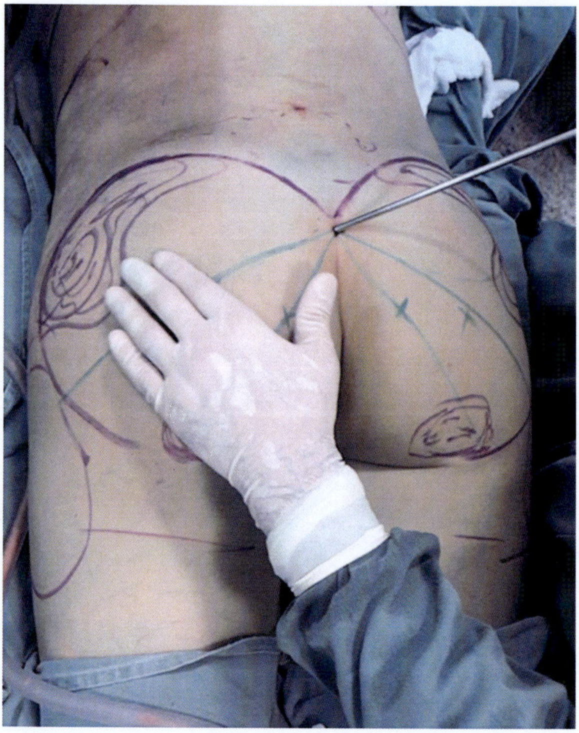

Fig. 39.11 Submuscular lipografting with number 5 cannula and 50 cc syringe, in retrograde and soft injection. Check before lipograft injection with syringe aspiration in order to avoid vascular damage

Complications and How to Prevent Them

The main complications are vascular (fat embolism) and neurological problems, lipograft infection, hematoma, and postoperative gluteal asymmetry. The neurological problems include leg pain and a temporary walking disability; this complication can be unilateral or bilateral. It is usually self-limited, and the problem is solved within 1 to 3 months. A sensitivity to cold, warmth, pricking, or paresthesia could result because the nerve is submitted a temporary inflammatory process (Vaccari-Mazzetti and Brock 2016). The identification of the danger triangle and lipografting care will prevent the cannula from producing a direct neurological lesion. Some patients have pain in their thighs, which indicates a sciatic nerve edema that can be confirmed via magnetic resonance at days 15 and 30. The symptoms decrease gradually and disappear within 3 months; at day 180, magnetic resonance exams show the disappearance of the sciatic nerve edema (Vaccari-Mazzetti and Brock 2016).

Infections can cause intense butt pain (usually the first clinical signal), fever, a walking disability, asymmetry in the two sides of the buttocks, and, in advanced conditions, inflammatory symptoms on the affected side. Usually, an infection leads to volume loss in all the lipografts, and it can become systemic in a few days if not properly treated (Vaccari-Mazzetti and Brock 2016). When the infectious agent is Gram positive, the intensity of infection is low, but in the majority of cases, the cause is a Gram-negative or anaerobic agent, and the intensity is high. In most cases featuring Gram-negative agents, the color of purulent secretions was brownish and had a fetid smell. Two or more surgical cleanings were necessary.

We observed two case of gluteus unilateral hematoma after submuscular lipografts. These two cases were related to a trauma history in the postoperative period. Both were drained under local anesthesia and via aspiration with a number 3 liposuction cannula, guided by ultrasound images (Vaccari-Mazzetti and Brock 2016).

The vascular complications include microscopic fat embolisms and macroscopic fat embolisms with thromboembolic pulmonary complications and consequent respiratory distress. Patients with such complications will need to be admitted to the intensive care unit (ICU). This complication could be avoided by using safety triangles, safety vectors, and putting nonintense pressure on the submuscular lipografts (Vaccari-Mazzetti and Brock 2016).

The Safety Triangles, Danger Triangles, and Safety Vectors of Lipoinjection to Prevent Neurovascular Complications and Macroscopic Fat Embolisms (MAFEs)

One of the most dangerous complications is the macroscopic fat embolism, according to a review by Cardenas-Camarena et al. (2018) which described that during the gluteal lipoinjection, the fat enters into the bloodstream through a lesion in a vein from the gluteal drainage system and causes a direct occlusion of the blood vessels. It is clinically very similar to a pulmonary thromboembolism secondary to a blood clot. The cardiorespiratory failure occurs immediately after the lipoinjection during the operation. To avoid MAFEs, use security vectors and avoid the muscular plane in the danger triangle area: in this area, only subcutaneous lipografts are recommended, and in the superior safety triangle, the deeper muscular plane (close to the bone) must be avoided.

Avoiding Microscopic Fat Embolisms

Microscopic fat embolisms can also result from microscopic vessel penetration. The presence of fat cells in the blood produces an irritative process in the microvascular circulation. This process allows the entry of fat particles into a microvascular system. The liquid fat is the most disruptive part and the most harmful when it enters into a microvascular system (Cardenas-Camarena et al. 2018). To avoid a microscopic fat embolism, the liquid part of the lipograft left over from the sieved fat must be removed. The presence of blood changes the naturally yellow color of the fat, and a wash procedure (of warm Ringer's lactate or saline solution) must be applied until the yellow fat color has been re-established.

High pressure inside a muscular compartment facilitates the vascular penetration of microscopic fat, the maximal limit of which is 30 mmHg (Chamosa 2004). High pressure can be detected when the fat reflows by the canula. This will also serve as the clinical signal to stop the lipograft procedure in this location, but the canula must be left until the reflow has stopped.

How to Avoid Buttock Asymmetry

All patients have asymmetric butts, though the asymmetry can be small. If both the surgeon and the patient don't mention it before the surgical procedure, it could cause an inconvenient situation for both, after the surgery, if the asymmetry remains. In other patients, the asymmetry is evident during the preoperative clinical exam and in the preoperative photographs (Avelar 1986b). This asymmetry must be considered in a preoperative evaluation, and different volumes of lipografts must be used for each side, with more volume injected into the smaller side. The average volume difference between the two buttock sides in our patients is usually 20% (Vaccari-Mazzetti and Brock 2016).

Discussion

The liposuction associated with lipograft in the butt improves the surgical results and promotes a very high level of patient satisfaction with the body contour after surgery (Cardenas-Camarena and Paillet 2007; Harrison and Selvaggi 2007; Murillo 2004). This technique avoids needing to insert implants into the gluteus to improve its size when the patient has fat reserves sufficient to increase the butt's size (Hwang et al. 2012). The advantages of this technique are as follows: It uses autologous tissue; it maintains the patient's ability to receive intramuscular medicine; there is no migration of the injected tissue; when there is a nerve damage, it is temporary; and if the patient's weight increases, more sessions might be booked (Cardenas and Muñoz Ahmed 2002; Mendieta 2007; Smith et al. 2006).

Anatomical studies provide not only anatomical information but also physiologic patterns of tension after subfascial augmentation (Hwang et al. 2012). In our studies, we focused on anatomical landmarks to avoid causing direct neurovascular damage. In our clinical series, we stopped performing a submuscular lipograft when the fat reflowed by the number five cannula injection. A high level of pressure in the submuscular layer was the signal that an intramuscular limit was reached, and at that point, no more lipografts should be performed at this location.

When a surgeon performs several procedures during the same surgery, the intraoperative and postoperative risks increase, and the care during the preoperative period must be more intense. Special care, such as controlling bleeding and corporal temperature control, must be taken during the entire surgery. In Brazil, the aspirated volume has a maximum limit of 7% of the corporal weight, and this limit can be reached only if all the clinical conditions are favorable (Cardenas-Camarena et al. 1999; Roberts III et al. 2001; Robles-Cervantes et al. 2005).

When everything proceeds as planned, we can try to enhance the results by combining a liposuction technique with the lipograft injection. Better results in terms of the maintenance of the fat volume have been demonstrated by using intramuscular techniques, but the studies have not exhibited a uniform pattern (Aiache 2006; Viterbo et al. 1994; Wolf et al. 2006) (Figs. 39.12, 39.13, 39.14 and 39.15).

Some authors have preferred inserting implants to achieve gluteal augmentation, but using the patient's autologous tissue is always better when possible. Fortunately, we have been able to use autologous tissue in almost all our cases (Aiache 2006; Cardenas-Camarena and Paillet 2007). When we used a lipograft in gluteal augmentation, it was important to understand what would happen to this fat. Other authors were also concerned about this and used magnetic resonance imagining to study lipograft survival (Aiache 2006; Murillo 2004; Viterbo et al. 1994; Wolf et al. 2006).

The difficulties in controlling the fat volume, such as having access to appropriate facilities, high costs, and varying results, have made the magnetic resonance imagining scans uncommon in clinical series with a high number of patients (Cuenca-Guerra and Quezada 2004; Murillo 2004; Roberts III et al. 2006; Wolf et al. 2006). Magnetic resonance is very useful to provide images of the soft tissues, such as the muscle, fat, and neurovascular structures. We needed to establish a method for analysis: In the sagittal view, we couldn't analyze the images, but in the axial views, the images could be studied, measured, and compared (Centeno et al. 2018; Murillo 2004; Wolf et al. 2006). In other magnetic resonance studies, the measurement methods were not described in sufficient detail for reproducibility. In this study, though, we provide the specific radiological details of our technique.

Our study includes a reasonable number of patients, who were studied immediately after surgery, 7 and 15 days after surgery, and when the lipograft biology was stable. We hoped to find differences between the three initial times (immediately after, 7 days after, and 15 days after) because there was a decrease in the inflammatory reaction. However, it was easier to observe after 30 days.

One of the serious complications is a neurovascular injury. It can result in a temporary or definitive neurological injury in the sciatic nerve, causing a walking disability. A vascular injury could result in a venous thrombosis. Consequently, resultant thromboembolic phenomena could occur, and they could result in a fatal prognosis (Cardenas-Camarena et al. 2018). To avoid neurovascular injuries, the danger triangle must be avoided when performing submuscular lipografts, and going through the two safety triangles is the best option. In the danger triangle, we recommend subcutaneous lipografts.

Complications from infections were the most important in our clinical series, and all efforts must be made to avoid this clinical condition. When the pain after the

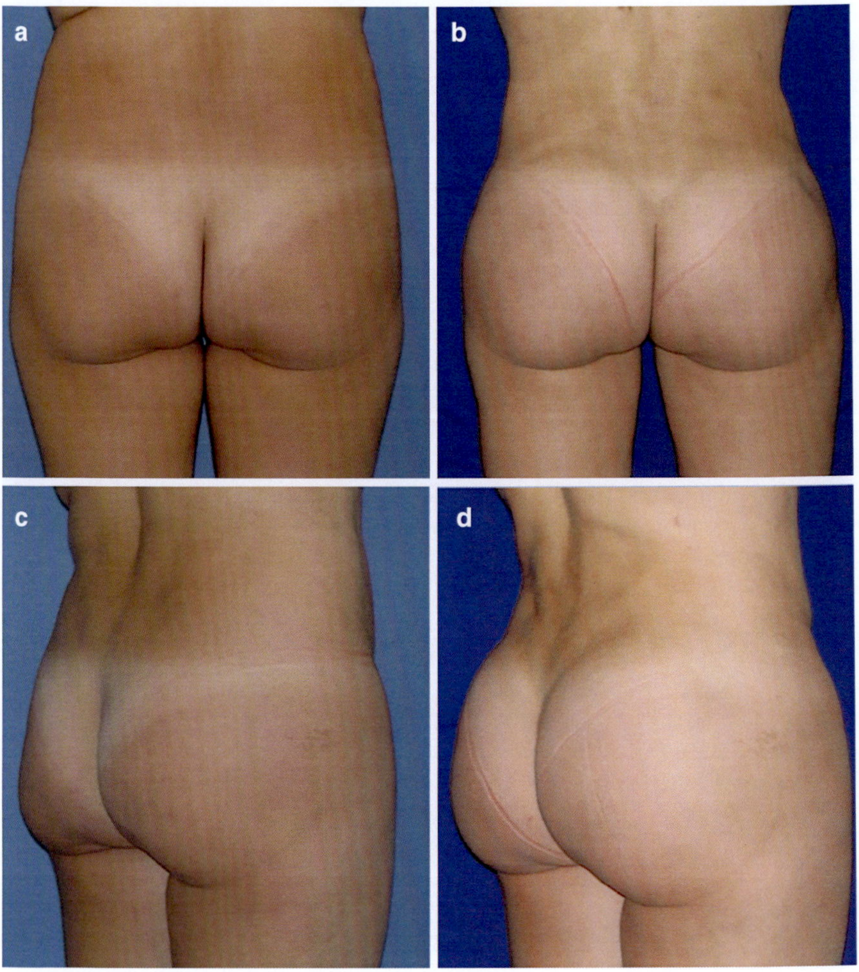

Fig. 39.12 Pre- and postoperative of a patient submitted to liposuction. It was injected 850 mL (760 mL of sub muscular fat graft: 430 mL in the right side and 330 in the left side and 90 mL at the subcutaneous). (**a**) Preop dorsal view: image with a quadrangular aspect and an asymmetry with more fat in the flank, (**b**) 16 months postop dorsal view: a concave format of the gluteus. (**c**) preoperative obliquos view, (**d**) 18 months postop obliquos view: a convex gluteus format

procedure remains specifically in the buttocks, it is a clinical signal of this complication (Vaccari-Mazzetti and Brock 2016). Two kinds of pain were observed: one that increases after day 3 and another that decreases until day 5 and increases afterward. Surgeons must distinguish between thigh pain, which has a neurological pattern, and butt pain, which indicates lipograft infection. The patient can usually indicate the precise site of pain, but the site of neurological pain is undefined.

The ultrasound was unable to show the infected area and was frequently normal in the first week. In our experience, the clinical symptoms were more important in

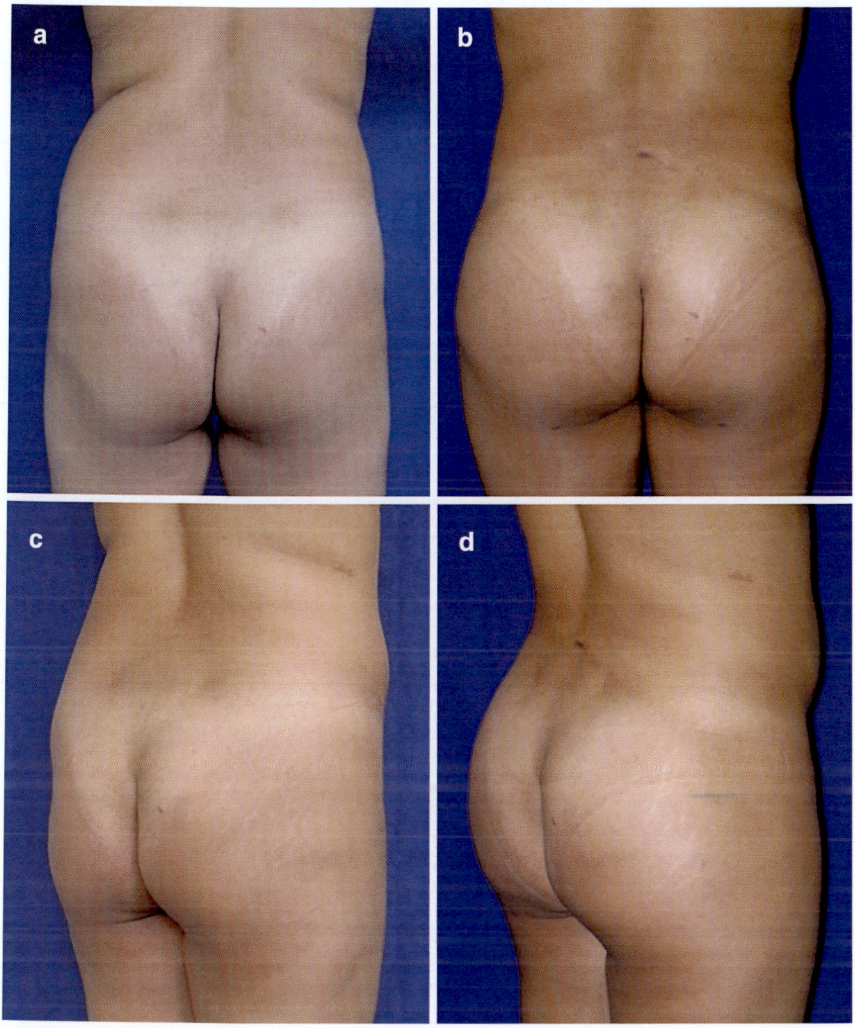

Fig. 39.13 Pre- and postoperative of a patient submitted to liposuction. It was injected 700 mL of submuscular fat graft and 100 mL at the subcutaneous. Patient submitted to submuscular lipografts with 800 mL, 450 mL in the right side and 350 in the left side. (**a**) Preop dorsal view: image with a quadrangular aspect and an asymmetry with left side bigger, (**b**) 16 months postop dorsal view: a concave format of the gluteus. (**c**) Preop obliquos view: image of the postoperative with a round format of the gluteus, (**d**) 16 months postop in obliquos view: a convex gluteus format

making a correct diagnosis and permitted a fast drainage intervention. After drainage, a vacuum drain was maintained for at least 2 days and until the seroma has diminished. A culture exam is necessary to diagnose the bacteria and guide the antibiotic treatment.

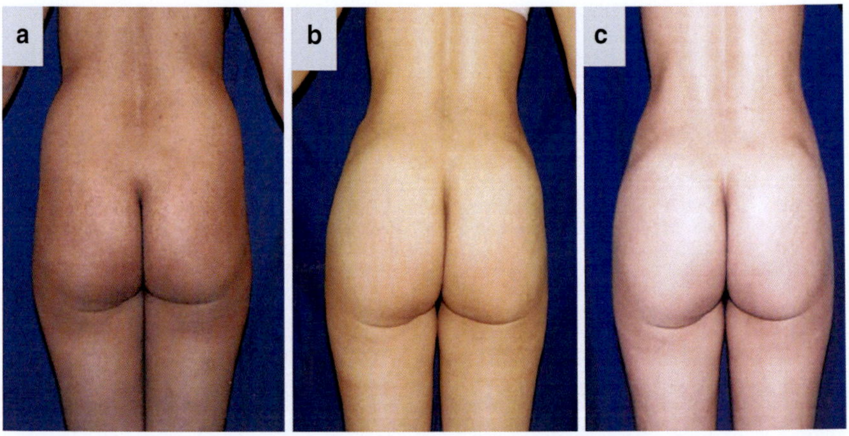

Fig. 39.14 Pre- and postoperative of a patient submitted to liposuction. It was injected 700 mL (300 mL in left side and 400 mL in right side) of submuscular fat graft and 100 mL at the subcutaneous. Patient submitted to submuscular lipografts with 800 mL, 450 mL in the right side and 350 in the left side. (**a**) Preop dorsal view: image with a quadrangular aspect and an asymmetry with more fat in the flank and a left side bigger, (**b**) 2 months postop dorsal view: a concave format of the gluteus, (**c**) 6 months postop dorsal view: a convex gluteus format looks like bigger than 2 months

The only complication that did not show a significant decrease with the experience of the surgeon was infection, maybe because it depends on the care given to the patient during postoperative period.

We took fundamental surgical steps to avoid infectious problems: trichotomy of all the anal regions with intense and careful degermation, the use of a closed system to collect fat, the maintenance of the fat almost without environmental air contact, a maximum limit of 40 min during which the fat was outside of the body, and repeating the degermation process every 2 h after the beginning of the surgical procedure.

The fat volume integrated very well into the muscle environment and showed a maintenance average close to 80%, and in some cases more than 90%, after 180 days.

Patients must maintain their corporal weight. A 3-L liposuction is expected to translate into an approximate 2 kg weight loss. When we reached this result and when the patient's weight did not change by more than 5%, we concluded that the increase or decrease in the gluteus would change not because of the fat graft volume but rather because fat cells are living tissues in the muscle. These results of lipograft insertion into the muscle reveal a good technique to improve buttock size and shape during a liposuction procedure with low rate of complications: insert the lipograft directly into the muscle (Fig. 39.16).

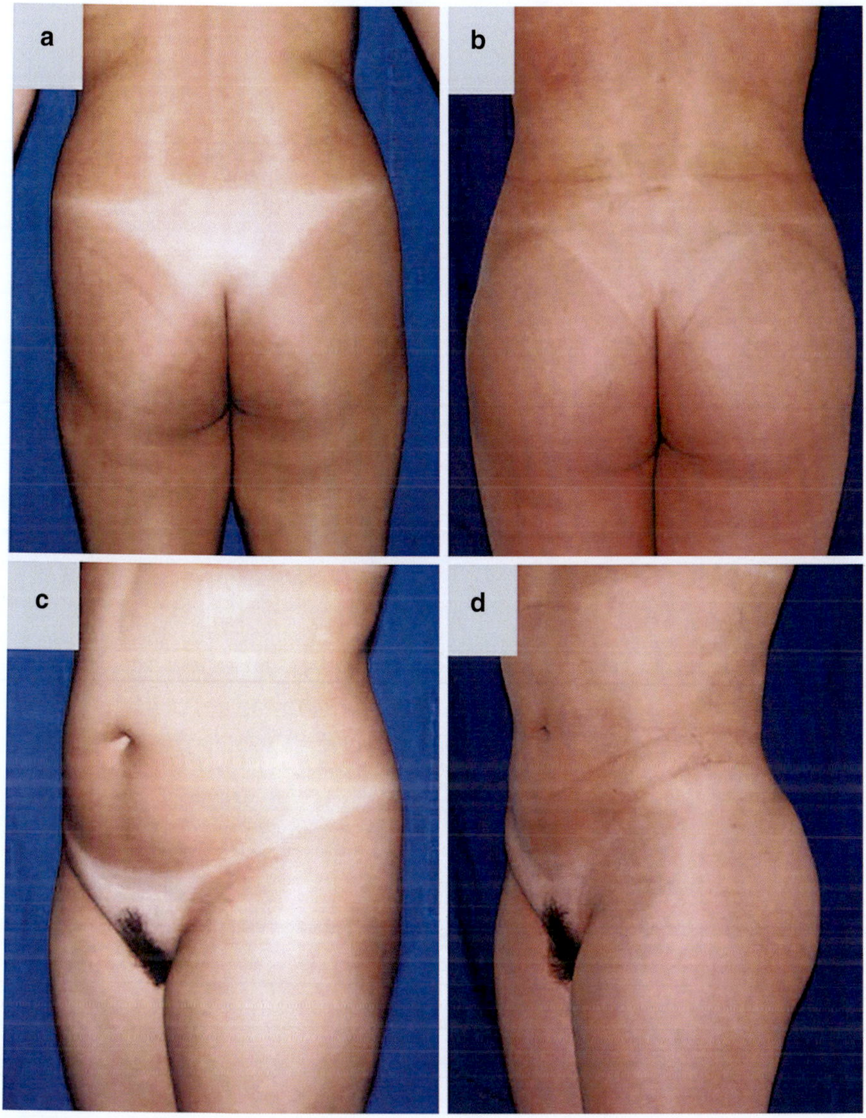

Fig. 39.15 Pre- and postoperative of a patient submitted to liposuction. It was injected 750 mL (700 mL of submuscular fat graft: 400 mL in the right side and 300 in the left side and 50 mL at the subcutaneous). (**a**) Preop dorsal view: image with a quadrangular aspect and an asymmetry with left gluteus bigger, (**b**) 16 months postop dorsal view: a round format of the gluteus. (**c**) Preoperative oblique view, (**d**) 18 months postop obliquos view: a convex gluteus format

Fig. 39.16 The complications present in our cases. Before the use of safety tringles and vectors we had one case of macroscopic fat embolism, but after that in almost 800 cases no more fat embolism was observed in our cases

Complications after Safety Triangles	Number of Cases and Porcentage	
	Number	Porcentage
Infection	12	1,5
Thigh Pain	250	31,6
Asymetria	5	0,6
Hematoma	2	0,25
Total cases	790	100

Conclusions

Smooth body contouring is the aim of plastic surgery. To achieve ideal gluteal contouring, the surgeon should opt for the gluteal submuscular lipograft because this surgical technique comes with the best results in maintaining fat, but the plastic surgeon must undergo adequate training in the technique to prevent (microscopic or macroscopic) fat embolisms and other complications. The collection and preparation of donor fat was detailed. The maintenance of the submuscular fat was studied. A preventive technique and various fat embolisms were explained. Other complications, such as infection, asymmetry, and nerve damage, and how to prevent them were described.

Conflicts of Interest The authors declare that they have no conflicts of interest.

Funding The study had no financial support.

References

Aiache AE. Gluteal recontouring with combination treatments: Implants, liposuction and fat transfer. *Clin Plast Surg*. 2006, 33:395–403.

American Society of Plastic Surgeons. National Plastic Surgery Statistics [Internet]. ASPS; 2019 [cited 2021 Dec 15]. Available from: https://www.plasticsurgery.org/documents/News/Statistics/2019/plastic-surgery-statistics-full-report-2019.pdf

Avelar J. Lipoaspiração da parede abdominal. In: Avelar J, Bolanho E. Lipoaspiração. 1. ed. Rio de Janeiro: Hipócrates; 1986a. p. 157–75.

Avelar J. Padronização fotográfica como método de documentação científica. In: Avelar J, Bolanho E. Lipoaspiração. 1. ed. Rio de Janeiro: Hipócrates; 1986b. p. 80–86.

Avelar J. Perfil psicológico do paciente. Introdução ao estudo. In: Avelar J, Bolanho E. Lipoaspiração. 1. ed. Rio de Janeiro: Hipócrates; 1986c. p. 8–12.

Caplan AI. Mesenchymal stem cells. *Journal of Orthopaedic Research*, 1991. 9(5):641–50.
Cardenas JC, Muñoz Ahmed JA. Large-volume lipoinjection for gluteal augmentation. *Aesthetic Surg J.* 2002, 22(1):33–8.
Cardenas-Camarena L, Duran H, Robles-Cervantes JA, Bayter-Marin JE. Critical differences between microscopic (MIFE) and macroscopic (MAFE) fat embolism during liposuction and gluteal lipoinjection. *PlastReconstrSurg.* 2018; 141(4):880–90.
Cardenas-Camarena L, Lacouture AM, Tobar-Losada A. Combined gluteoplasty: Liposuction and lipoinjection. *Plast Reconstr Surg.* 1999, 104(5):1524–31.
Cardenas-Camarena L, Paillet JC. Combined gluteoplasty: Liposuction and gluteal implants. *Plast Reconstr Surg.* 2007; 119(3):1067–74.
Centeno RF, Sood A, Young VL. (2018) Clinical anatomy in aesthetic gluteal contouring. Clin Plastic Surg 45: 145–57.
Chamosa M. Lipectomy of the ilio-lumbosacral region. *Plast Reconstr Surg.* 2004, 113(1):419–24.
Cuenca-Guerra R, Quezada J. What makes buttocks beautiful? A review and classification of the determinants of gluteal beauty and the surgical techniques to achieve them. Aesth Plast Surg. 2004, 28:340–7.
Fitzsimmons REB, Mazurek MS, Soos A, Simmons CA. Mesenchymal stromal/stem cells in regenerative medicine and tissue engineering. *Stem Cells International*, 2018. 1–18. https://doi.org/10.1155/2018/8031718.
Friedenstein AJ, Chailakhjan RK, Lalykina KS. The development of fibroblast colonies in monolayer cultures of Guinea-pig bone marrow and spleen cells. *Cell Proliferation*, 1970. 3(4):393–403.
Friedenstein AJ, Piatetzky-Shapiro II, Petrakova KV. Osteogenesis in transplants of bone marrow cells. *Development*, 1966. 16 (3):381–90.
Grambow F, Rutkowski R, Podmelle F, Schmoeckel K, Siegerist F, Domanski G, Schuster MW, Domanska G. The impact of lidocaine on adipose-derived stem cells in human adipose tissue harvested by liposuction and used for lipotransfer. *Int J Mol Sci.* 2020. 21:2869. https://doi.org/10.3390/ijms21082869
Harrison D, Selvaggi G. Gluteal augmentation surgery: Indications and surgical management. *J Plast Reconstr Aesthet Surg.* 2007, 60(8):922–8.
Heidekrueger PI, Sinno S, Tanna N, Szpalski C, Juran S, Schmauss D, Ehrl D, Ng R, Ninkovic M, Broer PN. The ideal buttock size: A sociodemographic morphometric evaluation. Plast Reconstr Surg. 2017, 140(1): 20e–32e.
Hwang SW, Nam YS, Hwang K, Han SH. Thickness and tension of the gluteal aponeurosis and the implications for subfascial gluteal augmentation. *J. Anat.* 2012, 221: 69–72.
International Society of Aesthetic Plastic Surgery. International survey on aesthetic / cosmetic procedures [Internet]. ISAPS; 2019 [cited 2021 Dec 15]. Available from: https://www.isaps.org/wp-content/uploads/2020/12/Global-Survey-2019.pdf
Lewis CM. Buttock augmentation: Case studies of fat injection monitored by magnetic resonance imaging. *Plast Reconstr Surg.* 2004, 1015–6.
Mendieta CG. Gluteal reshaping. *Aesthetic Surg J.* 2007, 27(6):641–55.
Murillo WL, Buttock augmentation: case studies of fat injection monitored by magnetic resonance imaging. Plastic Reconstr Surg. 2004, 114 (6): 1606–14.
Pitanguy I. Perspectivas Filosóficas e Psicossociais do Contorno Corporal. In: Avelar J, Bolanho E. Lipoaspiração. 1. ed. Rio de Janeiro: Hipócrates; 1986. p. 3–7.
Pittenger MF, Mackay AM, Becketal SC. Multilineage potential of adult human mesenchymal stem cells. *Science*, 1999. 284(5411): 143–7.
Pu LLQ, Coleman SR, Cui X, Ferguson REH, Vasconez HC. Autologous fat grafts harvested and refined by the Coleman technique: A comparative study. *Plast Reconstr Surg.* 2008, 122(3):932–7.
Roberts III TL, Toledo LS, Badin AZ. Augmentation of the buttocks by micro fat grafting. *Aesthetic Surg J.* 2001, 21(4):311–9.

Roberts III TL, Weinfeld AB, Bruner TW, Nguyen K. Universal and ethnic ideals of beautiful buttocks are best obtained by autologous micro fat grafting and liposuction. *Clin Plast Surg*. 2006, 33:371–94.

Robles-Cervantes JA, Martinez-Molina R, Cardenas-Camarena L. Heating infiltration solutions used in tumescent liposuction: Minimizing surgical risk. *Plast Reconstr Surg*. 2005, 116 (4): 1077–81.

Smith P, Adams Jr. WP, Lipschitz AH, Chau B, Sorokin E, Rorich RJ, Brown SA. Autologous human fat grafting: Effect of harvesting and preparation techniques on adipocyte graft survival. *Plast Reconstr Surg*. 2006, 117(6):1836–44.

Sociedade Brasileira de Cirurgia Plástica. Censo 2018 – Análise comparativa das pesquisas 2014, 2015, 2016 e 2018 [Internet]. SBCP; 2019 [cited 2021 Dec 15]. Available from: www2.cirurgiaplastica.org.br/wp-content/uploads/2019/08/Apresentação-Censo-2018_V3.pdf

Vaccari-Mazzetti MP, Brock RS. Buttock lipografting and augmentation combined with Avelar's abdominoplasty. In: Avelar JM. New Concepts on abdominoplasty and further applications. Springler. 2016, 329–44.

Viterbo F, Marques M, Valente M. Fat-tissue injection versus graft: Experimental study in rabbits. *Ann Plast Surg*. 1994, 33:184–92.

Wolf GA, Gallego S, Patron GAS, Ramirez ZF, Delgado BJA, Echeverri AA, Garcia GMM. Magnetic resonance imaging assessment of gluteal fat grafts. *Aesth Plast Surg*. 2006, 30 (4):460–8.

Chapter 40
Fat Grafting for Remodeling Gluteal Regions

Lybio Martire Junior

Abstract The gluteal region has great physiological importance for humans, as its musculature acts to support the body, but there is also a morphological importance, especially in females, since its shape and size are associated with fertility and seduction. Hence, there is a search for plastic surgery to achieve the increase and remodeling to give more grace to this region. Fat grafting in the gluteal region is an effective method that obtains excellent results with a minimum incidence of complications. This chapter describes the proper technique for introducing the fat graft and the precautions that must be taken to prevent complications. Late results are also presented showing that the fat in this region remains integrated.

Keywords Fat graft · Gluteal region · Liposuction · Adipose tissue

The gluteal region has great physiological importance for human beings. In addition to assisting in body support, posture, and protecting the hip structures, it protects the body itself when in a sitting position because it has a large amount of fat that works as a cushion. It also has the function of supporting the hip and helping the movement of the legs.

However, its importance goes further, morphologically and as an erogenous region, especially in females, since it is associated with fertility and seduction and, for this reason, it is a very erotic part of the female body.

L. M. Junior (✉)
Plastic Surgery, Surgical Clinic and History of Medicine at Itajubá Medical School (FMIT), Itajubá, MG, Brazil

Brazilian Society of Plastic Surgery, São Paulo, Brazil

International College of Surgeons, Brazilian College of Surgeons, Brazilian Society of History of Medicine, The Medical Academy of São Paulo, Instituto Prof. Lybio Junior Plastic Surgery and Health, São Paulo, Brazil

J. M. Avelar, R. Cavalcanti Ribeiro (eds.), *Body Contouring*,
https://doi.org/10.1007/978-3-031-42802-9_40

In addition, a beautiful body gives a woman more self-confidence (Pitanguy 1986).

The gluteal region of the female body has erotic appeal for males, who value it sexually. A wide hip and protruding gluteal region convey the information of "best reproducer" as nature seeks to preserve the species.

For all these reasons, the desire to have a protruding and graceful gluteal region is a frequent desire in females. Women in gyms do specific exercises for the gluteal region not only to strengthen it but also to make the region more beautiful and attractive. It is common for women to admire others who have improved their hips with exercise or have a protruding gluteal region due to genetics. Therefore, it is also common to see advertisements on the Internet for gyms or exercises that promise this transformation.

However, due to individual genetic compositions or other racial reasons, some women have a more enlarged and protruding region, while others do not have this privilege, and, in most cases, exercises alone are not enough to produce the desired increase and remodeling of the gluteal region.

In plastic surgery, there are basically two ways to increase the gluteal region satisfactorily: through the insertion of silicone prosthesis or the grafting of adipose tissue.

Fat grafting is a procedure capable of obtaining excellent results from an aesthetic point of view in the remodeling of the gluteal region. It has some advantages over the insertion of silicone prosthesis, such as being a more physiological procedure because it uses tissue from the body itself, allowing for a faster recovery and therefore less possibility of pain in the postoperative period. It is possible to inject medication into the gluteal region (an injection shot) after the surgery, so there is no need for potential future replacements. There is also a lower incidence of complications, such as seromas, dehiscence, double bubble etc. (Silveira 2018).

However, an obvious disadvantage is the need for the existence of a fat donor area to carry out a gluteal fat grafting.

The fat is usually obtained through liposuction of the abdominal, dorsal, and lower limbs. Very thin people with little body fat make this procedure impossible, since it is only feasible to use an autogenous graft.

Liposuction in the donor areas can be done using a liposuction device or syringe exerting negative pressure. I routinely prefer the use of a syringe, but it is just a matter of habit. However, in my opinion, the use of laser-assisted liposuction or ultrasonic liposuction is not recommended, as there is greater damage to the adipose tissue, which can compromise integration.

Special care is necessary and important for the fat grafting technique to be more efficient and safer, in order to obtain satisfactory results and prevent complications.

Performing liposuction in the dorsal region, just above the gluteal region, is a procedure that allows for better remodeling, favoring the result of fat grafting. Decreasing the volume above the gluteal region helps it seem more prominent. Liposuction should be more accentuated in the sacral region, accentuating the contour of the gluteal region. In this way, it is also possible to elevate the upper part of the gluteal groove, if necessary, which makes the region look more graceful (Fig. 40.1).

The access for performing a liposuction made in the upper part of the gluteal fold allows for treating the entire area (Figs. 40.1 and 40.2).

The aspirated fat can be prepared for use as a graft in various ways, through centrifugation, decantation, etc. I prefer to make the preparation by simply washing the fat with saline in a sieve. The material washed in a sieve is then packaged in syringes. This method has been shown to be very efficient in relation to the quality of the fat to be grafted, as we normally observe a high level of integration (Martire 2013).

The recipient site of the fat graft can be the adipose tissue of the gluteal region or the muscle in the region. It is not recommended, however, to perform fat grafting in muscle tissue because this approach increases the possibility of complications. The exuberant blood irrigation of the muscle tissue may even be a factor that favors the integration of the fat graft, but it increases the risk of fat embolism. Therefore, our recommendation is to perform the graft only (and always) in the adipose tissue, and this should be tended to with special care in the prophylaxis of complications (Martire 2019).

Another important precaution is to make the access for fat grafting in a place that does not coincide with the accesses used for liposuction. Moreover, the most cranial part of the gluteal region is the most preferrable where the action of gravity collaborates so that there is no contact of the fat graft with the access route or with the skin, thus reducing the risk of contamination, in addition to allowing a better distribution of the fat graft (Fig. 40.3).

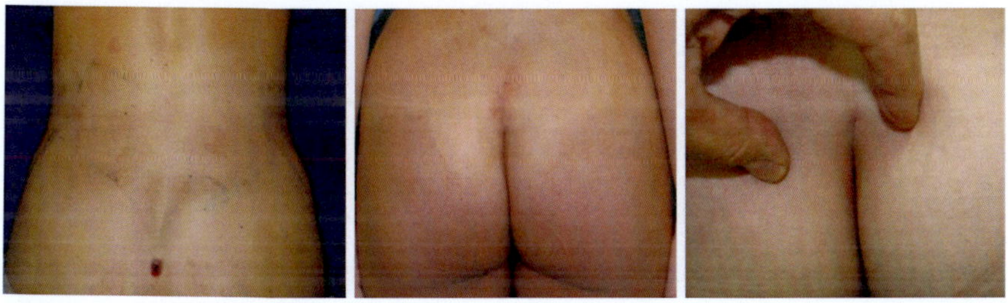

Fig. 40.1 The left image shows the depression produced by a liposuction in the sacral region, which will favor the result of fat grafting. It also shows the access site for liposuction in the gluteal sulcus. In the center and right image, notice the imperceptible scar it leaves after 6 months

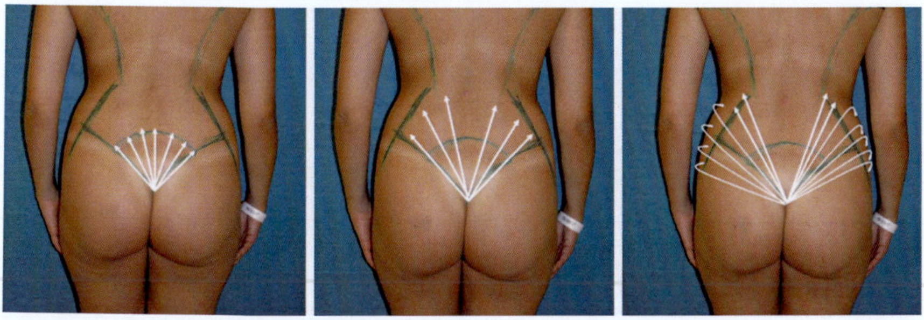

Fig. 40.2 Through the gluteal sulcus access, it is possible to treat the entire dorsal region above the gluteal region, favoring the projection of the gluteal region and the end result of fat grafting

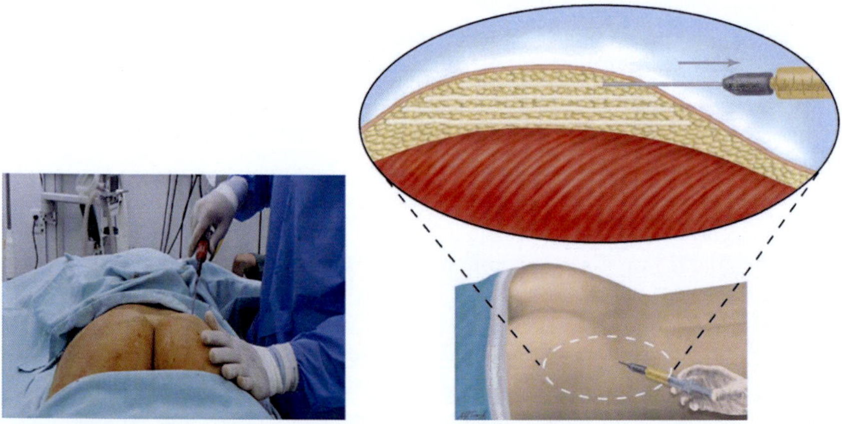

Fig. 40.3 The image shows the surgeon performing the fat grafting and, in detail, the access site for the fat grafting. The drawing shows the fat being introduced when the cannula is pulled back and in fillets which increases the possibility of integration

In the technique for introducing fat into the gluteal region, there is also a very special handling. A 3 mm cannula is used, measuring 25 cm in length, in the intimacy of the adipose tissue until the end, and then the fat is injected only by withdrawing the cannula. The fat is never injected when the cannula is introduced, only by retreating. This process makes the procedure very safe, with no possibility of vascular perforation, preventing fat embolism. In addition, the grafted fat is deposited in fillets within the adipose tissue of the gluteal region, which increases the possibility of integration and allows for a more homogeneous distribution of the fat (Fig. 40.3) (Martire 2016).

This special process, in addition to prophylaxis of complications, such as an eventual intravascular injection, causes the fat to be deposited in the intimacy of the adipose tissue of the gluteal region in fillets, which is a factor that will allow better irrigation, favoring integration and leaving a more homogeneous result.

The possible complications of fat grafting are infections, fat embolism, fat encystment, irregularities, and non-integration, but, taking the exposed precautions, the risk of these complications is practically negligible.

The immediate effect of fat grafting can be observed by the projection of the region in which it was performed (Fig. 40.4).

There are exceptional cases in which some patients in order to undergo a new fat grafting procedure to further enlarge the gluteal region, of their own volition, after having undergone a fat grafting, decide to gain weight in order to increase the fat donor region. The increase in the donor area then enables a new fat graft. This is what happened with the patient shown in Fig. 40.5; she was thin, a significant increase in the gluteal region was achieved in the first fat grafting, and she said she liked the result and asked if there was weight gain if she could undergo a new fat grafting. With the positive answer, she gained weight for 2 years, gained 5 kg of weight and returned to undergo new fat grafting. The result after the second surgery that finally left her completely satisfied is shown in Fig. 40.5.

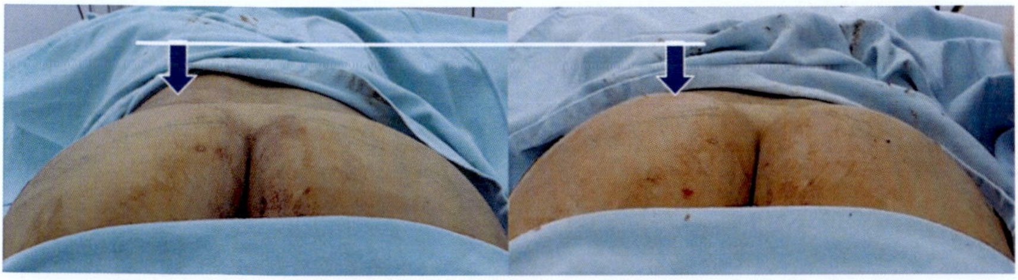

Fig. 40.4 The arrows compare the left gluteal region of the patient before and right after fat grafting, by which one can observe the immediate increase and projection obtained by fat grafting

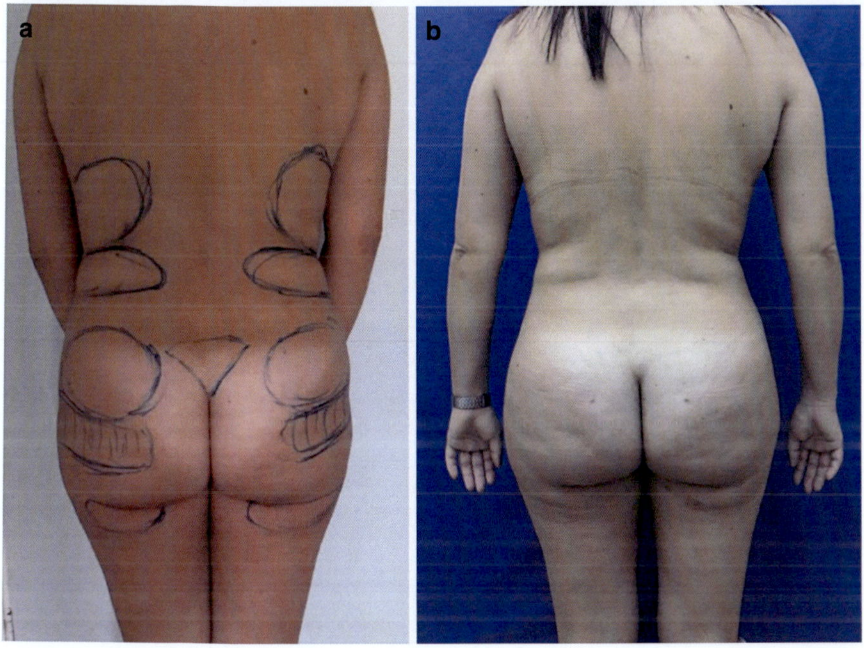

Fig. 40.5 Preoperative image on the left, with areas marked to be treated with body liposuction and fat grafting in the gluteal region. Right image, 1 year after the operation, showing the enlarged and remodeled gluteal region

Conclusion

Fat grafting is an effective method, capable of achieving satisfactory and permanent results, as long as the guidelines and special care described are followed. Its only contraindication is the absence of fat in the donor regions.

Results

The following Figs. 40.6, 40.7, 40.8, 40.9, 40.10, 40.11, 40.12, and 40.13.

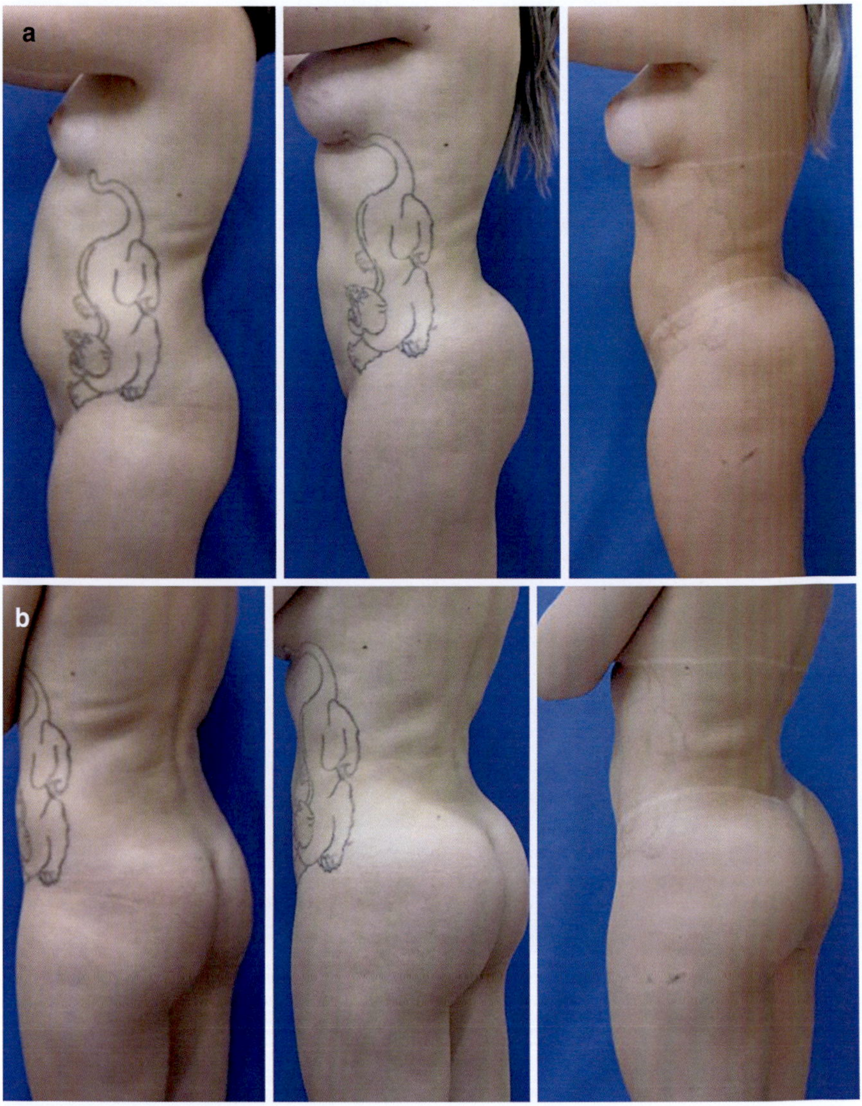

Fig. 40.6 (**a**) Body liposuction and fat grafting in the gluteal region. Left preoperative image (25 years old), center image 4 months after the operation, and the right image 4 years after the operation, showing the persistence of fat grafting. (**b**) Body liposuction and fat grafting in the gluteal region. Left preoperative image (25 years old), center image 4 months after the operation, and the right image 4 years after the operation, showing the persistence of fat grafting. (**c**) Body liposuction and fat grafting in the gluteal region. Left preoperative image (25 years old), center image 4 months after the operation, and the right image 4 years after the operation, showing the persistence of fat grafting. (**d**) Body liposuction and fat grafting in the gluteal region. Left preoperative image (25 years old), center image 4 months after the operation, and the right image 4 years after the operation, showing the persistence of fat grafting

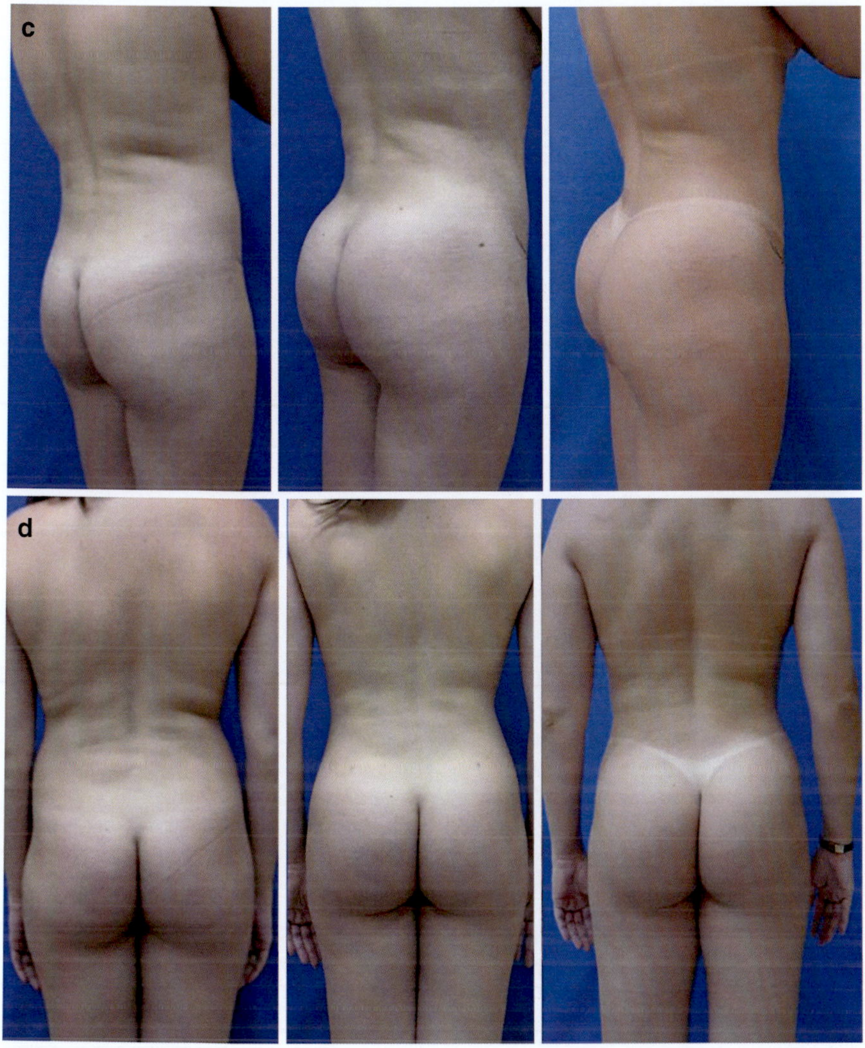

Fig. 40.6 (continued)

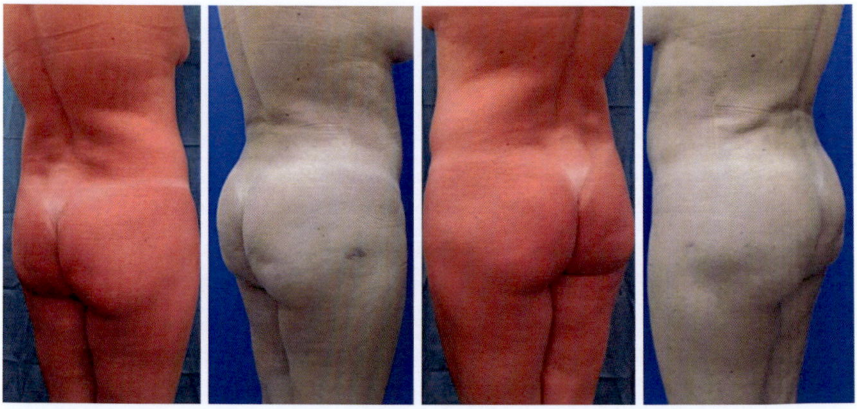

Fig. 40.7 (**a**) Preoperative and 6-month postoperative period in a 45-year-old patient

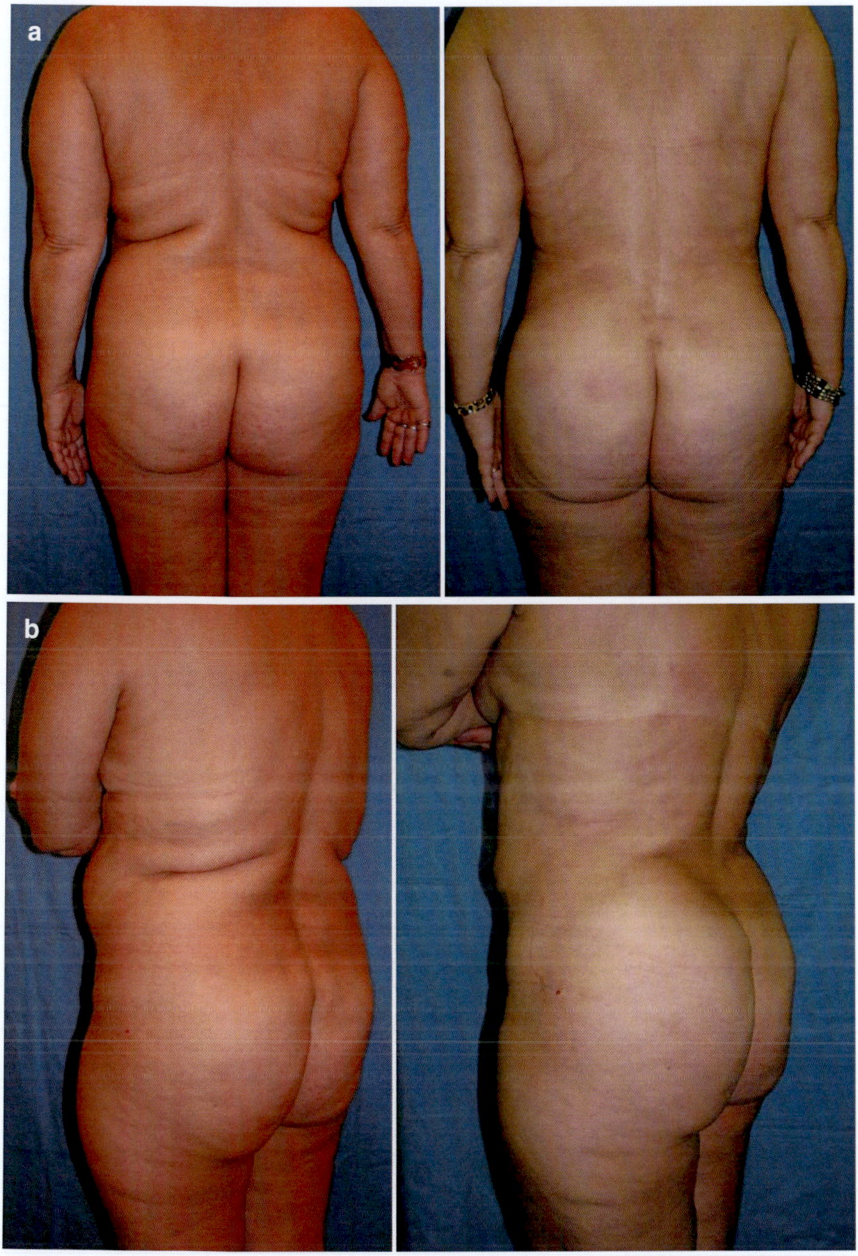

Fig. 40.8 (**a**) Preoperative and 1-year postoperative period in a 57-year-old patient, showing remodeling and elevation of the gluteal region. (**b**) Preoperative and 1-year postoperative period in a 57-year-old patient, showing remodeling and elevation of the gluteal region

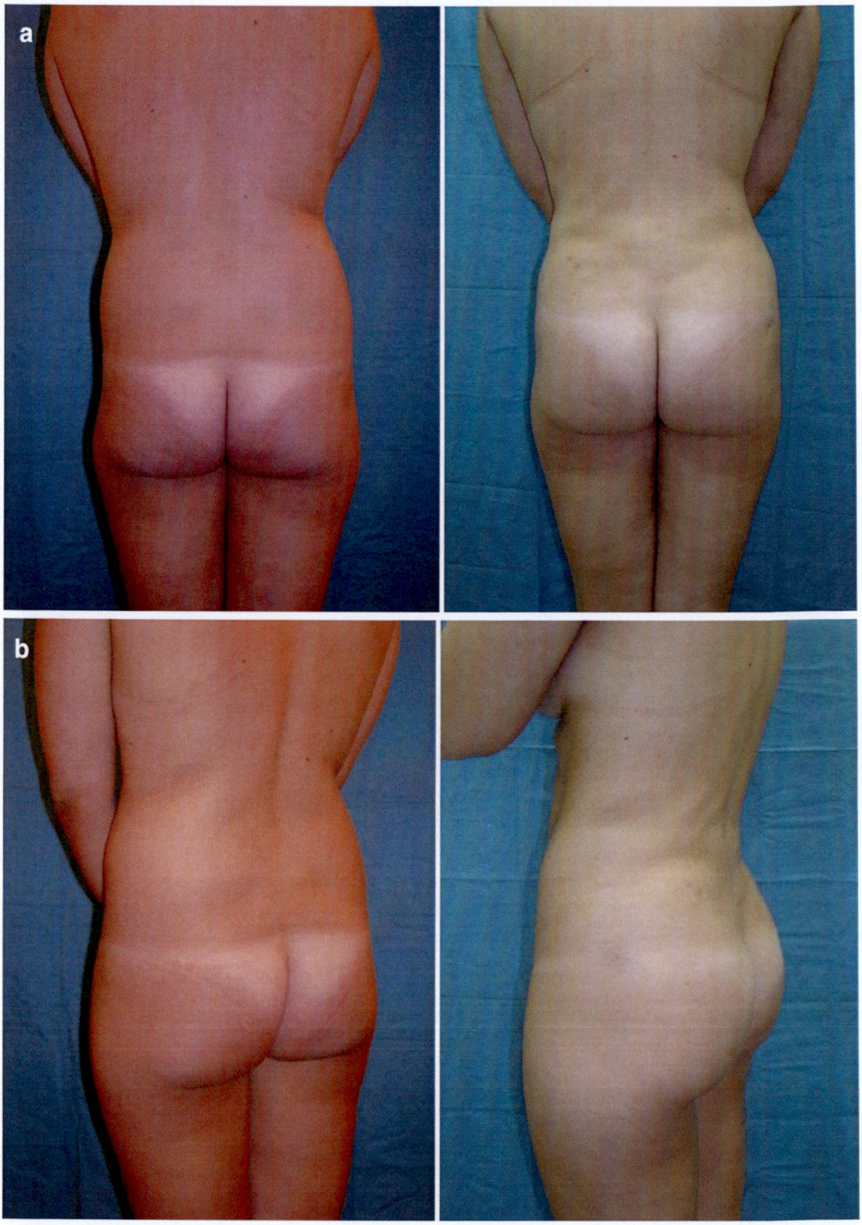

Fig. 40.9 (**a**) Preoperative and 1-year postoperative period in a 26-year-old patient, showing remodeling and projection of the gluteal region. (**b**) Preoperative and 1-year postoperative period in a 26-year-old patient, showing remodeling and projection of the gluteal region

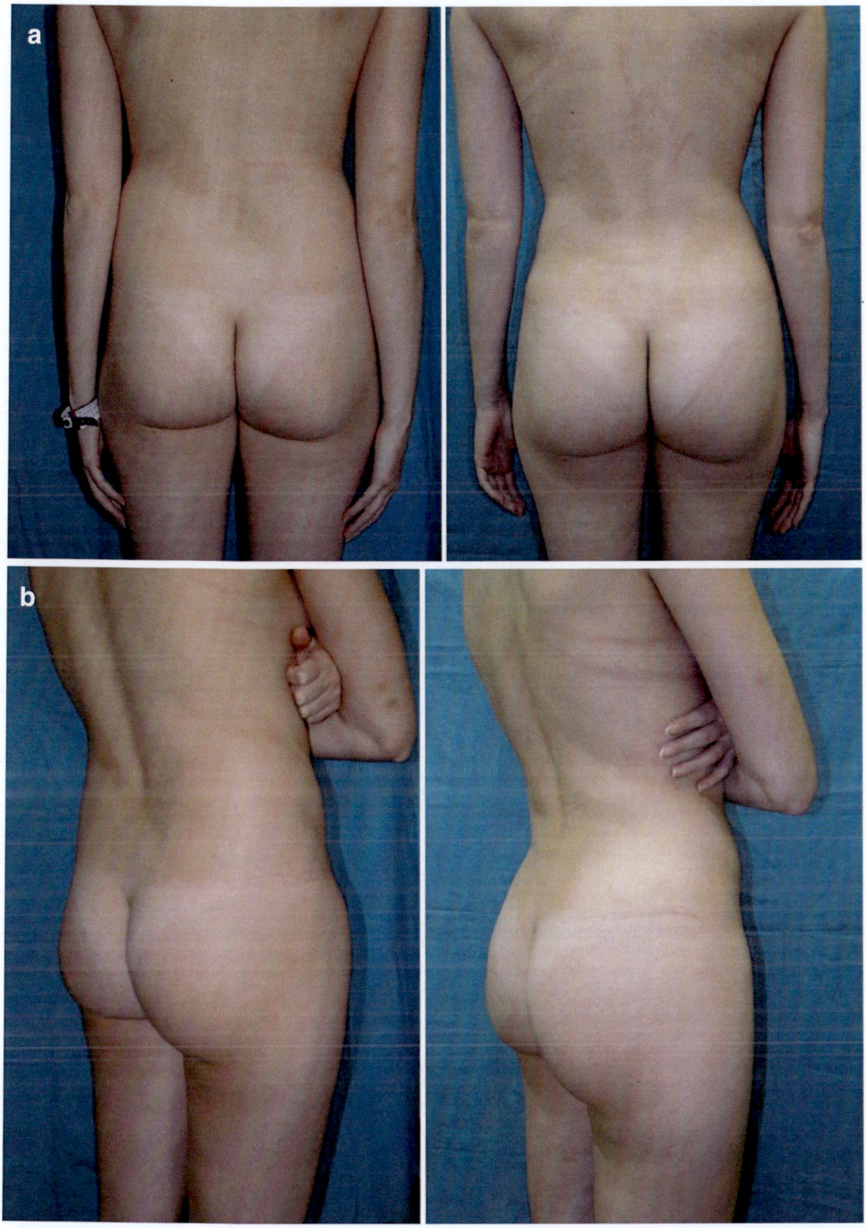

Fig. 40.10 (**a**) Preoperative and 1-year postoperative period in a 30-year-old patient, showing remodeling and projection of the gluteal region. (**b**) Preoperative and 1-year postoperative period in a 30-year-old patient, showing remodeling and projection of the gluteal region

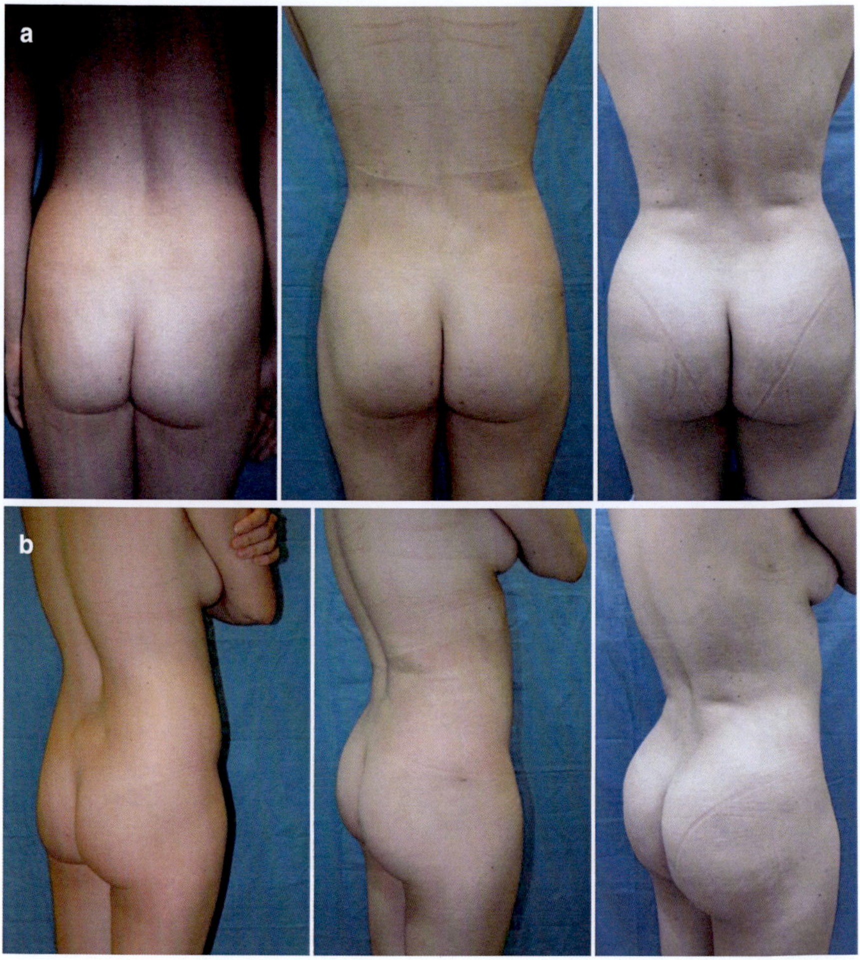

Fig. 40.11 (**a**) Left – Preoperative. Center – Postoperative, 1 year after fat grafting. Right - Postoperative, 1 year after second fat grafting, done two years after the first. The patient gained 5 kg in order to undergo a new fat grafting and further increase the gluteal region. (**b**) Left – Preoperative. Center – Postoperative, 1 year after fat grafting. Right - Postoperative, 1 year after second fat grafting, done two years after the first. The patient gained 5 kg in order to undergo a new fat grafting and further increase the gluteal region more

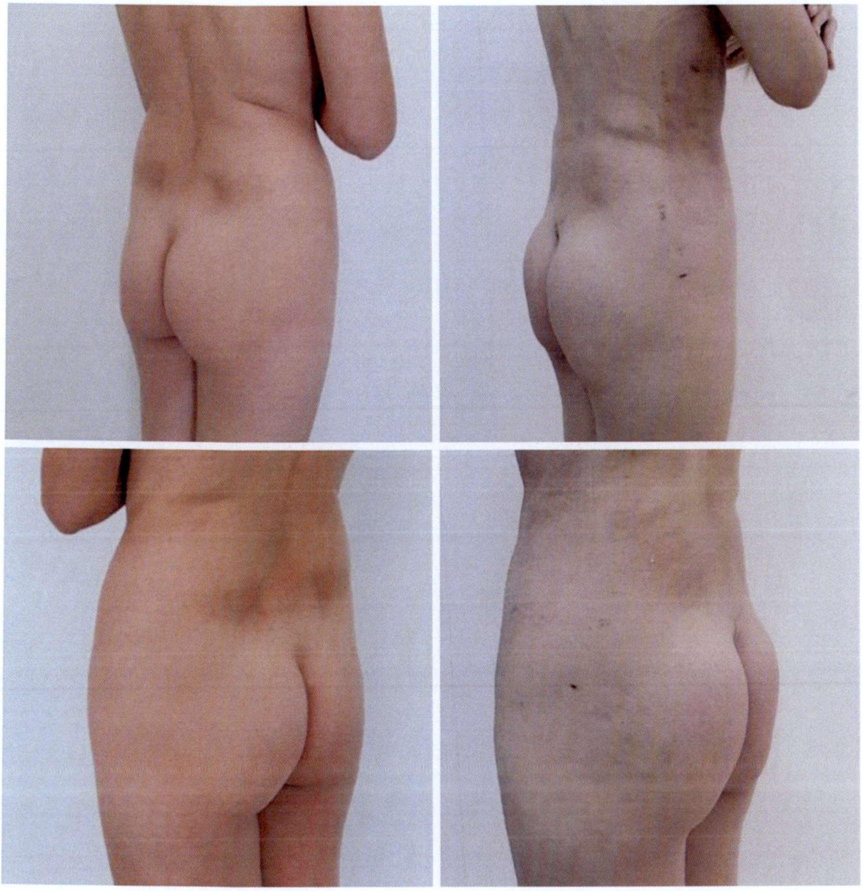

Fig. 40.12 Lipograft, preoperative and 4-month postoperative period in a 35-year-old, thin patient with little fat donor area. In this case, the result is limited by the small amount of fat present in the donor regions; however, it was possible to remodel and create a small increase in the gluteal region, giving it more grace

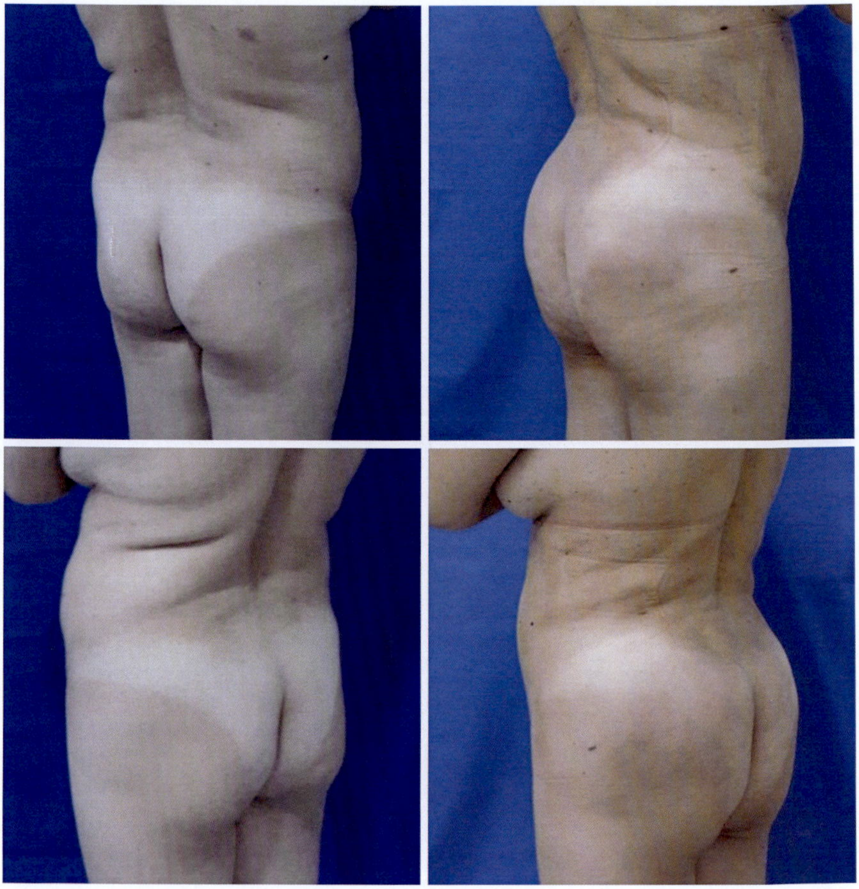

Fig. 40.13 Preoperative and postoperative period of fat grafting with 1-year evolution in a 60-year-old patient, showing remodeling and projection of the gluteal region

References

Pitanguy I (1986) Philosophical and Psychosocial Perspectives of the Body Contour in Avelar J, Illouz Y, Liposuction, São Paulo, Brazil

Silveira G D et al (2018) Double Bubble em Gluteoplastias com Implantes no Contorno Corporal Feminino: Como Prevenir e Tratar Rev. Bras. Cir. Plást. 2018;33(Supl. 1): 23–25

Martire Jr L (2019) Liposuction for body contouring - criteria and systematization, XII Sul Mineiro Congress of Plastic Surgery, University of Alfenas, Minas Gerais, Brazil

Martire Jr L (2016) Augmentation Gluteoplasty with Liposuction and Lipografting, X South Mineiro Congress of Plastic Surgery, FMIT, Itajubá, Minas Gerais, Brazil

Martire Jr L (2013) Liposuction of the Body Contour - Systematization to Improve the Result, VII South Mineiro Congress of Plastic Surgery, Alfenas, Minas Gerais, Brazil

Chapter 41
Liposculpture: Improving Results with Standard Lipografts and Mesenchymal Cells Lipografts

Marcelo Paulo Vaccari-Mazzetti, Juarez Moraes Avelar, Ryane Schmidt Brock, and Thalita Galdino de Oliveira

Abstract The association of stem cells with lipografts allows a better result in cases of tumor reconstructive surgeries of the buttock with poor vascularization and demonstrates a low rate of complications with submuscular associated with subcutaneous lipoinjection. The use of repeated sessions is required for an ideal aesthetic result.

In cases of breast augmentation during the corporal surgery, even in male and female, the results increased patient satisfaction with low rate of complications. Submuscular approach was used with limited volume, but it was enough to achieve a better breast shape.

Introduction

Since the first liposuction publication by Illouz in France and later by Avelar and Illouz, the liposuction technique had some changes that improved final results and gave more satisfaction to the patients and plastic surgeons (Avelar 1999, 2002, 2006; Illouz and Sterodimas 2009; Illouz 1986).

The basic principles remain the same; however, some current technical resources were added to the original one like lipografts. Scientific development and fat biology knowledge improvement resulted in better final aesthetic and reconstructive surgery results.

M. P. Vaccari-Mazzetti (✉) · R. S. Brock · T. G. de Oliveira
Brazilian Society of Plastic Surgery, Face Defects Research and Study Center, São Paulo, Brazil

J. M. Avelar
Brazilian Scientific Institute of Plastic and Reconstructive Surgery, São Paulo, Brazil

J. M. Avelar, R. Cavalcanti Ribeiro (eds.), *Body Contouring*,
https://doi.org/10.1007/978-3-031-42802-9_41

The technique demands professional training and appropriate physical hospital structure to be performed with security (Vaccari-Mazzetti and Brock 2016).

Liposuction has a high demand because it improves body contour with few scars and it can be associated with lipografts of the autologous adipose tissue to achieve better results on liposculpture. The most common are buttock and breast augmentation with submuscular combined with subcutaneous lipografts to improve body contour (Avelar 2006; Vaccari-Mazzetti and Brock 2016).

There are many techniques used to perform liposuction and this fat can be used to improve body contour or discarded. When the fat is used, the surgical procedure is usually called liposculpture (Harrison and Selvaggi 2007).

Liposculpture is an important technique to improve the results of liposuction and demands know-how in fat graft biology. The donor site, fat collection, fat treatment, and receiving site can change the result and decide the success or failure of the surgical procedure (Harrison and Selvaggi 2007).

The results in buttock shape are related to the fat graft volume, and sometimes the amount of available fat is less than we desire to improve a shape and transform it into a round and full buttock.

Studies demonstrate that the best choice to manipulate fat is to purify fat cells and put it into the muscle to give a better vascular supply and improve the maintenance of the fat volume (Lewis 2004; Mendieta 2007; Murillo 2004).

Nowadays, the regenerative medicine and tissue engineering gained an important participation at all fields of medicine. Mesenchymal stem cells are already known for its multipotential regenerative issues (Fitzsimmons et al. 2018; Grambow et al. 2020).

The use of stem cells in lipografts became of special interest in less vascularized areas like the breast and gluteus which have some deficiencies, like tumor resection deformities.

Technique

Mesenchymal Stem Cell Collection

The mesenchymal stem cell collection is made up of a small skin punch behind the ear, in aseptic technique, and it is sent to a culture stem cell laboratory (Brasil Cryogenic Center, CCB, São Paulo—SP, Brasil). The culture and these cells multiplication was made in 2 months in the protocol described by Ayoub and Lizier (Ayoub et al. 2013) (Fig. 41.1).

Radiological Studies

In the cases of gluteus deformities, angiotomography was done to give more information about the circulatory status of the gluteal area (Fig. 41.2).

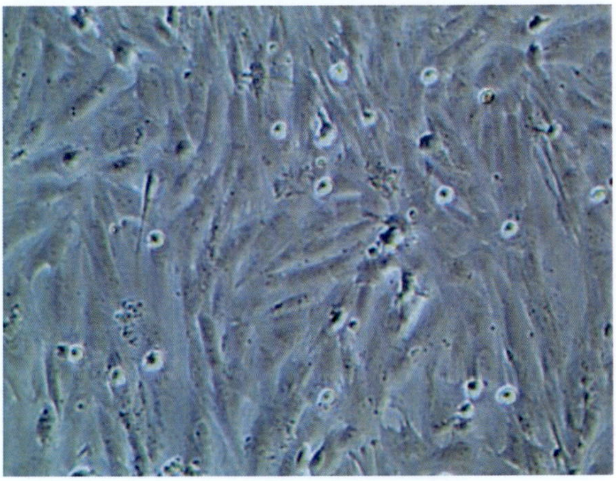

Fig. 41.1 Cultured stem cells from retroauricular cutaneous tissue, in the quantity of 100.000.000 (10^8). 100% viables with three positive markers: cd 73, cd 90, and cd 105. These cells will be mixed with fat graft immediately before the lipoinjection

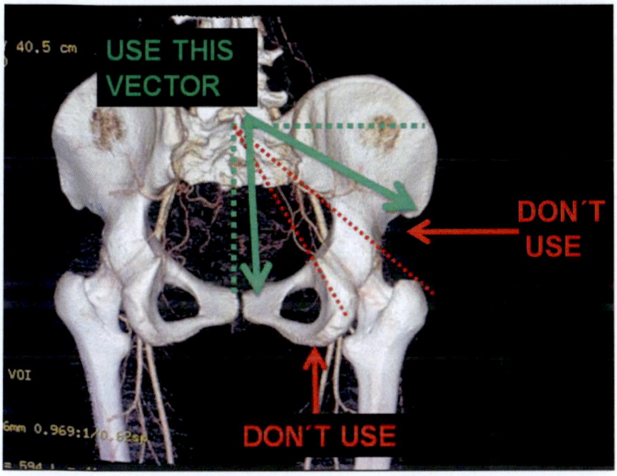

Fig. 41.2 Angiotomography with the circulatory status of the deformity gluteus and the safety triangles and vectors as described in other chapters of this book. Green arrows identify the safety vector to submuscular injection of the fat grafts. Others vectors are inadequate in red color. The red dotted line at the figure demonstrates the dangerous area to be avoided (for submuscular lipoinjection and the

Fat Surgical Technique Collection

The patients are submitted to general or peridural anesthesia. The operating room is prepared with warm temperature and the saline solution infusion is at 30 °C to avoid hypothermia. A thermal coat (warm touch®) is used to prevent loss of corporal temperature. The control of fluid reposition is based on urinary volume that must be 0.5–1.0 mL/kg/h (Vaccari-Mazzetti and Brock 2016).

The liposuction technique used is the wet technique, and the fluid contents are 1 L of Ringer's lactate, 20 mL of lidocaine 2%, and 3 ampoules of epinephrine. The volume is used at maximum of 3 L to the front and to the back. To perform liposuction, a number 4 Mercedes cannula connected to a vacuum aspirator is used, this

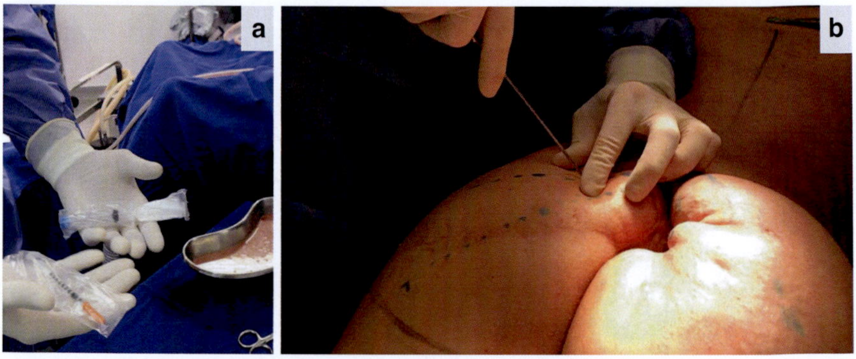

Fig. 41.3 (**a**) Stem cells in surgeon's hand ready to be mixed with the paste fat to be injected, (**b**) lipoinjection performed with 2 mm canula in the fibrous area of the gluteus

form, the fat aspiration and collection is done in a closed system (Vaccari-Mazzetti and Brock 2016).

The collected fat is filtered by sieving, and immediately after the fat became clear and macroscopic and free from blood, it is mixed with stem cells in a quantity of 10^8 cells per mL and stored in a 50 mL syringe to be used later for muscle injection.

Buttock Deformed Injection

The injection is done with a number 5 cannula, with three sequential roles, marked each 5 cm, deep in the muscle, according to the two safety triangles (lateral and medial) in the deformed side, and a subcutaneous injection is done with a 2 mm small cannula with a round hole in the tip (Fig. 41.3).

After cannula introduction, it is always important to aspirate and wait for a few seconds to identify possible minor vascular injury, and then after that, pressing softly the syringe is done associated with fat graft retro-injection for submuscular and subcutaneous tissue. It is done several times and for different parts of the gluteus, to complete depression areas and to improve gluteus size. The fibrous tissue is gently broken and after that lipoinjection is started (Fig. 41.3).

Usually, the deformed gluteus presents more limited area for lipografting, and the gluteus contour (border) could be done with subcutaneous grafting to improve the circle form of the gluteus.

Breast Injection

In female breast, liposuction is done at the lateral and superolateral side. In searching for a better breast contour, lipoinjection in two different planes is a solution, i.e., submuscular and subcutaneous planes, under the skin and under the mammary gland. Both planes can be used for breast fat injection.

The lipograft maintenance in the breast is lower when compared to the gluteus submuscular lipografts, and for this reason, we use fat enriched with mesenchymal stem cells.

In male breast, liposuction is associated with gynecomastia treatment in patients with excessive fat accumulation caused by excessive weight and hereditary, endocrinological, or senile factors. In some cases, it is necessary to resect the mammary gland.

After liposuction, the lipograft is injected into the pectoral major muscle and under it, at maximum volume of 250 mL for each side.

Complications

The complications observed were lipograft volume loss and mammary asymmetry.

Discussion

Liposuction associated with fat grafting in the buttocks increases the surgical results and promotes a very high level of patient's satisfaction with the corporal contour surgery (Cardenas-Camarena and Paillet 2007; Harrison and Selvaggi 2007; Murillo 2004).

We had three cases with gluteus deformities, two of them caused by tumor resection (teratosarcoma and teratoma at the first year of age) and other one caused by an infection after a medicine injection at the second year of age. These patients were submitted to a submuscular and subcutaneous lipograft only in one side of the buttock.

This technique avoids the necessity of implants into the gluteus to improve its size when the patient has a fat reserve sufficient to increase the buttock. The advantage of this technique is the use of autologous tissue, the possibility of receiving intramuscular medicine remains, and there is no migration of the tissue injected, but if this happens, a nerve damage is only temporary and if the weight of the patient increases, more sessions will possibly be done (Cardenas and Muñoz Ahmed 2002; Mendieta 2007; Smith et al. 2006).

The association of liposuction technique with fat graft injection can result in better form, and better results are demonstrated in the maintenance of fat volume with intra-muscle techniques, but the studies do not have a uniform technique pattern (Aiache 2006; Mendieta 2007; Wolf et al. 2006).

Autologous fat grafting in the buttock is a consolidated technique, and its use in cosmetic surgery, for example, breast augmentation, is effective, and when performed with stem cells, it became superior to conventional lipoinjection (Ghavami and Villanueva 2018; Yoshimura et al. 2008).

The autologous fat graft stem cells are enriched for reconstructive surgery, when repeated sessions are necessary, which demonstrated better aesthetic results. The

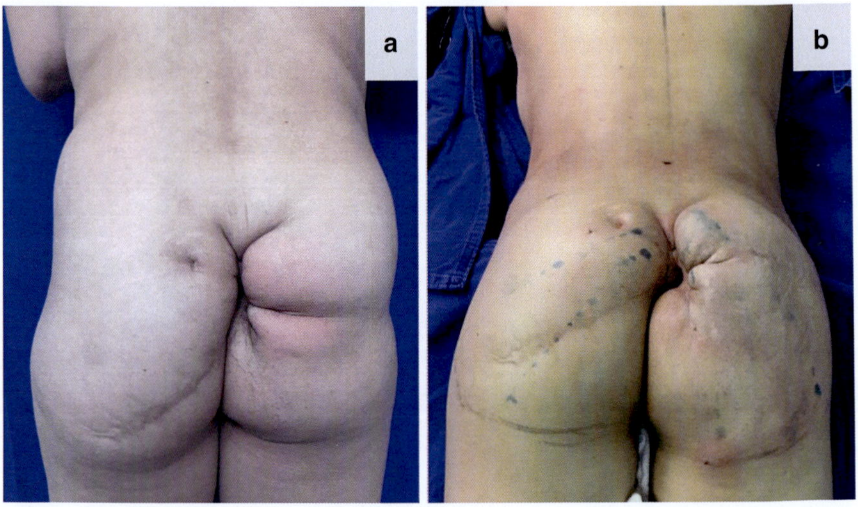

Fig. 41.4 (**a**) Preoperative view in prone position demonstrated the gluteal asymmetry with right gluteal hypoplasia, (**b**) postoperative prone view with submuscular and subcutaneous lipografts in the right gluteus muscle

stromal vascular fraction is fundamental in this refined technique (Gentile and Garcovich 2021; Sterodimas et al. 2012).

The cases previously described were submitted to the technique of Vaccari-Mazzetti and Brock with the addition of stem cells in only one side of the buttock (Vaccari-Mazzetti and Brock 2016). The interesting fact is that one of the patients had a diarrhea episode in the first postoperative day and remained contaminated for 4 h. When it was discovered, the patient was placed under the shower and was washed with chlorhexidine for 40 min. An infection was expected, but it did not happen and she had a normal evolution (Vaccari-Mazzetti and Brock 2016) (Fig. 41.4).

In the second case, the patient had lost the anal sphincter control because of the tumor treatment, and after the reconstructive treatment using stem cell and fat graft, he had a partial recovery of the anal sphincter control. There was no infection problems despite fecal incontinence (Figs. 41.5 and 41.6).

When using the fat graft for gluteal augmentation, it is important to understand what will happen to this fat graft. Some authors are also concerned about this and used magnetic resonance imaging to study fat graft survival (Aiache 2006; Murillo 2004; Viterbo et al. 1994; Wolf et al. 2006).

There were several difficulties to acess a useful exam to control the fat volume, like appropriate hospital facilities, high costs of exams and different possible results depending on the examining doctor, turned the magnetic resonance imagining an uncommon technique to study clinical case series with a high number of patients (Cuenca-Guerra and Quezada 2004; Murillo 2004; Roberts III et al. 2006; Wolf et al. 2006).

We used computed tomography scan to study our cases and it was possible to observe an increase in muscular tissue and soft tissue in the gluteus at the postoperative control imaging exam (Figs. 41.7 and 41.8).

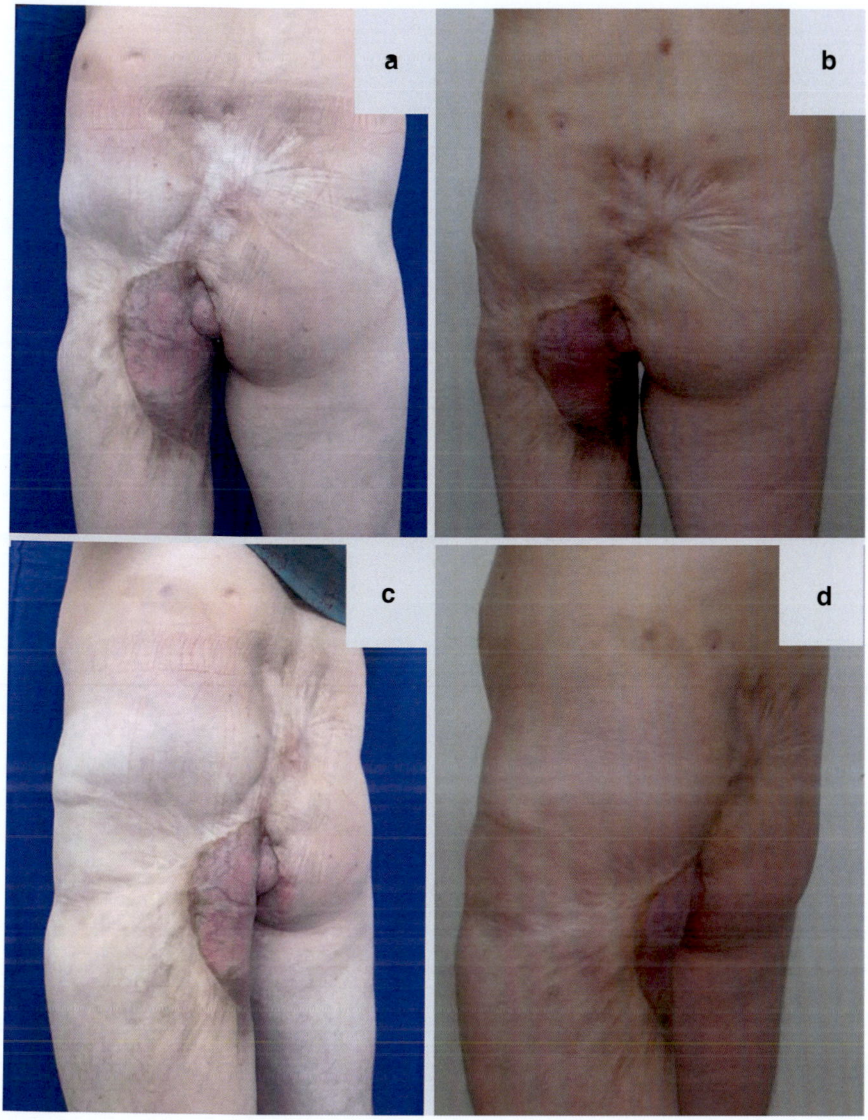

Fig. 41.5 (**a**) Preoperative dorsal view in a male patient with gluteal deformity and fecal incontinence, (**b**) postoperative dorsal view after submuscular and subcutaneous lipoinjection, (**c**) preoperative oblique view with skin graft over the deformity area, (**d**) postoperative oblique view with submuscular and subcutaneous lipografts and the increase of left gluteus, this patient demonstrated a better volume and a partial restored anal function

At some bibliographic references were exams like magnetic resonance were studied, the measurements methods were not described with sufficient details to provide reproducibility. In this study, we give specific radiological technique information (Wolf et al. 2006).

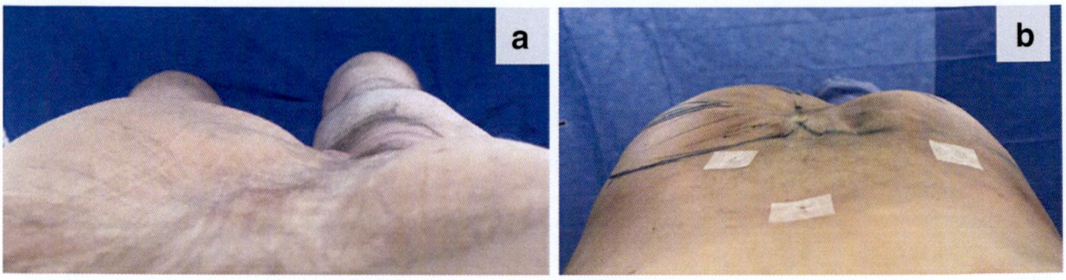

Fig. 41.6 (**a**) Preoperative prone view in a male patient with gluteal deformity and fecal incontinence, (**b**) immediate postoperative view after submuscular and subcutaneous lipoinjection included under the skin graft

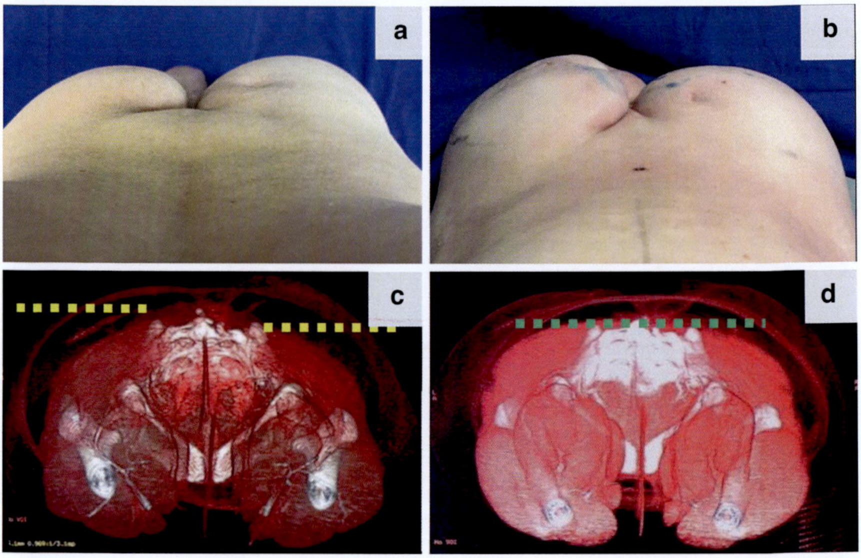

Fig. 41.7 (**a**) preop in supine position shows the gluteal asymmetry with hipoplasic in the right side, (**b**) postop with fill in the gluteal muscle right side, (**c**, **d**) 3D Tomographic image with prone position to study the gluteus muscle reconstruction with 350 mL of sifted fat in the right side only and 50 mL subcutaneous lipoinjection in the left side. (**c**) Preop with the yellow dotted lines show the difference between gluteal muscles. (**d**) Postop with the dotted green shows the filled right gluteus muscle

The small number of cases was not sufficient to conclude with certainty, but there were no complications after the use of stem cell and fat graft.

A vascular injury can result in a venous thrombosis. Consequently, resultant thromboembolic phenomena occur, and it could result in death. To avoid neurovascular damage, marking of the dangerous triangle must be done and avoided during the submuscular fat injection. Submuscular lipografts must be performed only at the two safety triangles (Vaccari-Mazzetti and Brock 2016) (Fig. 41.2).

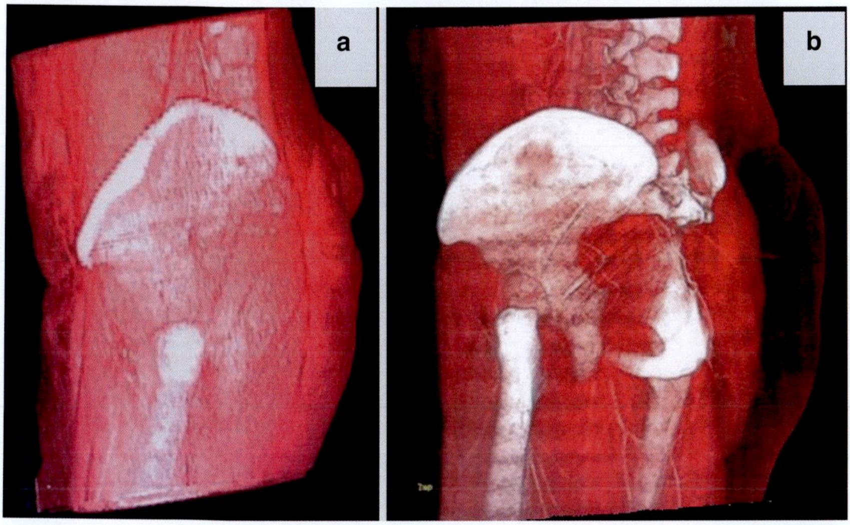

Fig. 41.8 3D Tomographic image with sagittal image to study the gluteus muscle reconstruction with 350 mL of sifted fat in the left side only. (**a**) Preop with the hypoplastic gluteus muscle. (**b**) Postop image with the muscular volume increase left gluteus

Patients with breast lipografts, both female and male, demonstrated a better corporal contour and there were no complications. The lipografted volume was small, but adequate to achieve a satisfactory result. The advantage is the use of viable and autologous tissue (Bayram et al. 2019).

In female patients, it was very important to have a previous information about the patient's desire and propose a small improvement of breast volume without mammary implants even though in some aesthetic cases, the volume improvement was similar to a breast implant. However, it is not an assurance due to unpredictable fat resorption.

When breast lipografts are superficially injected, there are risks of fat necrosis, and consequently clinical and radiological signs like nodules and cysts can also lead to a confusing diagnosis of mammary tumor. Other possible complications are persistent pain, hematoma, and palpable indurations. For this reason, injection in the right plane is necessary (Groen et al. 2016; Vasei et al. 2019).

In male patients, the satisfaction was increased because the aim of their surgery was to remove the excessive fat and the feminine breast aspect, the presence of a pectoral increase was an unexpected extra result (Figs. 41.9 and 41.10).

These results of buttock fat grafting in reconstructive surgeries with poor vascularization was promising, and the breast surgeries associated with lipograft demonstrated a good option to improve corporal contour in plastic surgery with a low rate of complications.

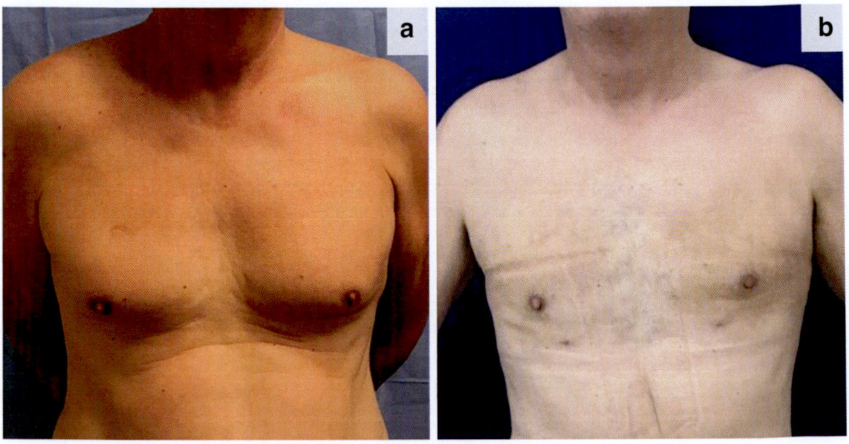

Fig. 41.9 (**a**) Preoperative frontal view in a male patient with senile gynecomastia, (**b**) postoperative frontal view after liposuction and submuscular (pectoral major) lipoinjection

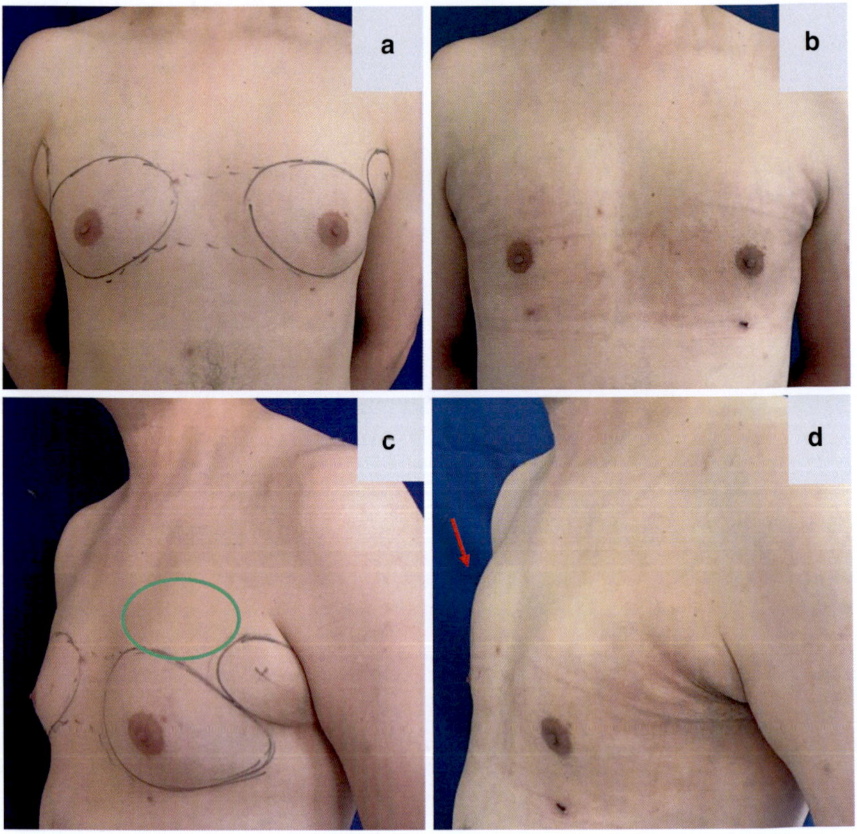

Fig. 41.10 (**a**) Preoperative frontal view in a male patient with predominant fat gynecomastia, (**b**) postoperative frontal view after liposuction and submuscular (pectoral major) lipoinjection, (**c**) preoperative oblique view with demarked liposuction areas in black and a lipoinjection in green, (**d**) postoperative oblique view with submuscular lipografts and the increase of muscle pectoral volume shown with red arrow

Conclusions

The association of stem cells with lipografts allows a better result in cases of tumor reconstructive surgeries of the buttock with poor vascularization and demonstrated a low rate of complications with submuscular associated with subcutaneous lipoinjection. The use of repeated sessions is required to achieve an ideal aesthetic result.

In cases of breast augmentation during the corporal surgery, even in male and female, the results increased patient satisfaction with low rate of complications. Submuscular approach was used with limited volume, but it was enough to achieve a better breast shape.

Conflicts of Interest The authors have no conflicts of interest.

Funding The study had no financial support.

References

Aiache AE. Gluteal recontouring with combination treatments: Implants, liposuction and fat transfer. Clin Plast Surg. 2006. 33:395–403.

Avelar JM. A new technique for abdominoplasty- closed vascular system of subdermal flap folded over itself combined to liposuction. Ver Bras Cir. 1999. 88/89(1/6):3–20.

Avelar JM. Abdominoplasty combined with lipoplasty without panniculus undermining: Abdominoplasty – a safe technique. Clin Plast Surg. 2006. 33(1).79–90.

Avelar JM. Abdominoplasty without panniculus undermining and resection. Analysis and 3 years follow up of 97 consecutive cases. Aesthet Surg J. 2002. 22:16–25.

Ayoub AC, Kerkis A, Lizier NF. Processo de produção de células tronco multipotentes e progenitors, células tronco e/ou progenitors, fragmentos de tecidos de nnct e concentrado de células tronco. 2013. INPI. BR10 2013 021202 4 A2.

Bayram Y, Sezgic M, Karakol P, Bozkurt M, Filinte GT. The use of autologous fat grafts in breast surgery: A literature review. Arch Plast Surg. 2019. 46:498–510.

Cardenas JC, Muñoz Ahmed JA. Large-volume lipoinjection for gluteal augmentation. Aesthetic Surg J. 2002. 22(1):33–8.

Cardenas-Camarena L, Paillet JC. Combined gluteoplasty: Liposuction and gluteal implants. Plast Reconstr Surg. 2007. 119(3):1067–74.

Cuenca-Guerra R, Quezada J. What makes buttocks beautiful? A review and classification of the determinants of gluteal beauty and the surgical techniques to achieve them. Aesth Plast Surg. 2004. 28:340–7.

Fitzsimmons REB, Mazurek MS, Soos A, Simmons CA. Mesenchymal stromal/stem cells in regenerative medicine and tissue engineering. Stem Cells International, 2018. 1–18. https://doi.org/10.1155/2018/8031718.

Gentile P, Garcovich S. Systematic review: Adipose-derived mesenchymal stem cells, platelet-rich plasma and biomaterials as new regenerative strategies in chronic skin wounds and soft tissue defects. Int J Mol Sci. 2021.22:1538.

Ghavami A, Villanueva NL. Gluteal augmentation and contouring with autologous fat transfer: Part I. Clin Plast Surg. 2018. 249–59.

Grambow F, Rutkowski R, Podmelle F, Schmoeckel K, Siegerist F, Domanski G, Schuster MW, Domanska G. The impact of lidocaine on adipose-derived stem cells in human adipose tissue harvested by liposuction and used for lipotransfer. Int J Mol Sci. 2020. 21:2869. https://doi.org/10.3390/ijms21082869

Groen JW, Negenborn VL, Twisk JWR, Ket JCF, Mullender MG, Smit JM. Autologous fat grafting in cosmetic breast augmentation: A systematic review on radiological safety, complications, volume retention and patient/surgeon satisfaction. Aesthet Surg J. 2016. 1–15.

Harrison D, Selvaggi G. Gluteal augmentation surgery: Indications and surgical management. J Plast Reconstr Aesthet Surg. 2007. 60(8):922–8.

Illouz YG, Sterodimas A. Autologous fat transplantation to the breast: A personal technique with 25 years of experience. Aesth Plast Surg.2009. 33:706–15.

Illouz YG. Estudo do adipócito nas lipodistrofias. In: Avelar JM, Illouz YG. Liposuction. Hipocrates, São Paulo, 1986. 19–23.

Lewis CM. Buttock augmentation: Case studies of fat injection monitored by magnetic resonance imaging. Plast Reconstr Surg. 2004. 1015–6.

Mendieta CG. Gluteal reshaping. Aesthetic Surg J. 2007. 27(6):641–55.

Murillo WL, Buttock augmentation: case studies of fat injection monitored by magnetic resonance imaging. Plastic Reconstr Surg. 2004. 114 (6): 1606–14.

Roberts III TL, Weinfeld AB, Bruner TW, Nguyen K. Universal and ethnic ideals of beautiful buttocks are best obtained by autologous micro fat grafting and liposuction. Clin Plast Surg. 2006, 33:371–94.

Smith P, Adams Jr. WP, Lipschitz AH, Chau B, Sorokin E, Rorich RJ, Brown SA. Autologous human fat grafting: Effect of harvesting and preparation techniques on adipocyte graft survival. Plast Reconstr Surg. 2006. 117(6):1836–44.

Sterodimas A, Faria J, Nicaretta B, Boriani F. Autologous fat transplantation versus adipose-derived stem cell-enriched lipografts: A study. Aesth Surg J. 2012. 31(6):682–93.

Vaccari-Mazzetti MP, Brock RS. Buttock lipografting and augmentation combined with Avelar's abdominoplasty. In: Avelar JM. New Concepts on abdominoplasty and further applications. Springler. 2016. 329–44.

Vasei N, Shishegar A, Ghalkhani F, Darvishi M. Fat necrosis in the breast: A systematic review of clinical. Lipids in Health and Disease. 2019. 18:139.

Viterbo F, Marques M, Valente M. Fat-tissue injection versus graft: Experimental study in rabbits. Ann Plast Surg. 1994. 33:184–92.

Wolf GA, Gallego S, Patron GAS, Ramirez ZF, Delgado BJA, Echeverri AA, Garcia GMM. Magnetic resonance imaging assessment of gluteal fat grafts. Aesth Plast Surg. 2006. 30 (4):460–8.

Yoshimura K, Sato K, Aoi N, Kurita M, Hirohi T, Harii K. Cell-assisted lipotransfer for cosmetic breast augmentation: Supportive use of adipose-derived stem/stromal cells. Aesth Plast Surg. 2008. 32:48–55.

Part VI
Body Lift After Weight Loss

Chapter 42
Brachioplasty in the Post-Bariatric Patient

Roberto Kaluf, Roberto Kaluf Filho, and Rafael Alves Tumeh

Abstract Brachioplasty, a body contouring method that redefines the brachial region, has been among the main surgical modalities for body rejuvenation sought by patients. In 2019 alone, 168,289 brachioplasties were performed in patients in the United States. Compared to the 2000s, when only 338 brachioplasties were performed, this number highlights a significant increase for this kind of surgery (Orpheu et al. 2009; Kornstein 2014; Han et al. 2014; ISAPS 2019).

Introduction

Brachioplasty, a body contouring method that redefines the brachial region, has been among the main surgical modalities for body rejuvenation sought by patients. In 2019 alone, 168,289 brachioplasties were performed in patients in the United States. Compared to the 2000s, when only 338 brachioplasties were performed, this number highlights a significant increase for this kind of surgery (Orpheu et al. 2009; Kornstein 2014; Han et al. 2014; ISAPS 2019; Kaluf 2006).

Several other brachial contour redefinition techniques have been used by plastic surgeons to treat brachial ptosis. Most of them run into the problem created by large areas of scars, since the arm occupies a substantial area of the body with a lot of visibility, which has made surgeons look for other ways to perform the incision and thus make the scar minimally evident as possible. These novel techniques have also sought to increase the safety of the procedure and reduce the possibility of complications (Lima Junior et al. 2013; Leclère et al. 2016).

R. Kaluf (✉) · R. K. Filho · R. A. Tumeh
São Paulo, Brazil

J. M. Avelar, R. Cavalcanti Ribeiro (eds.), *Body Contouring*,
https://doi.org/10.1007/978-3-031-42802-9_42

Aims

The aims are to learn how to do do the brachioplasty technique and its specificities, to describe the indications and to be aware of the possible complications, and to identify the pros and cons related to brachioplasty.

Diagnosis or Preoperative Assessment (General Considerations)

Planning and Surgical Technique

Planning to define the best surgical strategy to be prioritized is carried out through case-by-case analysis. There are several classifications that help the surgeon to decide which procedure is best for the patient, and the Pittsburgh scale is the most widespread worldwide (Lacerda et al. 2012; Fantozzi, 2014; Araújo, Kaluf, 2011).

First, to mark the resection regions, patients must be in a standing position with their arms extended. This delimitation is done through the bidigital tweezers respecting the linearity. It is guided according to the principle of sliding the liposuction flap. After liposuction and flap sliding, segmented resection and excess skin are guided to the axillary region (Kaluf et al. 2006). In 2006, Kaluf et al. published a classification that directed treatment according to four standard arm types, including Grade V as of 2014, as shown in Table 42.1.

Marking is performed with the patient standing, with the arms abducted at 90° and the forearms flexed at 90°. Three initial reference points are used, namely, the medial epicondyle of the humerus, the biceps sulcus, and the deltopectoral sulcus. These points are connected by a line that will serve as the basis for the resulting scarring. From this moment on, pinching maneuvers are performed to longitudinally define the excess skin that can be removed and thus form a half-moon image.

Table 42.1 Kaluf-Lisboa classification (modified) for post-bariatric arms according to deformities and proposed treatment

Kaluf-Lisboa classification (modified)		
Grade	Classification	Treatment
I	Excess adiposity without hanging skin	Liposuction
II	Excess adiposity with moderate hanging skin	Liposuction with an attempt to reduce the "L" or axillary scar
III	Excess adiposity with great hanging skin	Liposuction with an "L" skin resection
IV	Skin redundancy only	Skin resection without liposuction. Scar in "L"
V	Hanging skin with severe adiposity (batwing like)	Skin transfixation with stiches in places demarcated by bidigital tweezers and split resection. Scar in "L"

After that, traction is performed in the posterior proximal third of this half-moon, with pinching maneuvers, to define the excess skin in the axillary hollow region, thus forming a new compensation ellipse, in such a way that the result resembles an L- or J-shaped scar (Fig. 42.1).

In Grade V patients, in addition to the aforementioned principles, marking was developed using an instrument for transfixation and demarcation of the flap to be removed as shown in Figs. 42.2 and 42.3.

After the anesthetic procedure, the patient is placed in a supine position with arms abducted and forearms extended. It is suggested to avoid infusion of liquids in the venous system of the upper limb. The entire area not to be manipulated must be covered, strictly following all antisepsis and asepsis maneuvers in the surgical field.

Local infiltration is performed with 1:500,000 U adrenaline and 0.1% lidocaine, followed, after the time of vasoconstriction, by superficial and aggressive liposuction of the region to be resected, in addition to conservative liposuction in the posterior portion of the remaining flap, to release the dermis with minimal damage to the vascular and lymphatic components of the region. It is important to emphasize that the axillary hollow region can be considered a danger zone due to the local neurovascular bundle (brachial plexus and axillary artery and vein), and caution should be taken in the depth of liposuction and tissue resection in this region (preferably not to exceed Scarpa's fascia and never surpass the superficial muscular fascia).

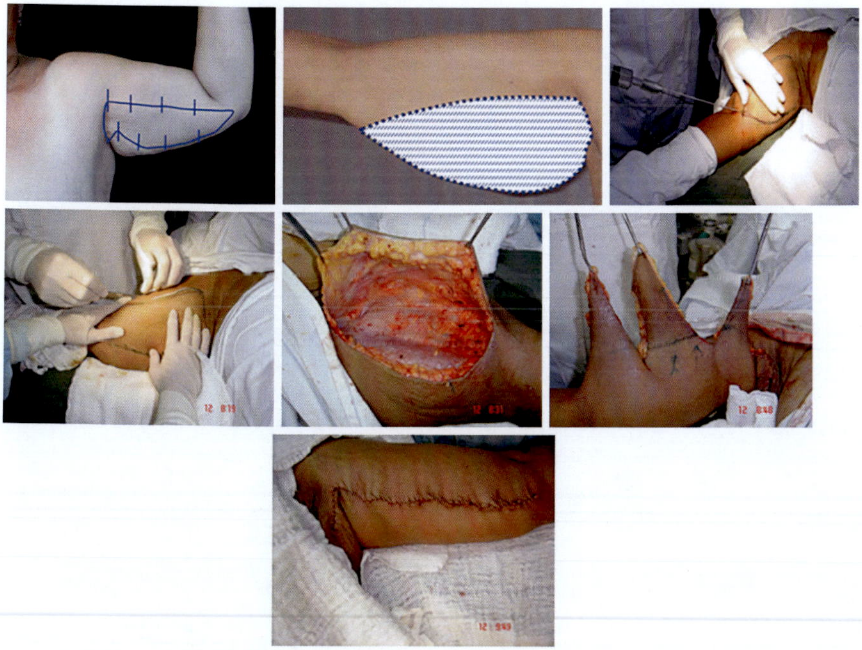

Fig. 42.1 Conventional brachioplasty marking

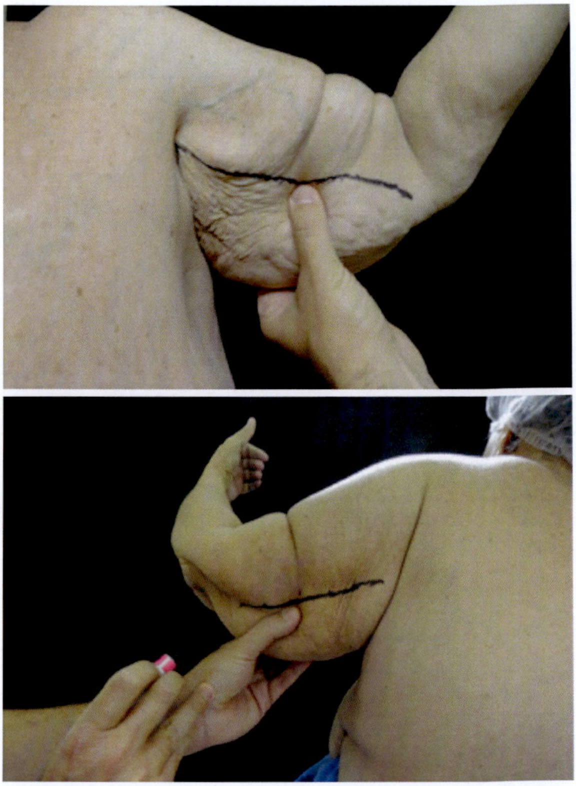

Fig. 42.2 Grade V brachioplasty marking

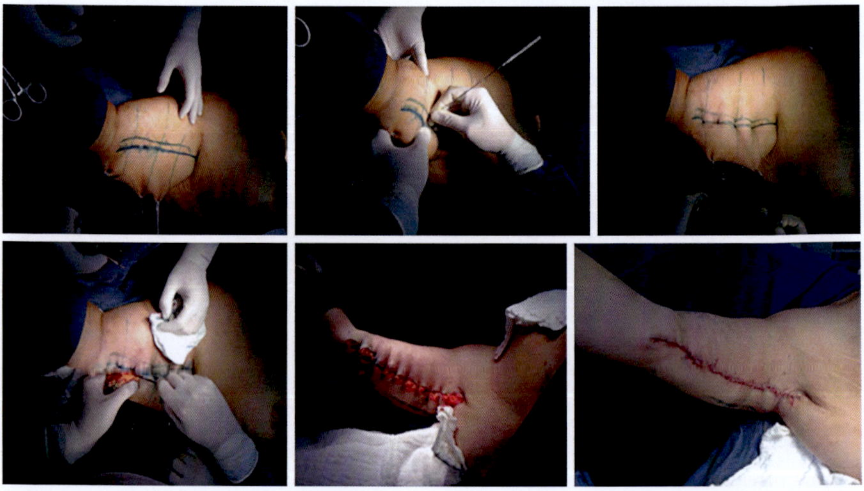

Fig. 42.3 Grade V brachioplasty marking

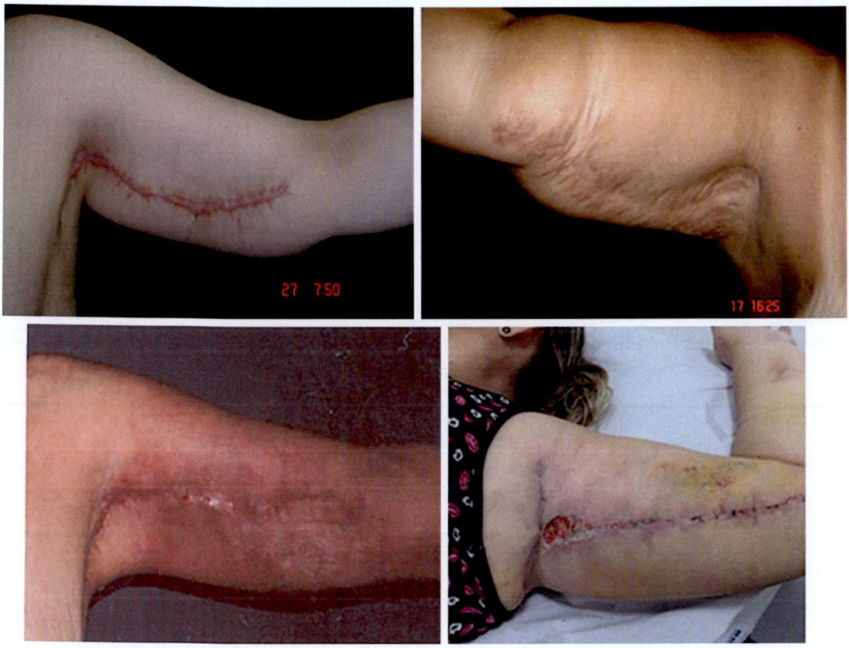

Fig. 42.4 Postoperative brachioplasty

The incision must follow the marked line, until it overcomes the dermis. It is prudent to initially make the incision in the biceps sulcus and release the flap in the demarcated area, dissecting it in the subdermal plane, pulling it, and making sure that the anterior and posterior edges are without excessive tension. Incisions are made in the flap, from distal to proximal, securely joining the edges. The compensation of excess skin occurs in the axillary region, in such a way that we have an L- or J-shaped scarring result. In those arms with flaccidity, without lipodystrophy, it is possible to remove a skin spindle that is limited to the extension of the arm, without entering to the armpit, according to Maciel (Lima Jr 2010).

Partial resection of excess skin occurs after all anchoring stitches have been performed. Then, hemostasis must be carefully reviewed, and vacuum suction drains can be maintained for 24–48 h to avoid collections that might force the suture lines, but it is not routine when hemostasis is rigorous.

The synthesis must take place in three planes. In the deeper plane, we suggest a colorless absorbable suture (e.g., Monocryl 3.0), with simple stitches and an inverted knot, approaching the deep subdermis from both edges and passing the suture through the loose areolar tissue that lines the raw area, in such a way to decrease dead space. In the second suture line, we suggest an absorbable suture (e.g., Monocryl 4.0), with simple stitches and an inverted knot, coapting the edges of the subdermis. Finally, the coaptation of the epidermis with an intradermal stitch is also with an absorbable suture (Monocryl 4.0).

The arms must be bandaged, avoiding compressive meshes in the first 3 weeks, to avoid traction forces on the suture and risk of dehiscence when putting them on.

Complications

The main complication is the hypertrophic scar. This problem goes against the essential objective of brachioplasty that is to redefine the brachial contour and make the patient satisfied with the result. In addition, the scar may be inadequately visible, residual contour deformities may remain even after combined liposuction and brachioplasty, and there may still be residual ptosis (Elkhatib 2013) (Fig. 42.4).

Other complications can also occur during the healing process and include retraction, scar enlargement, and seroma formation (Leclère et al. 2016; Orpheu et al. 2009). Regarding the surgical site, it is worth mentioning infections, surgical wound dehiscence, abscess formation, injuries to the medial cutaneous nerves of the arm and medial cutaneous nerves of the forearm and ulnar, lymphedema, and necrosis (Chowdhry et al. 2010; Han et al. 2014).

A 16.7% rate of complications was reported in patients who underwent brachioplasty after an average of 25.2 months of bariatric surgery. A case of seroma, treated by draining its content, one case of temporary paresthesia, and others related to scar imperfection that required revision were treated successfully by a new procedure (Modolin et al. 2011).

Considering that, some recommendations for the success of the procedure and the prevention of complications must be done.

As with the reconstruction of the brachial region performed by brachioplasty, an aesthetically pleasing, harmonious, and lasting result is expected in patients undergoing bariatric surgery, and the procedure should only be performed after the patient's weight is stable. Maintenance can be defined as a weight fluctuation of less than 1 to 2 pounds (approximately 0.91 kg) per month during the period of 3 to 6 continuous months (Shrivastava et al. 2008).

Furthermore, other precautions are also noteworthy. The first one concerns the need or not to perform pre-brachioplasty liposuction. In general, liposuction should be performed prior to brachioplasty in patients with a body mass index of less than 30 and who have not experienced massive weight loss, patients with mild to moderate brachial fat deposits, and patients with great weight loss (in the latter case, only conservative liposuction is performed). Very emaciated patients or with a small adipose layer do not need liposuction prior to brachioplasty (Elkhatib 2013).

The surgeon must also determine how much tissue must be removed during brachioplasty. He must decide if the patient needs only reduction of the arm, arm and lateral chest wall, or arm and breast tissue. For such purposes, he can make use of the truncated cone, a technique in which a cone is drawn on the patient's arm and all tissue that does not fit satisfactorily inside the cone is removed, based on the principle that it is not harmonious with the anatomy of the patient's chest and lower arm (Orpheu et al. 2009).

As for the care with the nerves of the brachial region, the surgeon should not perform the incision beyond the limit imposed by the elbow, as it may damage the medial cutaneous nerve of the arm. He should also not dissect the axilla too deeply, as he may injure the intercostobrachial nerve and the medial cutaneous nerve of the arm. The handling of structures to be moved, lifted, and pulled must be carried out with extreme care, especially when approaching the medial epicondyle, through which the nervous structures make their way (Han et al. 2014).

Therefore, complications, although common in medical practice, can be avoided or even minimized. By reducing excessive dissection, the risk of bruising is diminished, just as limiting the surgical time decreases swelling. This would hinder the healing process, as well as the achievement of the aesthetic result for both patients and surgeons (Shrivastava et al. 2008).

Result

Given the increase in the obese population worldwide and the popularity that bariatric surgery has gained as a form of treatment for obesity, patients who have experienced great weight loss have needed help from various medical areas in the period after bariatric surgery. With plastic surgery, it was no different, as these patients lose a large volume of weight, but the skin remains in excess due to changes in elastin inherent in the context of obesity. In this scenario, problems with body contour, intertrigo, and a greater propensity to infection related to hygiene difficulties arise, due to excess skin. These patients also face problems such as low self-esteem and difficulty in urination and sexual activity. One of the ways in which plastic surgery can help these patients is through brachioplasty, by improving the brachial contour in cases of brachial ptosis and thus helping the patient to return to their routine activities (Han et al. 2014; Orpheu et al. 2009). Examples of postsurgical results are shown in Figs. 42.4, 42.5, and 42.6.

Another application linked to brachioplasty is related to the normal aging process. With advancing age, the skin on the arm tends to have increased looseness and decreased elasticity and firmness. This ends up leading to flaccidity and the formation of so-called bat wings (areas of excess skin that are seen in the posterior area of the arm), characteristics considered unaesthetic and that can be circumvented by redefining the brachial contour which is achieved by performing brachioplasty.

Not only in bariatric surgery or senile elastosis, brachioplasty has also redefined the brachial contour in cases of systemic diseases that alter the body contour such as lipodystrophy, lipedema, hidradenitis suppurativa, and pseudoxanthoma elasticum, among others, which demonstrates the excellent connected versatility to this body contouring surgery technique (Bellini et al. 2017; Ching et al. 2017; Panettiere et al. 2013).

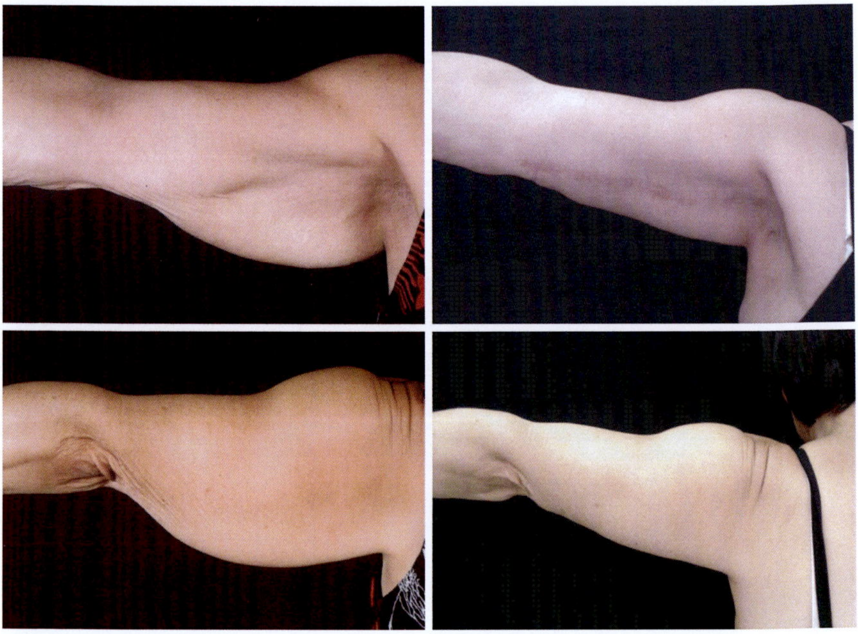

Fig. 42.5 Postoperative brachioplasty

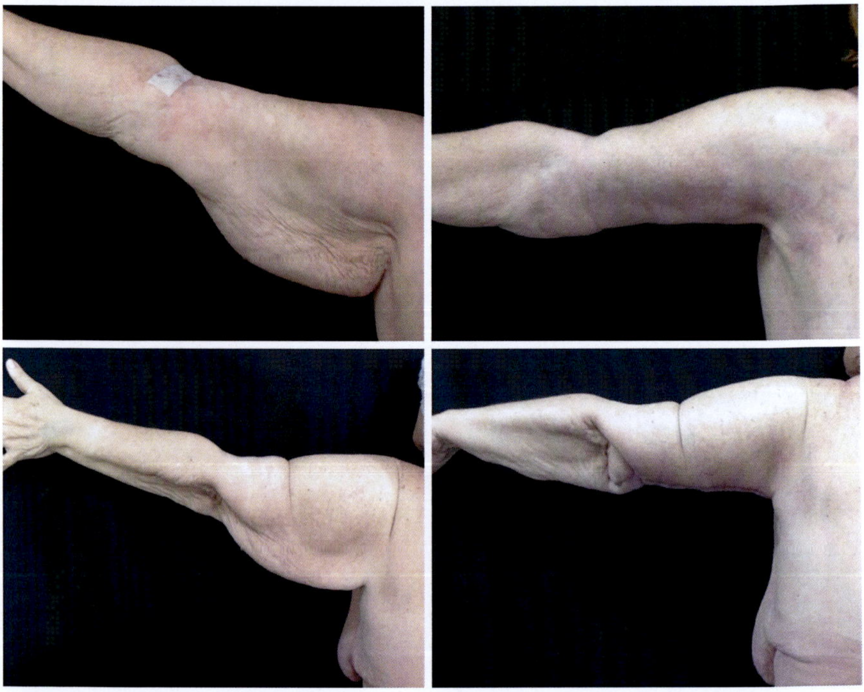

Fig. 42.6 Postoperative brachioplasty

Despite being a technique with excellent results, the main factor against its performance is the occurrence of complications, such as seroma; hypertrophic scarring; surgical site infection; wound dehiscence; nerve damage with hypoesthesia, paresthesia, or hyperesthesia; long-lasting edema, hematoma; lymphocele; and neuroma formation. However, although these complications exist, the trials carried out with brachioplasty have shown that their occurrence is infrequent and, for the most part, complications are amenable to treatment and may even have complete resolution without established treatment (Leclère et al. 2016; Orpheu et al. 2009).

Conclusions

As the advent of bariatric surgery has grown, the number of patients who experience massive weight loss and who develop excess skin, changing their body contour and leading to complications that hinder their well-being, has also increased. In this sense, body contouring surgeries bring quality of life to these patients, restoring their self-esteem and ability to perform their daily tasks (Cintra Junior et al. 2014).

Within the body contouring surgeries, there is brachioplasty, whose objective is to redefine the brachial contour. Several brachioplasty techniques have emerged with the aim of making the scar less visible and improving the aesthetic result, in addition to adapting the procedure to the specificities of each patient profile and avoiding complications. Among these, we can cite hypertrophic scars, lasting edema, nervous tissue damage, seroma, and infections as the main complications.

Thus, it is up to the surgeon to define the patient's profile and, based on that, choose the best method to be applied in his brachioplasty, always seeking the best aesthetic result and the maintenance of the patient's well-being.

References

Araújo BGO, Kaluf R. Sistematização e conduta do Hospital Geral de Goiânia nas dermolipodistrofias de membros superiores em pacientes ex-obesos. Rev. Bras. Cir. Plást.2011;26(3):95

Bellini E, Grieco MP, Raposio E. A journey through liposuction and liposculture: Review. Annals of medicine and Surgery. 2017; 24:53–60. https://doi.org/10.1016/j.amsu.2017.10.024.

Ching DL, Mughal M, Papas A, Soldin M. Axillary Reconstruction for Hidradenitis Suppurativa with an Inner-Arm Transposition Flap Creating a Brachioplasty Effect. Archives of Plastic Surgery. 2017;44(3):228–233. https://doi.org/10.5999/aps.2017.44.3.228.

Chowdhry S, Elston JB, Lefkowitz T, Wilhelmi BJ. Avoiding the Medial Brachial Cutaneous Nerve in Brachioplasty: An Anatomical Study. Eplasty. 2010;10:e16.

Cintra Junior W, Modolin M, Kasabkojian ST, Rocha RI, Zampieri L, Gemperli R. Braquioplastia pós-gastroplastia: avaliação da satisfação dos pacientes. Rev. Bras. Cir. Plást.2014;29(2):232–236

Elkhatib H. Posterior Scar Brachioplasty with Fascial Suspension: A Long-term Follow-up of a Modified Technique. Plastic and Reconstructive Surgery Global Open. 2013;1(6): e38. https://doi.org/10.1097/GOX.0b013e3182a71465.

Fantozzi F. Brachial lifting using the balanced triple-vector (BTV) technique with dual opposing flaps. European Journal of Plastic Surgery. 2014;37(2):95–102. https://doi.org/10.1007/s00238-013-0901-9.

Han HH, Lee MC, Kim SH, Lee JH, Ahn ST, Rhie JW. Upper Arm Contouring with Brachioplasty after Massive Weight Loss. Archives of Plastic Surgery. 2014;41(3):271–276. https://doi.org/10.5999/aps.2014.41.3.271.

ISAPS International Survey on Aeshetic /Cosmetic Procedures performed in 2019. https://www.isaps.org/discover/about-isaps/global-statistics/reports-and-press-releases/globalsurvey-2019-full-report-and-press-releases-english/OI.

Kaluf R, Azevêdo FN, Rodrigues LO. Sistemática Cirúrgica em Pacientes Ex-Obesos. Rev. Bras. Cir. Plást.2006;21(3):166–174

Kornstein AN. SERI Surgical Scaffold as an Adjunct to Conventional Brachioplasty. Plastic and Reconstructive Surgery Global Open. 2014;2(7):e190. https://doi.org/10.1097/GOX.0000000000000155.

Lacerda AMR, Torreão G, Pita P, Barreto RHC, Ramos AS, Ferreira Filho JRA. Braquioplastia: experiência do Serviço de Cirurgia Plástica do HC-UFPE com a utilização da técnica em "L". Rev. Bras. Cir. Plást.2012;27(3):90

Leclère FM, Alcolea JM, Vogt PM, et al. Laser-assisted lipolysis for arm contouring in Teimourian grades III and IV: A prospective study involving 22 patients. Plastic Surgery. 2016;24(1):35–40.

Lima Jr EM. Braquioplastia. In: Lima Jr. EM. Tratado de cirurgia plástica após grandes perdas ponderais. São Paulo: Editora Atheneu, 2010. pp.97–116

Lima Junior EM, Cavalcante HA, Lima VMM. Posicionamento da cicatriz da braquioplastia na região posterior do braço em pacientes ex-obesos. Rev. Bras. Cir. Plást.2013;28(4):538–543

Modolin ML, Cintra W Jr, Faintuch J, Silva MM, Moraes LB, Gemperli R, Ferreira MC. Improved double-fuse technique for post-bariatric brachioplasty. Rev Col Bras Cir. 2011 Jul-Aug;38(4):217–22. https://doi.org/10.1590/S0100-69912011000400003.

Orpheu SC, Coltro PS, Scopel GP, Saito FL, Ferreira MC. Body contour surgery in the massive weight loss patient: three year-experience in a secondary public hospital. Rev Assoc Med Bras (1992). 2009 Jul-Aug;55(4):427–33. https://doi.org/10.1590/S0104-42302009000400018.

Panettiere P, Marchetti L, Accorsi D. Arms Lift in a Case of Pseudoxanthoma Elasticum. Case Reports in Dermatological Medicine. 2013; 2013:870605. https://doi.org/10.1155/2013/870605.

Shrivastava P, Aggarwal A, Khazanchi RK. Body contouring surgery in a massive weight loss patient: An overview. Indian Journal of Plastic Surgery: Official Publication of the Association of Plastic Surgeons of India. 2008;41(Suppl):S114–S129.

Chapter 43
Body Lift and Gluteoplasty with Flaps

Marcelo Aniceto

Abstract Let's consider the opening paragraph of the chapter as an abstract.

Keywords Weight loss · Gluteal fat · Combined procedures · Body improvement · Sagging skin

Patients who lose excessive weight have a large excess of skin, requiring several surgeries to treat different body regions. Gonzales-Ulloa was the first professional who proposed an associated treatment of the anterior region, lateral region, and posterior region, since 1959, presenting the *belt lipectomy* (Gonzales-Ulloa 1959, 1961).

After the end of the 1980s, other authors show their concern with body contouring, mainly related to former obese people (Muhlbauer 1989; Baroudi 1989, 1991; Lockwood 1993, 1995). From the end of the 1990s, several surgeons published about their experiences and personal modifications, definitively naming the association of abdominoplasty and torsoplasty as *body lift* (Pascal and Le Louarn 2002; Hamra 1999; Hurwitz et al. 2004; Hurwitz and Zewert 2002; Aly et al. 2003; Cormenzana and Samprón 2004; Strauch et al. 2006; Wallach 2005; Aniceto and Claudio-da-Silva 2008; Aniceto 2009).

In addition to the great sagging skin, the gluteal region of these patients presents an *important loss of volume*, and, in most cases, it is necessary to associate *body lift* with some procedure for volumetric replacement.

M. Aniceto (✉)
Brazilian Society of Plastic Surgery, Rio de Janeiro, Brazil

Plastic Surgery Sector at the Federal University of Rio de Janeiro, Rio de Janeiro, Brazil

Alumni Association of Prof. Ivo Pitanguy, Rio de Janeiro, Brazil

Plastic Surgery Department of Santa Casa do Rio de Janeiro, Rio de Janeiro, Brazil

J. M. Avelar, R. Cavalcanti Ribeiro (eds.), *Body Contouring*,
https://doi.org/10.1007/978-3-031-42802-9_43

The gluteal region approach in former obese patients was performed in the form of different dermo- and adipose flaps, and the tissue from the posterior region which would be removed with the body lift was used as the donor area. Based on the abundant perforating vascularization of the gluteal musculature.

Pascal and Le Louarn in 2002 describe a semilunar-shaped flap to fill the upper part of the gluteal region (Pascal and Le Louarn 2002).

Sozer et al. (2005) present an ellipse flap with the base of the same diameter as the surface, which is caudally positioned (180° rotation); the authors report that more than one flap can be used, if necessary (Sozer et al. 2005) (Fig. 43.1).

Rodhe and Gerut (2005) use a randomized medial-based flap, in a ratio (base/length) of 1:2, with caudal rotation to the inferior gluteal fold (Rohde and Gerut 2005).

In 2006, Raposo-Amaral et al. published an article about the use of a long fusiform flap, where the medial and lateral edges are elevated at the level of the muscle fascia and undergo caudal rotation and fixation, keeping the flap pedicle in its medial portion (Raposo-Amaral et al. 2007) (Fig. 43.2).

In 2006, Mendieta describes the "upper base gluteal flap" where only its lower limit is incised (Fig. 43.3a) and the "central base gluteal flap," which is incised both at the upper and lower limits and fixed at a more caudal position (Fig. 43.3b),both filling only the upper portion of the gluteal region (Mandieta 2006).

Cowel et al. (2007) described an ellipse-shaped flap, pedicled in two perforating arteries of the superior gluteal artery (6 and 9 cm from the midline—intergluteal). Through an inferomedial rotation, this flap fills the inner lower quadrant (Colwell and Borud 2007) (Fig. 43.4).

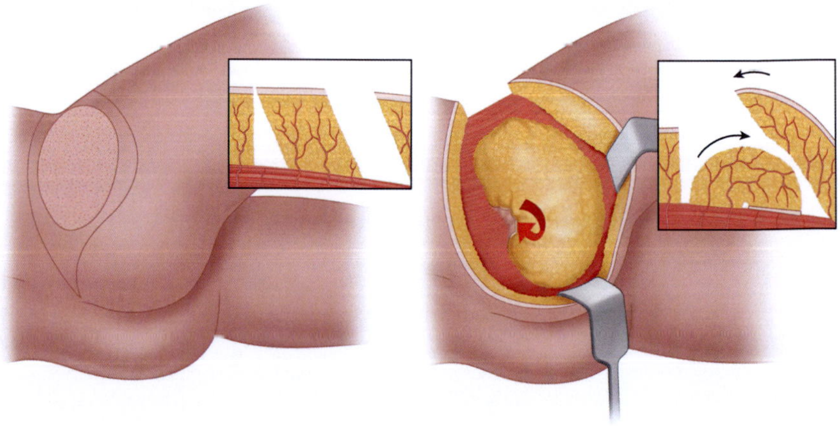

Fig. 43.1 Sozer et al. flap

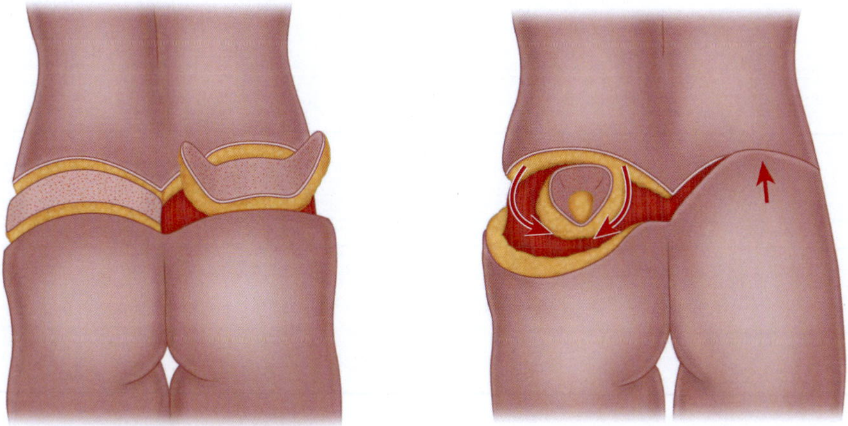

Fig. 43.2 Raposo-Amaral et al. flap

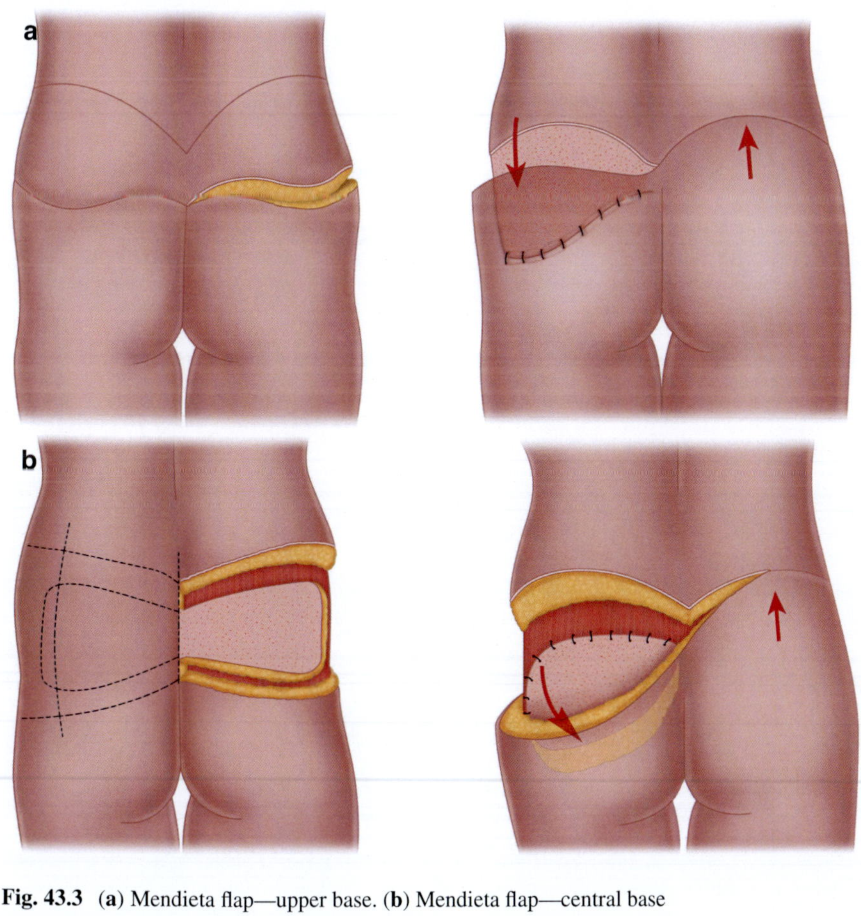

Fig. 43.3 (a) Mendieta flap—upper base. (b) Mendieta flap—central base

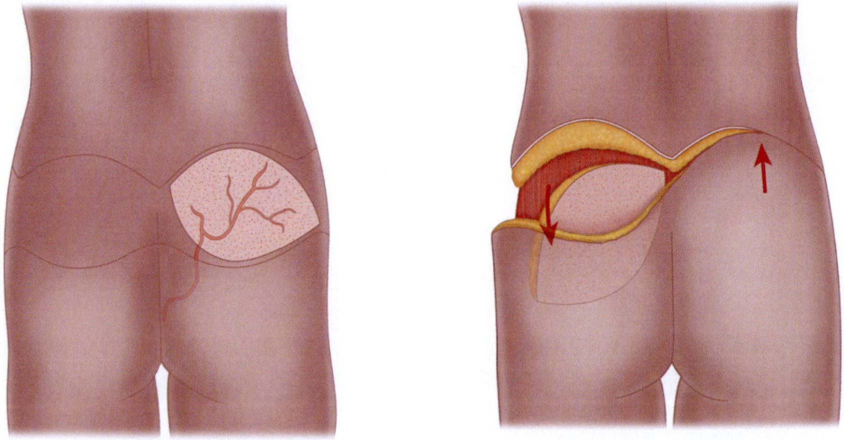

Fig. 43.4 Cowel et al. flap

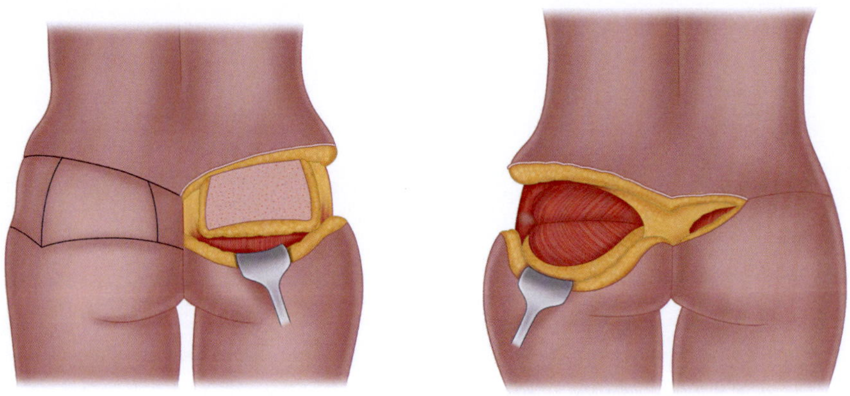

Fig. 43.5 Sozer flap (2012)

In 2012, Sozer proposed a flap in which the gluteus maximus muscle is divided in its thickness and, together with the dermal adipose flap, undergoes an inferior rotation, filling the distal portion of the gluteal region (Fig. 43.5)

There are also flaps of the inferior gluteal portion, which use the tissue of the region close to the inferior gluteal fold; as an example we have the (Toledo 2003; Coban et al. 2004; Huemer et al. 2005; Gonzales 2005) flaps.

Large-volume fat grafting and gluteal implants are other surgical options that will possibly increase the volume of the gluteal region.

Body lift treats the excessive skin in the gluteal region, but it does not correct the great loss of volume present in former obese patients. Sozer even emphasizes the early loss of projection of this region in cases where no dermoadipose flaps are used (Sozer et al. 2005).

In our routine, the lateral and posterior marking proposed by Le Louarn and Pascal for the body lift is used. In the abdominal region, both the vertical marking and the classic marking are performed, according to the needs of each patient. According to the specific approach to the pubic region, a dermoadipose flap is developed in order to avoid its early ptosis (Aniceto and Claudio-da-Silva 2008; Aniceto 2009).

Preoperative Marking of Body Lift

The body lift is a circumferential approach to treat regions of the lower body segment in a single surgical time—the pubic region, abdomen, flanks, lateral thighs, and gluteal region (Fig. 43.6). A circumferential scar is the result of this procedure, which is mostly associated with a vertical scar (Fig. 43.7)

The marking must be performed with the patient in an orthostatic position, aiming at symmetrical incisions that can be adequately hidden by the patient's bathing suit. The order below must be followed.

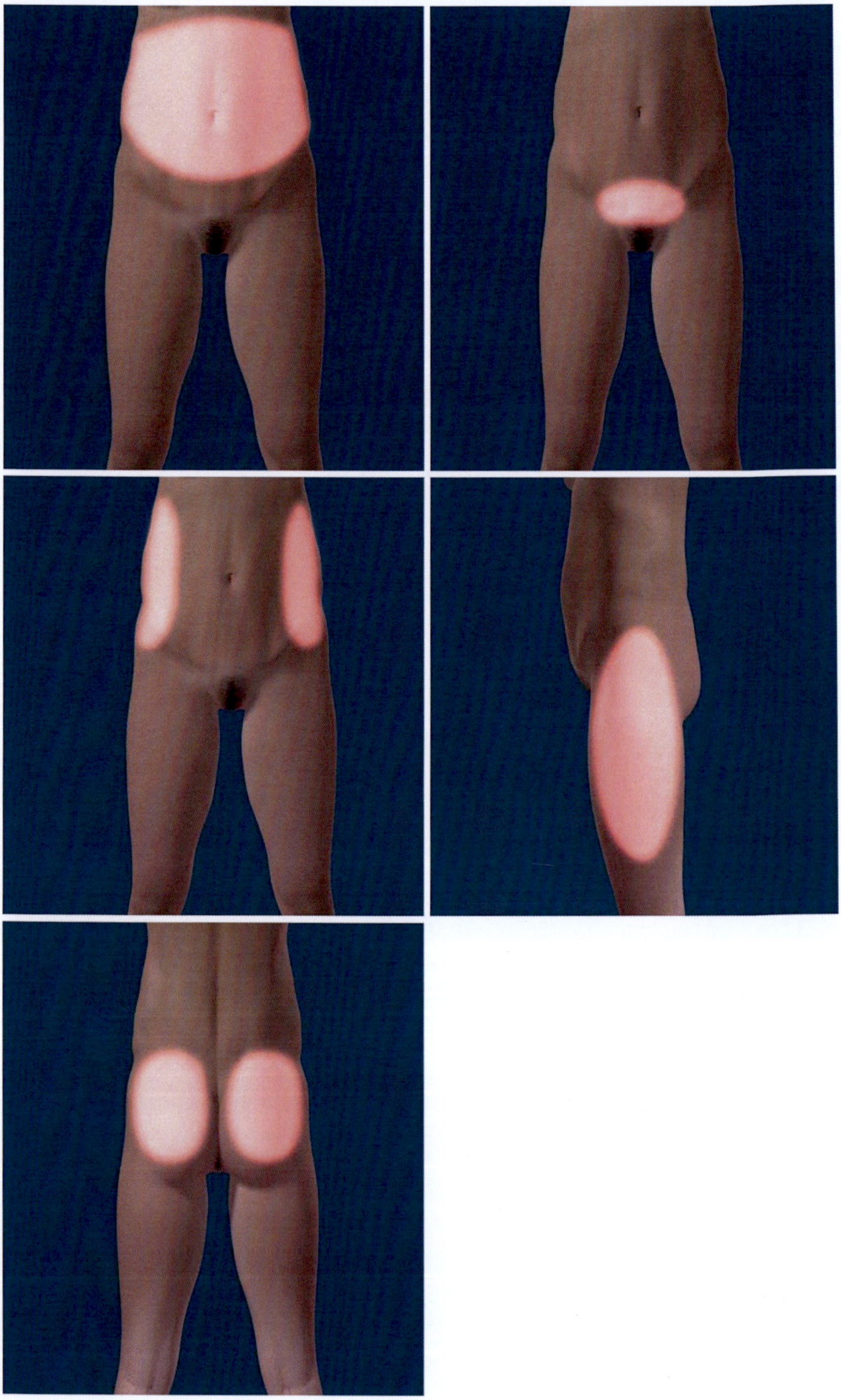

Fig. 43.6 Treated body regions

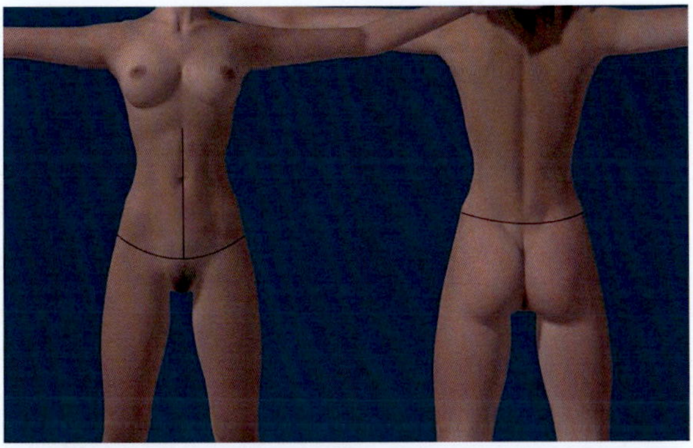

Fig. 43.7 Resulting scar

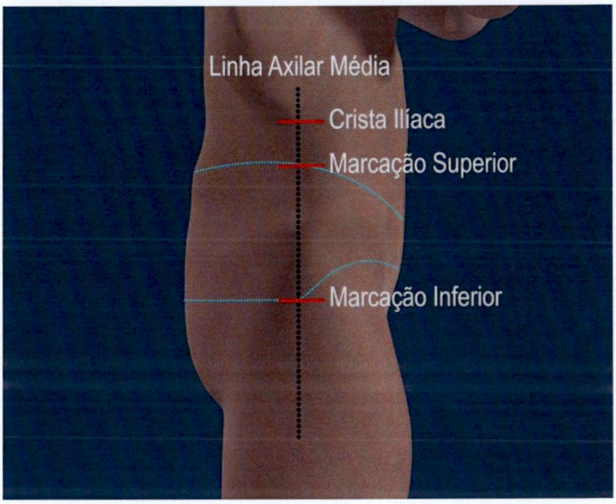

Fig. 43.8 Marking the lateral region

Lateral Marking (Fig. 43.8)

Initially, a vertical line is drawn following the middle axillary line, crossing the iliac crest to the lateral region of the thigh, where the next points are placed. Then the anterosuperior iliac crest is marked (by palpation). The next point determines the upper limit of the resection, and its marking can vary according to the patient's bathing suit. In most cases, this mark is located 4 cm below the iliac crest.

The lower limit of resection is positioned by digital clamping, remembering that the distance between the points determines the amount of tissue to be removed in the lateral region, which may vary according to the sagging skin of each patient.

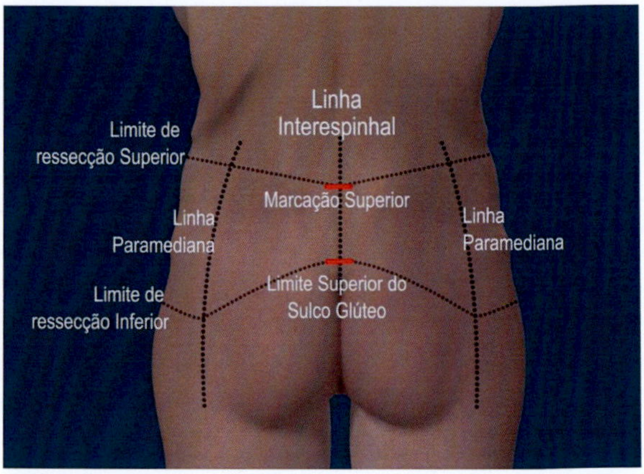

Fig. 43.9 Marking the posterior region

Front Marking (Fig. 43.9)

Marking starts with a median vertical line (interspinal line). Then, two more paramedian lines are drawn: those lines determine the boundary between the gluteal and trochanteric regions and symmetry must be maintained in relation to the interspinal line.

The lower limit of the interspinal line resection is marked at the upper limit of the intergluteal fold, and the upper limit of the interspinal line resection be determined by clamping. The distance between the points rarely exceeds 10 cm. The upper resection line is obtained with a straight or convex line joining the upper limit of resection on the interspinal line to the upper limit of resection on the midaxillary line. The inferior resection line is marked connecting the inferior limit of the resection on the interspinal line to the inferior limit of the resection on the midaxillary line, where the lower limit of this concave line is the paramedian vertical line.

Flap Marking for Gluteal Augmentation

Atrophy of the gluteal region is very common in patients who lost much weight. The correction of this alteration can be obtained using dermoadipose flaps, based on the abundant perforating vascularization of the gluteal region. Two different designs of flaps are used; those flaps are chosen according to the desired volume for the enlargement of this region.

Flap of Pascal and Le Louarn (Figs. 43.10 and 43.11)

This flap is indicated for patients who need a smaller volume and filling only the upper third of the gluteal region. The flap is designed within the area of the posterior marking; its inferior limit is the inferior resection line, and its lateral limits are the two posterior paramedian lines. The height of this flap can reach 10–12 cm and the horizontal axis 25 cm.

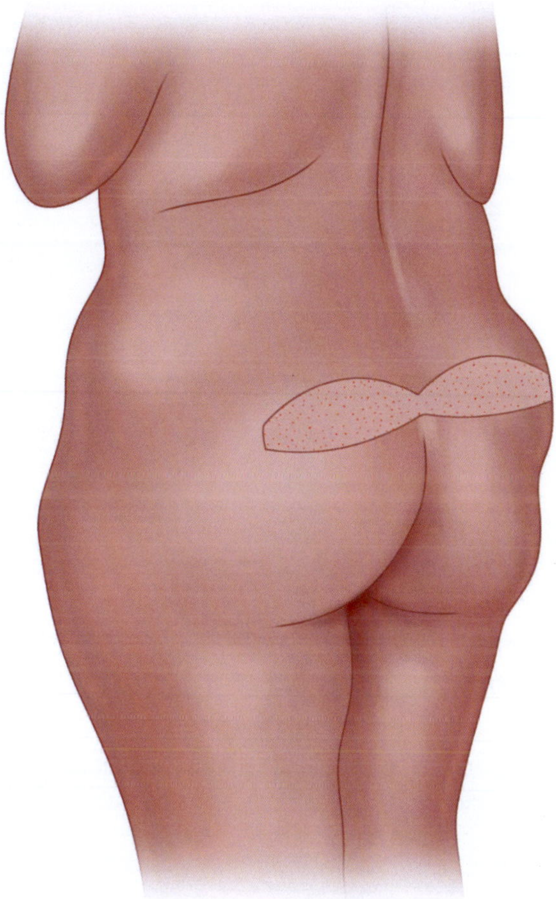

Fig. 43.10 Gluteal flap of Pascal and Le Louarn (in red)

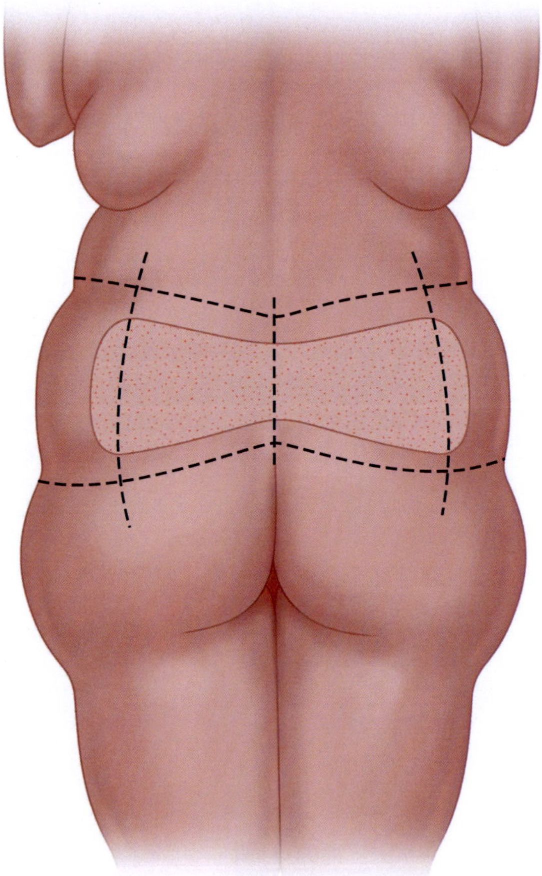

Fig. 43.11 Example of later booking of *body lift* with gluteal flap by Pascal and Le Louarn

Extended Flap (Figs. 43.10 and 43.12)

This flap makes possible to use a larger volume and fill the entire gluteal region, not just the upper third part. This marking can encompass the entire posterior area to be removed, both in height and in the horizontal axis, if necessary, in addition to the lines for medians (Fig. 43.13).

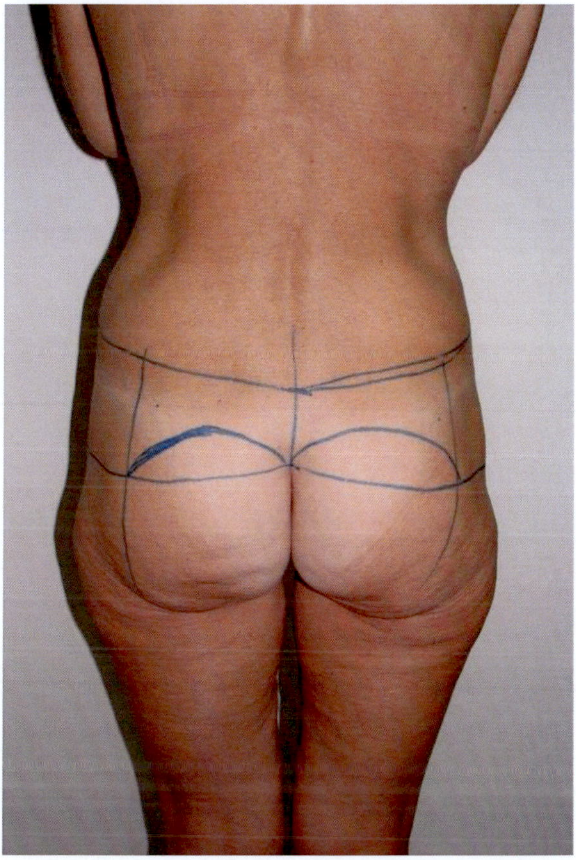

Fig. 43.12 Extended gluteal flap (red)

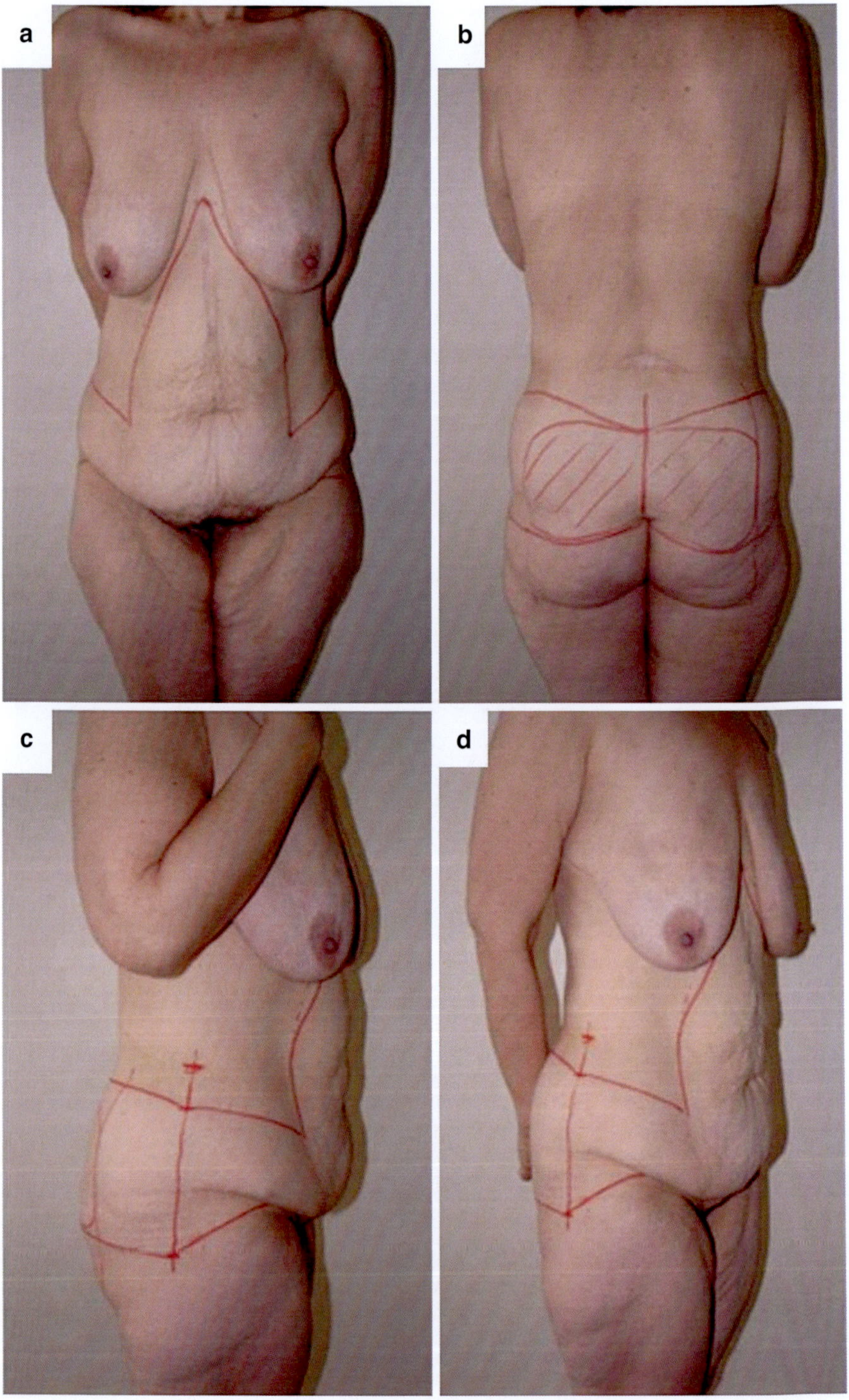

Fig. 43.13 Example of marking *body lift* with extended gluteal flap. (**a**) anterior, (**b**) posterior, (**c**) side, (**d**) oblique

Surgical Procedure

The surgery starts in the dorsal region; patient is in prone position, which allows two surgical teams to work simultaneously. Infiltration is carried out with adrenaline solution 1: 500,000 in the incisions and in the trochanteric areas to be liposuctioned (a procedure necessary in most patients).

The gluteal flap is de-epithelialized, and then all the excess tissue is removed at the level of the muscle aponeurosis (Fig. 43.14a). The flap is positioned following the upper contour of the greater gluteal muscle and fixed to its aponeurosis (Fig. 43.14b).

The Pascal and Le Louarn flap is slid inferiorly—vertical vector—without any detachment of it (Fig. 43.15); this flap increases the volume in the superior gluteal region. The extended flap is rotated in an inferomedial direction (Fig. 43.15a)—oblique vector toward the medial inferior quadrant—and the distal third of the flap is elevated, if necessary (Fig. 43.16), allowing its fixation in the aponeurosis of the greater gluteus muscle (detachment of the gluteal region above the muscle fascia), with filling of the entire gluteal region.

With the Pascal and Le Louarn flap, detachment in the gluteal region is performed below the superficial fascia, just enough for an adequate advance over the gluteal flap (Fig. 43.17). Detachment in the trochanteric region is performed at the same level, enabling the fixation of the superficial fascia to the muscle aponeurosis in a more superior position, to obtain adequate tension in this area and to prevent the creation of a "dead space."

Patients are maintained with suction drains (one for each side) until the output is less than 50 mL/day. In most cases, suction drains remain for 12 to 14 days.

The suture is performed in three planes: superficial, subdermal, and cutaneous fascia; it ends at the level of the midaxillary line, when the patient is then placed in the supine position (Fig. 43.18).

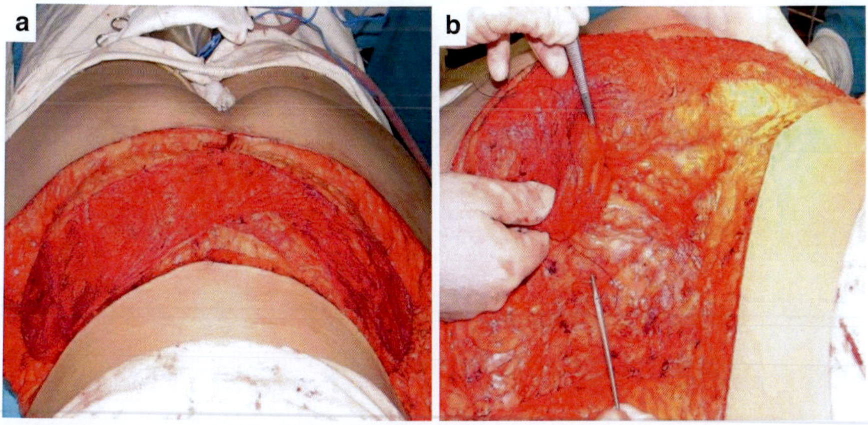

Fig. 43.14 (**a**) De-epithelialized gluteal extended flap. (**b**) Positioning and fixation of the gluteal flap at the level of the upper limit of the greater gluteus muscle

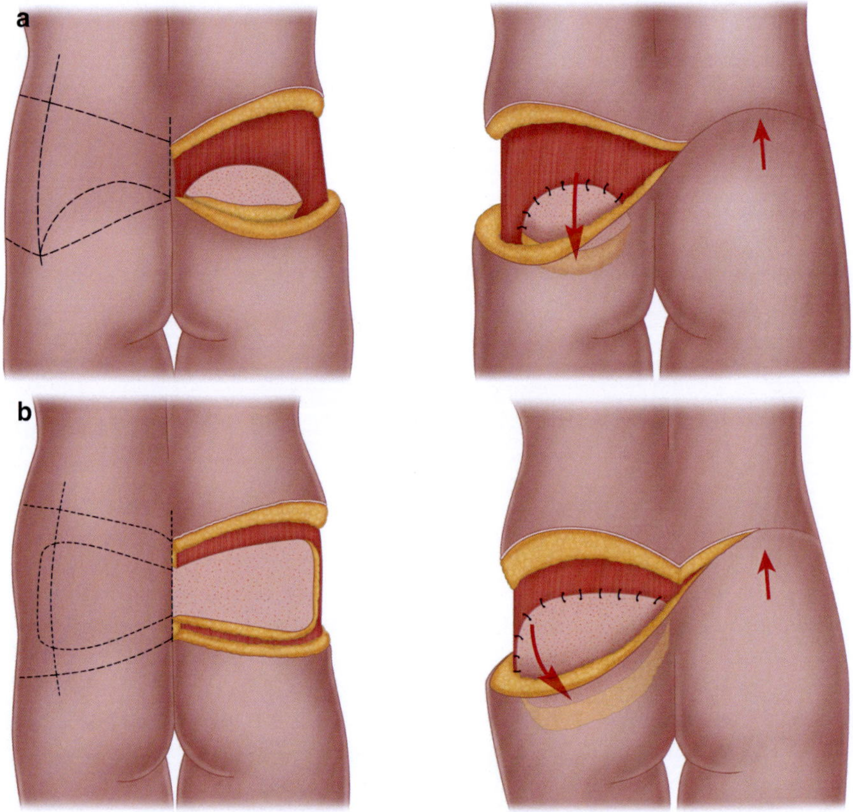

Fig. 43.15 (**a**) Pascal and Le Louarn gluteal flap—vertical vector. (**b**) Extended gluteal flap—oblique vector

Fig. 43.16 Extended flap—one third distally detached

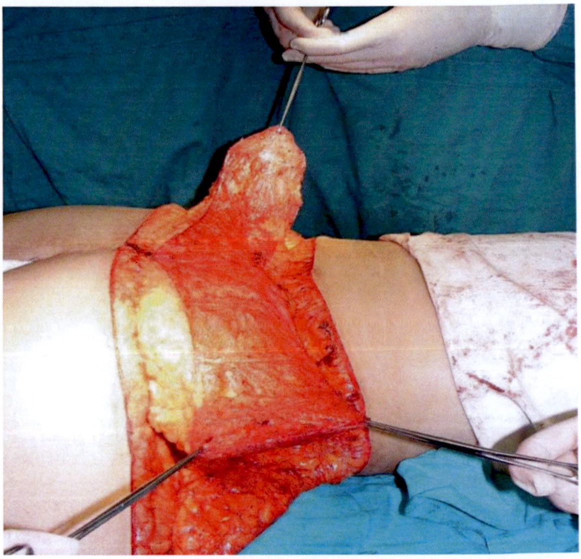

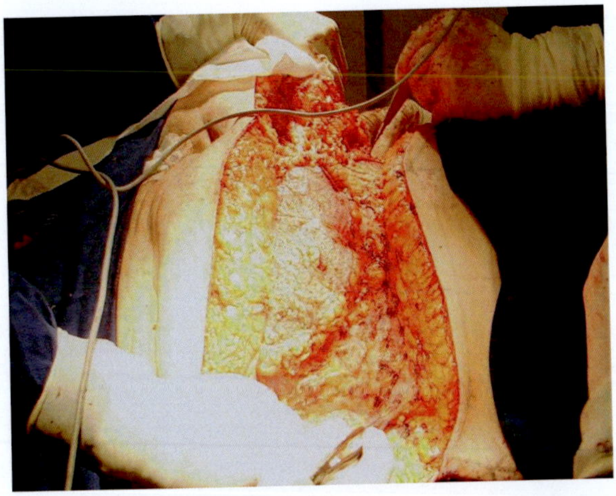

Fig. 43.17 Pascal and Le Louarn flap—positioned

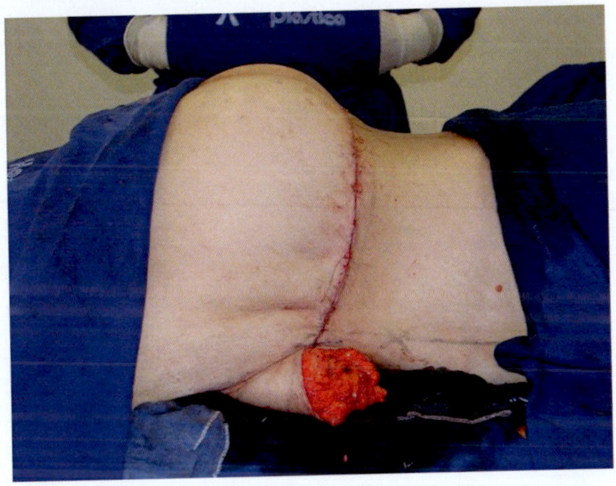

Fig. 43.18 Pascal and Le Louarn flap—end of posterior time of *body lift*

Below are some results of patients where gluteal flaps were used associated with *body lift* (Figs. 43.19, 43.20, and 43.21).

The volume obtained with the flaps used is limited by the area of posterior marking of the *body lift*. However, in cases where even the extended flap is not enough to obtain the desired projection, in a second surgical stage, another method of increasing the volume of the gluteal region can be associated, such as fat grafting or gluteal implants.

Complications reported in the literature regarding the *body lift* are seroma, hematoma, suture dehiscence, and scar hypertrophy. The occurrence of fat necrosis is rare. However, Cowell, using the pedicled flap, describes two cases (out of 18): one case of minimal necrosis characterized by hardening located in a segment of the flap and another of more than 50% of the flap (Sozer et al. 2005; Rohde and Gerut 2005; Raposo-Amaral et al. 2007; Mandieta 2006; Colwell and Borud 2007).

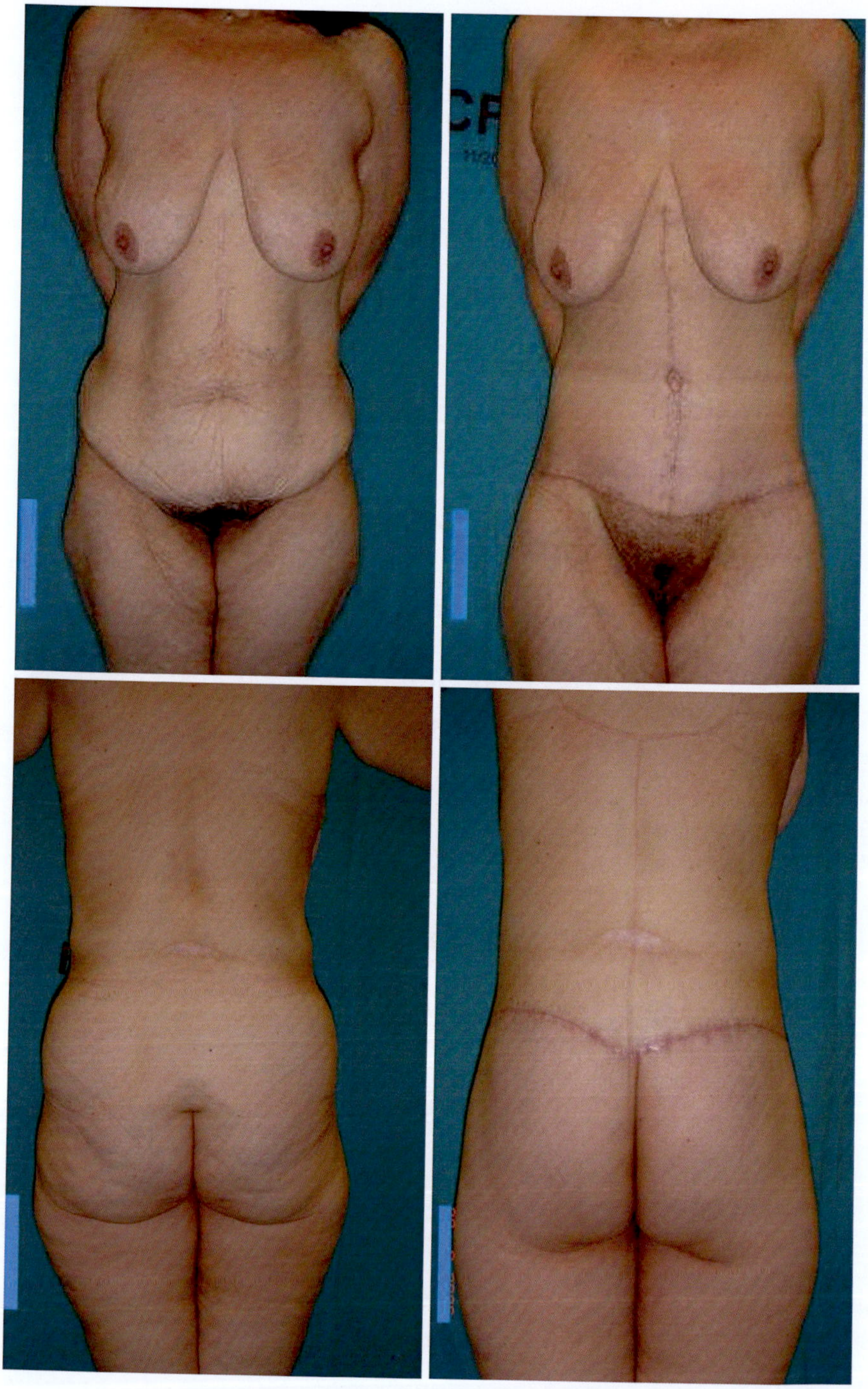

Fig. 43.19 *Body lift* with extended gluteal flap, 36 years old, loss of 62 kg, 3 months after surgery

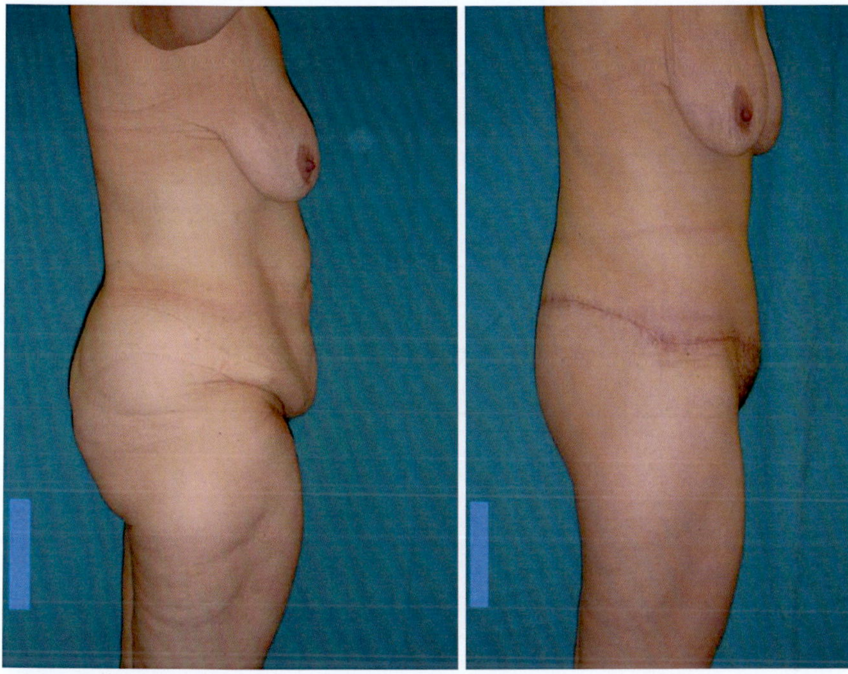

Fig. 43.19 (continued)

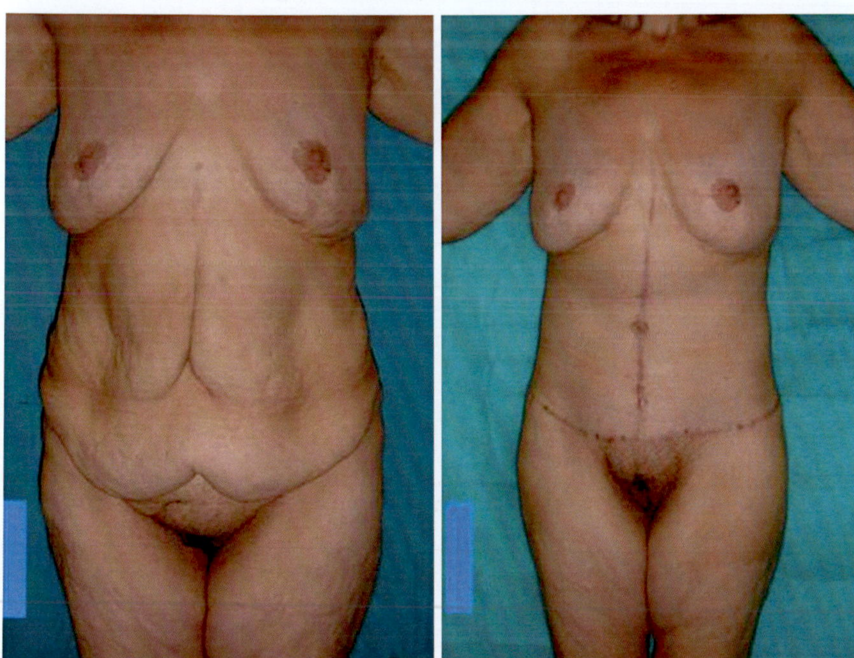

Fig. 43.20 *Body lift* with gluteal flap by Pascal and Le Louarn, 50 years old, loss of 35 kg, 8 months after surgery

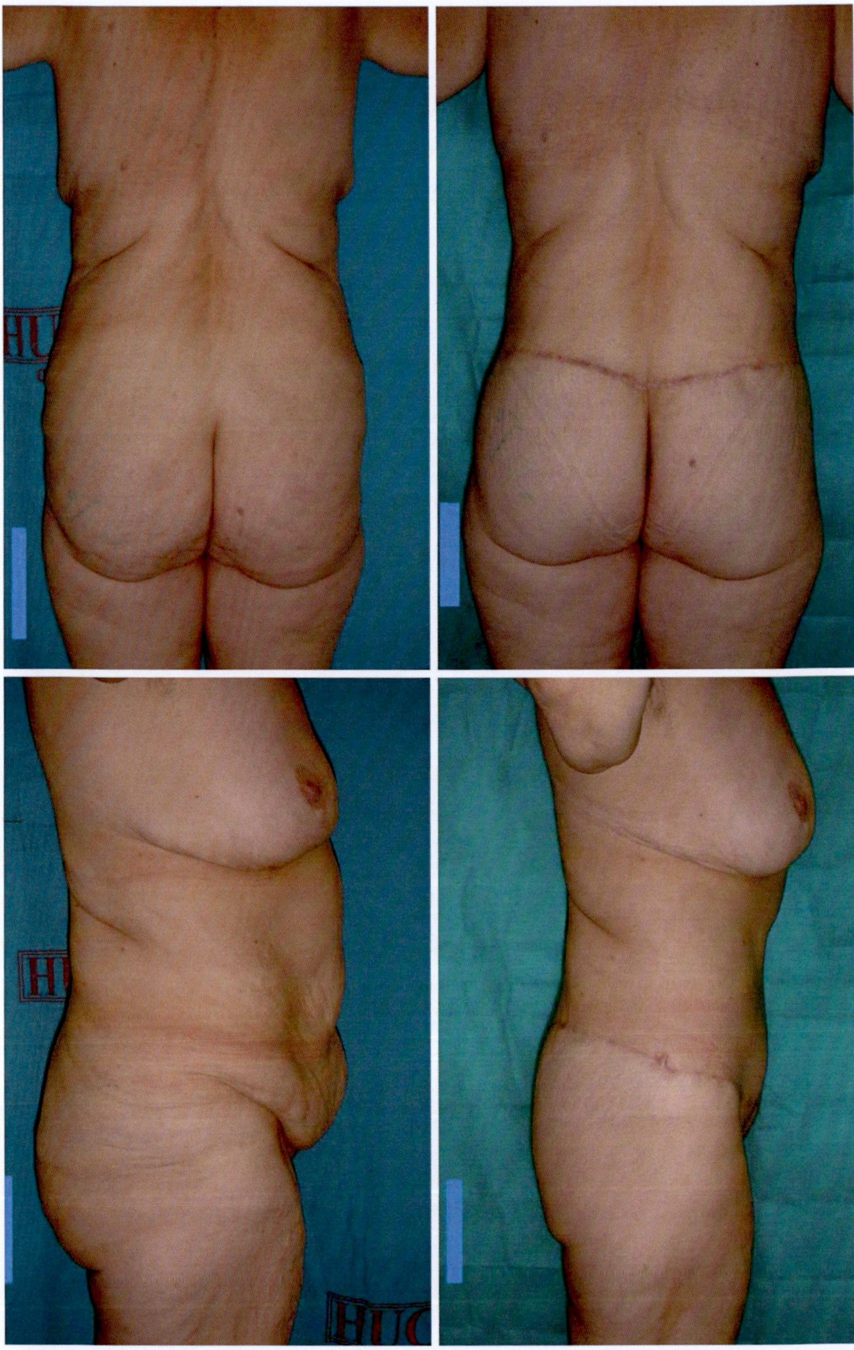

Fig. 43.20 (continued)

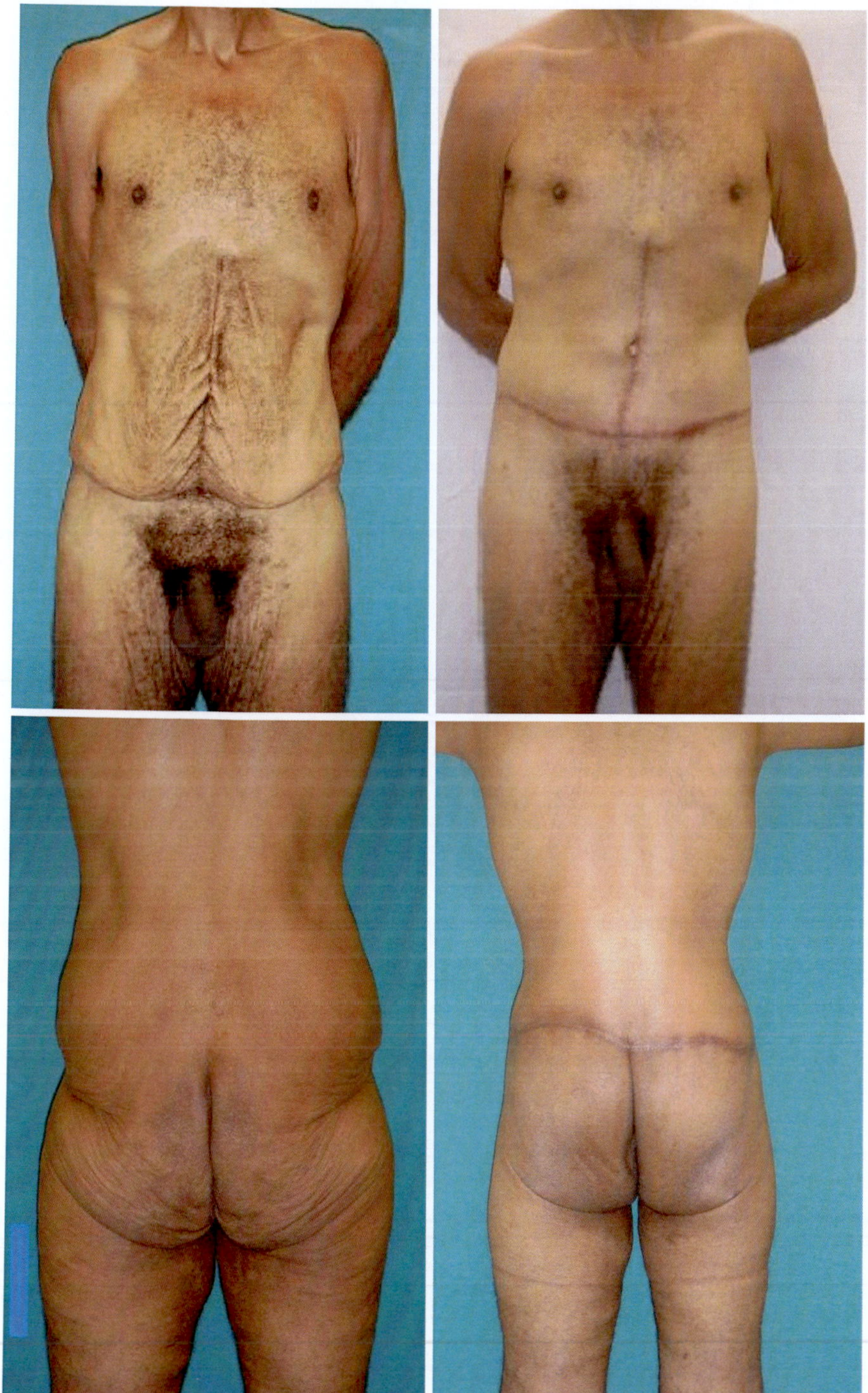

Fig. 43.21 *Body lift* with extended gluteal flap, 45 years old, loss of 90 kg, 1 month after surgery

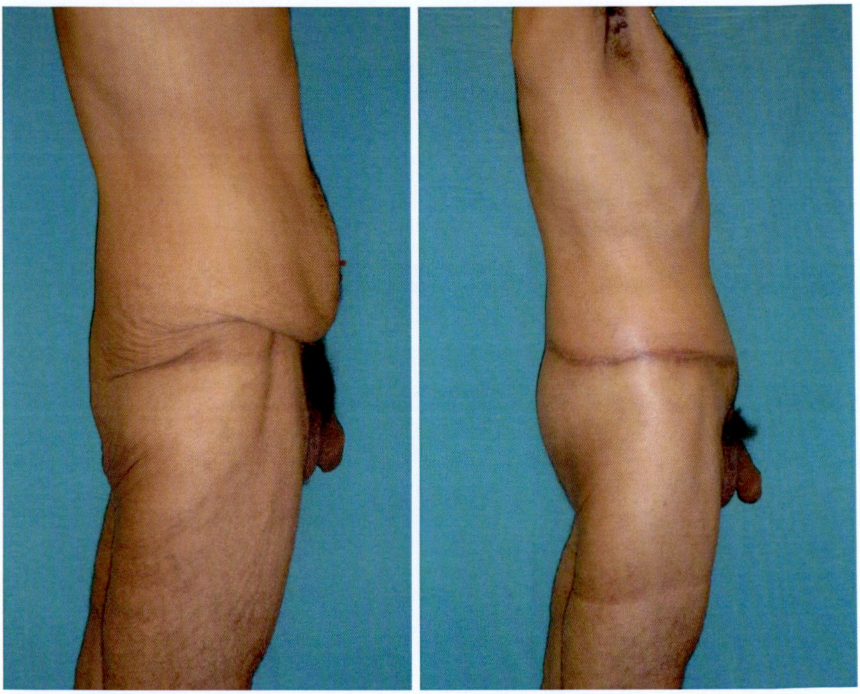

Fig. 43.21 (continued)

In our experience, no patient had problems related to the gluteal flap, as this proved to be quite safe and highly vascularized (large number of perforating vessels of the greater gluteus muscle), providing a definitive increase in the region's volume and great patient satisfaction.

References

Gonzales-Ulloa M. Circular lipectomy with transposition of the umbilicus and aponeurotic plastic technic, Cirurgia 1959 Sep; 27:394–401.

Gonzales-Ulloa M. Belt lipectomy. Br J Plast Surg 1961 Jul; 13:179–185.

Muhlbauer W. Radical abdominoplasty, including body shaping: representative cases. Aesthetic Plast Surg.1989;13:105–110.

Baroudi R. Body countoring surgery. Cin Plast Surg. 1989;16:263–271.

Baroudi R. Flankplasty: a specific treatment to improve body contouring. Ann Plast Surg. 1991;27: 404–410.

Lockwood T. Lower body lift with superficial fascial system suspension. Plast Reconstr Surg. 1993;92:1112–1122.

Lockwood T. High lateral tension abdominoplasty with superficial fascial system suspension.Plast Reconstr Surg.1995;96:603–615.

Pascal J, Le Louarn C. Remodeling body lift with high lateral tension. Aesth Plast Surg.2002;26:223–230.
Hamra S. Circunferncial body lift. Aesthetic Surg J.1999;19:244–250.
Hurwitz D J, Rubin P, Risin M, Sajjadian A, Sereika S. Correcting the saddlebag deformity in the massive weight loss patient. Plast Reconstr Surg. 2004;114:1313–1325.
Hurwitz D J, Zewert T. Body contouring after bariatric surgery. Op Thech Plast Reconstr Surg.2002;8:87–97.
Aly A,Cram A, Chao M, Pang J,McKeon M.Belt lipectomy for circumferential truncal excess: the University of Iowa experience. Plast Reconstr Surg,2003;111:398–413.
Cormenzana P, Samprón MN. Circumferential approach to contouring of the trunk. Aesthetic Sur J.2004;24:13–23.
Strauch B, Herman C, Rohde C, Baum T. Mid-body contouring in the post-bariatric surgery patient.Plast Reconstr Surg.2006;117:2200–2211.
Wallach S. Abdominal contour surgery for the massive weight loss pactent: the fleur-de-lis approach. Aesthetic Surg J.2005;25: 454–465.
Aniceto M, Claudio-da-Silva CS. *Body Lift*: tratamento do contorno corporal em pacientes ex-obesos. Rev. Bras. Cir. Plast. 2008; 23(4): 294–301.
Aniceto M. Associação de abdominoplastia vertical e torsoplastia no tratamento de ex-obesos mórbidos. Tese de Mestrado.Universidade Federal do Rio de Janeiro, 2009.
Sozer SO, Agullo FJ, Wolf C. Autoprosthesis buttock augmentation during lower body lift. Aesthetic Plast Surg 2005 Maio-Jun; 29(3): 133–7.
Rohde C, Gerut ZE. Augmentation buttock-pexy using autologous tissue following massive weight loss. Aesthetic Surg J 2005 Nov-Dez; 25(6): 576–81.
Raposo-Amaral CE, Cetrullo Jr CL, Guidi MC, Ferreira DM, Raposo- Amaral CM, Bilateral Lumbar hip Dermal fat rotation flap: A novel technique for autologous augmentation gluteoplasty. Plast Reconst Surg. 2007 Maio; 117(6):1781–1788.
Mandieta CG. Buttock's aesthetics: shaping, contouring and enhancing. In: Body contouring after massive weight loss. Aly AS. 1st ed. S.Louis,Missouri 2006. 237–301.
Colwell AS, Borud LJ. Autologous gluteal augmentation after massive weight loss: aesthetic analysis and role of the superior gluteal artery perforator flap. Plast Reconstr Surg 2007 Jan; 119(1): 345–56.
Toledo LS. Sculpting the buttocks after major weight loss. Aesth. Surg. J. 2003; 23:125–127.
Coban YK, Uzel M, Celic M. Correction of buttock ptosis with anchoring deepithelialized skin flaps. Aesth. Plast. Surg. 28:116–119,2004.
Huemer GM, Dunst KM, Schoeller T. Restoration of the Gluteal fold by a deepithelialized skin flap: Preliminary observation. Aesth. Past. Surg. 29:13–17,2005.
Gonzales R. Buttocks lifting: the dermo-tuberal anchorage technique. Aesth. Surg. J. 2005;25:15–23.

Chapter 44
Combined Surgeries in Massive Weight Loss Patients

Carlos del Pino Roxo and Luigi Losco

Abstract Body contouring procedures following massive weight loss (MWL) continue to increase as a result of the rapidly growing number of patients undergoing bariatric procedures. Unlike traditional plastic surgery patients who present with specific anatomical complaints, massive weight loss patients often have multiple regions of concern (Wallach 2008).

Introduction

Body contouring procedures following massive weight loss (MWL) continue to increase as a result of the rapidly growing number of patients undergoing bariatric procedures. Unlike traditional plastic surgery patients who present with specific anatomical complaints, massive weight loss patients often have multiple regions of concern (Wallach 2008).

To avoid extreme disappointment that they may experience with their body contour after massive weight loss, obese patients should also be familiarized with the expected changes their body will undergo as they lose weight.

If patients present during the weight loss process, they should be educated about what changes to expect in body contour after massive weight loss surgery, because it does not return to "normal." Bariatric surgeons have a different emphasis from that of plastic surgeons when treating obese patients, and they may neglect to inform patients about body changes after weight loss. Patients will benefit from the information about the variety of body contour procedures available. Patients must also be familiarized with the costs of these operations. Patients should be aware of these

C. del Pino Roxo (✉)
Head of Carlos Roxo Clinic, Rio de Janeiro, Brazil

L. Losco
Department of Medicine, Surgery and Dentistry, University of Salerno, Baronissi, Salerno, Italy

J. M. Avelar, R. Cavalcanti Ribeiro (eds.), *Body Contouring*,
https://doi.org/10.1007/978-3-031-42802-9_44

issues early on the process. In today's healthcare climate, this is particularly true because third-party payors are generally unlikely to cover most body contouring surgeries conducted after bariatric surgery. If patients are informed, they will be able to better plan for the future. Many patients report interference with proper fitting of clothes, social interactions, or hygienic issues. Almost all patients present with more than one area of their body that they would like to improve. It is important to ascertain patient priorities and discuss staging scenarios (Wallach 2008).

The most common order for treating problems is to address the lower trunk first, followed by the arms or overall thoracic region with the thighs treated last. Facial rejuvenation is often dealt with after completion of body contour work.

No single procedure can address the whole-body deformities associated with massive weight loss. Accordingly, patients frequently seek to have multiple procedures performed concomitantly to reduce costs and recovery time.

The decision to combine procedures requires careful preoperative consideration. Factors that need to be evaluated include the patient's overall medical condition, surgeon experience, length of surgery, vectors of tension, and cost to the patient. Numerous authors have advocated strategies for approaching this problem; however, there is relatively little evidence assessing how staging and different combination strategies affect clinical outcomes (Borud 2007; Hurwitz et al. 2008; Coon et al. 2010). We sought to report our experience with combined procedures.

Patient Selection and Assessment

We currently perform multiple procedures on over 75% of our MWL patients with around 30% undergoing three procedures during the same stage.

We consider adult patients for operation after a 12-month period after bariatric surgery and their weight loss had plateaued over a 3-month period. Selection criteria included American Society of Anesthesiologists (ASA) classification I or II, minimal medical comorbidities, and no significant cardiac or pulmonary disease. Patients who are smokers are asked to stop smoking 1 month before and after surgery. Patients are rated eligible to surgery with ≥12 Hb and ≥ 37 Hct.

The plastic surgeon and the nutritionist who are managing the postbariatric patient have to confirm that the patient has reached his/her plateau weight for several months and is nutritionally optimized before plastic surgery should be offered.

It is reasonable to assume that a patient who undergoes both upper and lower body contouring procedures simultaneously will have a more demanding postoperative recovery course. Patients that have gone through it point out frequently the burden of limited arm mobility coupled with abdominal and lower extremity pain.

Preoperative Assessment

Cutaneous folds are the most evident sequelae of massive weight loss. Consequently, many patients report interference with proper fitting of clothes, social interactions, or hygienic issues; aesthetic concerns might be, among others, the abdomen, mons pubis, hip region, gluteal region, arm, and breast (Poodt et al. 2016).

Circumferential tightening procedures of the lower trunk could address the most lateral extent of loose skin; they have the goal to restore skin and improve the body shape including the abdominal, flank, upper thigh, and gluteal region; then those procedures are willing to address the most part of deformities in our patients.

These patients usually have skin excess in a trunk-wide distribution. Attempts to manage the postbariatric patient with abdominoplasty alone are likely to result in an unsatisfactory outcome. Likewise, lengthening an abdominoplasty incision without completing a circumferential procedure gives rise to poor results.

For patients with multiple saddlebags and laxity of the lower trunk, thighs, and buttock region, a lower body lift is, in our practice, the gold standard. We found that combining a circumferential contouring procedure with arm lift and mastopexy addresses the upper and lower trunk that satisfies both patients and surgeons. Fleur-de-lis approaches were reserved for patients with severe supraumbilical excess instead of lower body lift.

We typically avoid combining lower body lifts with a medial thigh or upper back lift because of the opposing vectors of tension, although we have performed them together on occasion of extremely redundant skin folds without adverse results. In a second stage, a medial thigh lift and upper back lift could be accomplished. A facial lifting is performed in few patients in the third stage. The second stage and third stage are also employed for aesthetic refinements, scar revision, and postsurgically acquired subtle deformities.

One week before the surgery, patients were provided with a detailed description of the operation and were informed about postoperative care. Clinical photographs were taken preoperatively before and after surgical markings.

A final issue of importance early on treatment is obtaining informed consent for the procedures. Informed consent ultimately includes the aforementioned information about staging, length of time, expectations, and limitations, but should also discuss other pertinent issues such as the likelihood and number of scars and the potential for complications.

One useful suggestion is not only showing photographs of previous work but also making sure that the photographs represent a range of results, from problematic to desirable. This might temper unrealistic expectations and prepare patients for the realities of body shape and scarring after body contouring.

Preoperative markings should be performed in standing position. We usually mark our patients on the evening before the surgery. This offers several potential advantages, including (1) a more contemplative marking period (more relaxed than the surgery day—free of the numerous interruptions by perioperative personnel typical of the preoperative holding area), (2) not exposing the patients to hypothermia immediately before a long procedure, (3) surgeons having approximately 12 h to think about the planned incisions, and (4) providing an opportunity for the patients to question their surgeon about incision patterns and expected outcomes while they are less anxious than they might otherwise be immediately before their surgery. Surgeons who elect to mark their patients the night before surgery should be advised to use heavy permanent marker that will not easily fade due to cleansing before the next day.

Preoperative Markings

We will describe our most common surgical combination: lower body lift for lower body defects and brachioplasty and mastopexy for upper body contouring (Fig. 44.1).

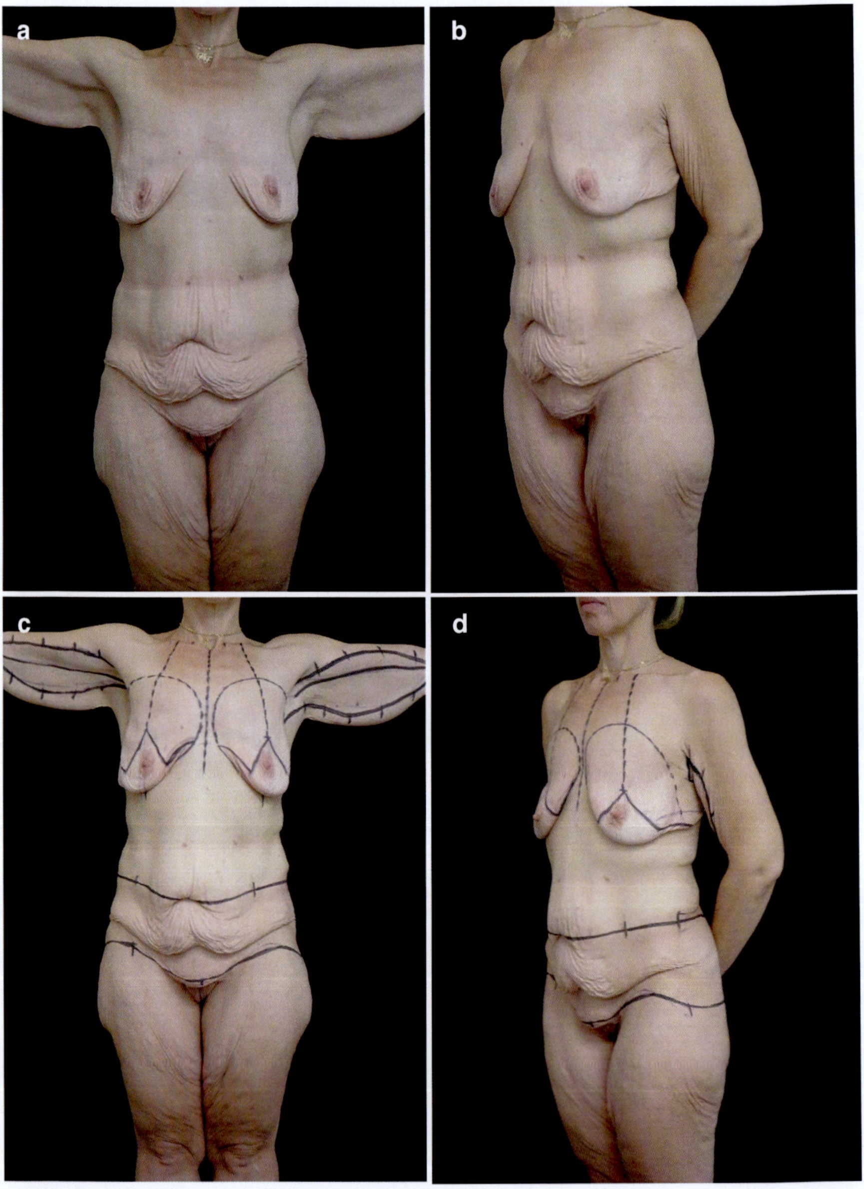

Fig. 44.1 (**a–b**) Preoperative pictures of a MWL female patient undergoing combined procedure: lower body lift, mastopexy with implants and brachioplasty. (**c–d**) Preoperative drawings. (**e–f**) 6-month postoperative pictures

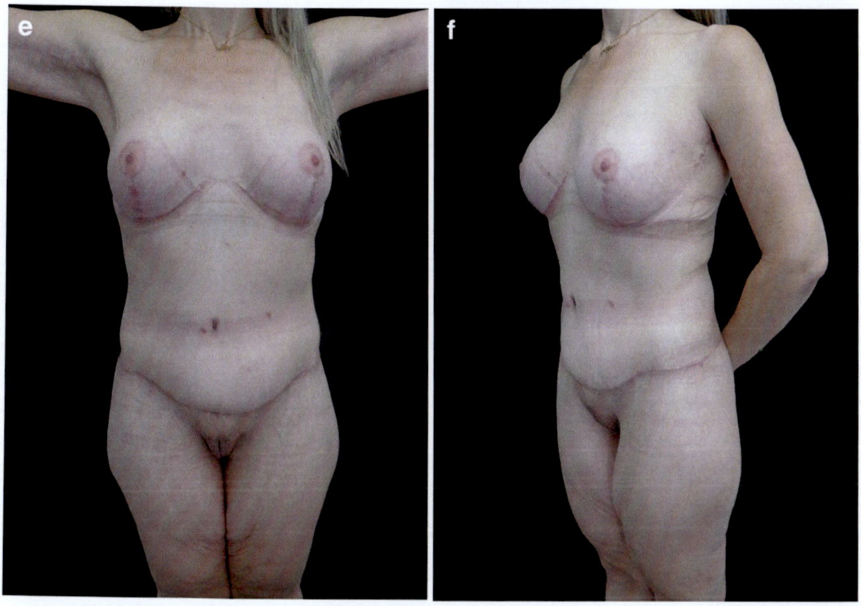

Fig. 44.1 (continued)

However, depending on patients' desires and expectations and if the patients had already undergone a surgical step, only two of the surgeries could be combined (i.e., lower body lift and mastopexy).

When the upper and lower body should be marked, we usually start with lower body markings. The drawings are performed in standing position. Firmly pulling the lower abdomen upward, a point was marked 5.5–6.5 cm to the upper vulvar commissure (or base of the penile shaft) (point A). The "pinch test" was used to assess the amount of median skin excess: The cutaneous fold was held between the thumb (point A) and forefinger-middle finger (point B), simulating skin closure under maximum tension. Another point (B1) was marked slightly below it (1–2 cm). Next, from point A, a line was drawn on both sides of the inguinal region, laying 1 cm above the inguinal ligament or just on it (accordingly with pinch test assessment and upper thigh expected improvement) and angulated upward toward the anterior superior iliac spine. Planning a low inferior incision, we obtained improvement in upper thigh contour and prevented the scar from being visible above the swimwear.

Again, the pinch test was used to evaluate the amount of lateral laxity at the flank; here, points C and D were drawn as superior and inferior borders of the lateral excess; on the contralateral side, the drawings were specular.

The anterior marking was completed connecting point A with C and point B (B1) with D. The choice about using either the B or B1 pathway was made intraoperatively depending on the degree of the flap advancement. The posterior drawing started marking the midline inferior extent of excision at the buttocks crease. The superior extent was assessed by performing the pinch test and asking the patient to flex the waist; this maneuver helped to prevent posterior dehiscence.

The superior line connecting the mid-back line to lateral marks (point C) was drawn slightly above the planned scar position (underwear line). The inferior marking was designed with a pinch test using the superior line as a starting point. On the contralateral side, the drawings were specular (Fig. 44.2). The posterior back excision was planned to be more aggressive laterally than medially to address the upper buttocks and thigh deformity improving shape and contour in women. An assistant checks every point of the preoperative marking for symmetry right to left and to the midline. A grid that connects the upper and inferior marking could be designed to help the surgeons intraoperatively.

Then the upper body is marked. The arm is abducted (90° with the trunk) and the expected scar position is drawn in the bicipital sulcus. The more distal extent is not

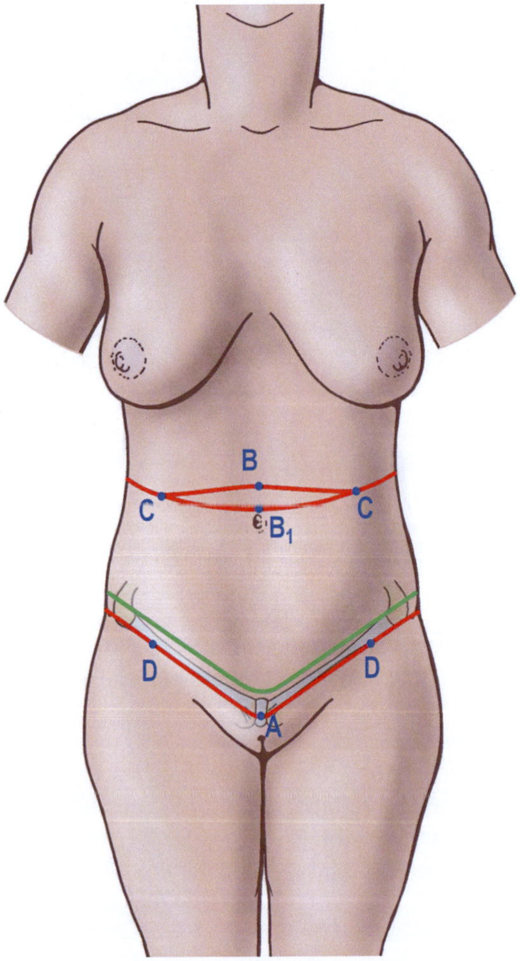

Fig. 44.2 Illustrative drawing of surgical markings

farther than the elbow crease. The width of the skin excision is defined through a pinch test from the elbow to the axilla. The more proximal end of the drawings is performed asking the patient to raise the arm further: in this way, the medial bicipital sulcus line can be continued into the axilla and the incision lines are easily completed. The surgeon should be very careful during the preoperative markings; it is important to check also at the forearm to avoid that after the surgery, the arm has a smaller circumference than the forearm (especially for dramatically deflated arms).

The mastopexy, in our series, has a T-inverted design with retro-glandular implant placement. The preoperative markings follow the Pitanguy's description with areola diameter of 4 cm and areola to inframammary crease distance of 5 cm. If the lateral thorax has a conspicuous saddlebag, the horizontal lateral excision can be prolonged using a pinch test to assess the amount of skin excision. The final scar should lie in the bra line.

Lower Body Lift vs. Belt Lipectomy

Patients are considered for a circumferential lower body procedure if presenting with lateral abdominal tissue besides an undesirable abdominal contour and redundant skin circumferentially.

To reverse the changes caused by massive weight loss, a circumferential wedge of tissue needs to be excised from around the lower trunk, whether through a lower body lift or belt lipectomy. The position of the wedge in the vertical dimension, especially laterally and posteriorly, is different in a lower body lift than in a belt lipectomy.

A lower body lift treats the lower truncal subunit and the thigh as one unit. The position of the wedge to be excised, laterally and posteriorly, is more inferiorly located in a lower body lift when compared to the wedge excision in a belt lipectomy.

With the lower body lift, tissues from the upper thigh must lift. The zone of adherence at the junction of the lateral thigh and hip fat deposits is destroyed. Along with the inguinal fascia attachments lateral to the femoral triangle, the destruction of these fascial attachments allows the thigh tissues to be lifted mid-thigh and cranial to it.

Surgical Technique and Surgical Timing

In our practice, undermining is never performed, and when combining two or three surgical procedures, no liposuction is performed.

There are several logistical barriers to organize this type of surgical team. In an academic surgical setting, a primary surgeon may have the support of residents and fellows, but in a private practice with two physicians, those types of surgical combination should be avoided due to the prolonged timing. In our series, only the epidermis and upper part of the dermis are incised by a scalpel, and the rest of the procedure is carried out by cautery minimizing blood loss and shortening the operative time.

In our practice, surgery starts with lower body contouring with a prone-to-supine approach. Surgery is performed by two surgeons and two assistants divided into two teams on the right and left side of the patients. A methylene blue-dipped scalpel should be used to avoid loss of markings during the procedure. In an extensive combined procedure, it is paramount to avoid any unnecessary blood loss and lengthening of the operative times. After a drain is placed, the wounds are closed. The patient is turned to the supine position, re-prepped, and draped including the breast and arms if surgery has to be performed. One surgical team is completing the anterior dissection of the lower body lift and the second team is approaching the brachioplasty. The arm is incised at the proximal side of the drawings and the skin-subcutaneous excision is carried at the level of the Scarpa's fascia till the middle third of the arm to avoid any possible injury to the main lymphatic and blood vessels. In the middle distal third, the excision can be deeper, always respecting the muscular deep fascia.

If more assistants are available, surgery on both arms could be performed simultaneously. Once the lower body lift and brachioplasty are concluded, mastopexy could be started.

Perioperative Care

Graded compression stockings and pneumatic calf compression boots were worn throughout the operative procedure, and the stockings also postoperatively. The drains were removed when the output was less than 40 cc in a 24-h period. In our practice, early ambulation is mandatory. We encourage ambulation on the first postoperative day, by the second postoperative day, and upon discharged home on the day after. Postoperative garments were worn for 12 weeks postoperatively night and day; from this time, an adequate rehabilitation program was allowed.

Photographs were taken 1 day postoperative and during the follow-up period between 1 and 12 months postoperatively. Surgeons should stress the importance of weight maintenance and explain how weight regain can negatively affect body contouring.

Combined Versus Staged Surgery

For plastic surgeons who do not have a large team, two to three stages may be required to perform three procedures in postbariatric patients. Advantages of staging procedures include the potential for decreased blood loss and the avoidance of opposing tension vectors. Staging also allows for the correction of any contour irregularities and skin laxity that may have occurred as a result of previously performed procedures.

After massive weight loss, many areas of the body usually require body contouring surgical procedures. If only a single body area is treated per operation, several surgeries are necessary for deformity correction and improvement in patient well-being. In our recent study on 323 patients, the lower body lift was safely combined with another surgical procedure (Losco et al. 2020). Many authors stated that the overall complication rate increased with the increase in procedures performed (Wallach 2008; Winocour et al. 2015; Michot et al. 2016). We believe that combination of surgical procedures in patients with MWL must be carried out carefully by an experienced surgeon/team. Operating time showed to be the most important factor in triggering the metabolic response to trauma in body contouring surgery. Therefore, it seems that if the surgical team does operation in a systematic manner, thus optimizing time, it is possible to associate procedures without adding risks for the patients (Roxo et al. 2019). Having a short operative time for such an extensive surgical procedure is important, and these findings confirm our directions to treat MWL patients with the safest and most resolutive surgery; many body areas can be addressed within the same procedure.

We recommend that surgeons consider the following criteria when deciding to combine procedures: the medical condition of the patient, the operative team and the anesthesia team (i.e., number of surgeons and extenders), the surgeon's experience with major body contouring procedures, and the operative facility and resources (i.e., outpatient center vs hospital). Staging is a good alternative for patients who are not ideal candidates for combined procedures or who desire combinations that cannot be safely performed.

References

Wallach SG. Treating the abdominotorso region of the massive weight loss patient: An algorithmic approach. *Plast Reconstr Surg.* 2008;121:1431–1441.

Borud LJ. Combined procedures and staging. In: Rubin JP, Matarasso A, eds. *Aesthetic Surgery in the Massive Weight Loss Patient.* Philadelphia: Elsevier; 2007.

Hurwitz DJ, Agha-Mohammadi S, Ota K, Unadkat J. A clinical review of total body lift surgery. *Aesthet Surg J.* 2008;28:294–303; discussion 304–305.

Coon D, Michaels J 5th, Gusenoff JA, Purnell C, Friedman T, Rubin JP. Multiple procedures and staging in the massive weight loss population. Plast Reconstr Surg. 2010 Feb;125(2):691–698. 1

Poodt IG, van Dijk MM, Klein S, Hoogbergen MM (2016) Complications of lower body lift surgery in postbariatric patients. Plast Reconstr Surg Glob Open.

Losco L, Roxo AC, Roxo CW, Lo Torto F, Bolletta A, de Sire A, Aksoyler D, Ribuffo D, Cigna E, Roxo CP. Lower Body Lift After Bariatric Surgery: 323 Consecutive Cases Over 10-Year Experience. Aesthetic Plast Surg. 2020 Apr;44(2):421–432

Winocour J, Gupta V, Ramirez JR, Shack RB, Grotting JC, Higdon KK (2015) Abdominoplasty: risk factors, complication rates, and safety of combined procedures. Plast Reconstr Surg 136:597e–606e

Michot A, Alet JM, Pe'lissier P, Grolleau-Raoux JL, Bodin F, Chaput B (2016) Morbidity in combined-procedure associating abdominoplasty and breast surgery: a systematic review. Ann Chir Plast Esthet 61:e9–e19

Roxo ACW, Roxo CDP, Marques RG, Rodrigues NCP, Vigna Carneiro D, Souto FMDC, Nahas FX (2019) Endocrine-metabolic response in patients undergoing multiple body contouring surgeries after massive weight loss. Aesthet Surg J 39:756–764

Chapter 45
Abdominoplasty in Post-Bariatric Patients

Roberto Kaluf, Roberto Kaluf Filho, and Rafael Alves Tumeh

Abstract Obesity is considered an epidemic disease and most often associated with other comorbidities which causes a high morbidity and mortality rate. Because of that, more people are seeking for obesity treatment nowadays. The clinical treatment of obesity is complex because it is not only about weight loss but also about maintaining the weight achieved. Recurrence rates are high, and success rate is low. Therefore, surgical treatment has been improving over the years. Its effectiveness in weight loss has been confirmed by several studies. Today, with laparoscopy and robotic surgery technologies, the mortality rate has been dropping exponentially. Post-bariatric patients constantly complain about the great skin redundancy, which interferes with the practice of exercises and appropriateness of clothes, which not only represent an aesthetic problem but also cause posture and mobility problems. This excessive tissue can affect hygiene and cause dermatitis and fungal infections.

Introduction

Obesity is considered an epidemic disease and most often associated with other comorbidities which causes a high morbidity and mortality rate. Because of that, more people are seeking for obesity treatment nowadays. The clinical treatment of obesity is complex because it is not only about weight loss but also about maintaining the weight achieved (Karlsonn et al. 2007). Recurrence rates are high, and success rate is low. Therefore, surgical treatment has been improving over the years. Its effectiveness in weight loss has been confirmed by several studies. Today, with laparoscopy and robotic surgery technologies, the mortality rate has been dropping exponentially. Post-bariatric patients constantly complain about the great skin redundancy, which interferes with the practice of exercises and appropriateness of

R. Kaluf (✉) · R. K. Filho · R. A. Tumeh
São Paulo, Brazil

J. M. Avelar, R. Cavalcanti Ribeiro (eds.), *Body Contouring*,
https://doi.org/10.1007/978-3-031-42802-9_45

clothes, which not only represent an aesthetic problem but also cause posture and mobility problems. This excessive tissue can affect hygiene and cause dermatitis and fungal infections (Zannis et al. 2012).

Aims

To learn the abdominoplasty technique and its specificities, along with its indications and possible complications.

Diagnosis or Preoperative Assessment (General Considerations)

Abdominal dermolipectomy in post-bariatric patients is correctly indicated 12–18 months after gastroplasty associated with weight stability in the last 6 months, which guarantees a better metabolic/nutritional balance, reduces the risk of complications, and allows for better aesthetic results (Kaluf et al. 2008).

In the preoperative period, a complete clinical evaluation of the patient is performed, including imaging tests to investigate abdominal wall defects, laboratory tests, and cardiac evaluation. For most patients, the procedure is performed under

Risk factors	Score
1. Age ≥ 40 years	1
2. Age ≥60 years	2
3. Smoking	1
4. Obesity	1
5. Estrogens or contraceptives	1
6. Neoplasm	2
7. Pregnancy and puerperium	1
8. Immobilization	2
9. Thrombophilia	2
10. Nephrotic Syndrome	1
11. Polycythemia	2
12. Autoimmune disease	1
13. Leukemia	1
14. Uncomplicated AMI	1
15. Complicated AMI	2
16. CVA I	2
17.Previous DVT / PE	2
18. Edema, varicose veins, ulcer, and stasis of the lower limbs	2
19. Diabetes mellitus	1
20. CHF	2
21. Family history DVT / EP	2
22. Major surgery in the last 6 months	1
23. Extensive burns	2
24. Antiphospholipid antibody present	2
25. Infections	1
26. General surgery ≤60 min	1
27. General surgery > 60 min	2
28. Surgery of the hip, knees, prostheses, fractures of long bone or multiples and polytrauma	>4

Fig. 45.1 Risk factors for thromboembolism

Prophylaxis of DVT

Physical methods
Graduated compression stockings (GCS)
Early walking
Intermittent pneumatic compressions (IPC)
Trendelenburg position

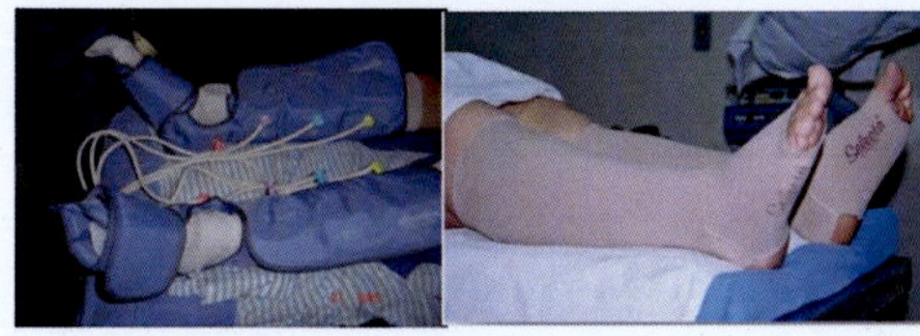

Drugs	Risk	Score	Dosage schedule
Enoxaparin sodium	Moderate	2-4	20mg / 2h before, and 20mg qd for 5 days after surgery
	High	> 4	40mg / 12h before, 40mg / 12h after surgery
Nadroparin calcium	Moderate	2-4	0.3mL / 2h before, 0.3mL qd for 5 days after surgery
	High	> 4	0.6mL / 12h before, 0.6mL qd for 5 days after surgery

Fig. 45.2 Prophylaxis of DVT

general anesthesia with the use of fast dissolving drugs. Prophylaxis of venous thromboembolism (VT) is routinely performed according to the criteria of the Brazilian Society of Angiology and Vascular Surgery (Kaluf et al. 2008) (Figs. 45.1 and 45.2).

Technique Options

Relief Surgeries

The most common presentation of this type of disabling condition in obesity is located at the level of the lower abdominal wall, with different degrees of intensity of the sized panniculus. Igwe proposed a classification based on panniculus that covers the pubic hairline, but not the entire mons pubis (grade 1), the genitals (grade 2), upper thigh (grade 3), mid-thigh (grade 4), and knees and beyond (grade 5). In addition to the amount of abdominal ptosis, it is necessary to evaluate trophic skin and subcutaneous tissue conditions. Relief surgeries must have a restorative character, and the technique must be safe and faster (Zannis et al. 2012; Friedrich et al. 2008).

Marking the lower and central portion of the ellipse to be resected should start with the patient in the supine position when the presentation of the suprapubic region is facilitated. On the other hand, the lateral portions of the ellipse, including its entire upper portion, must be performed with the patient in an orthostatic position, since the action of gravity will collaborate in determining the area to be demarcated. In cases of grades 3, 4, and 5 of Igwe, the positioning of one of the hands under the ptosis tissue, at the level of the inferior marking of the ellipse, allows us to identify its projection on the anterior wall (Kaluf et al. 2008; Donnabella 2013).

A preoperative bath with 4% chlorhexidine, rigorous antisepsis, and antibiotic prophylaxis is performed. The incision lines are infiltrated with a vasoconstrictor solution (1:200,000), which start at the lower pole of the ellipse with detachment in a supra-aponeurotic plane and cranial direction. Dissection is performed with an electric scalpel and the larger vessels are identified, separated, and connected with nonabsorbable sutures. The umbilical stump is identified and connected at its base with nonabsorbable suture, remembering that the neo-omphaloplasty should be postponed for a second surgical time, in the same way we waive the abdominal plication. On the other hand, if ventral hernias are seen, correction is indicated with the use of plications or meshes made of alloplastic material (Donnabella 2013; Franco et al. 2006).

Once the flap is fully lifted, we make the upper incision after checking the possibility of closing the wound. No tissue will be resected apart from the ellipse which is resected en bloc. Strict hemostasis is performed, negative pressure drains are positioned, and flap synthesis is completed in three planes.

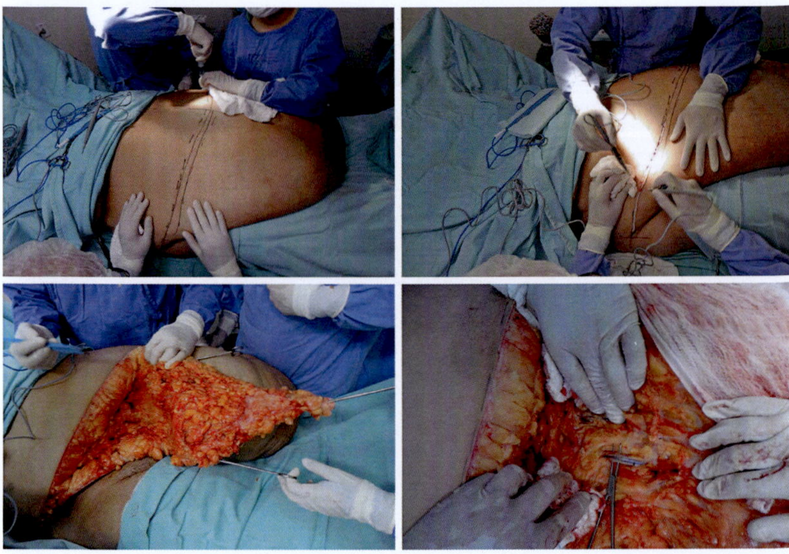

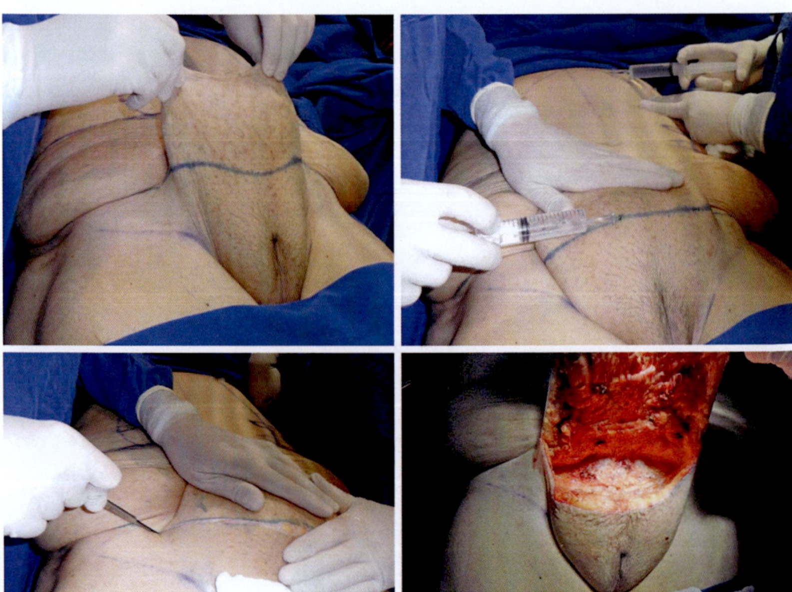

The patient is maintained with an indwelling urinary catheter for 24 h and drains for up to 1 week, being removed when they reach a flow rate of less than 40 mL/day. Encouraging early ambulation is essential, and the use of an elastic abdominal band starts on the first postoperative day, together with daily dressing changes (Brown et al. 2014).

In superobese (BMI > 50) and super-superobese (BMI > 60) patients, the extremely high rates of complications have led some authors to indicate resection of the morbid panicle with treatment of the surgical wound by secondary closure, with the use of negative pressure dressings (Brown et al. 2014).

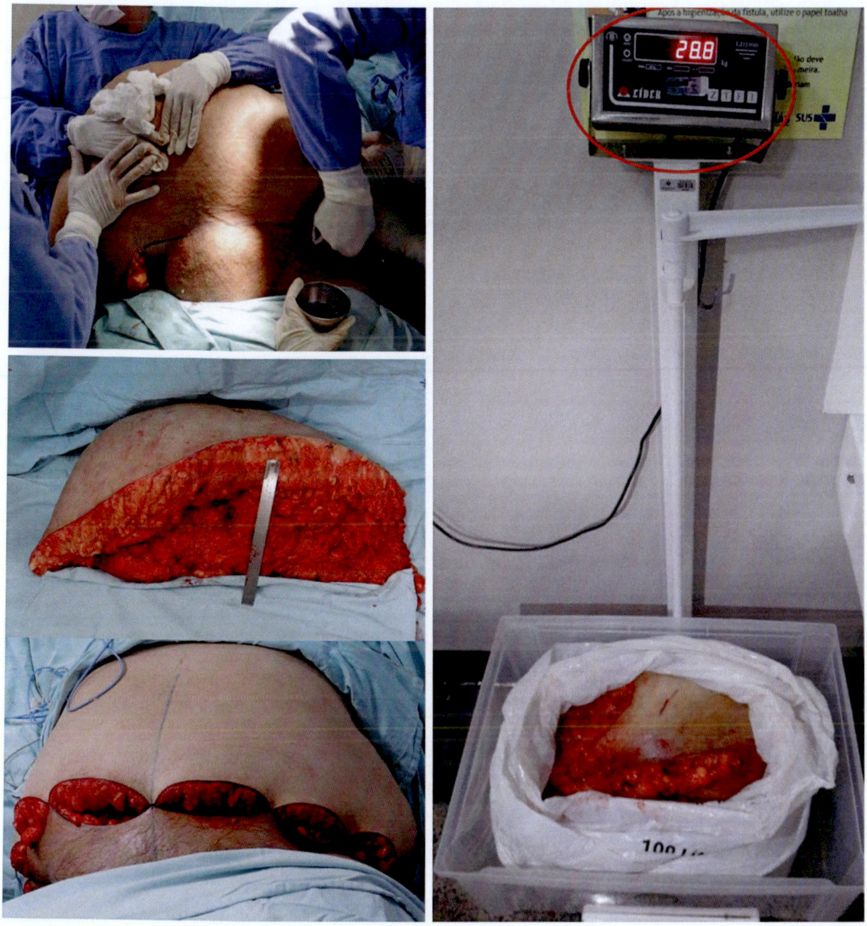

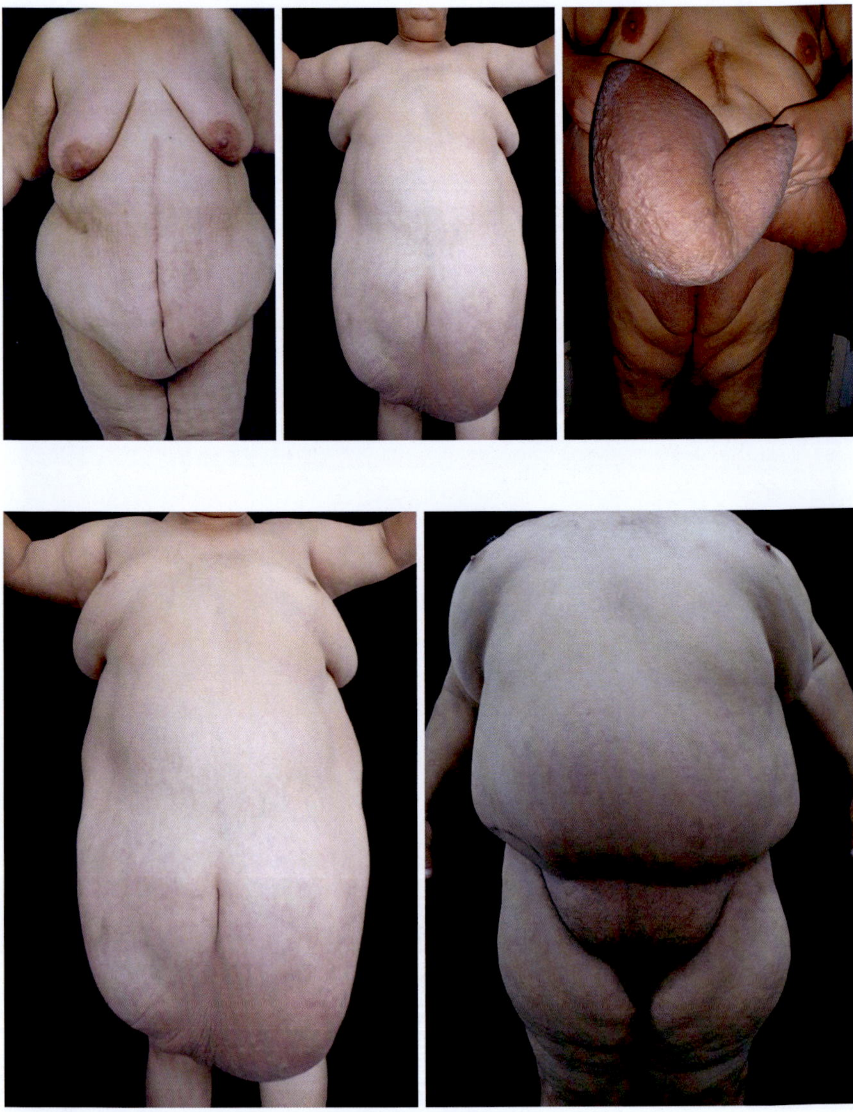

Classic Abdominal Dermolipectomy

This is the technique normally used in conventional patients, with little indication for post-bariatric patients. In patients with massive weight loss undergoing this technique, there is usually an aspect of amputation of the abdomen in the vertical direction, with extra skin around flanks and back that looks unsightly, also involving the thighs' roots and the buttocks (Baroudi 1984; Shermak et al. 2006).

The transverse anterior approach does not correct the horizontal excess of tissues at the level of the waist and upper abdomen, resulting in residual laxity that is extremely uncomfortable in the postoperative period, when the body contour is evaluated. Most patients want this approach because of the restricted and hidden scars, especially those who underwent video gastroplasty and who do not have vertical scars. In these cases, it is important to highlight in preoperative consultations regarding the horizontal abdominal flaccidity in the postoperative period (Baroudi 1984; Shermak et al. 2006).

For pre-surgical marking, we positioned the patient in horizontal dorsal decubitus. It starts with a vertical line from the xiphoid process to the vulvar commissure (xx′). Two straight lines are transverse and parallel to each other: (A) crossing the pubis of about 6–7 cm above the vulvar commissure and (B) at the upper pole of the umbilicus. Over the line (A), points 1 and 2 are marked and bilaterally positioned on the external limits of the pubis. Starting from the anterior superior iliac spines, an arcuate line reaches the navel. Once again, from points 1 and 2, two vertical and parallel lines bilaterally with respect to xx′ are applied on the arcuate line A, with the numbers 3 and 4 and with the numbers 5 and 6 at line B. Stitching1–3–5 as well as 2–4–6 should be bilaterally level to obtain maximum symmetry in the final suture line of the surgery. Provisional stitches are applied about 1–2–5–6 at the start of surgery to serve as a reference. At the end of the skin markings, there will be a medium segment over the pubic region with a variable length of 10–12 cm according to its limits, 6 to 7 cm away from the vulvar commissure. Two slightly arcuate lateral lines run from the ends of the pubic segment to the anterosuperior iliac spines. The skin to be dissected is infiltrated with saline and epinephrine (1:500,000) and the incision with epinephrine (1:200,000) (Baroudi 1984; Shermak et al. 2006).

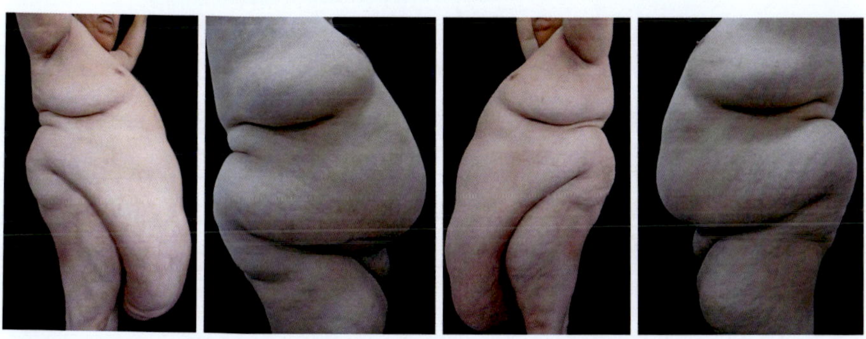

The skin is incised, and the flap is dissected and lifted in the entire internal region of the marking. In the supraumbilical region, detachment should be measured and in the form of a tunnel up to the xiphoid appendix, just enough to allow plication of the anterior abdominal wall, using nonabsorbable 2–0 sutures. After plication, we fixed the flap in the pubis to measure the resection, and the new umbilical scar was marked using the Avelar technique. Bipartite flaps are resected, and bilaterally, we perform rigorous hemostasis and Baroudi stitches along the entire length of the supraumbilical tunnel. (Donnabella 2013; Kaluf et al. 2008; Franco et al. 2006).

After flap resection, the puboplasty is marked, where the pubis in its deep fascia is detached, and it is reattached to the aponeurosis with U stitches and nonabsorbable suture. Then, a tubular drain is placed in the infraumbilical region and synthesis is performed in three planes. (Donnabella 2013; Kaluf et al. 2008; Franco et al. 2006).

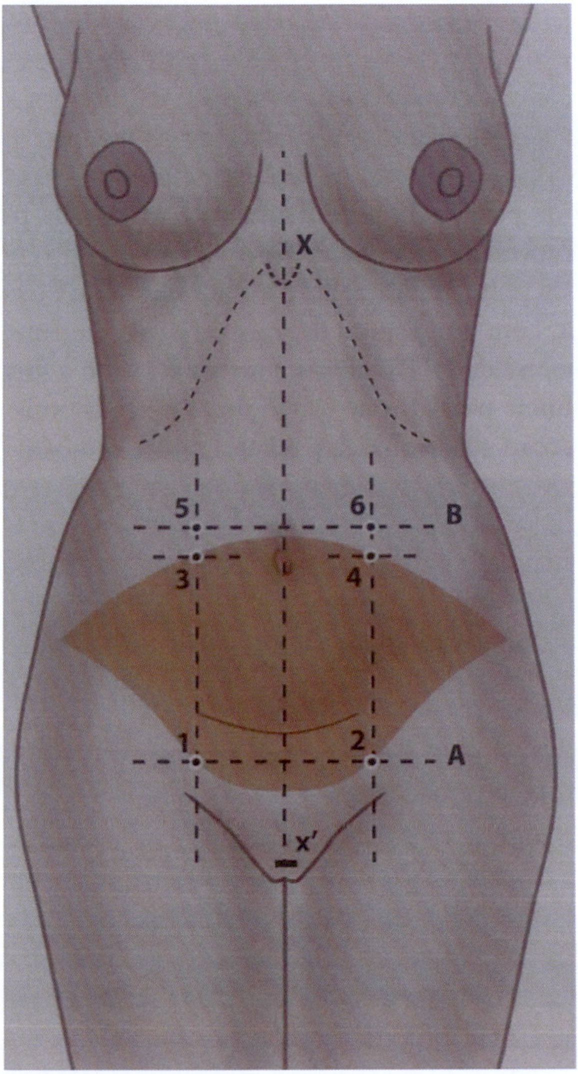

Early walking may be stimulated as soon as possible, preferably in the immediate postoperative period or on the first day after the procedure. The drain is maintained until the second postoperative day, when the patient is discharged from the hospital, except in some cases where the output is still high. The first dressing change is performed on the second postoperative day (Donnabella 2013; Kaluf et al. 2008; Franco et al. 2006).

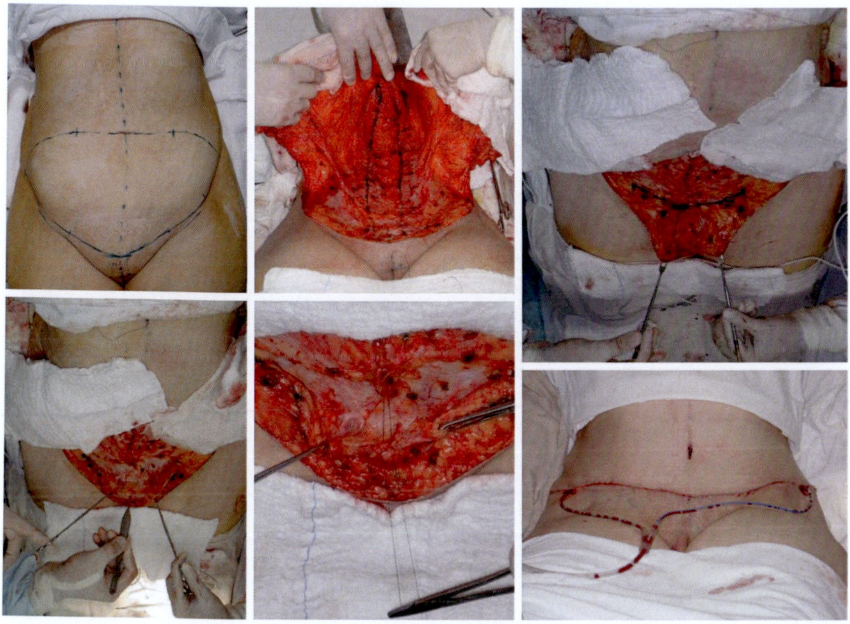

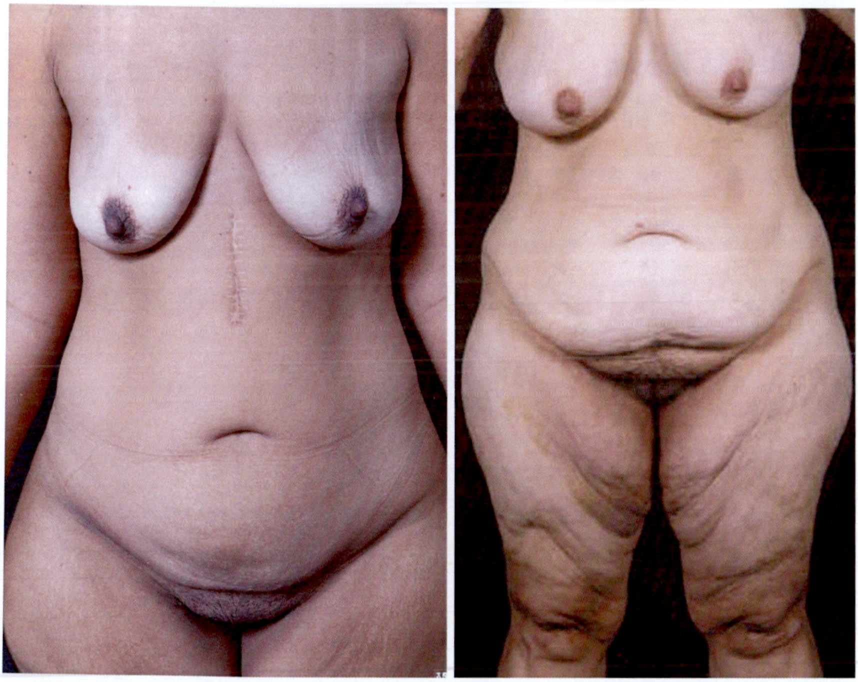

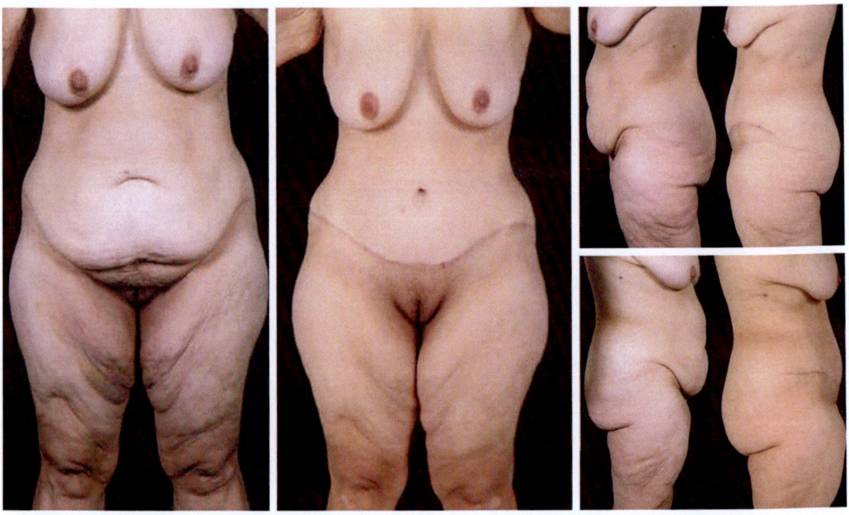

Anterior Anchor-Line Abdominoplasty Approach

The technique is indicated for patients who have a large amount of excess skin, in which resection with vertical traction alone will not be able to produce a satisfactory result. Many of these patients have a vertical scar on the abdomen (open gastroplasty), which could impair the irrigation of the abdominal flap with only horizontal resection and could not be resected by this technique, which would maintain the stigma of an apparent scar in the abdominal region in these patients. Although video gastroplasties are increasingly frequent, the benefits that the vertical component of the scar can bring despite its scarring sequel should be discussed with patients after major weight loss (Donnabella 2013; Kaluf et al. 2008).

Surgical marking is performed with the patient standing, marking the xiphopubic midline, taking due care for possible deviations that excess tissue may cause. We marked the patient's horizontal creases at the level of the iliac spines to guide the horizontal resection. With the patient in the supine position, we performed the bimanual crease to mark the limits of vertical resection (like Pitanguy's maneuver in breasts). Attention should be paid to the symmetry of the markings to avoid distortions in the midline and possible deviations from the umbilicus. Another important precaution is not to exceed the limit of the xiphoid process so that the scar does not reach the intermammary region. In our routine, we use the Donnabella neo-omphaloplasty technique, with marking of two lateral flaps in the vertical incision, the flaps are marked 17 cm from the upper vertical limit and measure 2.5–3.0 cm in width by 2.5 cm in length. For the horizontal marking, we make light traction on the pubic mound and mark a point 6 cm from the vaginal rim. We continue the horizontal markings for about 5 to 6 cm from the midline, left and right, and then make the marking slightly arched so that the resulting line is parallel to the patient's creases. We perform the puboplasty technique in all patients with pubic ptosis (Donnabella 2013; Kaluf et al. 2008)

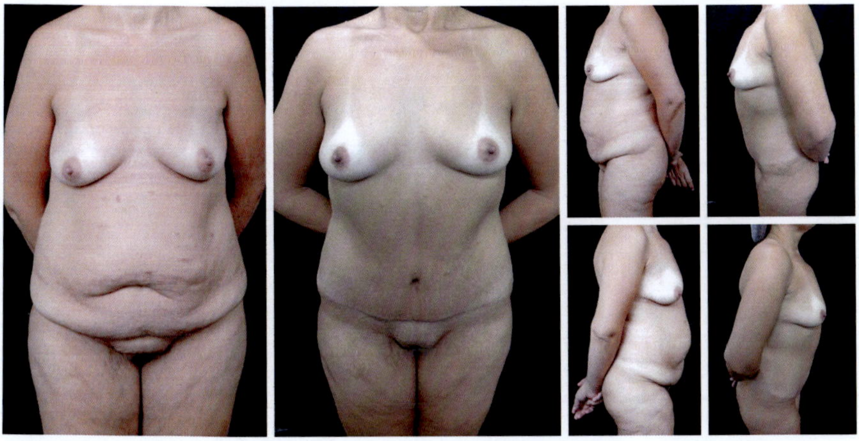

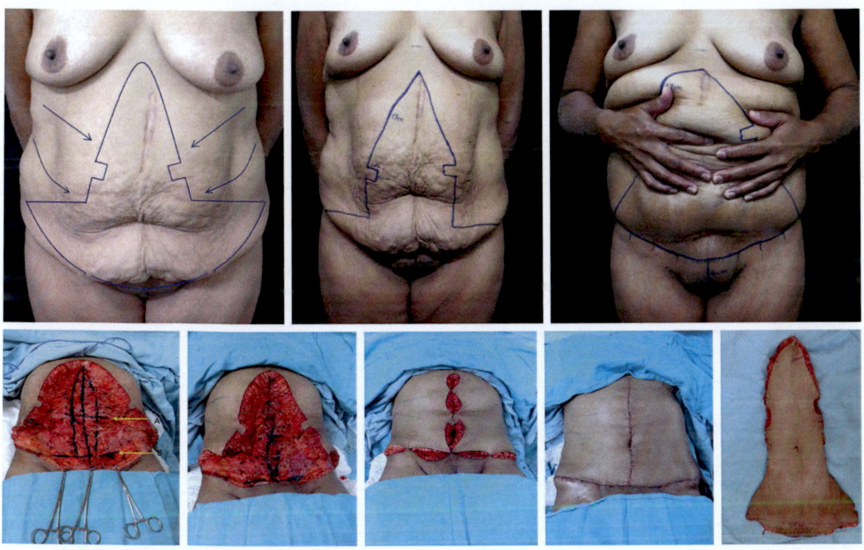

The surgical procedure begins with infiltration of an epinephrine solution (1:200,000) in the incision marks. The entire skin is scratched so as not to lose the marking, and the dissection is performed from lateral to medial and from cranial to caudal in the plane of the aponeurosis, and the flap is resected as a block. During the dissection, care must be taken with the lateral traction of the abdomen to avoid perforating vessel damage. Larger vessels should be stitched with nonabsorbable sutures. Careful amputation of the navel was performed, checking for the presence of umbilical hernias, and umbilical scar suture with nylon 3–0, and then we performed the plication of the rectus abdominis with continuous suture with 2–0 or 0–0 nylon (Donnabella 2013; Kaluf et al. 2008).

The hemostasis is rigorously reviewed and then the patient is placed in the Fowler position; hence, we proceeded to position the drains and synthesis in three planes.

After that, we do the Donnabella neo-umbilicoplasty using three suture stitches (Nylon 4–0) between flaps and the aponeurosis of the rectus abdominis muscle, and two more subdermal stitches (Monocryl 4–0) on the cranial and caudal ends of the flaps (Donnabella 2013; Kaluf et al. 2008).

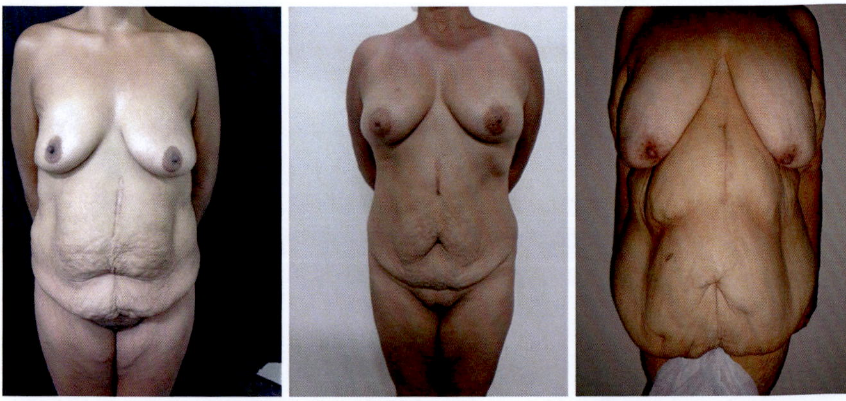

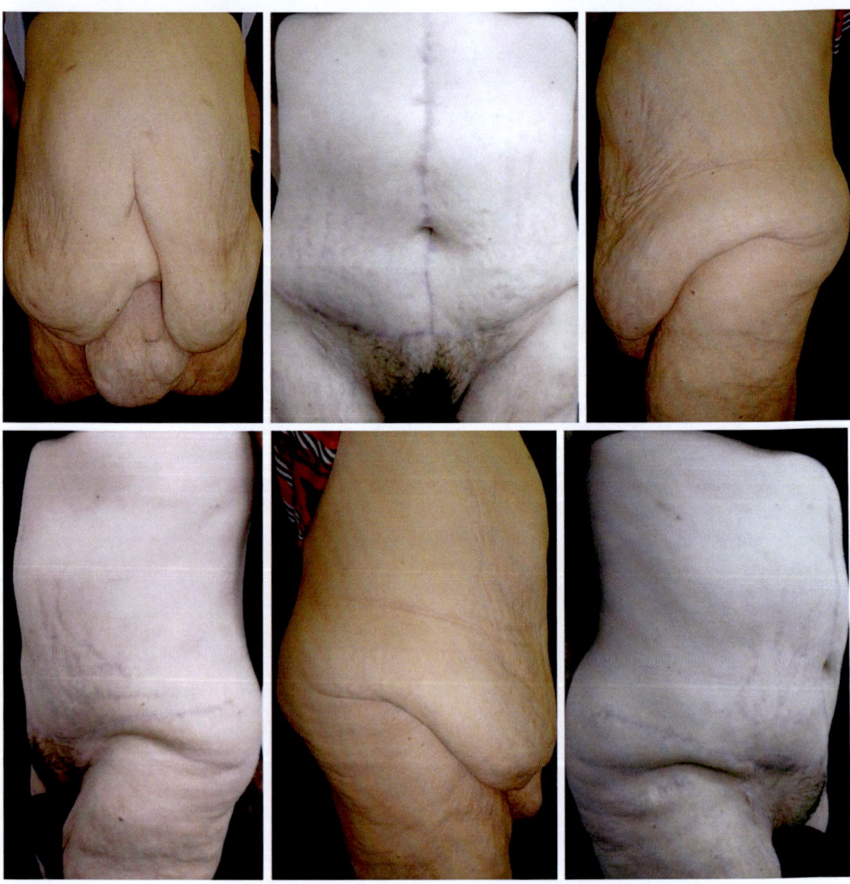

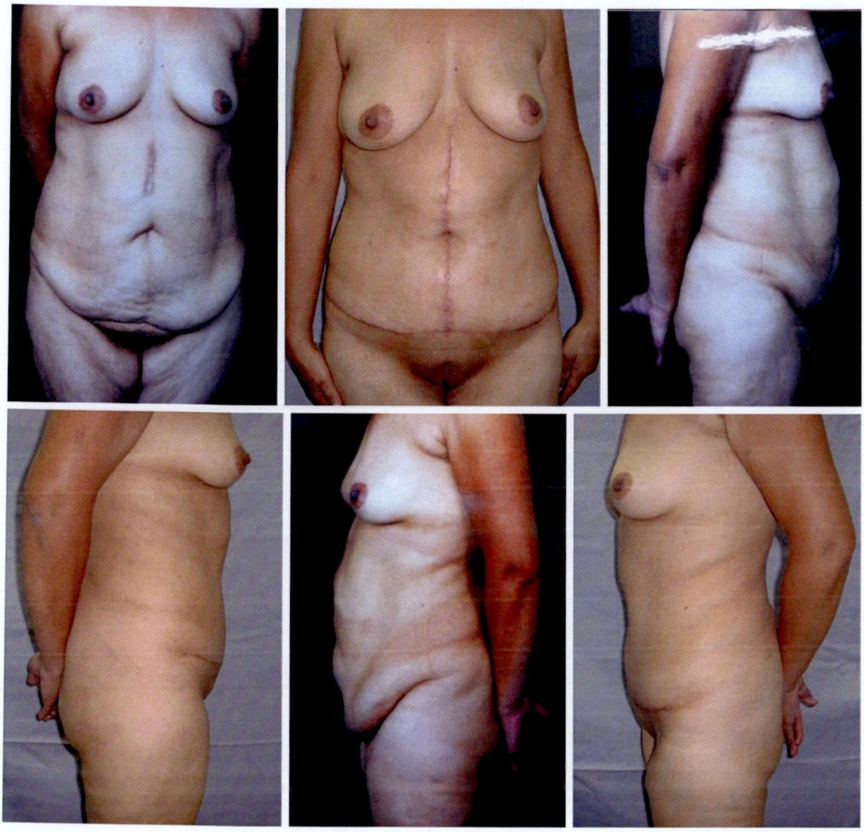

Complications

Seroma is the most frequent complication in post-bariatric abdominoplasties; however, the treatment is usually effective through serial aspiration punctures. Hematomas, flap necrosis, and suture dehiscence may also occur, but are rarer. Good planning including adequate nutritional preparation and technical care with the limitation of detachments prevents seroma formation and other complications. Navel stenoses are no longer a problem after the adoption of the neo-umbilicoplasty (anchor) technique (Kaluf et al. 2008; Zannis et al. 2012).

Conclusion

In the current and variable scenario of post-bariatric patients, the surgeon must evaluate and decide together with the patient what technique is the best indication for each case, considering all the pros and cons of each technique explained above.

References

Karlsson J, Taft C, Rydén A, Sjöström L, Sullivan M. Ten-year trends in health-related quality of life after surgical and conventional treatment for severe obesity. the SOS intervention study. Int J Obes (Lond). 2007;31(8):1248–61.

Shermak MA, Chang D, Magnuson TH, Schweitzer MA. An outcomes analysis of patients undergoing body contouring surgery after massive weight loss. Plast Reconstr Surg. 2006;118(4):1026–31.

Petty P, Manson PN, Black R, et al. Panniculus morbidus, Ann Plast, Surg 1992;28:442–452.

Zannis J, Woods BC, Griffin LP, et al. Outcome study of the surgical management of panniculitis. Ann Plast Surg 2012;68: 194–197

Friedrich JB, Petrov RV, Askay AS, et al. Resection of panniculus morbidus: A salvage procedure with a steep learning curve. Plast Reconstr Surg 2008; 121:108–114

Brown M, Adenuga P, Soutanian H. Massive Panniculectomy in the super obese and super obese: Retrospective Comparison of Primary Closure versus Partial Open Wound Management. Plast Reconst Surg 2014(133): 32–39

Baroudi R. Body Sculpting. Clin Plast Surg. 1984; 11(3): 119–143

Kaluf R, et al. Tratamento da região pubiana na abdominoplastia de pacientes após grande perda ponderal. Rev Soc Bras Cir Plast 2008;23(4):302–304

Donnabella A. Reconstrução anatômica da cicatriz umbilical. Rev Soc Bras Cir Plast 2013;28(1):119–123

Franco D, Medeiros J, Farias C, et al. Umbilical reconstruction for pacientes with midline scar. Aesthetic Plast Surg 2006; 30(5): 595–598.

Chapter 46
Neo-Omphaloplasty in Anchor-Line Abdominoplasty

Alfredo Donnabella

Abstract The change in eating habits in the last years has accompanied the increase in obesity on a global scale. Technological advances have permitted techniques and materials used in bariatric surgeries to improve. Gastroplasties are one of the treatments for obesity, though always accompanied by changes in lifestyle and eating habits.

Introduction

The change in eating habits in the last years has accompanied the increase in obesity on a global scale. Technological advances have permitted techniques and materials used in bariatric surgeries to improve. Gastroplasties are one of the treatments for obesity, though always accompanied by changes in lifestyle and eating habits (Abreu Ng 2010).

The improvement in surgical results and the population's increased access to procedures have added a new category of patients to plastic surgery. After having gastroplasties, patients lose a large quantity of adipose tissue. These patients have bodily changes due to the excess skin. Due to the increasing number of patients who chose to have reparatory plastic surgery to treat dermatolipodystrophy, new studies were required. In addition to new studies, techniques to improve the reestablish the quality of life of these patients had to be developed (Abreu Ng 2010; Song et al. 2005).

A. Donnabella (✉)
Alfredo Donnabella, Belo Horizonte, Brazil

Cristina Oliveira Ribeiro, Belo Horizonte, Brazil

Letícia Abramo Ribeiro, Belo Horizonte, Brazil

Fernanda Pinheiro Manhães, Belo Horizonte, Brazil

J. M. Avelar, R. Cavalcanti Ribeiro (eds.), *Body Contouring*,
https://doi.org/10.1007/978-3-031-42802-9_46

Table 46.1 Pittsburgh scale for the classification of abdominal dermatolipodystrophy

Scale	Characteristics	Proposed treatment
I	Normal	No surgery is required
II	Excess skin Wrinkles Moderate excess of fat, Lack of skinfolds	Mini abdominoplasty or liposuction
III	Paraumbilical skinfold	Classic abdominoplasty
IV	Multiple skinfolds with excess skin in the epigastrium	Modified abdominoplasty, including the fleur-de-lis (anchor-line) or upper body lift

The abdomen is a region that is highly affected by weight loss. Excess skin and folded skin, also known as paraumbilical skinfold, are very common. This makes abdominoplasty in even higher demand with patients after they have undergone bariatric surgery (Barbosa et al. 2009; Cavalcante 2010). A change in anatomy in the genital region is also very common, along with a distortion of the umbilicus. To evaluate patients and treatment programs, we can use the Pittsburgh classification, as proposed by Hurwitz, Rubin, and others who classify the abdomen in four parts (Table 46.1):

This scale is used as a basis to discuss treatment for each patient. A large percentage of patients, post-bariatric surgery, are classified on the scale of III and IV. That means that the appropriate treatment would be anchor-line abdominoplasty. This is a surgery that requires a medium, or conventional, scar. The definition of the best surgery technique takes the Pittsburgh scale into consideration, including an excess of skin in the supraumbilical region, and does not consider a medium scar after having gastroplasty surgery via laparotomy (Song et al. 2005; Craig et al. 2000). The symmetry and esthetics of the abdomen are linked to the placement of the navel. This has been a main factor in abdominoplasty surgery.

The navel should have an anatomical format, be well positioned, without strictures or widenings, so that it seems natural. Approximately 20–30% of patients who undergo bariatric surgeries via laparotomy develop incisional hernias. Often, the abdominal wall's weakness includes the umbilicus. Individuals who have umbilical hernias have an increased risk of ischemia and umbilical necrosis. In those cases, primary neo-omphaloplasty may be a good alternative. This technique has been used a lot by surgeons who do this procedure, not only because it is safe but also due to its esthetic results. The proposal in this chapter is to review and develop abilities to do neo-omphaloplasty and anchor-line abdominoplasty surgeries.

Abdominal/Navel Anatomy

The top of abdominal wall ends at the osteocartilaginous framework of the thorax, at the sides it is hemmed in by anterior axillary line and iliac crest, and at the bottom it is hemmed by inguinal ligaments and the pubic tubercle. The umbilicus is located in the lower middle abdomen (Sisti et al. 2021).

The umbilicus is anatomically defined as a depressed scar, surrounded by a natural fold of skin of approximately 1.5 to 2.5 cm in diameter. Normally you find it described as the height of the line that connects the highest points of the anterior superior iliac crest, between the third and fourth lumbar disks. There can be either upward or downward variation wherein the umbilicus is located, but the consensus is that its most cranial location gives the most attractive esthetic result. The mamelon, the wrinkled part, surrounded by a ring, is the base of the navel, while the cushion consists of an upper part that surrounds the depressed area (Craig et al. 2000; Rohrich et al. 2003).

The umbilicus is a rounded shape, similar to an ellipse, and is normally located between 9 and 12 cm from the pubic symphysis, characterized as important in abdomen esthetics. Its vascularization comes from septocutaneous and musculocutaneous perforating branches of the medial branch of the inferior epigastric artery and the median umbilical ligament. There is an intimate relation of these perforations with the rectus abdominis muscle and its aponeurosis to the base of the navel (Mendes et al. 2019; O'Deya et al. 2004).

Due to the loss of a large part of the adipose tissue and its support, ex-obese people often have a large umbilicus. The larger the vascular pedicle, the larger the chance of having necrosis in this area. This risk increases when there are incisional and umbilical hernias.

Material and Method

So that the reconstruction can be as close to ideal as possible, all anatomical units (mamelon, umbilical ring, and cushion) must be reconstructed step by step. The umbilicus can be completely removed during surgery. To reconstruct the umbilicus, due to the hernias, destroyed by previous surgeries, or esthetic reasons, two flaps in the form of parallel trapeziums are sutured together and fixed to the aponeurosis of the rectus abdominis muscles. These trapeziums should measure 1.5 cm in height by 2.0 cm in width at their distal positions and 3.0 cm at their base, but they can be slightly larger (Donnabella 2013; Donnabella et al. 2016). The transition of the flaps with the skin must be done not in a straight line but curvilinear. This is because the same curvilinear form must be kept in the distal (Fig. 46.1).

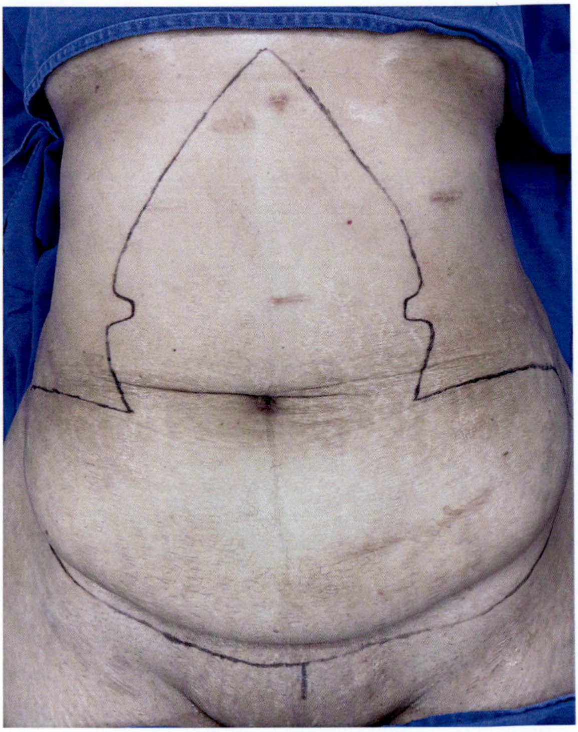

Fig. 46.1 Preoperative marking of the whole area to be removed. Definition of two trapezoidal flaps that will shape the neoumbilicus

Surgical Marks

In a classic abdominoplasty, the navel is an important reference point, but in an anchor-line abdominoplasty, it is isn't used as a parameter at all. In a didactic way, the abdomen is divided into two geometric figures, an ellipse and an isosceles triangle. The final figure will be an ellipse with a triangle in the upper portion. All abdominal marks must be done to promote tissue traction, in the direction that they will remain after the surgery. For instance, the pubic region should be done cranially and the epigastric region caudally and medially.

The most caudal point of the ellipse, denominated point C (Fig. 46.2) should be 5–7 cm from the anterior commissure of a woman's labia and 6–8 cm from the base of a man's penis. Normally, this spot coincides with the pubic symphysis. From this spot, a slightly arched lateral line is traced to the left and right (this line is more arched on a woman, less on a man). The final point of this line is defined by the surgeon; in some cases the left and right parts can be on the midline of the back, creating a mark in circumferential abdominoplasty. This is the lower limit marking in an abdominoplasty.

Next, the lateral excess is then marked. With a bidigital maneuver of tissue approximation, traction is carried out on the excess tissue of the supraumbilical region in the medial direction. The overlapping of the excess tissue must be made, avoiding a maneuver that promotes their pinching (Fig. 46.2). In this way, you can define the excess tissue and feel the tightness of the skin that you aim to reach at the end of the surgery. A bidigital maneuver increases the closing of the wound

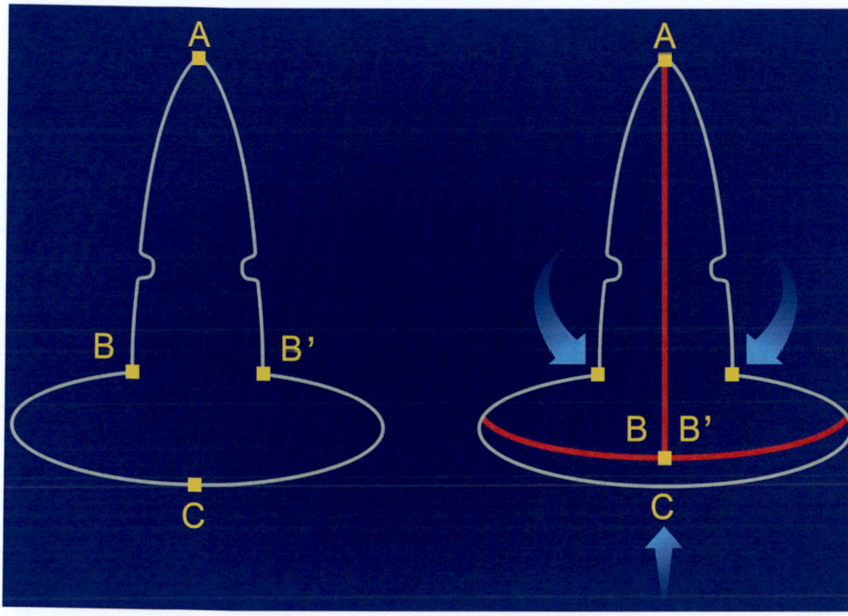

Fig. 46.2 Surgical marking scheme simulating the movement of tissues. Observe the union of points B, B′, and C creating a sole stitch at the end of the surgery

side-to-side, protecting against excess drying. On approaching the tissues, the points of contact between them are marked. Repeating this down the abdomen, there are several points down each side of the middle line, linking the points on each side by tracing an oblique, or curvilinear, line. The two lines will unite in their most cranial portion, the final point of these lines we will call point A. These two lines make up the identical sides of the isosceles triangle.

The definition of the two inferior points on these two lateral lines, points named B and B′, are the most difficult parts of the marking. We will call these lateral lines AB and AB′. At the end of the markings of B and B′, they meet point C.

Since A and C were defined earlier and knowing that B and B′ will meet C, the distance between A and C is measured. This measurement is transferred to the lines AB and AB′, defined by B and B. As the descent of the lateral flaps isn't done only in the caudal direction, and is instead done in the caudal and medial directions, it's necessary to add a few centimeters in the measurement between points A and C. However, the measurement between lines AB and AB′ will be measurement between the points A and C plus 3 cm. Remembering that those measurements will always be done pulling the tissues in the direction, they will be in after the surgery.

Marking the space where the new navel will be is done in a distance of 10 cm between the points B and B′, though in elongated patients this distance may be a bit larger (Fig. 46.2).

Often these patients have a large excess of tissue to be treated. The distortion caused by the weight of these surgical pieces is common. A marking that has been well done and re-enforced pre-surgery and that doesn't go away during surgery is absolutely necessary. If new markings are needed, they must be traced on the tissue trying to keep them in the position they should be after the operation. Unfortunately, even with careful planning to keep symmetry, irregularities in the form and position of the scars are common. The same can be said about the positioning of the new navel. It must be centralized and should avoid using the line of stitches to correct the diastasis as a reference. This is because the diastasis may be to the side, which leads to an incorrect positioning of the navel.

The approximation of the flaps after the resection of excess tissue must be done without tension. The use of adhesion sutures is essential to prevent seromas, delimit hematomas, and fix the tissues, avoiding distortions in the position of the scars or the new navel (Figs. 46.3 and 46.11).

The fixing of the flaps is done on the midline of the aponeurosis, then the flaps are joined from one side to the other with two parallel stitches that reach the dermis (Figs. 46.4, 46.5, 46.6, and 46.7).

In this way, there is a light compression on the distal part of the flaps when they are joined, creating the shape and reconstructing the mamelon. The inclusion of the dermis of the shortened suture will give a wrinkled appearance, similar to the umbilical indent (Fig. 46.8).

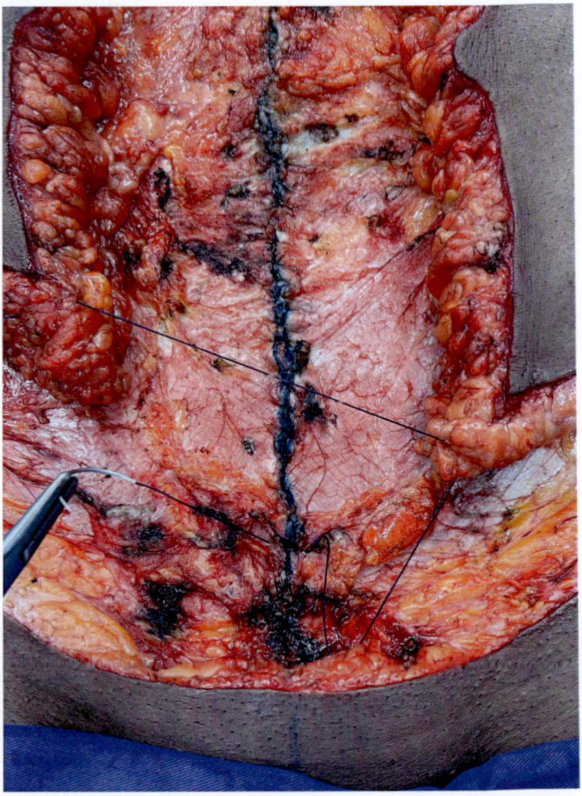

Fig. 46.3 Union of points B, B′, and C through the Scarpa's fascia, including the aponeurosis of the rectus abdominis muscle creating an adhesion stitch. All the suturing line will be made with this type of adhesion stitch

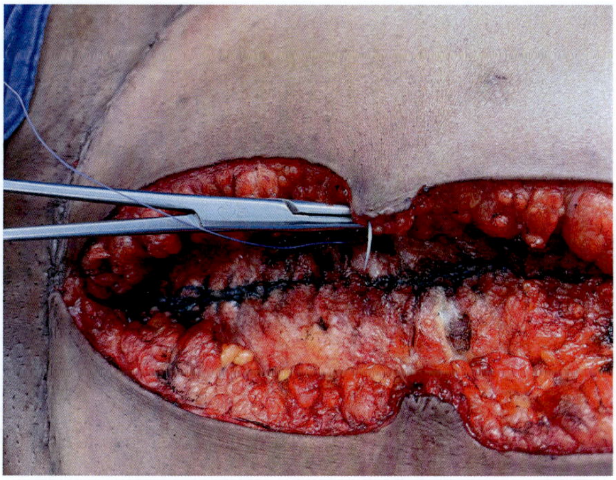

Fig. 46.4 Stitch of Vicryl 2–0 that will make the fixation of flaps in order to create the neoumbilicus. This stitch includes the dermis in order to achieve a better fixation for the flaps to the aponeurosis

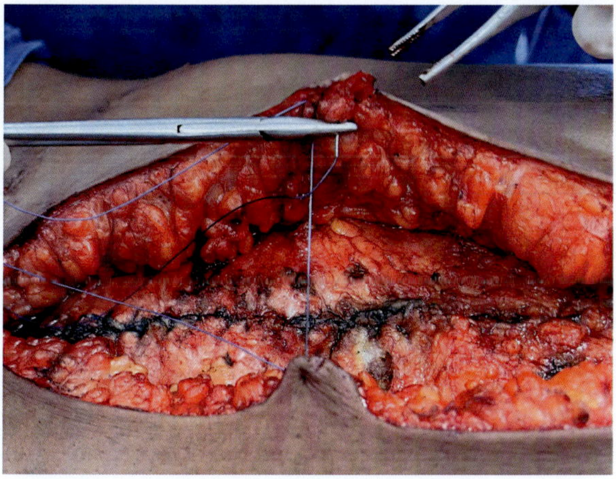

Fig. 46.5 Second stitch of suture parallel to the first, uniting the two opposite trapezoidal flaps

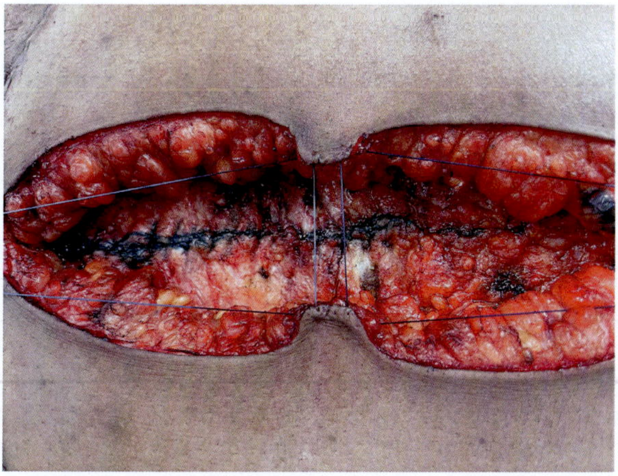

Fig. 46.6 View of both parallel suture stitches. Observe the stitches of depression in the patches caused by the suture encompassing the dermis. This inclusion of the dermis in the suture stitches will provide a better fixation of the flaps allowing the creation of the ring

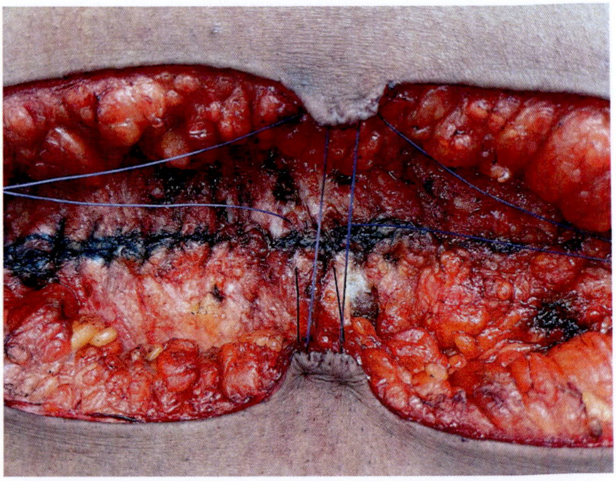

Fig. 46.7 View of two parallel suture stitches encompassing the aponeurosis. Observe that the distance between two parallel stitches in the patch is the same of the aponeurosis

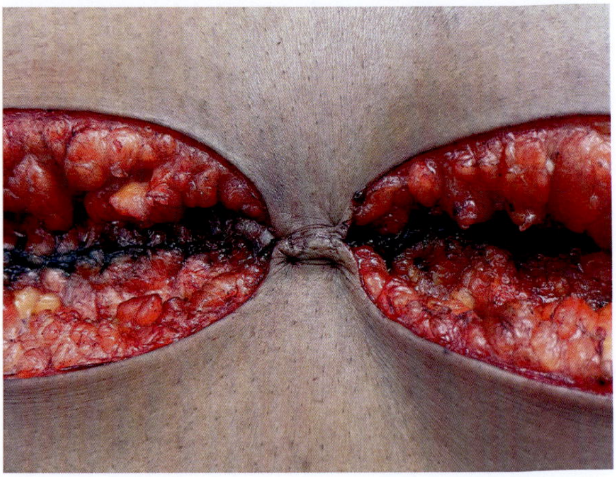

Fig. 46.8 Final aspect of the fixation of the flaps to the aponeurosis. Discrete compression between both flaps. Beginning of the formation of the ring and the mamelon

Afterward, an approximation of the fatty tissue around the new umbilicus is created with Vicryl®1 (polyglactin) and a 4-cm needle (Fig. 46.9). This elevates the sides of the umbilicus so that the correct depth can be achieved. Ideally, a large needle would be used to encompass and tighten the fatty tissue as much as possible. Once it is no longer possible to deepen the mamelon further than the aponeurosis, it is possible to obtain the effect of depth by increasing the tissue around the neo-navel. The main tissue available to move is the fatty tissue, so moving the periumbilical fat is essential to define the depth of the neo-navel. The technique is delicate, and a lot of care is required to move it, as there is the risk of tissue injury (Figs. 46.10 and 46.11).

Bringing the stitches together must be done with caution, because if they are done too tightly, liponecrosis may occur. Consequently, there is a higher risk of tissue dehiscence and the loss of the correct format. The procedure is finished when

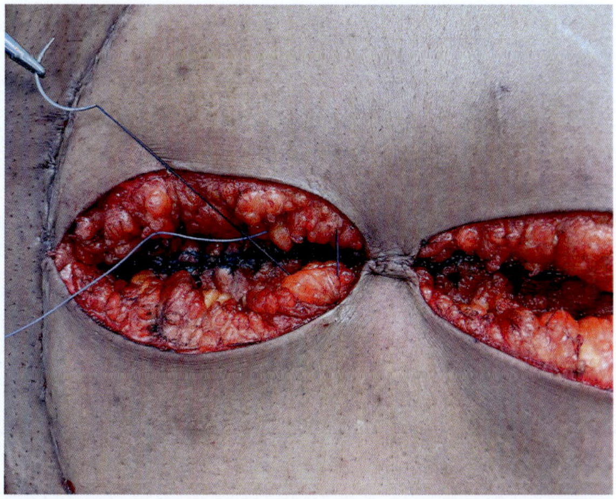

Fig. 46.9 Creation of a stitch point to approach the periumbilical fat to promote elevation of the borders of the neoumbilicus and provide better depth for it

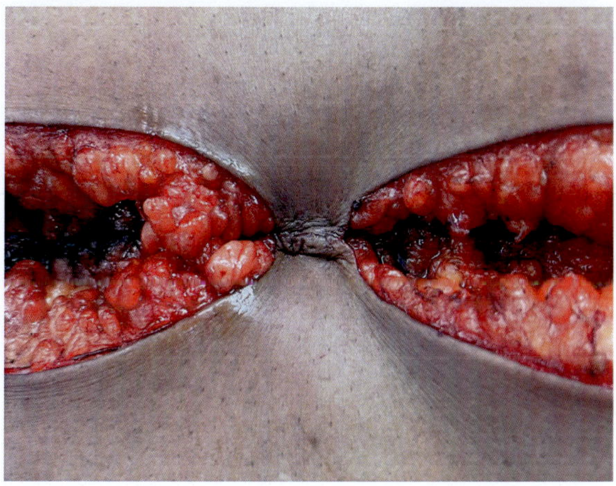

Fig. 46.10 Avoid tightening the suture too much in order to avoid liponecrosis. Stitches supra and infraumbilical are made

the skin is sutured (Fig. 46.12). With the final suture, once the flaps are cut, there will be a curving of the skin around the new umbilicus, creating its rounded shape (Fig. 46.13).

The figures below show the pre- and postoperative period of patients undergoing the technique. Patients have a natural-looking abdomen, with scars well positioned in natural folds of the body and good definition of the neoumbilicus (Figs. 46.14 and 46.15).

In a late postoperative period, we can observe the neoumbilicus with good depth, good positioning, and natural appearance. One of the great advantages of this technique is having a new navel without the stigma of an operated abdomen (Fig. 46.16).

One can observe the complete social reintegration of the patients with the new appearance of the abdomen, having a neoumbilicus without apparent scars and with all its anatomical units reconstructed (Fig. 46.17).

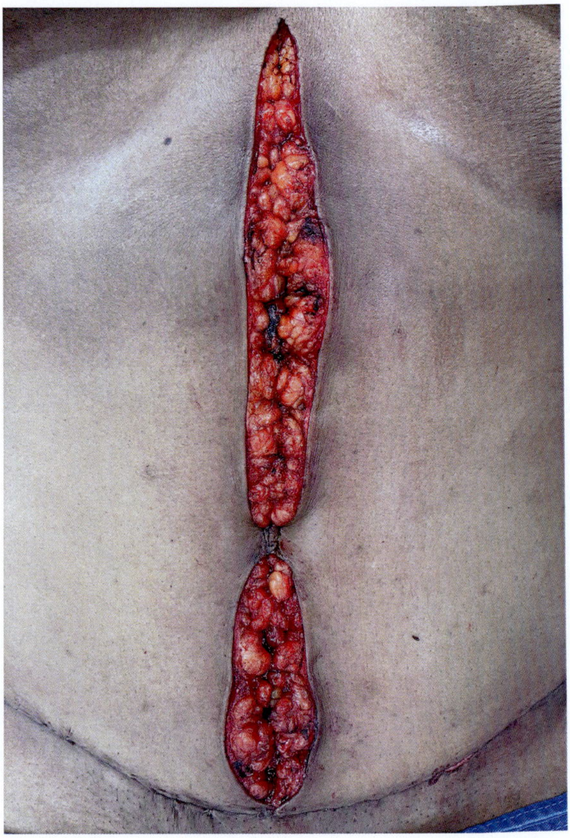

Fig. 46.11 Approximation of all the fat with closure of the spaces and use of adhesion stitches

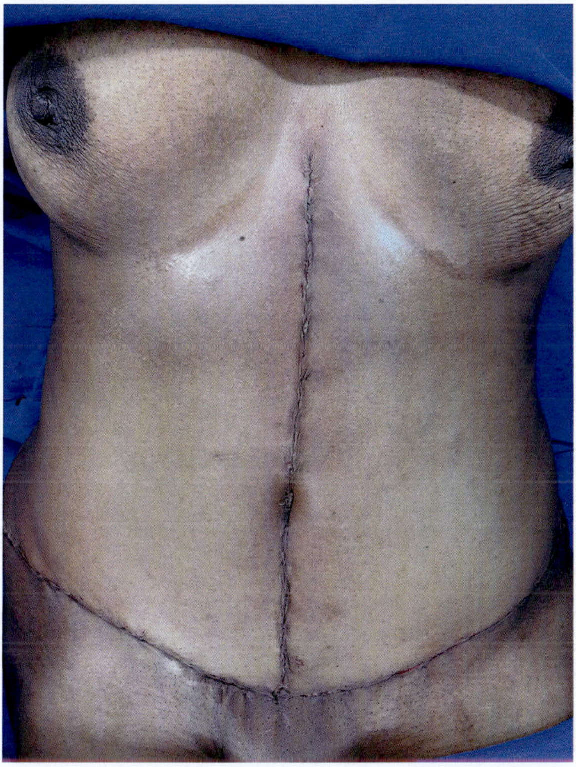

Fig. 46.12 Final aspect of the surgery

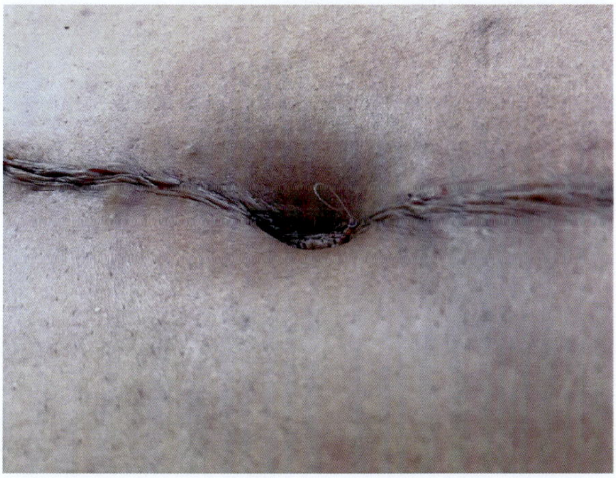

Fig. 46.13 Neoumbilicus with a good conformation. The reconstruction of all anatomic units of the navel was complete providing a good depth

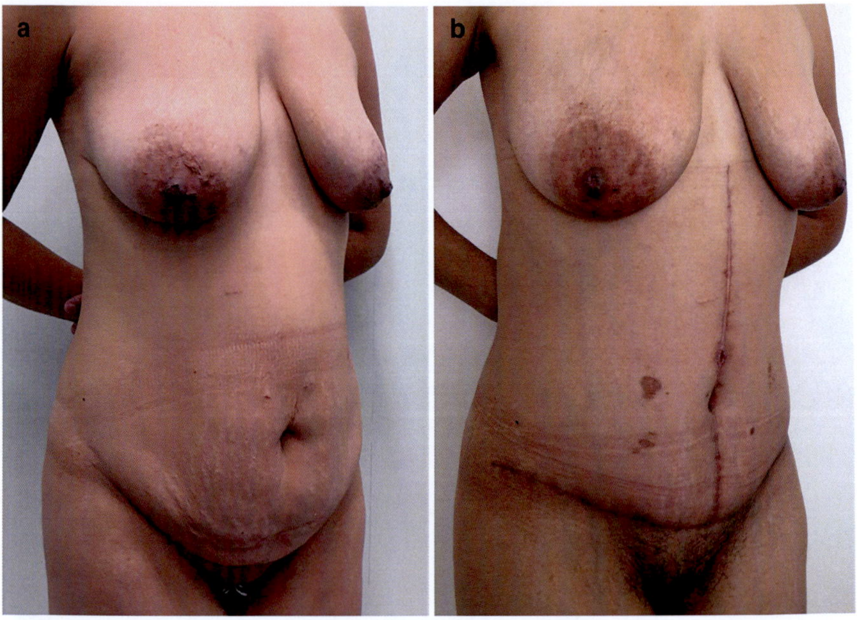

Fig. 46.14 (**a**) Preoperative aspect of the abdomen. (**b**) Postoperative aspect of the abdomen

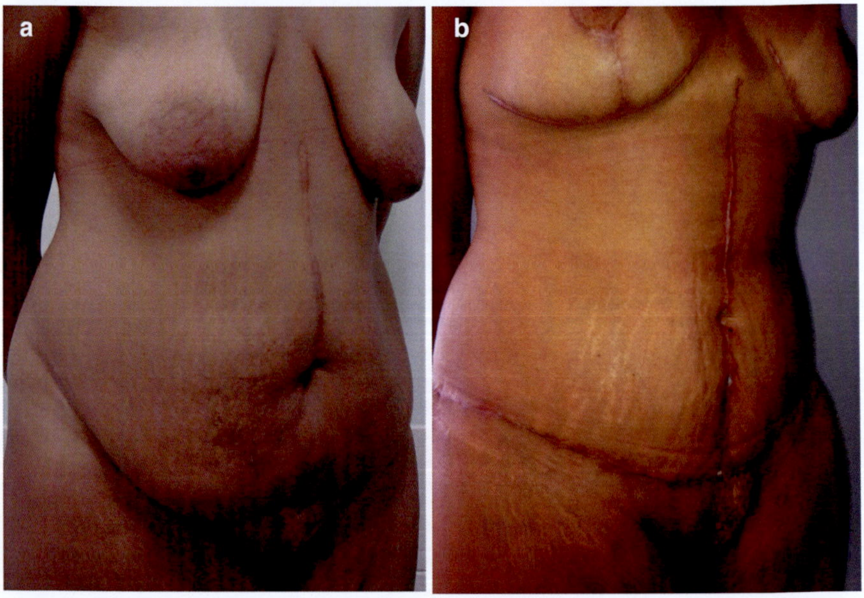

Fig. 46.15 (**a**) Preoperative aspect of the abdomen. (**b**) Postoperative aspect of the abdomen

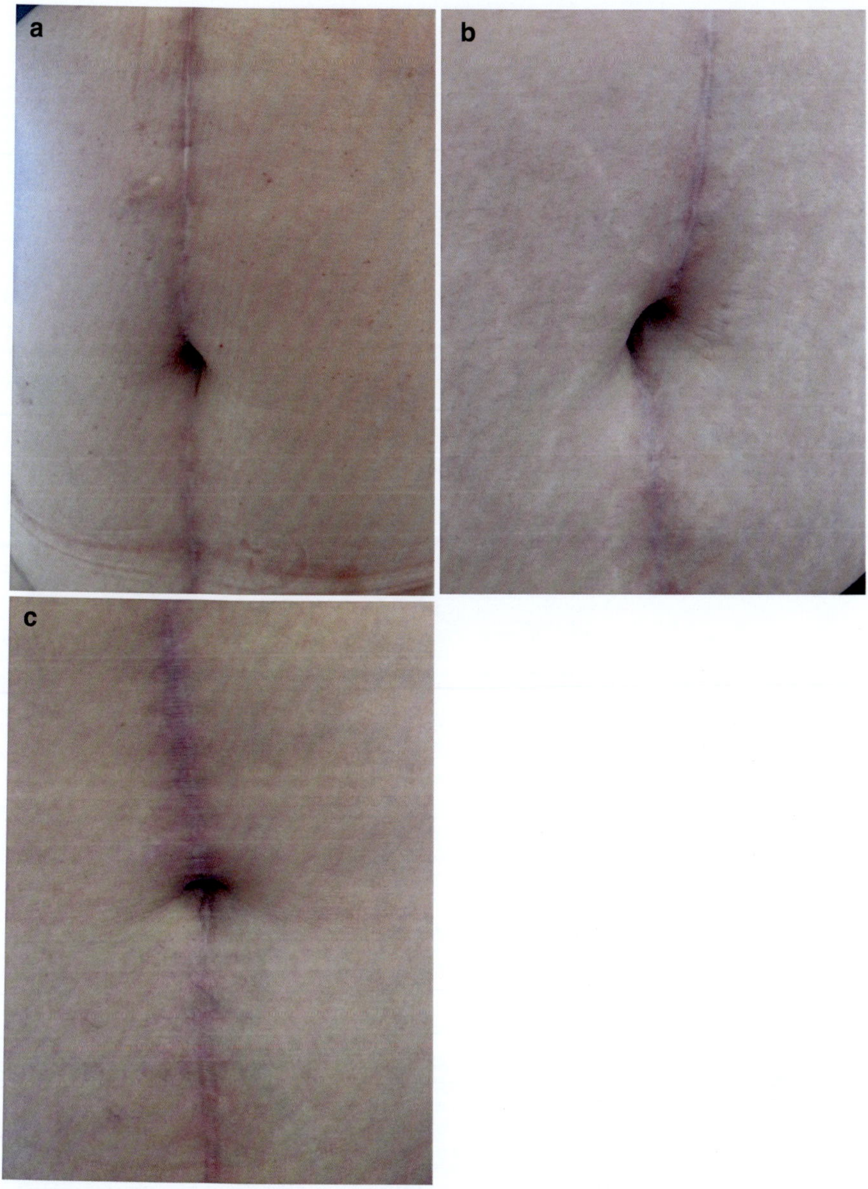

Fig. 46.16 (**a**) Postoperative aspect of the neoumbilicus. (**b**) Postoperative aspect of the neoumbilicus. (**c**) Postoperative aspect of the neoumbilicus

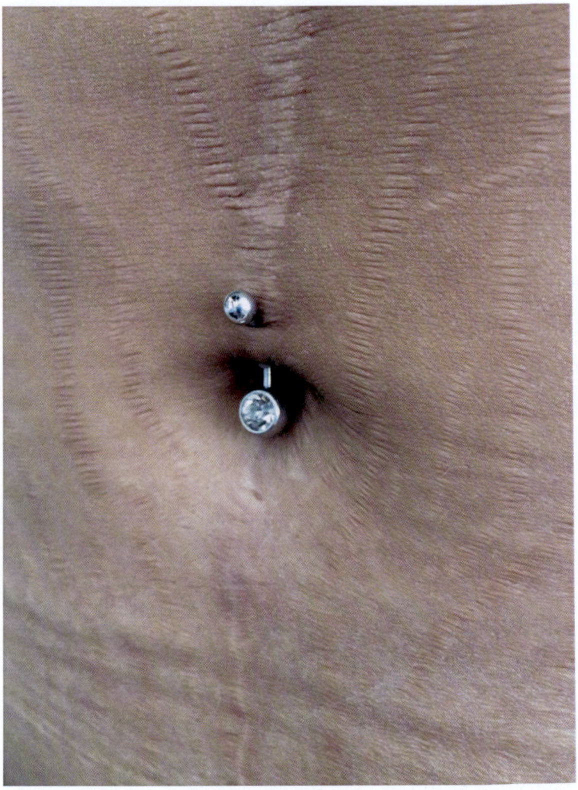

Fig. 46.17 Natural aspect of the neoumbilicus allowing the use of piercing. This aspect enables the patients' full social integration

Discussion

Our objective is to delve into the proposed technique, which is to obtain all the anatomical parts (mamelon, ring, and cushion), as well as have the right depth in the reconstructed navel scars. Once the new umbilicus doesn't have a circular scar around it, a possible stenosis is avoided, along with the stigma of an operated abdomen.

Even though pathological scarring can occur on the vertical supra- or infraumbilical scar, normally a hypertrophic scar or keloid shouldn't form on the new umbilicus. The reconstruction becomes even more natural over time. It's expected that after a few months skin ptosis occurs in the cranial portion of the reconstructed umbilicus. This creates a discrete pleat which gives the final reconstruction a more natural look.

The flaps should be kept at 1.5–2.0/3.0 cm so that the umbilicus stays small and esthetically pleasing. Other indications for the use of this technique include a post-navel resection reconstruction due to endometriosis or post-omphalocele. Then, it can be used for the correction of different parts and defects of the umbilicus.

Silva and Abramo (2010) and Vallim et al. (2017) contributed with a strategy to determine the height of the umbilicus on the abdomen, which can be used with this new technique of reconstruction in anchor-line abdominoplasty surgeries. The aforementioned technique is to leave a larger flap of skin to later define the flap of 1.5–2.0/3.0 cm safely.

In particular, patients with a large weight loss and a scarcity of adipose tissue may have difficulties obtaining the depth of the neo-navel (Marconi 1995; Mendes and Viterbo 2018; Silva and Oliveira 2017). In the technique set out here, because it is concerned with contemplating and approaching the adjacent fatty tissue, this issue can be resolved. It's important to keep the curve at the base of the flap and to avoid straight lines. This stops the sides getting too close and, in this way, creates a rounded navel, rather than a long, closed scar. Silva and Abramo (2010) later changed their original technique and also suggested that a 90° angle should be avoided at the base of the flaps to try to improve the final aspects of the new navels. The reconstruction of the mamelon requires an open bottom in a "U" shape, to avoid a close navel in the shape of a "V."

In anchor-line abdominoplasty, there is a medium scar that extends to the xiphoid appendix, or above it, to the pubic region (Mendes et al. 2019; Guerrerosantos et al. 1980). When the umbilical stump is preserved and is externalized through the median scar, this scar is crossed with an upper and lower rectilinear portion interrupted by a rounded scar corresponding to the outward navel. When the neo-navel is done, this situation doesn't occur, what does happen is there is a single, straight scar with a depression that corresponds anatomically with the new navel in a more natural way.

Conclusion

The reconstruction based on anatomical parts is the principle of plastic surgery. The technique described for the reconstruction of the navel respects the characteristics of the umbilical scar and is presented as a good alternative. It corresponds with the harmonious shape of the new navel which becomes more natural over time, when a portion of skin drops over the top part. Therefore, with this technique we can obtain an umbilicus with a good depth and size and that looks natural. This moves away from the classic image of an operated navel, as you only have a slight scar only in the upper portion of the neo-navel.

References

Abreu Ng JA. Abdominoplastias: neo-onfaloplastias sem cicatriz e sem excisão de gordura. Rev. Bras. Cir. Plást. 25(3): 499–503,2010

Angela Y. Song, M.D., Raymond D. Jean, M.D., Dennis J. Hurwitz, M.D., Madelyn H. Fernstrom, Ph.D., John A. Scott, M.S., J. Peter Rubin, M.D. A classification of contour deformities after bariatric weight loss: the Pittsburgh rating scale. Plast Reconstr Surg 116:1535–1544,2005.

Barbosa, M.V.J.; Nahas, F.X.; Neto, M.A.S.; Ferreira, L.M. Strategies in umbilical reconstruction. Journal of Plastic, Reconstructive & Aesthetic Surgery 62:e147–e150, 2009

Cavalcante ELF. Neo-umbilicoplasty as an option in umbilical reconstruction in abdominal anchor dermolipectomy post gastroplasty. Rev. Bras. Cir. Plast. 25(3):509–18,2010

Craig SB, Faller MS, Puckett CL. In search of the ideal female umbilicus. Plast Recontr Surg 105:389–392,2000

Sisti A, Huayllani MT, Boczar D, Restrepo DJ, Cinotto G, Lu X, Cuomo R, Grimaldi L, Nisi G, Forte AJ. Umbilical reconstruction techniques: a literature review. Aesth Plast Surg. 45:1078–96,2021

Rohrich RJ, Sorokin ES, BrownSA, Gibby DL. Is the umbilicus truly midline? Clinical and medicolegal implications. Plast Recontr Surg 112:259–263,2003

Mendes FH, Donnabella A, Moreira ARF. Fleur-de-lis abdominoplasty and neo-umbilicus. Clinics in Plastic Surgery. 46(1):49–60,2019

O'Deya, D.M.; Heimburga, D.V.; Prescherb, A.; Palluaa, N. The arterial vascularisation of the abdominal wall with special regard to the umbilicus. The British Association of Plastic Surgeons 57:392–397,2004

Donnabella A. Anatomical reconstruction of the umbilicus. Rev. Bras. Cir. Plást. 28:119–123,2013

Donnabella A, Neffa L, Barros BB, Santos FP. Abdominoplasty after bariatric surgery: experience in 315 cases. Rev. Bras. Cir. Plast. 31(4):510–515,2016

Silva FN, Abramo E. Neo-onfaloplastia na abdominoplastia vertical. Rev Bras Cir Plast 25:330–336,2010

Vallim MG, Calderoni DR, Bueno MA, Motta MM, Basso RC, Kharmandayan P. Patient versus surgeon preferences between traditional and neo-omphaloplasty in post-bariatric abdominoplasty. Aesthet Plast Surg 41:102–107,2017

Marconi F. Reconstruction of the umbilicus: a simple technique. Plast Recontr Surg 95:1115–1117,1995

Mendes FH, Viterbo F. Inner scar umbilicus: new horizons for vertical abdominoplasty. Plast Reconstr Surg. 141(4):507e–16e,2018

Silva FN, Oliveira EA. Neo-umbilicus in vertical abdominoplasty. Adult umbilical reconstruction principles and techniques. 144–57,2017

Guerrerosantos J, Dicksheet S, Carrillo C, Sandoval M. Umbilical reconstruction with secondary abdominoplasty. Ann Plast Surg 5:139–144,1980

Chapter 47
Post-Bariatric Cruroplasty

Moacyr Pires de Mello Fillho, Rolf Gemperli, Otávio Machado de Almeida, Fernando José Gatto Ribeiro de Oliveira, and Marcos Bandiera Paiva

Abstract Patients with major weight loss after treatment for obesity have significant body contour deformities in the inferior limbs due to flaccidity and loss of skin turgor, especially on the medial surface of the thigh, which can cause great discomfort to the patient, in addition to the possibility of developing dermatitis and recur-

M. P. de Mello Fillho (✉)
Brazilian Society of Plastic Surgery, São Paulo, SP, Brasil

University of Sao Paulo School of Medicine, São Paulo, SP, Brasil

Brazilian Society for Bariatric and Metabolic Surgery, São Paulo, SP, Brasil

De Mello Plastic Surgery, São Paulo, SP, Brasil

R. Gemperli
Disciplina de Cirurgia Plástica da Faculdade de Medicina da USP, São Paulo, SP, Brasil

Departamento de Cirurgia do Hospital das Clínicas da FMUSP, São Paulo, SP, Brasil

O. M. de Almeida
Especialista da SBCP, São Paulo, SP, Brasil

Cirurgia Plástica Pela FMUSP, São Paulo, SP, Brasil

Ciências Médicas Pela Fundação Antônio Prudente, São Paulo, SP, Brasil

F. J. G. R. de Oliveira
Head and Neck Surgery Beneficencia Portuguesa Hospital, São Paulo, SP, Brasil

Plastic Surgery Beneficencia Portuguesa Hospital, São Paulo, SP, Brasil

Former Member of the Plastic Surgery Technical Chamber of the Sao Paulo State Regional Council of Medicine, São Paulo, SP, Brasil

Clínica Gatto, São João da Boa Vista, SP, Brasil
e-mail: fernando@gatto.com.br

M. B. Paiva
Brazilian Society for Head and Neck Cancer, São Paulo, SP, Brasil

Head and Neck Surgery Federal University of Sao Paulo, Paulista School of Medicine, São Paulo, SP, Brasil

J. M. Avelar, R. Cavalcanti Ribeiro (eds.), *Body Contouring*,
https://doi.org/10.1007/978-3-031-42802-9_47

rent infections in the region. Guided physical exercises associated with a well-oriented diet may obtain a satisfactory esthetic result. However, in order to obtain an esthetic result, crural dermolipectomy may offer the best therapeutic alternative. This surgery requires from the plastic surgeon a great knowledge of the local anatomy and the possible techniques that are used to obtain an adequate result, minimizing the risk of complications.

Introduction

Patients with significant weight loss after treatment for obesity have significant body contour deformities in the inferior limbs due to flaccidity and loss of skin turgor, especially on the medial surface of the thigh, which can cause great discomfort to the patient, in addition to the possibility of developing dermatitis and recurrent infections in the region. Guided physical exercises associated with a well-oriented diet may obtain a satisfactory esthetic result. However, in order to obtain an esthetic result, crural dermolipectomy may offer the best therapeutic alternative. This surgery requires from the plastic surgeon a great knowledge of the local anatomy and the possible techniques that are used to obtain an adequate result, minimizing the risk of complications.

As in other parts of the body, the deformity of the thighs depends on the individual pattern of fat deposit and the quality and quantity of the skin in the area. Thus, patients who did not have excessive fat volume in the lower limbs may not need treatment after weight loss, while individuals who had a large increase in the volume of fat on the thighs will probably present sagging skin after weight loss, justifying surgical treatment. Several surgical techniques may be used in plastic surgery of the lower limbs, depending on the location, pattern of lipodystrophy, and skin flaccidity.

In Brazil, about 10% of the longitudinal crural dermolipectomy (**LoCr**) performed solves the sagging of the inner thigh from its root to the level of the knee. Helicoidal crural dermolipectomy (**HeCr**) is performed in 8% to 10% of cases of flaccidity and lipodystrophy of the upper internal and external third of the thigh, while lateral crural dermolipectomy (**LaCr**) solves flaccidity and lipodystrophy in the trochanteric region. This last procedure is less used and performed in about 2% of cases. Other techniques still used, but with reservations, are called atypical dermolipectomy (**AtCr**), which are responsible for approximately 2% of cases and would be indicated for patients (cases) who present flaccidity and lipodystrophy located throughout the extension of the thigh. In these cases, we find a true aberration of form and flaccidity, which is considered by some authors as lymphedema of the lower limbs and occasionally will require several surgical procedures (Fig. 47.1).

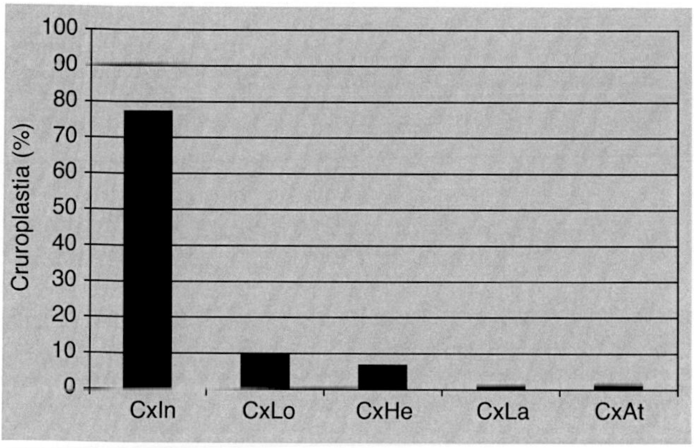

Fig. 47.1 Comparing different cruroplasty techniques. InCr (thigh suspension): dermolipectomy of the upper inner third of the thigh, 78%. LoCr (longitudinal dermolipectomy): inner thigh dermolipectomy, 10%. HeCr (helicoidal dermolipectomy): dermolipectomy of the upper inner and outer third of the thigh, 8%. LaCr (lateral trochanteric dermolipectomy): dermolipectomy of the upper outer third of the thigh, 2%. CxAt (atypical dermolipectomy): varied dermolipectomy over the entire length of the thigh, 2%

Historic Evolution

Surgical techniques involving resection of sagging skin in the lower limbs were initially described by Lewis in 1957 (REWIS 1957). Despite this, the medial suspension of the thighs was not well accepted, as it presented unreliable results and important scarring sequelae. The suspension of the thighs and gluteal region using the technique of Pitanguy (1964) excised only the ptotic tissues, without suspending and fixing them for better positioning, resulting in flattening and decreased spinal lordosis, characteristic signs of the aging process. Moreover, the scars resulting from the initial techniques were positioned outside the usual line of the swimsuits currently used, in addition to their enlargement, and, in many cases, distortions of the vulva were observed.

In 1982, Teimourian and Adam (1982) described the crural dermolipectomy technique with a medial incision extending to the iliac crest for periosteal fixation, in order to obtain the lifting of the anterior and medial thigh. Based on this author's work, Lockwood (1988) in 1988 introduced a new concept for the suspension of the medial surface of the thighs, by anchoring the skin flap to Colles' fascia, contributing to solving the problem of maintaining the final outcome, mainly addressing the mobility of the scar tissue. This very resistant fascial layer, described by Colles in 1811, represents the superficial fascia of the perineum. In 1990, Lockwood (1992) spread the concept of the superficial fascial system, which is the dominant support structure within the subcutaneous cellular tissue. The superficial fascial system

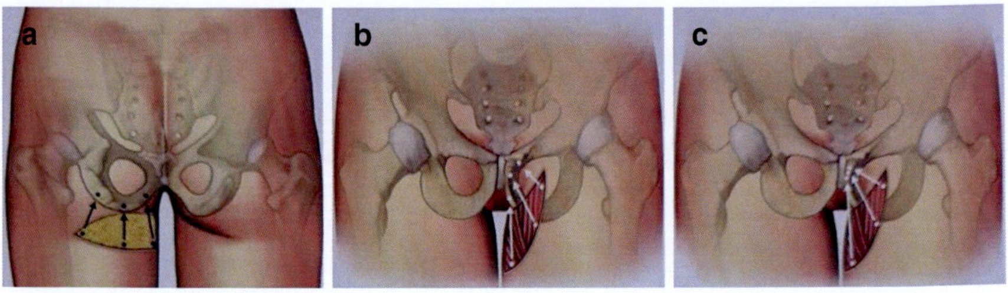

Fig. 47.2 Crural suspension. (**a**) Posterior view of the crural suspension with fixation to the periosteum of the sciatic bone. (**b**) Anterior view of the crural suspension with fixation to the periosteum of the pubis with separate stitches. (**c**) Anterior view of the suspension with fixation to the pubic crest in a single location

would be a highly organized collagen structure responsible for supporting the weight of the subcutaneous cellular tissue. Relaxation of the superficial fascial system results in loss of skin tone. Skin stretching is achieved by attaching this system to rigid structures using permanent suture threads which stabilizes the resulting scar and improves body contour.

Based on this concept, new options for the surgical treatment of the lower limbs emerged, e.g., flancoplasty and abdominoplasty, associating with some situations in a single operative time. Depending on the amount and location of skin laxity in the lower limbs, different types of incisions and resections have been suggested, aiming at the best body contour in this region (PASCAL and LOUARN 2002; LOEB 1979; GUERREROSANTOS 1984; LOUARN and PASCAL 2004; MORALES GARCIA 2003). Some authors recommend the fixation of the skin flap to the periosteum of the pubic and sciatic bones, and in some cases with three distinct points on the flap inferior to three separate points on the periosteum of the pubis, which is an important step in this type of procedure. Because it presents a more complicated and painful postoperative period, De Mello et al. (2002) suggested a technical variation in which the inferior flap was directed and fixed with three different points to a single point in the periosteum of the pubic bone, with similar results and a more comfortable postoperative period (Fig. 47.2).

Physical Examination

With the patient in the orthostatic position and the feet slightly apart, the direction in which there is greater skin excess on the thigh is determined during the physical examination, that is, longitudinal or transverse, in addition to the presence of local infection and presence or absence of localized edema and excess skin.

In this same position, bimanual and digital palpation is performed as a more accurate assessment of the degree of flaccidity. Alternatively, the patient may be positioned in lateral decubitus and with abduction of one of the lower limbs, evaluating in this way, with the presence of gravitational force, the flaccidity in all its extension.

After a thorough physical examination and broad disclosure of the proposed surgical procedure including an extensive orientation regarding the postoperative care, the plastic surgeon will determine the best technique to be used in order to obtain a satisfactory result.

Preoperative Procedures

Preoperative tests are routinely requested consisting of complete blood count and coagulogram, blood glucose, total proteins and fractions, total cholesterol and fractions, T3 + T4, serum iron, ferritin, urea and creatinine, type I urine, electrocardiogram, and chest X-rays.

When there is a need for more specific assessment, the patient is referred to specialists, who will determine the additional care to be taken.

All patients are submitted to a detailed analysis of the weight loss treatment, date of the surgical procedure, maximum weight reached, current weight, calculation of the ideal weight for the patient, body mass index (BMI), height, weight stabilization time, occupation, diet, physical activities, and individual and family history, in addition to esthetic, functional, and psychological complaints.

The analysis of expectations regarding the result can be obtained through psychological assessment and assessment by the plastic surgeon, thus avoiding compromising the result and the doctor-patient relationship. It is known that patients with a BMI below 30 have the best esthetic-functional results, and complications are rare. Strict perianal and genital trichotomy is essential, and patients should bathe with antiseptic soap a few days prior to surgery and before demarcation. Care in the operating room must be rigorous, performing asepsis and antisepsis before positioning the patient on the operating table, with sterile drapes and in the proper position for each type of cruroplasty.

Thigh Suspension (InCr)

This technique is also known as dermolipectomy of the upper third of the inner thigh.

Demarcation

With the patient in orthostatic position, point "A" on the inguinal crease is demarcated in a location that depends on the degree of flaccidity. Point "B" must be at a distance from the inguinocrural crease that is determined by the traction of excess skin when it is pulled upward with the fingertips towards the inguinal region at the height of the vulvar crease, with the corresponding "C" point in the crease close to

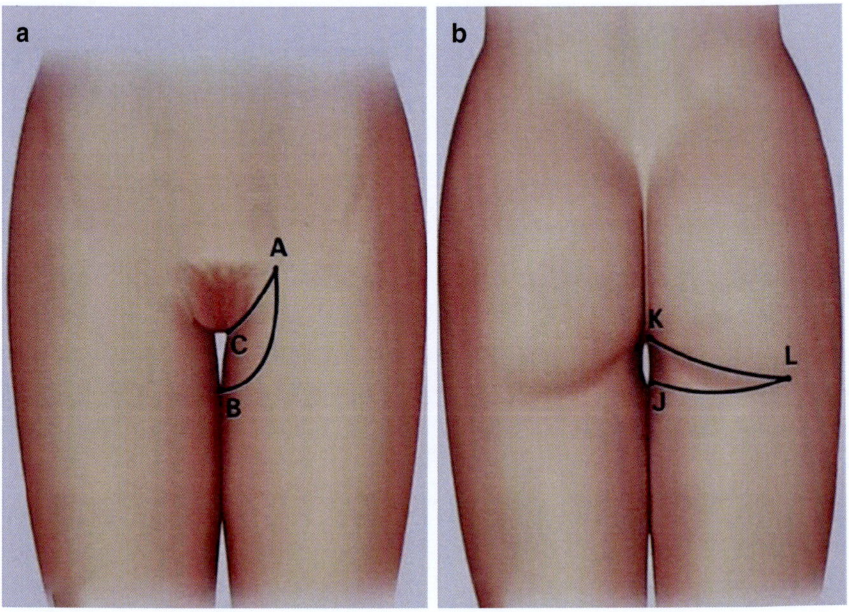

Fig. 47.3 Crural suspension. (**a**) Anterior demarcation. (**b**) Posterior demarcation

the vulvar. Next, segments “AB” and “AC” are joined, demarcating the area to be resected.

With the patient in orthostatic position, point “L” is subsequently demarcated posteriorly, which is located at the end of the gluteal sulcus, close to the trochanteric region, which will depend on the degree of skin flaccidity. Then, point

“J” is demarcated by means of traction and further suspending with bidigital and manual maneuvers that will also determine point “K.” Therefore, point K is located a little above the gluteal groove, corresponding to the projection of point “J.” All points are connected demarcating the area to be resected (Fig. 47.3).

Surgical Technique

Having the patient in horizontal ventral decubitus (HVD), a pad of approximately 10 cm in diameter is placed under the hip. The incision is made over the demarcated lines, deepening to the level of the superficial fascia from point “L,” extending upward to approximately 5 cm beyond points “K” and “J.” Lastly, the entire demarcated cutaneous extension is resected (Fig. 47.4).

Thorough hemostasis using an electrocautery and closing of the surgical wound by segment, that is, separate stitches in the subcutaneous cellular tissue using Polyglactin® 4–0 threads, subdermal separated stitches with Poliglecaprone® 4–0 thread, intradermal suture anchored with continuous thread Poliglecaprone® 4–0, and finally, braided bandage with porous adhesive tape 2.5 cm in diameter.

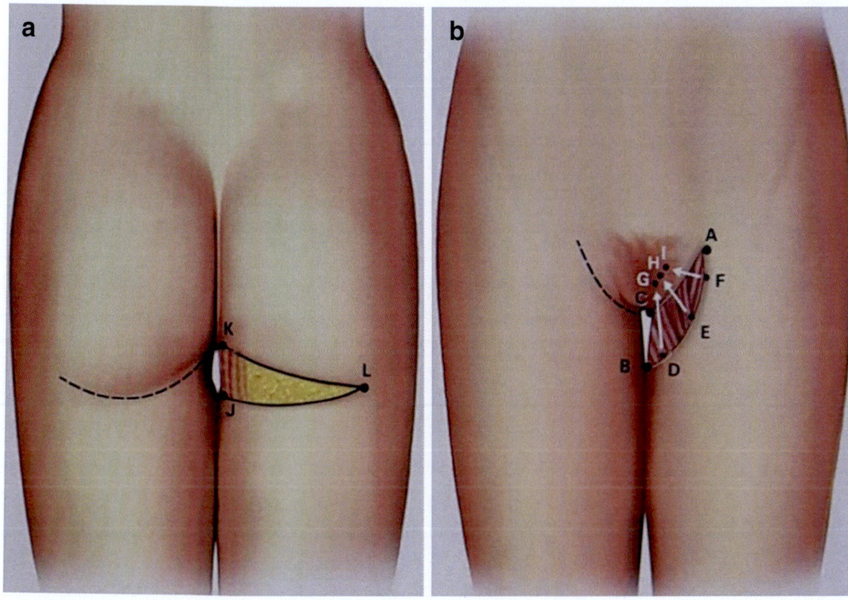

Fig. 47.4 (**a**, **b**) Surgical technique for crural suspension. (**a**) Patient in HVD: on the left, resulting scar; on the right, posterior dermolipectomy. (**b**) Patient with DD: on the right, suspension with fixation on the pubic thigh; on the left view of the resulting scar

Change of Decubitus

With the patient in horizontal dorsal decubitus (HDD), an incision is made over the previously marked lines and dermolipectomy is performed at the level of the deep fascia. Next, the elliptical dermofat flap is removed and hemostasis with an electric scalpel is implemented.

Having the operating table in Fowler's position, the deep fascia of the cutaneous-distal flap is fixed to the periosteum of the pubic crest by means of three stitches with 2–0 monofilament nylon joining the stitches "FI," "EH," and "DG."

Closure of the surgical wound is done in the same fashion as described in the posterior region and braided dressing with porous adhesive tape measuring 2.5 cm in diameter.

Thigh Helicoidal (ThHe)

This technique combines crural dermolipectomy of the inner thigh (suspension) with lateral crural dermolipectomy.

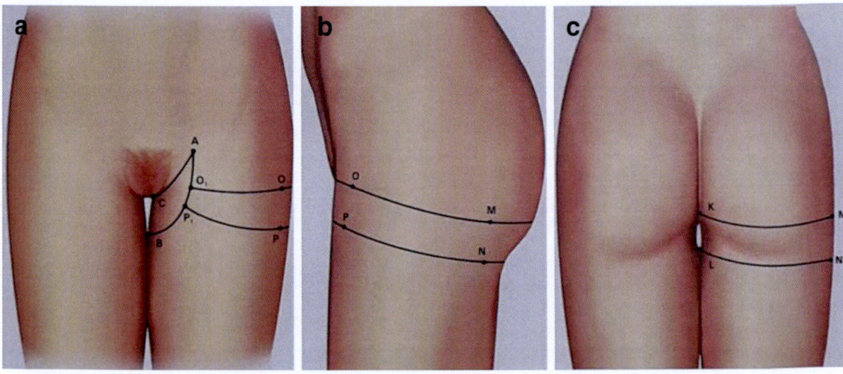

Fig. 47.5 Demarcation in helical thigh dermolipectomy. (**a**) Anterior view, (**b**) lateral view, and (**c**) posterior view

Demarcation

Having the patient with a frontal view in the standing position, and with a slight distancing of the feet, the demarcation is carried on in the same way as for the suspension of the thighs. Hence, on the anterolateral surface of the thigh by means of bidigital and manual clamping, the "O" point is demarcated, which is located in the anterosuperior region of the femoral trochanter, and the "P" point, which is the lower projection of the "O" point.

With the patient in lateral orthostatic position, points "M" and "N" are demarcated posteriorly to the femoral trochanter.

In a posterior orthostatic position, point "K" is demarcated, located medially 2 to 3 cm above the gluteal sulcus. With a digital antigravity maneuver pressing the skin at a point inferior to the gluteal sulcus in the superior direction toward the "K" point superimposing them, the "L" point is demarcated.

The distance from point "K" to point "L" depends on the degree of sagging skin specific to each case (Fig. 47.5).

With the patient in an anterior orthostatic position, points "A," "B," and "C" are demarcated in a similar way to the crural suspension. In segment AB, points "O_1" superior and "P_1" inferior are demarcated, whose distance will depend on the degree of flaccidity presented by the patient.

The following points will be joined.

Surgical Technique

With the patient in the horizontal prone position (HPP), a cushion of approximately 10 cm is placed under the hip.

The incisions are carried out on the lines demarcated from points "K" and "L" to points "O" and "P," passing through points "M" and "N," deepening until the *fascia*

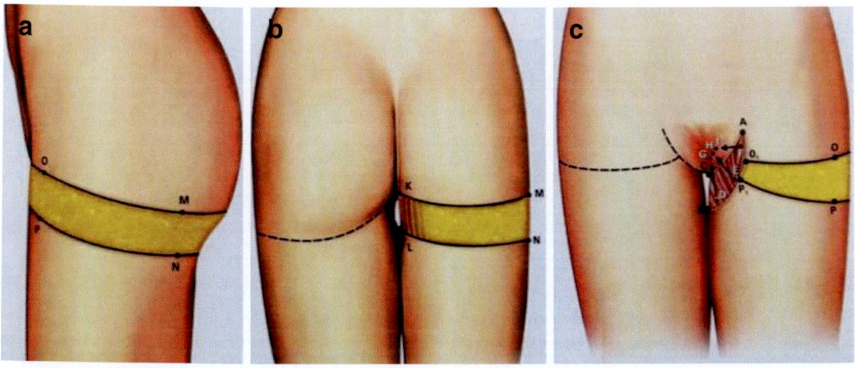

Fig. 47.6 Helicoidal dermolipectomy of the thigh associated with trochanteric dermolipectomy. (**a**) Lateral view, (**b**) posterior view: to the right the level of detachment is deep at the height of points "K" and "L." To the left: the resulting scar. (**c**) Anterior view: right helical dermolipectomy completed with patient in DDH, in Fowler's position. Note the concentric suspension of points "G," "H," and "I." To the left, the resulting scar

superficialis, followed by dermolipectomy and detachment at the level of the *fascia superficialis* in the lateral and posterior regions, at the level of the deep fascia, when points "K" and "L" are surpassed. This step should be followed rigorously with electrocautery.

Next, the operative incision is closed starting with the subcutaneous cellular tissue through separate stitches with Polyglactin® 4–0 threads, subdermis with separate stitches with Poliglecaprone® 4–0 threads, and the skin through an anchored continuous intradermal suture with 4–0 Poliglecaprone® threads. Finally, a braided dressing is applied using a 2.5 cm porous adhesive tape.

Decubitus Change

With the patient in horizontal dorsal decubitus (HDD), the demarcated lines are incised from points "O" and "P" to the segment "AB" (Fig. 47.6a–c).

Then, proceed with dermolipectomy with detachment at the level of the superficial fascia.

Suspension of the distal skin flap is performed by means of three stitches ("G," "H," and "I") fixed to the periosteum of the pubic crest using 2–0 monofilament nylon threads that will support stitches "D," "E," and "F," separated in the deep fascia of the interior flap, corresponding to segment "AB." Through these points, the "AB" segment is elevated, and a final scar is positioned in the inguinocrural region.

The remaining surgical incisions are sutured in planes, with separated stitches in the subcutaneous cellular tissue using Polyglactin® 4–0 threads, subdermal separated stitches with Poliglecaprone® 4–0 threads, and continuous intradermal suture anchored with Poliglecaprone® 4–0 threads.

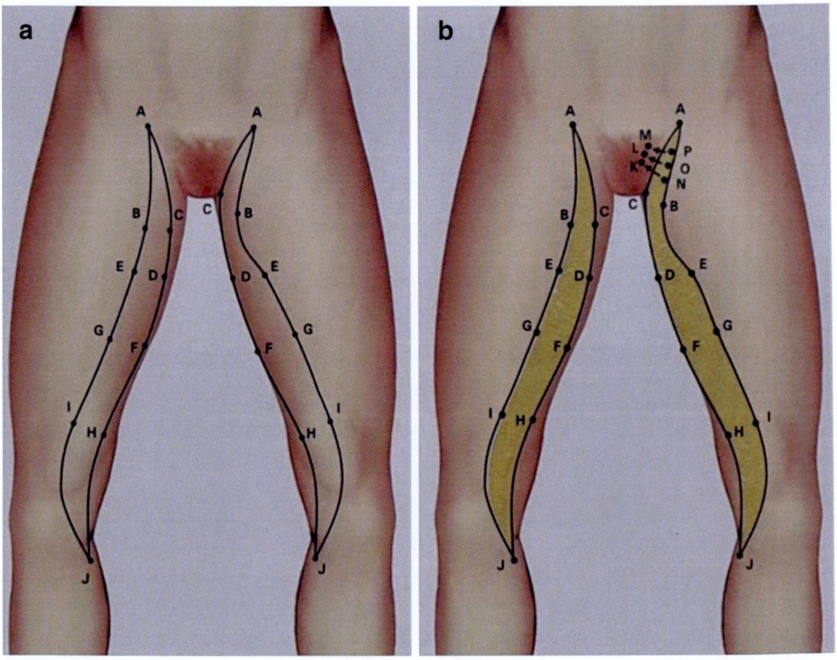

Fig. 47.7 Crural dermolipectomy longitudinal demarcation. (**a**) On the right, in women. Note: points "A," "B," and "C" are similar to points "A," "B," and "C" on the crural suspension. On the left, longitudinal dermolipectomy demarcation, for men. Points "B" and "C" are placed anteriorly since there is no need for suspension. (**b**) On the right, observe on the inguinal area the same type of fixation used on the suspension of the thighs

Longitudinal Thigh (LoTh)

Demarcation

With the patient in an orthostatic position, points "A," "B," and "C" are demarcated, similar to those of the thigh suspension with a slight modification.

In female patients, points "B" and "C" are demarcated more posteriorly, and in male patients more anteriorly. The "J" point is located inferiorly to the medial region of the knee, inferiorly to the popliteal fold.

Points "E," "F," "G," "H," and "I" are determined by a bidigital pinch maneuver, which determines the area of sagging skin to be resected. The stitches are then joined, determining the ellipse to be resected (Fig. 47.7).

Surgical Technique

The patient is positioned in dorsal decubitus (DDH) and with a slight abduction of the thigh to be operated, and slight flexion of the leg, and in order to improve the presentation, a small lateral rotation of the thigh is performed.

Incision is carried on the lines previously demarcated from point "A" to point "F," proceeding to a crural dermolipectomy with detachment at the level of the superficial fascia. After resection, rigorous hemostasis is performed, and then three separate stitches are applied with 2–0 monofilament nylon threads on the pubic crest ("K," "L," and "M"), elevating and securing the inferior skin flap through points "P," "O," and "N" at the level of the deep fascia.

Therefore, segment "AB" of the flap is suspended toward the inguinal crease.

The closing of the surgical incisions is performed in planes starting with the subcutaneous cellular tissue through separate stitches with Polyglactin® 4–0 threads, then the subdermal plane with separate stitches of Polyglactin® 4–0 threads, the skin through continuous intradermal suture anchored with 4–0 Poliglecaprone® threads, and, finally, a braided dressing with 2.5 cm diameter porous tape.

Atypical Thigh Dermolipectomies

These types of procedures are performed in less than 2% of cases, in which crural dermolipectomy is indicated. The main procedures are as follows:

Oblique dermolipectomy: generally used in male patients to correct sagging of the inner thigh between the middle and upper thirds. The elliptical dermofat segment is excised starting in the anterior region of the upper third and descending obliquely to the posterior region of the medial third of the thigh. It is a dermolipectomy at the level of the fascia superficialis. Sometimes, it is associated with liposuction.

Some patients, due to preexisting hyperpigmentation in the upper flap and the absence of hair in the region, request its removal, which solution is suspension. This surgical procedure is performed in a second time and it is not always possible to completely eliminate the pigmented area.

Dermolipectomy of the inner thighs combined with longitudinal dermolipectomy: technique used in female patients who initially present a BMI > 40, later reaching a BMI < 25, and presenting significant flaccidity.

Helical dermolipectomy combined with longitudinal dermolipectomy: procedure generally used in female patients, in one or two surgical stages. Technique used when lipodystrophy and flaccidity are severe. It is often performed in two surgical stages.

Mixed dermolipectomies: procedure used in men and women with significant lower limb lipodystrophy in which some liposuction sessions are previously performed before the classically employed dermolipectomy. In these cases, extra dermolipectomy may occur, depending on the deformities presented.

Postoperative Crural Dermolipectomies

During the first 24 h, the patient is kept at bed rest, in Fowler's position, wearing elastic stockings and sequential pressure boots, in order to reduce the possibility of deep vein thrombosis and pulmonary thromboembolism. The use of enoxaparin will depend on the background or guidance of a vascular surgeon. Antibiotics (cefazolin) and analgesics are routinely used.

The patient is removed from bed on the first day after surgery, to walk, and positioned with a slight flexion of the trunk on the hip.

On the second postoperative day, the patient is discharged from the hospital, after changing the surgical dressings. The use of elastic stockings remains for a week; boots are removed when the patient starts to walk.

In the first week of the postoperative period, rest is strongly recommended, walking slowly only a few times a day, in flat areas and always with compressive meshes that help in the rest of the scar area, keeping the flap with less gravitational action.

Dressings are changed weekly at the clinic. One month after the surgery, guided physical exercises and freer and more prolonged walks are recommended, with the patient being able to drive.

Sexual intercourse must be done carefully and after medical release so that they do not compromise the surgical area and do not cause severe pain, especially in sudden movements.

Three months after the surgery, the patient will be discharged, but still under medical orders.

References

REWIS, J.R. The thigh lift. *J Int Coll Surg,* v. 27, p. 330, 1957.

PITANGUY, l. Trochanteric lipodystrophy. *Plast Reconstr Surg,* v. 34, p. 280, 1964.

TEIMOURIAN, B; ADAM MN. Anterior periosteal dermal suspension with suction curettage for lateral thigh lipectomy. Aesth Plast Surg, v. 6, p. 207, 1982.

LOCKWOOD, T.E. Fascial anchoring technique in medial thigh lifts. *Plast Rec Surg,* v. 82, p. 229,1988.

LOCKWOOD TE. Lower body lift with superficial fascial system suspension. *Plast Reconstr Surg, v. 92, p. 1112,1992.*

DE MELLO, M.P.; WADA, A. Técnicas de Cirurgia Plástica pós-cirurgia bariátrica. *In:* SZEGO, T. (Ed.) *Vídeo atlas of obesity surgery.* São Paulo: Editora Atheneu, 2002.

PASCAL, JF.; LOUARN CL. Remodeling body lift with high lateral tension. *Aesth Plast Surg,* v. 26, p. 26, p. 223, 2002.

LOEB, R. Narrowing of the mons pubis during thighs lifts. *Ann Plast Surg,* v. 2, p. 290, 1979.

GUERREROSANTOS, J. Secondary hip-buttock-thigh plasty. *Clin Plast Surg, v. 11, p. 491, 1984.*

LOUARN CL; PASCAL JF. The concentric medial thigh lift. *Aesth Plast Surg,* v. 28, p. 20, 2004.

MORALES GARCIA, H.J. Circular lipectomy with lateral thigh-buttock lift. *Aesth Plast Surg, v. 27, p. 50, 2003.*

Chapter 48
Panniculectomy in Morbidly Obese and Post-Massive Weight Loss Patients

Horacio F. Mayer

Abstract An apron-like deformity, called panniculus, is usually present in morbidly obese or post-massive weight loss patients preventing adequate hygiene and reducing the functional capacity and mobility, and also determining significant psychosocial stress. Panniculectomy is a major surgical procedure by which this lower abdominal apron is removed followed by direct closure. This is not a traditional abdominoplasty, and as such, it is not associated with rectus abdominis plication and often the navel is not repositioned. Although the abdominal contour is modified, panniculectomy is not performed to improve the abdominal contour. Actually, its indication is purely functional to alleviate the associated problems. This chapter deals with the current indications, classification, preoperative and postoperative care, surgical technique, and complications of panniculectomy.

Keywords Panniculus · Panniculectomy · Fatty apron · Morbid obesity · Massive weight loss · Apronectomy

Introduction

The incidence of obesity, defined as a body mass index (BMI) greater than 30 kg/m^2, has increased significantly in recent years among adult men and women in Latin America (Webber et al. 2012). According to recent studies, the prevalence of obesity among adults in Argentina is 26.7% in men and 30% in women (Panorama de la Seguridad Alimentaria y Nutricional en América Latina y el Caribe 2014). Weight

H. F. Mayer (✉)
Plastic Surgery Department, Hospital Italiano de Buenos Aires, University of Buenos Aires School of Medicine, Buenos Aires, Argentina

Hospital Italiano de Buenos Aires University Institute, Buenos Aires, Argentina
e-mail: horacio.mayer@hospitalitaliano.org.ar

J. M. Avelar, R. Cavalcanti Ribeiro (eds.), *Body Contouring*,
https://doi.org/10.1007/978-3-031-42802-9_48

loss, whether due to diet, exercise, or bariatric surgery, can produce excess skin and hanging fat in the lower abdomen, a true apron, which creates a moist environment that encourages bacterial and fungal colonization, which can result in intertrigo, infections, edema (panniculitis), ulcers, and even fistulas (D'Ettorre et al. 2017).

The incidence of the formation of an abdominal apron after bariatric surgery is higher in older operated patients with a previous higher BMI. Therefore, bariatric surgery in younger patients and in patients who have reduced their BMI before bariatric surgery would help to prevent the formation of an apron after bariatric surgery (Chung et al. 2014).

The apron-like deformity, called panniculus, prevents adequate hygiene and reduces the functional capacity and mobility of the patient, making it difficult to walk or work and also determining significant psychosocial stress (Michaels et al. 2017; Richter et al. 2013). On the other hand, this cutaneous-adipose apron often complicates the surgical management of patients who must undergo abdominal surgeries such as hernioplasties (Bailey et al. 2015; Mundra et al. 2018; Giordano et al. 2017; Koolen et al. 2014).

Definition

Panniculectomy is the transverse resection of the lower abdominal apron, between the umbilicus and the pubis, followed by direct closure. Except for more severe cases, the umbilicus is not transposed through the superior epigastric flap. There is no undermining or this is minimal, so when direct closure is performed, there is usually a difference in thickness between the upper flap and the pubis and an abnormal position of the navel that is pulled down. The upper abdomen and mons pubis which are not treated remain protruding in contrast to the lower abdomen, which looks flattened.

Panniculectomy is not a traditional abdominoplasty, and as such, it is not associated with rectus abdominis plication and often the navel is not repositioned. It is important to note that, although the abdominal contour is modified, panniculectomy is not performed to improve the abdominal contour. Actually, its indication is purely functional to alleviate the associated problems. This is why it is usually covered by social security and prepaid medical insurance.

While the procedure alleviates functional disturbances, traditional panniculectomy provides cosmetically poor results. Indeed, clothes usually fit very poorly. In order to obtain superior aesthetic results, a more complex and high-risk lipoabdominoplasty would be necessary, including flap thinning with liposuction, undermining of the upper abdominal flap, plicating the rectus abdominis muscle, and transposing the umbilicus (Hurwitz 2017).

Indications

Some morbidly obese patients may present with a giant fat apron before bariatric surgery and may be candidates for panniculectomy. These obese patients have more comorbidities than patients who achieved normal weight or are just overweight after bariatric surgery. These comorbidities include cardiovascular disease, respiratory

Table 48.1 Classification of obesity according to BMI by the US National Institutes of Health

Class		
Normal	18.5–24.9	
Overweight	25.0–29.9	
Obesity	30.0–34.9	I
	35.0–39.9	II
Extreme obesity	40.0+	III

disease, high blood pressure, diabetes, and metabolic syndrome (Pasulka et al. 1986). On the other hand, sometimes after bariatric surgery, some patients do not reach the ideal weight or the ideal deflated appearance for a post-bariatric tummy tuck. On the contrary, they remain obese and develop a heavy apron with the functional disorders that it entails, being only candidates for a panniculectomy.

According to the US National Institutes of Health (NIH), obesity is classified into three classes (Table 48.1) (National Institute of Health n.d.). Class III obese patients (BMI 40 or more) have a higher risk of comorbidities compared to other obese patients (class I and II), and the incidence of postoperative complications is double in patients with BMI ≥ 30 kg/m^2 compared to those with BMI < 30 kg/m^2 (Van der Beek et al. 2011). Usually, these patients have, after panniculectomy, a higher risk of readmission at 30 days, early reoperation, sepsis, wound infection, and medical complications such as kidney failure, urinary tract infection, pneumonia, re-intubation, and myocardial infarction (AlQattan et al. 2017).

For safety purposes, a patient with criteria for bariatric surgery (BMI 40, BMI 35–39.9 with at least one obesity-related comorbidity, or BMI 30–34.9 with uncontrolled diabetes or metabolic syndrome) (Phillips and Shikora 2018) is always referred to a bariatric surgeon before attempting a panniculectomy. Panniculectomy should be indicated only in highly selected patients, with a severely disabling cutaneous-adipose apron, in whom weight loss is not possible (patients with a BMI of 35 or more and a panniculus of 13.6 kg) (Michaels et al. 2017).

The potential benefits of panniculectomy must be weighed against the surgical risks in the group of patients where it may prove to be a lifesaving procedure (National Institute of Health n.d.). For the remaining patients, various measures must be taken to reduce the risk of postoperative complications.

Frequently, those patients who have lost weight in preparation for a kidney transplant develop a fat apron which represents an additional obstacle to being candidates for the expected transplant. The apron is usually located over the iliac fossa, in the lower abdominal quadrants, where the incision for renal transplantation is made (Bailey et al. 2015). The panniculus is frequently hypovascularized, with intertrigo and dermatitis being commonly associated, which if combined to the immunosuppression necessary for transplantation can be catastrophic for wound healing. Currently, there is a growing demand to perform panniculectomy in patients candidates for kidney transplantation (Bailey et al. 2015; Mundra et al. 2018). These patients have a higher risk of deep vein thrombosis (DVT) and severe medical complications, prolonged hospital stays, and a higher mortality rate (Mundra et al. 2018).

The absolute indication for panniculectomy, the recommended indications, and the relative and absolute contraindications have been recently proposed by Thaller et al. (see Table 48.2) (AlQattan et al. 2017).

Table 48.2 Indications and contraindications for panniculectomy

A. Indicated
• Persistent dermatological disorders (ulcers, intertrigo, fistulas) refractory to medical treatment
• Apron produces functional impotence interfering with daily activities, thus reducing quality of life
• Presence of the apron prevents a procedure that saves the patient's life (e.g., kidney transplant)
B. Recommended
• Associated with abdominal wall or gynecological/obstetric surgery (e.g., hernioplasty, eventroplasty, caesarean section), provided there are no risk factors that increase the risk of complications
C. Not recommended
• Cases of massive weight loss as they are better candidates for a tummy tuck
• Non-modifiable disorders that adversely affect wound healing (e.g., immunodeficiency, wound healing disorders)
• Medical disorders that determine a high risk of postoperative complications (e.g., diabetes mellitus, renal insufficiency)
D. Contraindicated
• Modifiable conditions that adversely affect wound healing or increase the risks of postoperative complications (e.g., malnutrition, smoking, active wound infection)
E. Absolutely contraindicated
• Various severe comorbidities that would put the patient at prohibitive surgical risk

Classification

According to the degree of ptosis of the apron with respect to the mons pubis and the thigh, the American Society of Plastic Surgeons (ASPS) has proposed the classification in 5 degrees, with grade 5 being the most severe (Table 48.3 and Fig. 48.1) (American Society of Plastic Surgeons 2007a). Clinical examples of the different grades are presented in Fig. 48.2.

Due to its functional nature, the procedure is usually covered in Argentina by social security and prepaid medical insurance. In the USA, health companies have established a series of criteria that must be met for panniculectomy to be authorized, based on the ASPS grade classification (grade 3 or more) (Table 48.4) (American Society of Plastic Surgeons 2007b). According to a survey of North American plastic surgeons, the most common criteria for medical coverage of panniculectomy was stable weight for 6 months and for 18 months after bariatric surgery. For medical insurers, the most common requirement was chronic skinfold maceration without response to oral or topical treatment for 3 months (Dreifuss and Rubin 2016).

Table 48.3 Classification in degrees according to the severity of ptosis of the fatty apron

Grade 1: The apron covers the pubic hair and the Mons pubis, but not the genitals
Grade 2: The apron covers the genitals and inguinal fold
Grade 3: The apron covers upper parts of the thigh
Grade 4: The apron covers the mid-thigh
Grade 5: The apron covers the knee and below it

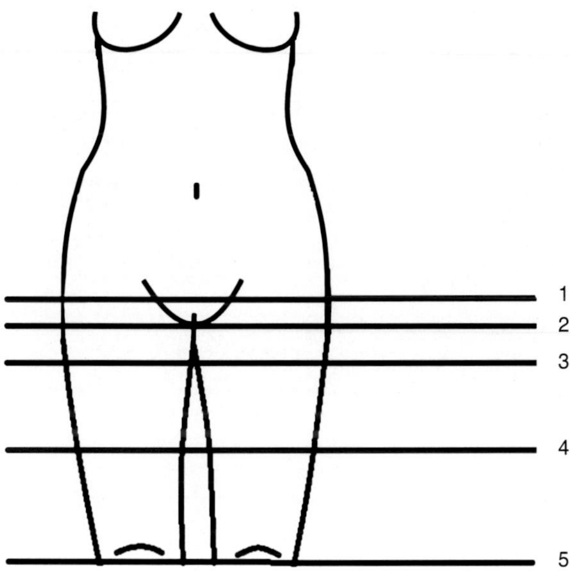

Fig. 48.1 Classification in degrees according to the severity of ptosis of the fatty apron

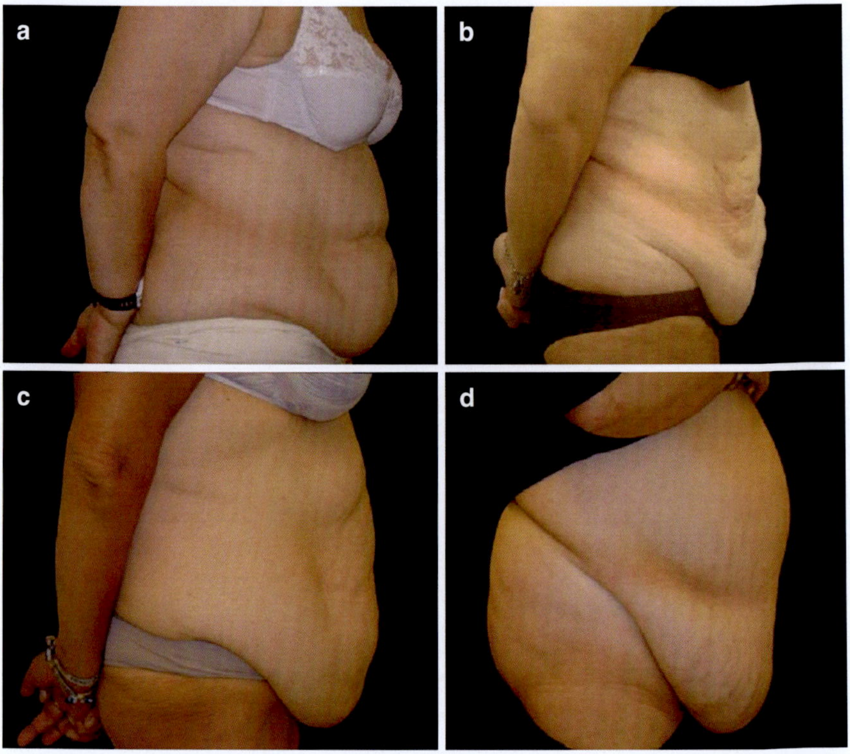

Fig. 48.2 Clinical examples of panniculus of different severity: (**a**) grade 1, the apron covers pubic hair and the mons pubis; (**b**) grade 2, the apron covers the genitals and inguinal folds; (**c**) grade 3, the apron covers the upper part of the thigh; and (**d**) grade 4, the apron covers the middle part of the thigh. In grade 5, the most severe, the apron reaches and covers the knees

Table 48.4 Criteria for medical coverage of post-bariatric panniculectomy or abdominoplasty

1. Weight loss of at least 45 kg (100 lbs)
2. Fatty apron covering genitalia and upper or mid-thighs, knees or below (grade 3 or greater)
3. Weight loss due to medical treatment or lifestyle change (diet or exercise) and stable weight for at least 6 months Weight loss after bariatric surgery and stable weight for at least 18 months after surgery
4. The apron causes all of the following: Functional impotence that interferes with daily activities including physical exercise Intertriginous ulcerations or persistent symptomatic macerations refractory to good hygiene Supervised local medical treatment for several months Recurrent skin infections (at least two episodes in 12 months) requiring systemic antibiotics

Preoperative Preparation

Patients are instructed to shower with a chlorhexidine solution for 5 days prior to surgery (Veiga et al. 2009). If the patient is a smoker, smoking cessation is indicated for at least 6–8 weeks before surgery (Deliaert et al. 2012). All nonsteroidal anti-inflammatory drugs or vitamin supplements that include vitamin E and herbal compounds that include ginkgo biloba should be discontinued for at least 1 week beforehand to avoid further intraoperative bleeding (Chang and Whitaker 2001; Shalom and Wong 2003; Spencer 2000).

The patient is marked using indelible markers on the day of surgery while standing and sitting. Correct marking is essential to achieve a symmetrical scar that is as well positioned as possible and to avoid the formation of lateral dog ears. The usual marking is a transverse ellipse that may include the umbilicus if it has been decided to sacrifice it. During the anesthetic induction, the bladder catheter, graduated compression stockings, and pneumatic compression boots are placed. All of them will remain throughout the surgery and till the moment the patient is able to walk on their own.

Surgical Technique

In order to reduce surgical times as much as possible, two surgical teams are always involved, operating simultaneously on both sides of the patient. This allows us to keep the surgical time always below 2 h. This strategy, also reported by Richter et al., makes it possible to reduce postoperative complications by reducing surgery time (Reichenberger et al. 2008). It is known that the longer the surgical procedure, the higher the incidence of complications (Rambachan et al. 2013). We always perform a predetermined resection, which facilitates surgery and allows for symmetrical resection and closure. As a means to reduce blood loss, the incision line is infiltrated with a solution of adrenaline (1:100,000). With a similar purpose, while the epidermis and dermis are incised with a scalpel and the adipose plane is incised with electrocautery. Undermining is also performed with electrocautery, progressing cephalad while preserving the distal portion of the Scarpa fascia to reduce the incidence of seroma (Costa-Ferreira et al. 2013). All vessels whose diameter is equal to or greater than the width of the cautery tip are usually ligated or clipped.

Different methods of suspending the apron from an orthopedic or Balkan frame using hooks have been described (Bonnet et al. 2015; Janakiramanan and Dowling 2009; Knight et al. 2009).This maneuver not only makes the procedure more expeditious but also allows blood and lymphatic drainage by gravity from the flap. The navel is usually not incised and as a consequence, it might look pulled inferiorly after closure. Sometimes, it can be directly sacrificed or it can be repositioned as in a traditional abdominoplasty. If this is the case, a minimal undermining is performed at the midline to reposition the navel in a higher position, being afterward exteriorized through a "Y"-shaped incision. Once the resection of the apron is completed, a meticulous control of the hemostasis is carried out and two silicone drains are left in place. Then, we proceed to wound closure layer by layer with sutures. The use of barbed sutures and adhesives derived from cyanoacrylate, associated or not with mesh, allows suture times to be reduced, thus further optimizing surgical time (Duscher et al. 2016; Richter et al. 2012). The maintenance of normothermia throughout the procedure is of great importance. Perioperative hypothermia has been associated with an increased risk of seroma, blood loss, and the need for transfusion (Coon et al. 2012). In order to prevent it, routine use of warmed fluids and thermal blankets is indicated, and very low temperatures are avoided at the operating room. Representative surgical results are presented in Figs. 48.3, 48.4, 48.5 and 48.6.

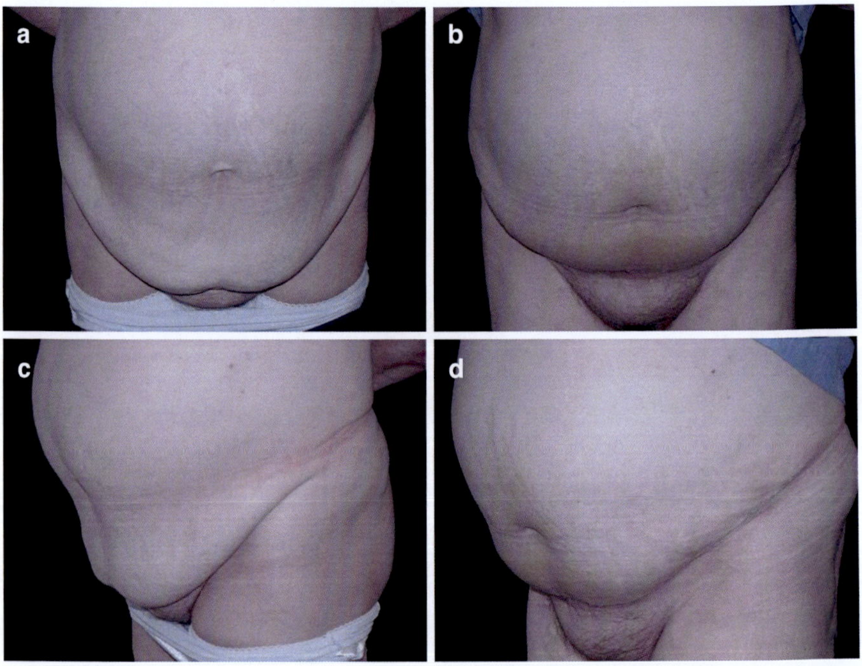

Fig. 48.3 A 69-year-old morbidly obese female patient with severe heart disease and diabetes who underwent panniculectomy without umbilical transposition: (**a**) preoperative frontal view, (**b**) postoperative frontal view at 30 days, (**c**) preoperative oblique view, and (**d**) postoperative oblique view at 30 days

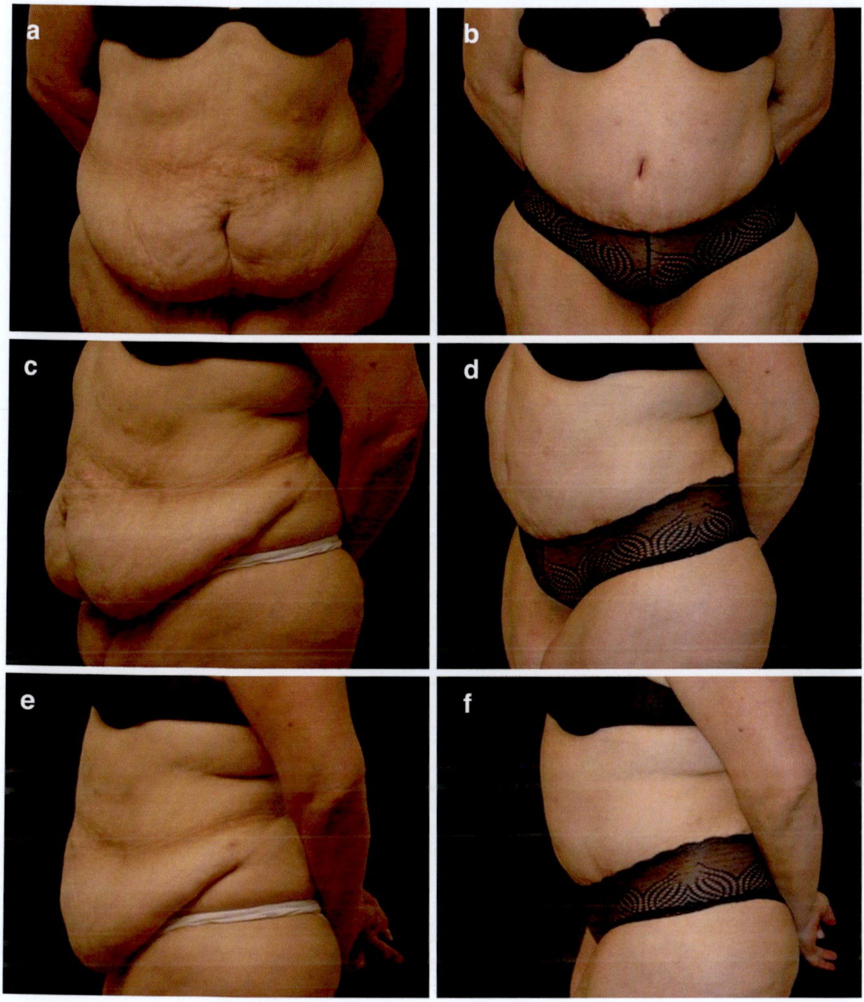

Fig. 48.4 A 62-year-old female patient, ASPS classification grade 2, who underwent panniculectomy with umbilical transposition and without rectus plication: (**a**) preoperative frontal view, (**b**) postoperative frontal view at 12 months, (**c**) preoperative oblique view, (**d**) postoperative oblique view at 12 months, (**e**) preoperative lateral view, and (**f**) postoperative lateral view at 12 months

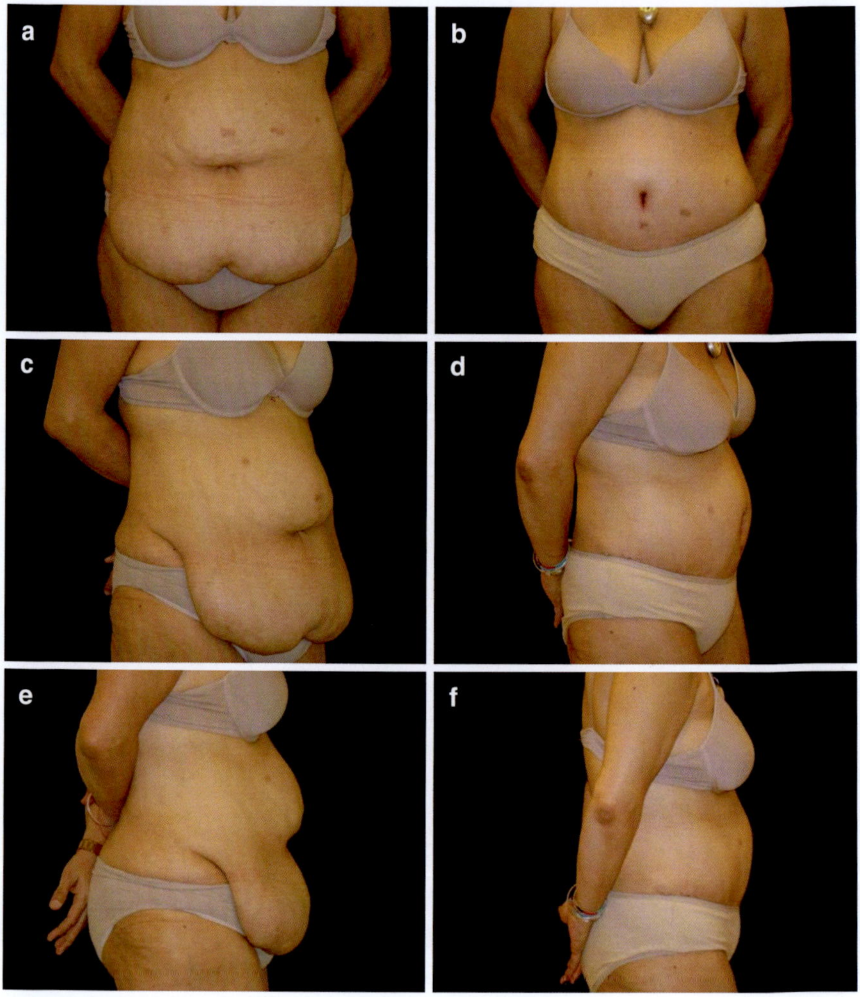

Fig. 48.5 A 57-year-old female patient with a history of deep vein thrombosis, ASA III, ASPS grade 2 classification, who underwent panniculectomy with umbilical transposition and without rectus plication: (**a**) preoperative frontal view, (**b**) postoperative frontal view at 3 months, (**c**) preoperative oblique view, (**d**) postoperative oblique view at 3 months, (**e**) preoperative lateral view, and (**f**) postoperative lateral view at 3 months

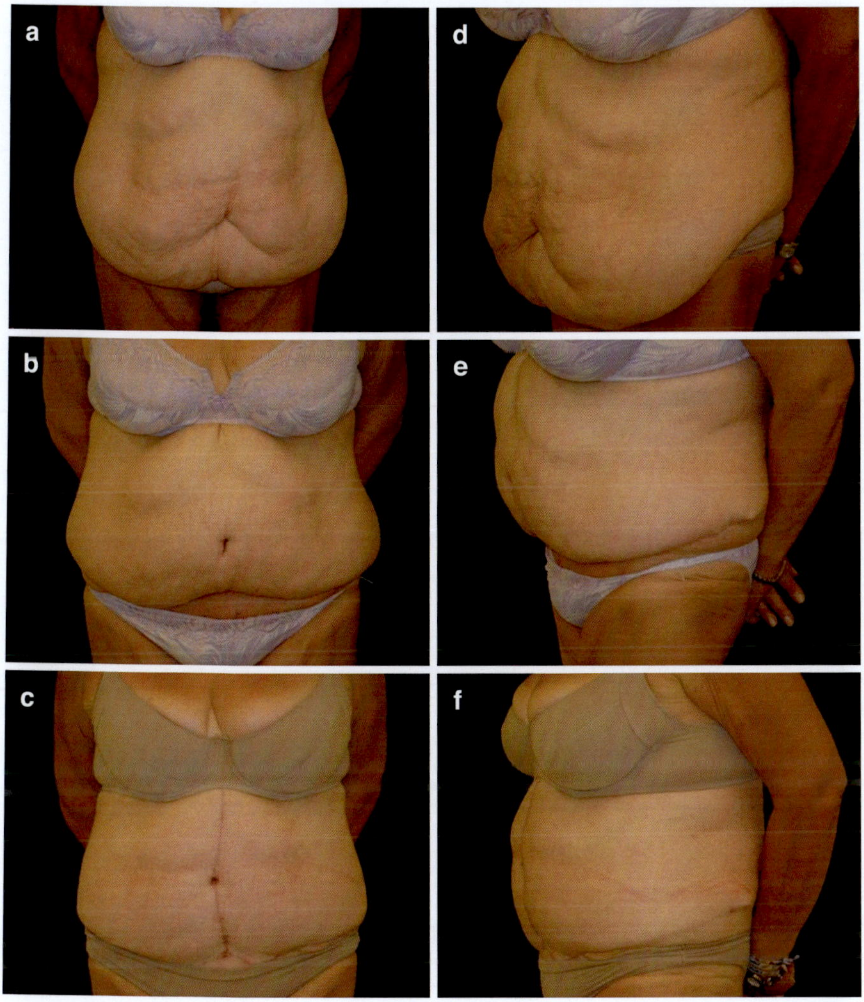

Fig. 48.6 A 49-year-old female patient, type II diabetic, with a history of coronary artery disease, ASA III, ASPS grade 3 classification, underwent classic panniculectomy with umbilical transposition and without rectus plication. In a second time, 18 months later, a vertical dermolipectomy was performed: (**a**) preoperative frontal view, (**b**) postoperative frontal view at 3 months, (**c**) frontal view post vertical dermolipectomy at 12 months, (**d**) preoperative oblique view, (**e**) postoperative view at 3 months, and (**f**) oblique view post vertical dermolipectomy at 12 months

Postoperative Care

The first postoperative day can be spent in a regular recovery room, at the intensive care unit or coronary care unit, depending on the associated comorbidities and the consequent surgical risk. As a large fatty apron can contain between 500 and 700 ml of blood, the procedure could be associated with great blood loss, determining postoperative hypovolemia. In order to avoid this, adequate postoperative fluid management and diuresis rhythm control are essential. Hematocrits are requested immediately after surgery and the day after surgery, monitoring the drain output through the abdominal drains. Postoperative pain management aims to minimize patient discomfort and facilitate early mobilization and functional recovery and includes administering paracetamol, without the antiplatelet effect of most nonsteroidal anti-inflammatory drugs, and opioid analgesics such as tramadol.

The incidence of deep vein thrombosis (DVT) is 1.2–1.6% and of pulmonary thromboembolism is 0.8–3.2%, being directly linked to the duration of the surgical procedure (Kim et al. 2015). High-risk patients according to the Caprini index (7 or higher) usually receive low-molecular-weight heparin (LMWH) 12 hours after the surgery and are encouraged for early mobilization (Geerts et al. 2008). Although the use of LMWH effectively reduces DVT incidence after body contouring surgery, this might increase the risk of bleeding and hematoma formation. We recently evaluated the incidence of DVT in body contouring surgery after massive weight loss patients in whom mechanical prophylaxis alone was indicated. According to our findings, DVT incidence was deemed acceptable in this cohort of patients if compared to the incidence reported in the literature. Therefore, the use of mechanical prophylaxis alone could be an attractive alternative for patients with a low Caprini score (<7) (Petersen et al. 2022).

As in panniculectomy cases, no plication of the rectus abdominis muscles is usually involved, and the patient is indicated to mobilize the same day of surgery. On the other hand, not performing the rectus abdominis plication avoids the consequent increase in intra-abdominal pressure and compression of the inferior vena cava, thus reducing the risk of thromboembolic complications (Geerts et al. 2008). Graduated compression stockings and pneumatic compression boots are kept in place till the moment the patient is able to walk on their own. In order to encourage continued mobilization, patients are discharged as soon as possible, usually within the first 24 h. In some centers, by protocol they recommend the placement of a removable inferior vena cava filter on the day of surgery to minimize the risk of pulmonary embolism (Piano et al. 2007). However, there is no consensus on the systematic use of the inferior vena cava filter. For example, the American College of Chest Physicians (ACCP) does not recommend the use of these filters for PTE prophylaxis (Geerts et al. 2008). However, the American Society for Metabolic and Bariatric Surgery (ASMBS) only recommends it in high-risk patients such as those with BMI 55 kg/m^2, history of deep vein thrombosis, hereditary thrombophilia, or preoperative immobility (Vaziri et al. 2011).

Complications

Comorbidities are not uncommon in patients undergoing panniculectomy. Obese patients are particularly prone to developing metabolic syndrome defined as the association of obesity and at least two variables: diabetes, hypertension, hypertriglyceridemia, or reduced high-density lipoprotein (Zavlin et al. 2017). All of them constitute risk factors for postoperative complications. We must be aware of the high morbidity and mortality of these patients, and we need to consider the optimization and adequate preoperative management of these patients. A very high BMI influences postoperative cardiac and respiratory complications because obesity alters cardiorespiratory physiology. Obesity specifically alters respiratory mechanics by reducing lung volume and increasing airway resistance (Agarwal et al. 1982). A study by Bell et al. revealed that obese patients are more prone to respiratory distress syndrome, heart failure, deep vein thrombosis, pulmonary embolism, and unscheduled intubation (Bell et al. 2017).

Patients with a BMI > 30 are 1.6 times more likely to develop an infectious complication during their hospitalization, including pneumonia, catheter septicemia, urinary tract infection, and surgical wound infection (Bell et al. 2016). Different theories have been proposed to explain the increased risk of infection. Obesity promotes a low-grade chronic inflammatory state that alters metabolism and the immune system. Proinflammatory cytokines, tumor necrosis factor alpha, and interleukin 6 and 1b are produced in high amounts in the adipose tissue of obese patients, leading to an altered immune response to infection (Bell et al. 2016; Green and Beck 2017).

In addition to cardiorespiratory and infectious complications, obese patients have a higher incidence of other postoperative complications, including wound healing problems, dehiscence, skin necrosis, hematoma and seroma, need for blood transfusion, and death (D'Ettorre et al. 2017; Zuelzer et al. 2010). Manahan et al. reported a 56% wound healing complications and a 28% incidence of seroma in a series of 24 patients undergoing panniculectomy by a single surgeon at an academic center (Manahan and Shermak 2006). The incidence of wound complications is also associated with high BMI. Coon et al. showed that those patients with a BMI between 40 and 49 were 3.4 times more likely to develop wound complications. Patients with a BMI between 50 and 59 were 12.1 times more likely, and those with a BMI >60 were 15.5 times more likely. Thus, this study shows a linear relationship between increased BMI and incidence of complications (Coon et al. 2009). Arthurs et al. conducted a retrospective study of 126 patients undergoing post-bariatric panniculectomy, reporting a 40% incidence of complications that included hematoma, seroma, wound infection, transfusions, skin necrosis, and re-exploration. Using multivariable logistic regression analysis, the authors showed that a BMI >25 before panniculectomy represents a 3.3-fold increased risk of postoperative complications. Thus, despite weight loss, pre-panniculectomy BMI still predicts the risk of postoperative complications (Arthurs et al. 2007).

Mioton et al. investigated whether panniculectomies performed by surgeons not specialized in plastic surgery affected postoperative results, detecting 2.09 times more likely to suffer from postoperative complications such as pneumonia, deep vein thrombosis, urinary tract infections, kidney failure, bleeding requiring transfusions, and myocardial infarction and 1.73 times more chances of developing wound infection (Mioton et al. 2013). Similar results were found by Koolen et al. when they compared panniculectomy performed by plastic surgeons and general surgeons. Surgeries performed by plastic surgeons suffered fewer postoperative complications, whether or not they were associated with simultaneous hernioplasties (Koolen et al. 2014). In the study carried out by Taller et al., it was shown that, in the USA, one third of panniculectomies are performed by general surgeons and that this was associated with a high risk of complications in wounds, sepsis, blood transfusions, return to the operating room, and medical complications in general. On the other hand, the average hospital stay for general surgeons was also higher (4.6 vs. 3.5 days) (AlQattan et al. 2017). In other words, those morbidly obese patients who require panniculectomy should be referred to plastic surgeons considering the substantial reduction in the risk of postoperative complications.

Despite the high incidence of complications, patient satisfaction with the procedure is high. In a mail survey, Cooper et al. demonstrated 81% satisfaction in a cohort of patients who underwent panniculectomy with an incidence of complications of 43% (Cooper et al. 2008). Similarly, a recent study by Rubin et al. demonstrated significant improvements in quality of life and health. Patients reported improvements in their ability to walk, dress, and perform their own personal hygiene (Michaels et al. 2017).

Conclusions

The growing incidence of obesity in Latin America and the rise of laparoscopic bariatric surgeries have contributed to increasing the demand for panniculectomy in both morbidly obese and post-bariatric patients. Although panniculectomy continues to be a surgery with a high risk of complications, the long-term improvement in quality of life justifies its indication.

It is the surgeon's obligation to inform the morbidly obese patient on the increased risks and preoperatively control the comorbidities detected. If weight loss is not possible, higher-risk surgery may be considered when it alters lifestyle and puts life at risk or when adequate access is required for other operations. Morbidly obese patients requiring panniculectomy should be referred to specialized plastic surgeons considering the substantial reduction in the risk of postoperative complications. The careful selection of patients, the adequate preoperative preparation of the patient, and the reduction of surgical times minimize complications and contribute to optimizing results in this high-risk population.

References

Webber L, Kilpi F, Marsh T, Rtveladze K, Brown M, McPherson K. High rates of obesity and non-communicable diseases predicted across Latin America. PLoS One. 2012;7(8): e39589.

Panorama de la Seguridad Alimentaria y Nutricional en América Latina y el Caribe (2014). Organización de las Naciones Unidas para la Alimentación y la Agricultura (FAO). http://www.fao.org/3/a-i4018s.pdf. Visitado 14 de enero de 2018.

D'Ettorre, M., Tambasco, D., Mingrone, G. et al. Predictive value of biochemical and tissue modifications for wound healing in post-bariatric patients. Eur J Plast Surg (2017) 40: 549.

Chung CW, Kling RE, Sivak WN, Rubin JP, Gusenoff JA. Risk factors for pannus formation in the post-bariatric surgery population. Plast Reconstr Surg. 2014 May;133(5):623e–627e.

Joseph Michaels 5th , Coon D, Calotta N, Rubin JP. Surgical management of the giant Pannus: indications, strategies, and outcomes. Aesthetic Plast Surg. 2017 Dec 21. https://doi.org/10.1007/s00266-017-1041-6.

Richter DF, Lampe H, Wolters M (2013) Panniculectomy in patients with super obesity, Chapter 27. In: Rubin JP, Jewell ML, Richter DF, Uebel CO (eds) Body contouring and liposuction. Elsevier, p 265-277.

Bailey CM, Troppmann C, Kuo J, Wong MS (2015) Panniculectomy in end-stage renal disease: six-year experience of performing panniculectomy in preparation for renal transplant. Ann Plast Surg 74(Suppl 1):S9–11

Mundra LS, Rubio GA, Al Qattan HT, Thaller SR. (2018) Panniculectomy Outcomes in Patients with End-Stage Renal Disease in Preparation for Renal Transplant. Aesthetic Plast Surg https://doi.org/10.1007/s00266-017-1043-4

Giordano S, Garvey PB, Baumann DP, Liu J, Butler CE. Concomitant Panniculectomy Affects Wound Morbidity but Not Hernia Recurrence Rates in Abdominal Wall Reconstruction: A Propensity Score Analysis. Plast Reconstr Surg. 2017 Dec;140(6):1263-1273.

Koolen PG, Ibrahim AM, Kim K et al (2014 Patient selection optimization following combined abdominal procedures: analysis of 4925 patients undergoing panniculectomy/abdominoplasty with or without concurrent hernia repair. Plast Reconstr Surg 134:539e–550e

Hurwitz DJ. Discussion: Abdominal Contouring Outcomes in Class III Obesity: Analysis of the ACS-NSQIP Database. Aesthetic Plast Surg. 2017 Dec 21. https://doi.org/10.1007/s00266-017-1033-6.

Pasulka PS, Bistrian BR, Benotti PN, Blackburn GL 1986 The risks of surgery in obese patients. Ann Intern Med 104:540–546

Classification of Overweight and Obesity by BMI, Waist Circumference, and Associated Disease Risks. National Institute of Health n.d.

Van der Beek ES, van der Molen AM, van Ramshorst B. Complications after body contouring surgery in post-bariatric patients: the importance of a stable weight close to normal. Obes Facts 2011; 4: 61 – 6.

AlQattan HT, Mundra LS, Rubio GA, Thaller SR. Abdominal Contouring Outcomes in Class III Obesity: Analysis of the ACS-NSQIP Database. Aesthetic Plast Surg. 2017 Oct 12. https://doi.org/10.1007/s00266-017-0976-y.

Phillips BT, Shikora SA. The history of metabolic and bariatric surgery: Development of standards for patient safety and efficacy. Metabolism. 2018 Jan 5. pii: S0026-0495(17)30357-8. https://doi.org/10.1016/j.metabol.2017.12.010.

Practice parameter for surgical treatment of skin redundancy for obese and massive weight loss patients. American Society of Plastic Surgeons Web site. http://www.plasticsurgery.org. Publicado 2007a. Visitado 14/01/18.

ASPS recommended insurance coverage criteria for third-party payers: surgical treatment of skin redundancy for obese and massive weight loss patients. American Society of Plastic Surgeons. http://www.plasticsurgery.org. Publicado en 2007b. Visitado 14/01/2018.

Dreifuss SE, Rubin JP. Insurance coverage for massive weight loss panniculectomy: a national survey and implications for policy. Surg Obes Relat Dis. 2016 Feb;12(2):412-6

Veiga DF, Damasceno CA, Veiga-Filho J. Randomized controlled trial of the effectiveness of chlorhexidine showers before elective plastic surgical procedures. Infect Control Hosp Epidemiol. 2009;30:77-9.

Deliaert AE, Van den Kerckhove E, Tuinder S, Noordzij SM, Dormaar TS, van der Hulst RR. Smoking and its effect on scar healing. Eur J Plast Surg. 2012 Jun;35(6):421-424.

Chang LK, Whitaker DC. The impact of herbal medicines on dermatologic surgery. Dermatol Surg. 2001 Aug;27(8):759-63.

Shalom A, Wong L. Outcome of aspirin use during excision of cutaneous lesions. Ann Plast Surg. 2003 Mar;50(3):296-8.

Spencer AP. Vitamin E: cautionary issues. Curr Treat Options Cardiovasc Med. 2000 Apr;2(2):1-3.

Reichenberger MA, Stoff A, Richter DF (2008) Dealing with the mass: a new approach to facilitate panniculectomy in patients with very large abdominal aprons. Obes Surg 18(12):1605–1610

Rambachan A, Mioton LM, Saha S et al. The impact of surgical duration on plastic surgery outcomes. Eur J Plast Surg, 2013, 36 (11), 707-14.

Costa-Ferreira A, Rebelo M, Silva A et al. Scarpa fascia preservation during abdominoplasty: randomized clinical study of efficacy and safety. Plast Reconstr Surg 2013;131(3):644-51.

Bonnet A, Mulliez E, Andrieux S, Duquennoy-martinot V, Guerreschi P (2015) Suspension of abdominal apron in massive panniculectomy: a novel technique. J Plast Reconstr Aesthet Surg 68(2):272–273

Janakiramanan N, Dowling GJ (2009) A simple apparatus for pannus suspension during exceptionally large panniculectomy procedures. Plast Reconstr Surg 124(5):272e–273e

Knight, R.J.W., Rtshiladze, M.A., Reddy, C. et al. Looking at bariatric surgery with a different 'frame' of mind. Eur J Plast Surg (2009) 32: 115.

Duscher D, Pollhammer MS, Wenny R et al. Barbed Sutures in Body-Contouring: Outcome Analysis of 695 Procedures in 623 Patients and Technical Advances. Aesthetic Plast Surg. 2016 Dec;40(6):815-821.

Richter D, Stoff A, Ramakrishnan V, et al. A comparison of a new skin closure device and intradermal sutures in the closure of full-thickness surgical incisions. Plast Reconstr Surg 2012;130(4):843-50

Coon D, Joseph Michaels 5th, Gusenoff JA, Chong T, Purnell C, Rubin JP. Hypothermia and complications in postbariatric body contouring. Plast Reconstr Surg. 2012;130(2):443-8.

Kim JY, Khavanin N, Rambachan A, et al. Surgical duration and risk of venous thromboembolism. JAMA Surg 2015;150(2):110-7.

Geerts WH, Bergqvist D, Pineo GF et al. (2008) Prevention of venous thromboembolism: American college of chest physicians evidence-based clinical practice guidelines (8th Edn). Chest, 133(6 Suppl):381S-453S

Petersen ML, Vázquez FJ, Mayer HF. (2022) Mechanical Thromboprophylaxis Alone in Body Contouring Surgery for Post Massive Weight Loss Patients: Is this Good Enough?. *Aesthetic Plast Surg* 46(1):248-254.

Piano G, Ketteler ER, Prachand V et al (2007) Safety, feasibility, and outcome of retrievable vena cava filters in high-risk surgical patients. J Vasc Surg 45(4):784–788

Vaziri K, Devin Watson J, Harper AP et al (2011) Prophylactic inferior vena cava filters in high-risk bariatric surgery. Obes Surg 21(10):1580–1584

Zavlin D, Jubbal KT, Balinger CL, Dinh TA, Friedman JD, Echo A. Impact of Metabolic Syndrome on the Morbidity and Mortality of Patients Undergoing Panniculectomy. Aesthetic Plast Surg (2017) 41:1400–1407

Agarwal N, Shibutani K, SanFilippo JA, Del Guercio LR (1982) Hemodynamic and respiratory changes in surgery of the morbidly obese. Surgery 92:226–231

Bell T, Stokes S, Jenkins PC, Hatcher L, Fecher AM (2017) Prevalence of cardiovascular and respiratory complications following trauma in patients with obesity. Heart Lung. https://doi.org/10.1016/j.hrtlng.2017.05.010

Bell TM, Bayt DR, Siedlecki CB et al (2016) Infectious complications in obese patients after trauma. J Surg Res 204:393–397

Green WD, Beck MA (2017) Obesity altered T cell metabolism and the response to infection. Curr Opin Immunol 46:1–7
Zuelzer HB, Ratliff CR, Drake DB. Complications of abdominal contouring surgery in obese patients: current status. Ann Plast Surg. 2010;64(5):598-604
Manahan MA, Shermak MA (2006) Massive panniculectomy after massive weight loss. Plast Reconstr Surg 117:2191–2197
Coon D, Gusenoff JA, Kannan N et al. Body mass and surgical complications in the post bariatric reconstructive patient: analysis of 511 cases. Ann Surg 2009; 249: 397 – 40.
Arthurs ZM, Cuadrado D, Sohn V et al (2007) Post-bariatric panniculectomy: pre-panniculectomy body mass index impacts the complication profile. Am J Surg 193:567–570
Mioton LM, Buck DW II, Gart MS, Hanwright PJ, Wang E, Kim JY (2013) A multivariate regression analysis of panniculectomy outcomes: does plastic surgery training matter? Plast Reconstr Surg 131:604e–612e
Cooper JM, Paige KT, Beshlian KM, Downey DL, Thirlby RC (2008) Abdominal panniculectomies: high patient satisfaction despite significant complication rates. Ann Plast Surg 61(2):188–196

Part VII
Behavior of Torsoplasty for Body Contouring

Chapter 49
Body Contouring: Concepts, Evolution, and Patient Engagement. Plastic Surgery: Concept of Stretching X Working Volumes

Jose Carlos Daher and Leonardo Daher

Abstract Plastic surgery assumed the position of medical specialty very recently. Major technical changes came supported by two major tools: silicone prostheses and liposculpture. In a short period of time, changes in social habits, digital media, and surgical procedures themselves demanded from plastic surgeons a great ability to adapt to technical, social, and ethical concepts. This revolution demanded from professionals improvements in the procedures, concepts, lowering costs, and increasing the quality of services provided, as requirements of modern capitalism. The demands of our clients and consumers supported by legal structures in defense of the consumer have had an impact not only on market competition but also on the patrimonial integrity of surgeons. All these factors together are analyzed, offering a broad view of concepts, techniques, and behavioral issues, addressing psychological aspects of patients as well as suggestions regarding defensive medicine.

Keywords Plastic surgery history · Volume recovery · Silicone protheses · Plastic surgery psychology · Bariatric surgery · Defensive medicine · Liposuction · Liposculpture

---

J. C. Daher (✉)
Brazilian Plastic Surgery Society (SBCP), International Society of Aesthetic Plastic Surgery (ISAPS), Hospital Daher's Plastic Surgery Residency Program, Brasilia, Brazil
e-mail: daher@hospitaldaher.com.br

L. Daher
Brazilian Plastic Surgery Society (SBCP), Hospital Daher Plastic Surgery Residency Program, Lago Sul, Brazil

J. M. Avelar, R. Cavalcanti Ribeiro (eds.), *Body Contouring*,
https://doi.org/10.1007/978-3-031-42802-9_49

Introduction

At its origins, plastic surgery focused on the conception of covering tissues. Correcting and reconstructing the deformities for covering function, otherwise, the outcome of scars and tissue texture would be poor. These were the reasons and motivations to the surgeons who were dedicated in treating the covering tissues.

Sometimes these concepts migrate to restoration of volumes, when the body prominences substance loss occurs. The nose amputations lead to a rich period of new surgical flap descriptions to its restoration (Penfield 1969).

The surgical advent of breast reduction was an important milestone in volume performance: the search was about an organ's volume reduction, one that interferes directly in the body contouring design (Thorek 1924).

Several authors evolved within different techniques in mammoplasties, and it culminated into Ivo Pitanguy's versatile technique for mammoplasty (Pitanguy 1961). Although there were different technical and tactical aspects between these surgeries to reach breast reduction, the one thing tha was extracted from this period is the aspect of body contouring modification, using not only covering tissues but also interfering on the organ's size and projection upon the body's surface, in order to comply with the individual patient's requests and achieve the whole-body harmony.

Discussion

The mammoplasties were a milestone in the volume work conception, adding up the previous knowledge of merely "tissue continuity" (Fig. 49.1).

Observe that the abdominoplasty ("tummy tuck surgery") pursuit normality in a post-pregnancy abdomen, in the predominant conception of tissue tension: repositioning the anatomical elements back to the pre-pregnancy body status, correcting umbilical hernias and others, and pulling the rectus abdominis muscle to its previous position. The increased abdominal continent is adjusted in the postpartum period into a smaller continent. The flaccid skin is stretched and distributed, and the excess is removed, etc.

The volume modification happened but the "volume treatment" wasn't the central idea of the surgical planning motivation. The foundation of the early plastic surgery was **stretching**: stretch the naturally expanded abdominal skin after pregnancy and stretch the aged face skin or the flaccid and saggy breasts.

The volume work acting on the continent was a challenge of mental posture in the plastic surgeon's creativity. The skin "stretch" is an additional surgical period in each operative act, where the continent is adjusted, the skin wrapper, to the created volume.

In this evolving phase of plastic surgery, the rebuilding of the amputated breasts was intended, after Halsted in 1882 (Halsted 1894), which systematized and popularized his technique of breast cancer surgical treatment, with total and radical amputation of the organ. From that era emerged a huge legion of mutilated women by this treatment that was necessary but caused profound psychological and social damage to these patients.

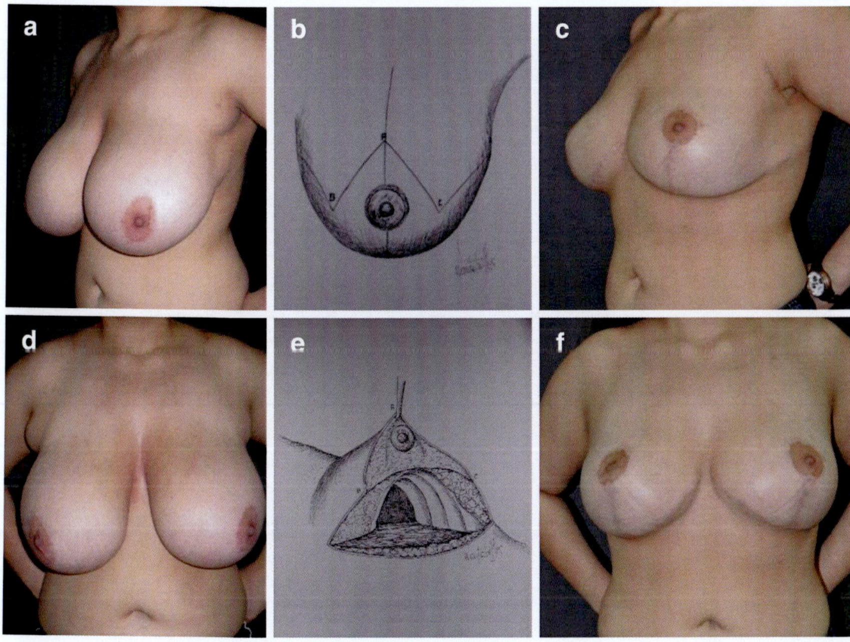

Fig. 49.1 Reduction mastoplasty performed by Pitanguys technique. Photos (**a**, **d**) before surgery showing large breasts; schems (**b**, **e**) surgical demarcation and mamary glandular resection accordind the technique; photos (**c**, **f**) after surgery

It can be said that the breasts are for women as the penis are for men, in sexual perception terms of each one's body image.

Back in the 1960–1970s, the plastic surgery field already knew how to reduce breasts but was extremely unguarded about breast reconstruction knowledge and techniques. The 1970s dwelled on this major challenge.

Many creative and curious surgeons used all engineering implanting, such as foams, rubber balls, etc., so they created volume to reconstruct or shape the breasts.

The Silicone Prosthesis Advent

Applied engineering in medicine produced the first silicone prosthesis that progressively evolved until nowadays, looking for the best long-term results and minimum complications.

In 1962, Cronin developed, along the industry, the first **silicone implants**. It was a great progress, but implants had very low projection, low viscosity silicone, and a thin envelope coverage, which allowed rupture/leaking, culminating to high rates of capsular contracture cases. In 1969, Ashley achieved a significant reduction on the contracture cases, using anatomical implants coated by polyurethane. These industries progressed, with viscosity adequation and non-permeable coating, which remain until today (Fig. 49.2) (Cronin and Gerow 1964; Ashley 1970).

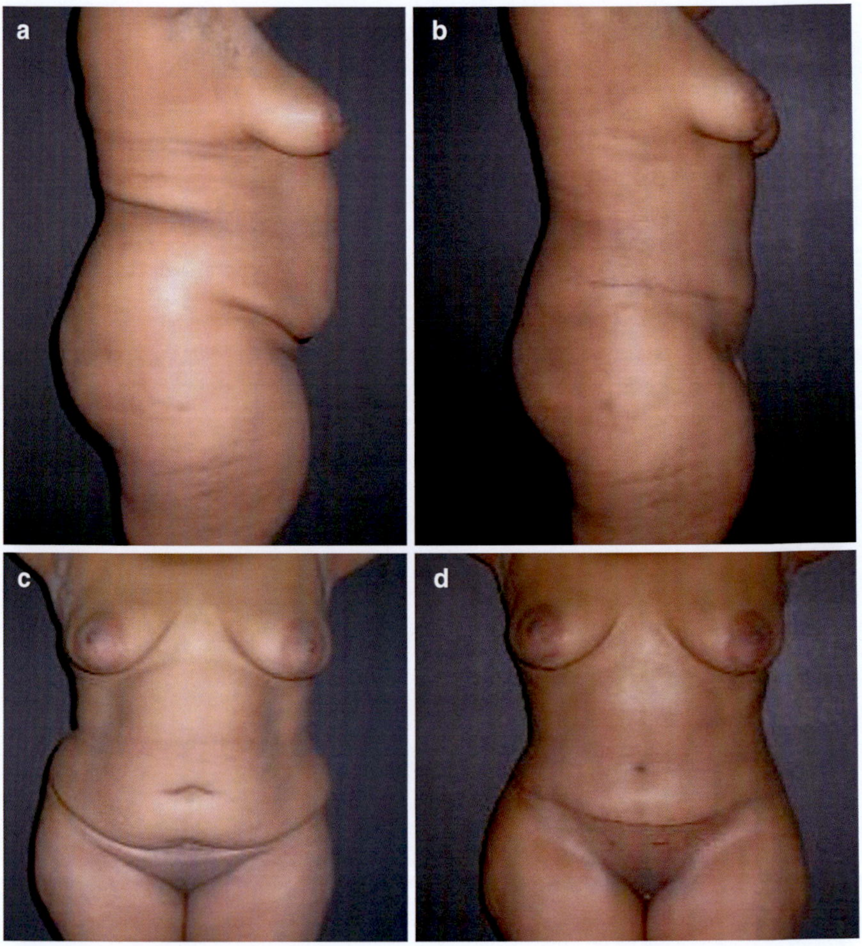

Fig. 49.2 Abdominoplasty combined with liposuction. Photos (**a**, **c**) before operation; (**b**, **d**) after surgery

Observe that we spoke about volume reduction, and now, we speak about creating them. So, we already had the silicone prosthesis that could enlarge small breasts, but the absence of skin coverage in amputated breasts was still an issue. In 1970s, an intense pursuit for new procedures and techniques was built, to achieve these goals.

The Expanders and Myocutaneous Flaps

As it happens during pregnancy, Radovan (1977) conceived the idea that every area in the body could "get pregnant." Intimately placed in subcutaneous tissue, an empty bag that progressively gets filled generates skin cell multiplication. The skin got expanded, grew, and so it remained. With this, it was possible to create the needed skin coverage for silicone implants and reconstructing breasts. The expanders were a big enhancement on body contouring.

This proposal was very beneficial for its applicability in any area of the human body where covering tissues were needed, not only in the mammary region.

And this brilliant idea was accompanied by the systematization and study of myocutaneous flaps (Vasconez, Mathes and Nahai) (Mathes and Nahai 1997). Several new flaps were created, and the anatomical bases of myocutaneous flaps used in the past were explained, which had no description or explanations of their anatomical bases (Tansini's flap for reconstruction of the anterior chest wall) (Tansini 1906).

The Geniality of Yves-Gerard Illouz: Liposculpture

Geniuses are those who see the obvious. Thus, I classify Yves-Gerard Illouz as a genius who revolutionized everything about body contouring with the creation of liposuction, a new tool. Hence, we evolved to the aspirated fat graft in places, which lacked volume. We have seen the evolution of liposuction into liposculpture. The obvious was there and no one saw it.

This one had been thought by Schrudde previously, a German physician who used an intrauterine aspiration device to aspirate subcutaneous fat and was later innovated by Kesselring, who was already using aspiration devices (Kesselring 1983).

Devices had the same purpose but didn't get ahead. It was up to Illouz to simplify the process using a simple cannula with negative pressure. We could now decrease undesirable prominences and increase depressed ones. If they are contiguous, we create curves that did not exist and an almost perfect harmony (Illouz 1996, 2014).

Liposculpture has been adopted around the world by thousands of surgeons, accompanied by innovators on the subject such as Pierre Fournier and others (Figs. 49.3 and 49.4).

We have arrived, therefore, at the historical moment to work on the body contour. Not just in breast reductions, then breast augmentations, in abdominoplasty, but throughout the entire body, decreasing or increasing volumes. It became the most performed plastic surgery in the world, since most of the times, it is not the main operative act; it became an additional act associated to many other surgeries.

An important watershed has been consolidated. Plastic surgery stopped thinking only about stretching tissues; we started thinking about first defining the volume and then adapting the tissues to continent, resecting/stretching the skin, or not.

If we look for an analogy, we can take, for example, rhinoplasty, where the basis and main tool is to work the volume of the content.

The dissemination of liposculpture in social media, among the numerous positive aspects, led to mishaps: unprepared physicians or individuals who were not qualified, misjudged the process as a simple procedure, or promoted several complications. But it was a small and transitory period in face of the importance of the liposculpture conquest.

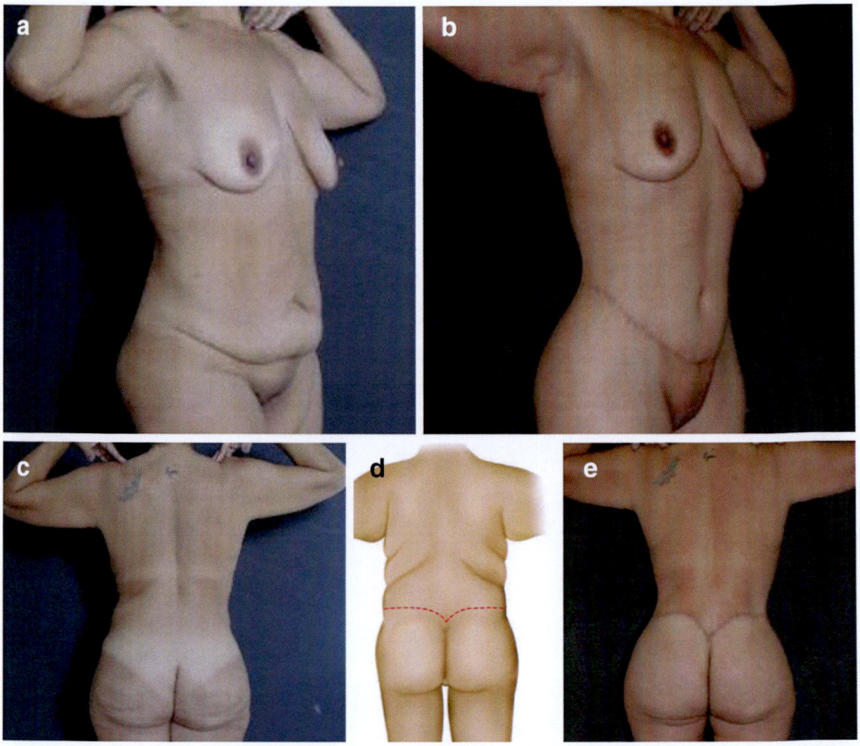

Fig. 49.3 A female patient after weight loss underwent belt abdominoplasty with modeling of the gluteal regions. Photos (**a**, **c**) before surgery; (**b**, **e**) after operation; (**d**) schem of the technique showing the posterior aspect of the torso for remodeling the gluteal regions

The procedure with the cannula allowed surgeons accustomed to using a scalpel or scissors to intervene on previously unreachable areas, using a simple negative pressure cannula, such as the back, flanks, inner face of the knees, arms, inner thighs, and abdomen.

We have come to the moment of re-reading the body-contouring chapter for both plastic surgeons and patients.

The surgeon used to say: "I can only operate you, ma'am, if you lose that much weight." Nowadays, he will tell his patient that losing weight is ideal, and liposcu-lpture is not a weight loss procedure, instead, he will tell that the intervention can be immediate and intervene in the areas where the deformity is established and where weight loss is known to not be enough to resolve. There is the localized fat, which will be treated immediately (Fig. 49.4).

The visceral fat that will keep your abdomen still bulging cannot be vacuumed and will improve only through weight loss. Although liposuction doesn't resolve all the deformities, it has benefits, by reducing the abdominal fat layer. The surgeon can deliver the benefits of liposuction by reducing the fat layer and by removing the hanging abdomen tissue, for example. This creates a new psychological moment

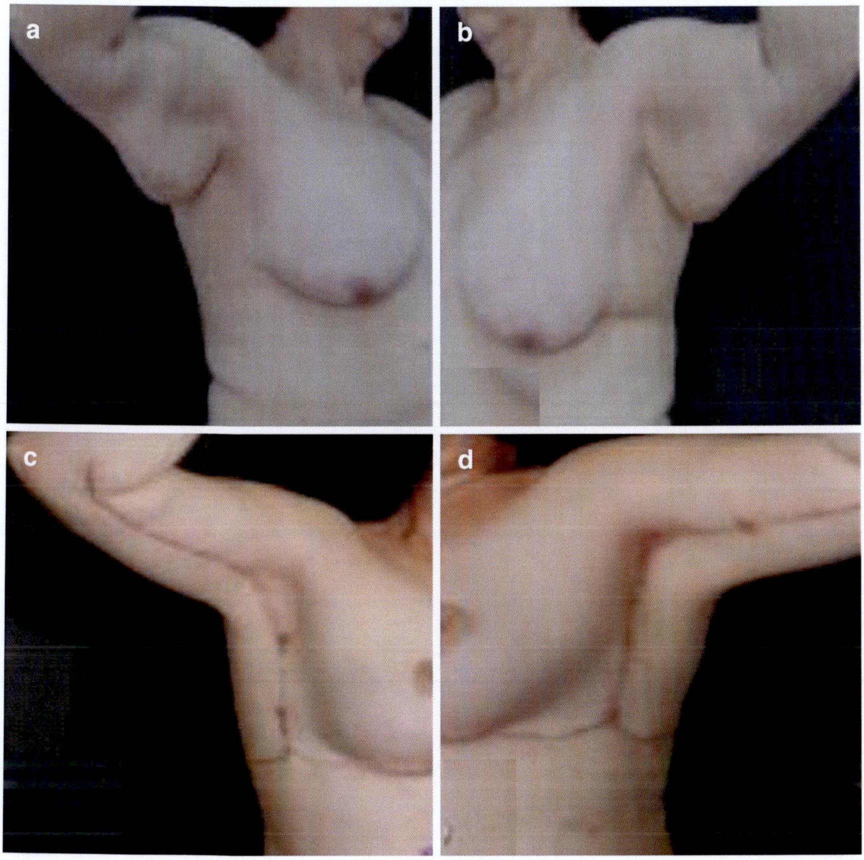

Fig. 49.4 Improving contour of the arm, axila, breast and lateral side of the chest in a female patient after weight loss performed by Pitanguys technique. Photos (**a**, **c**) unaesthetic appearance showing redundant and flebby cutanoeus covering; photos (**b**, **d**) 8 months after one stage operation

that stimulates the patient to improve continuously, gaining strength for a difficult change in eating habits.

Post-Bariatric Surgery: A New Chapter in the Contemporary Plastic Surgery

The history of body contouring treatment takes another step of great medical and social meaning: post-bariatric surgeries.

Bariatric surgery, after curing or improving several comorbidities brought by obesity (diabetes, hypertension, dyslipidemias, etc.), usually leaves leftover tissue sequel (the continent that became large in relation to the reduced content), associated with residual localized fat deposits, those that do not disappear, with a conventional weight loss: regions of the flanks, back, lateral extensions of the breasts, arms, culottes, thighs, and inner face of the knees (Mendes and Viterbo 2016).

Plastic surgery, already extremely advanced in techniques for adjusting the skin in all body regions, is associated with the liposculpture genius technique to reduce these continents and offer maximum improvement of results to post-bariatric patients.

The scars in post-bariatric surgeries, as in all plastic surgery, must be as small as possible, but as extensive as necessary to achieve the best body contouring results. We should never allow ourselves to compromise a maximum result of the body contour to avoid a few centimeters of scar. It would be insane because patients care less about these scars, in view of the gain from recovering a normal contour, especially because, in general, post-bariatric scars tend to be hypotrophic and almost disappear within months.

When we talk about bariatric surgery with our eyes always focused on the maximum results, which is also the expectation of our patients, it is necessary to reflect on a more rational planning, with maximum results and lower material and social costs.

A post-bariatric patient, excluding facial deformities that will be approached in another context, has to undergo the following surgeries: in the lower body segment, abdomen and genitals, lower back, buttocks, and thighs. In the upper part of the body, you will have to treat the breasts, arms, and upper back. Therefore, there are from seven to eight regions to be operated.

The very important matter of planning must be considered. Health insurance or the patients' own resource costing must be seriously considered, since we are talking about expensive procedures that demand a specific hospital infrastructure and support. These are patients debilitated by the disabsortive syndrome caused by bariatric surgery.

Operating surgery by surgery presupposes seven to eight operative acts. The material and social cost would be very onerous, in addition to limiting results. The optimization of results is only achievable when the simultaneous correction of contiguous regions is associated. For instance, abdominoplasty associated with flank treatment is almost mandatory.

In our service, we chose to perform as many associated surgeries as possible in each operative act. Nowadays, we are able to perform all the surgeries of the lower body segment (abdomen, flanks, lower back, buttocks, thighs, and inner face of the knees) in a single surgical procedure, when indicated, and all surgeries of the upper body segment (breasts, upper back, arms) are also in a single operative act (Fig. 49.4).

With a highly engaged and trained team, each of these two operations can be performed in 4 and a half hours. The intervals of these operative acts will be dictated by the patient's desire and analysis of the new preoperative period. Normally the minimum interval is 30 days.

With this modern systematization, the patient who heals faster from all his deformities gains time, and with the social benefits of being hospitalized only twice, the surgeon benefits, rewarded with beautiful results that can be offered to his clientele, and the society also benefits, with lowering the cost of these surgeries either for the patient or for health insurance.

Psychological Aspects

Patients with severe body contouring disorder are psychologically complex. It is extremely important to discuss with them the real expectations and possible results. Many of these patients have fanciful perceptions awaiting results that will never be achieved, so it is our obligation to show and deconstruct this idea when it exists.

Body dysmorphism or body dysmorphic disorder is a condition in which the patient is extremely dissatisfied with their appearance, which does not match the physical examination findings. In these cases, psychological and/or psychiatric treatment should be considered before any surgery, considering that this disorder may be a contraindication for purely aesthetic intervention (Dornelas et al. 2019).

For post-bariatric patients, multidisciplinary follow-up is essential. One of the most performed surgeries in these patients is the gastric bypass, a restrictive and disabsorptive surgery. Due to the nature of this surgery, it is common for some patients to have low levels of hemoglobin, and proteins, among other changes, so a periodic follow-up with the physician, and/or nutrology can be beneficial. Emotional stability is also a major milestone for successful treatment. Weight regain and/or exchange of eating compulsion to other addictions such as alcoholism or smoking is frequent, so periodic psychological and/or psychiatric follow-up would be prudent.

The Defensive Medicine

Physicians must be prepared to defend themselves against eventual result contestations, generally unfounded contestations, which are a harmful spin-off of the current legal structure in physician-patient relationships. A poorly conducted or lost lawsuit can represent very important financial losses, sometimes destroying assets accumulated in a lifetime of toil and hard struggle to exercise the profession. You must have the most detailed consent terms and an excellent prior discussion with your patients. Once well briefed in the presence of witnesses and signed terms, groundless challenges are discouraged.

Conclusion

Plastic surgery is an extraordinary specialty in which the surgeon's skill and creative ability are paramount. The concept of working with volumes grew, especially after the advent of the important reliable tools as silicone prostheses and the ingenious liposculpture. Our medical practice is increasingly linked to the needs of cost optimization within the indisputable need for better results. The treatment purposes must be combined with the complete patient engagement, psychologically well prepared and enlightened, and the surgeons must be attentive, taking preventive measures on their own legal defense.

References

Thorek M. Plastic surgery of the breast and abdominal wall. Springfield, IL: Charles C Thomas; 1924

Pitanguy I. Mamoplastias: Estudo de 245 casos consecutivos e apresentação de técnica pessoal. Rev Bras Cir. 1961;42:201

Halsted WS. I. The Results of Operations for the Cure of Cancer of the Breast Performed at the Johns Hopkins Hospital from June, 1889, to January, 1894. Ann Surg. 1894;20(5):497–555

Penfield W. Halsted of Johns Hopkins. JAMA. 1969 Dec 22;210(12):2214–2218

Cronin TD, Gerow FJ. Augmentation Mammaplasty: A New 'Natural Feel' Prosthesis : Transactions of the Third International Congress of Plastic Surgery. Amsterdam: Excerpta Medica; 1964

Ashley FL. A new type of breast prosthesis. Preliminary report. Plast Reconstr Surg 1970;421–424

Radovan C: Adjacent flap development using expandable silastic implants. Annual Meeting of American Society of Plastic and Reconstructive Surgeons, Boston, Mass, USA, Sept. 30, 1977

Mathes SJ, Nahai F. Reconstructive surgery: principles, anatomy, and technique. London: Churchill Livingstone; 1997. p. 61742

Tansini I. Sopra il mio nuovo processor di amputazione della mammella. Gazz Mal Ital. 1906;57:141

Illouz YG. Body contouring by lipolysis: a 5-year experience with over 3000 cases. Plast Reconstr Surg 1983;72:591–7

Illouz YG. History and current concepts of lipoplasty. Clin Plast Surg. 1996;23:721

Illouz YG. Liposuction – the evolution of classical technique. PMFA News. 2014; vol 1 No. 4

Kesselring U. Regional fat aspiration for body contouring. Plast Reconstr Surg 1983;72:610–19

Dornelas MT, Corrêa MPD, Corrêa LD, Dornelas GV, Soares AA, Dornelas LV, et al. Transtorno dismórfico corporal sob a perspectiva do cirurgião plástico. Rev. Bras. Cir. Plást.2019;34(1):108–112

Mendes F, Viterbo F. Cirurgia Plástica Pós-Bariátrica. Rio de Janeiro: Di Livros; 2016

Chapter 50
Torsoplasty Improving Body Contouring

Marcelo Daher and Alvaro Daher

Abstract The authors make a semantic allusion to the trunk in which it is put in synonymy with the torso. So any plastic surgery on the torso would then be a torsoplasty, from the arms to the thighs, to correct deformities caused by obesity, pregnancy, and massive weight loss, to improve body contour or even to repair congenital problems. They consider the various associations and the current trends of performing less combined surgeries and the contradiction of the modern era when patients want to do as many associations as possible. A careful work of pros and cons, adapting to the patient's clinical condition and the technical-surgical conditions of the team, can reach a situation of optimal surgical planning, precisely defining the type of surgery, whether combined or not. The results have been satisfying and the complications are minimal when patients follows the postoperative recommendations.

Keywords Torso · Torsoplasty · Obesity · Massive weight loss · Tissue aging · Bariatric surgery, Body contouring · Mammaplasty · Abdominoplasty

Introduction

The torso is the most voluminous part of the human body and is also referred to as the trunk; human body is excluded from the head and limbs (Ferreira n.d.).

M. Daher (✉)
Interclínica—Centroplástica, R. Jardim Botânico, Brazilian Society of Plastic Surgery (SBCP), Rio de Janeiro, Brazil

A. Daher
São Paulo, Brazil

J. M. Avelar, R. Cavalcanti Ribeiro (eds.), *Body Contouring*,
https://doi.org/10.1007/978-3-031-42802-9_50

The Greek term from which the word torso derives means “wand” or “stem”; the torso is the portion of the body that extends from the upper part of the arms to the upper part of the thighs (González-Ulloa 1979).

The surgical treatments of areas of the torso can be done either alone or in combination, when a greater number of operations are performed at once, allowing a partial or complete plastic surgical reshaping of the torso, which generated the term torsoplasty.

Some authors cite torsoplasty as a surgical intervention to adjust the skin and fat over the dorsal region of the torso (Wakefield et al. 2014; Boswell 2010), which in our assessment would be called “dorsoplasty,” one of the procedures that includes a torsoplasty. This fact can generate some confusion when researching and studying this subject, especially in Portuguese. Sometimes, we can also find this procedure as “lumboplasty” (González-Ulloa 1979) (Figs. 50.1 and 50.2).

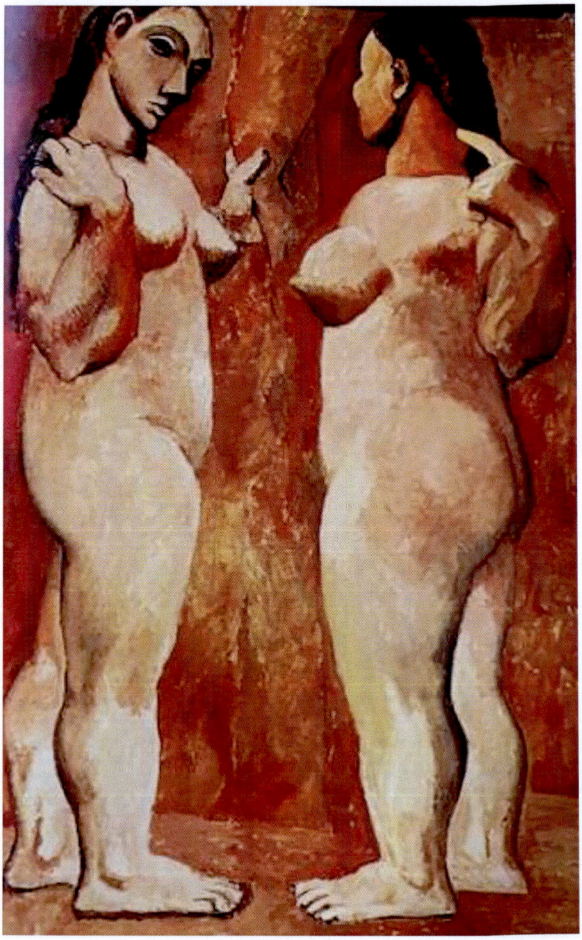

Fig. 50.1 Pablo Picasso Deux 2 Nudes, 1906. Source: Interclínica-Centroplástica Image Bank – Marcelo Daher

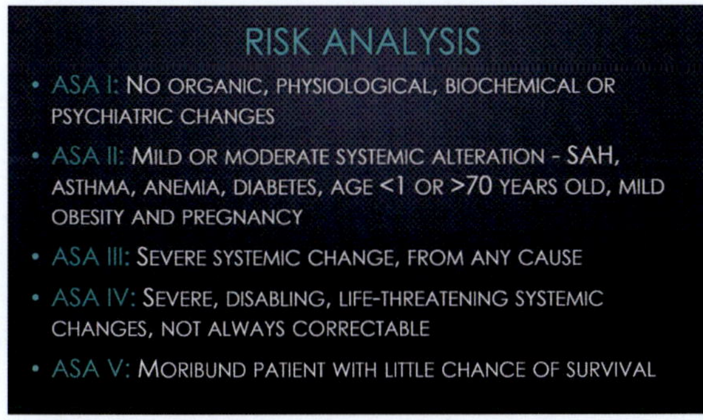

Fig. 50.2 The American Society of Anesthesiologists (ASA) classification

Current Concepts

Torsoplasty has currently encountered some resistance among surgeons, who increasingly tend to reduce the number of surgeries performed in combination, given the increased morbidity that these surgeries provide (Roxo et al. 2019; Resende 2008).

In our experience, two or three surgical combinations on the torso are allowed at the same time, the most common association being mammaplasty with abdominoplasty. This is still frequently associated with liposuction of the flanks or even the entire waist (surgery in two decubitus), which we also try to avoid in order to reduce morbidity and operative risk. In these cases, the procedures in the dorsal region (performed in the prone position) end up being left for a second surgery, unless they are a continuation of the abdominoplasty, as the circular abdominoplasty (Modarressi et al. 2016).

Torsoplasty includes main procedures, namely, (1) brachioplasty (in various degrees, depending on the deformity), (2) mammaplasty to increase or decrease volume and reshape, (3) abdominoplasty (various modalities), (4) gluteoplasty to increase or decrease volume and correct ptosis, (5) cruroplasty to improve the thighs or to reduce the volume of the trochanteric region, and (6) dorsoplasty to improve excess skin and adipose tissue in this region (González-Ulloa 1979).

However, there may be combinations including other procedures, such as (7) gynecomastia surgery; (8) reverse abdominoplasty, often performed together with mammaplasty; (9) liposuction of the anterior abdomen; (10) liposuction of the subscapular region; (11) liposuction of the "bat wing" (posterior region of the arm reaching the scapular area); (12) resection of the subscapular skin (bra-line back lift); (13) supragluteal skin resection; (14) gluteal fat grafting; and (15) the "Cinta-liga" surgery (abdominoplasty with cruroplasty) (Pontes 2004; Roxo et al. 2008; Aly and Nahas 2019; Rocha et al. 2012).

Indications/Contraindications

The complaint of the female public is very often linked to pregnancies. There was an increase in weight, the "breasts fell out," there was diastasis of the rectus abdominis muscles, there was an increase in fat on the sides and back, and they make the characteristic gesture using their hands and pinching the tissues of the flank to demonstrate their dissatisfaction. It is a classic indication of torsoplasty, which is currently called the "mommy makeover."

The surgeon must be skilled to achieve their goals, which are the patient satisfaction and safety.

The patient's complaint must flow freely and gradually and must be respected. The surgeon must be careful not to (inadvertently) induce any operation that is not very well established in the patient's imaginary. Patients often give an idea of "general catastrophe" of their condition when they expose the problem to the surgeon. Special care must be taken with this type of patient to strictly comply with their main complaint, remembering that the patient is layman and does not know about the increasing morbidity with the increase in the number of procedures in the same surgical intervention (Resende 2008).

However, the surgeon must explain the possibilities and advantages of performing more procedures in the same surgical act, aiming to take advantage of the same anesthesia and hospitalization, in a clear and objective exposition of the pros and cons to the patient.

In view of the patient's decision, patient's clinical conditions and the preparation of the surgeon and the surgical team must be evaluated to define whether the surgery can be combined or not.

Post-Bariatric Plastic Surgery

In the last three decades, there has been great progress in bariatric techniques and treatments, leading the population with a BMI greater than or equal to 40 (morbid obesity), or greater than or equal to 35 (grade II obesity) with comorbidities, to seek specialized medical services (Resende 2008).

Current techniques were reborn, and re-edited from the 1960s/1970s when only the jejunal shunt was performed for the techniques that, in addition to the shunt, also include gastroplasty, reducing the gastric lumen. They are mixed techniques, that is, they are disabsorptive and restrictive (Anon n.d.).

This was motivated by the unrestrained growth of obesity around the world, particularly in the western population, associated with the continued increase in collective anxiety. The uninterrupted demand for success in all areas of existence, associated with the very large and easy supply of food (mainly carbohydrates, represented by sugars and farinaceous), in addition to a weak or nonexistent infant nutrition education, when mothers confuse that "eating a lot" is healthier than "eating well"—all of this contributed a lot to this increase in obesity in the world's population.

When undergoing bariatric surgery, these individuals with grade II or morbid obesity present significant weight loss of 50 to 100 kg, sometimes even more, and as a consequence, post-bariatric patients appear. There is another category of patients with a normalized BMI or close to it, but with immense amounts of skin and fat excess. This situation often causes dysfunction of the arms and legs, in addition to psychological disturbance due to the unaesthetic body contour and consequent loss of self-esteem and human dignity (Resende 2008; PEC et al. 2006; Cannistra et al. 2006).

Some plastic surgeons were mainly dedicated to this chapter of plastic surgery and became specialists in post-bariatric surgeries.

Torsoplasty currently has much more complex treatments, especially in post-bariatric cases, going around the abdomen (circular abdominoplasty) or in mammaplasties, completing with a body lifting. In the last one, the incision is made over the bra-line and goes to the anterior axillary incisions, perpendicular to the posterior axillary pillar. These incisions are often unsightly and do not solve the problem of great tissue redundancy (Downey and Gross 2008).

There are surgeons who defend the total transformation of the torso in the same surgical procedure, the surgery being performed in several positions, and also including brachioplasty and cruroplasty, with numerous and well-trained teams (Roxo et al. 2019). Others preserve the step-by-step approach, more cautiously but with a longer treatment.

Preoperative

The patient needs to be seen the day before or a few days before the surgery, when we check the requested preoperative exams, the free and informed consent documents are signed, the preoperative photographs are taken, and the doubts are clarified again. In this preoperative consultation, a new physical examination will also be performed, at which time we use a resource that we created a few years ago—the CSP (consolidated surgical plan)—as complaints and demands often change at the time of surgery, which causes a psychological disturbance both for the team and for the patient himself, who is insecure and hesitant about the surgery. So these issues must be resolved first! The CSP is nothing more than the verification of the surgical plan that had been made in the first consultation, together with the team, the patient, and his companion, when we can make the last changes, add or remove small associated procedures, and that the patient signs at the end, showing that it is in accordance with the surgical plan, now consolidated.

The photographs are taken within the same pattern, always in the same room with the same lighting and distance; its limits go from the lower lip to the middle of the thighs, which matches all the pre- and postoperative photos regarding the torso. The views are the classic ones: front, bilateral three-quarters, bilateral profile, bilateral posterior three-quarters, and back.

Reference points should be marked with the patient in an orthostatic position, e.g., beginning and end of the lower abdominal, suprapubic fold. It is an important reference, even if it has to be exceeded in some cases. Scoliosis is marked, hip unevenness and tissue accumulation greater on one side than the other (usually on the lower side). The patient must be informed of this very gently, as he often does not receive this observation well. The use of a corrective insole for the shoe of the shorter limb is recommended, and the patient is ideally referred to a postural physiotherapist

Prior marking brings great savings in surgical time and greater precision. The patient is recommended not to rub these demarcated areas when bathing, leaving the marker ink for up to 2 or 3 days. The final design can be made on the operating table, now with a compass and ruler.

Make sure that the patient does not use anticoagulant/antiplatelet drugs such as Acetilsalicilic acid, Clopidogrel, Aspirin, and Warfarin, as well as some herbal medicines such as arnica, garlic (Cannistra et al. 2006; Woodbury & Sniecinski 2016), ginseng, gingko biloba, kawa-kawa, green tea, vitamin E, cascara sagrada, ginger, and St. John's wort, among others. It is quite common for patients to think that these are not considered drugs, or that they are "unimportant" drugs, and do not mention them in the anamnesis, which can cause serious problems for the surgeon (Bedi et al. 2016; Destro et al. 2006; Teixeira et al. 2010).

Other medications that may interfere with the operation are oral contraceptives, hormone replacement therapy, nonsteroidal anti-inflammatories, and the monoamine oxidase inhibitor antidepressants.

If any of these drugs are detected, we must suspend the surgery and reschedule it at least a week in the future.

Create an environment of friendship and trust with the patient and focus on follow-up issues, omitting some issues and details of the surgery itself. This greatly reduces the patient's anxiety.

Some of the risk factors that are considered by the cardiologist for the release of surgical risk (ASA classification) and also to be considered by the surgeon are as follows:

- Age > 40 years.
- Obesity.
- Oral contraceptive.
- Diabetes.
- Deep vein thrombosis (DVT)/pulmonary thromboembolism (PTE).
- Autoimmune disease.
- General anesthesia.
- Prolonged surgery (> 6 h).
- Prolonged immobilization in bed.

Surgical Technique

The anesthesia that we normally use in our practice is the peridural block, which can be low or high, or both. When performing the double puncture, the anesthetist has the option of leaving a catheter in one of the blocks so that he can reinforce it during the surgery if this part of the operation is the last to be performed and, therefore, it may take longer time.

Another option widely used by colleagues who perform surgeries combined with three or more procedures is the general anesthesia, which is currently performed safely. Even so, the surgeon must be concerned about completing the surgery within the allotted time, ideally less than 6 h. This can be achieved with fewer procedures in the same surgery, or with a larger and well-trained team to perform the procedures almost concurrently.

The placement of an indwelling urinary catheter is essential to control diuresis, as well as to avoid bladder distension causing local dysmorphism (lower abdomen), in addition to pain stimulus and consequent increase in blood pressure, which can occur even with the anesthetized patient (Fig. 50.3).

Surgery lighting should be well suited with at least three different sources. The team must be composed of five to seven people directly involved in the surgery, being one senior surgeon, two assistant surgeons, one or two scrub technicians, and one anesthesiologist, sometimes two (Fig. 50.4).

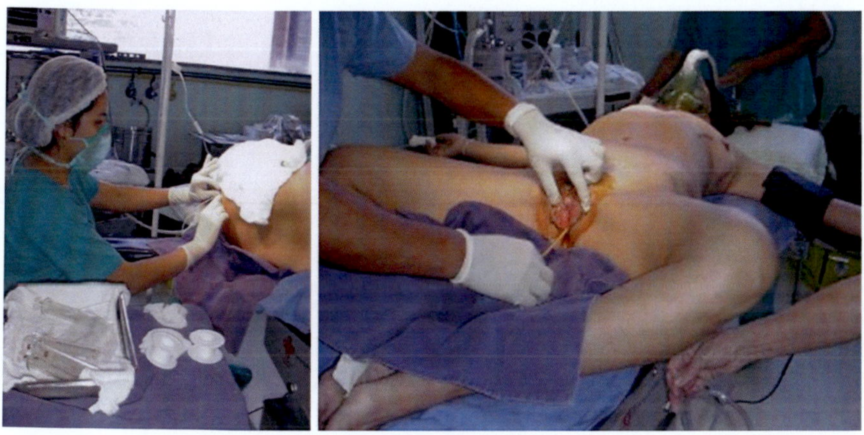

Fig. 50.3 The preoperative procedures: peridural anesthesia and urinary catheterism

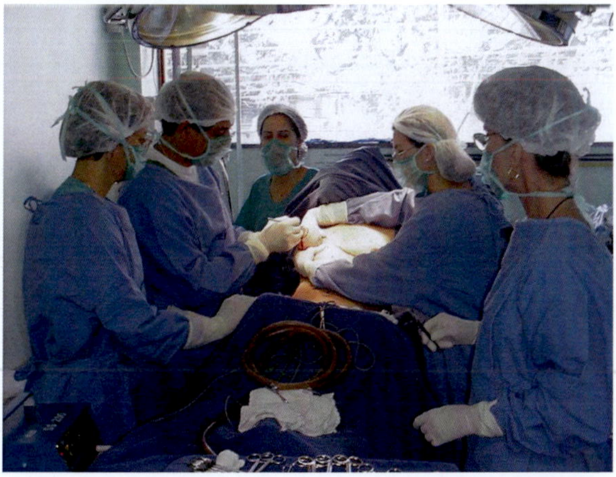

Fig. 50.4 The surgical team performing a combined surgery (five people)

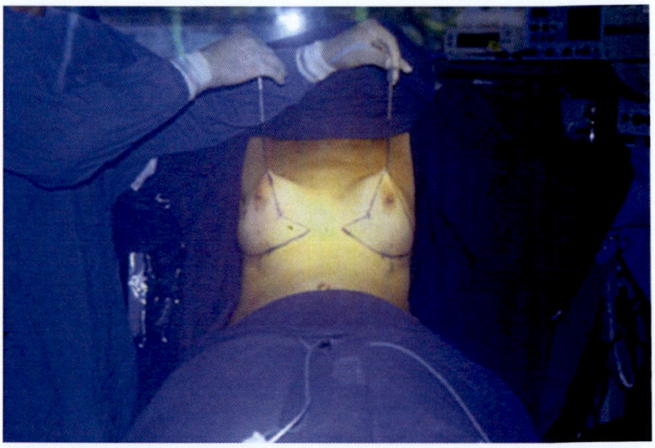

Fig. 50.5 A torsoplasty, starting with the breast. On the anterior torso, the author did in this case a modified Pitanguy's technique. Semi-sitting position, 45°

The time of combined surgeries must be carefully planned, including calculating the overlap of operative times.

For example, for this team, a reduction mammaplasty or mastopexy surgery takes approximately 3 h, including dressings, etc. When associated with abdominoplasty, the times do not add up, but they overlap in part, demanding about 4:30 h. And, curiously, when liposuction of the flanks and anterior abdomen is associated (in the same decubitus), the time remains at the same level of 4:30 h.

In the most common complete torsoplasty, breast + abdomen + liposuction type (two positions), we recommend starting in the ventral decubitus, proceeding with liposuction of the back and flanks, and then changing to the supine position. We usually perform mammaplasty in a semi-sitting position, 45° or with a low angle, or even horizontally during the suturing phase. While the breasts are sutured, liposuction of the anterior abdomen and flanks is performed, followed by abdominoplasty itself, finishing all the sutures (breast + abdomen) almost simultaneously (Fig. 50.5).

It is important to remember that, as in an orchestra, nothing should go out of rhythm; otherwise, the planning fails.

The patient, in addition to wearing medium compression elastic stockings, must wear intermittent pneumatic compression boots in the lower limbs, which are worn throughout the surgery to avoid blood stasis in the calves. In major surgeries, boots are used even after the surgery is over, while the patient is bedridden in the ward, until ambulation can begin (Fig. 50.6).

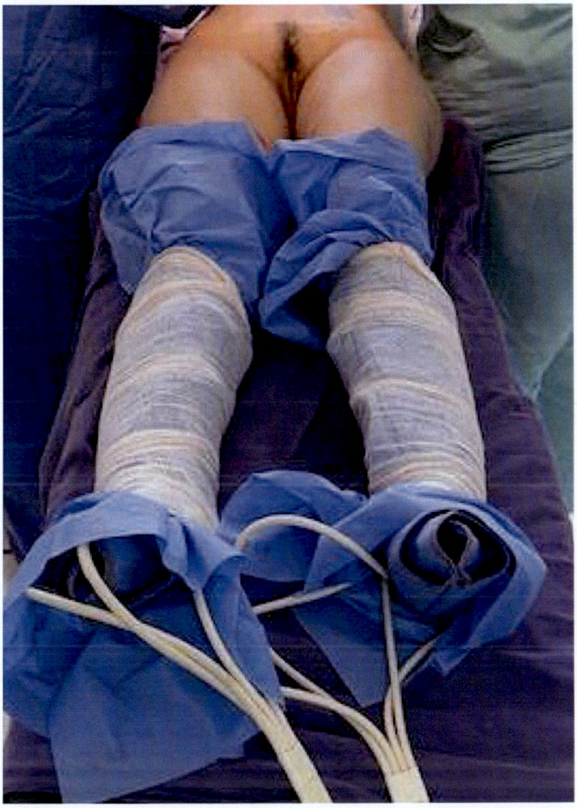

Fig. 50.6 The intermittent pneumatic compression boots being used during the surgery

The operating room temperature should not deviate from the range of 21–22 °C, reminding the patient that he/she will be naked for long hours. Do not hesitate to increase the room temperature if necessary.

Postoperative and Follow-Up

Greatly important is this part of the treatment. In the immediate postoperative period, ensure good hydration and moderate movements of intermittent dorsiflexion of the feet to ensure the "blood pump" is working on the calves. Early ambulation (very moderate), and usually with flexed torso until 2 weeks postoperative. Restrictive diets should not be started at this stage and should be hyperproteic and normoglycidic, with some restriction of in natura fats.

The long-term follow-up is also very important to ensure a good evolution, to photograph all of the stages of evolution, and to accompany the healing process. The patient must feel safe being closely monitored by the surgeon, not only the team.

DVT/PTE Prevention

The DVT is prevented by all means, starting with a good anamnesis and a preoperative color Doppler study of the deep venous system of the lower limbs. We use elastic stockings and intermittent pneumatic compressors during surgery (and in the immediate postoperative period), foot exercises (in bed) and moderate early ambulation in the immediate postoperative period, and low molecular weight heparin (Clexane®), which is made according to the Caprini protocol (Caprini et al. 2001; de Azevedo et al. 2010; Paiva Rita et al. 2013).

Do not forget about obsessively controlled hydration, which prevents dehydration with increased blood viscosity. The anesthesiologist will certainly perform intravenous hydration in a moderate and cautious manner in patients of advanced age and/or known to have heart disease, in order to avoid the risk of cardiovascular events due to volume overload.

When DVT is discovered, start immediate treatment with the help of an angiologist or vascular surgeon (Fig. 50.7).

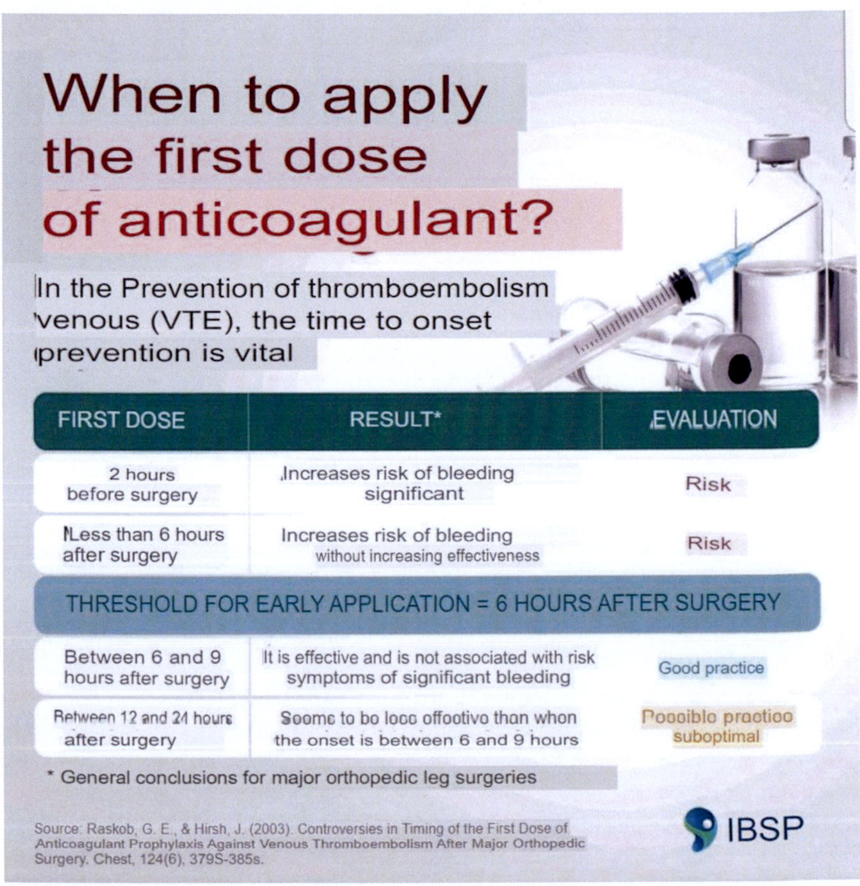

Fig. 50.7 A protocol for the prevention of deep venous thrombosis and pulmonary thromboembolism

Complications

The most frequently observed postoperative complication is the seroma formation. Other complications are ecchymosis, suture dehiscence (especially in areas of greatest tension), prolonged edema, operative site infection, and, more rarely, hematomas. Poor quality hypertrophic, hyperchromic, and retractable scars can occur mainly in melanodermic patients.

If the surgery is performed in a good technique and the patient follows the recommendations right, the complications are usually minimal (González-Ulloa 1979; Boswell 2010; Resende 2008).

Results

Associated surgeries such as torsoplasty must be performed by highly qualified surgeons acquainted with associated surgeries (Figs. 50.8, 50.9, 50.10, 50.11, 50.12, 50.13, 50.14, 50.15, 50.16, 50.17, 50.18). The time set aside for surgery should be as comfortable as possible and the hospital facilities appropriate, i.e., good lighting and electronic tables that allow several maneuvers with a simple touch. The team must be very well planned with elements neither lacking nor in excess.

The senior surgeon should not have any appointment to the immediate postoperative period. Unforeseen events can occur and stress is the enemy of excellence.

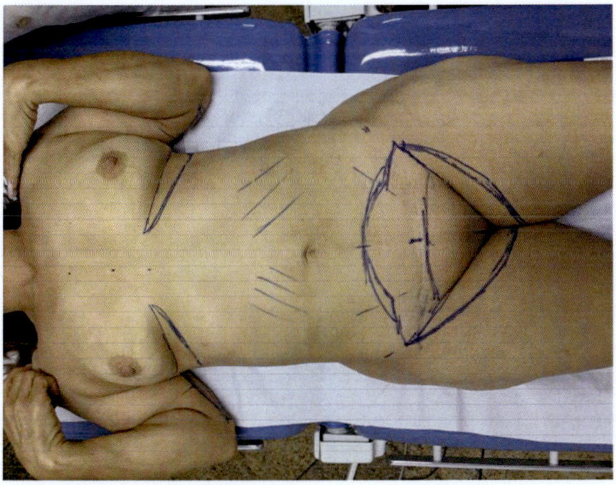

Fig. 50.8 A combined surgery of mastopexy, "Cinta-liga" (abdominoplasty and cruroplasty), brachioplasty, and abdominal liposuction (preoperative markings)

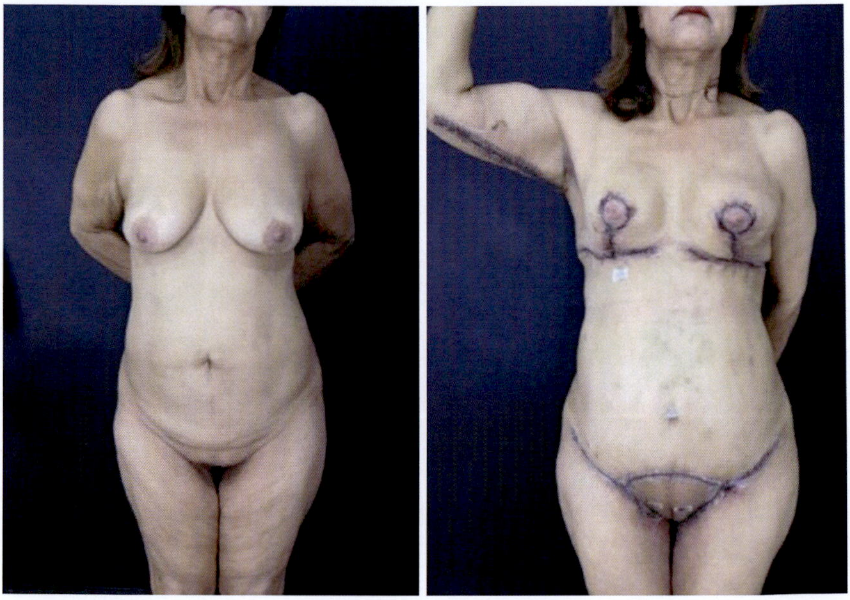

Fig. 50.9 A combined surgery of mastopexy, "Cinta-liga" (abdominoplasty and cruroplasty), brachioplasty, and abdominal liposuction (postoperative, 3 weeks)

Fig. 50.10 A combined surgery of mammaplasty and abdominoplasty (postoperative, 5 days)

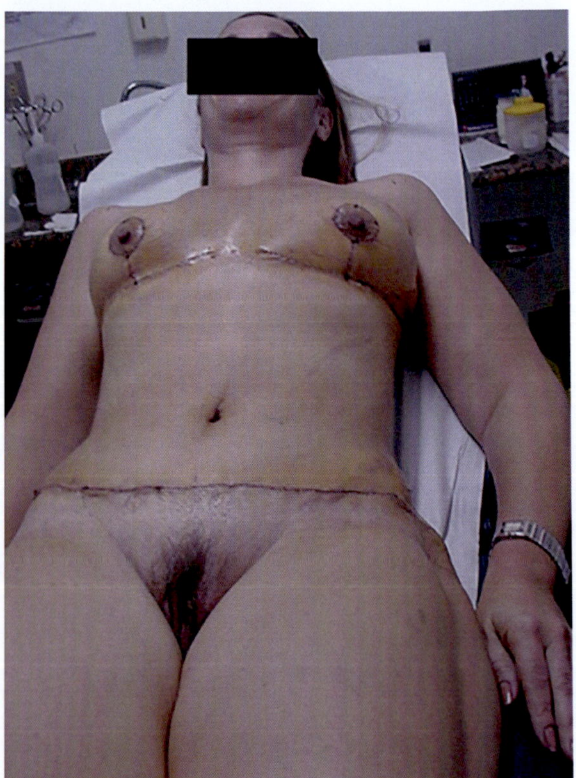

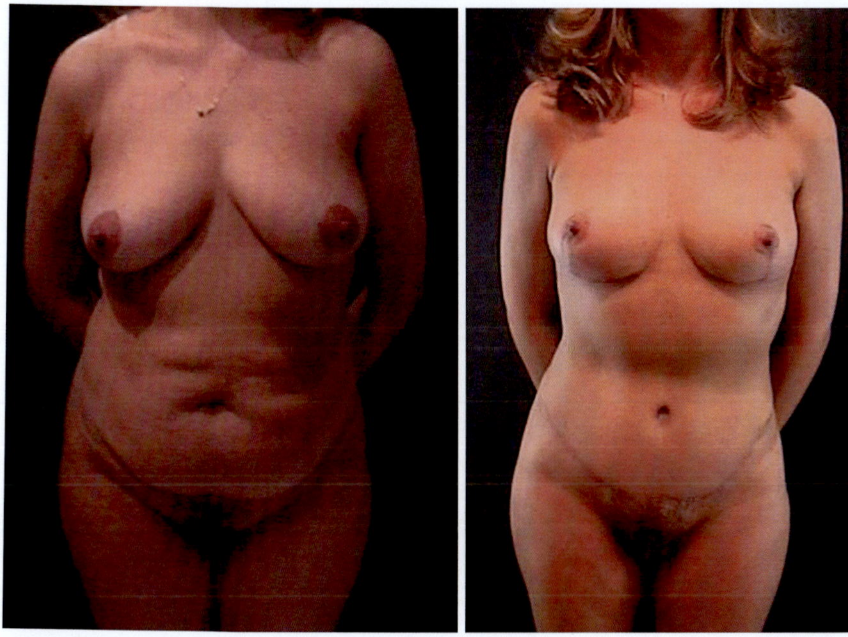

Fig. 50.11 A combined surgery of mammaplasty and abdominoplasty (pre- and postoperative pictures)

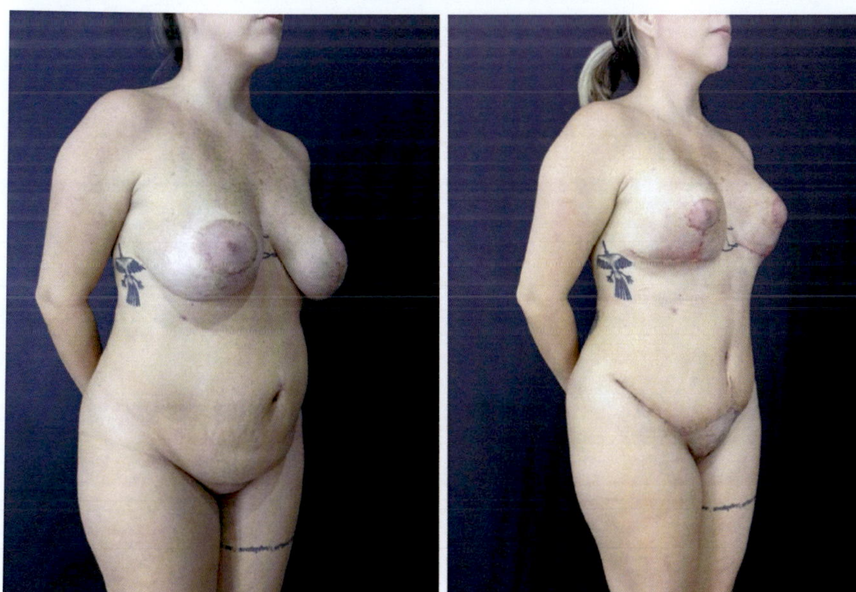

Fig. 50.12 A combined surgery of mammaplasty, abdominoplasty, and abdominal/flank liposuction—the "mommy makeover" surgery (pre- and postoperative pictures)

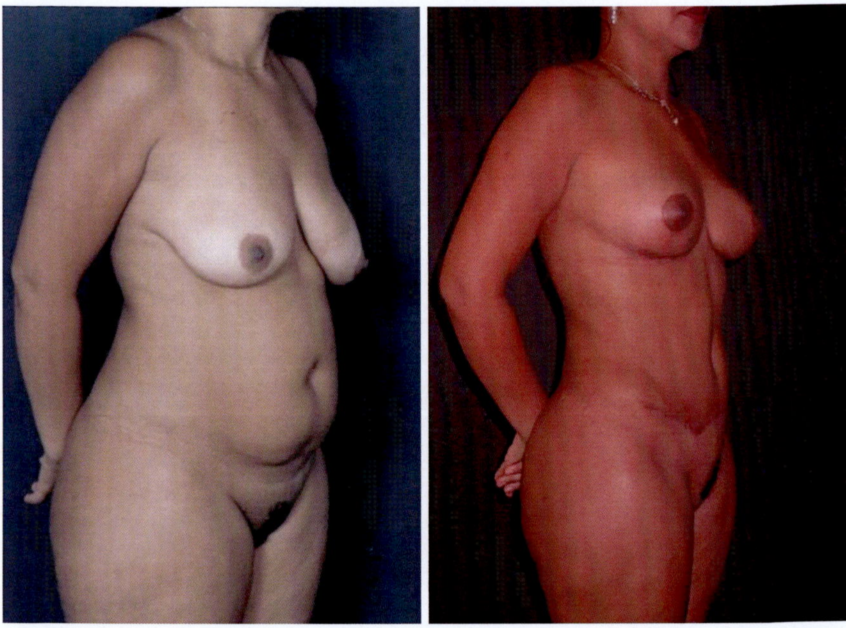

Fig. 50.13 A combined surgery of mastopexy, abdominoplasty, and waist liposuction (pre- and postoperative pictures)

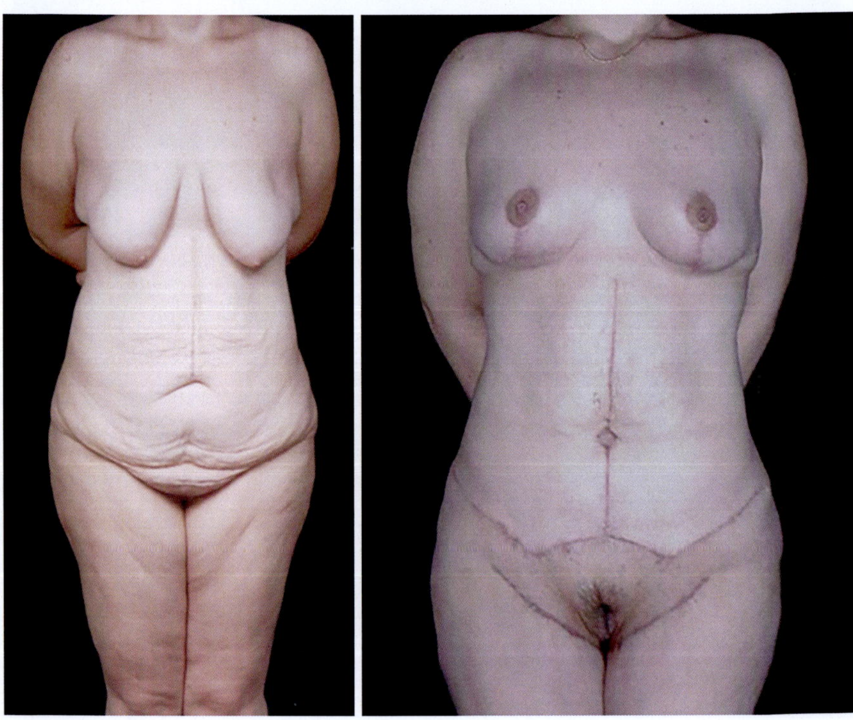

Fig. 50.14 A post-bariatric combined surgery of mammaplasty, "T" abdominoplasty, and cruroplasty (pre- and postoperative pictures)

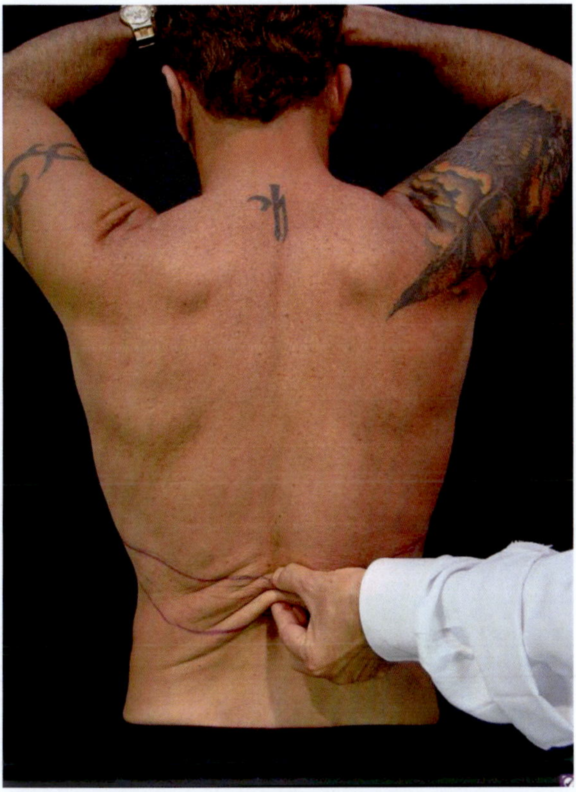

Fig. 50.15 Dorsoplasty on a male patient (preoperative demarcation)

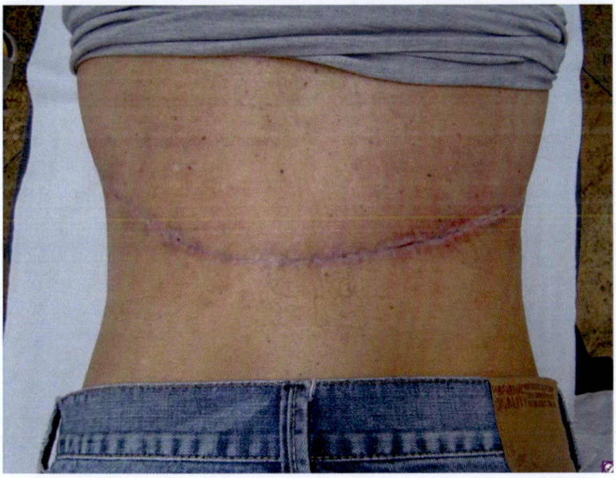

Fig. 50.16 Dorsoplasty on a male patient (postoperative scar, 1 month)

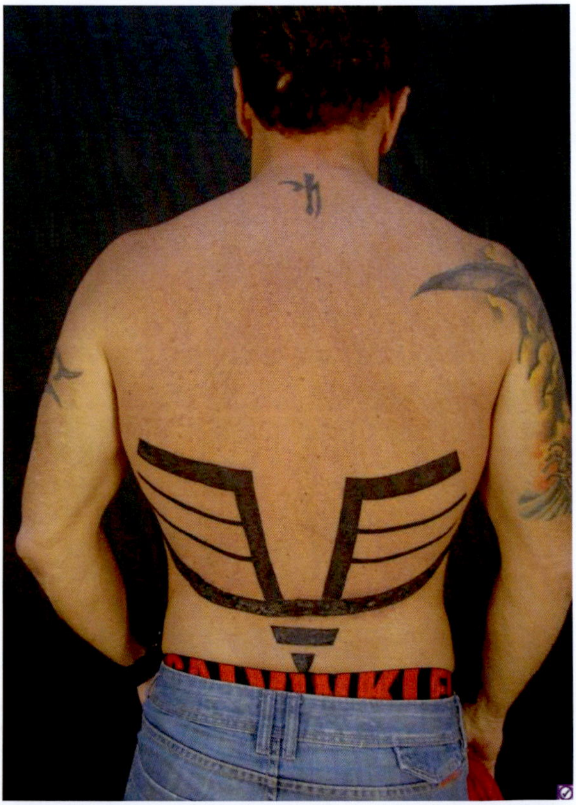

Fig. 50.17 Dorsoplasty on a male patient (late postoperative, scar hidden by a tattoo)

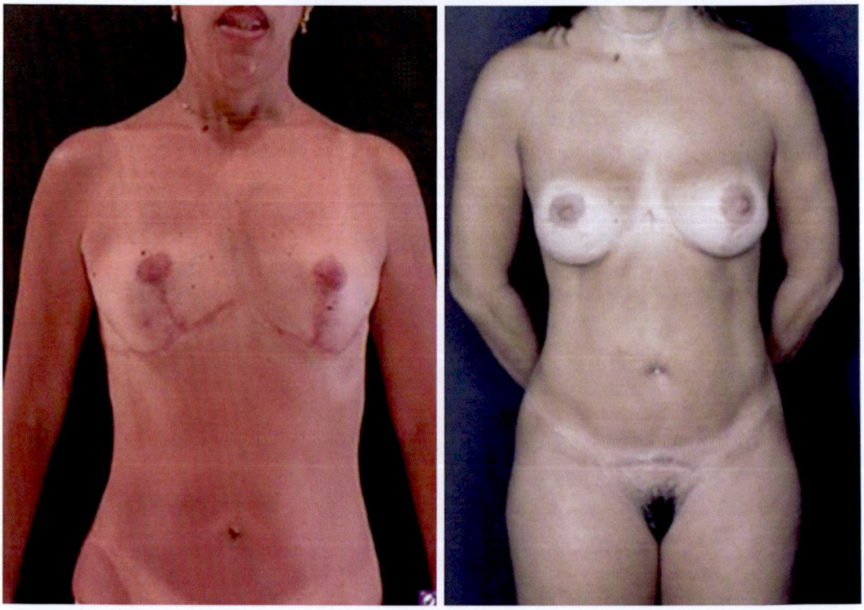

Fig. 50.18 Patient operated elsewhere with dissatisfaction due to asymmetry; submitted to mastopexy with silicone implant, abdominoplasty, and a flank liposuction

Discussion

The contrast between the initial concepts of torsoplasty, in which a greater number of surgical procedures are performed, and the current concept, in which many advocate for smaller associations, must be evaluated by the operator, of course, considering the patient's tendencies.

Curiously in recent times, there has been a movement opposite to that of surgeons, by patients, who increasingly choose to perform everything at once, defending the idea that they will "operate only once," as is the case of the "mommy makeover." At this point, concepts inherent to the current era of the speed of media and information from Google® end up opposing the doctor's guidelines and considerations!

Currently, it is also very important to mention the need to document all this, with careful and detailed informed consent, in addition to a specific consent form for each patient, about the step-by-step decisions taken, in a gentle and careful way, thereby not harming the doctor-patient relationship, which is most sacred in medicine!

Conclusion

Torsoplasty is a current-day procedure. On the one hand, there is a tendency to perform a greater number of surgeries on the torso simultaneously. On the other hand, there are considerations about limiting the number of surgeries to reduce morbidity.

A careful work of pros and cons, adapting to the patient's clinical condition and the technical-surgical conditions of the team, can reach a situation of optimal surgical planning, precisely defining the type of surgery, whether combined or not.

Annex

I declare that all patient's pictures are from my personal archive in the Interclinica—Centroplastica Image Bank, and I allow their publication.

References

Ferreira, ABH; J.E.M.M. New Dictionary of the Portuguese Language, Nova Fronteira Edithor, page 139;

González-Ulloa M. Torsoplasty. Aesthetic Plast Surg. 1979; 3(1): 357–68;

Wakefield W., Rubin JP, Gusenoff JA. The life program after weight loss: a paradigm for plastic surgery care after massive weight loss. Plast Surg Nurs. 2014; 34(1): 4-9; 10–1 quis;

Boswell CB. Body contouring after major weight loss. Mo Med. 2010; 107 (3): 189–94;
Roxo, AC, Roxo, CDP, Marques, RG, Rodrigues, NCP, Carneiro, DV Souto, FMDC, Nahas, FX. Endocrine-Metabolic Response in Patients Undergoing Multiple Body Contouring Surgeries After Massive Weight Loss, Aesthetic Surgery Journal, Volume 39, Issue 7, 2019, Pages 756–764;
Resende, JHC. Treatise on plastic surgery in obesity. Rio de Janeiro 2008; Edithor Rubio, page 14/109 to 339;
Modarressi A, Meia Rüegg E, Bezzola T, Pittet-Cuénod B. Circular abdominoplasty after massive weight loss: Is it a risky procedure? J Plast Reconstr Aesthet Surg. 2016 Nov;69(11):1497–1505;
Pontes, R. (2004) Abdominoplasty. Thigh Lift; pages 154/183;
Roxo C, Roxo A, Almenares M. Multifunctional abdominoplasty: retrospective study of 5 years of experience with 108 patients. Cir Plast Iberolatinoam. 2008; 34(3): 201–210;
Aly, AS. & Nahas FX. The art of body contour. 2019. Rio de Janeiro; Thieme Revinter Publications, 2019.
Rocha, Rodrigo Itocazo; Gemperli, Rolf: Modolin, Miguel L.A. Et Al. Plastic surgeries to readjust the body contour of patients undergoing bariatric surgery during adolescence, Revista Brasileira Cir. Plast, 27, 2012.
Anon (n.d.) https://www.sbcbm.org.br/historia-da-cirurgia-bariatrica-no-brasil/;
Zantut PEC, Boiler AML, Tournieux TT, Longo FH. Torsoplasty. In: Stocchero I; Tournieux AAB. Update on Aesthetic and Reconstructive Plastic Surgery. Sao Paulo: Santa Isabel, f. 502, 2006. 1004 p. ch. 81, p. 665-679;
Cannistra C, Rodrigo V, Marmuse J.P. Aesthetic Plast Surg , Torsoplasty after important weight loss 2006;30(6):667–71;
Downey SE, Gross JE. Lateral thoracic excisions in the post massive weight loss patient. Clin Plast Surg. 2008 Jan;35(1):115–20;
Woodbury A, Sniecinski R. Garlic-Induced Surgical Bleeding: How Much Is Too Much? A A Case Rep. 2016 Dec 15;7(12):266–269;
Bedi HS, Tewarson V, Negi K. Bleeding risk of dietary supplements: A hidden nightmare for cardiac surgeons. Indian Heart J. 2016;68 Suppl 2(Suppl 2):S249–S250
Destro, Marco Williams Baena et al. Study of preoperative use of medicines or herbal drugs that alter blood clotting. Journal of the Brazilian College of Surgeons [online]. 2006, v. 33, no. two;
Teixeira, RR; Mandin, BL; Fonseca, NM; Ruzi, RA. Regional anesthesia and anticoagulation. Rev Med Minas Gerais 2010; 20(4 Suppl 1): S17–S23;
Caprini JA, Arcelus JI, Reyna JJ. Effective risk stratification of surgical and nonsurgical patients for venous thromboembolic disease. Semin Hematol 2001; 38 (2 Suppl 5):12–9;
de Paiva Rita Azevedo et al. Venous thromboembolism in plastic surgery: prevention protocol at Clínica Ivo Pitanguy. Rev. Bras. Cir. Plastic 2010; 25(4): 583–8;
Paiva Rita A. et al. Venous thromboembolism prevention protocol at Instituto Ivo Pitanguy: efficacy and safety in 1,351 patients. Rev. Bras. Cir. Plastic 2013; 28 (1): 3–9;

Chapter 51
Flankplasty

Barbara Helena Barcaro Machado

Abstract Contour deformities in the lower back including flank tissue redundancy, hip rolls, buttocks, and thigh ptosis can accrue either from genetic conditions, the natural aging process, or massive weight loss. Histopathologically, these contour deformities arise from changes in the soft tissue envelope due to major modifications in the skin layers accompanied by subcutaneous volume deficiency.

These alterations can lead to skin irritation, mycotic infections, and/or self-imaging problems. Interestingly, patients searching for flankplasty aim at aesthetic enhancement, significant improvement of self-esteem, and social performance.

From circumferential excisions to flankplasties based on oblique scars, several techniques have been described to address the skin excess in the lower back. The reproducible and reliable flankplasty presented in this chapter provides a simplified, flank skin resection and simultaneous outer thigh lift and partial correction of the gluteal ptosis.

As for technical considerations, patients undergoing flankplasties have their body examined and marked, and patients can discuss and confirm the acceptance concerning the final scar.

The surgery must be planned in advance to determine the areas to be suctioned and those that should be kept, because candidates to flankplasty usually present supratrocantheric volume deficiency and/or some degree of gluteal ptosis in conjunction with volume reduction and loss of tissue consistency.

Whenever indicated, the surgical incision is limited to the skin, and the subcutaneous tissue is spared to be used as an advancement flap for the correction the aforementioned contour deformities. As dissection proceeds, a superior, cutaneous flap created by the flank skin resection provides volume for the superior part of the buttocks and corrects insufficient buttock projection. The preserved, local fascia

B. H. B. Machado (✉)
Rio de Janeiro, Brazil
e-mail: barbara@barbaramachado.com.br

J. M. Avelar, R. Cavalcanti Ribeiro (eds.), *Body Contouring*,
https://doi.org/10.1007/978-3-031-42802-9_51

allows the fixation of the superior gluteal flap and variable degrees of gluteal ptosis correction. The gluteal fat grafting is the final step of the procedure and aims at providing gluteal augmentation and avoiding the postoperative flattened buttock contour which is referred to as a frequent shortcoming of flankplasties.

Keywords Body contouring · Autologous gluteal augmentation · Fat grafting · Buttocks · Lipectomy · Flankplasty

Key Points
- The flankplasty technique described in this chapter includes the liposuction of eventual fat excess, the excision of the skin from the flanks, buttocks, and lateral thigh. It addresses the flank skin redundancy and the ptosis of the lateral thigh and the buttocks.
- The technique provides buttocks lift and creates a subcutaneous flap that acts as an autologous buttock implant that provides gluteal projection in a single-stage procedure.
- The advancement flap does not increase morbidity as vascularity, innervation, and function of the underlying tissues such as gluteus maximus muscle are not compromised.

Flankplasty

Introduction

A sensible alteration of skin composition and subcutaneous tissue anatomy is observed in the senescence process and in post-obese patients and includes the decrease of tissue protein content, hydroxyproline, and biochemical substances involved in wound healing. Macroscopically, the areolar layer fat consists of small, well-defined lobules firmly contained by dense vertical fibrous septa connected to the deepest dermal layer. The lamellar fat layer comprises large lobules of fat loosely packaged in poorly delimitated spaces bound by oblique fibrous septa. In the lumbar area, the anatomy of the superficial areolar layer is thicker than the lamellar layer in patients who underwent spontaneous weight loss, while post-bariatric patients present lamellar layer hypertrophy. Besides, the disarrangement of the superficial fascial system consisting of small, ill-defined lobules in poorly delimitated spaces leads to the absence of fibrous septa and loss of the connections to the deep dermal layer (Levy et al. 2011).

The elastic fibers can reveal overgrowth, disarray, and greater dimensions, whereas collagen fibers can be thickened, hypereosinophilic, and sclerodermic. Sclerosis involving the subcutaneous tissue with collapsed adipocytes, fibrous septum thickening, and pseudocysts and persistent inflammation extracellular matrix was observed (D'Ettorre et al. 2010).

All these alterations are linked to the challenging skin laxity observed in the ever-growing number of post-obese patients. The body contour alterations contribute to problems concerning local infections and self-esteem and surgical approaches which target the correction or mitigation of the resultant skin laxity and body-contouring improvement.

Flank Aesthetic Importance: Contemporary Concepts and Current Trends

Flanks are a watershed between the upper and lower back. Lying between the woman's tapering ribs and flared iliac crests, flanks are the posterolateral contribution to the waist. Attractive waists vary greatly and are appreciated in the context of gender and personal preference. Female patients present subtle reflections of the posterior spine and sensuous curves with tight skin even after massive weight loss. By a recent population survey, the most desirable female waist-to-hip ratio is 0.65. In contrast, male waists form a uniform narrowing, from a barrel-like chest through narrow pelvic rims (Hurwitz et al. 2019).

Circumferential body lift or belt lipectomy was initially created to treat circumferential excess skin of the lower trunk. As the surgical incision crosses the midline, some tactical modifications included the preservation of a skin bridge in the midline of the lumbar region to minimize the risk of elongation of the gluteal cleft (plumber's crack deformity) and to avoid placing an incision directly over a pressure point (Carloni et al. 2016).

As a preference of several authors for avoiding the circumferential procedure, and because several patients have already undergone abdominoplasties, there is a current trend toward the indication of flankplasties. Flankplasty has been established as an useful technique that can be associated with the improvement of flank redundancy and gluteal laxity.

In the technique presented in this chapter, gluteal ptosis and loss of volume are addressed by means of combined flank skin resection, tissue avulsion, flap advancement, and concomitant fat grafting. The technique must be adequately planned and executed to overcome the skin laxity, soft tissue descent, or deflation (Isakson et al. 2020). The surgery results in a simplified step-by-step flank and gluteal improvement.

Indications and Contraindications

The outer thigh/buttock lift or flankplastyis usually indicated in patients with genetic conditions or those who have developed skin laxity from aging process or massive weight loss whether after an effective dieting or after bariatric surgery. Redundant flank and hip rolls, buttocks, and thigh ptosis can lead to skin irritation, mycotic infections, and self-imaging problems.

Eligible Patients

Patients presenting for body contouring due to senescence or after massive weight loss, whether spontaneous or by gastrointestinal bypass surgery or gastric banding, often present for an extensive series of body-contouring procedures to restore a functional and satisfactory body contour. As a common sense, the patient must have achieved a stable body weight for at least 6 months to be eligible to such procedures. In addition, the blood loss, duration of hospitalization, and the length of the surgical procedures must be balanced against the rate of possible complications.

Preoperative Markings

Therefore, accurate preoperative markings are preferably drawn with patients in stand-up position and with open arms as this facilitates the identification of landmarks and establishment of anatomic planes. The marking must include areas in the back, the volume depletion, and buttock contour alteration. Liposuction of remote areas that need to be addressed so that the result can be refined must be planned and designed at the same moment of incision markings. However, patient's safety must be safeguarded as well as precise technique execution.

For the skin resection, firm bimanual gathering of excess tissue at the junction of the lower back and gluteal area outlines the excess of flaccid tissue laxity. An undergarment or a bikini can be used to project the ideal position for the resultant scar after the skin resection. While designing the incisions and skin resection, curve lines are aesthetically preferable to straight ones.

The superior marking of the incision is made at the superior apex of the back skin and is slightly reduced in the midline through inferior angulation toward the buttock crease. The inferior incision is continued from anterior and marked below the flank skin excess, crossing the midline just above the buttock crease.

Surgical Technique

Patients are given intravenous antibiotic during the anesthetic induction. General anesthesia is preferred although other techniques can be applied. The patients are placed in the supine position, and bedsore protection must be placed under the chest, iliac crests, knees, ankles, and toes.

As a comprehensive flankplasty includes the lower body lift, the outer thigh lift, and the improvement of the gluteal region, the procedure lasts over 3–4 h. A urinary catheter is inserted after the anesthetic procedure and kept during surgery to monitor hydration.

The surgical field is disinfected with chlorohexidine from scapular area toward the knees where stockinettes are used to drape the patient. Change of gowns and gloves or instrument sets can be performed whenever necessary, but without lengthening the operating time.

The areas to be liposuctioned are infiltrated with a blunt cannula. The tumescent solution is composed of saline solution and adrenalin diluted to a concentration of 1:1,000,000. The maximum vasoconstriction can be achieved 10 min after tissue infiltration, which permits for reduced bleeding.

The procedure is initiated by traditional liposuction to harvest the fat tissue in a sterile glass to be grafted by the end of the procedure. Fat is left to decant to be used to remodel the buttock or fill areas of volume deficiency of areas presenting contour deformity. Blunt 4 and 5 mm cannulas are preferably used. Digital pinch testing confirms the effective evacuation of the subcutaneous tissue, but excessive tissue trauma must be avoided. If the flanks and/or lateral thighs present lipodystrophy, judicious liposuction decreases the tension on the wound closure.

The markings concerning skin resection are confirmed, and the tumescent infiltration is extended to the area corresponding to the planned resection. The superior incision is started at the right flank, crosses the midline, and continues toward the left flank. However, in the center, the dermis is preserved in order to keep the integrity of the deep adhesions that give this area a nice curvature. The preservation of this dermal bridge avoids the interference with the natural back depression. The incision can be extended toward the anterior flank, whenever necessary.

The incision is usually limited to the cutaneous layers although it may include a small amount of subcutaneous tissue (Fig. 51.1a). The excess fat above the superior incision must be removed from the areas neighboring the incision site.

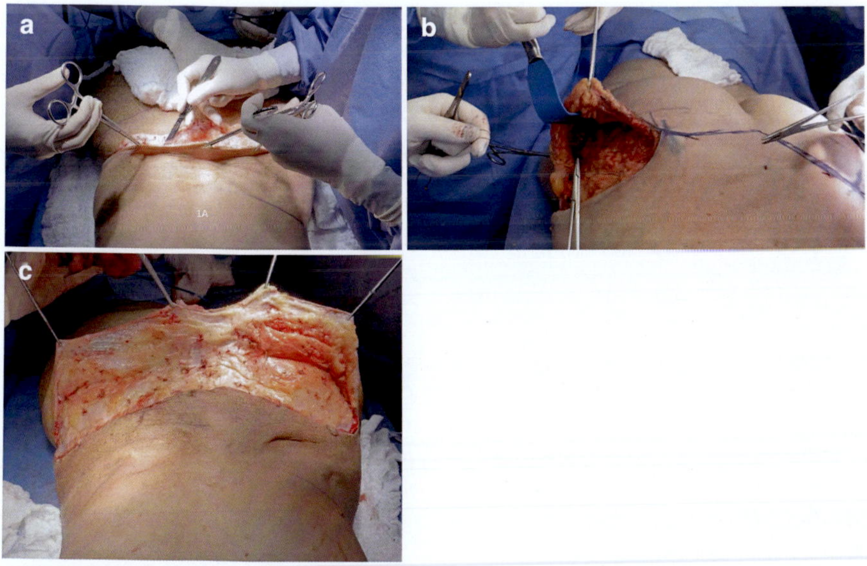

Fig. 51.1 After confirming the marking of the final scar, the incision is initiated and includes preferentially only the skin layers (**a**). The subcutaneous tissue is spared superiorly and/or inferiorly whenever necessary to be used as advancement flaps to fill contour deformities such as supratrocantheric deficiency (**b**) and gluteal deflation (**c**)

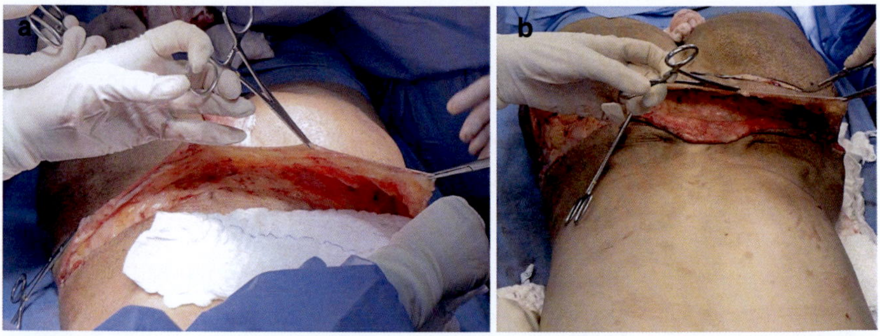

Fig. 51.2 The skin excess must be confirmed (**a**) before the skin resection (**b**) to avoid hypertrophic scars or scar migration

The skin resection provides the lifting of the gluteal region and the outer thigh area. The subcutaneous tissue is spared for volume restoration and the local fascia is preserved to allow the fixation of cutaneous flaps.

If some volume depletion over the lateral trochanteric area is detected, an advancement subcutaneous flap obtained from below the resected skin excess can be fixed inferiorly to fill the deformity (Fig. 51.1b). As dissection proceeds, a cutaneous flap is created by the flank skin resection extends at the level of the lower. This flap provides volume to the upper buttocks and supports the correction of insufficient buttock projection (Fig. 51.1c).

Ensuing, buttock augmentation can be achieved through the confection of a gluteal flap supplied by perforators from the superior gluteal artery, lateral sacral arteries, and lumbar artery (Carloni et al. 2016; Sozer et al. 2005).

The mobile flap is advanced and sutured to the fascia. These structures play the role as secure anchors in an attempt to support the local tissue lifting and avoid recurrence of skin laxity, scar drifts, or subcutaneous thinning.

Tissue undermining is reduced as most as possible and scalpel dissection is preferred to diminish the risk of seroma (Swanson 2019). In some cases, gluteal implants can be inserted under the gluteus maximum during the procedure.

At completion of the dermal and gluteal flap procedures, hemostasis is carefully performed by electrocautery, and the flap is anchored superiorly to the fascia with permanent sutures. The skin excess must be confirmed (Fig. 51.2a) before the skin resection (Fig. 51.2b) to avoid hypertrophic scars or scar migration. The edges of the wound are pulled to cover the flap, and the wound closure is performed by layers. Deep absorbable interrupted sutures, followed by subdermic running polyglactin (3/0), and subcutaneous running poliglecaprone (3/0).

If more severe gluteal ptosis is observed, skin can be resected in the inner thigh and infragluteal fold (Fig. 51.3).

As the last surgical step, fat is grafted into the supratrocantheric depression and the subcutaneous plane of the buttock for gluteal augmentation (Fig. 51.4a, b). Fat graft can avoid the postoperative loss of gluteal projection and flattened buttock

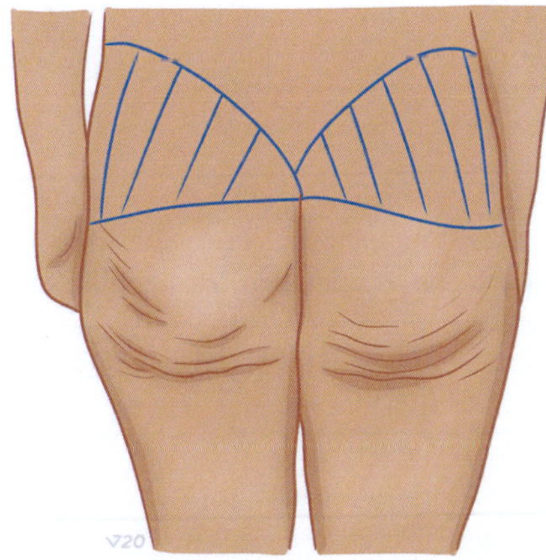

Fig. 51.3 If severe gluteal ptosis is verified, the procedure can be complemented by inner thigh skin resection

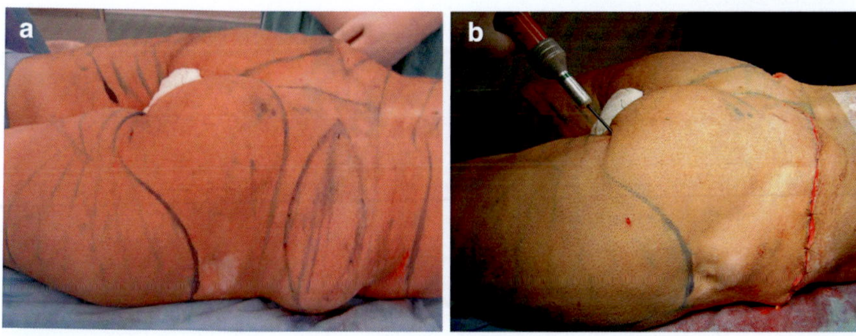

Fig. 51.4 A 39-year-old patient presenting neurofibromatosis in the flanks. The surgical planning was reinforced by the preoperative demarcation including areas to be liposuctioned and the skin resection (**a**). The flank resection included the skin and the histopathologically modified subcutaneous tissue. The supratrocantheric deficiency was filled with fat graft (**b**)

contour which is referred as a frequent shortcoming of this procedure. Obtention of maximal gluteal projection is the goal, and the fat grafting is performed in several layers of the subcutaneous layer. However, the volume of fat grafting is restricted to 450 ml per side maximum to avoid excessive pressure, tissue congestion, and reduction of fat graft integration rate (Sozer et al. 2005).

The incisions are finally closed with Prineo® Dermabond® skin closure system (Ethicon, Inc., Somerville, New Jersey, USA). The cyanoacrylate liquid adhesive seals the wound and permits the patient to shower precociously. No drains are necessary as minimal undermining of the non-resected tissues is performed.

The surgical dressing consists of placing adhesive tapes over the treated area, cushion sterile pads, and slight compression by means of appropriate elastic bandages or garments.

Postoperative Care

Antibiotics are intravenously again administered 4 hours after the initial dose is given at beginning of the anesthetic procedure. Thromboprophylaxis includes early ambulation, the use of compressive stockings (placed below the knees during the anesthesia induction), and pneumatic intermittent devices (Carloni et al. 2016). Prophylactic low-molecular-weight heparin subcutaneously is initiated from 12 to 24 h after the completion of the surgical procedure until patient's discharge (usually 24–48 h after the surgery). Ambulation must be encouraged on the same day of the procedure. Before patient's discharge, a Doppler ultrasound examination is advisable if the patient presents history of thrombophilia or has not been able to walk on the day of the surgery.

On the next day, dressings are changed and the patient is discharged. An elastic garment, below the knee, must be worn for 1 month, 24 h per day. Standard postoperative instructions are given including activity restrictions and avoidance of sitting on buttocks. Yet, lying on supine positioning must be avoided so as to avoid pressure on the sacral area.

The patient is allowed to shower 48 h postoperatively. Physiotherapy begins on the third to fifth postoperative day or earlier.

After 10 days, patients are allowed to gradually increase physical activities. However, restriction to flexion of the waist and legs is advised for 2 months to avoid scar enlargement. Free exercising can be started 2 months after surgery. The patient is regularly followed up to 1 year after surgery so that scars and the body shape can be observed.

Results

Eleven female patients underwent the flankplasty technique described in this chapter in the last 10 years. The median age was 43 years (range: 27–53 years). One of the post-obese patients lost 41 kg and presented bulimia. The patient was under psychological treatment.

The average total volume of fat grafting was 500 mL per patient (range: 250–900 mL).

No pulmonary embolism or functional alteration resulted from the surgery. No major blood loss, seroma, or hematoma were detected. No fat or skin flap necrosis was detected, but two patients presented small wound dehiscence. One patient required a secondary procedure to remove a slight residual skin excess in the lateral thighs.

As for the aesthetic result, all patients referred significant improvement of soft tissue excess, gluteal ptosis and shape, projection, and body contour (Figs. 51.5 and 51.6). Although gluteal cleft elongation and some disruption of skin adhesions by transverse incisions have been described after lower body lift (Swanson 2019), the

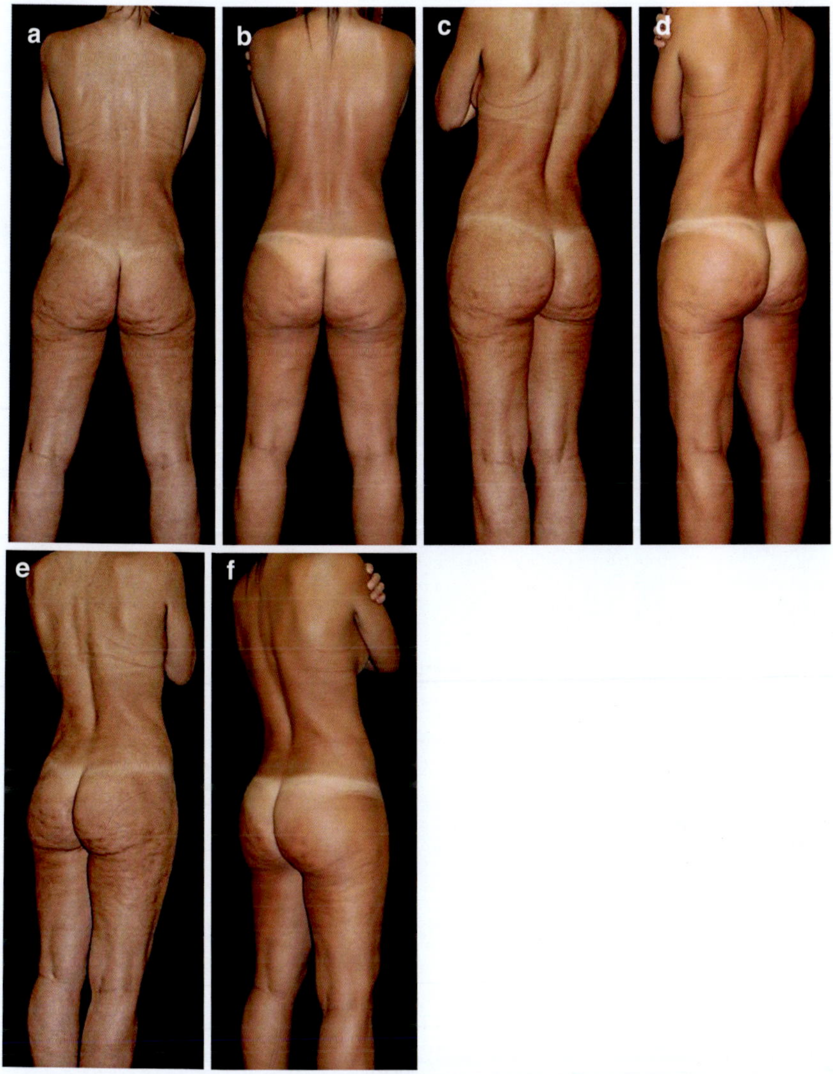

Fig. 51.5 A 42-year-old patient presenting gluteal and thigh skin flaccidity due to a genetic condition. Flankplasty included advancement flaps that allowed the gluteal projection and improvement of the lateral thighs. (**a**, **c**, **e**) display the preoperative views and (**b**, **d**, **f**) depict the result. The final scar was located inside the bikini line and presented good quality

sinuous female contour has been preserved and no gluteal cleft elongation was observed. All patients showed reduction of gluteal ptosis and better gluteal projection and contour apart from the major improvement of the lateral thighs.

Despite wound closure tensions were moderate and some patients may have presented predictors of poor outcome, namely, high pre-body contouring BMI,

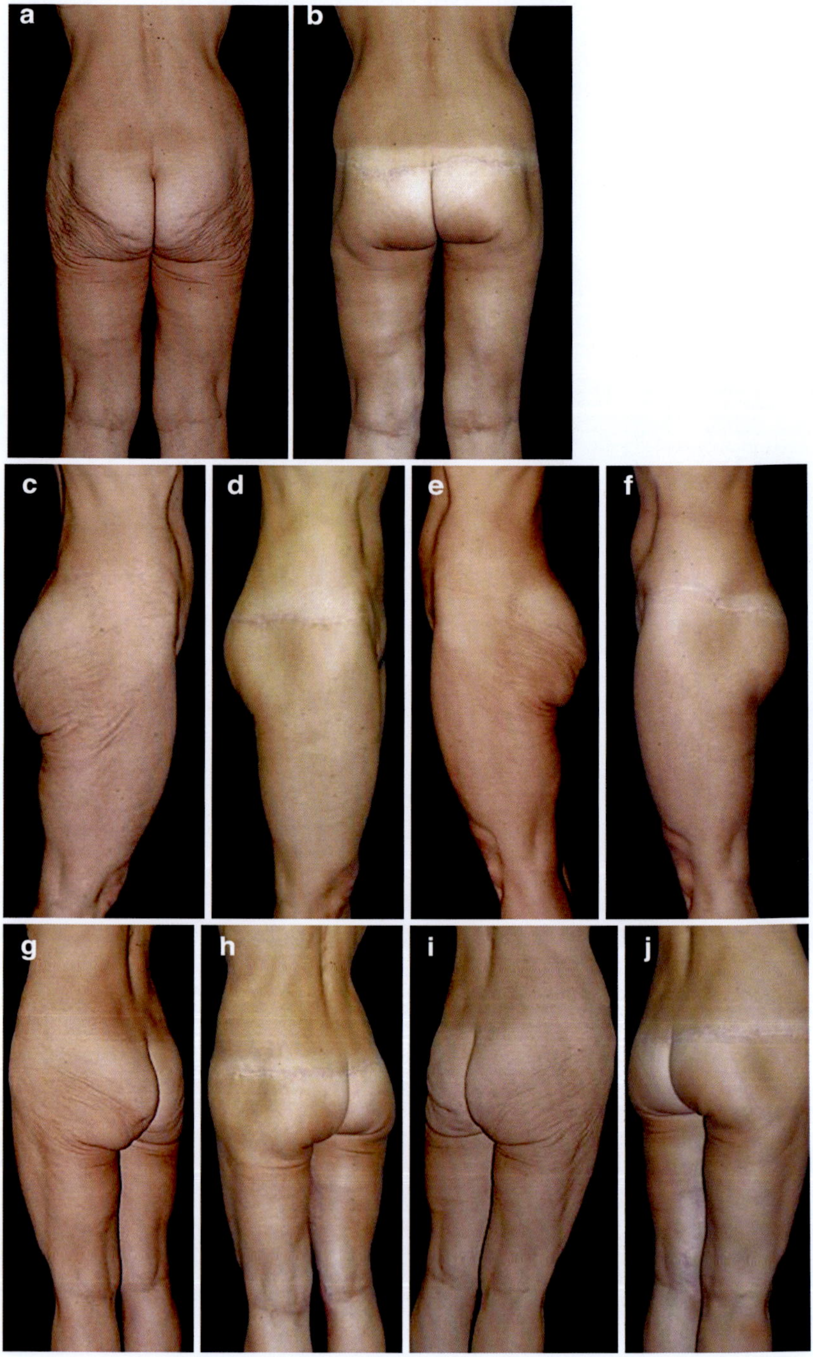

Fig. 51.6 A 48-year-old patient who underwent massive weight loss (45 kg). Note the gluteal ptosis severe skin flaccidity. The flankplasty technique described in this chapter permitted the improvement of the flanks and lateral thighs and shortening of the gluteal crease and gluteal projection. Gluteal fat grafting was limited due to the restricted donor areas. (**a**, **c**, **e**, **g**, **i**) are preoperative views and (**b**, **d**, **f**, **h**, **j**) show the result of the procedure

smoking, diabetes mellitus and/or hypertension, and nutritional deficiency (Hurwitz et al. 2019), no major complication has been observed. However, wound dehiscence limited to the sacral area was observed in two patients. Although gluteal hypoesthesia has been reported in patients treated with auto-augmentation flaps, this occurrence was not observed in the case series reported in this chapter.

Discussion

Contour deformities in the lower back, flanks, and gluteal area can accrue either from massive weight loss or the natural aging process. The visible aesthetic alterations arise from subcutaneous volume loss or deficiency, skin changes, and consequent ptotic soft tissue envelope.

After massive weight loss, plastic surgery procedures can lead to a significant quality of life improvement, especially in domains such as physical and psychosocial wellbeing, social/cultural performance, and self-esteem (Cintra Jr et al. 2008). In fact, patients searching for flankplasty aim at aesthetic enhancement in the first place.

The flankplasty addresses the ptosis of lateral thigh and provides satisfactory suspension of the loose skin of the buttocks. Loose skin is excised directly and closed by minimal undermining. As deep undermining is not necessary, superficial lymphatic and neurovascular structures are preserved. As consequences, healing is facilitated, and lymphedema or other fluid collections are rare.

Despite the preferred scar placement within the line of the underwear or a swimsuit, the potential of scar dehiscence or poor scar healing must be discussed in advance with patients undergoing flankplasty. Suture suspension of the dermis and the advancement flaps to the fascia, an anchor that stabilizes the scar positioning and avoids its stretching. However, the weight of the gluteal region added to the action of gravity can lead to partial recurrence of ptosis and widening of the scars.

Mild to moderate gluteal ptosis in conjunction with volume reduction and loss of consistency is usually involved, and gluteal volume restoration is required to achieve satisfactory projection and optimize flankplasty results.

To overcome the decreased projection in the buttocks contour accruing from conventional flankplasties, no adipose tissue should be resected across the skin resection as this fat must be used as an advancement flap to fill the gaps. There are a variety of reliable adipose fascial flaps harvested from the lower body excision site for buttock augmentation and to correct supratrochanteric deformities (Hurwitz et al. 2019; Isakson et al. 2020). The technique described herein creates a subcutaneous flap that acts as an autologous buttock implant that provides additional projection and buttocks lift in a single-stage procedure (Sozer et al. 2005). The local advancement flaps for the repair of volume deficiencies do not increase morbidity as it does not sacrifice the vascularity, innervation, or function of the underlying tissues such as gluteus maximus muscle (Sozer et al. 2005; Kitzinger et al. 2013).

Flankplasty can include the liposuction of eventual fat excess, the excision of the skin from the flanks, buttocks, and lateral thigh. The fat obtained through liposuction fat grafting can be safely injected to the gluteal area. Despite the regenerative possibilities offered by fat grafting, the aesthetic result is limited by the skin quality and complex contour deformities eventually presented by the patient. End points for successful fat grafting include the obtention of smooth convexity and shortening of the infragluteal crease that must end as medial as possible to the vertical line passing through the middle of the thigh as seen from the back.

Besides, if major gluteal ptosis is verified, additional skin removal in the inner thigh and in the gluteal crease can improve the result. The analysis of the degree of gluteal ptosis supports the decision-making to include these surgical steps in order to provide satisfactory results (Gonzalez 2006).

The low complication rate and the high subjective patient satisfaction demonstrated by this case series make this procedure suitable for the management of flank deformities and gluteal volume loss and moderate ptosis. Nonetheless, if severe gluteal ptosis is involved, an excisional procedure with incisions in the inguinal area extending to the infragluteal fold must be considered.

As for the resulting scars, Hurwitz et al. (Hurwitz et al. 2019) described, in 2020, an oblique flankplasty in combination with lipoabdominoplasty as an alternative to a lower body lift that provides a tighter skinned lower torso with gender-appropriate contours. Despite the satisfactory results, the flank scars proposed by those authors course obliquely above the bikini line which is an important issue to consider. As Brazil has an extensive littoral and hot weather throughout the year, the greatest advantage of the technique described in this chapter is the final scar which can be properly hidden in a swimsuit. Unfortunately, the lateral aspect of the scar often drifts inferiorly under the stress of heavy lateral thigh and the action of gravity which tends to pull the gluteal region downward. The lack of secure underlying anchor fascia which undergoes laxity, alongside with alterations of the subcutaneous tissue, may also be responsible for the poor tissue fixation and scar stretching or migration. Even so, patients felt more attractive and declared that the scars were not a cause for embarrassment nor were they visible all times if patients were not naked.

As a limitation to further conclusions, the number of candidates to flankplasty including outer thigh/buttock lift is small, and the data reported cannot demonstrate superiority over other flankplasty techniques. On the other hand, the greatest advantages of the flankplasty technique described encompass the following: (1) the low complexity of the procedure, (2) the duration of the procedure is not protracted as the structures involved are anatomically interconnected, and (3) thighs and buttocks are approached as a whole unit, which provides better aesthetic outcome.

Hints for Better Results

- Rigorous patient selection by analyzing preoperative body mass index and nutrition.
- Ask for physiological evaluation to detect dysmorphia or possible setbacks such as unrealistic expectations.
- Advise patients for possible additional surgical procedures to correct residual skin laxity or scar enlargement.
- Plan fat harvesting from fat deposits that can be easily accessible in the prone position to optimize operating time.
- Design of the incisions to place the final scar inside the limits of swimsuits.
- Slightly underestimate skin resection to avoid wound closure under excess tension.
- Use superwet infusions to reduce blood loss.
- Limit undermining to reduce seromas and preserve vascularity.
- Augment buttocks with neighboring flaps and fat grafting.
- If severe gluteal ptosis is verified, shape the inferior buttocks and posterior thigh with a thighplasty and infragluteal skin resection.

Conclusion

The popularity of body contouring procedures has increased over the past years, in parallel with the worldwide prevalence of obesity, and this has boosted the indication of procedures such as flankplasty. Flankplasty is a body contouring surgery that consists of removing flaccid skin and subcutaneous fat preservation, followed by tissue suspension. The technique described in this chapter is an effective, reproducible, and low-risk variation of the lower body lift technique that permits for lifting the lateral thigh and buttock.

As for gluteal ptosis and supratrochanteric defects, the flank and/or gluteal deepithelialized advancement flaps can provide an implant-like shape volumization while preserving superficial lymphatics and neurovascular structures. The tissue lift and skin tightening can be safely combined with fat grafting to provide gluteal volume, projection, and better body contour.

Although no guidelines exist for indicating flankplasty, accuracy is required concerning preoperative assessment of patients, selected BMI ranges, and preoperative risk evaluation so that satisfactory outcomes can be obtained. Complication rates are low, and the incision is easily concealed with clothing.

References

Levy, S., Gomes, F. R., & Sterodimas, A. (2011). Macroscopic anatomic changes of subcutaneous fat tissue in massive-weight-loss patients. *Aesthetic plastic surgery*, *35*(5), 814-819.

D'Ettorre M, Gniuli D, Iaconelli A, Massi G, Mingrone G, Bracaglia R. (2010). Wound healing process in post-bariatric patients: an experimental evaluation. Obes Surg. Nov;20(11):1552–8. doi: https://doi.org/10.1007/s11695-010-0224-x. PMID: 20628832.

Hurwitz, D. J., Beidas, O., & Wright, L. (2019). Reshaping the oversized waist through oblique flankplasty with lipoabdominoplasty. *Plastic and reconstructive surgery*, *143*(5), 960e-972e.

Carloni R, De Runz A, Chaput B, Herlin C, Girard P, Watier E, Bertheuil N. (2016). Circumferential Contouring of the Lower Trunk: Indications, Operative Techniques, and Outcomes-A Systematic Review. Aesthetic Plast Surg. Oct;40(5):652-68. doi: 10.1007/s00266-016-0660-7. Epub 2016 Jun 10. Erratum in: Aesthetic Plast Surg. 2016 Oct;40(5):669. PMID: 27286851.

Isakson MH, Vasilakis V, Kortesis BG, Hunstad JP, Bharti G. Avulsion Fat Graft Gluteoplasty: Technique Overview. Ann Plast Surg. 2020 Jun;84(6S Suppl 5):S375–S381. doi: https://doi.org/10.1097/SAP.0000000000002274. PMID: 32149851.

Sozer SO, Agullo FJ, Wolf C. (2005). Autoprosthesis buttock augmentation during lower body lift. Aesthetic Plast Surg. May-Jun;29(3):133–7; discussion 138-40. doi: https://doi.org/10.1007/s00266-005-0024-1. PMID: 15948016.

Swanson, E., 2019. Near-circumferential Lower Body Lift: A Review of 40 Outpatient Procedures. *Plastic and Reconstructive Surgery Global Open*, *7*(12).

Cintra Jr W, Modolin ML, Gemperli R, et al. (2008), Quality of life after abdominoplasty in women after bariatric surgery. Obes Surg 2008;18:728e32.

Kitzinger HB, Cakl T, Wenger R, Hacker S, Aszmann OC, Karle B. (2013). Prospective study on complications following a lower body lift after massive weight loss. J Plast Reconstr Aesthet Surg. Feb;66(2):231–8. https://doi.org/10.1016/j.bjps.2012.09.006. Epub 2012 Oct 4. PMID: 23040202.

Gonzalez R. (2006). Etiology, definition, and classification of gluteal ptosis. Aesthetic Plast Surg. May-Jun;30(3):320–6. doi: https://doi.org/10.1007/s00266-005-0051-y. PMID: 16733776.

Chapter 52
Lipotorsoplasty: A Novel Body-Contouring Surgical Technique

Wilson Novaes Matos, Ricardo Cavalcanti Ribeiro, Paola Martinez, and Luis Fernandez de Córdova

Abstract Torsoplasty is indicated for patients who have great flaccidity and circumferential excess of the skin of the trunk, including the back and abdomen.

Lipotorsoplasty is a combination of liposuction in the flanks, trunk, and hips with skin resection to shape the female or male silhouette of individuals when in presence of major skin excess and sagging. The basic principles are the lipoplasty procedure that removes the excess of remaining fat and allows what we call "lipoundermining," dissecting the adipose tissue and enabling the preservation of the vascular and lymphatic systems, following Avelar's philosophy. The aspirated fat is treated and used as a fat graft to volumize, increase, project, and shape the gluteal region. Lipoabdominoplasty may be associated for better results of trunk contouring.

This technique is indicated for patients with great skin excess and sagging around the circumference of massive-weight-loss or post-bariatric patients, but we also use it for sagging and excess of skin of any origin, caused by excessive sun exposure, aging, intense fibrosis in the subcutaneous tissue, and secondary and tertiary liposuction corrections.

Keywords Lipoabdominoplasty · Torsoplasty · Liposuction · Massive weight loss

---

W. N. Matos
Plastic Surgery, Plastic Day Hospital, São Paulo, Brazil

Plastic and Reconstructive Surgery, Federal University of the State of Rio de Janeiro, Rio de Janeiro, Brazil

R. Cavalcanti Ribeiro (✉) · L. F. de Córdova
Plastic and Reconstructive Surgery, Federal University of the State of Rio de Janeiro, Rio de Janeiro, Brazil

Plastic Surgery, Global Plastic Surgery, Rio de Janeiro, Brazil
e-mail: rribeiro@centroin.net.br

P. Martinez
Plastic Surgery, Global Plastic Surgery, Rio de Janeiro, Brazil

J. M. Avelar, R. Cavalcanti Ribeiro (eds.), *Body Contouring*,
https://doi.org/10.1007/978-3-031-42802-9_52

Introduction

The first published papers were of Somalo "Dermolipectomy of the Trunk" (1940), Gonzalez-Ulloa described Circular Lipectomy in (1959), and Baroudi in (1989; 1991) presented body contouring as another option for circular surgery. Lockwood published "Transverse Flank-Thigh-Buttock Lift (1991) and Lower-Body Lift (1993, 2001). Based on this concept, numerous works have been published: Circumferential Torsoplasty (Carwell and Horton 1997), Circumferential Body Lift (Hamra, 1999), Circumferential Torsoplasty, Al Aly – Belt Lipectomy (Van Geertruyden, 2003), and Total Body Lift (Hurwitz, 2004). These surgeries aim to treat the body contour circumferentially involving the abdomen, flanks, back, and gluteal regions. These en bloc resections to remove the skin and fat (superficial and deep) are performed in the aponeurotic plane; trauma and bleeding are characteristic of this type of approach. The elevation of the gluteal region improves flaccidity; however, there is a loss of volume and projection of this region as multiples studies to trear body contour and obesity have shown (Correa-Iturraspe 1952; Lockwood 1996; Modolin et al. 2003; Baroudi & Carvalho 1981; Navarro et al. 2002).

Pascal presented "Remodeling Bodylift with High Lateral Tension" in 2002, a dermal fat flap to provide volume and projection of the gluteal region, the "buttocks lift." The high rate of post-bariatric patients with massive weight loss generating sagging skin has resulted in a growing interest in refining these major body-contouring resections. Current studies describe the use of dermal fat flaps to fill, improve, and shape the gluteal region. From this surgery, other authors published studies with different flaps (Sozer, Autoprosthesis Buttock Augmentation During Lower Body Lift (2005), Autologous Augmentation Gluteoplasty with a Dermal Fat Flap (2008); Richter 2007, Centeno/Mendieta, Gluteal Contouring Surgery in the Massive Weight Loss Patient (2008); Rubin, Plastic Surgery After Weight Loss: Current Concepts in Massive Weight Loss Surgery (2008); Gonzalez Raul, Butterfly Flap (2008)).

Subcutaneous tissue preservation in skin flaps was a great advance for torsoplasties, and the results of the buttocks have improved and evolved; however, they have some disadvantages: longer surgical time, longer learning curve, ingenuity in making greater pockets, longer recovery time, and other complications of skin flaps such as oily inclusion cysts, steatonecrosis, abscesses, and infections.

Lipotorsoplasty is a combination of liposuction in the flanks, trunk, and hips with skin resection to shape the female or male silhouette of individuals when in presence of major skin excess and sagging. The basic principles are the lipoplasty procedure that removes the excess of remaining fat and allows what we call "lipoundermining," dissecting the adipose tissue and enabling the preservation of the vascular and lymphatic systems, following Avelar's philosophy. The aspirated fat is treated and used as a fat graft to volumize, increase, project, and shape the gluteal region.

Lipoabdominoplasty may be associated with a lipotorsoplasty to treat the abdominal region in a lipotorsoabdominoplasty.

We started using lipotorsoplasty in 2005. By 2020, 325 patients had been operated in our service. These patients ranged between 28 and 72 years, 80% were female, 60% underwent bariatric surgery, and in 85% of the cases another surgery was performed in combination (mammoplasty, lipolift of thighs and arms), of which 65% lipoabdominoplasty was the combined procedure.

This technique is indicated for patients with great skin excess and sagging around the circumference of massive-weight-loss or post-bariatric patients, but we also use it for sagging and excess of skin of any origin, caused by excessive sun exposure, aging, intense fibrosis in the subcutaneous tissue, and secondary and tertiary liposuction corrections.

Patient Evaluation

During the preoperative physical examination, the entire circumference of the trunk should be examined: the anterior, lateral and posterior trunk, hips, flanks, and gluteal region.

The amount of excess skin and the distribution of remaining fat in these regions should be observed. The type, quality, elasticity of the skin, presence of scars, striae biotype and global lipodystrophies, body asymmetries, and biotype are important in this evaluation.

Gluteal Region

In the gluteal region, the volume, shape, excess skin, degree of ptosis, gluteal groove, asymmetry, cellulite, irregularities, adhesions, and musculature should be evaluated.

The pinch test must be performed in all regions and especially in areas to be resected.

Abdomen

In the abdominal region, we evaluate the amount of excess skin in the upper and lower abdomen, pubis, fat deposits, scars, and diastasis of the rectus abdominis muscles.

It is important to examine patients in various positions: supine, lateral, prone, and seated.

Markings

The markings for both procedures must be performed before the surgery, starting with the liposuction areas in the trunk, back, waist, flanks, hips, and upper thigh region, where fat excess will be treated and the detached with cannulas,"lipoundermining."

Through pinch test, we mark the incisions for resection of skin. Starting in the sacral region up to the iliac crest, continuing with flanks and lateral trunk and followed by the markings of the abdomen for lipoabdominoplasty according to the bathing suits of the patient to keep the scar hidden.

The fat grafting areas are previously marked using the pinch test maneuver to correct the excess and ptosis of the glutes where the fat graft will be performed. At the end of the surgery, these markings will be reassessed to allow the fat graft to be placed in the right position.

Surgical Technique

The patient is positioned in a slightly hyperextended supine position. Wet liposuction (adrenaline – 1:500,000) is performed on the upper, lower, lateral, and anterior flanks.

With the patient positioned in the prone position, liposuction of the lateral regions, flanks, back, and lateral lower limbs is performed.

Liposuction reaches both the superficial and deep layers in these regions; in the areas of skin resection marking, the superficial layer must be completely removed. The deep plane fat of these regions is partially preserved in order to avoid trauma to the lymphatic vessels located above the muscular aponeurosis.

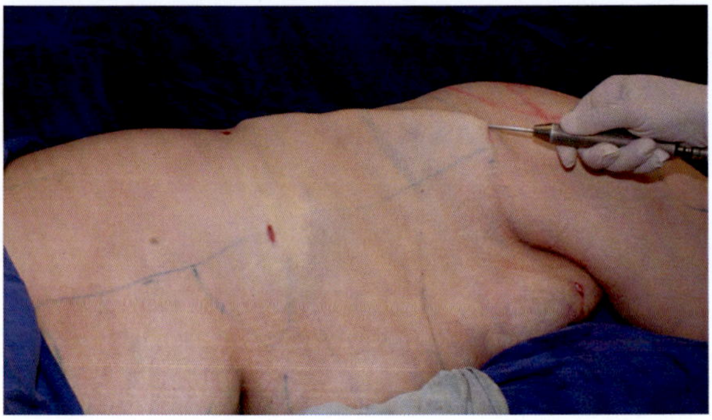

Skin excess is removed and flap movement is performed through lipoundermining. Fat excess can be removed with "open liposuction," and Scarpa's fascia is removed without reaching the aponeurotic plane. We create a tunnel in the lateral region of the trunk until the middle of the back to facilitate the traction of the trunk flap and to loosen the adhesions and folds and to reposition the skin and subcutaneous of the back. The gluteus is tractioned from lateral to medial to gain more projection. The back, flanks, and lateral thigh are tractioned.

Closure is performed by anatomical planes, up to the skin, and suction drains are placed.

The fat graft is washed with saline solution and grafted onto the previously marked gluteal areas. The volume varies from 300 to 600 ml of fat on each side, depending on the needs of each case. We perform a manual massage for better distribution and homogenization of the grafted fat.

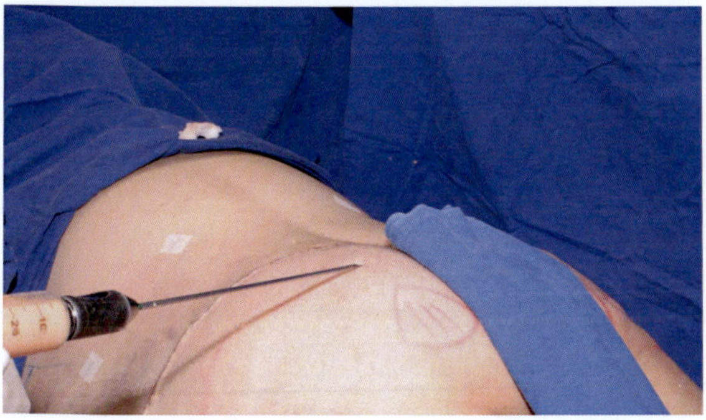

The patient is positioned again in the supine position, and the lipoabdominoplasty is completed with skin resection, plication of the rectus abdominis muscles, and omphaloplasty. Pubis lifting is always performed to aesthetically improve this region.

UAL, VAL, and PAL are routinely used technologies that help and facilitate the execution of the technique.

We can use lipoabdominoplasty variations according to the needs of each case, following the classification of the case at hand.

Aspiration drains are used, and then closed, followed by dressings and compression garments.

Torsoplasty can be divided into three phases. The first involves en bloc resections of skin in addition to superficial and deep fat in the supra-aponeurotic plane, causing major trauma to the vascular and lymphatic systems. Complications such as seroma, hematoma, and skin necroses were frequent. Until the 1990s, liposuction was not performed and the gluteus region was treated only with skin and subcutaneous traction lift.

With the increase in post-bariatric and massive-weight-loss patients, there was an increase in torsoplasty indications. Pascal's work with the dermal fat flap to treat the gluteal region represents the second phase, offering excellent results with increased volume, greater projection, and better shape of the buttocks.

Aiming to reduce the rate of complications of this surgery led us to use the same principles of lipoabdominoplasty, a technique developed and improved by us from 2000 to the present. This technique proposes a complete liposuction of the entire body contour associated with isolated skin resection as opposed to en bloc resections mentioned in other previously published techniques. Dissection with lipoundermining cannulas is less traumatic for anatomical structures, arteries, veins, and lymphatics, generating a flap with greater viability and blood supply, reducing the risk of hematoma necrosis and reduction of dead space. The preservation of lymphatic vessels, which are anatomically above the aponeurotic plane, is essential for seroma prevention.

The large amount of fat removed through liposuction is used for gluteoplasty.

We managed to obtain the desired volume to improve the projection, shape, firmness, and shaping of the buttocks, completing the "buttocks lift." Its execution is simpler and faster without the need for large gluteal dissection when compared to large skin flaps.

We observed numerous advantages of this technique including reduction of surgical time and trauma, consequently a significant decrease in complications such as seroma, necrosis, hematomas, oily cysts, abscesses, and infections. The recovery period is shorter and faster; the patient returns to their routine activities between 15 and 20 days per operative.

Due to the preservation of the vascular anatomy, arteries of the abdominal and dorsal region, the combination with lipoabdominoplasty, that is, "lipotorsoabdominoplasty" to treat the abdomen at the same surgical stage, is safe and ideal, providing a complete change and harmonization of the contour silhouette involving the back, flanks, hips, abdomen, and glutes.

Patients with severe liposuction sequelae and marked fibrosis in the subcutaneous tissue and tertiary and often quaternary liposuctions can be resolved with lipotorsoplasty.

The preoperative evaluation defines the liposuction regions and the amount of skin to be removed. We must make a prediction of the aspirated volume so as not to exceed the limit of 7% of the body contour.

The positioning of the scar in women and men should follow its anatomy so that it is camouflaged inside the bathing suit. In the feminine silhouette, we outline the waist, hips, and buttocks.

The surgical technique follows a pattern that begins with liposuction of the abdominal region followed by posterior liposuction of the trunk. The lipoplasty procedure reaches the superficial layer, overlapping Scarpa's fascia. After skin resection, the fat underlying Scarpa's fascia can be aspirated and partially resected in a fuse to correct its redundancy.

Assisted lipoplasty (PAL) and ultrasonic lipo "VASER LIPO" are used, further decreasing bleeding, facilitating liposuction. The fat graft must be inserted after the end of the posterior surgery when the gluteus and waist are correctly positioned.

The effectiveness of this new approach can be verified by the good results and the low rate of complications. We believe that lipoundermining is the main factor for this reduction due to the decrease in trauma and the preservation of anatomical structures.

We always use anticoagulant prophylaxis.

Results

Lipotorsoplasty results point to a significant reduction in circumference measurements, harmonization of the body contour with a defined abdomen and waist, and firm and voluminous buttocks with better shape.

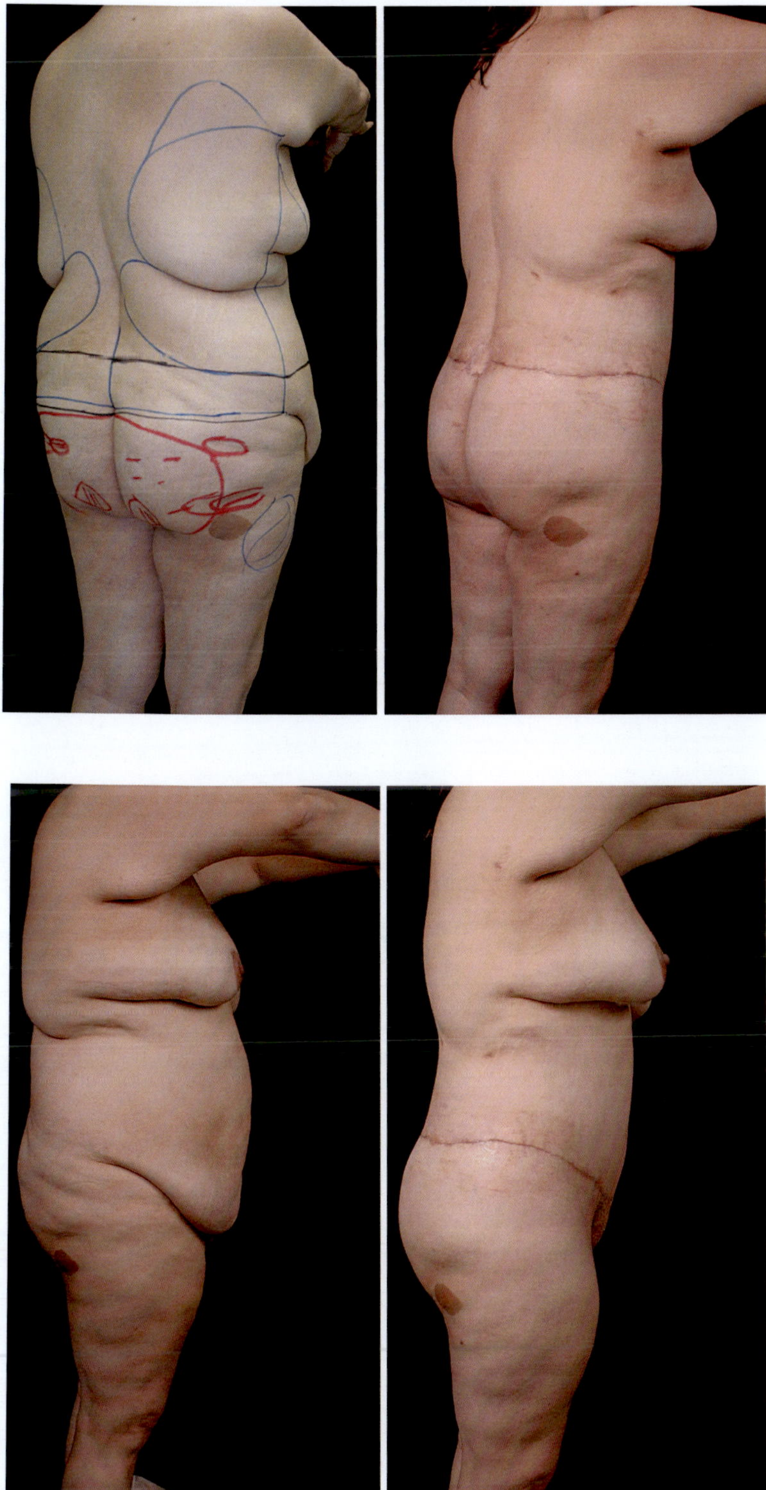

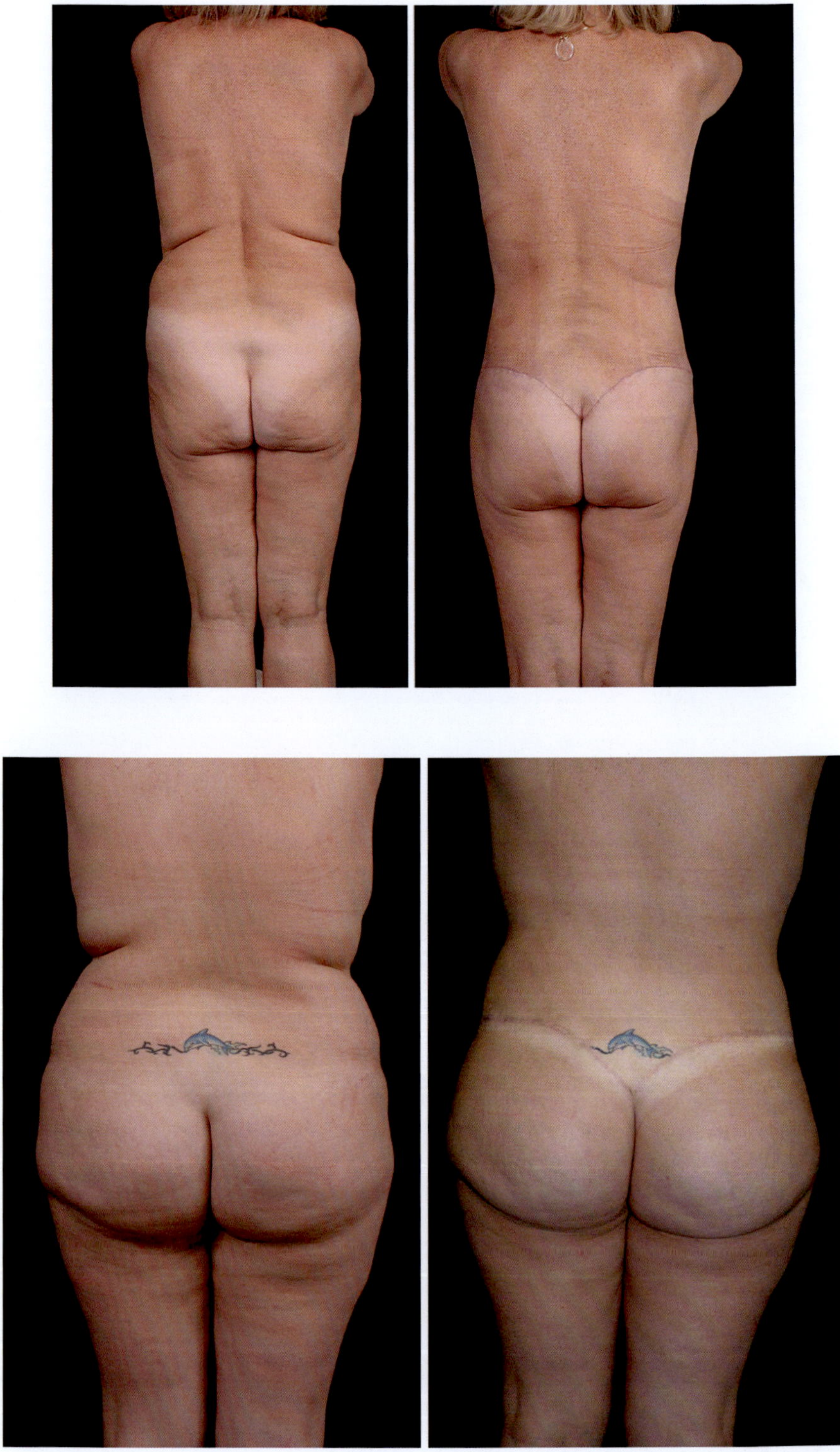

Patients achieved an ideal contour. It is important to emphasize the significant functional and aesthetic improvement in patients who had a large excess of skin, fat, and flaccidity of the circumferential trunk.

The overall complication rate is very low compared to a case study. We observed two cases of skin dehiscence (both patients were post-bariatric).

Conclusions

The association of the liposuction procedure with skin resection modifies the approach to the trunk which, through lipoundermining, is less traumatic and preserves the vascular and lymphatic systems, reducing the rate of complications.

The combination of torsoplasty and lipoabdominoplasty, "lipotorsoabdominoplasty," is safe due to the preservation of the abdominal and trunk blood supply, becoming an ideal option for the circumferential treatment of the body contour.

The fat graft completes the buttock lift, and it is simpler and faster in its execution to balance the gluteal shape.

References

Somalo M (1940) Circular dermolipectomy of the trunk. Semin Med 1:1435

Gonzalez-Ulloa, M. Lipectomia circular com transposição do umbigo e tecnic plástico anatântico. *Cirurgia,* 27:394, 1959.

Baroudi, R. Cirurgia de contorno corporal. *Clin Plast Surg,* 16:263–77, 1989.

Baroudi, R. Flankplastia: um tratamento específico para melhorar o contorno corporal. *Ann Plast Surg,* 27:404–20, 1991.

Correa-Iturraspe, M. Tratamiento quirurgico de la obesidad. *Rev Assoc Med Argent,* 66:340–45, 1952.

Lockwood, T. Parte inferior do elevador corporal. *Oper Tech Plast Reconstr Surg,* 3:132–44, 1996.

Carwell, GR, Horton, CE. Torsoplastia circunferencial. *Ann Plast Surg,* 38: 213–16, 1997

Modolin, M; Cintra Junior WCIC.; Ferreira, MC. Abdominoplastia circunferencial para tratamento sequencial após obesidade mórbida. *Obes Surg,* 13:95–100, 2003.

Lockwood, TE. Elevador transversal flanco-coxa-nádega com suspensão fascial superficial. *Plast Reconstr Surg,* 87:1019–27, 1991.

Sozer SO, Agullo FJ, Wolf C. Authoprose na nádega durante o levantamento inferior do corpo. *Cirurgia Plástica Estética*, 29:133–40, 2005.

Baroudi R, Carvalho CGS. Elevação do terço interno das coxas. Uma análise dos resultados imediatos e mediatos. *Cir Plast Iber Lat Am,* 7: 275, 1981.

Navarro RJ, Fajardo M, Mariscal R, Pérez, R. Levantamiento de glúteos com hamaca subdérmica. *Cir Plást*, 12: 80–84, 2002.

Pascal JF, Le Louarn C. Bodylift remodelando com alta tensão lateral. *Estética Plast Surg*, 26:223–30, 2002.

Chapter 53
Thoracobrachioplasty

Francesco Mazzarone, Raphael Schemberk Chamma,
and Márcio Mendes Manente

Abstract Obesity is a chronic and multifactorial disease characterized by excessive accumulation of body fat. Its continuous increase around the world has led patients and physicians to seek mechanisms for its treatment.

Introduction

Obesity is a chronic and multifactorial disease characterized by excessive accumulation of body fat. Its continuous increase around the world has led patients and physicians to seek mechanisms for its treatment.

Due to the popularization of bariatric surgery (reduction gastroplasty), a considerable increase in patients with significant weight loss was seen. Those patients have a great skin flaccidity, which became a wide field of action for plastic surgery, requiring a complex approach, associating multiple surgical procedures to reestablish the body contour (Pitanguy et al. 2016; Neligan & Járrewend 2015; Rohrich et al. 2020).

Although skin flaccidity is widespread in these patients, the dysmorphism evidenced in the upper segment of the body is of greater concern to patients due to its visibility during daily activities. Morbidly obese patients tend to have greater accumulation of fat along the anterior and posterior armpit and medial regions of the arms (Pitanguy et al. 2016). After accentuated weight loss, a marked ptosis of the arms is found, and it can cross the armpit and extend to the chest wall, causing the so-called bat wings (Neligan & Járrewend 2015). The greater the variation in BMI, the more prominent will be the individual's tissue laxity.

F. Mazzarone (✉) · R. S. Chamma · M. M. Manente
Rio de Janeiro, Brazil

J. M. Avelar, R. Cavalcanti Ribeiro (eds.), *Body Contouring*,
https://doi.org/10.1007/978-3-031-42802-9_53

Indications and Contraindications

The treatment of excess brachial and thoracic skin can be performed in a single combined procedure, and it is indicated for cases in which the benefit of the correction of dysmorphia is greater than its scar. Even in the correct location and with a good appearance, the scars are apparent, and the patient should be aware of and oriented toward this aspect. It is essential to ensure full understanding to avoid unrealistic expectations regarding the potential benefits of surgery.

Thoracobrachioplasty should be avoided in patients with severe comorbidities, who have not achieved the planned total weight loss, smokers, or with a history of previous axillary lymphadenectomy and/or lymphedema in the upper limbs.

Preoperative preparation follows the principles presented in the brachioplasty chapter.

Surgical Technique: Thoracobrachioplasty-Pitanguy Technique

Surgical Marking

This technique was first described in 1975 by Pitanguy, and it allows the correction of lipodystrophy and excess skin in the arms, extending to the lateral aspect of the chest (Pitanguy et al. 2016).

The marking is made in the patient in an orthostatic position, with the arms in lateral abduction and elbows flexed at 90° to show the amount of skin to be resected and the internal biceps sulcus.

A sinuous line is drawn around the posterior edge of the brachial biceps, which starts from the region immediately proximal to the medial epicondyle of the humerus and extends to the axillary hollow. In the armpit, the smooth and sinuous course of the marking is interrupted to prevent the occurrence of scar contracture that can impair the mobility of the shoulder joint. The marking follows the posterior axillary line until finding the lateral limit of the inframammary fold. The length of the incision is determined by the digital clamping maneuver of the cutaneous redundant, as shown in Fig. 53.1.

Operative Technique

General anesthesia is given, and the procedure is performed with the patient in the supine position, arms in abduction. Asepsis, antisepsis, and placement of sterile fields are performed.

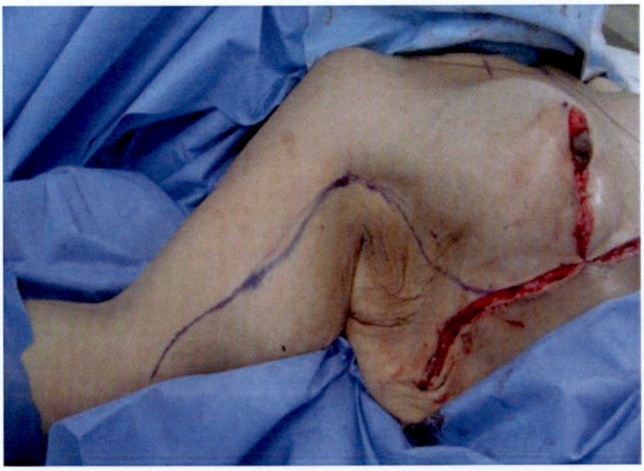

Fig. 53.1 Demonstration of intraoperative marking

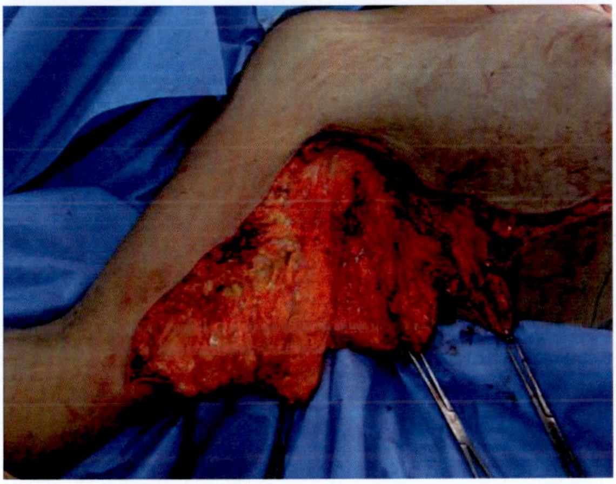

Fig. 53.2 Dermal fat flap detachment

After infiltration with a vasoconstrictor solution (0.9% SF + adrenaline – 1:200,000), the skin is incised over the previous marking and opening in layers to the subcutaneous fat, followed by detachment of the redundant tissue.

The detachment is performed later, in a superficial plane, preserving the subcutaneous from the supra-aponeurotic plane, and its extension will depend on the degree of flaccidity presented (Fig. 53.2). Precise hemostasis is essential at this time.

Traction of the posterior flap is conducted toward the anterior axillary line, for posterior splitting of the flap and delimitation of the axillary fold. Subsequently, the posterior flap is pulled over the anterior flap, with no excessive tension; the excess dermal fat is marked with Pitanguy's forceps soaked in methylene blue. Excessive tension on the flap must be avoided to prevent complications. This process is repeated throughout the entire incision, resulting in a dotted line (Fig. 53.3).

The flap is incised along this line, and the edges are brought together with temporary sutures to ensure its correct alignment.

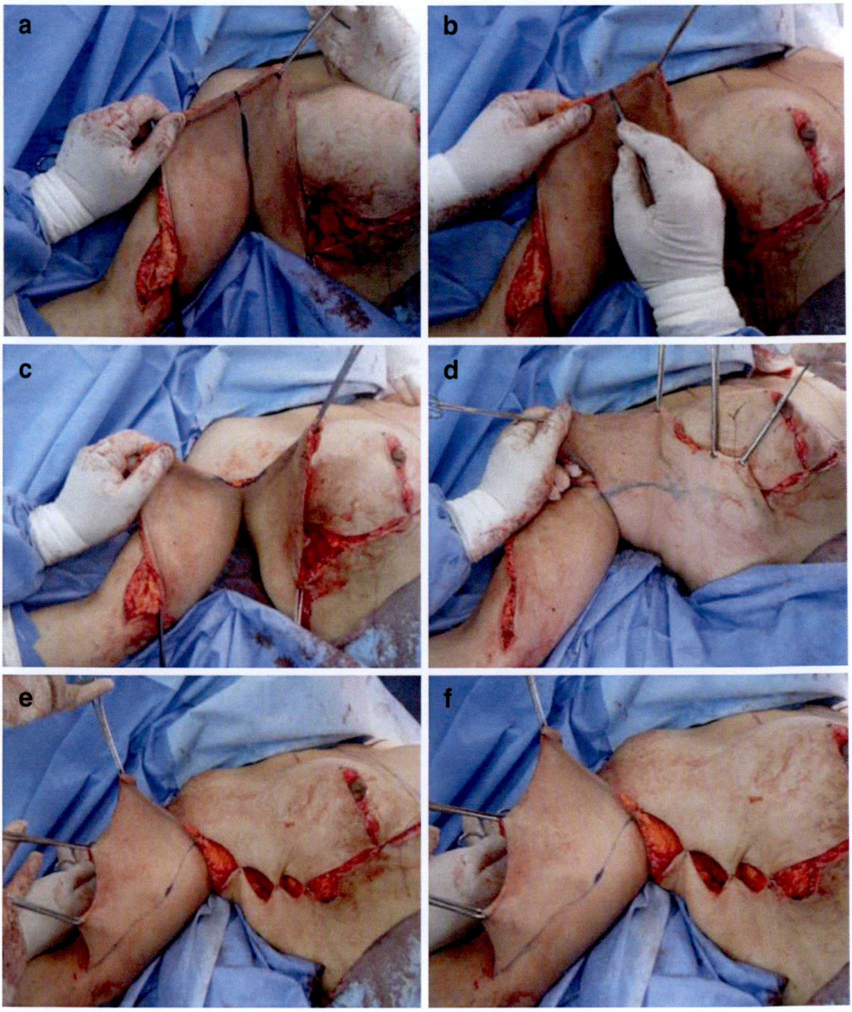

Fig. 53.3 (**a**) Demonstration of flap traction and demarcation of the axillary fold. (**b**) Incision under previously marked splitting of the flap. (**c**) Split flap in the axillary fold. (**d**) Flap distribution and accommodation. (**e**, **f**) Accommodation and distribution of the flap with temporary sutures

The synthesis is performed with stitches separated in two planes: superficial fascia and subdermal plane. The intradermal plane is continuously sutured with absorbable suture.

Adhesive tapes are placed along the incision and then a compressive bandage.

Postoperative Care

The bandage is changed after 24 h and then the use of compressive meshes is started.

Early movement of the arms should be encouraged, taking care to avoid sudden movements and flexions above the line of the shoulders. Weightlifting is contraindicated in the first weeks.

Patients should be instructed to perform specific exercises with the arms to avoid the formation of axillary scarring bands.

Physical activities are allowed 12 weeks after the procedure.

Lymphatic drainage can be started 48 h after the procedure and should be encouraged to reduce edema.

Protocols for the treatment of scars are initiated after 15 days.

Results

Preoperative and postoperative comparison 1 year after the procedure.

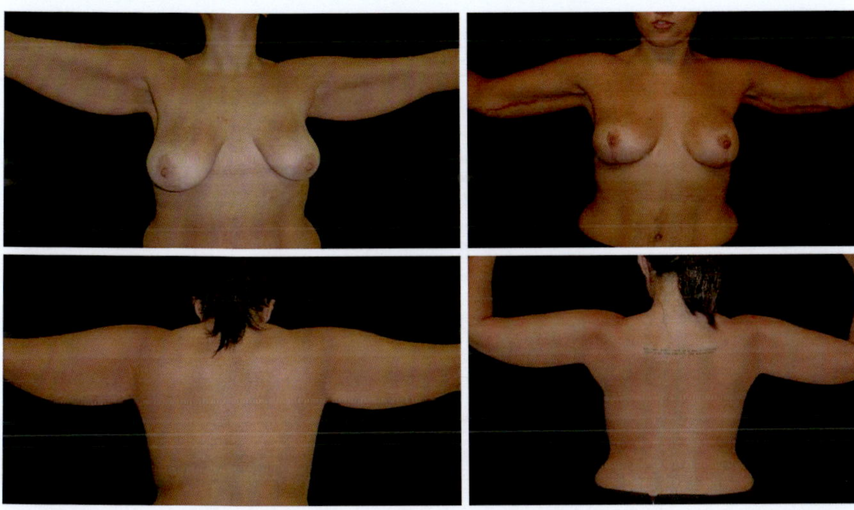

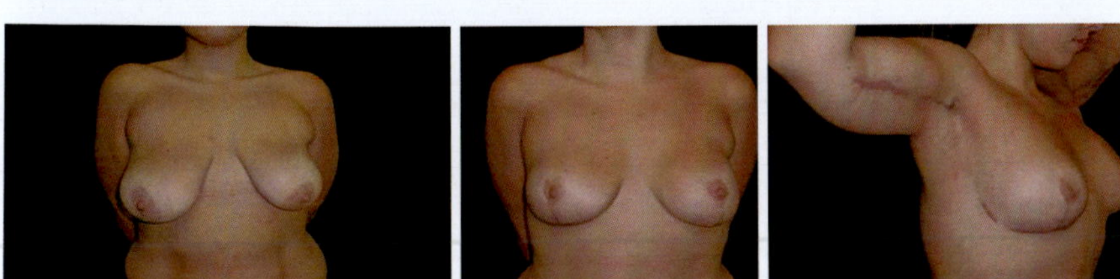

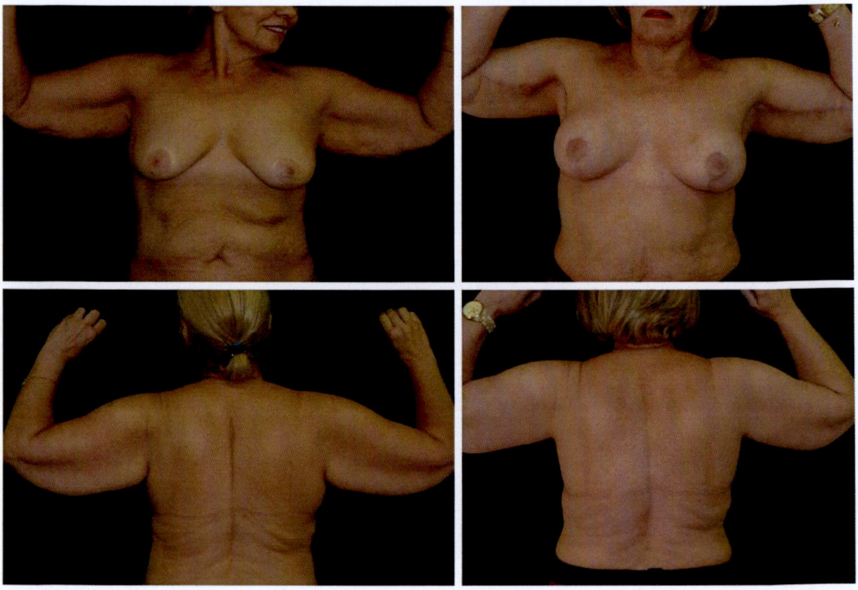

References

Pitanguy I, et al. Cirurgia plástica: uma visão de sua amplitude. São Paulo: Atheneu; 2016.

Neligan PC, Járrewend R. Contorno dos membros superiores. In: Neligan PC, et al. Cirurgia plástica. v. 2. Rio de Janeiro: Elsevier; 2015.

Rohrich RJ, Mohan R, Durand PD. Brachioplasty Refinements. Plast Reconstr Surg. 2020 Apr;145(4):754e-756e.

Part VIII
Upper and Lower Extremities

Chapter 54
Brachioplasty

Francesco Mazzarone and Raphael Schemberk Chamma

Abstract Brachioplasty is the restoration of the contour of the upper limbs. According to the American Society of Plastic Surgery (ASPS), from 2000 to 2020, there was a substantial increase of 4174% in the number of brachioplasties in the USA.

Introduction

Brachioplasty is the restoration of the contour of the upper limbs. According to the American Society of Plastic Surgery (ASPS), from 2000 to 2020, there was a substantial increase of 4174% in the number of brachioplasties in the USA.

Flaccidity of the upper limbs is usually a frequent complaint after the progressive and natural aging process, but especially in obese patients with significant weight loss. Distension and flaccidity of the skin and superficial fascia associated with a reduction in elastin and collagen seem to be the phenomena related to this condition, generating an irreversible condition requiring surgical intervention for correction. The arms lose their cylindrical shape due to tissue ptosis in the inner and lower region, extending from the armpit to the elbow, and eventually to the side chest wall. These changes are especially evident when the arms are in 90° abduction (Pitanguy et al. 2016).

Surgical treatment of brachial flaccidity is one of the challenges of plastic surgery; due to the extension and apparent location of the scars, acceptance by patients limits its indication. Even if healing occurs properly, scars remain visible on the medial face of the upper limb. Patients should be carefully evaluated, with further skin resection indicated only in selected cases (Neligan & Járrewend 2015).

F. Mazzarone (✉) · R. S. Chamma
Plastic and Reconstructive Surgery, Instituto Superior de Ciências da Saúde Carlos Chagas, Rio de Janeiro, Brazil

J. M. Avelar, R. Cavalcanti Ribeiro (eds.), *Body Contouring*,
https://doi.org/10.1007/978-3-031-42802-9_54

In 1954, Correa and Fernandez initially proposed correction of brachial lipodystrophy. Since then, improvements in the technique have been described, as modifications regarding the placement of the incisions and associated to liposuction (Nguyen et al. 2016).

Among the various techniques described, the following techniques stand out: straight incisions in the internal brachial sulcus with resection of excess dermal fat in the longitudinal direction; superficial detachment of the subcutaneous cell tissue to preserve the lymphatic vessels, with z-plasty in the axillary cavity to avoid retraction; making a quadrangular flap and closing the axillary scar in "T" shape; making an L-shaped scar; W-plasty incision; and suspension of the superficial fascia system, among others (Pitanguy et al. 2016; Neligan & Járrewend 2015; Rohrich et al. 2020).

Preoperative Evaluation

Clinical History

Several comorbidities can have a negative impact on the recovery of patients undergoing brachioplasty. These patients must undergo preoperative investigation of diseases such as hypertension, type 2 diabetes, dyslipidemia, coronary artery disease, obstructive sleep apnea, and characteristics of metabolic syndrome frequent in patients with obesity. Patients with hypertension are classified at greater risk for postoperative bleeding; hypertension may be associated with coronary artery disease and kidney failure. Anemia is frequent in formerly obese patients and red cell counts should be closely monitored. Other factors that can affect healing and predispose to complications and should therefore be investigated include smoking history, autoimmune diseases, and endocrine disorders. It is important to emphasize that patients who have already undergone axillary lymph node resection are at increased risk of developing lymphedema. All medications that the patient uses regularly should be evaluated and, if necessary, dose or suspension adjustments should be made.

Nutritional Assessment

It is important to emphasize the need for a body mass index less than or equal to 30 kg/m^2, in addition to weight stabilization for at least 6 months. The nutritional status of patients must be evaluated prior to surgery, especially in patients with great weight loss, due to the elevated risk of nutritional and vitamin deficiencies.

Table 54.1 Classification of arm deformities and treatment strategies. Adapted according to the classification of El Khatib (2007)

El Khatib		
Types	Presentation	Treatment
I	Minimal fat accumulation (<300 mL) without ptosis	Circumferential liposuction
IIa	Moderate lipodystrophy + grade I ptosis (<5 cm)	Staged circumferential liposuction
IIb	Intense lipodystrophy + grade I ptosis (5–10 cm)	Liposuction +/− axillary skin excision
III	Generalized obesity and intense skin sagging	Liposuction + "short scar" brachioplasty
IV	Absent or minimal lipodystrophy + grade III ptosis (>10 cm)	Brachioplasty

Physical Exam

The patient must undergo a complete physical examination, with special attention to conditions identified in the clinical history. The assessment of the degree of lipodystrophy and skin excess, skin quality, and lymphedema and general assessment of healing are fundamental elements and must be documented.

The use of classification systems is valuable for the stratification of patients who will undergo brachioplasty. These systems include the assessment of the degree of lipodystrophy, skin flaccidity, and location of the deformity (proximal, entire upper limb, arm, and chest). Table 54.1 shows the El Khatib classification, proposed for the stratification of patients who will undergo brachioplasty (El Khatib 2007).

Initial stages can be managed by liposuction alone, dermal lipectomy complemented by liposuction, or mini brachioplasty. The most advanced form will require extensive brachioplasty.

Marking and Surgical Technique

Surgical Marking

Patient is in an orthostatic position, arms in lateral abduction and elbows flexed at 90°, and the marking of the amount of skin to be resected begins. This position allows tissue ptosis and flaccidity to be evident.

A sinuous line is drawn around the posterior edge of the brachial biceps, which starts from the region immediately proximal to the medial epicondyle of the humerus and extends to the axillary hollow. Abduction and flexion maneuvers can be useful for defining the muscle contour.

In the armpit, the smooth and sinuous course of the marking is interrupted to prevent the occurrence of scar contracture that can impair the mobility of the shoulder joint. The length of the incision is determined by the digital clamping maneuver of the cutaneous redundant.

The scar position is related to the degree and extension of skin flaccidity, as well as the excessive amount of local adipose tissue. This will be confirmed during the surgical procedure with the Pitanguy marker.

Operative Technique

The procedure is started with the patient under general anesthesia in the supine position, with the arms in abduction, free to allow mobility during the procedure. Asepsis, antisepsis, and placement of sterile drapes are performed.

Infiltration is performed with a vasoconstrictor solution with saline and adrenaline in the proportion of 1:200,000.

The skin incision is made over the previous marking, opening up to the subcutaneous fat. Detachment of the redundant tissue is performed.

The detachment is performed later, in a superficial plane, preserving the subcutaneous from the supra-aponeurotic plane, and its extension will depend on the degree of flaccidity presented. Precise hemostasis is essential at this time.

The posterior flap is pulled over the anterior flap, with no excessive tension; the excess dermal fat is marked with Pitanguy's forceps. This process is repeated throughout the entire incision, resulting in a dotted line.

The flap is incised along this line and the edges are brought together with temporary sutures to ensure its correct alignment.

The synthesis is performed with stitches separated in two planes: superficial fascia and subdermal plane. The intradermal plane is continuously sutured with absorbable suture.

Adhesive tapes are placed along the incision and then a compressive bandage.

Postoperative Care

The early movement of the limbs, in a controlled and moderate manner, should be encouraged, and active movement of the arms is recommended as soon as the patient is awake. However, large movements should be avoided, as well as lifting weights.

Physical activities with loads are allowed 3 months after the procedure.

Bandages are changed the following day and the surgical site must be evaluated to identify hematoma, which, if identified, must be promptly drained.

The use of compressive meshes is indicated during the first 4 weeks in order to avoid the formation of seroma, ensuring uniform controlled pressure on the flap. Its use can be postponed individually, according to clinical evolution.

In general, lymphatic drainage massage can be started 48 h after the procedure, after evaluation by the surgeon.

Complications

Surgical wound complications are frequent and include seromas, dehiscence, infection, and hematomas and occur in patients with comorbidities (Nguyen et al. 2016). Flap necrosis may also occur, and in this case, the devitalized tissues must be debrided in order to accelerate healing and reduce the risk of infection (Table 54.2).

Seroma

A fluid collection can develop under widely detached tissue or in places where substantial amounts of skin have been removed. It clinically presents with discomfort, fullness, or burning sensation, and a fluid fluctuation may be palpated. In these cases, the patient must undergo drainage of the seroma, associated with compression therapy. Repeated drainages may be necessary until complete resolution.

Infection

Bacteria present in the skin's microbiota typically cause infection. Antimicrobial treatment, preferably guided by cultures, should be used.

Bruise

Patients with comorbidities or who use anticoagulants are at higher risk of developing hematomas. These occur in the immediate postoperative period, and the patient must return to the operating room for adequate drainage and hemostasis.

Lymphedema

Lymphedema may occur due to interruption of the lymphatic drainage of the upper limbs by scar tissue. Treatment consists of compression therapy, massage, and physical therapy.

Table 54.2 Frequency of surgical wound complications in patients undergoing brachioplasty (Neligan & Járrewend 2015)

Skin dehiscence	25%
Seroma	10%
Infection	2.6%
Bruise	0.6%
Skin necrosis	0.6%

Unaesthetic Scar

Scar enlargement seems to be related to suture tension and flap weight. We believe that it is difficult to find a balance between the risk of tension and undercorrection, with little expressive results.

Dermolipectomy of the upper limbs can result in disharmony around the arm, with excessive resection of the skin and subcutaneous tissue in the middle portion of the flap and excesses in the extremities. Some authors cite surgical alternatives to avoid this complication. Baroudi and Ferreira proposed incision and detachment of the posterior flap, analyzing intraoperatively how much tissue could be respected. Similarly, Júri et al. describe a quadrangular arm flap and "T" closure to compensate for excess axillary skin.

Results

See Figs. 54.1 and 54.2.

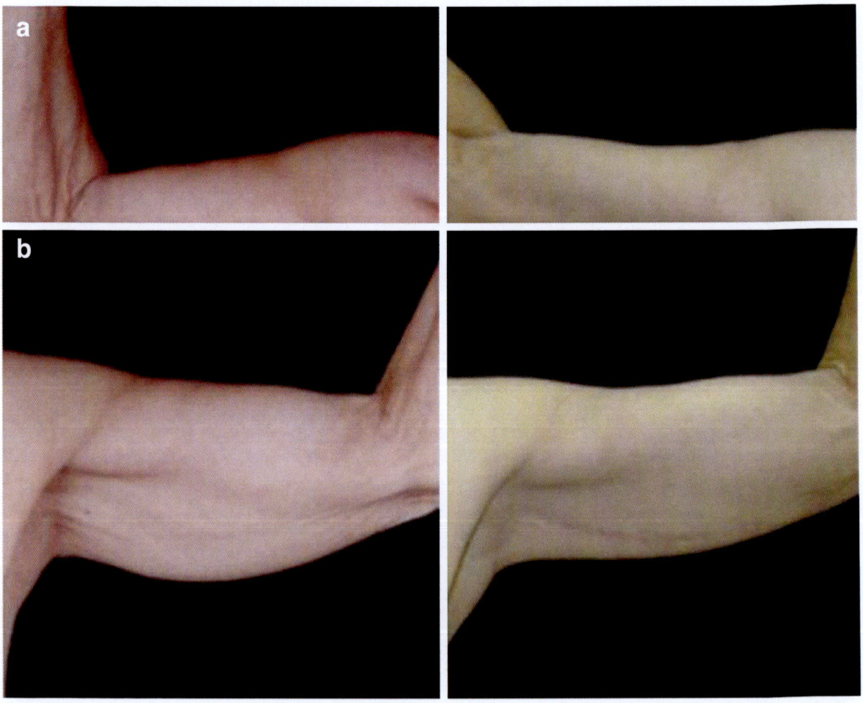

Fig. 54.1 (**a**) Comparison before and after the operation of 1 year – right arm. (**b**) Comparison before and after the operation of 1 year – left arm

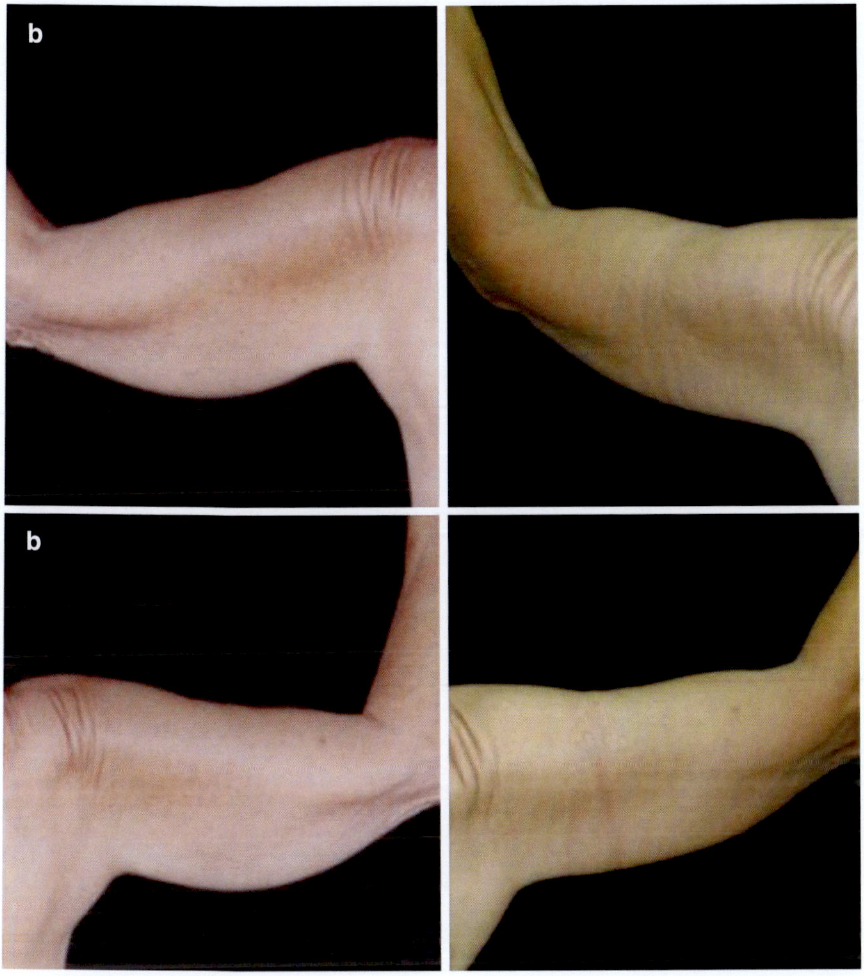

Fig. 54.2 (**a**) Comparison before and after the operation of 1 year – right arm. (**b**) Comparison before and after the operation of 1 year – left arm

References

Pitanguy I, et al. Cirurgia plástica: uma visão de sua amplitude. São Paulo: Atheneu; 2016.

Neligan PC, Járrewend R. Contorno dos membros superiores. In: Neligan PC, et al. Cirurgia plástica. v. 2. Rio de Janeiro: Elsevier; 2015.

Nguyen L, et al. Incidence and Risk Factors of Major Complications in Brachioplasty: Analysis of 2,294 Patients. Oxford University. Aesthet Surg J Advance Access published May 23, 2016. 2016 mai 23; p. 1–12.

Rohrich RJ, Mohan R, Durand PD. Brachioplasty Refinements. Plast Reconstr Surg. 2020 Apr;145(4):754e–756e

El Khatib HA. Classification of brachial ptosis: strategy for treatment. Plast Reconstr Surg. 2007 Apr 1;119(4):1337–1342.

Chapter 55
Block Resection in Tight Lift

Gisela Hobson Pontes, Ronaldo Pontes, and Clara Pontes

Abstract Large amounts of weight loss can generate excess tissue in all areas of the body, especially in the abdomen and thigh region. To correct such deformities, several surgical techniques were created. The four techniques described in this chapter are derivatives of the surgical concept of en bloc resection, created by Ronaldo Pontes in the early 1960s. These include the block thigh lift, the anteromedial thigh lift without suprapubic resection, the orbital block lift, and the vertical block lift. Each technique is indicated for a specific type of patient, and the proper selection of the candidate for each procedure is the first step toward surgical success. Indications for the thigh lift are adiposity, flaccidity, cellulite in the thigh, and contour irregularity, which may be associated with flaccidity in the abdomen, flanks, and gluteal region. In general, thigh lifting techniques have a low complication rate, the most common being related to seroma formation and scar decency. Regardless of the technique chosen, one should always bear in mind the importance of removing the tissue in one piece and the principle of supporting the thigh through the abdomen.

Keywords Body contouring · Excess skin · Inner thigh lift · Medial thigh lift · Plastic surgery · Surgical technique

---

G. H. Pontes (✉)
Plastic Surgery Department, Serviço de Pós-Graduação Ronaldo Pontes, Hospital Niterói D'or, Niterói, Rio de Janeiro, Brazil

R. Pontes · C. Pontes
Fundação Técnico-Educacional Souza Marques (FTESM), Rio de Janeiro, Brazil

J. M. Avelar, R. Cavalcanti Ribeiro (eds.), *Body Contouring*,
https://doi.org/10.1007/978-3-031-42802-9_55

Introduction

The block abdominoplasty technique was created by Ronaldo Pontes in the early 1960s. In 1964, he presented all variations of the technique at the III Regional Conference of.

Petrópolis, of the International College of Surgeons, and later at the VIII Brazilian Congress of Plastic Surgery, held in 1971 in Salvador, Bahia. The technique is described in our book *Abdominoplasty: Block Resection and Its Application in Thigh Lifting and Torsoplasty*.

The first concept of the thigh lifting technique described in this chapter was conceived in 1981 by Professor Ronaldo Pontes. Since its conception, several variations of the technique have been improved over the years, finally being summed up as an extension of the block abdominoplasty technique, adopting the ideals of this kind of surgery (Pontes 2004); (Maciel and Júnior 2010).

The thigh lift surgery had already been described in the works of Lewis (1957),

Lockwood (Lockwood 1988, 1991, 1995, 2000); Hakme (1982), and Baroudi (Baroudi and Moraes 1991). However, it was rare, given the small range of execution of the procedure. In the current context, the obesity epidemic is a concern in the world health scenario. This has been countered with the advent of new bariatric surgery techniques that, along with drastic changes in the patient's lifestyle, can lead to sudden weight loss with significant fat loss. Although the massive weight loss provides a huge health benefit, it generates a new problem: large amounts of excess skin in areas that are difficult to correct, leading people to consider having the previously unpopular thigh lift surgery.

The loss of a large volume of fat, especially in the subdermal mesh, causes accentuated flaccidity in the most diverse areas of the body, having a greater impact on the torso, thighs, and arms (Lewis 1957). Nevertheless, regardless of the technique used, the repair of these deformities results in substantial scarring, caused by the extensive surgical approach required. Usually, the type of patient who seeks this correction is already in the process of accepting their new physical shape, and the mechanical and functional benefits tend to outweigh the concerns about the scars left by the treatment. Overlapping surgeries should be avoided in post-bariatric patients, especially those who have certain comorbidities prior to weight loss (Ramsy 1993). However, with adequate patient selection and correct preoperative preparation, en bloc resection without any type of lateral or inferior flap detachment is associated with rapid patient recovery. It is important to emphasize the need for a multidisciplinary team to tend to all of the patient's needs, including physical therapists for the patient's early mobilization and ambulation, as well as clinicians (Fig. 55.1).

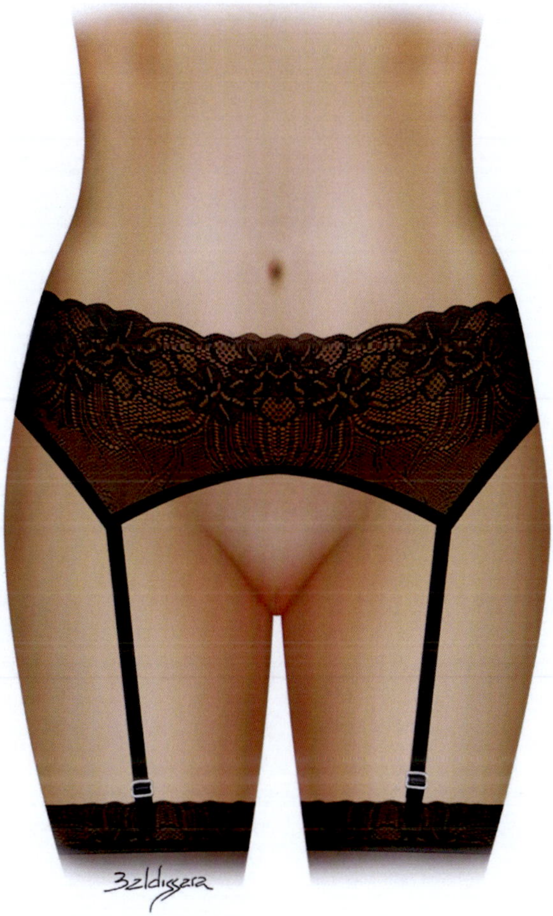

Fig. 55.1 Illustrative image of a garter belt on a female body, representing the support of the thigh by the abdomen, performed by a garter belt

The Anatomy of the Thigh and Inguinal Region

Knowing the anatomy of the inguinal region is extremely important when performing the techniques described below. This region is where the femoral triangle is located, in which the lymphatic vessels responsible for draining the lower limbs are located, whose preservation is essential when treating the deformities with a thigh lift. During surgical resection, it is always essential to maintain the natural shape of the thighs, which is an inverted cone, thus removing more skin from the medial region than from the distal region (Aly 2008) (Fig. 55.2).

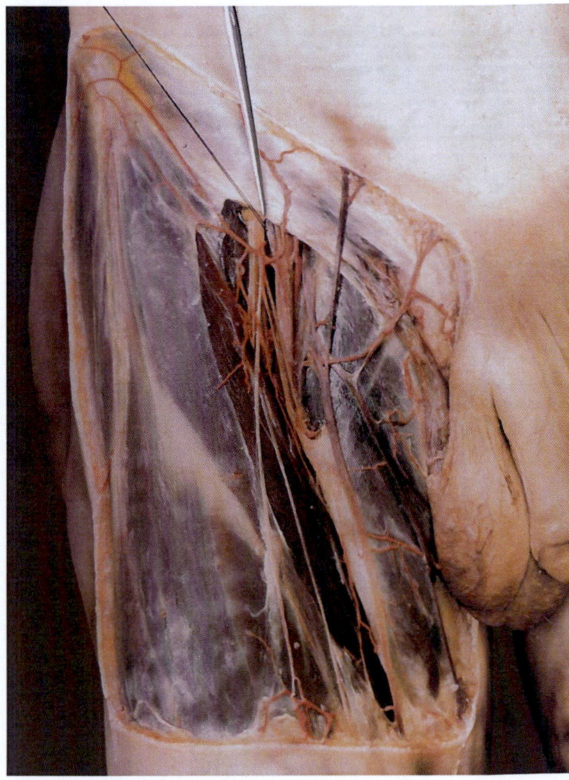

Fig. 55.2 Anatomical image of the femoral triangle region

Technique Description: Block Thigh Lifting

Before addressing the surgery in question, it is necessary to understand the concept of the block technique. This essentially consists of tracing a flap through imaginary lines acquired by the pinch test and removing just one piece of excess tissue without any type of lateral detachment. The flap is resected en bloc, and after hemostasis, the lesion is closed. There are several benefits in performing the technique en bloc, including easy reproducibility, reduced operative time, ease of detachment, greater possibility of overlapping with other surgical procedures, symmetrical scars, and a general improvement in results. In addition to these advantages, the absence of lateral detachment allows the patient to walk earlier which reduces recovery time as well as the incidence of thromboembolic problems (Aston et al. 2009).

In thigh lifting surgery, the first step for a successful result is the proper selection of the patient, with the correct indication being evaluated for such a procedure. This evaluation must present flaccidity, adiposity, and cellulite in the thigh, which may be associated with flaccidity of the abdomen, flanks, and gluteal region, as well as irregularity of contour. Regarding the patient's complaint, it is essential that the most impaired area be located in the cranial and middle third of the thigh, because as this flaccidity moves away from the inguinal region, the flap traction force decreases. Even if initially in the recent postoperative period the result is positive, over the course of 6 months to 1 year, it may be lost almost completely. Among the contraindications for surgery are obesity, poor acceptance of the scar, and absence of flaccidity or mobility. In our practice, we invariably perform the marking on the day before the surgery. This is performed as follows: we place the patient in an orthostatic position, the patient's midline is demarcated with a guide wire, and then, from the medial point at around 5 cm above the anterior vaginal commissure or around 7–8 cm above the base of the penis, a semi-arched line is drawn up to the lateral limit of the pubis. From there, cranially, by means of tissue clamping, we verify how much of the thigh flaccidity can be corrected, tracing a semi-arched line above the anterior line whose lateral limits, defined with the patient in a seated position, extend up to the lateral crease of the abdomen. Subsequently, in dorsal decubitus with the patient in "frog leg position," from the perineal fold to the infra-gluteal crest (infrabuttocks crease) and with a clamping maneuver, the extension of the tissue to be resected in the region between the thighs is delimited, taking care not to cause any deformities in the patient's labia majora or in the male perineal region. It is important to point out that with this technique the thigh tension is sustained by the abdomen, similar to a garter belt for women, decreasing the chances of vulvar or perineal stretching, due to the lower tension in the medial scar region between the thighs. These measurements are checked with a pair of compasses and a tape measure (Figs. 55.3 and 55.4).

See Figs. 55.5 and 55.6.

This technique is indicated in cases of flaccidity on the anterior and lateral faces of the thighs in patients who have already had a previous abdominoplasty and/or do not have tissue flaccidity in the suprapubic region. It follows the same principle of the thigh being supported by the abdomen. With the patient in an orthostatic position, we perform the marking of the inguinal crease, and through manual clamping of the lateral face of the thigh and flanks and performing cranial traction, the complete correction of the flaccidity is observed. Then, from the initial line, an upper line is drawn according to the need for resection to achieve the desired result, as ascertained by the previous maneuver. Both demarcations are limited by the extension of the posterior axillary line. For the demarcation of the dorsal region, the midline is delimited, the beginning of the intergluteal sulcus is demarcated, and, based on these reference points, a semi-curved convex line is drawn to meet the previous marking. The marking is done one side at a time in the following order: front 1, front 2, back 1, back 2. After marking each side, it is necessary to check the symmetry of the markings with the help of a compass, ruler, and tape measure, always using the floor as a reference point (Figs. 55.7–55.9).

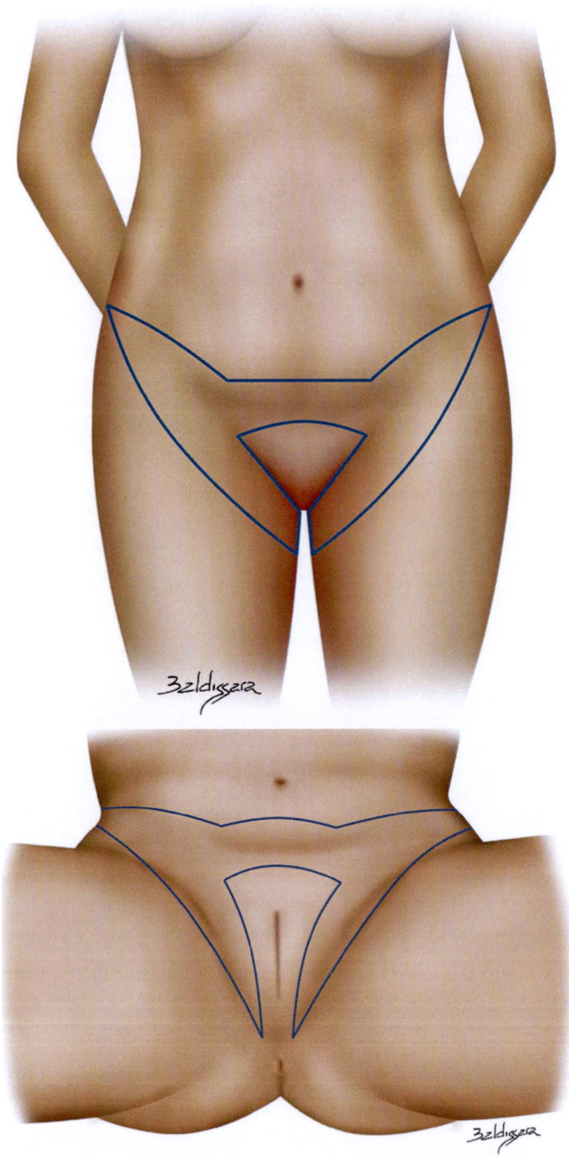

Figs. 55.3 and 55.4 Drawings of the Thigh lift Marking Based on Abdominal Support

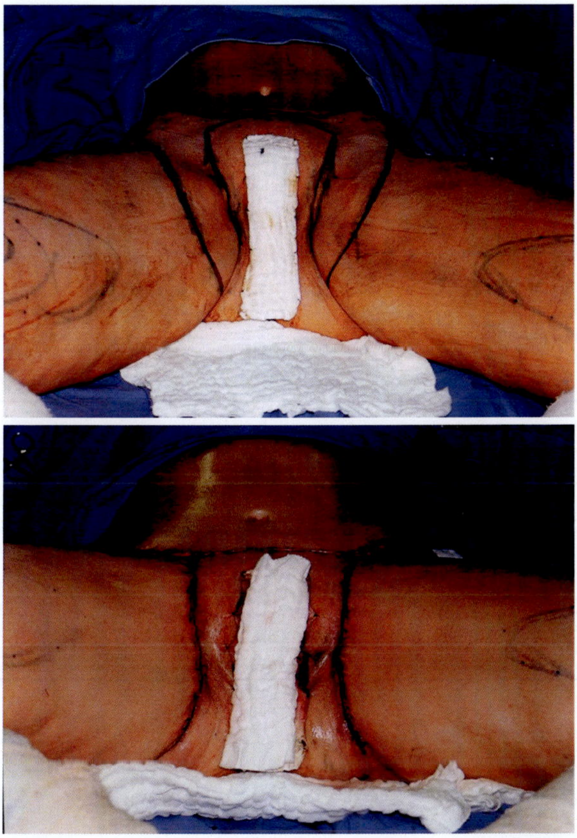

Figs. 55.5 and 55.6 Patient pre- and post-surgery Technique description - Anteromedial Thigh Lift Without Suprapubic Resection

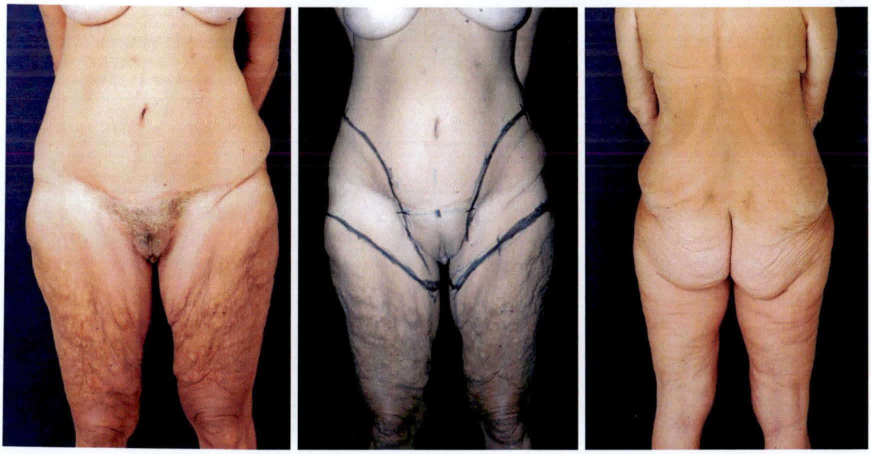

Figs. 55.7–55.9 Pre- and postoperative period of a 66-year-old patient after bariatric surgery, with a 50 kilos weight loss

Technique Description: Orbital Block Thigh Lift

To perform the markings for this technique, we start with the patient in the supine position. A midline is drawn with the help of a guide wire. Then, around 5–6 cm from the anterior vaginal commissure or around 7–8 cm above the base of the penis, with the region tractioned, a semi-lateral line is drawn up to the posterior axillary line. After that, the arched line is marked on the dorsal region, with the patient in a standing position, finishing at the beginning of the upper gluteal fold. The drawing of the upper arched lines is delimited by a pinch test, which determines the amount of excess tissue to be resected. The marking is mirrored on the opposite side following the same logic, and then all markings are checked using a compass, ruler, and measuring tape to ensure the maximum possible symmetry in the design. It is essential that the distance between the inverted peaks of each posterior arcuate line not be too great in order to reduce the risk of cranial stretching of the intergluteal sulcus (Figs. 55.10 and 55.11).

See Figs. 55.12–55.15.

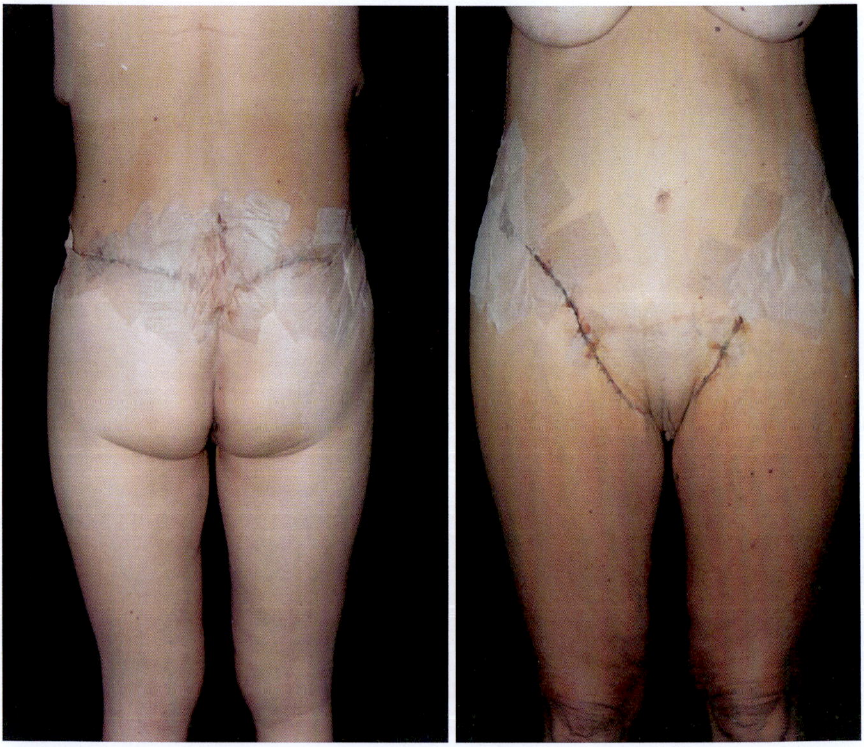

Figs. 55.10 and 55.11 Drawings of the orbital block thigh lift

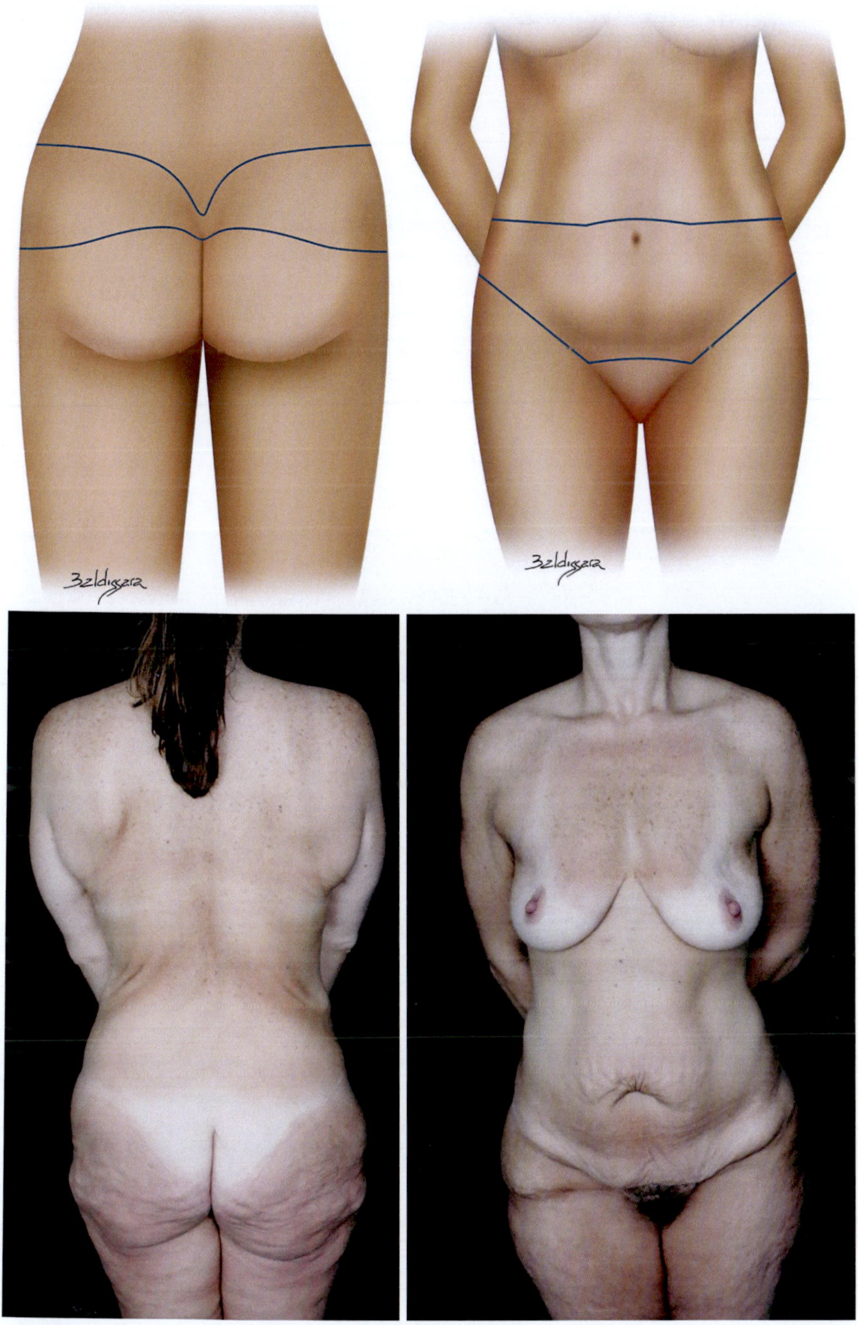

Figs. 55.12–55.15 Pre- and postoperative patient after a 60 kilos weight loss

Description of the Technique: Vertical Block Lift

The marking is initially done in dorsal decubitus with the patient in "frog leg position," and the perineal fold is marked up to the posterior gluteal crease. The marking is then made immediately after the gracilis tendon, extending to the area of skin laxity to be corrected; this line will be the center of the ellipse that will be resected. A "pinch test" is performed on the areas with skin laxity in order to delimit the ellipse. To finish the marking, the patient is placed on a standing position in order to conclude the ellipse and to trace equidistant horizontal lines inside the ellipse that will guide the wound closure without distorting it. Remember that the surgeon's keen sensitivity is essential so that no more tissue is removed than necessary. Complementing the technique with liposuction of the medial surface of the knee and resection of the ellipse from distal to proximal (with proximal resection being as superficial as possible in order to preserve the lymphatic and venous structures in the region) are also of great importance (Figs. 55.16 and 55.17).

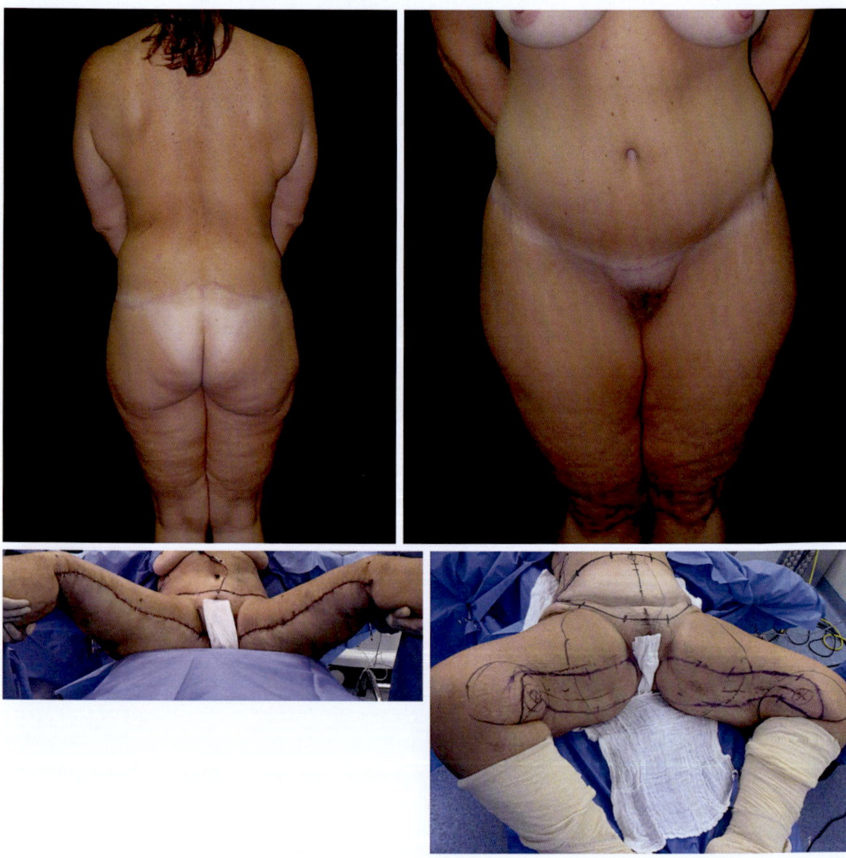

Figs. 55.16 and 55.17 Pre and postoperative patient

Intraoperative Phase

In the operating room, general anesthesia is administered, which allows for greater hemodynamic control of the patient, asepsis of the patient, and reinforcement of the demarcation. Then the procedure begins. With the patient in dorsal decubitus, we perform the isolation and protection of the perineum fixed with stitches. The skin is incised with a 15 blade along the marking so that it does not get erased. Then the region to be resected is infiltrated with a solution of 1 ampoule of 20 mL of xylocaine 2%, 20 mL ropivacaine 7.5%, and adrenaline 1% diluted in 500 mL of saline solution. Next, the flap detachment from the lateral to the medial region, or distal to proximal (in the case of the vertical thigh lift), is started with an electric scalpel, performing rigorous hemostasis, up to the midline. This flap is resected en bloc, and while the assistant performs the wound closure by planes using mononylon 2.0, 3.0, and 4.0, anchoring the dermis with colorless mononylon 4.0 and finishing the skin with dermabond-premium R, the main surgeon starts the detachment of the other side in the same way. Afterward, with the patient in "frog leg position," the same resection and closure process is performed for the medial flap. In the abdominal portion, a compensation is made in the medial direction of the flap in order to avoid tissue leftovers and "dog ears." In the mid-thigh portion, the flap rotation is done in the posteroanterior direction, in order to avoid deformities in the infrabuttocks crease.

Complications

Complications from thigh lift surgery can be both local and systemic, with local complications being more frequent. Among the systemic complications, deep vein thrombosis and pulmonary embolism can be cited. These are serious complications, but with early diagnosis performed by angiotomography, they present a good prognosis. These problems may be prevented by using injectable Clexane® 12 h after the end of the surgery and maintained for 7 days. Bearing in mind the specificities of each patient, a single daily dose can be used for prevention. In addition to medication, the use of pneumatic compression boots is indicated in the intraoperative and immediate postoperative periods, associated with the stimulation of early ambulation. It is essential to seek diagnosis if the patient presents any changes in the clinical and laboratory tests. Regarding local complications, hematoma, seroma, infection, and poor scar evolution with scar hypertrophy and/or keloid may occur. Regarding seroma, since the inclusion of adhesion points ("Baroud points") in the technique, this has become less frequent. Special attention should be paid to the supra-trochanteric region so that there is no dead space. Although this surgery does not routinely present cases of necrosis, we use a Meticorten 12 mg IV during the induction of anesthesia and wet oxygen at 5 L in the first postoperative hours to decrease the endocrine-metabolic response to trauma.

Pearls and Pitfalls

- In the region near the sacrum, avoid a wide resection and position the caudal scar close to the end of the intergluteal sulcus. This is because positioning the scar cranially can give the buttocks an elongated and aged appearance, the opposite of what the technique aims to accomplish.
- Preferably this surgery should not be overlapped with abdominoplasty, since every time there is detachment of the abdomen, there is a relative loss of cranial tension force. This force is used in thigh lift surgery, as the thigh is supported by the abdomen.
- This approach corrects the proximal third and the first half of the distal third, with accentuated flaccidity of the distal third being a contraindication, in which case a vertical lift would be the best choice, not only for the possibility of a greater correction but also to avoid risking a complication of vulval distortion. Warning the patient about the limitation of the technique is very important to adjust expectations and thus increase the chances of patient satisfaction with the surgical result.
- The use of immediate postsurgical tape is indicated for this type of surgery. This is performed by physical therapy professionals and can be of great help in patient recovery. Among the benefits of taping are prevention of edema, aid in tissue recovery, and maintenance of tension under the tissue, thus relieving scar traction (Chi et al. 2018).

Final Considerations

With the advent of these techniques, it is possible to successfully treat the wide variety of deformities resulting from drastic weight loss. When approaching thigh lifting, it is important to always bear in mind the principle of en bloc resection, with the removal of the flap in one piece, applying abdominal support in almost all variations as the basis of the technique.

References

Pontes, R. Abdominoplastia - Ressecção em Bloco e sua Aplicação em Lifting de Coxa e Torsoplastia. Rio de Janeiro: Revinter, 2004.

Maciel LIMA Júnior, E. Tratado de Cirurgia Plástica Após Grandes Perdas Ponderais. 1a ed. [s.l.] Atheneu, 2010. cap. 16, p. 159–173

Lewis JR. The thigh lift. J Int Coll Surg 1957; 27: 330.

Lockwood T. Transverse Flank. Thigh. Buttock lift with superficial fascial suspension. Plast Reconstr Surg 1991; 87: 1019–27.

Lockwood T. Fascial anchoring in medial thigh lifts. Plast Reconstr Surg 1988; 82: 299–304.

Lockwood T. High lateral tension abdominoplasty with superficial fascial system suspension. Plast Reconstr Surg 1995; 96; 603–15.
Lockwood T, Contouring of the arms, trunk and thighs. In Guyuron b. Achaur BM, Eriksson E, Coleman III JJ, Russell Rc, Vander Kolk CA. Plastic Surgery: indications, operations and outcomes. St. Louis, MI: Mosby, 2000: 2839–57.
Hakme F. Evolução histórica das abdominoplastias e contribuição pessoal. Anais do simpósio Brasileiro de abdominoplastias 1982. p. 3.
Baroudi R, Moraes M. Philosophy, technical principles, selection and indications in body contouring surgery. Aesthetic Plast Surg 1991; 15: 1–18.
Aly, A. Body contouring after massive weight loss. Philadelphia: W.B. Saunders, 2008; cap 7, 214–236.
Aston, S. J.; Steinbrech, D. S; Walden J. L. Aesthetic plastic surgery. Vol. 2. [s.l.] Philadelphia Saunders, 2009; cap 66, p.791–803.
Chi A, Lange A, Guimarães MVTN, Santos CB. Prevenção e tratamento de equimose, edema e fibrose no pré, trans e pós-operatório de cirurgias plásticas. Rev. Bras. Cir. Plást.2018;33(3):343–354

Chapter 56
Calf

Nicola Menichelli

Abstract Silicone implants have been reported to correct the contour of the legs since 1977, according to publications by Glitzenstein (France) and Carlsen (Canada). We suggest the placement of implants according to the patient's need, namely, thin legs, arched legs, and legs that do not look graceful due to silhouette disorders or due to congenital or acquired deformities. In general, women wish for more elegant legs, and men wish for more muscular legs.

The implant location is sub-fascial, and the approach coincides with the popliteal groove. The detachment is smooth and atraumatic, obeying the pre-established limits. The suture is made in planes, always with internal, absorbable stitches, including the cuticular ones.

The procedure has an exceptionally low morbidity.

The adverse results are dependent on the poor planning of the surgery.

Fat grafts are used, always as a complement to the silicone implant. When multiple implants must be applied, the treatment should be scheduled in multiple procedures, with a minimum interval of 1 year between one surgery and another. Simultaneous placement of tissue expanders is another option to be considered.

Keywords Calf · Calves · Silicone prosthesis · Leg increase · Leg augmentation · Thin legs · Arched legs

The first reports on the augmentation of legs with silicone implants were published in 1977, written by Glitzenstein (Glitzenstein 1979), in France, and Carlsen (Carlsen 1979), in Canada.

The surgery aims to recover or improve the contour of the legs, in some way harmed by congenital or acquired deformities, or simply because they were not favored by nature.

N. Menichelli (✉)
São Paulo, Brazil

J. M. Avelar, R. Cavalcanti Ribeiro (eds.), *Body Contouring*,
https://doi.org/10.1007/978-3-031-42802-9_56

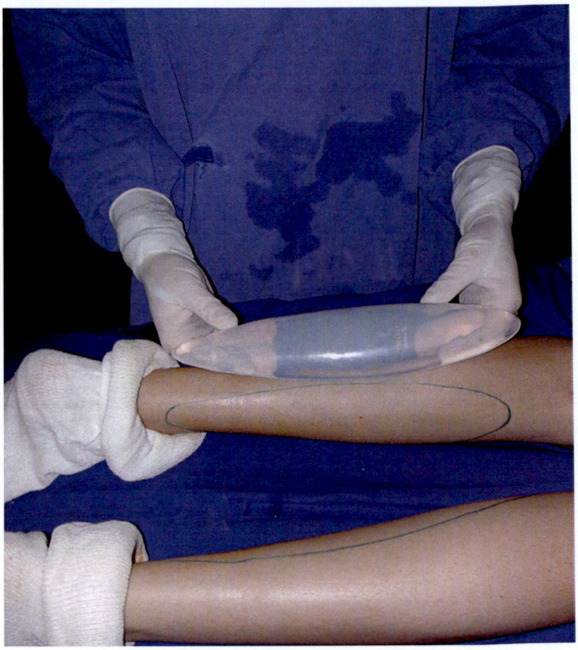

Fig. 56.1 Silicone elastomer implant, 290 mL, custom made

According to Menichelli (Menichelli Netto 1999), we found four basic types of complaints regarding the legs:

1. Thin legs, out of harmony with the rest of the body.
2. Arched legs, because of the lack of volume in the territory of the medial gastrocnemius muscle, whether genu varum or not.
3. Diverging legs, caused by genu valgum.
4. Asymmetric legs, caused by trauma or multiple pathologies, congenital or acquired, such as polio and clubfoot.

Thin or arched legs, excessively thin ankles, and silhouette impaired by muscular atrophies (difficult or impossible to be corrected through physical exercises) can benefit from the placement of silicone implants, specially designed for this purpose (Fig. 56.1).

Medical consultation on this procedure is just as important as performing the procedure itself.

Almost all patients report a great inhibition in wearing short clothes, bathing suits, or any clothing that exposes their legs. Instead, they opt for the constant use of long pants. This ends up bringing severe limitations to living in society. It is not uncommon for a patient to report never having gone to the beach, so as not to show his legs.

In the absence of a worldwide consensus on how attractive legs should look, attention should be focused on the intimate desires of each patient.

Since the surgical proposal is to provide volume in the parts where it is considered insufficient (a general increase would not alter the silhouette), these points should be discussed very well with the patient. A good idea to start with is to ask him to point out the place he dislikes most with his hand.

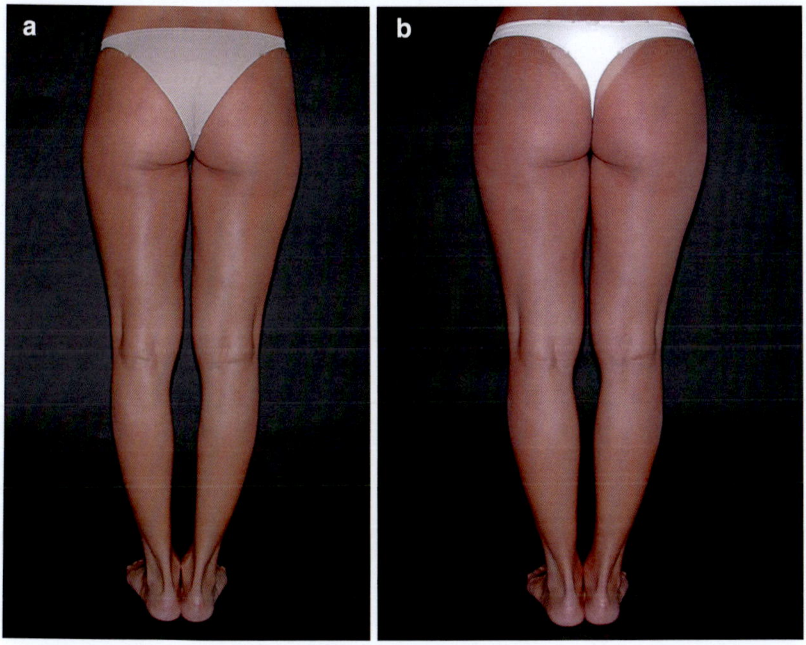

Fig. 56.2 Thin legs. (**a**) Preoperative appearance. (**b**) Two years after inclusion of 140 ml prostheses, type Glitzenstein

If possible, discuss in a subsequent consultation the simulated correction of the procedure.

Women aim for a more beautiful contour on the whole leg (not only on the calf), so we use long (26 cm) and thin implants (Fig. 56.2).

Men, on the other hand, usually look for a muscular aspect, for which we use shorter implants (20–23 cm) although bulkier (140, 180 mL or even larger) (Fig. 56.3).

For arched legs we suggest placing more bulky implants on the medial side of the leg. This increase simulates correcting the longitudinal axis of the legs (Fig. 56.4).

When the lack of volume affects both sides of the leg, we do not hesitate to place two implants, one medial and one lateral, the only way to obtain a pleasant silhouette in the leg in question (Fig. 56.5).

There are situations in which the thinning of the leg occurs only in the lower third, in the region of the malleoli, being the upper thirds (gastrocnemius) and medium (soleus + gastrocnemius) normal in volume and silhouette. In these cases, we must apply an implant only in the lower third. This placement requires a certain locking of the implant in this place, due to the risk of it returning through the tunnel through which it was introduced, losing correction in the desired location. A long implant can also be used, whose projection becomes evident only in the lower third, hiding the upper projection behind the muscle volume (oblique situation of the implant, where the distal end faces forward and the proximal end backward) (Fig. 56.6).

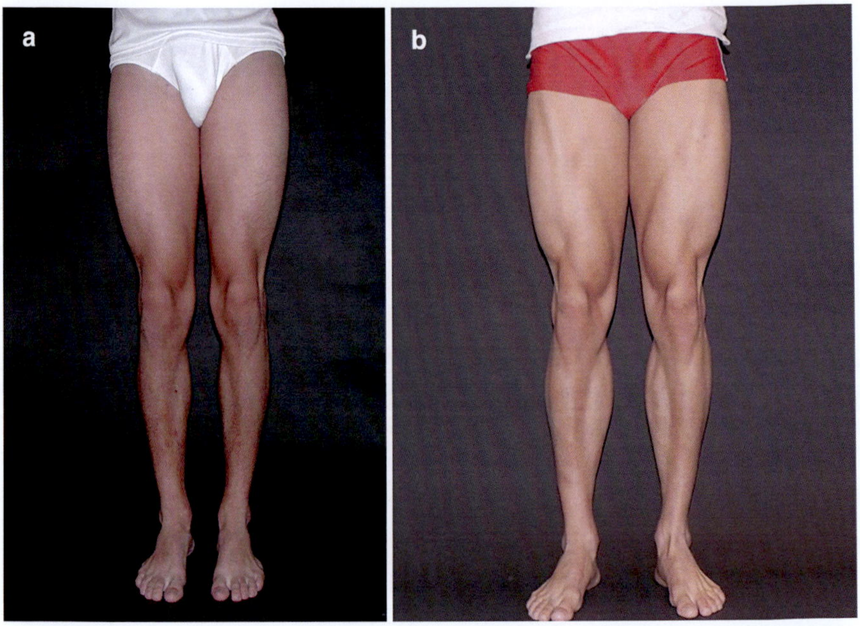

Fig. 56.3 Muscular hypotrophy of the legs, refractory to physical exercises. (**a**) Preoperative appearance. (**b**) Five years after placing 290 mL implants, only on the medial side of the legs. The thighs were hypertrophied thanks to weight training

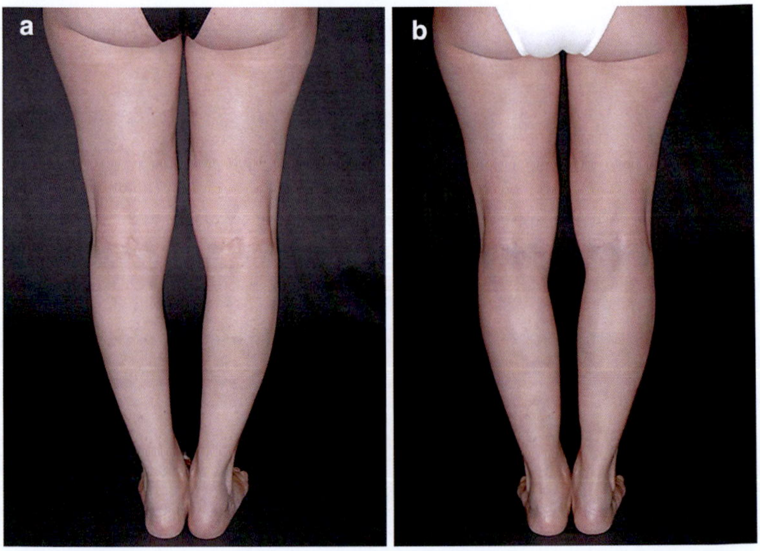

Fig. 56.4 Arched legs. (**a**) Preoperative appearance. (**b**) One year after inclusion of 180 mL Montellano-type prostheses (Montellano 1991) in the medial aspect of the legs

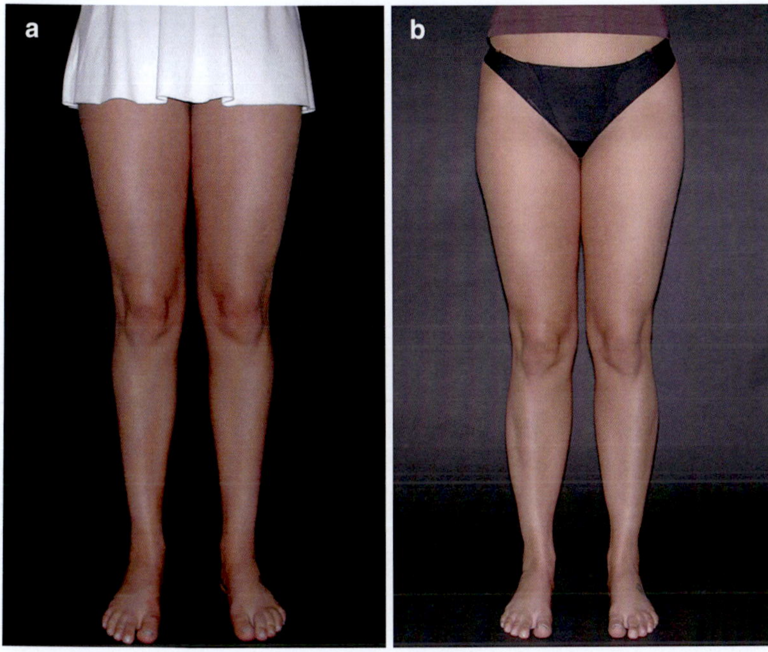

Fig. 56.5 Thin legs due to hypo development of both gastrocnemius muscles, medial and lateral. (**a**) Preoperative appearance. (**b**) Seventeen months after implantation of Glitzenstein-type prostheses, 140 mL on the medial side and 120 mL on the lateral side of the legs

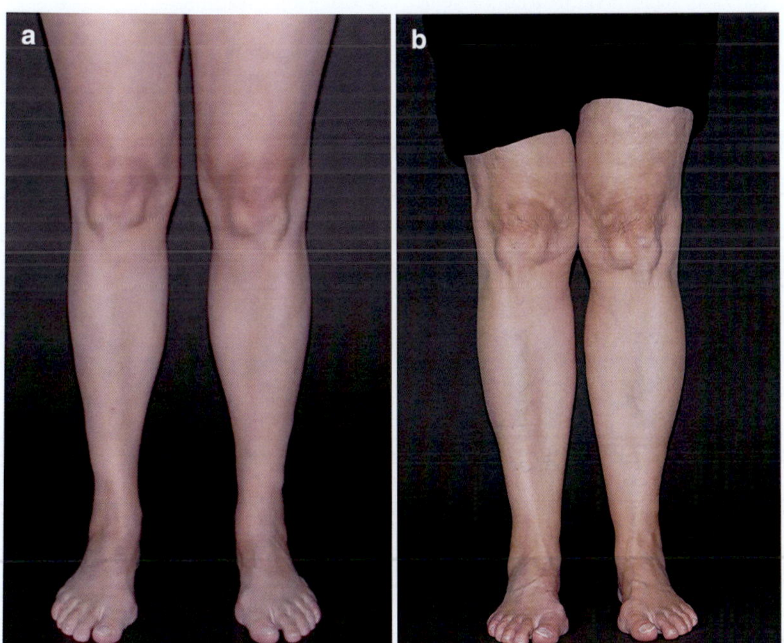

Fig. 56.6 Implants treating only the lower third of the leg. (**a**) Preoperative appearance. (**b**) Postoperative with 12 years of evolution

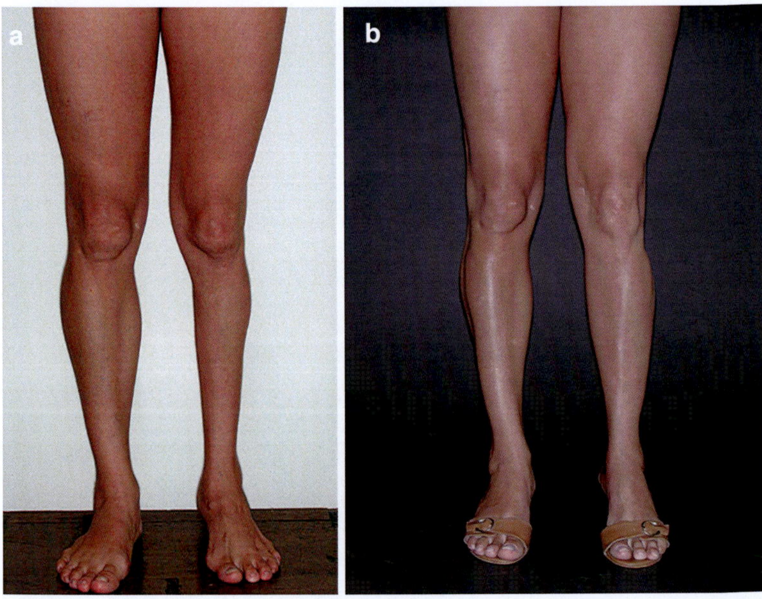

Fig. 56.7 Patient with polio sequelae in left inferior limb. (**a**) Preoperative appearance. (**b**) Two years after placing a 180 mL implant on the medial side of the thigh, 140 mL on the medial side of the leg, and 120 mL on the lateral side of the leg

Finally, in atrophies produced by congenital pathologies (e.g., clubfoot) or acquired (polio, other neurological syndromes, various trauma on the lower limb), it is necessary to place as many implants as needed, in the appropriate places, to approach the silhouette of the contralateral leg (Fig. 56.7).

Surgical Technique

Surgery is performed in prone position, under epidural block or general anesthesia.

Asepsis of the entire lower limb is important, using brushing with surgical soap (for 5 min) and pure alcohol at the end, in the same way that we perform asepsis of our hands before any procedure.

The site is approached through a skin incision, from 3 to 4 cm, coinciding with the popliteal groove, in the median and posterior portion of the knee.

This first incision goes through the skin and subcutaneous cell tissue, until the fascia is visualized.

If, during the incision, we see a larger caliber vein (saphenous vein branch), it should be gently detached, and then lay aside, instead of simply sectioned.

The incision on the fascia is previously dyed (3–4 cm, parallel to the skin incision) with methylene blue or bright green, to better identify its edges at the time of closure.

The careful suturing of the fascia, performed with the semi-flexed leg (approx. 30 °) to relieve tension, is essential for a less painful postoperative and a natural aspect of the entire suture.

Once the fascia is sectioned, a variable amount of fatty tissue is visualized, which must be divulsed with scissors, until the clear and clean visualization of the gastrocnemius muscle mass.

This incision can be used for both the medial and lateral placement of the implants.

After visualizing the muscle, we begin the detachment, now digital, of the subfascial space, toward the medial or the lateral portion of the leg, according to our purpose.

(Obs.: In the lateral detachment, avoid the fibular head, where the fibular N. passes.)

Detachment must be quite easy; this is an indication that you are in the right plane. Turning the digital pulp upward, one can feel it is under an inelastic screen, with a slightly striated internal surface, which does not offer any resistance to detachment. This detachment progresses distally, as far as the finger reaches. From there, it is continued with a wire cannula mandrel (for its delicacy) up to the pre-established limits,

marked in the patient's room, in a standing position.

These first detachments, atraumatic, determine the placement plan, always subfascial. Then, these tunnels become confluent by using malleable retractors 30 × 3 cm, 40 × 3 cm, and even 50 × 3 cm.

Once the cavity has been created, which should comfortably accommodate the implant, the introduction is made directly, if the implant is made entirely of silicone elastomer, or with the help of the same wire cannula mandrel, if it is gelatinous (gelatinous implants have a small pouch at the lower end, which supports the rod that will push it into the cavity).

Check the contour obtained, to evaluate if we have achieved what we wanted.

If constrictions appear along the leg, the detachment in these regions should be conducted once again, expanding the cavity laterally. This can be done with the implant already placed or, preferably, after its temporary removal, a simple procedure to be performed which guarantees the integrity of the implant, if gelatinous. The tissue planes are sutured, initially from the fascia, with absorbable thread (Vicryl 3.0), four separate stitches, flexing the leg 30 ° to bring the edges together. Then, three or four separate stitches (Vicryl 4.0) were conducted on the subcutaneous cellular tissue, and finally few intradermal separate stitches (Vicryl 5.0) to perfectly approximate the epidermis.

The entire suture is stabilized by covering it with Micropore tape directly on the skin. In this way, the obtained scar will become inconspicuous in a few months.

Postoperative Care

A soft compression elastic pantyhose will be used immediately or at hospital discharge.

The patient is encouraged to walk, without assistance, taking care not to overextend the knee, in order to protect the fascia suture.

The use of a heel, not too high, provides more comfort in the initial walking. In the absence of this, a discreet elevation can be created under the heel, with folded socks inside the shoe.

We do not use heparin post-operatively.

The patient is discharged the next day, prescribed with painkillers, anti-inflammatories, and extra antibiotic coverage of Cefadroxil 500 mg 12/12 h, for another 4 days.

Complications

This surgery has, in our experience, an exceptionally low morbidity rate. The adverse results have to do with the inadequate planning of the procedure, generating unpleasant and/or artificial-looking silhouettes, which requires surgical revision. We were able to bring these adverse results down to almost zero as we progressed on our learning curve.

Common complications inherent to surgical procedures, such as hematomas, seromas, infections, and dehiscence, are rare, not to say non-existent. Capsular contractures were also never found.

Compartmental syndrome, the greatest fear of the novice surgeon in the technique, has no reason to occur if the undermining plan – sub-fascial – is respected.

Discussion

Fat grafts, applied in a more superficial plane to that of the implant (suprafascial, in the subcutaneous tissue) can be particularly useful for finishing the contour, always in small quantities and at selected points. In my experience, the fat graft does not satisfactorily replace the silicone implant (for promoting irregularities in the skin), but it works very well in attenuating the edges of the implant, when the subcutaneous tissue is very scarce, or to increase areas where the implant cannot reach, such as the lateral side of the knees or surrounding the malleoli.

Patients with genu valgum, with a normal contour of the legs, except for the divergence of the longitudinal axes, do not benefit much from silicone implants, although they often ask for it.

The difficulty in achieving satisfactory results only with the traditional way of placement (over medial side of the leg) when hypotrophy is bilateral has led us to develop a new location for the implant, on the lateral side of the leg. The indication is clear when a rectification of the lateral contour of the leg is observed, from below the fibular head to the malleolus. This contour is, however, very responsive to volume increases, and thin implants with low projection should be used for its correction, under the risk of going from hypotrophy to hypertrophy, which is unusual in this area.

When aiming to use more than one implant per leg, at the same surgical time, it is necessary to pay attention to the possibility of increasing dangerously the pressure in the muscular compartments. A simple and immediate way to measure the existence or not of pressure's excess is to assess the perfusion and saturation in each operated limb by means of the oximeter. If on a toe the values are identical to those on the hand, everything goes as planned. On the other hand, if a decrease or even absence of perfusion is detected, or saturation is decreased, it is time to remove one or more implants and check it again.

Large atrophies require large volume implants, a proposal that usually cannot be performed in a single surgical procedure. In these cases, we use tissue expanders or, preferably, we schedule the procedures, with the placement of the implant possible, and after obtaining the tissue distention caused by the implant (which occurs after 1 or 2 years), we place other implants, in the missing locations, and may even replace the first with a larger one.

Fasciotomies, used at first to gain space for the placement of implants, do not have a good evolution in the long run.

It is worth remembering that the use of elastic stockings, recommended for providing greater comfort, as well as prevention of venous thrombosis (combined with early ambulation), must be of mild or medium compression. The high compression, at the level of the ankles, will favor the rise of the implant, requiring later external maneuvers to return to its original position. If necessary, a circular bandage on the knee, from the second or third day of ambulation, helps to keep the implants in place.

References

Glitzenstein J (1979) Correction of the amyotrophies of the limbs with silicone prosthesis inclusions. Rev Bras Cir; 69:117

Carlsen LN (1979) Calf augmentation – A preliminary report. Ann Plast Surg; 2:508

Menichelli Netto N (1999) Correction of limb deformities with silicone prosthesis. Aesth Plast Surg; 23:134

Montellano L (1991) Calf augmentation. Ann Plast Surg 27: 429

Chapter 57
Thigh Implant: Its Importance to Achieve Harmony of Lower Extremities

Nicola Menichelli

Abstract Silicone implants to increase the thighs started to be used more frequently after the good results obtained with the calf implants.

At first, they were placed with the patient in prone position (the same position for the calf implant) to correct deformities on the medial surface of the thighs, which were the most frequent complaints.

With the emergence of new cases, requiring corrections in other points of the thigh (even exclusively in the thighs), new sites and new implants for these corrections were developed.

We describe here the indications and surgical techniques for the introduction of implants in the antero and posteromedial sides of the thighs, lateral face, posterior face, and intermediary placements, in order to contemplate the patients' desire for more harmonious legs.

Interventions have low morbidity. Details of the surgical technique that can facilitate the procedure are discussed.

Examples of harmony between segments are given.

Keywords Thigh · Arching thighs · Silicone prosthesis · Limb increase · Lower extremity augmentation · Thin legs · HIV seroma · Body contour · Multiple implants · CT · Computerized tomography

The surgery to increase the volume of the thighs with silicone implants is contemporary with its similar one, which increases the volume of the calves. Its indication, however, was timid, being used mainly to correct amyotrophies (Glitzenstein 1979). The implants were the same ones used for the calf. At first, they were introduced in the areas of the thighs where there was markedly lack of volume due to congenital or acquired pathologies (Fig. 57.1) or to mutilating traumas (Fig. 57.2).

N. Menichelli (✉)
São Paulo, Brazil

J. M. Avelar, R. Cavalcanti Ribeiro (eds.), *Body Contouring*,
https://doi.org/10.1007/978-3-031-42802-9_57

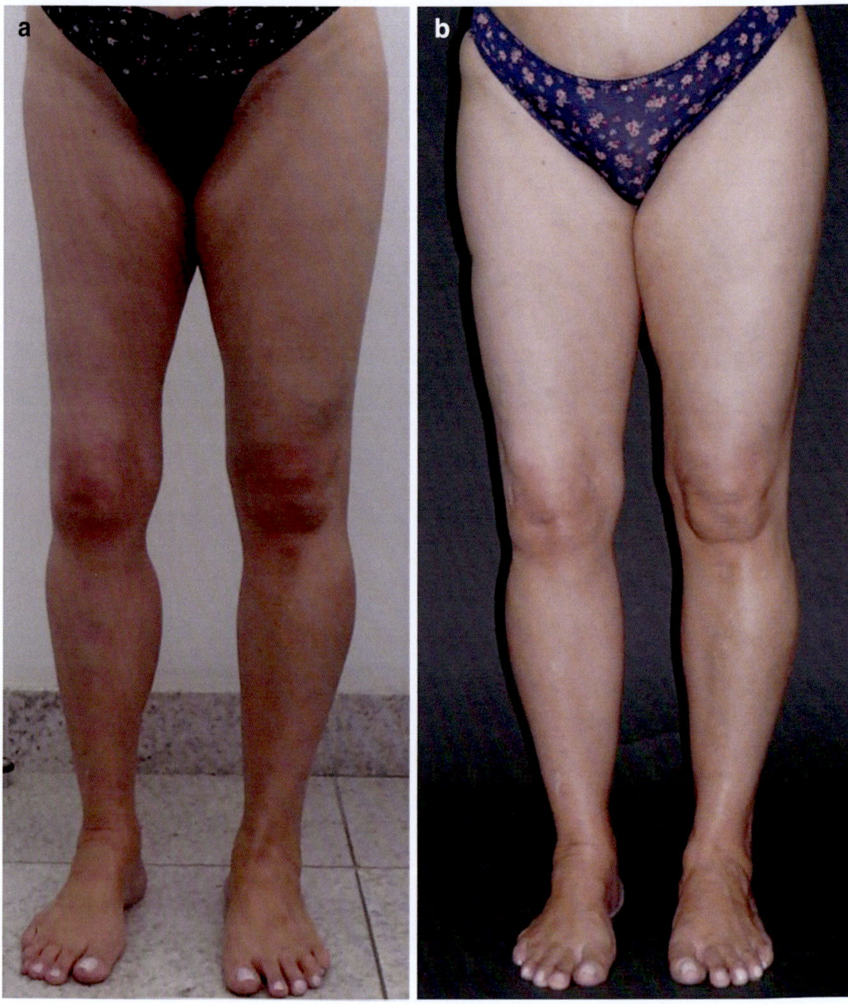

Fig. 57.1 A 51-year-old patient with poliomyelitis in the entire right lower limb. Correction with prostheses had already been attempted, without success. (**a**) Preoperative appearance. (**b**) Two years after the inclusion of new implants in the right thigh, namely, 375 mL on the lateral face and 180 mL on the medial face (the calf implant was also changed to improve symmetry between the calves)

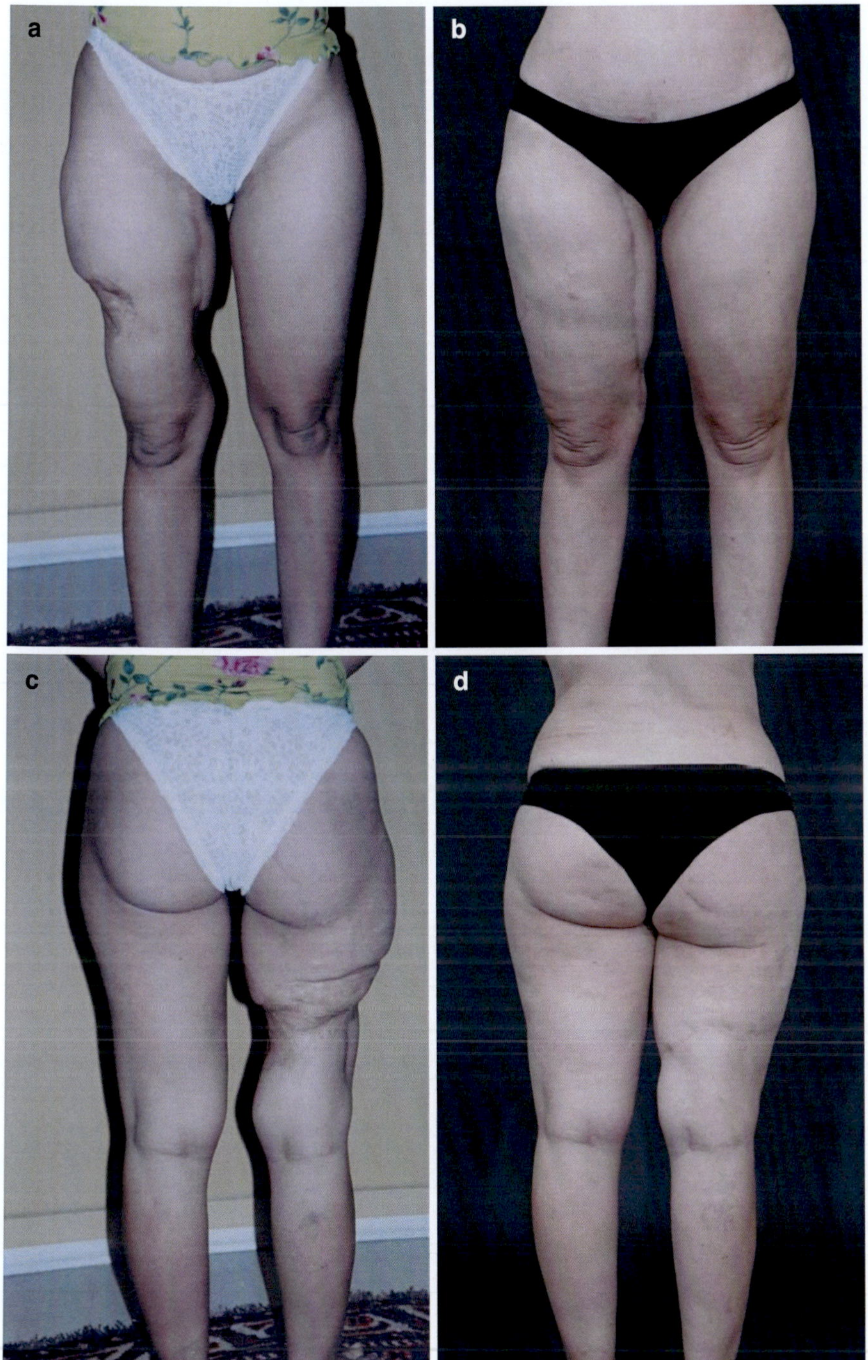

Fig. 57.2 (**a**, **c**) Patient victim of being run over, 10 years after emergency care to save her life, and covering raw areas of muscle and skin loss with skin grafts. (**b**, **d**) 17 years after treatments with tissue expanders, flap rotation, and placement of silicone implants in the lower third of the right thigh

Technique Evolution

With the refinement of calf surgery with implants, more patients began to desire the correction of the thighs' contour, now seeking pure aesthetic improvements.

Implants started to be used in the posteromedial aspect of the thighs to correct an arching in this location.

Montellano (1991) frequently presented, combined with calf implants, procedures on the medial surface of the thighs, in the prone position, with an approach through a small incision coincident with the sub-gluteal sulcus, close to the perineum. Anger (2005) demonstrated, through anatomical dissections, the location of these implantations – submuscular – between the gracilis and adductor magnus muscles.

We also used to use the prone position for these procedures (Fig. 57.3), but with the emergence of patients who clearly needed volume in the anteromedial area of the thigh, we developed, after dissections in a cadaver, a better location for these

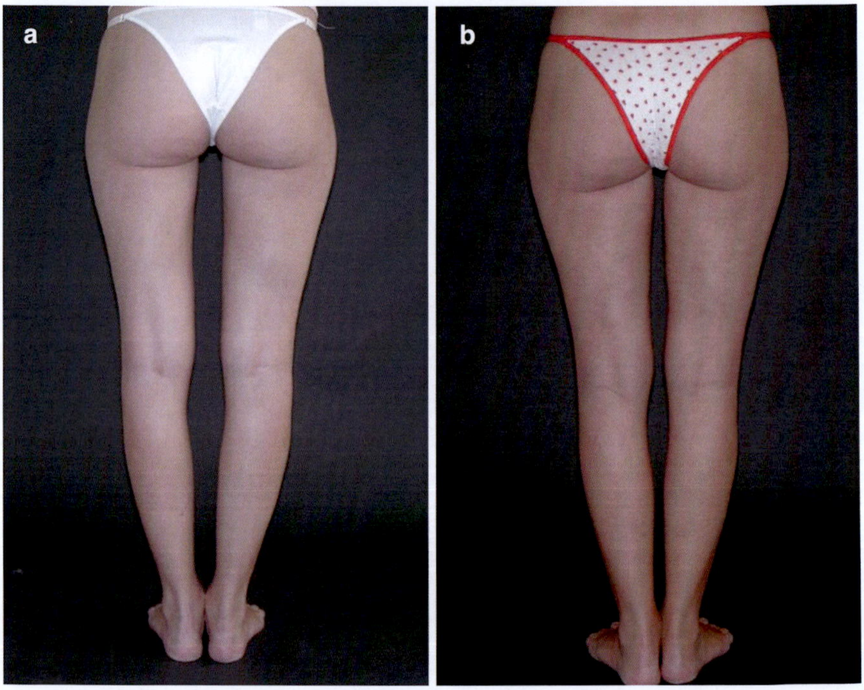

Fig. 57.3 Patient complaining of exaggerated distance between the thighs. (**a**) Preoperative appearance. (**b**) Two years after placement of large (330 ml) custom-made implants on the medial aspect of the thighs. The purpose of the surgery was to bring the thighs close together. There was no arching between them

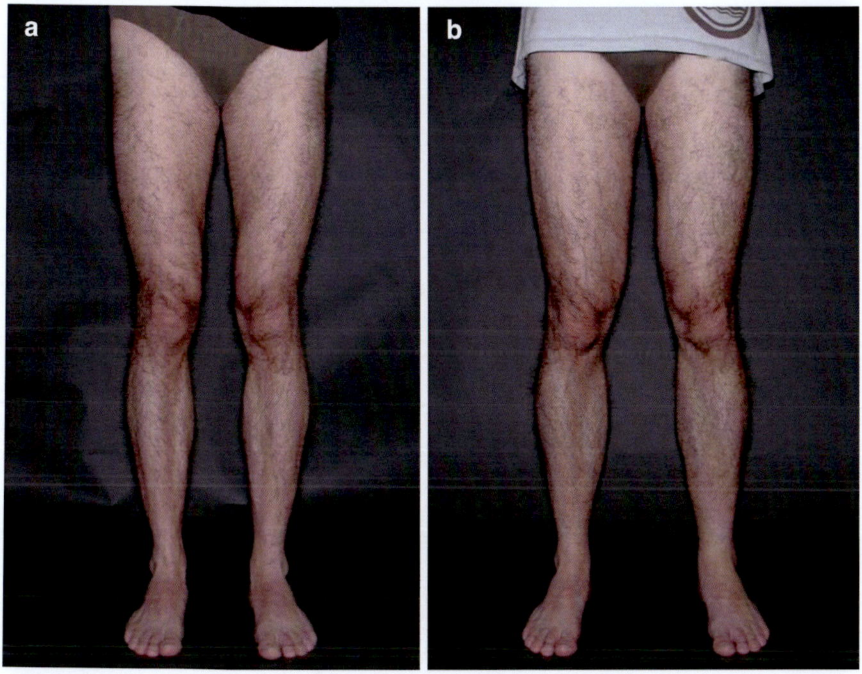

Fig. 57.4 Patient with severe muscle atrophy in the adductor area, probably resulting from antiretroviral treatment. (**a**) Preoperative appearance. (**b**) Six months after inclusion of a 290 ml silicone implant in the anteromedial aspect of the thighs

cases. It is coincident with Scarpa's triangle and the incision being now in the inguinal crease, with the patient in the supine position (Fig. 57.4).

Challenged by new cases, we developed different locations for implantation, namely, the lateral aspect of the thighs, the posterior aspect, and intermediate locations between all previously mentioned. We have also developed new, larger implants with different textures to meet the growing demand from patients for bolder results (Menichelli Netto 2011).

New Indications and their Surgical Techniques

We will describe the multiple locations where implants can be placed, with their entry ports and placement plans. The basic condition inherent in all of them is that they must always lay deeply, covered at least by the fascia, in the manner of the calf. In the thigh, there are a variety of possibilities due to the greater complexity of the muscle's compartments.

Medial and Anterior Face of the Thigh

The arching of the medial surface of the thighs, which causes an unsightly separation between them, was the most frequent complaint. This configuration seems to be due to an unsatisfactory balance (in aesthetic terms only), between the adductor muscles and the sartorius, causing this arching.

In this place is the so-called Scarpa triangle, formed by the gracilis, the sartorius, and the inguinal ligament. The floor of this triangle is given by the pectineus and adductor longus muscles. Through the gutter thus formed, the femoral vessels and nerves descend. In this delicate location, we placed our implant, through a small incision (3–4 cm) coinciding with one of the skin folds that occur parallel to the inguinal ligament, approximately in the median portion of the groin. This incision should not be located too medial (approaching the perineum), in order to obtain an adequate entry axis for the implant, which will progress obliquely from the median portion of the groin to the medial aspect of the thigh, in its inferior third (Fig. 57.5).

The incision reaches the skin and subcutaneous cellular tissue, then the superficial fascia, and after the other muscle fascia. At this point, detachment can be done with scissors or scalpel, depending on the fragility of the tissues. It is important to

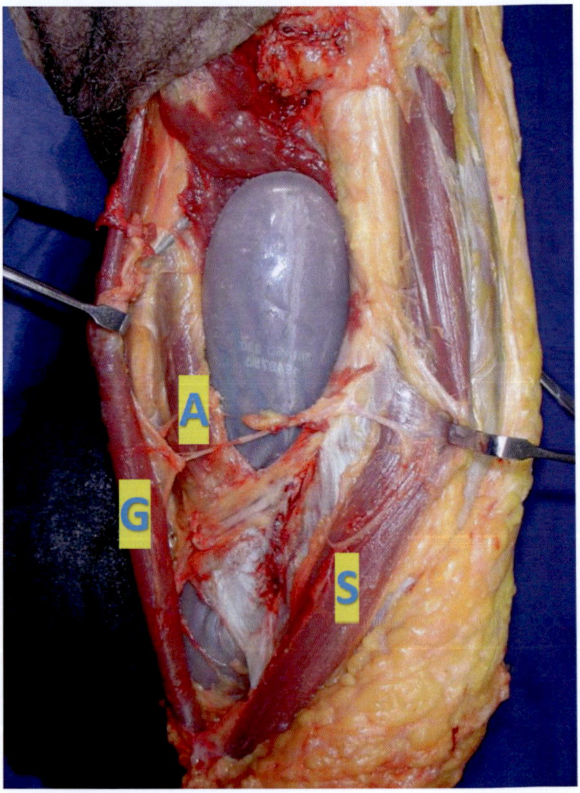

Fig. 57.5 Anatomical dissection showing an implant placed in the left thigh, following Hunter's canal. The retractors separate the gracilis (G) and the sartorius (S), while the adductor magnus (A) embraces the distal third of the implant

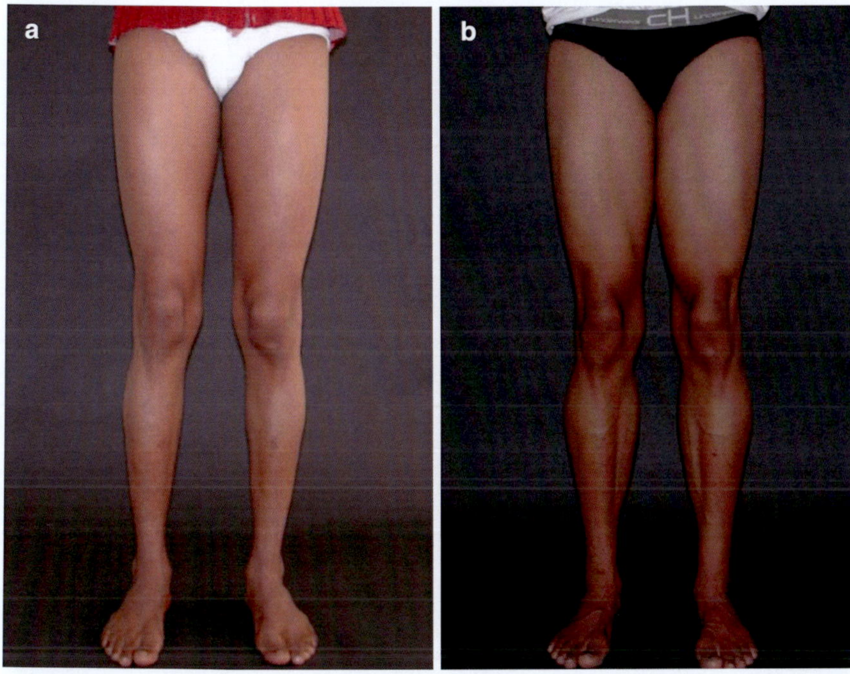

Fig. 57.6 Patient complaining of underdeveloped thighs. (**a**) Preoperative appearance. (**b**) 18 months after placement of large implants (290 mL) in the anteromedial aspect of the thighs (implants also in the calves)

visualize, at the end, the muscular bellies. Any interposed fascia must be previously dyed before being sectioned, in order to allow its repair when the cavity is closed. Detachment starts with the finger and proceeds with malleable retractors.

This results in a pocket, coincident with the lack of volume that evoked the surgery, which can now be corrected with the inclusion of the implant (Fig. 57.6).

Lateral Face of the Thigh

The lateral aspect of the thigh usually does not present deformities that require correction with prostheses. A wider hip can, however, give the impression that there is a narrowing below it. This aspect, or the fact that the musculature is not satisfactorily developed in this location, has encouraged patients to request correction for this area.

A positive fact is that there are no anatomical elements susceptible to trauma in this location, as in Hunter's canal, thus facilitating the procedure (Fig. 57.7).

The contour of the lateral aspect of the thigh is basically due to the vastus lateralis muscle. This muscle is crossed from top to bottom by the tensor fasciae latae

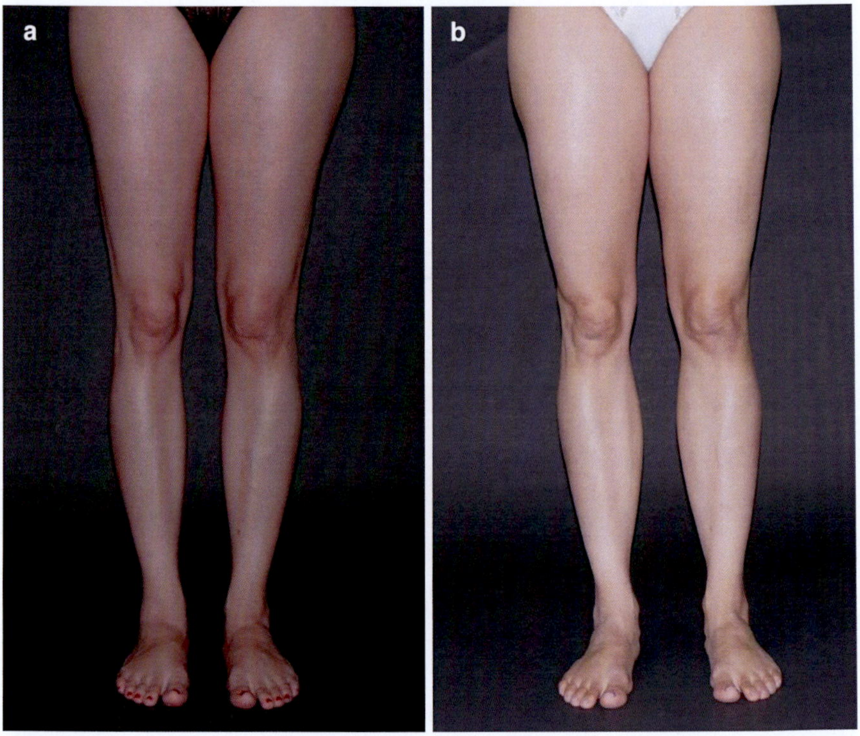

Fig. 57.7 Patient does not like the conical shape of her thighs. (**a**) Preoperative appearance. (**b**) Two years after placement of large implants (290 mL) on the lateral aspect of the thighs, improving the contour (implants also in the calves)

muscle, which offers little volume, as it is just fibrous to a good extent, but plays an important role in stabilizing the knee.

In this area, we find an excellent place for the insertion of an implant, even if it is of great size and volume, since there is a very wide virtual space between both muscles, without any objection to placement, and with excellent coverage provided by the Iliotibial tract.

The access to this compartment is through an incision in the lateral aspect of the thigh (Fig. 57.8).

Although this site is more exposed, this visibility can be bypassed with a neat skin suture.

The incision, measuring 4 cm, is made horizontally in the middle portion of the thigh, on its lateral surface. The attempt to reduce the exposure of the scar, placing it upper, where it could be covered by short garments, results in a more difficult access to the deep planes, due to the subcutaneous fat, which is abundant in this location.

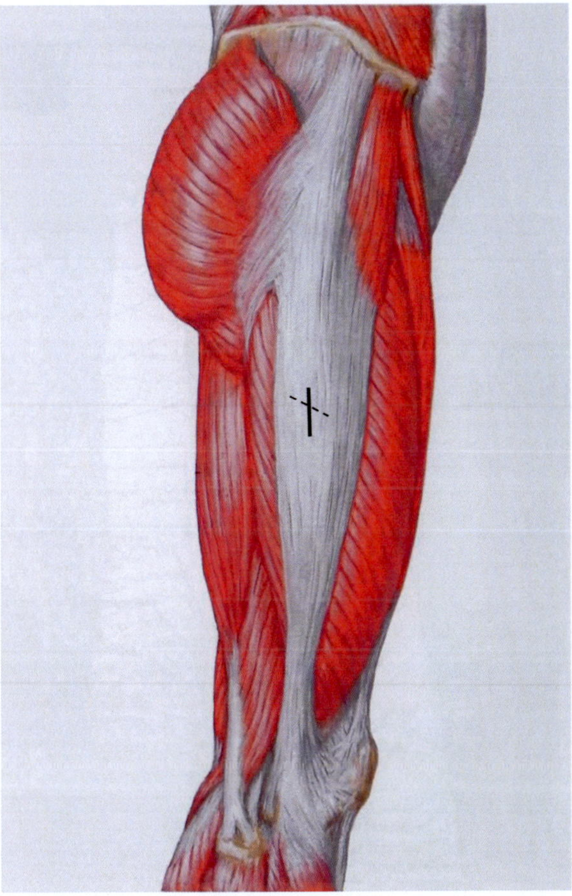

Fig. 57.8 Lateral aspect of the thigh (In Netter, Atlas of human anatomy, fifth ed., Netter 2011). In the foreground, tensor fasciae latae muscle with its aponeurotic thickening (Iliotibial tract) that goes to the knee. Underneath it, the vastus lateralis muscle. In between them, the implant will be placed. The skin incision is represented by the dashed line, and the aponeurosis incision by the solid, vertical line

Once the skin and subcutaneous fat are cut, the fascia lata is visualized. Then it is marked with ink in a vertical way, transversely to the skin incision, and incised around 4 cm. After that, the muscle bundles of the Vastus lateralis m. are seen.

Nothing joins one to another: vastus lateralis and tensor fasciae latae muscles. The detachment must, therefore, be very judicious, so as not to enlarge too much the cavity, favoring the free transit of the implant that could, in some way, hinder its desirable position.

The implant is introduced freely, first into one half of the pocket and then into the other, after gentle pressure.

Carefully suture the fascia lata, then the subcutaneous tissue, and finally the skin, always with absorbable suture, done with separated stitches.

Posterior Face of the Thigh

The purpose of the placement in this location is always a volumetric increase, in order to balance (in lateral view) the thigh contour with the buttock projection, or the symmetry between the two thighs, when they are different.

The implant will fit naturally in between the posterior muscles of the region (semitendinosus, semimembranosus, and biceps femoris long head muscles). The approach is made through an incision in the sub-gluteal sulcus, at any point of its extension (Fig. 57.9).

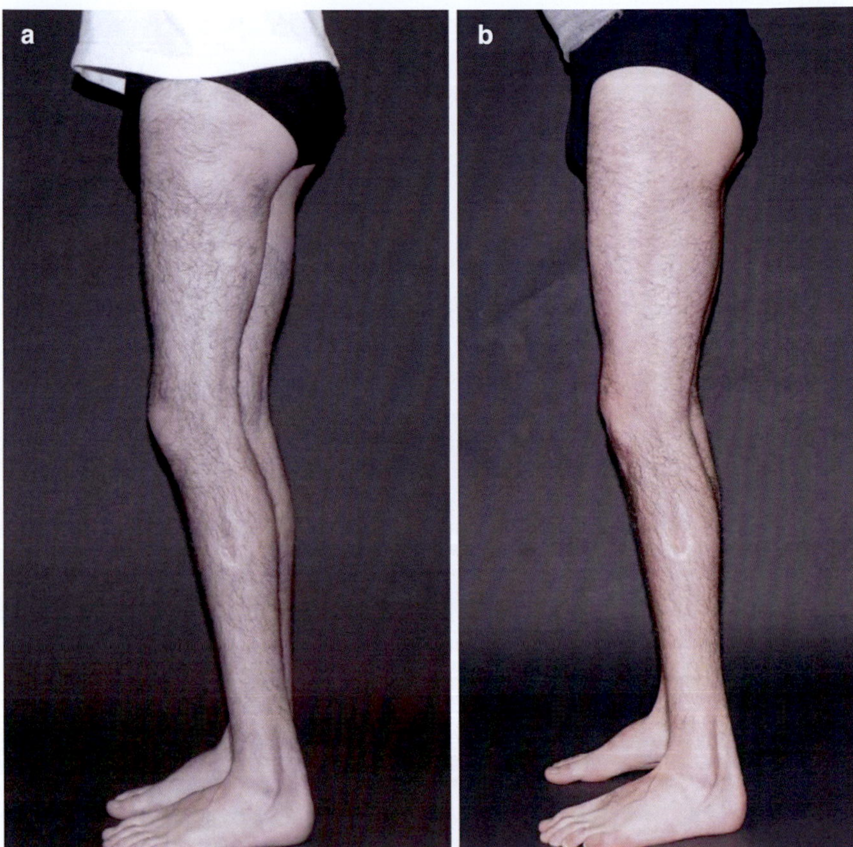

Fig. 57.9 (**a**) Patient with poliomyelitis sequelae in the left lower limb. (**b**) Six years after the operation, after placing an implant on the posterior surface of the thigh (in addition to others in different positions). The right leg is no longer visualized when looking from the left side

Intermediary Placements

If necessary, more implants can be placed, alongside the previously existing ones, without prejudice to function and to the benefit of shape, respecting the same planes, and avoiding the confluence of the cavities (Fig. 57.10).

In this way we can obtain the so desired symmetry between the limbs (Fig. 57.11).

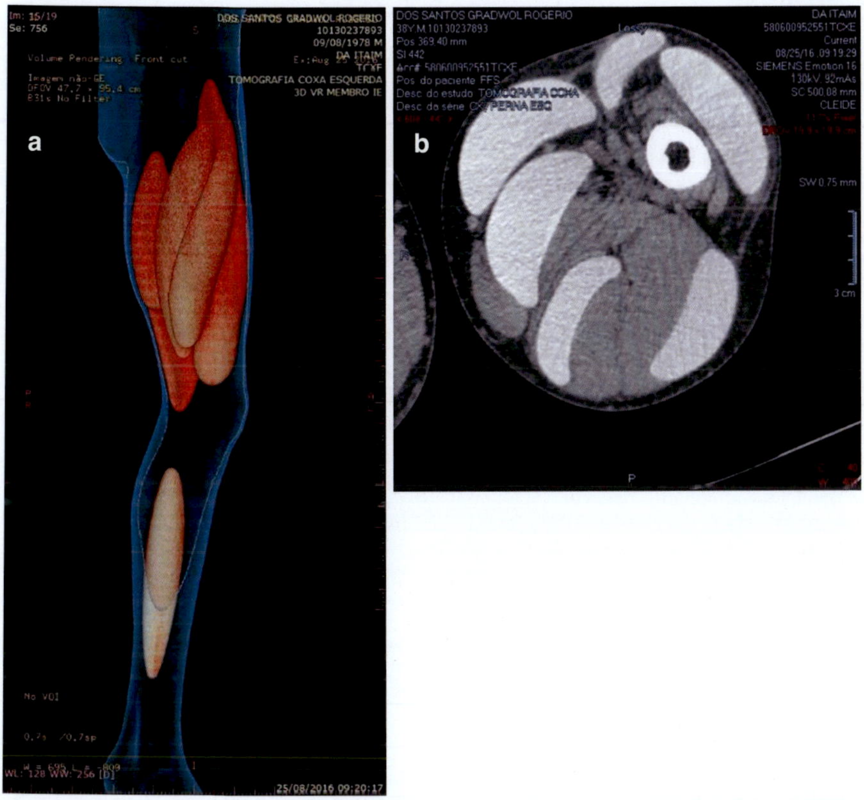

Fig. 57.10 (**a**) Three-dimensional tomography image reconstruction and (**b**) its cross-section on the thigh, showing the implants' proper distribution

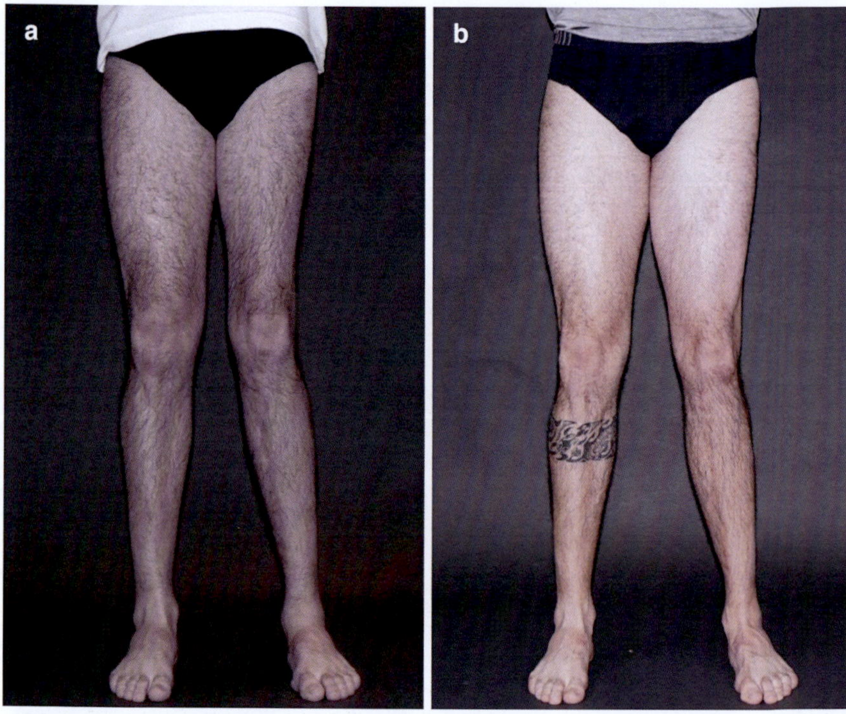

Fig. 57.11 Patient with poliomyelitis sequelae in the left lower limb. (**a**) Preoperative appearance. (**b**) Eight years after four surgical interventions to place six implants in the left thigh, with intervals of approximately 2 years between them (the CT of this patient is shown in Fig. 57.10)

Complications

Hematomas have already happened in our initial cases, but they did not happen again, since there are no tissue lacerations on fascia or muscles beyond the surgical wound, thus avoiding any vascular injury.

Seromas occurred in few patients (<0.1%). Despite the profusion of operated areas (silicone prostheses in both calves, thighs, and biceps), he developed a seroma only in the left thigh. In this same place, tumoral and inflamed lesions appeared on the skin, with rapid growth. The patient was HIV+ with no viral load, being treated with antiretroviral drugs. We chose to remove the implant, simultaneously with the resection of the skin tumors.

Neuropathic pain. More frequent than the previous ones, these episodes of stabbing pain in the knee appear in the immediate postoperative period or after 2–4 days. They affected approximately 2% of the operated thighs.

The pain manifests itself in the territory of the accessory saphenous nerve, when the patient assumes the orthostatic position, and is most likely due to a traumatic injury to this nerve branch at the time of detachment, which is repeated each time the patient stands up and the implant forces the traumatized site.

In a patient who presented this symptom next day after surgery and was still hospitalized and suffering crisis of very intense pain (sic), we opted for immediate removal of the implants. The symptoms also ceased immediately.

In other cases, where the symptom was unilateral, beginning after the discharge with bearable pain, we treated them conservatively, and the symptoms improved or ceased within a week.

Implant malpositioning. Adverse results arising from the unwanted migration of the implants, with the consequent asymmetries and loss of naturalness, were the most frequent issues in our series.

On the medial aspect of the thighs, the desired position is usually a few centimeters distal to the incision. However, the movement of muscles during the act of walking, and even unsuitable attitudes, such as raising the legs to improve drainage, can cause the newly placed implant to rise. Even if one tries to occlude the tunnel, in order to maintain the implant in its definitive place, muscular sutures cannot be quite strong, and therefore easily breakable. The definitive fixation of the implant only occurs when the organic capsule materializes. Until then, there is a risk of ascending.

In the early postoperative days, it is still possible to reposition the implant through external maneuvers and keep it in place using elastic bands.

Discussion

When placing the implant on the anteromedial surface of the thigh, we find, on several occasions, difficulty in progressing the detachment, at the point where the sartorius muscle is overcome. The malleable retractor blade must gently seek the way, without force, in order to prevent the detachment from becoming superficial, which would compromise the result by making the implant visible at this point (Fig. 57.12), or which would traumatize the adjacent noble structures, such as the femoral vessels and nerves, especially the saphenous nerve.

Once the cavity is created, another difficulty could appear, now when inserting the implant (at the same point where we tentatively prospected the path). A quite simple and efficient way to avoid this difficulty is never to remove the retractor from the obtained cavity. Instead, add one more retractor, juxtaposed to the first, and between them, moving one blade away from the other, place the implant inner as possible. Fixing the implant with the finger (so as not to follow the movement of the retractors), one and then the other blade are pulled out a few centimeters, taking care the distal end does not go beyond the point of difficulty, and back to introduce the set (blades and implant) until the end of the cavity. This maneuver is repeated as many times as necessary for the implant to gradually migrate to its definitive place, without ever losing the path initially acquired (Fig. 57.13).

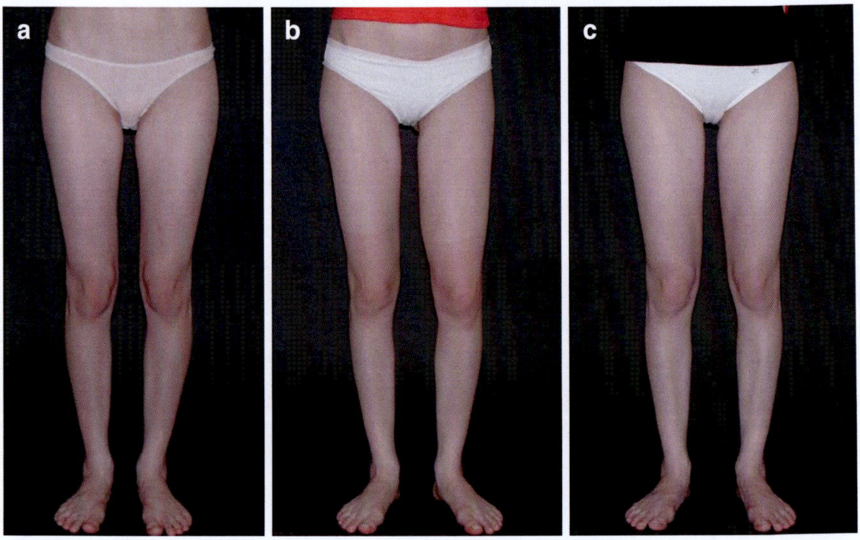

Fig. 57.12 (**a**) Arching of the inner thigh. (**b**) Six months after placement of 180 mL implants in the anteromedial aspect of the thighs. The left implant became superficial at the lower third. (**c**) One year after revision, with removal of the implant from the left thigh, creation of a new space, now deeper in the lower third, and replacement of the same implant in the new cavity

Fig. 57.13 Placement of the implant with the aid of two malleable detachers, juxtaposed, which will guide it into the newly formed cavity

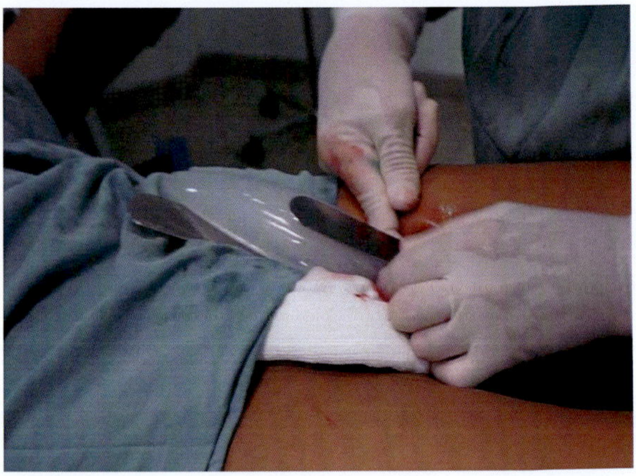

Harmony Between Segments

In some patients it happens that, once operated with calf implants, they also dislike their thighs, either because they are in fact very thin or because this thinness has become more evident, compared to the calves, which are now to their liking. Therefore, they ask for implants in the thighs as well, and then they finally become satisfied with the contour of their lower limbs (Fig. 57.14).

Liposuction of the thigh, when indicated, helps in harmonizing the limb, regardless of the placement of implants (Fig. 57.15).

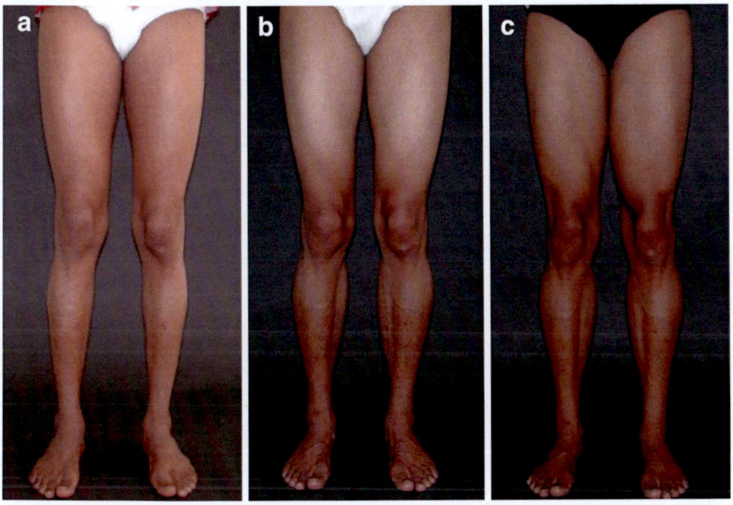

Fig. 57.14 Patient who requested calf augmentation and then thigh augmentation. (**a**) Preoperative appearance. (**b**) Two years after placement of 180 mL implants in the posteromedial aspect of the calves. Note that from then on, the patient does not expose their thighs to the sun. (**c**) Eighteen months after placement of 290 mL implants in the anteromedial aspect of the thighs. Now sun exposure is integral

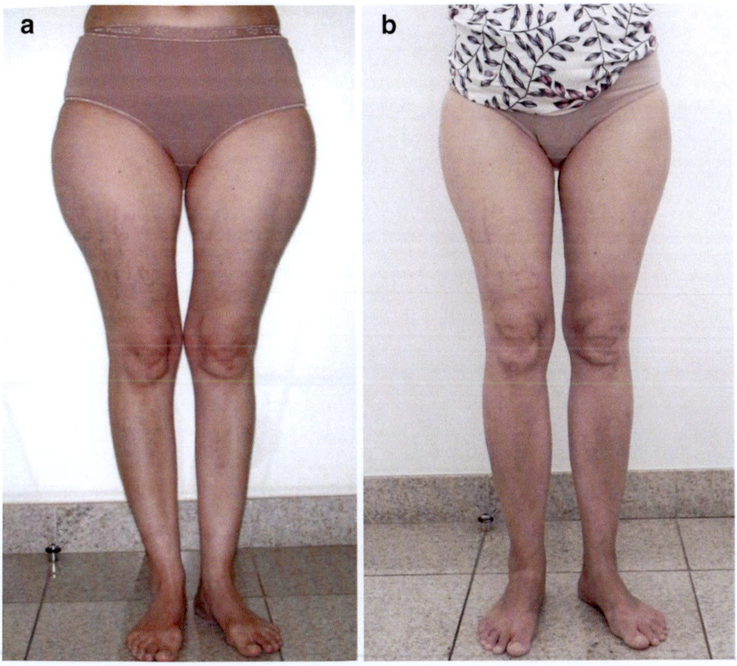

Fig. 57.15 (**a**) Patient with less graceful silhouette of the lower limbs, notably due to the exaggerated deposition of supratrochanteric fat, arching of the medial surface of the thighs, and flattening of the medial contour of the calves. (**b**) Seven years after liposuction of the outer thighs, placement of large implants (290 mL) in the anteromedial aspect of the thighs, and moderate and long implants (140 mL, 26 cm long) in the posteromedial aspect of the calves

References

Glitzenstein J (1979) Correction of the amyotrophies of the limbs with silicone prosthesis inclusions. Rev Bras Cir; 69:117

Montellano L (1991) Calf augmentation. Ann Plast Surg; 27: 429

Anger J (2005) Thigh augmentation: submuscular placement of a silicone gel-filled prosthesis. Aesthet Surg J; 25: 44

Menichelli Netto N (2011) Aumento das coxas com implantes de silicone. Rev Bras Cir Plast; 26: 306

Netter, F.H (2011) Atlas of human anatomy 5th ed

Chapter 58
Body Implants

Ivan Abadesso, Ricardo Cavalcanti Ribeiro, Marcos D. Pumarol N, Emir Duquela S, and Luis Fernandez de Córdova

Abstract
Background

Plastic surgeons have long dealt with congenital anomalies that produce degeneration of the muscle and leave asymmetry between two members of the body. The implants have been used in these cases to help maintain the shape of the muscle and achieve greater symmetry between affected and unaffected sides. Body beauty highlights the importance of well-defined muscles. But sometimes this musculature does not develop as it would have been thought and desired. Patients with aesthetic reasons seek bilateral placement of implants.

Objectives

The purpose of this chapter was to provide information about the muscular implants, the different types of prothesis, the complications, surgical planning, and aesthetic outcomes.

Patient Selection

The ideal patients for this procedure are those older than 18 years of age, without health comorbidities, who want to increase the volume of the muscles and who is not contraindicated the use of prosthesis. It is also indicated for patients who have suffered a malformation or accident in a member of the body and have not developed the muscle (unilateral or bilateral).

I. Abadesso · M. D. Pumarol N · E. Duquela S
Plastic and Reconstructive Surgery, Casa de Portugal, Rio de Janeiro, Brazil

R. Cavalcanti Ribeiro (✉) · L. F. de Córdova
Plastic and Reconstructive Surgery, Casa de Portugal, Rio de Janeiro, Brazil

Plastic and Reconstructive Surgery, Federal University of the State of Rio de Janeiro, Rio de Janeiro, Brazil
e-mail: rribeiro@centroin.net.br

J. M. Avelar, R. Cavalcanti Ribeiro (eds.), *Body Contouring*,
https://doi.org/10.1007/978-3-031-42802-9_58

Conclusions
Body implant surgery is a relatively straightforward procedure that affords great results. They can correct asymmetry and deformity, and it also gives great aesthetic results, increasing the patient's self-esteem. Prudent dissection of the pocket for the implant is essential for optimal cosmesis and to prevent implant malposition and complications.

Keywords Body implants · Body contour surgery · Silicone implants

Introduction

Changing the body contour with implants is nothing new. After breast surgeries, it was a natural process to expand them to other areas of the body such as gluteus, calves, thighs, etc. to the present day, with deltoid and trapezoid implants.

In this chapter, all body implants performed today will be addressed, except for breasts and buttocks, which have chapters apart. Some of these surgeries are already widely known and others are not. Therefore, it is necessary to know a little of the evolution to get to what we have today.

Most of these surgeries started with the corrective purpose of congenital and acquired deformities. Aesthetic use came after the successes achieved. It was so with calves and pectorals, for example. And of the body implants to be addressed here, the oldest and perhaps, therefore, the most accomplished by plastic surgeons, is that of calf, with a history of more than 50 years. There were several models of implants used, different placement plans, until reaching what is most often used today.

The history of pectoral implants here in Brazil began in 2000, with the placement of the first case in Latin America by Dr. Ivan Abadesso, in Rio de Janeiro. After the diffusion of this surgery, some people who could not develop muscle in the brachial region showed a willingness to increase the volume of this region. After much study and planning, in 2006, the first biceps and trapezoid implant surgery were performed also by Dr. Ivan Abadesso. Silicone gel implants called "baby calf," small 30 cc implants for the calf, were used. However, the increase was very small and unsatisfactory. The idea then arose of using "baby calf" elastomer, which had the same size, but with 100 cc of elastomer. To achieve the desired volume, it was necessary to combine the two types of baby calf implants, as in a sandwich. In this way the result was very good, and the patient felt satisfied. Less than a year later, the first female patient underwent surgery to correct triceps sagging, not for the purpose of volume increase and the result was equally excellent.

Ten years and several surgeries later, the contour curving blocks replaced the baby calf. There are several advantages in using them, such as the use of only one implant, instead of two joined, the appropriate hardness for the musculature, and the main: the possibility of shaping, sculpting the implant according to the needs of each patient. And the use of elastomer implants proved so rewarding that it eventually extended to pectoral, thighs and, in some patients, calves.

This type of implant was also very important in the correction of malformation, such as in the Poland syndrome, by Sprengel, and in pectus excavatum, because the possibility of shaping them as needed, both before and in the perioperative period, allowed the results to become increasingly natural. Traumas with sequelae affecting the musculature, either due to loss of muscle tissue or nerve lesions that lead to muscle hypotrophy, or even iatrogenic diseases such as hypercorrection of gynecomastia may also benefit from aesthetic correction by implants.

These are surgeries procured by both genders. But it is interesting to realize that most male patients want to have a body with defined and bulky musculature. Female patients, on the other hand, usually prefer a softer contour, maintaining their delicacy, only correcting the sagging, especially of the arms and thighs. In the planning of surgery, it is very important to have this vision, so that the volume used is in accordance with the patient's expectation.

Regardless of the purpose of use, implants should always be placed in a safe and reproducible anatomical dissection plane.

As in any other surgeries, preparation begins with a good preoperative anamnesis. In addition to the data traditionally researched, it is of paramount importance to understand the patient's expectation of body change. If the expectation is higher than the possibility, it is essential that the surgeon makes clear how far can be reached, both in relation to physical abilities and aesthetic harmony.

It is also essential to perform preoperative photographs, the measurement of muscle groups to be treated, the detailed examination of skin quality, the analysis of the degree of sagging existing, and, finally, the palpation of muscle insertions, which will provide us with an idea of the size of the store where the implant will be inserted and, consequently, its size, predicting asymmetries and proportions. The quality of operated skin should also be observed and evaluated. The better the turgor, the better the result.

To give a result as natural as possible, the edges of the implants cannot be palpable, and we must produce the greatest possible symmetry to the region. The key to the success of these surgeries is the proportionality between the appropriate dissection, with the manufacture of an implant suitable for the store, and the size of the muscle and the amount of volume that is to be increased.

The search for the best body contour is a frequent goal in both genders. Whether for correction of asymmetries or deformities, or for muscle volume gain and sagging correction, body implants can meet expectations. They can be used in almost all regions of the body, with great versatility and safety, especially when it comes to silicone elastomer implants, which can be molded as needed, giving individuality to surgery. Body implants are the current response to body symmetrization and increased muscle volume.

Pectoral Implants

History

The first publication on silicone implants in the pectoral region occurred in 1965, by Murray (1965), who used solid silicone implants for the reconstruction of pectus excavatum. Since then, several plastic surgeons have used elastomer implants for chest wall reconstruction. They were initially used for correction of birth defects, especially Poland syndrome and pectus excavatum. Sorensen (1988) described in 1988 the use of implants in the subcutaneous plane also for the correction of pectus excavatum. In 1991, Aiache (1991) and Novack (1991), separately, published their papers on pectoral muscle enlargement with purely aesthetic purpose with the use of implants. In 1997, Hodkingson (1977) reported his 15-year experience using a solid implant to correct several thoracic deformities, evidencing the versatility of his use. On the other hand, Chugay (1999), in 1999, published the cases of 16 patients using solid implants for aesthetic purposes only.

It was in 2002 that the silicone gel implant was described, with Horn's publication (2002). These implants have been specially developed for the pectoral region. In 2003, Ruiz (Benito-Ruiz 2003) described the use of glute implants to increase the pectoral region, using the same technique described by Aiache, with good results.

Anatomy

The pectoral muscles major and minor and the anterior serratus muscles constitute the anterior and lateral walls of the thorax. The fan-shaped pectoralis major has three points of origin: clavicular, sternocostal, and abdominal. It is in the proximal end of the arm, in the intertubercular groove of the humerus. This muscle forms the anterior wall of the chest and the axillary fold, where the surgery of pectoral implants is made. The pectoralis major is the main muscle of this surgery.

The pectoralis minor is a thin triangular muscle in the upper portion of the chest and below the pectoralis major. It originates from the third, fourth, and fifth ribs, near its cartilages and intercostal aponeurosis and is part of the coracoid process of the scapula. Innervation of both pectorals is done by the medial and lateral thoracic nerves. The anterior serratus occupies the side of the thorax and the medial wall of the armpit and innervated by the long thoracic nerve. These two muscles are not related to this surgery.

Indications, Contraindications, and Limitations

The placement of pectoral implants should be performed in men after 18 years, so that hormonal maturation is already completed. It is indicated for correction of congenital anomalies (Poland syndrome and pectus excavatum) and for correction of iatrogenic as hypercorrection of gynecomastia. However, as in other implant placement surgeries, it began to be used for purely aesthetic purposes to increase muscle volume in the region and greater definition.

Patients with body dysmorphic syndrome and patients with unrealistic expectations regarding the results of this surgery are contraindicated, in addition to those with formal contraindications to a surgical procedure.

Consultation/Choice of Implants (Types of Implants)

During the patient's history, in addition to traditional history collection assessments, it is important to investigate traumas in the region, nerve lesions, and formal contraindications to surgical procedures. It should also be asked about the patient's desire and expectation.

During the physical examination, the evaluation of the patient's pectoral musculature dynamically and statically is important to verify the thickness of the pectoral muscles. And it is essential to measure the thoracic circumference and abdominal insertion of the muscle and observe asymmetries. In patients with Poland syndrome, normal side measurements will be used to evaluate the dimensions of the implants to be used. Usually, implants are used on both sides, which facilitates symmetry. In certain cases, it may be necessary to use custom implants. In this case, computed tomography images assist in the development of the implant.

As in all plastic surgery, it is essential to make preoperative photographs. They must comply with the general protocols of imaging, and the patient should be facing diagonally (3/4) on both sides and profile on both sides.

After the physical examination, it is very important that the surgeon makes clarifications about the possible change to be obtained. You should also understand if there was a complete understanding on the part of the patient of our limitations. This understanding of what is possible, aligned with the surgeon's understanding of the patient's expectations, leads to a fully satisfactory result.

Types of Implants

There are specific implants for the thoracic region in the national and international market. In the domestic market, only implants filled with silicone gel are available. In the international market, we have elastomer implants, which can be customized pre- or perioperatively.

Gel Implants

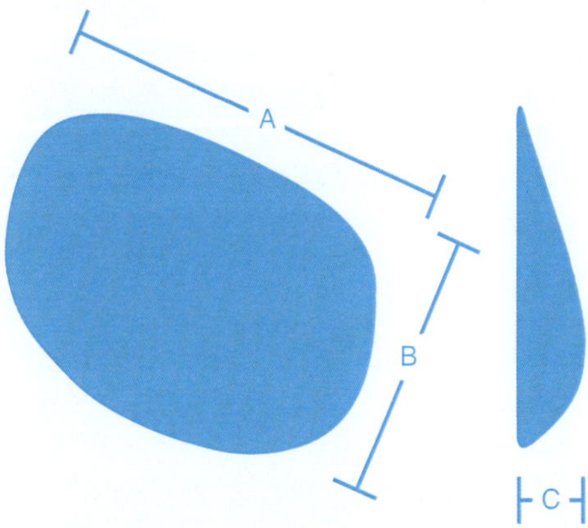

Silicone gel pectoral implant (Silimed)

Elastomer Implants

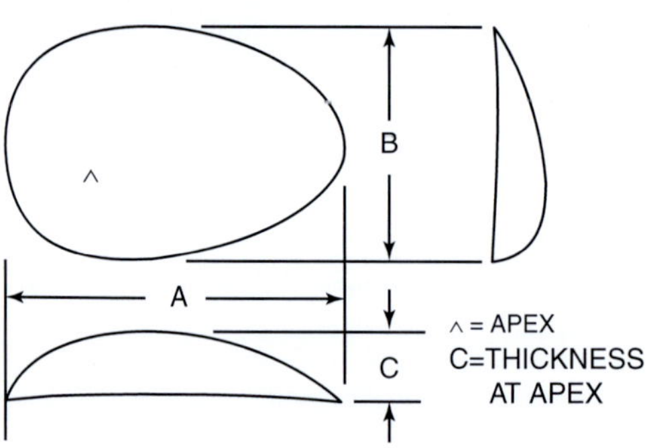

Pectoral PowerFlex (Implantech)

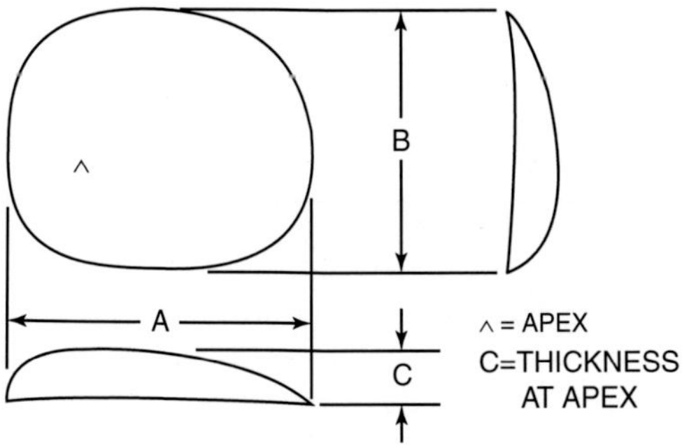

PowerFlex Pectoral II (Implantech)

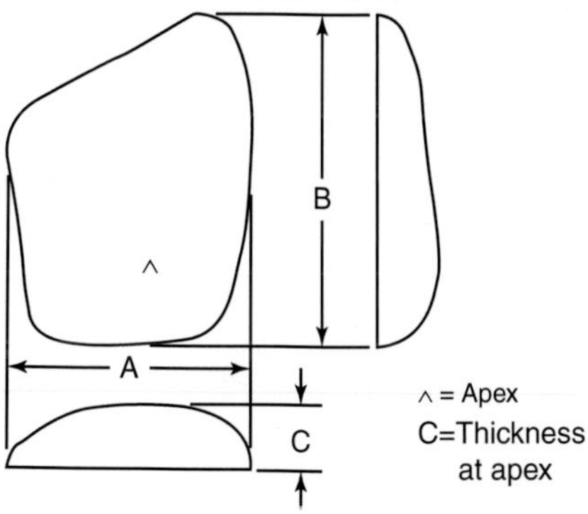

PowerFlex Plus Pectoral (Implantech)

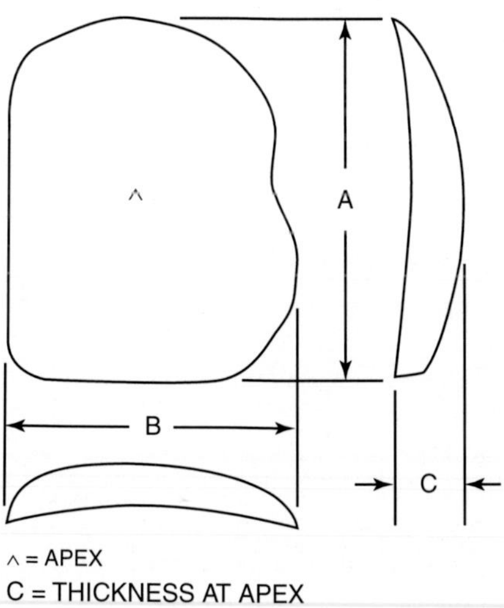

Novack Pectoral Implant (Implantech)

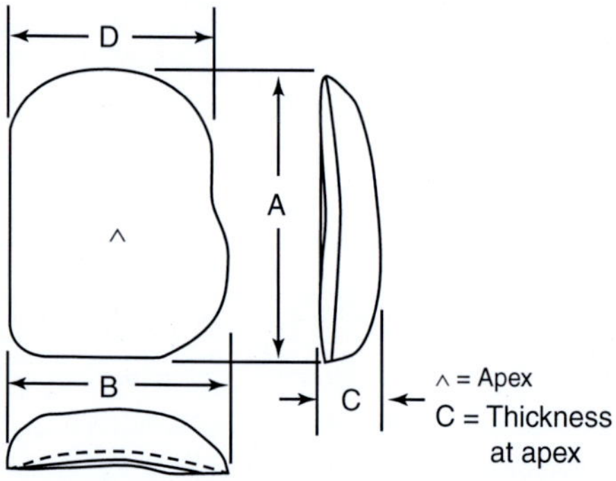

Novack Pectoral Implant Style II (Implantech)

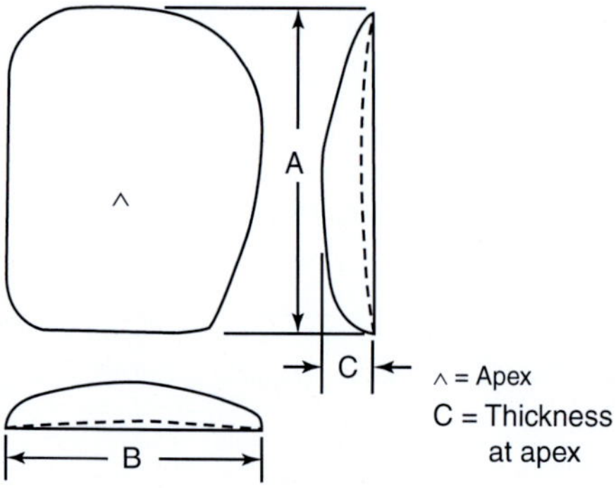

Novack Pectoral Implant Style III (Implantech)

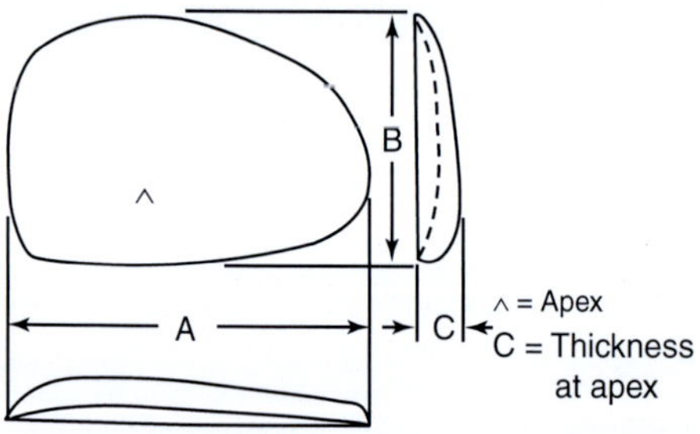

Aiache Pectoral Implant Style IV (Implantech)

With experience, the surgeon can determine the most appropriate implant for each patient. Measurements help the surgeon choose volume and format. The determination of the style used depends on the desire and need of each patient, either to increase the volume of the musculature or to correct a deformity. It is a surgery of reasonable ease of execution, which improves with surgical practice. Silicone elastomer implants can be modeled and confer customization of the surgery, increasing the degree of satisfaction.

Surgical Technique

This surgery is preferably performed under general anesthesia and may also be epidural. After the asepsis and antisepsis procedures, the italic “S”-shaped incision line is marked at the lateral edge of the muscle to be manipulated, close to the axillary hair line or axillary line. It follows with the marking of detachment limits, always keeping the muscle insertions intact, to avoid feminization of the pectoral region. This limit should be approximately 3 cm below the lower line of the nipple-areolar complex (NAC). The marking proceeds to the insertions of the pectoral musculature in the line of the true ribs and in the sternum line.

Infiltration is made with 1:160,000 adrenaline solution in the incision line and throughout the region to be taken off. The incision is made to the fascia of the pectoral, then in the fascia itself and, with digital maneuver, we start the detachment of the musculature, creating the space where the implant will be introduced. It is very important to keep this cool space restricted to the size of the implant to be used, due to the possibility of implant displacement. The implant is then positioned in the submuscular plane. The pocket closure is made with nylon thread 2–0 or Stratafix 2–0, reducing the possibility of herniation of the implants to the supramuscular plane. This is followed by intradermal suture with PDS 3–0, subcutaneous with PDS 4–0, and skin with intradermal suture with PDS 4–0.

Tips

- Care in detachment, keep within the limits of implants and patient, avoid “over-dissection.”
- Do not perform the disinsertion of the pectoral muscles of your abdominal insertions, the true ribs, and the sternal region.
- Perform a suture with high strength threads, due to the characteristics of the musculature of the region.
- Compressive dressing for 24 h to avoid seroma and displacement of implants.
- Attention to the patient’s complaints, especially postoperative pain. Because it is a surgery that involves muscle detachment, pain in the immediate postoperative period can be intense.

Step by Step

- Markings of the incision and submuscular detachment area.
- Marking of the desired store for the implant.
- Infiltration of the site with adrenaline solution 1:160,000.
- Avoid traumatic dissection.
- Do not uninsert the musculature.
- Resistant sutures in the fascia to prevent herniation of implants.
- Use of suitable material for the manufacture of the implant pocket.
- Pay close attention to the symmetrization.

Postoperative Care

Early ambulation, still in the first 24 h of surgery, should be encouraged. Use compressive dressing for 24–48 h. After this period, the patient may wear compressive mesh or medium compression shirts. As there may be pain, the use of analgesic, anti-inflammatory, and muscle relaxant is regular in the first 72 h. Measures should be taken to avoid thromboembolism, such as the use of compression stockings and the use of anticoagulants in the first 24 h after surgery. Patients should lie in supine position for a period of at least 10 days. The return-to-work activities take place in approximately 6 days, drive in 7–10 days, and light exercises in 2 weeks. Total release occurs between 20 and 30 days, depending on the patient's recovery, including for heavier exercises.

Complications

Complications are rare; however, among them, the most frequent is the formation of seroma in the immediate or even late postoperative period. Asymmetry is much less common, and to avoid it, it is necessary to observe carefully in the perioperative period. Other possible complications are hematoma, infection, and suture dehiscence.

Arm Implants

Biceps and Triceps

Like other body implants, bicep implants were initially used to reconstruct soft tissue deformities in the region, such as trauma sequelae, postoperative oncologic surgeries, and nerve damage, whether due to surgeries or anesthetic blocks or traumas.

Although they did not return the movement of the arms to the patients, it significantly improved the appearance, with lasting aesthetic results.

Hodkingson (2006a), in 2006, reported a case of using solid silicone implants to restore arm volume after rupture of the biceps and triceps tendons. In the same year, Chugay (2006; Chugay and Chugay 2009) published his work on the use of solid silicone implants in the arms. Dini and Ferreira (2010), from the University of São Paulo (USP), evaluated the short head size of the biceps for the use of implants in the region in 2010. In 2012, Abadesso and Serra (2012) published a series of 32 cases of increased biceps and triceps region using silicone gel implants added to silicone elastomer implants with purely aesthetic purposes.

Anatomy

The anterior face of the arm is formed by three muscles: the brachial biceps, the coracobraquial, and the brachial. The brachial biceps muscle is responsible for the convex surface of the anterior region during forced flexion of the arm. That's why it's the focus of increasing the region by silicone placement. The biceps originates from two heads in the scapula: the long head in the supraglenoidal tubercle and the short head in the coracoid process. The two heads move caudal and join together forming a single tendon that attaches to the tuberosity of the radio and the fascia of the forearm, through the aponeurosis of the biceps.

The other two muscles of the anterior region are the coracobrachial with origin in the coracoid process of the scapular and is part of the middle third of the medial face of the humerus and the brachial, with origin in the medial face of the humerus and insertion in the coronoid process and tuberosity of the ulna. However, these do not interfere with the procedure.

The shape of the posterior region of the arm is mainly given by the triceps brachial muscle. It has three origins: the long head, in the infraglenoidal process of the scapula; the lateral head, on the posterior face of the humerus, superior to the juice of the radial nerve; and the medial head, with origin in the posterior face of the humerus, inferiorly to the groove of the radial nerve. The insertion of the brachial triceps takes place at the proximal end of the olecranon of the ulna and also opens in the fascia of the forearm.

The other muscle of the posterior region is the anconeus originates from the lateral epicondyle of the ulna and insertion and on the lateral face of the olecranon.

Indications, Contraindications, and Limitations

This surgery has aesthetic indication in the arms with mild to moderate sagging, especially in the triceps region and in cases of desire for increased muscle volume of the region. It also has corrective indication in the sequelae of arm trauma and brachial plexus nerve lesions, with consequent muscle hypotrophy.

It is not indicated for sharp sagging, nor for correction of excessive skin after large weight loss. As in other surgeries, patients with body dysmorphic syndrome and patients with unrealistic expectations regarding results should not be operated. Classically, patients with formal contraindications for performing surgeries are also excluded.

This surgery is limited in the volume to be introduced. A large volume can cause compartment syndrome and should not be performed.

Consultation/Choice of Implants (Types of Implants)

During the patient's history, in addition to the common evaluation, the surgeon should investigate traumas in the arm region, history of nerve lesions, or formal contraindications to surgical procedures. It is important for the surgeon to understand if there was an understanding of the patient about the limitations of the surgery. It is also important that the surgeon understands the patient's expectations.

On physical examination, measurements of the circumference of both arms should be taken, in addition to the distance between their insertions, both from the anterior and posterior region of the arms to predict the size of the implant. The arm is palpated for lesions or anatomical changes. The evaluation of the muscles of the region dynamically and statically is important to verify the degree of sagging and the volume of pre-existing musculature.

In addition to standard preoperative examinations, computed tomography of the arms with 3D reconstruction should be requested for better evaluation of the region.

Preoperative photographs are fundamental. The postures for the photos should be with the patient standing, with arms in 90 degrees with the chest and forearms bent toward the shoulder, at 90 degrees. The arms should be relaxed to observe the sagging of the triceps region. Anterior and posterior view photos should be taken on both sides.

Types of Implants

There are no specific implants for the upper limb region in the national and international market. Abadesso and Serra (Novack 1991) reported the use of the association between implants of the baby calf type of 30 cc volume silicone gel and 100 cc volume elastomer. They were united and inserted into the Currently, the use of elastomer implants, the so-called "contoured carving blocks," brought greater practicality and facilitated the reproducibility of the technique. In addition, there are different degrees of hardness of these elastomer implants, which gives greater similarity to the natural muscle. Another advantage of the use of this type of implant is the possibility of sculpting them according to the need of surgery. For this, in addition to physical examination, tomography assists in the analysis.

Contoured Carving Blocks

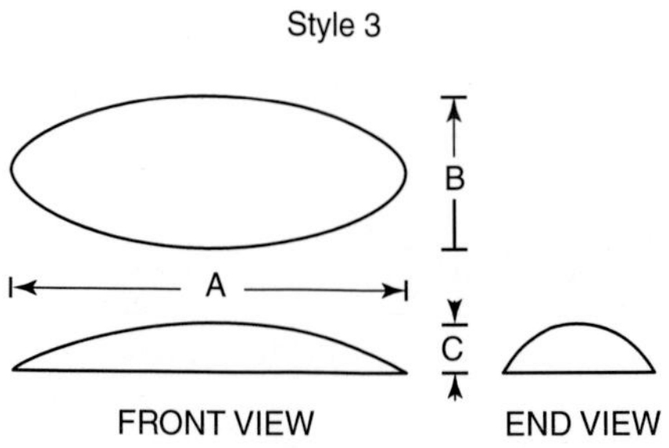

Contoured carving block style 3 (Implantech)

During surgery, after designing the pocket, these implants are customized. Scissors and scalpels are used for this. The edges of the implants should be without tips and protrusions. This prevents implants from being perceived visually and by palpation, giving a more natural result.

Surgical Technique

For this surgery, the best option is that the patient is under general anesthesia. However, it is possible to perform it with sedation and regional block after the initial preparations, with asepsis and antisepsis, markings of the muscle insertion are performed, which helps us in determining the area to be taken off. The biceps are then individualized with the fingers in the form of tweezers, aiming to identify the space between it and the triceps. An Itelic "S" of 3cm in average, is performed. At the lower edge of the biceps, careful dissection is performed until the neurovascular bundle is reached. It should be isolated with caution, and, with digital dissection maneuvers, the triceps fascia is exposed; this is the first muscle where the implant will be inserted. After opening the fascia, a dissection is performed with digital maneuver of the previously demarcated region followed by placing the implant in the submuscular plane. After placement of the triceps implants, it is proceeded in the same way to the biceps, with incision of its fascia, detachment, and introduction of the implant.

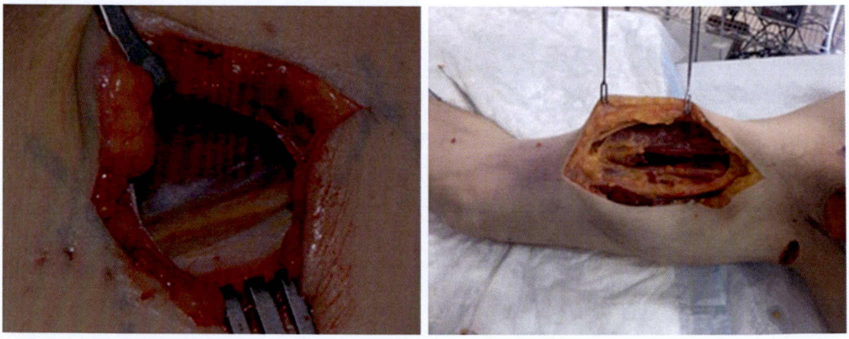

Pocket Design and Implantation

This surgery is entirely monitored by pulse oximetry in the two upper limbs to notice compartment syndrome. A fall in oxygenation should be evaluated. Possibly the implant should be removed, reduced, and reintroduced. The size of the implants should be evaluated during placement, and, if necessary, adjustments in their customization should be made.

After the hemostasis, the closure of the area is performed in the three suture planes. The fascia suture should always be reinforced, with the use of nylon 2–0 or Stratafix 2–0, for vigorous closure of the muscle pocket. For the intradermal plane, 3–0 nylon is used and, in the subcutaneous, PDS 4–0. Surgical glue should be used for skin closure.

Tips

- Care in detachment, keep within the limits of implants and patient, avoid "over-dissection."
- Perform a suture with high strength threads, due to the characteristics of the musculature of the region.
- Compressive dressing for 24 h to avoid seroma and displacement of implants and use of compressive sleeves for a minimum period of 10 days.
- Attention to the patient's complaints, especially pain and paresthesias in the postoperative period. Because it is a surgery that involves muscle detachment, pain in the immediate postoperative period can be intense.
- Due to the characteristics of the region, special care should be given to complaints related to hypoesthesias, decreased strength and sensitivity throughout the upper limb.

Step by Step

- Markings of incisions and submuscular detachment area.
- Marking of the desired store for the implant.
- Infiltration of the site with adrenaline solution 1:160,000.
- Avoid traumatic dissection.
- Be careful when you reach the vasculonervous bundle; move it away with retractors covered with sterile gloves.
- Do not uninsert the musculature.
- Resistant sutures in the fascia to prevent herniation of implants.
- Cautious detachment of the entire region, always seeing the vasculonervous bundle.
- Careful beam clearance for muscle detachment.

Postoperative Care

Ambulation should be encouraged on the first 24 h. Compressive dressings in the first 24 h, and after this period, the patient should wear compression sleeves. In the first 72 h, analgesic, anti-inflammatory, and regular muscle relaxant should be made. The return-to-work activities usually take time in 7 days, release to drive in 10–12 days, and the performance of light exercises in 20 days. Complete release occurs in 30–40 days, including intense physical exercises.

Complications

The major and most important complication of this surgery is compartment syndrome, which should be evaluated in the perioperative period. In rare cases, limb hypoesthesia occurs due to nerve compression due to edema resulting in surgical trauma. Hematoma, seroma, and suture dehiscence are rare. Another possibility is the displacement of the implants, but the attentive suture of the muscular fascia prevents this displacement.

Deltoid and Trapezoid Implants

Like most body implants, the primary use of deltoid and trapezoid implants was for the correction of deformities in the shoulder and trapezoid region. Deltoid asymmetry due to brachial plexus injury and Sprengel syndrome, which causes shoulder asymmetry due to scapular malformation and periscapular muscles, are two of the main corrective indications. With the positive results in these cases, the surgery began to be used to confer increased muscle volume.

This surgery has a short history of publications. The first occurred in 2000, by Saray (2000), with the report of a case of Sprengel deformity with hypotrophy of the trapezoid, in which a calf implant was used in the subfascial space to correct the asymmetry. In 2006, Hodkingson (2006b) published a series of 11 patients with arm and deltoid trauma in which solid silicone implants were used, modeled for the region, introduced by previous scars in the submuscular space of the deltoid.

It was in 2011 that Chugay (2014a) created a customized implant for the deltoid, with purely aesthetic purpose, encouraged by the previous success obtained in the correction of deltoid with implant in a patient with Sprengel deformity.

Anatomy

The musculature of the scapular region is composed of the trapezoid, deltoid, and latissimus dorsi. The deltoid muscle arises from a V-shaped fixation of the anterior margin of the lateral part of the clavicle, the lateral margin of the acromion. Innervated by the axillary nerve and irrigated by the posterior circumflex artery which is branch of the third part of the axillary artery, it covers and gives the shoulder a smooth and convex contour.

The deltoid is divided into three parts: clavicular or anterior part, acromial or middle part, and spinal or posterior part. Together, they insert themselves laterally into the deltoid tuberosity of the humerus.

The trapezoid is a flattened triangular muscle and located superficially on the back of the neck. It is innervated by the accessory nerve (cranial nerve XI) and cervical plexus from C2 to C4 and is involved in the movements of the shoulder girdle, being functionally considered a muscle of the upper limb and not of the back. The trapezoid has its origin in the occipital bone, nuchal ligament, and spinous apophyses from C7 to T12 and is inserted into the spine of the scapula and the lateral third of the clavicle. Its vascularization is given at the upper part by the occipital artery, in its middle part by the cervical artery and in the lower part by the dorsal scapular artery.

Indications, Contraindications, and Limitations

Indicated for correction of shoulder asymmetries by congenital or acquired defects and for increased muscle volume of the region.

Cases in which the patient has an expectation above the surgical possibilities, body dysmorphic syndrome and individuals who have formal contraindication to surgery are contraindicated.

This surgery does not provide improvement of the functionality of the region, only aesthetic gain.

Consultation/Choice of Implants (Types of Implants)

At the first moment of the consultation, the anamnesis should be clearly done, searching for the history of procedures and traumas in the region, in addition to the traditionally collected data. The surgeon needs to make clear the function of these implants and realize the patient's expectation.

On physical examination, it is necessary to pay attention to the quality of the skin and the pre-existing musculature. The thinner the musculature and the skin, the greater the chance of the implants being perceived postoperatively, both tactilely and visually. The necessary measurements are made vertical and horizontal distance of the deltoid and trapezoid, both at rest and in strength.

The photographs are essential, taken following the protocols, with the patient standing, in anatomical position, front, back, at 45-degree angle, and profile on both sides.

Types of Implants

There are no implants suitable for these regions, so elastomer implants are used since they can be molded and sculpted during surgery. In the trapezoid, the silicone elastomer blocks of symmetrical fusiform shape are used. For deltoides, elastomer glute implants are more indicated.

Contoured Carving Blocks

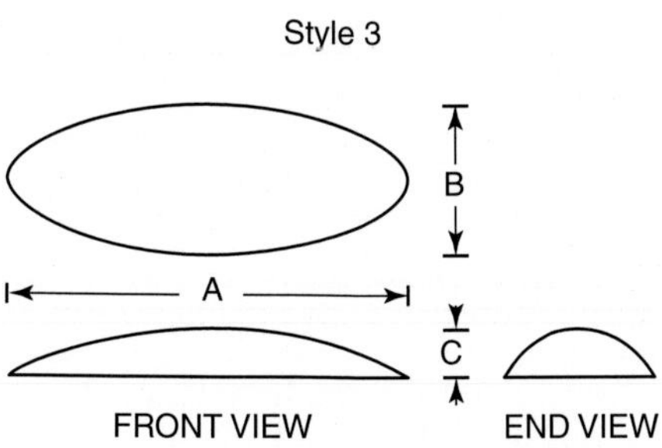

Contoured carving block style 3 (Implantech)

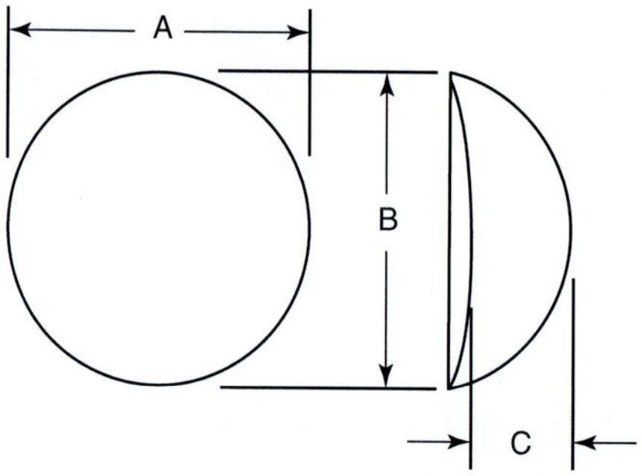

ContourFlex gluteal round natural contour (Implantech)
Implants should be treated capriciously so that the edges are delicate and without protrusions. Thus, the implant is not apparent, and the result becomes natural and satisfactory.

Surgical Technique

Under general anesthesia, asepsis and antisepsis performed, the detachment area is marked, and deltoid infiltration with 1:160,000 adrenaline solution is initiated. An incision of approximately 4 cm to 2 cm of the coracoacromial ligament is made. From the incision, a subcutaneous detachment is made to the fascia of the muscle. At this moment, a division of the deltoid is made in the direction of its fibers and a detachment ed. size such that it receives the implant previously customized for the region. This customization is performed intraoperatively. The muscle pocket suture is performed with nylon 2–0 or Stratafix 2–0. Then, the closure of the anatomical planes with PDS 3 and 4–0 is performed.

For the placement of the implant in the trapezoid, an incision of approximately 3 cm is made in the scapular region, 2 cm from the coracoacromial ligament, the same access route for the deltoid. However, it continues until the fascia of the trapezoid, which is incised and dissected in the less traumatic way possible in order to create a subfascial pocket. Before placing the implants, hemostasis should be performed; these implants are also customized intraoperatively. Fascia closure is done with 3–0 nylon and other anatomical planes with PDS 3 and 4–0.

Tips

- Care in detachment, keep within the limits of implants and patient, avoid "over-dissection."
- Perform the closing of the muscle pocket with resistant sutures.
- Perform fascia closure independently and separately from the skin suture line
- Attention to symmetry and care in the customization of implants.

- Attention to the patient's complaints, especially pain and paresthesias in the postoperative period.
- Due to the characteristics of the region, special care should be given to complaints of hypoesthesia, tingling and decreased strength throughout the upper limb.

Step by Step

- Markings of incisions and submuscular detachment area.
- Marking of the desired pocket for the implant.
- Customization of implants, attention to symmetry.
- Infiltration of the site with adrenaline solution 1:160,000.
- Avoid traumatic dissection.
- Resistant sutures in the fascia to prevent herniation of implants.
- Cautious undermining from the entire region.

Postoperative Care

The patient should start ambulation in the first 24 h postoperatively. The use of analgesic, anti-inflammatory, and muscle relaxant is regular in the first 72 h. Return to work activities in about 5 days, drive with 8–10 days, and practice light exercises in 20 days. The patient will be fully released in 30–40 days, including for more intense exercises.

Complications

The most common complication is hypoesthesia by nerve compression. Hematoma, seroma, and suture dehiscence are rare. Implant displacement may occur in cases of fragile suture of the muscular fascia.

Thigh Implants

The beginning of the use of implants to correct the volume of the lower limbs comes from more than 40 years. Glitzenstein (1979) and Carlsen (1979a) were the introducers of the technique, initially proposed for the calf region and later adapted for use in the thighs.

Based on his experience with calf and glute implants, Kon (1995), in 1995, designed a new type of implant to increase the thighs, presenting a case.

In 1997, Montellano (n.d.) published in the Brazilian Journal of Plastic Surger his work of calf implants in thighs. In 1995, Menichelli (2011), in São Paulo, began to use calf implants in thighs, for patients who wanted only to increase muscle volume, having published their work in 2011. In both studies, symmetrical calf implants with volumes higher than those existing at the time on the market are presented, that is, manufactured especially for the patients in question.

Chugay (2014b), in 2014, reports in his book his experience of more than 10 years of using implants for increase, from the quadriceps region of the thigh.

Anatomy

The thigh is topographically divided into three regions: adductor or medial, anterior, and posterior. The one that most often receives implants is the previous one; however, all can receive, and later placement is rare. Thus, the most important muscle for thigh implants is the quadriceps, formed by four muscles (femoral rectus, vastus lateralis, vastus medial, and vastus intermediate) that join and insert themselves into the tuberosity of the tibia.

The second area that receives the most implants is the adductor or medial. It is formed by the long adductor, gracilis, adductor magnus, and short adductor.

The posterior region is formed by the biceps femoris muscles of the thigh, semimembranosus and semitendinosus.

The most important point of attention for the surgery of thigh implants is the femoral triangle, through which nerve, artery, and femoral vein pass toward the thigh. Therefore, the incision for implant placement should preserve this region.

Indications, Contraindications, and Limitations

Initially idealized for correction of thigh deformities due to birth defects or sequelae of surgeries or traumas, currently its most frequently seen indication in plastic surgery offices is for increased muscle volume, either for definition purposes or for decreased sagging skin in the region.

Unrealistic expectations and body dysmorphic syndrome are the most important contraindications of this surgery, in addition to formal contraindications for performing surgeries. The patient should be alerted to severe postoperative pain. Those who do not wish to go through the phase of pain should be encouraged to give up surgery.

As the thigh is a large area addressed, it may be necessary to place several implants to obtain the volume and result desired by the patient. In certain cases, up to six implants are used on only one side. However, if the patient's musculature is not ideal for receiving these implants, the result may not be satisfactory. Sharp sagging of the skin may also not be corrected to the satisfaction with the use of implants. Sometimes it is necessary to intervene more than once to give the long-awaited result. It's a painful postop surgery. Patients with low pain resistance may need more hospital stay for intravenous analgesia and sometimes become individuals with contraindication scan so far.

This surgery limits the pre-existing muscle mass and, if little developed, may need to receive several implants on each side in order to achieve the symmetry or volume desired by the patient. Sometimes it requires more than one surgical intervention.

Consultation/Choice of Implants (Types of Implants)

The case history should follow the usual questions, in addition to factors that may interfere with the surgery in question, such as previous surgery or trauma of the region, history of previous surgery, vascular diseases such as varicose veins and femoral insufficiency, diabetes, and any other conditions that lead to a risk of decreased venous circulation in this region.

Patients who have congenital or traumatic anomalies should be alerted to the risk of requiring more than one surgical intervention to achieve the desired and satisfactory symmetry between the limbs.

The quality of the skin, subcutaneous tissue, and musculature should be evaluated before surgical planning.

The choice of the type of implant and the amount of implants to be used vary according to the patient's desire, skin, and musculature quality. The maximum size of the implants to be used is predicted by the measurement between muscle insertions.

Types of Implants

In addition to symmetrical and asymmetric gel-filled implants, silicone elastomer implants can be used.

Gel Implants

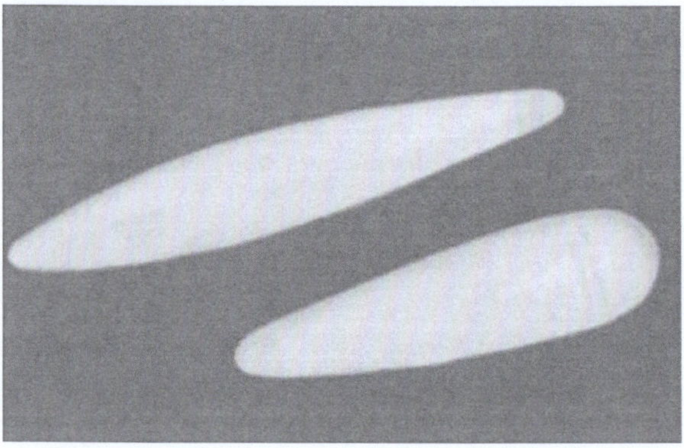

Symmetrical and asymmetric Silimed Implants (designed for the calf)

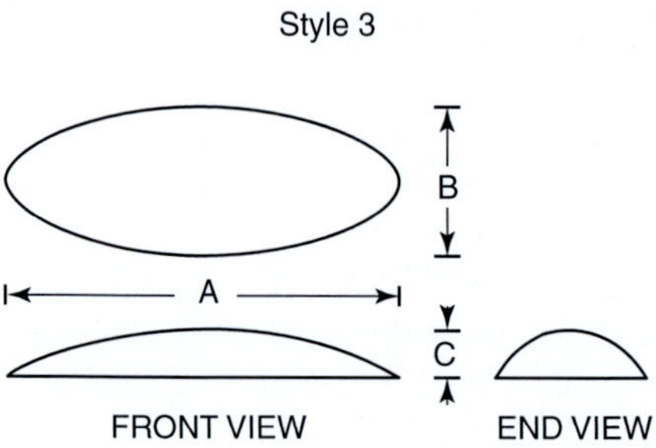

Contoured carving block style 3 (Implantech)

With experience, we were able to determine the most appropriate implant for each patient. What determines the choice between the available styles is the joint of the desire, need, and purpose of the surgery, whether to increase the volume, or to correct an asymmetry, or to correct sagging.

Surgical Technique

Usually, this surgery is done under general anesthesia with constant epidural block by catheter, which helps in the management of postoperative pain. After the asepsis and antisepsis procedures, the incision line is marked varying according to the muscle group to be treated. Incisions can be used in the gluteus groove and on the lateral and medial sides of the thighs, depending on the amount and placement of the implants. The incision site and the store where the implants will be placed infiltrate. The incision is made until the fascia of the chosen muscle group. With long hipsters, such as calf scoffs, the space where the implant will be inserted is created. It is important to keep this space restricted to the size of the implant to be used.

After the implants are allocated in the submuscular plane, the store is closed with 2–0 nylon wires or Stratafix 2–0, reducing the possibility of herniation of the implants to the supramuscular plane. It then proceeds with the closure by anatomical planes with PDS and nylon wires.

Tips

- Care in detachment, keep within the limits of implants and patient, avoid "over-dissection."
- Perform a suture with high strength threads, due to the characteristics of the musculature of the region.
- Compressive dressing for 24 h and half of medium compression for 7 days, to avoid seroma and displacement of implants.
- Attention to the patient's complaints, especially postoperative pain, because it is a surgery that involves a large number of muscle groups, and pain in the immediate postoperative period is usually very intense.

Step by Step

- Markings of incisions and submuscular detachment area.
- Marking of the desired store for the implant.
- Infiltration of the site with adrenaline solution 1:160,000.
- Avoid traumatic dissection.
- Resistant sutures in the fascia to avoid herniation of implants, use nylon 2–0 or Stratafix 2–0.
- Use of suitable material for the manufacture of the implant shop.
- Pay close attention to symmetrization.

Postoperative Care

As postoperative care, it is important that the patient begins to walk on the second postoperative day and that he/she uses anticoagulant for 24 h. Compressive dressings are kept for 24–48 h. It is important to use analgesic, muscle relaxant, and anti-inflammatory in the first 72 h. To stay lying down, the patient should keep a pillow under his ankles. Return to work activities and driving take place in approximately 5–7 days, depending on pain, light exercise in 2 weeks, and total release in 30–40 days.

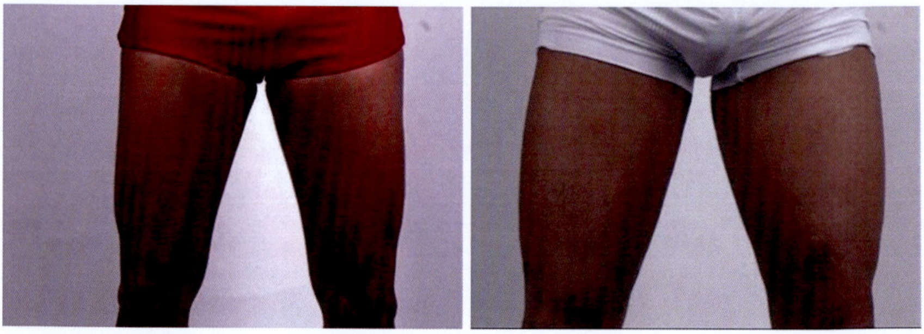

Before and after surgery: 3 months postop

Complications

The most common complication of this surgery is severe pain in the immediate postoperative period. Asymmetry, implant displacement, and seroma may also occur. Compartment syndrome and infection are rare.

Calf Implants

History

Calf implant surgeries have a long history, begun more than 50 years ago. There have been several proposals for formats and various placement plans throughout this time. Currently, the most used formats are the symmetrical, fusiform, proposed by Glitzenstein (1979) and the asymmetric, proposed by Montellano (1985), both filled with silicone gel. The surgical plans proposed were the subfascial, by Glitzenstein (1979), Carlsen (1979b), and Montellano (1985); submuscular by Kalixto and Vergara (2003), and supraperiostal, by Nunes and Garcia (2004), who proposed this plan associated with intraoperative fasciotomy. The subfascial plane is commonly used today.

Anatomy

The muscle groups of the leg are classified by four regions that work separately: anteromedian, anterolateral, lateral, and posterior regions, object of the present study. Calf is the name given to the upper half of this region and is formed by the two heads of the gastrocnemius muscle and the soleus muscle. In the middle of the leg, the gastrocnemius merges with its tendon that narrows rapidly. The soleus muscle remains below the middle of the leg, but during contraction, its lateral margin is projected slightly ahead of the gastrocnemius. Below the calf, the calcaneus tendon (Achilles tendon) is projected. In the groove between the two heads of the gastrocnemius the small saphenous vein runs. Both irrigation and innervation of the region run in a deeper plane than the incision made to place the prostheses in the calves. Vascularization is given by the popliteal artery, through its anterior and posterior tibia branches, released after the passage of the popliteal artery through the tendinous arch of the soleus muscle and anastomose freely. The calf is irrigated by the posterior branch and innervated by the tibial nerve, which walks alongside the posterior tibial vessels. These structures descend medially to the fibula, then pass to the medial malleolus, and end at the ankle.

Indications, Contraindications, and Limitations

Calf implants were initially developed to correct congenital and acquired defects, such as sequelae of cerebral palsy, poliomyelitis, and osteomyelitis and repair after oncological surgeries. However, today the increase in aesthetic volume of the region is the most frequent indication in plastic surgery offices. The calf is formed by a muscle group difficult to grow with physical exercises; thus, implant placement is an option for harmonization of the lower limbs.

Unrealistic expectations and body dysmorphic syndrome are the most important contraindications of this surgery, in addition to formal contraindications for performing surgeries.

The main limitation of this surgery is the impossibility of correction of the ankle region.

Consultation/Choice of Implants (Types of Implants)

During anamnesis, special attention should be paid to factors that may interfere with surgery: history of trauma or previous surgeries in the ankle and Achilles tendon, congenital left foot, previous vascular surgeries, vascular insufficiency, diabetes, and any other conditions that lead to the risk of decreased venous circulation in this region. In the case of congenital or traumatic anomalies, patients should be alerted to the possibility of performing more than one surgery in order to achieve a satisfactory symmetry between the limbs. At this time, attention should also be paid to the patient's desire and their expectations of results.

On physical examination, we should evaluate the quality of the skin, subcutaneous tissue, and musculature. These factors form the points that define the quantity, location of the store, and the size of the implants. To guide the choice of size, in addition to the patient's desire, the distance between the popliteal fossa and the insertion of the Achilles tendon is used. This measure defines the maximum size of implants that can be used. On the other hand, the quality of the skin guides the possibility of increasing the region safely. It is also observed the need to increase only one region of the calf (medial or lateral) or both, which gives the amount of implants to be used.

As in all plastic surgery, photos are essential. One should follow with all imaging protocols, doing front, back, and profile poses. Profile ones should be done first with one leg in front of the other (in a walking position, with both heels resting on the ground) and then alternating the position of the legs.

Types of Implants

In addition to the symmetrical and asymmetric gel-filled implants, we have silicone elastomer implants.

Gel Implants

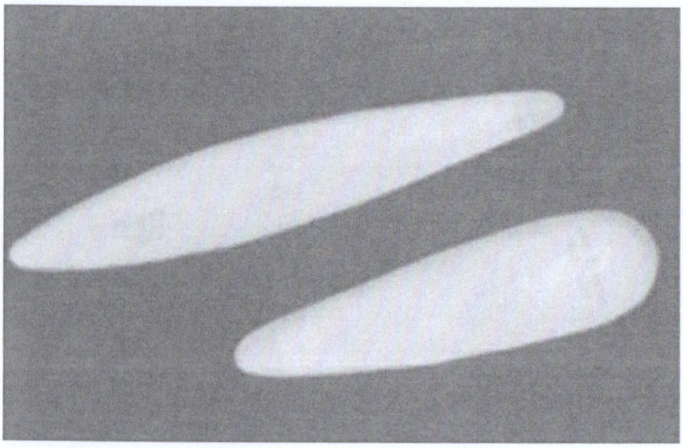

Symmetrical and asymmetric Silimed implants

Elastomer Implants.

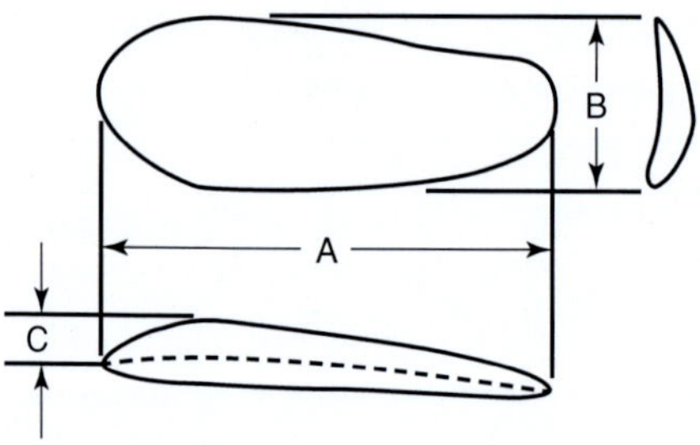

Carlsen Style (Implantech)

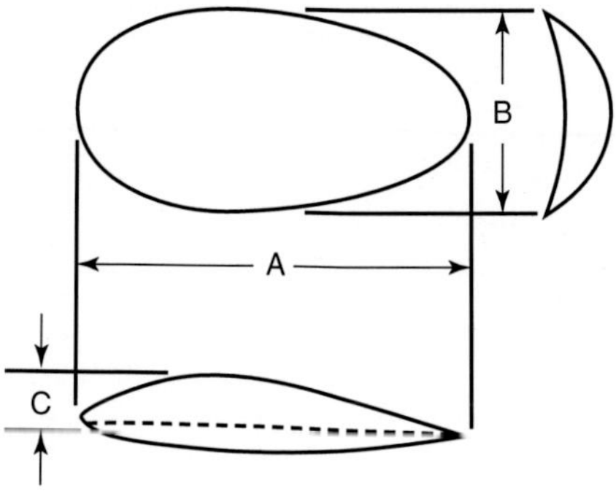

Aiache Style (Implantech)

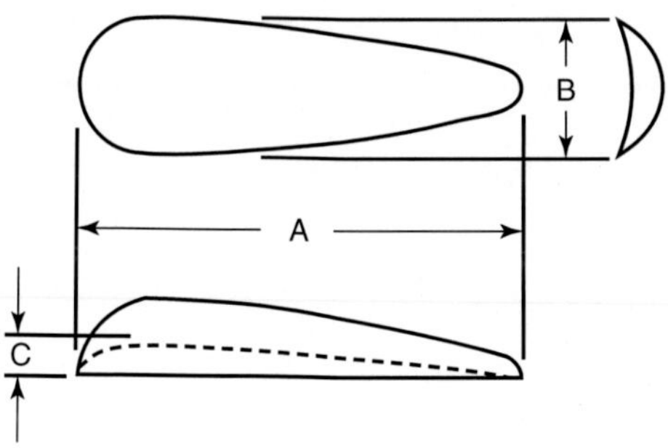

ContourFlex Style (Implantech)

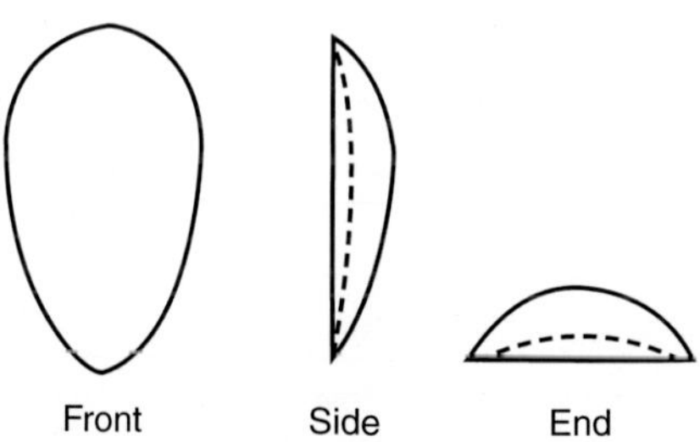

Alpha Aesthetic Style 1

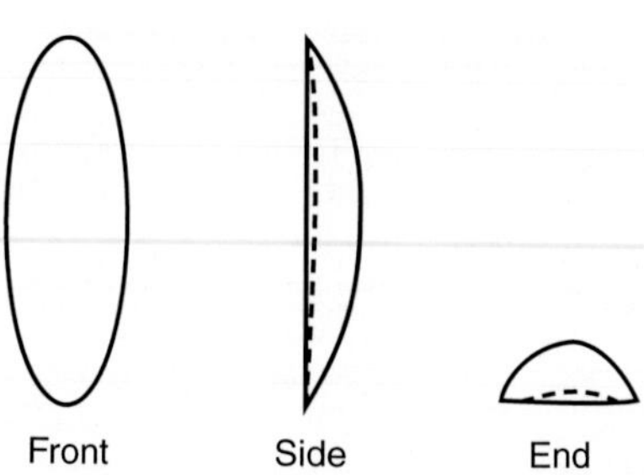

Alpha Aesthetic Style 2

Determining the most appropriate implant for each patient is a learned ability from experience and knowledge. Knowing what is available in the market gives the breadth of possibility of modeling the calf. What determines the chosen model and type is the desire and need of each patient, either to increase the volume of the musculature or to correct an asymmetry. In addition, there is the possibility of designing and sculpting an implant entirely customized using elastomer implants. All this range of choices makes this surgery easy to perform and have a certain complexity.

Surgical Technique

For the placement of silicone implants in the calves, the patient may be under general or epidural anesthesia and in ventral decubitus. After the procedures of asepsis and antisepsis, the incision line is marked in the popliteal fossa of approximately 5 cm. Infiltration is performed with 1:160,000 adrenaline solution in the incision line plus a semicircle with a radius of approximately 4 cm, in the caudal direction.

The incision is made in the marked line, and a suprafascial detachment is made in the area of the infiltrated semicircle. In the apparent fascia, its incision line is marked 4 cm long, 2–3 cm from the skin incision line.

Through this incision, the detachment of the aponeurotic fascia with scissors begins, moving on to the use of the calf detachment to make the implant(s) store. The implants are positioned in the subfascial plane, always looking at the positioning of the medial and lateral implants, depending on the case. Attention to symmetry between the legs is of paramount importance, being one of the major causes of dissatisfaction in this surgery, especially when we use two implants in each leg.

After correct positioning of the implants in the store, the fascia was sutured with nylon 2–0, followed by intradermal suture with PDS 3–0, subcutaneous with PDS 4–0, and skin with intradermal suture with PDS 4–0.

Tips

- Care should be taken with detachment, remaining within the limits of the implants and the patient. Avoid over-dissection.
- The two suture lines, skin and fascia, should always be on different planes.
- In the immediate postoperative period, compressive dressing for 24 h and then half compression medium for 7 days, to avoid seromas and displacement of the implants.

Physical exercises are partially released after 10 days and completely after 30–40 days. Early return or excess load can generate seroma, hematoma, and even implant displacement.

Step by Step

- Markings of the incision and subcutaneous detachment area.
- Marking of the desired pocket for the implant.
- Infiltration of the incision site and subcutaneous detachment with 1:160,000 adrenaline solution.
- Avoid traumatic dissection.
- Resistant sutures in the fascia to prevent herniation of implants.
- Use of suitable material for the manufacture of the implant pocket.
- Pay close attention to the symmetrization.

Postoperative Care

Although it varies according to the professional, some postoperative care should be followed for better recovery. Walk in the first 24 h, maintain compressive dressings for 24–48 h, and, after this period, make use of medium compression stockings for 7 days. Pain control is necessary, and, for this, the administration of analgesic, anti-inflammatory, and muscle relaxant is done regularly in the first 72 h. Caution should be taken with thromboembolism, hence the use of compression stockings in addition to an anticoagulant in the first 24 h after surgery. When lying down, the patient should keep the lower limbs elevated with one or two pillows under the ankle. The return-to-work activities take approximately 6 days, the release to drive in 7–10 days, light exercises in 2 weeks, and total release in 30–40 days for heavier exercises.

Complications

The most common complications in calf implant surgery are (1) postoperative pain, which can be controlled with medications; (2) seroma, which should be treated with lymphatic drainage and/or puncture; (3) asymmetry, sometimes requiring further intervention; (4) herniation, requiring a new approach for suture reinforcement; (5) hypertrophic scar, which should be treated with infiltration or resection of the scar or other due treatments; more rarely, (6) compartment syndrome, which is the most severe of complications and should be treated with partial or total fasciotomy; and (7) infection.

References

Murray JF., Correction of pectus excavatum by synthetic subcutaneous implants. Presented at American Society of Plastic and Reconstructive Surgery. Philadelphia.PA, 1965

Chugay NV., Quach Q., Pectoral augmentation. Int. J. J. It's cosm. Surg. 1999;7(1):23–5

Sorensen JL., Subcutaneous silicone implants in pectus excavatum. Scan. J. J. Plast. Reconst. Surg. Hand Surg. 1988:22(2):173–76

Aiache AE. Male chest correction. Pectoral implants and gynecomastia; Clin Plast Surg 1991;18(4):823–8

DJ Hodkingson. Chest R., wall implants: their use for pectus excavatum, pectoralis muscle tears, Poland's syndrome and muscular insufficiency. Aesthetic Plast Surg. 1977;21(1):7–15

Novack BH, Alloplastic implants for men. Clin Plast Surg. 1991:18(4):829–55

Horn G., A new concept in male chest reshaping: anatomical pectoral implants and liposculpture. Aesthetic Plast Surg. 2002;26(1):23–5

Benito-Ruiz J., Buttock implants for male chest enhancement. Plast reconstr. Surg. 2003;112(7):1951

Pereira LH., Sabatovich O., Santana KP., Picanço R., Sterodimas A. Surgical correction of Poland's syndrome in males – a proposed designed implant. J. J. Plast reconstr. Surg. 2008;61(4):393–9

DJ Hodkingson . Contour restoration of upper limb using solid silicone implants. Aesthetic Plast Surg. 2006a;30(1):53–8

Chugay NV, Racnelli J., Hsu J., Chugay P., Bicipital augmentation. Am J cosm Surg. 2006;23(1):33–6

Chugay NV, Chugay YP., Bicipital Augmentation: A retrospective review of 94 patients cases. Am J Plast Surg. 2009;26(4):241–5

Dini GM., Ferreira LM., Augmentation brachioplasty with cohesive silicone gel implants. In: Shiffman MA, Di Giuseppe A. Editors. Body contouring: art, science and clinical practice. Berlin: Springer; 2010 p.:327–30

Abadesso I., Serra F., Augmentation brachioplasty: surgery for improving the appearance of the arms. Rev Bras Cir Plast. 2012;27(1):97–101

Saray A., Metin E., Oztuna V., Augmentation of the shoulder using a calf implant. Aesthetic Plast Surg 2000; 24:386–388

Hodkingson DJ., Contour restauration of the upper limb using solid silicone implants, Aesthetic Plast Surg 2006b; 30:53–58

Chugay NV., et al., Body Sculpting with Silicone Implants, Springer, 2014a; 9:229–245

Gliztenstein J. Correction of limb amyotrophy by inclusion of silicone prostheses. See. Bras. Cir. 1979; 69:177

Carlsen L., calf Augmentation: The preliminary report. Ann. Plast. Surg. 1979a;2(6):508–510

Kon, M., Christ'l MW., Marjolein Y., Thigh augmentation, Ann Plast Surg 1995;35:519–521

Montellano L., Aesthetic correction of leg deformations. In: Mélega JM, ed. Plastic Surgery Fundamentals and Art - Aesthetic Surgery. Rio

Menichelli, NN., Thigh augmenting with silicone implants, See. Bras. Cir. Plast. 2011; 26(2):306–313

Chugay Nicolas V., Chugay Paul N., Shiffman Melvin A., Body Sculping. With Silicone Implants, Springer 2014b; (7): 167–192

J. Glitzenstein Correction the amyotrophies of the limbs with silicone prosthesis. Rev. Bras. Cir. 1979; 69: 117

Montellano L., Zenteno S. Calf Augmentation Surgery – Paper presented at the XVI National Meeting of the Mexican Association of Plastic Surgeons – La Paz, Baja California, February 1985

Carlsen LN. Calf augmentation – The preliminary report. Ann. Plast Surg. 1979b; 2(6): 508–510

Kalixto MA; Vergara R. Submuscular calf implants. Aesthetic Plast Surg 2003; 27(2):135–138

Nunes GO, Garcia DP. Calf augmentation with supraperiostic solid prosthesis associated with fasciotomies. Aesthetic Plast Surg. 2004;28(1):17–19

Chapter 59
Calves and Ankle Liposuction: Advanced Concepts

Guilherme Miranda De Freitas

Abstract The anomalous accumulation of fat in the calves and ankles is a very dissatisfying factor. Many patients avoid exposing their legs because they are ashamed of the disproportion and simply cannot wear boots that fit on their legs. In addition, many patients with lower limb lipedema suffer from frequent pain and edema in this region. Liposuction of the lower limbs is extremely valuable in adjusting the body contour in harmony with the other areas of the body, generating great satisfaction in the patients, besides relieving painful symptoms.

However, since this is a terminal body extremity region, an adequate knowledge of the surface anatomy and special care is required in order to avoid complications, especially vascular ones.

We present modern concepts with a systematization of the surgical approach to liposuction in this region, with the definition of specific cutaneous stab-perforation points; use of specific material, multi-angled cannulas specially designed for use in this surgery; as well as the determination of particular areas of hyperdefinition, in order to promote better results with better ergonomics, safety, and increased accuracy, achieving the appropriate anatomical contour of the lower legs.

Keywords Liposuction · Lipedema · Calves · Ankles

G. M. De Freitas (✉)
Head of Department of Plastic and Reconstructive Surgery on Galeão Air Force Hospital, Rio de Janeiro, Brazil

Carlos Chagas Institute, Rio de Janeiro, Brazil

J. M. Avelar, R. Cavalcanti Ribeiro (eds.), *Body Contouring*, https://doi.org/10.1007/978-3-031-42802-9_59

Introduction

Liposuction of the lower limbs is extremely valuable for the global aesthetic balance and adequacy of body contour, and its importance and performance have been described by Illouz himself since his first publications on the subject (Illouz 1983). In his initial reports, however, Illouz drew attention to the need to improve the approach and special care when intervening in this region due to its peculiar characteristics, in order to avoid complications. The tragic case of a ballerina who underwent an attempt of a kind of leg liposuction in 1927 by the French surgeon, Charles Dujarier, still lingers in the collective memory, which resulted in the death of the patient due to serious local complications of the surgery (Dujarier 1919). Nowadays, liposuction of the lower limbs is performed quite safely, but many surgeons are afraid to intervene aesthetically in the calves and ankles, limiting themselves to the culottes and, at most, to the inner thighs. This fear is probably due to the historical warning and due to the peculiar characteristics of being a terminal body extremity, a frequent site of circulatory problems in the region, for fear of generating greater circulatory damage (Illouz 1985).

However, it is necessary to remember that, at the time of Illouz, the subcutaneous fat anatomy knowledge was not very widespread and the liposuction technique was just in the beginning, with much thicker and traumatic cannulas than the ones used today. Moreover, the surgery was mostly performed in a dry mode or merely wet, characteristics that determined a tissue trauma considerably greater than today (Mladick 1999).

With the advent of the concepts of tumescent infiltration by Klein (Klein 1987) combined with the progressive reduction of the caliber of the cannulas and the development of ogival-shape tips, it has been possible to reduce tissue and vascular trauma, less blood loss, allowing a considerable advance in accuracy and detailing of liposuction in general, as well as safety improvement and increasing the number of areas covered in a single surgical event.

The work of Hoffman and collaborators in 2002 brought important evidence on the subject, since they concluded, with the study of fresh cadavers and lymphatic stains, that liposuction performed in a tumescent fashion greatly reduces the degree of lymphatic injury (Frick et al. 1999).

Other authors, especially Mladick (1990) and Watanabe (1990) over the subsequent years, have divulged their experience and technique of specific calf and ankle liposuction, perfecting the liposuction approach in the region, with a large number of cases operated without major complications, demonstrating the safety of the procedure.

Watanabe (1987) found that, compared to abdomen and face liposuction surgeries (98% satisfaction), for example, calf and ankle liposuction surgeries results were less satisfactory by the patients (84% satisfaction) than in those areas. He listed the factors he attributed the causes of what was observed in his report, as follows (Table 59.1).

However, it is important to emphasize that these factors were presented as causes of dissatisfaction of patients compared to liposuction in other areas of the body, but despite

Table 59.1 Factors described by Watanabe (1987) for causes of dissatisfaction of patients with calf and ankle liposuction surgery compared to liposuction of other areas

1	Less slender than anticipated
2	Irregular skin surface
3	Asymmetry in shape
4	Prolonged edema
5	Pigmentation of skin
6	Postoperative pain
7	Dysesthesia

this fact, liposuction of the calves and ankles still has a high degree of patient satisfaction, especially in the change of behavior, for the use of short clothes to expose the legs, possibility of using boots, as well as pain reduction in patients with lipedema (Buck 2016).

Thus, the current techniques aim to reduce these postoperative effects in order to achieving grater patient satisfaction.

We therefore believe that one should not promote an equal reduction of calf and ankle areas but work to define transitions and contour surface anatomy rather than just overall volume reduction. The concepts of superficial anatomy visibility of shadows, interleaving positive and negative spaces, hightlightened by Alfredo Hoyos described in his high-definition liposuction technique, enligthened us about these goals in order to not only reduce the global volume of localized fat, but also highlight normal anatomic underlying contour (Hoyos and Prendergast 2016).

However, over the years we have noticed a technical difficulty in performing liposuction in lower legs due to the specific anatomical contours. This led us to develop a special cannula to work in this region which, with a multi-angled shape, allows for better ergonomics and greater accuracy for the procedure.

In addition, we proposed a sistematic positioning of ideal points for skin puncture stabs for cannula access.

The procedure is indicated for patients who present accentuated fat accumulation in the calf and ankle region, generating increased volume and blurring of the anatomical contours. The North Americans have nicknamed this condition as "cankles" in an allusion to the conjunction of calf plus ankle, as if ankle and calf were a single structure, one thing only, usually with a continuous tubular aspect (Fig. 59.1).

Another condition that often accompanies this condition is the so-called lipedema, which is basically defined as the enlargement and hypertrophy of fat cells located in the lower and upper limbs. We put the term "lipedema" in quotation marks because we believe that although the name is well known, it is not appropriate. The reason for this questioning is because, in fact, a truly primary edema of fat cells does not occur in these cases, but rather the development of hypertrophied, inflamed and enlarged fat cells that can result a secondary edema by mass effect, compressing surrounded lymphatic vessels. So, that is the main reason why we think this condition should be better named, trying to follow the pathophysiological way and because it can be easily confused with lymphedema. However, lipedema still the stablished name used today for this condition. As the disease progresses, with prolonged and persistent edema over the years, there will be an increase in type III collagen deposits, and the edema becomes persistent, generating pain on local palpation or mechanical compression, leading to another condition named lipolymphedema.

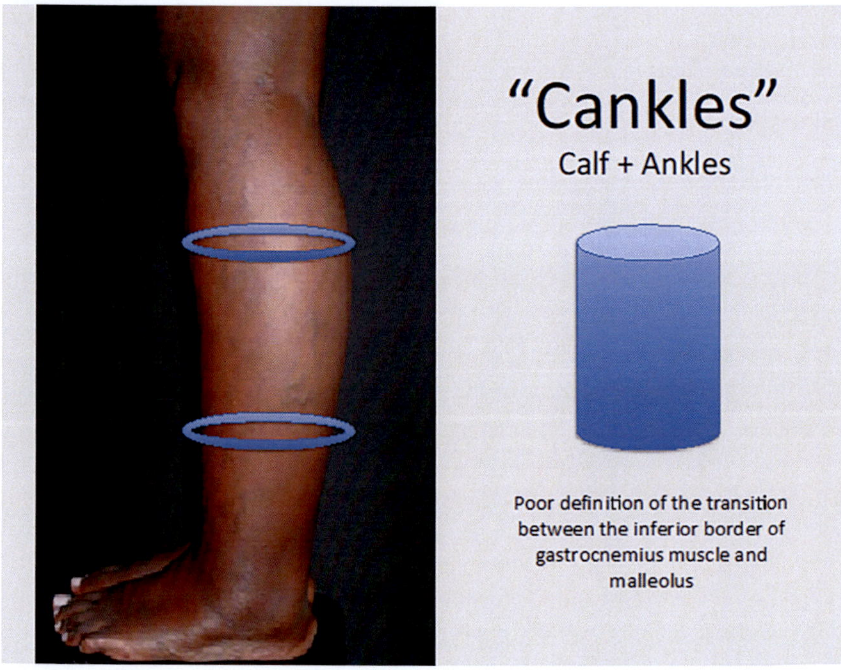

Fig. 59.1 Cankles

So, It is very important to differentiate lipedema from the classic lymphedema. The latter one appears due to other causes, and the occurrence of the edema is primary, caused by a directly involvement of the lymphatics vessels and/or lymphatic nodes, normally affecting the entire limb, including hands or feet. It usually occurs unilaterally (such as filariasis, lymph node damage of groin or axilary nodes) but sometimes both sides can also be compromised.

Treatment for those different conditions will be different as well. For cases of "cankles" and lipedema, there is formal treatment indication by fat removal under liposuction. However, liposuction is contraindicated in lymphedema, leading the differential diagnosis between these condition mandatory before proceeding any surgical approach.

The main sign of difference is so the presence of selective edema of the feet and hands. In lipedema feet and hands are preserved, free of edema. In addition, lipedema has aways a bilateral presentation. lymphedema, on the other hand, presents edema in the feet and hands of the affected limb, and is usually can unilaterally.

In more advanced cases, with higth-grade obesity there could be diagnostic difficulty because of fat acummulation also in hands and feet and testing for Stemmer's sign can valuable for differential diagnosis. The test consists of pinch the skin of the second toe, making a pleat. If the examiner cannot pinch the skin, the sign is present (positive) and the condition is associated with lymphatic disese (Table 59.2).

The preoperative investigation should include MRI of the lower limbs to evaluate the amount of subcutaneous fat and should also be carried out post-operatively to assess how much fat has been removed. The MRI also helps to analyze the

Table 59.2 Adapted from Bauer, A.T. New Insights on Lipedema: The Enigmatic. Disease of the Peripheral Fat. Plast Reconstr Surg 1475:84, 1990

Differential diagnosis between obesity, lipedema, lymphedema, and lipolymphedema				
Characteristic	Obesity	Lipedema	Lymphedema	Lipolymphedema
Gender	Male or female	Almost exclusively female	Male or female	Almost exclusively female
Time at onset	Childhood onward	Typically at age 10–30 years	Childhood (primary); adult (secondary)	Typically at age 30 years onward
Family history positive	Common	Common	Only for primary lymphedema	Occasionally
Effect of dieting on condition	Positive	None	None	None
Effect of elevation	None	Minimal	None	Helpful until fibrosis occurs
Pitting edema	Absent	Minimal	Pitting may stop as fibrosis progresses	Usually present to some degree
Bruises easily	No	Yes	No	Yes
Pain	None	Present in legs	None in the early stages	Present in legs
Area affected	All parts of the body	Bilateral legs, thighs, buttocks (feet spared); arms sometimes (hands spared)	Feet affected first, then progressive leg involvement; unilateral more common than bilateral	Feet affected eventually with positive Stemmer's sign; usually lower extremities (bilateral)
Stemmer's sign	Absent	Absent	Present	Present

component of muscle hypertrophy that may contributing to the increase in the caliber of the leg, information that must be taken into account in predicting the expected postoperative result.

In addition, in cases where venous insufficiency is suspected, a dopplerfluxometry must be requested for the study of the superficial and deep venous plexus.

Planning and Markings

The patient is positioned in dorsal decubitus and the feet are isolated, keeping a complete exposure of the both malleoli. The cutaneous projection of the transition between the lower border of the gastrocnemius muscles to the lower leg, we named the infra gastrocnemius inflection, is then analyzed. This transition zone is very important for the anatomical design of the region. In cases of "cankles" and lipedemathis transition zone is usually erased, undefined by excess of fat accumulation and must be redone in order to highligth the normal anatomy shape and improve contours of this area. Normally, a proportion of 1:1.6 between those landmarks is

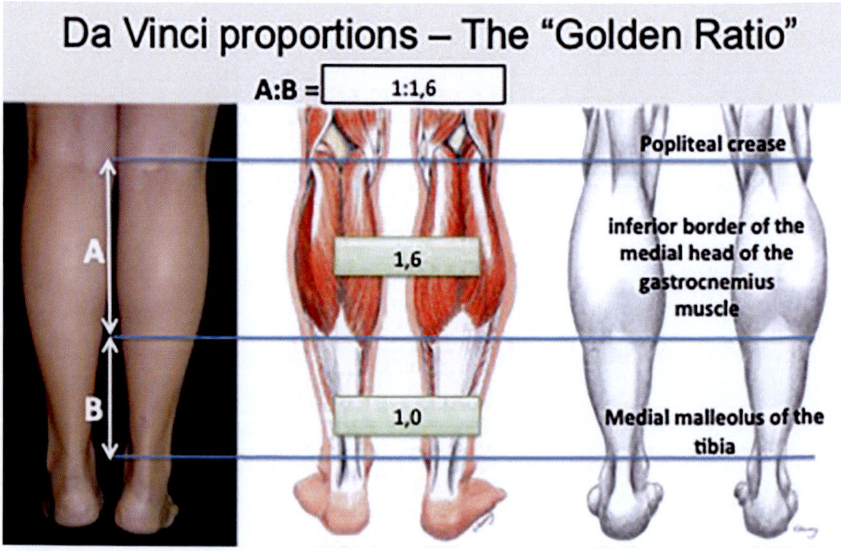

Fig. 59.2 Leg proportions and measures

respected, the golden ratio that is also observed in anatomic relation in other several parts of the body (Fig. 59.2).

We proposed a 7-point positioning of the skin stab-incisions in order to facilitate access to the liposuction cannulas, as well as the removal of the excess fat in a more ergonomic way, with better accuracy and safety, according to the following scheme (Fig. 59.3).

Three puncture points are marked anteriorly: slightly lateral to the projection of the extensor hallucis longus (1); a point anterior to the lateral malleolus (2); and a point posterior to the medial malleolus (3). These points are positioned this way, in order to avoid inadvertently perforation of the great and small saphenous veins and to allow a circumferential liposuction of the ankles. After these markings, two other markings are made, upper in the anterior projection of the posterior gastrocnemius inflection, one lateral and one medial (4 and 5), following the design lines of the desired fat removal.

Subsequently, two more points are marked: inferiorly, a point lateral to the Achilles tendon (6), and superiorly, a central point on the cutaneous projection of the posterior gastrocnemius inflexion (7), directing the movement of the cannula slightly obliquely downward, that mimic the design of the muscles.

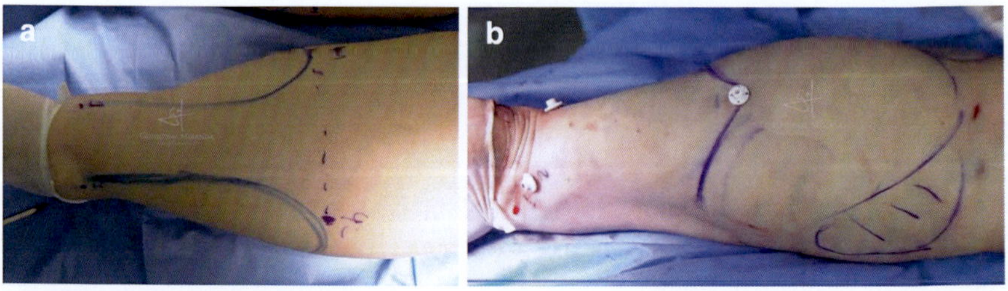

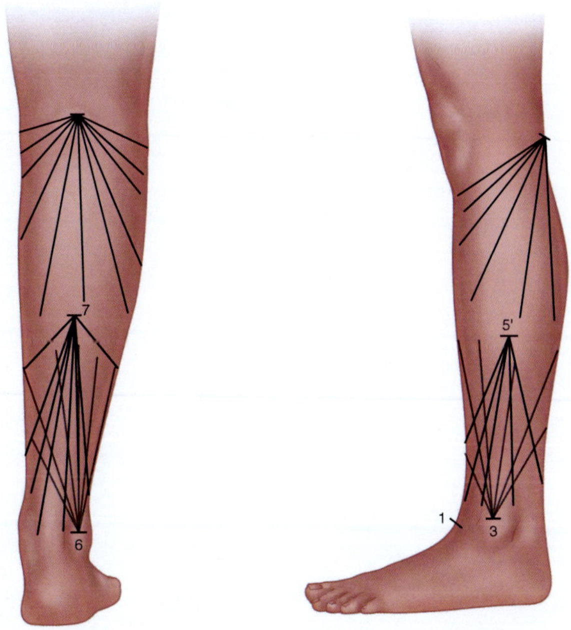

Fig. 59.3 Drawing scheme

In more complex cases if necessary, other puncture points can be made, but with these basic points, it is already possible to perform a complete and well-defined liposuction effectively.

Through the central superior posterior point, it is also possible to promote a volumetric reduction of the calves in the suprajacent projection of the gastrocnemius muscles. In some cases, it is necessary to perform liposuction on the upper sides of the leg, just below the popliteal region and knees. The removal of the fat located in these regions will give a more rounded shape to the calves, reducing the upper tubular aspect, mimicking the underlying muscle projection.

Special Cannulas

The cannulas desgined specifically for this procedure have three angulations, and after the last angulation there are variations in the cannula's length, allowing to act according to the range required, reaching more or less distance. We use a 3.5 gauge, with two lateral and one posterior orifice. The advantage observed of this triple angulation is that it easily allows the perform of a straight and parallel liposuction, avoiding collision with the feet and ankles, and allowing angling the direction exactly as desired, according to the surgeon's need for that movement, a maneuver that is very difficult to do with the conventional straight or curved cannulas.

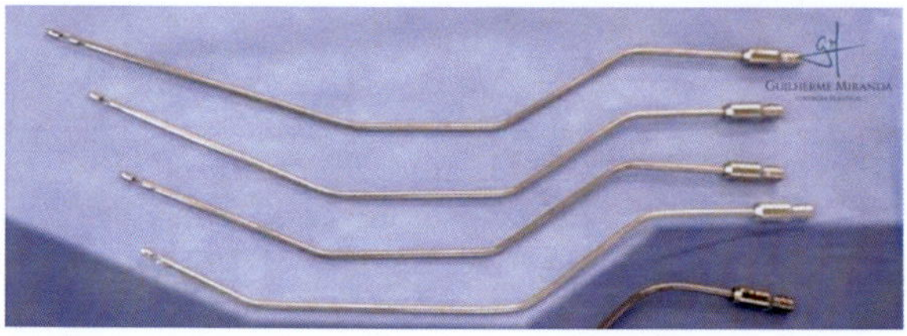

These cannulas were properly patented, being part of the conclusion of a master's in science project concluded at the Federal University of the State of Rio de Janeiro (UNIRIO).

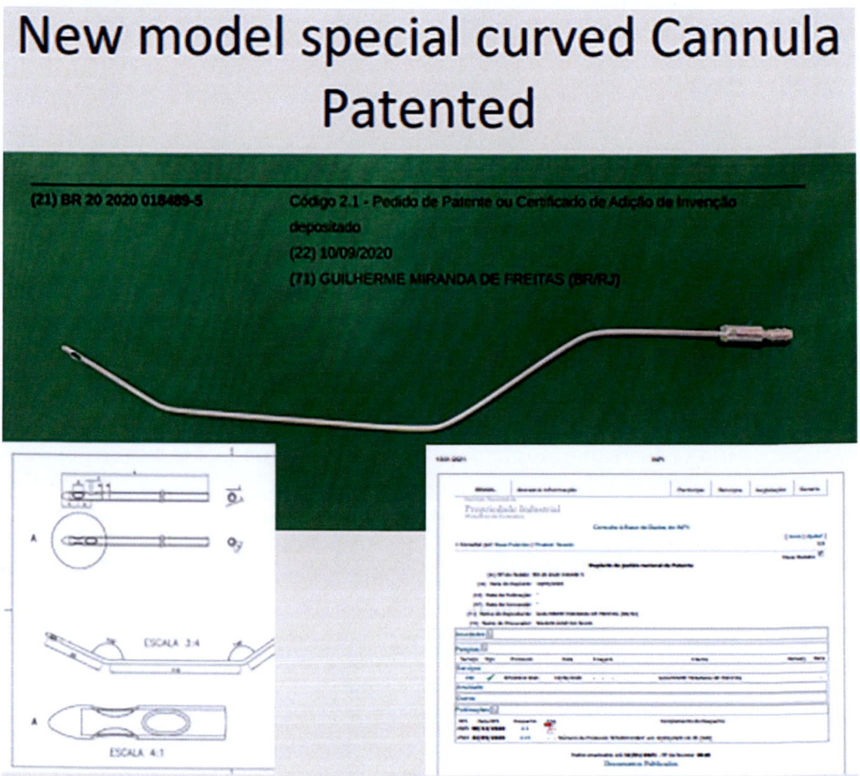

Surgical Procedure

After anesthetic induction with epidural block or general anesthesia, the surgery begins by making the stab-incisions on the previously marked points using a number 11 blade, insertion of small cutaneous protective trocars to avoid skin burns by friction, followed by tumescent infiltration of the areas to be liposuctioned with saline solution with adrenaline 1:500,000 and tranexamic acid 2 ampoules/500 mL and lidocaine 0.5%.

The liposuction is started with the patient in dorsal decubitus, first from the bottom up, through the lower incisions, numbers 1, 2, and 3. We start with the multi-angled cannula with 5 cm final length in the region around the ankles and progressively evolve to those of greater final length, in order to reach the entire length of the leg. Starting with shorter cannulas can offer greater accuracy and control of liposuction around the ankles.

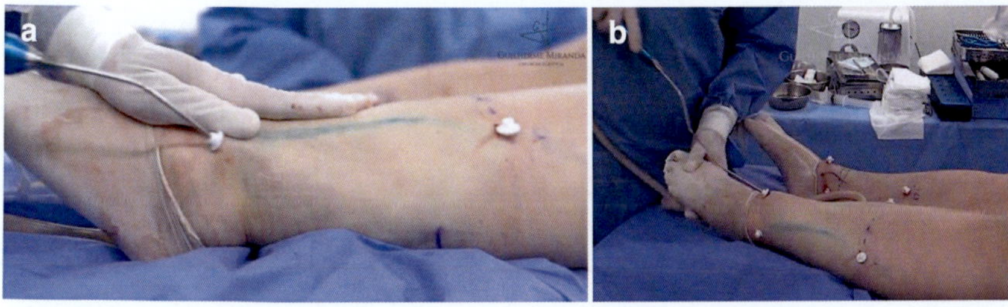

After this region, we cross the liposuction tunnels through the upper incisions (4 M and 5 L), finishing the definition of the lower leg anteriorly.

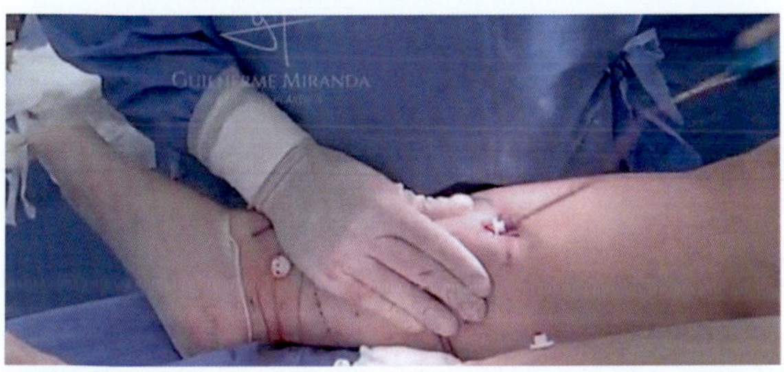

The patient is then changed from supine to prone position. The liposuction is restarted through the stab-incision lateral to the Achilles tendon (6), promoting the removal of fat in the lower leg posteriorly through this hole and also through the already existing posterior medial malleolar hole (3). This is followed by crossing of the tunnels from top to bottom through the central point of the infragastrocnemius inflection (7). This maneuver, in addition to, promoting this crossing, will make a transition zone between the lower portion of gastrocnemius muscle and the lower leg, through a slightly oblique high-definition liposuction in this region, mimicking the muscle contours, highlighting the infragastrocneius inflection.

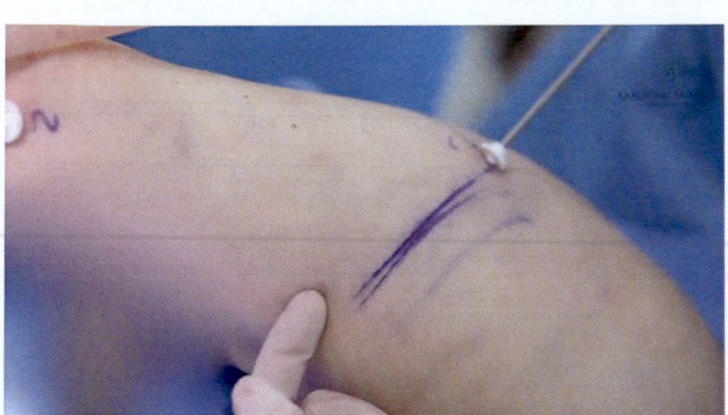

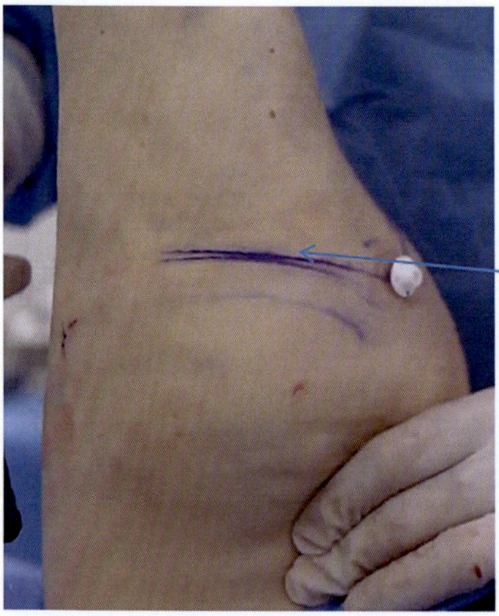

After adequate liposuction, the trocars are removed and a "milking" is performed to eliminate the excess of liquid and accumulated blood, and the incisions are closed with mononylon 5.0 thread. Immediately, Kinesio Tape is applied by a physical therapist still in the surgical room with the legs elevated, followed by the application of medium compression elastic stockings.

Results

Hospital discharge occurs in 24 h. The patient is oriented to keep her limbs elevated whenever possible and encouraged to walk. We recommend avoiding prolonged static standing in the postoperative period. The stitches are removed after 10 days, and the return to daily activities and driving is permitted after 15 days. Light physical activities are allowed after 30 days. Prolonged edema is the most common inconvenience of this surgery and patients are advised about this issue and must maintain dermato-functional physiotherapy follow-up and lymphatic drainage for at least 30 days after the procedure and the use of medical compression stockings for at least 2 months postsurgery.

Case 1

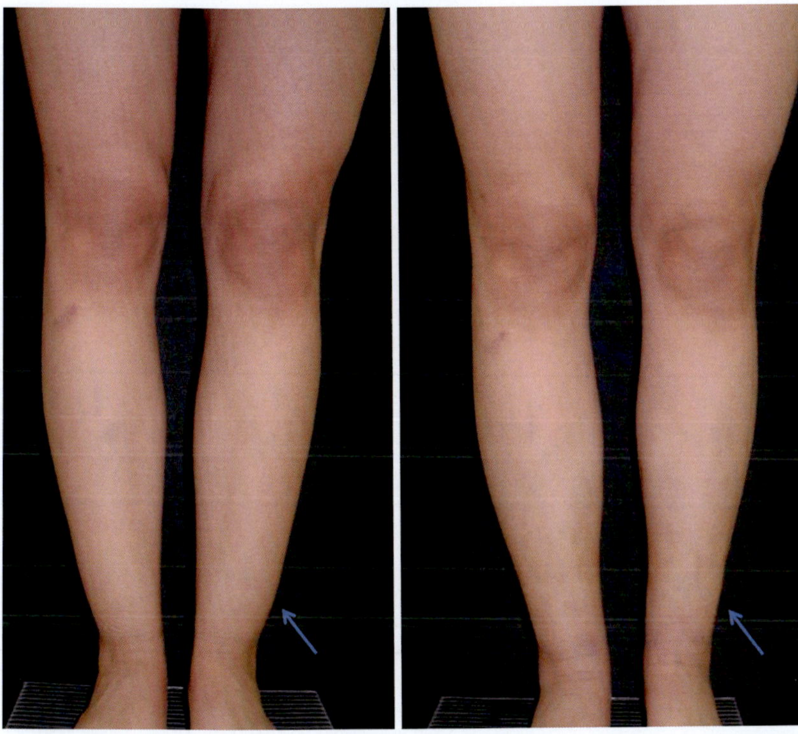

Case 1

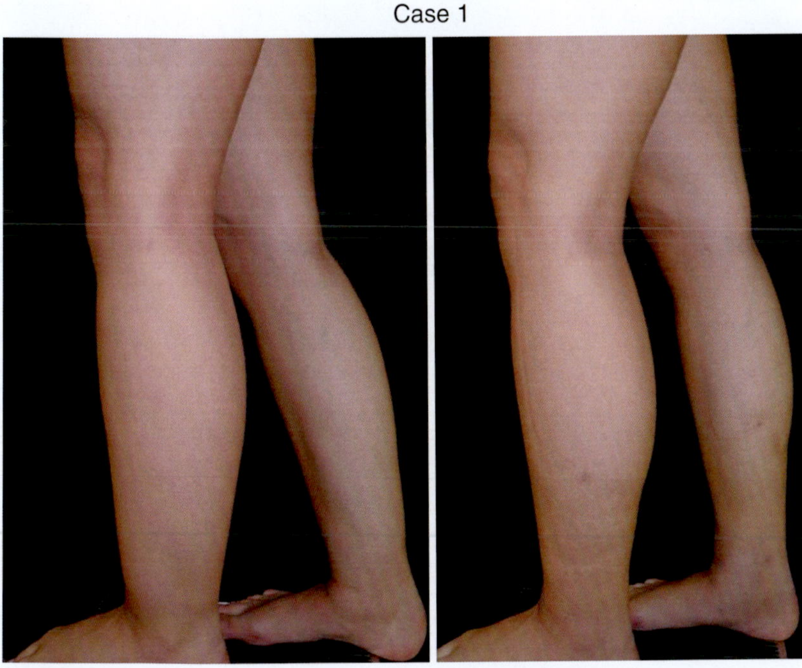

Case 2

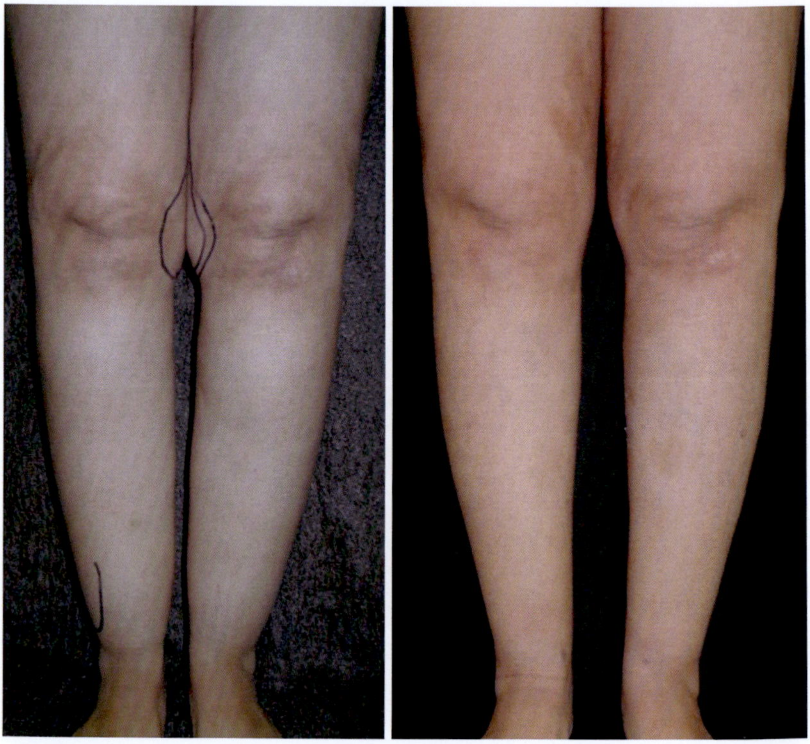

Case 2

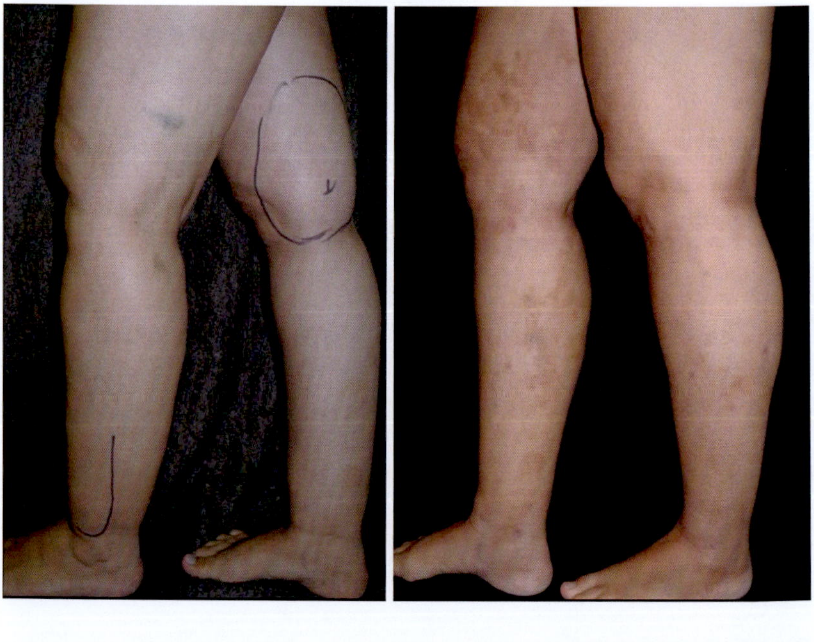

Case 3

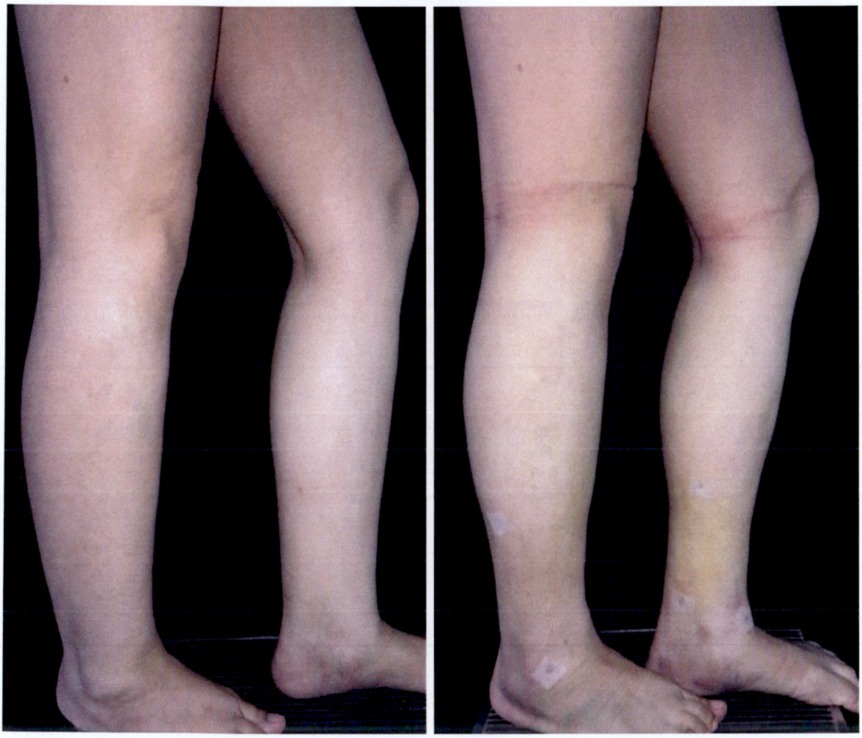

Case 4 – Lipodistrophy ("cankles") – 1 year PO

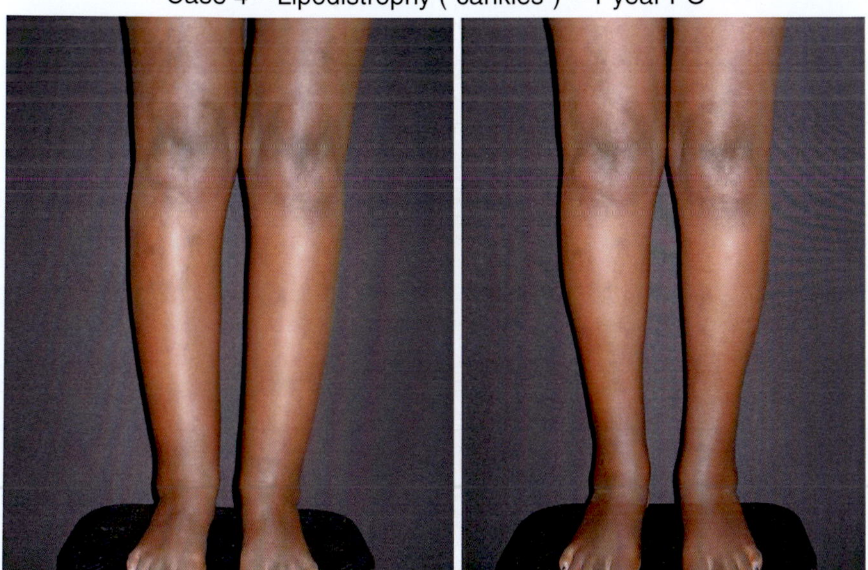

Case 4 – Lipodistrophy ("cankles") – 1 year PO

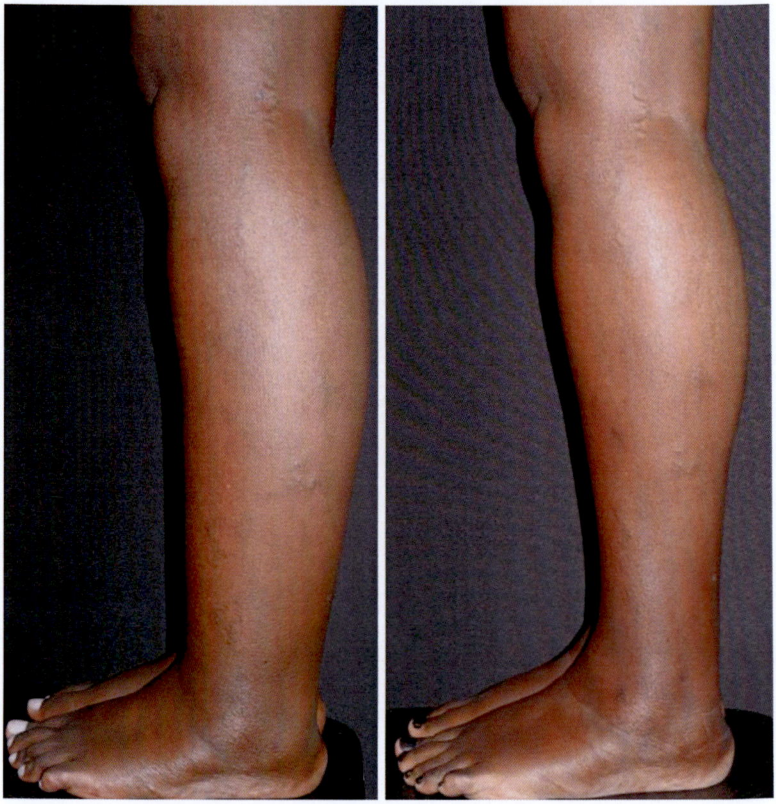

Case 4 – Lipodistrophy ("cankles") – 1 year PO

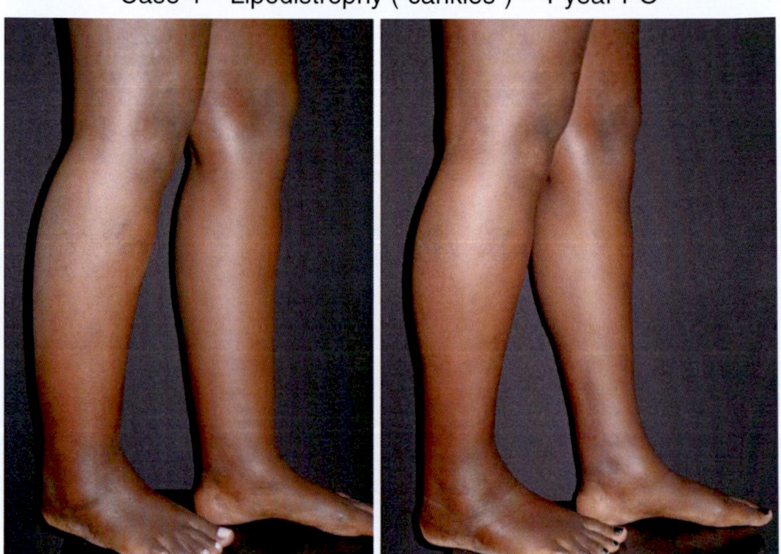

Complications

The possible complications of this procedure are those common to any liposuction, surgery, such as hematomas, infection, skin pigmentation and excessive fat removal at inappropriate areas generating unsighly retraction. Specific complications or unwanted effects of calf and ankle liposuction are those listed by Watanabe in the first part of this chapter (Table 59.1). Of these, prolonged edema is the most common, different from liposuction of other body areas, lasting on average four to five months, and there may be intermittent edema (especially at the end of the day) for up to 8–10 months after surgery. However, once the superficial lymphatic network is restored, there is a return to a presurgical lynphatic drainage capacity, with remission of the intermittent and prolonged edema. Inadequate skin retractions can occur if liposuction is performed too superficial in areas where this aspct is not desireble, or due to excessive damage to superficial subdermal plexus. This condition can be corrected later by releasing skin adhesions followed by lipografting. Skin pigmentation can occur in some cases because of the rupture of superficial vessels followed by blood extravasation, and subsequent formation of hemosiderin deposits. This complication can be reduced or avoided with the use of tranexanic acid diluted in the infiltration solution and the early use of heparin-based ointments or gels in local post-op massages. However, when skin pigmentation is unfortunately established, specific dermatological treatments should be used, in order to minimize its appearance.

Unsatisfactory results are specially related to patients expectations of contour improvement. The analysis of the amount of accumulated fat should be done carefully, including MRI, in order to differentiate muscle hypertrofy from lipoacummulation. In some cases the increase in leg volume is partially due to a constitutional muscular hypertrophy, mainly of the gastrocnemius, which can lead to the legs remain thicker even after the procedure. This aspect of the preoperative assessment should be thoroughly discussed whith the patient. In addition, the intensification of the infragastrocnemius transition allows for greater definition, reducing dissatisfaction regarding contour. This is because, if the calf has a tubular, undefined shape and we liposuction all the areas equally, it will continue to have a tubular aspect, only thinner.

Discussion

Liposuction of the calves and ankles has been performed since the beginning of the development of liposuction. However, since this is a terminal body extremity region, being a frequent site of vascular insufficiency, many surgeons are afraid of performing liposuction in these regions, making it a relative taboo. However, the adequate knowledge of local anatomy as well as the adoption of less traumatic techniques, such as tumescent infiltration, and the use of specific cannulas with adequate caliber and multiple angulations have provided greater accuracy and safety to the procedure. Even skinny patients can present fat accumulation in the lower legs, making it difficult to use boots, distorting the local anatomical contour. In addition, in some cases, the problem is accompanied by pain and feelings of haviness of legs, making its treatment a necessity, in order to improve the quality of live of these patients.

The need for specific cannulas for liposuction in this region is not new, and some authors already have tried to develop different cannula types that facilitate the work in this area (Bruno 2000). The development of the multi-angled cannulas have been shown to allow a more accurate targeting of liposuction, with greater range of motion and desired angular positioning, proving to be ergonomically more appropriate.

The proper positioning of the skin stab-perforations also aids in performing a more homogeneous liposuction, reducing the possibilities of asymmetries and allowing access to the various areas in a circumferential fat removal in the lower half of the leg and high definition in the transition of the posterior muscle groupings—infragastrocnemius inflection.

In addition, the intensification of the infragastrocnemius transition allows for greater anatomic definition, reducing dissatisfaction regarding contour. The concept of selectively liposuctioning certain areas to the detriment of others seeks to achieve a more anatomical appearance of the region. One of the most common mistakes in this surgery is to liposuction all areas equally. This simply ends up transforming a tubular-looking leg into a thinner tube rather than a leg with enhanced anatomical contours. Finally, adequate postoperative physiotherapy follow-up controls the expected prolonged intermittent edema and reduces the formation of subcutaneous fibrosis, that is a cause of residual volume maintenance (Wenczl and Daróczy 2008; Buck II and Herbst 2016; Bauer 1990).

Conclusions

- Liposuction of the calves and ankles is a valuable therapy for achieving a balance in body proportions.
- Even though it is an area surrounded by old taboos, surgery is now performed very safely.
- An adequate preoperative analysis of the excess fat deposits must be done, including with MRI.
- The liposuction areas must be properly marked, respecting the appropriate and desired anatomical contour, taking into account the golden ratio of 1:1.6 between the lower and upper leg.
- Marking of the seven entry points of the cannulas for a complete, comprehensive, and balanced liposuction.
- Tumescent infiltration using adrenaline 1:500.00 and tranexamic acid 2 amp/500 ml and lidocaine 0.5%.

- Use of special multi-angled cannulas to facilitate ergonomics and accuracy of liposuction.
- High-definition liposuction in the posterior muscle transition—infragastrocnemius inflection.
- Use of Kinesio Tape/elastic stockings and dermato-functional physiotherapy follow-up and postoperative lymphatic drainage.

References

Illouz, Y.-G. Body contouring by lipolysis: 5 years experience with over 3,000 cases. Plast. Reconstr. Surg. 72:591–597, 1983.

Dujarier, Charles. Medical Record (1866-1922); New York Vol. 96, Iss. 8 (Aug 23, 1919): 323

Illouz, Y.-G. Surgical remodeling of the silhouette by aspiration lipolysis by selective lipectomy. Aesth Plast Surg 9:7, 1985.

Mladick, R. A. Advances in liposuction contouring of calves and ankles. Plast. Reconstr. Surg. 104: 823, 1999.

Klein, J. A. The tumescent technique for liposuction surgery. Am. J. Cosmetic Surg. 4: 263, 1987.

Frick, A., Hoffmann, J. N., Baumeister, R. G. H., and Putz, R. Liposuction technique and lymphatic lesions in lower legs: Anatomic study to reduce risks. Plast. Reconstr. Surg. 103: 1868, 1999.

Mladick, R. A. Liposuction of the calves and ankles. Plast. Reconstr. Surg. 86: 84, 1990.

Watanabe, K. Circumferential liposuction of calves and ankles. Aesth Plast Surg, 14:259–269, 1990

Watanabe, K. Suction assisted lipectomy for lower extremities. Trans IX congr Plast Reconst Surg 530, 1987.

Buck II, D. W. Lipedema: A Relatively Common Disease with Extremely Common Misconceptions Plast Reconstr Surg Glob Open 2016;4:e1043; doi: 10.1097/GOX.0000000000001043, Published online 28 September 2016.)

Hoyos, Alfredo, and Peter M. Prendergast. *High definition body sculpting*. Springer-Verlag Berlin An, 2016.

Bruno, G. Lipoplastics of Legs: Our Experience with a New Cannula Compared with Classical Technique Aesth. Plast. Surg. 24:401–405, 2000

Wenczl E, Daróczy J. Lipedema, a barely known disease: Diagnosis, associated diseases and therapy (in Hungarian). Orv Hetil. 2008;149:2121–2127.

Buck DW II, Herbst KL. Lipedema: A relatively common disease with extremely common misconceptions. Plast Reconstr Surg Glob Open 2016;4:e1043.

Bauer, A.T. New Insights on Lipedema: The Enigmatic Disease of the Peripheral Fat. Plast Reconstr Surg 1475:84, 1990.

Index

J. M. Avelar, R. Cavalcanti Ribeiro (eds.), *Body Contouring*, https://doi.org/10.1007/978-3-031-42802-9

B

M

T

SPRINGER NATURE

GPSR Compliance

The European Union's (EU) General Product Safety Regulation (GPSR) is a set of rules that requires consumer products to be safe and our obligations to ensure this.

If you have any concerns about our products, you can contact us on ProductSafety@springernature.com

In case Publisher is established outside the EU, the EU authorized representative is:

Springer Nature Customer Service Center GmbH
Europaplatz 3
69115 Heidelberg, Germany

The manufacturer's authorised representative in the EU is Springer Nature Customer Service Centre GmbH, Europaplatz 3, 69115 Heidelberg, Germany. If you have any concerns regarding our products, please contact ProductSafety@springernature.com

Printed and bound by CPI Group (UK) Ltd, Croydon, CR0 4YY

30/09/2026

02224059-0014